Author's Personal Communications with Giants of Medicine

Regarding errors in renal clearance test

Dr. John Macleod

13 Merchiston Avenue
Edinburgh, Scotland, EH10 4PJ
13/7/83

It was good of you to take the trouble to write to me about the 13th edition of Davidson.
Thank you for your kind comments.
You are, of course, correct about the typographical error on page 428. It should have been C = U × V/P; the printer omitted the division sign. This is now being adjusted.
Again many thanks for writing. With best wishes.

Regarding some clinical methods & apex beat localisation

Dr. J G Douglas

Chest Clinic, Clinic C
Aberdeen AB25 2ZN 02/11/2005
Ref: MacLeod's Clinical Examination, 11th edn

Thank you very much for your recent e-mail .... I am an editor of this edition..... I am responsible for writing much of the Respiratory Chapter and was most interested in your comments. In response:

Examining for Tracheal Shift................. Clearly this technique could also be performed with the patient standing or sitting.

Technique of Percussion – I entirely agree with your comment that to obtain the loudest percussion note ideally the other fingers, apart from the middle finger, should not touch the skin surface. Figure 4.19 is ambiguous and I will make a note of this for the next (12th) edition.

... Vocal Resonance........... However I agree that as written in the first paragraph of page 143 there is some confusion ....Again I will make a note to clarify this for the next (12th) edition.

Aegophony (page 144) .... However I agree that it's position is a little confusing and again I will make a note of this when redrafting the next (12th) edition.

Examination Sequence (page 97 .... palpation of apex beat) – I entirely agree with you that the second half of the statement under the 3rd arrow: "If you cannot feel it, ask the patient to roll on to their left side" is incorrect and references the wrong figure! I will make sure this is removed at the next reprint.

We are enormously grateful to you for your attention to detail in pointing out these points.
With best wishes. Yours sincerely.

Regarding errors in serum-ascites albumin gradient

Kurt J. Isselbacher, MD

Director, Massachusets General Hospital Cancer Center, Boston, Mallinckrodt Professor of Medicine, Harvard Medical School
Editor: Harrison's Principles of Internal Medicine, 13th edn 23/2/98

I must commend you for your astute and thorough reading of the Harrison's textbook and in addition, thank you for pointing out two obvious typographical errors. In fact, this was already done in the second printing of the 14th edition............................ *Again, many thanks for your thoughtfulness in bringing these two typographical errors to our attention.*

A compliment from Chief Editor of Harrison's book

Dennis L Kasper, MD

William Ellery Channing Professor of Medicine and Professor of microbiology and Molecular genetics, Harvard Medical School. Director, Channing Laboratory, Brigham and Women's Hospital, Boston, MA 02115
Editor: Harrison's Principles of Internal Medicine, 16th edition 7/10/2006

................I very much appreciate your interest in contributing to Harrison's. I have looked up your publications on PubMed, and I can see that you are active and productive in your field..........................., and I wish you all the best in your ongoing studies and clinical practice.
Best regards.

Regarding some queries on clinical medicine

Laurence Hunter

Senior Commissioning Editor, Elsevier
Ref: Hutchison's Clinical Methods, 22 edn
11/9/2008

Once again I am most grateful to you for taking the trouble to contact us with queries about the content of this textbook. I shall pass on to the Editors the comments and ask them to take full account of these in the revision of the book.
Thank you once again for your interest in our publishing programme.
With all good wishes.

Regarding erythema nodosum, & pulmonary stenosis

Keith A A Fox

Duke of Edinburgh, Professor of Cardiology and Head of Department, Cardiovascular Research Unit, The University of Edinburgh, Hugh Robson Building, George Square, Edinburgh EH8 9XF, 5/12/1995

Re: Davidson's Principle and Practice of Medicine: 17th Ed. 1995

On behalf of Editors of this textbook I have been asked to respond to you in view of the fact that this chapter was written by Dr. Boon and myself.

In response to your first question we have obtained source material which indicates erythema nodosum is a manifestation of acute rheumatic fever.

In conjunction with pulmonary stenosis, the only reason why the thrill may be best palpated in expiration is because of the fact that the heart moves closer to the anterior chest wall. We entirely agree that the velocity of blood flow across the pulmonary valve is increased in inspiration and this is demonstrated using echo Doppler techniques. However, for the reasons mentioned above palpation of thrill may be more obvious in held expiration when the heart and vessels are closer to the chest wall. I hope that these comments help to clarify the situation.
Yours sincerely.

Regarding contribution in "Kumar & Clark's" Textbook on Medicine

Ellen Green

Senior Commissioning Editor Elsevier, 1-3 Baxter's Place, Leith Walk, Edinburgh EH1 3AF
23/6/2005

Firstly, on behalf of Kumar & Clark, I would like to thank you for your contributions to the Online Appendix for Clinical Medicine 6e .... I hope you are pleased with the book ....
Kind regards.

In their Esteemed Opinion About the Book

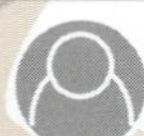

Prof BM Hegde

Ex-Professor & Dean of Medicine, Kasturba Medical College, Mangaluru (Ex-Vice-Chancellor, MAHE University, Manipal)

"Your book is an excellent replicative educational medium for exam-going students. Congratulations ....". ".......I am proud of you as you are a THINKER. May your tribe increase. Many students make you their role model. God will bless you always.........".

Dr AP Jain

Professor & Head, Department of Medicine, MG Institute of Medical Sciences, Sevagram, Maharashtra

"The monograph on *Bedside Clinics in Medicine* is very well written, studded with your long experience as clinical teacher. Such monograph was a long felt need. You have really done an excellent job. The monograph will be very well received not only by undergraduate and postgraduate students but by clinical teachers as well."

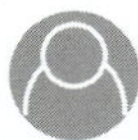

Dr SB Agarwal

Professor & Head, Department of Medicine, BJ Medical College and Civil Hospital, Ahmedabad, Gujarat

"I highly appreciate the efforts, hard work and sincerity in bringing up this publication in a beautifully designed manner with rich clinical material inside".

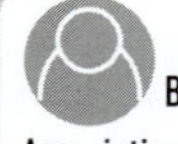

Book review (Part I) in Journal of the Indian Medical Association (JIMA)

"........ Examinees who wish to anticipate routine questions and to avoid long embarrassing silences would do well to read these pages. .... important points have received appropriate emphasis. .... The text is closely written and the amount of information provided is truely gross. Every line and word has to be remembered. ....".

Prof (Dr) DK Hazra

Director, Professor & Head, Department of Medicine, SN Medical College, Agra, Uttar Pradesh.

"...... I have gone through this book and found it most suitable for the students. I will definitely recommend this book to the students........"

Dr PC Bhattacharyya

Ex-Professor of Medicine, Gauhati Medical College, Assam.

" .... is an excellent book for junior students in Medicine. This book, very simply written in a concised and rational manner will greatly help the undergraduate students to establish the foundation of Clinical Medicine with ease and confidence."

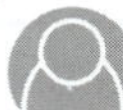

Dr PS Shankar

Dean, KJ Somiya Medical College, Mumbai

Book review in Journal of the Association of Physicians of India (JAPI)

Dr. Kundu has brought out a book based on bedside clinics on 26 model long cases and 74 short and spot cases oriented to clinical and oral examinations with special stress on clinical methods. .... He discusses the history, diagnosis, signs, differential diagnosis and management in the form of questions and answers. The answers are given in detail. .... There is an exhaustive coverage of the subject and Dr. Kundu has to be congratulated for bringing out such a wealth of knowledge. ......The book is very helpful to the students of clinical medicine while revising the subject before examination. Dr. Kundu has discussed the various questions which student may encounter during the examination and he has done it admirably".

Final year MBBS student, NRS Medical College, Kolkata.

"......It is a poetry on Clinical Medicine."

Dr PK Rathor

PG trainee, MKCG Medical College, Berhampur, Odisha.

".........I congratulate you for bringing out this book. ...."

Prof (Capt.) G Nagaiah

Professor & Head, Department of Medicine, Thanjavur Medical College & Hospitals, Tamil Nadu.

".....The book is good and very useful to undergraduates & postgraduates in Medicine .... I shall continue to recommend your book............congratulation to the author for his concentrated effort."

Dr BT Tukol

Professor of Medicine, KMC, Hubli, Karnataka

".......*Bedside Clinics in Medicine* by Dr. Arup Kumar Kundu is a good book for undergraduate medical students. It is helpful for preparing for final MBBS Examination. Students can guess as what type of questions may be asked in the practicals. ...."

in http://stupidsid.com

"Kundu's *Bedside Clinics in Medicine*, Part I & II are mesmerising books for Medical students. Every student should possess these books to have knowledge in Basic Clinical Medicine"

Dr AP Jain

Professor & Head, Department of Medicine, MG Institute of Medical Sciences, Sevagram, Maharashtra.

"The second revised edition of *'Bedside Clinics in Medicine'* contains information at one place which postgraduates in Medicine aspire to assimilate in order to learn art and science of Medicine. Really an excellent job by Dr Arup Kundu".

Dr K Gandhi

Assistant Professor of Medicine, Thanjavur Medical College, Tamil Nadu.

"........It is so nice that all clinical problems are completed in so small a volume. ......".

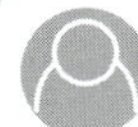

Dr Kiranmoy Mitra

Ex-Assoc. Professor & Head, Department of Medicine, Burdwan Medical College and Hospital, West Bengal.

"........This is not a book but something more than that. This is self-explanative and could be one of the best books in the field of Clinical Medicine required for our students. The book is indispensable for not only undergraduates and postgraduate students but also for teachers and practitioners in Medicine as well. This book is a living Clinical Tutor".

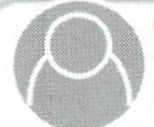

Prof (Dr) CR Maity

Ex-Dean, Faculty of Medicine, Burdwan University; Principal, Burdwan Medical College, Burdwan, West Bengal (Ex-DME, WBMES, Government of West Bengal).

"In keeping with the expanding horizon of medical sciences and the gallant gallops of a plethora of newly emerging methodologies, Dr Arup K Kundu has very meticulously and ingenuously architectured his master creation *Bedside Clinics in Medicine*, Parts I and II. A purist pedagogue, a massive mentor, and an exemplary exponent engrossed with an expansive professional expertise and competency, he has probed deeply into several cases along with history, diagnosis and management invariably in an easy-to-understand question-answer form......... The diagnostic procedures and methodologies are nicely delineated. This book will be a constant concise companion for all, students and teachers alike, in different Indian Universities and Medical Colleges as this treasure will elicit the clinical spirit of approach from a modest conventional way to highly sophisticated method."

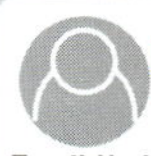

Dr V Venugopal

Professor of Medicine, Perundurai Medical College, Tamil Nadu.

I can recommend the book to my students as a ready reckoner........."

Col AS Kasthuri
Professor and Head, Department of Medicine, AFMC, Pune, Maharashtra.

"The book *Bedside Clinics in Medicine*, Part I and II is comprehensive with wide coverage of all systems and attractively produced. .... it is informative and beneficial not only to the UGs/PGs, but also to the physicians."

Dr K Ramachandran
Visiting Professor of Radiology, MG University School of Medicine, Gandhi Nagar, Kottayam, Kerala.

"....... I found that there is a wealth of information in the book which is difficult to get from other books. ....you must have gone through several journals and the whole of encyclopedia of medicine .... Congratulations."

Dr Saif Omar
Internee, Katihar Medical College, Katihar, Bihar

"....... I have been an ardent reader of both of your textbooks on clinical medicine, since the first day of my ward duty. To be very honest I have learnt more from your books than from........"

Dr Kamaalchand M
PG trainee in Pediatrics, JNMC, Aligarh Muslim University, Aligarh, Uttar Pradesh.

"....... many congratulations for writing an ultimate manuscript in medicine. ...."

Prof (Dr) PR Nath Barbhuiya (Retd.)
Professor & Head, Department of Medicine, Silchar Medical College & Hospital, Assam.

"....... *Bedside Clinics in Medicine*, Part I & Part II is a 'Treasure Island" for students of Medicine both undergraduates & postgraduates. .... The book has in fact satisfied the need of a long awaited reference book for examinee being complete by itself in all respects. ....recommend this book strongly for students of medicine........"

Dr NS Neki
Associate Professor of Medicine, Government Medical College, Amritsar, Punjab.

"....... *Bedside Clinics in Medicine*, Part I, which is highly informative, well-written with latest additions ...."

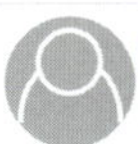

Dr Keerthana Karumbaiah K
Internee, Bangalore Medical College, Bengaluru, Karnataka.

"....... the joy of reading the book is so overwhelming that, by far, medicine has never seemed so pleasurable........ . It is unequivocal opinion that the book is outstanding and entirely removes the need to study multiple books in clinical medicine. .... For my final year exams .... the questions that were asked during discussion were entirely based upon the facts given in your book. I just had to quote them to be appreciated by the examiners........"

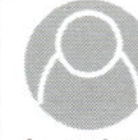

Book review (Part II) in Journal of the Indian Medical Association (JIMA)

"....... this 'made easy', if assimilated properly by the students, will help to learn many aspects of medicine. ..... The chapters on radiological diagnosis and ECG interpretations will certainly help all concerned. Emergency tackling of different cases also, will help the young professionals. ...... The book is likely to be well accepted and the second edition of the book supports that expectation."

Dr Pradeep Kumar Shenoy C
Ex-clinical fellow and registrar, Department of Rheumatology, Manipal Hospital, Bengaluru, Karnataka.

"....... its really the eighth wonder in the world. Looking back, recollecting my MD days, I repeat my words ....I owe you my MD."

Dr Bhushan Madke
student of Indira Gandhi Govt. Medical College, Nagpur, Maharashtra.

"......I am very happy to inform you that I have got selected for MD........... I owe my success to your book, and your in time valuable suggestion and advice. You have been my behind the scene teacher and educator and inspiration.........."

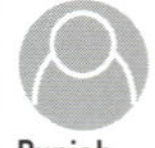

Jagroop Singh
Student of Guru Gobind Singh Medical College, Faridkot, Punjab.

".....You have donated breath to me.........."

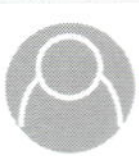

J Mahammad Sadiq
Government Medical College, Salem, Tamil Nadu.

"I am a final year medical student. I read your book on bedside clinical examination........ The book is really wonderful. Hats of sir......"

Ramchandra Chaudhary
Student of SRTR Medical College, Ambajogai, Maharashtra.

".....I am highly impressed with clarity and concept of your book. The book is not only helpful for clinical exams but also for theory. The book is really a wonderful book....."

Dr Amit Sharma,
(DM cardiology student), and passed MD (medicine) from KGMC, Lucknow, Uttar Pradesh.

"Sir, its really great whatever you write, I have read your book in final year to clear exam, that helped very much to pass final prof......"

Parvathy Rajmohan
Sree Gokulam Medical College, Thiruvananthapuram, Kerala.

"First of all, thank you for writing this book. It is truly a lifesaver......"

C. Manpa Phom
Intern, Agartala Govt. Medical College, Tripura.

"Sir, thanks for the wonderful book of yours of *Bedside clinics in Medicine* part I & II............ have passed my final mbbs finally and sir your book was the only book I read for my practical examination......."

Ashwin Joshi
Intern, Agartala Govt. Medical College, Tripura.

".............I must say that the book '*Bedside Clinics in Medicine*' which you have authored is extremely useful, exam oriented and very relevant. I can vouch and say that all 180 students from final year in our college will be preparing from it, especially for the practical exam ....Highest regards and respect."

Dr. Rakesh Das
1st year PGT, Agartala Govt. Medical College, Tripura.

"....Thanks a lot to you for gifting such a nice book "*Bedside Clinics in Medicine*". Its a must read book for both UG & PGT Medicine...."

Dr Abhishek Sachdeva
DNB student, Videocon Group of Hospitals, Maharashtra.

"...........Sir your books are a great help for students learning medicine. Sir,..... I would like to tell you that its my dream to have a teacher like you some day. I also feel proud that such an amazing piece of work is done by an Indian Author."

Om Prakash Mishra
Final year MBBS student, Institute of medicine, Kathmandu, Nepal.

"First of all I would like to thank you for producing such a marvellous book, the only one of its kind, for Clinical Medicine. This book is beyond comparison. It is helping to raise the standard of clinical examinations in students' as well as doctors worldwide."

Dr Jalal Ahmed
Kasturba Medical College, Manipal, Karnataka

"Thanks for writing a great book for postgraduates ......"

Final year MBBS student, GMERS Medical College, Gotri, Vadodara, Gujarat.

"I thank you a lot for bringing out this book. I never felt medicine too interesting although I'm in final year..... credit goes to you..... Thanks sir"

Mina Aziz
Ain Shams University, Cairo, Egypt.

"Thank you for your great book. It really helped us a lot......".

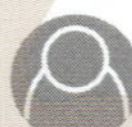

Pawon Goel
Final year MBBS student, Maulana Azad Medical College, New Delhi.

".....Here in our college your book is recommended by everyone, even the senior residents. I enjoyed your book very much....."

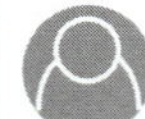

Gopal Yadav
MBBS 3rd year student, BP Koirala Institute of Health Sciences, Dharan, Nepal.

"Sir Namaste! Your book on bedside medicine has become a part and parcel of medical students......."

Dr Sagar Tandel
MD student, Shri MP Shah Medical College, Jamnagar, Gujarat.

"First of all I would like to congratulate you on immensely informative '*Bedside Clinics in Medicine* - Edition 7th'. You would be happy to know that we, residents, are considering it as a principle book for preparation of case presentations in our MD Medicine curriculum....."

Dr Vivek Agarwala
Dept. of Medicine, GSVM Medical College, Kanpur, Uttar Pradesh.

".........I would like to congratulate you and thank you for your wonderful book and your efforts towards making the subject of medicine easier to learn for us."

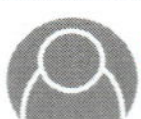

Soumya Roy
Student of Calcutta Medical College, West Bengal.

"......I had been a die-hard fan of your book. Lots of respect...."

Dr Milind Patil
BJ Medical College, Pune, Maharashtra.

"I have used your book ..... during my undergraduate (MBBS) and postgraduate exam (MD) in internal medicine. Its a very good book for both exams. It saves a lot of time of students in preparing for exams. Thanks for spending your valuable time in writing such excellent book"

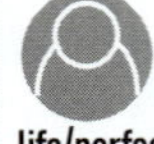

http://medchrome.com/medicalcolleges/student-life/perfecting-yourselfclinical-examination/

"Kundu's *Bedside Clinics in Medicine* — another wonder book for medicine. It has almost everything and even things found no where else. Will help students a lot. ...."

www.quora.com

"......Casewise the best in Kundu"

http://medcosmosbaroda.blogspot.com/2008–09–01–archive.html

"*Bedside Clinics in Medicine* by Dr Arup Kundu is really nice to crash all the viva Q-A in your clinical viva......... also it helps to clear basics.......It teaches you how to think medicine"

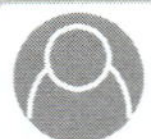

in www.doctorshangout.com/profile/peuishsugathan

"....Favorite medical books: Harrison's principle's of internal medicine, Kundu, de Gruchy, John Patten...."

www.xmail.net/wfmustudents/medicalbooks.htm

Website in China (Weifang Medical University, Shandong, China) recommends this book for their students

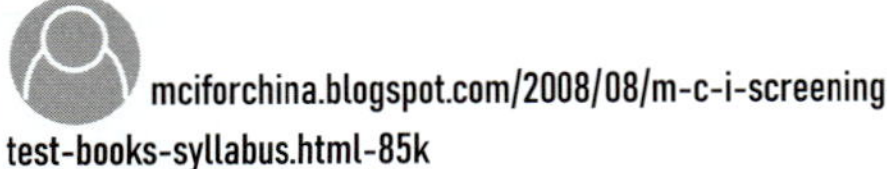

mciforchina.blogspot.com/2008/08/m-c-i-screening-test-books-syllabus.html-85k

....recommended Bedside Clinics in Medicine, Part I & II for MCI screening test books for students passed MBBS from aborad.

www.quora.com

"....Kundu: the book is in question answer format. Any and all question that will ask in viva by externals in the exam comes from this book. It has part B which gives the necessary details for charts, tables, ECG, etc......"

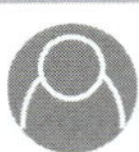

www.quora.com

"We read Arup Kumar Kundu's *Bedside Clinics in Medicine* for Medicine practicals. It has all Long, Short cases and Instruments, ECGs, X-rays, etc...."

www.quora.com

".......Kundu helps you to understand the cases better and helps you to stand in good position to answer the questions"

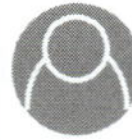

www.quora.com

".....For practical, "*Bedside Clinics in Medicine*—Kundu" (it's an unparallel clinical medicine book worth to read)......"

in www.cafemedico.com

".......I m using Kundu.........all casewise clinical study is very fine.......I really like it...."

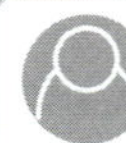

www.quora.com

"..........Most answers in the book were based on sound concept rather than mere dumping of facts....... Level of recommendation: VERY VERY HIGH..."

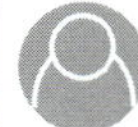

in https://desimedicos.com

"........Many seniors recommend it for differential diagnosis (D/D). The book is excellently detailed. Students should go through this book .... call it best book for clinical medicine and practicals"

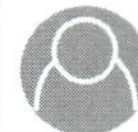

www.aippg.net

"......also Arup Kundu if you want to dash answers in ward round cases. I would recommend Kundu as a must buy over and above one basic book like Hunter....."

in www.doctorshangout.ning.com/ profile/DrMansi

".....Favorite Medical Books: Guyton's Physiology & Kundu's Medicine...."

Rajkishor Singh
Nalanda Medical College & Hospital, Patna, Bihar.

"I am very grateful to you that you bestow such a nice material for understanding a huge subject of medicine which made very easy for both clinical examination as well as theory exam, and best supplement for PG entrance exam. Thanks a lot"

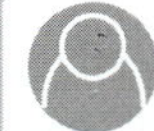

Apildev Neupane
Final year medical student at Institute of Medicine, Kathmandu, Nepal.

".....It is a well known fact among medical professionals, that your book on bedside medicine has proved to be a holy gift to the generations of medical students in this part of the world...."

Dr Nidhish Chandra M
(DM) Rhumatology Sr. Resident, King Georage MU, Lucknow, Uttar Pradesh.

"I read your book during my MD times and was very useful as a bedside tool.......I always felt that you are teaching us from the patient's bedside. Thanks a lot for providing us with such a powerful tool...."

Abhishek Raj A
Student of Chettinad Medical College, Tamil Nadu

"..... Your book *'Bedside Clinics in Medicine* Part I' has offered the eager n thirty medical student child with in me! Kudos n power to u Sir! N may your tribe increase!...."

Part I

Ninth Edition

Bedside Clinics in Medicine

with COLOUR Photos and Clinical Integration

Long, Short and Spot Cases

As per the latest NMC Guidelines | Competency Based Medical Education (CBME) Curriculum under Graduate Medical Education Regulation

- **Clinical Methods All-in-One**
- **Step-wise Approach to Cases**
- **Extra Edge in Practical Exam**

The Best Text for NExT Examinations—Thoroughly Revised and Updated

"Medicine is to be learned only by experience; it is not an inheritance; it cannot be revealed. Learn to see, learn to hear, learn to feel, learn to smell, and know that by practice alone can you become expert. Medicine is learned by the bedside and not in the classroom. See, and then reason and compare and control. But see first."

—Sir William Osler (1849–1919)
Professor of Medicine, Oxford, UK

Other Books/Chapters by the Same Author

- *Bedside Clinics in Medicine*, Part II (9th Ed), 2024
- *Kundu's Practical Medicine* (2nd Ed), 2024
- *MCQs in Internal Medicine* (6th Ed), 2022
- *Pearls in Medicine for Students* (3rd Ed), 2024
- *Memorable Memoirs of a Medico* (on Amazon portal), 2023

Chapters in:

- *API Textbook in Medicine*, 8th Ed, 2008
- *Postgraduate Medicine*, 2009
- *Rheumatology: Principles and Practice*, 2010
- *Medicine Update*: 2010–15, 2017, 2018, 2021–24
- *Progress in Medicine*: 2016, 2019, 2020, 2023, 2024
- *Manual of Rheumatology*: 5th Ed, 2018; 6th Ed, 2024
- *Rheumatology Clinics: Clinical Scenarios*, 2024
- Online appendix of "Kumar & Clark's", *Clinical Medicine:* 6–10th Ed

Biography (Author)

Included in Marquis Who's Who in the World 2014, 2015 and 2016
Who's Who in Science and Engineering 2016–17, and in
Wikipedia & WikiVisually

'Gifted Teacher' Awardee in 2022 (by Association of Physicians of India)

Fellow/Member of

- Fellow, Indian College of Physicians (India)
- Fellow, Royal College of Physicians (Edinburgh)
- Member, New York Academy of Sciences (USA)
- Member, International Advisory Panel of "Kumar & Clark's" textbook, *Clinical Medicine*, 7–10th Ed (Edinburgh)
- Life-member, Association of Physicians of India (API)
- Life-member, Indian Rheumatology Association (IRA)
- Life-member, Indian Medical Association (IMA)

Part I

Ninth Edition

Bedside Clinics in Medicine

with COLOUR Photos and Clinical Integration

Long, Short and Spot Cases

As per the latest NMC Guidelines | Competency Based Medical Education (CBME) Curriculum under Graduate Medical Education Regulation

Arup Kumar Kundu MD FRCP FICP MNAS
Ex-Visiting Faculty and Consultant Rheumatologist
IQ City Medical College
West Bengal, India

Formerly
Professor, Department of Medicine and
In-charge, Division of Rheumatology
NRS MC, KPC MC, IQ City MC, and
RG Kar Medical College, West Bengal, India
and
Author of five other books with chapters in different books on medical sciences
Thirty years of teaching experience in Govt and private medical colleges
UG and PG examiner in different Indian Universities
Prestigious 'Gifted Teacher' Awardee in 2022 by API
Mentor and Instructional Coach, pan-India for teaching in MBBS, MD, DNB

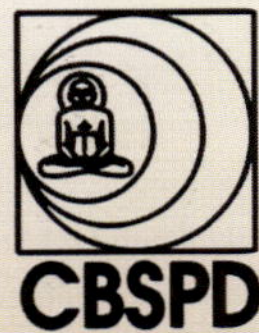

CBS Publishers & Distributors Pvt Ltd

New Delhi • Bengaluru • Chennai • Kochi • Kolkata • Lucknow • Mumbai
Gujarat • Hyderabad • Jharkhand • Nagpur • Patna • Pune • Uttarakhand

Disclaimer

Science and technology are constantly changing fields. New research and experience broaden the scope of information and knowledge. The author has tried his best in giving information available to him while preparing the material for this book. Although all efforts have been made to ensure optimum accuracy of the material, yet it is quite possible some errors might have been left uncorrected. The publisher, the printer and the author will not be held responsible for any inadvertent errors, omissions or inaccuracies.

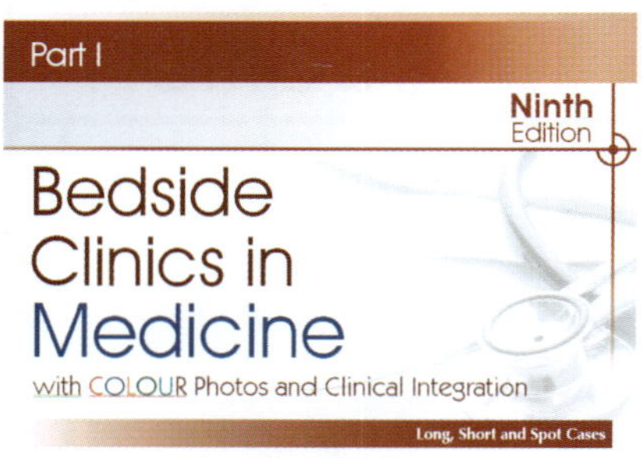

ISBN: 978-93-5466-771-8

Ninth Edition 2024

Reprint 2025

First Edition 1996
Second Edition 1997
Third Edition 1999
Fourth Edition 2002
Fifth Edition 2006
Sixth Edition 2010
Seventh Edition 2014
Eighth Edition 2019

Published by Satish Kumar Jain and produced by Varun Jain for

CBS Publishers & Distributors Pvt Ltd

4819/XI Prahlad Street, 24 Ansari Road, Daryaganj, New Delhi 110 002, India

Ph: 011-23266838, 23289259 Website: www.cbspd.com
e-mail: delhi@cbspd.com

Corporate Office: 204 FIE, Industrial Area, Patparganj, Delhi 110 092, India

Ph: 011-49344934 Fax: 011-49344935
e-mail: publishing@cbspd.com; publicity@cbspd.com

Branches

- **Bengaluru:** Seema House 2975, 17th Cross, K.R. Road, Banasankari 2nd Stage, Bengaluru 560 070, Karnataka, India
  Ph: +91-80-26771678/79 Fax: +91-80-26771680 e-mail: bangalore@cbspd.com
- **Chennai:** 7, Subbaraya Street, Shenoy Nagar, Chennai 600 030, Tamil Nadu, India
  Ph: +91-44-26680620, 26681266 Fax: +91-44-42032115 e-mail: chennai@cbspd.com
- **Kochi:** 42/1325, 1326, Power House Road, Opposite KSEB, Power House, Ernakulum 682018, Kochi, Kerala, India
  Ph: +91-484-4059061–67 Fax: +91-484-4059065 e-mail: kochi@cbspd.com
- **Kolkata:** 147, Hind Ceramics Compound, 1st Floor, Nilgunj Road, Belghoria, Kolkata 700056, West Bengal, India
  Ph: +91-33-25330055/56 e-mail: kolkata@cbspd.com
- **Lucknow:** Basement, Khushuma Complex, 7 Meerabai Marg (behind Jawahar Bhawan), Lucknow 226001, UP, India
  Ph: +91-522-4000032 e-mail: tiwari.lucknow@cbspd.com
- **Mumbai:** PWD Shed, Gala No. 25/26, Ramchandra Bhatt Marg, Next JJ Hospital Gate No. 2, Opp. Union Bank of India, Noorbaug, Mumbai 400009, Maharashtra, India
  Ph: +91-22-66661880/89 e-mail: mumbai@cbspd.com

Representatives

- **Gujarat** 0-9879558667 • **Hyderabad** 0-9885175004 • **Jharkhand** 0-9811541605
- **Nagpur** 0-8692091830 • **Patna** 0-9334159340 • **Pune** 0-9664372571
- **Uttarakhand** 0-9716462459

Printed in Goyal Offset Works Pvt. Ltd., Haryana (INDIA)

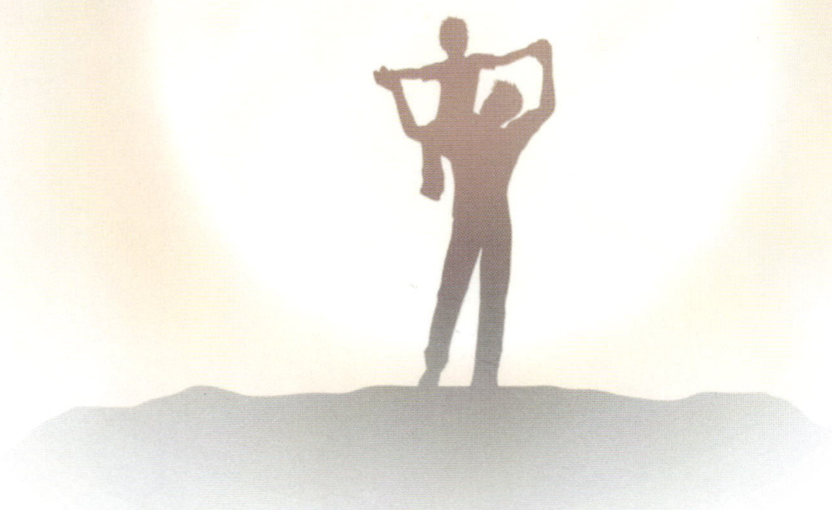

to

my father

Late Professor (Dr) Amiya Kumar Kundu MD (Cal)

a great physician

who has taught me clinical medicine

Preface to the Ninth Edition

I have great pleasure in presenting the Ninth Edition of *'Bedside Clinics in Medicine, Part I'*. The first Edition was published in the year 1996, and thereafter it was revised and edited from time to time in order to make the same up-to-date. In view of the wide acceptance of the previous editions by the medical fraternity, by the God's grace, I have ultimately succeeded to bring out the present edition of the book in a new layout. The overwhelming success of previous editions boosted me to bring out the new edition. Virtually all the chapters have been rewritten, appreciably revised and updated, maintaining the previous style and tradition intact. The book reviews a wide range of common clinical cases in general medicine with elaborate discussion on core topics. Many new photographs have been included for easy and better understanding of the concepts of clinical medicine. I have wholeheartedly tried to present here all clinical topics required for a modern, clinical curriculum. This 'magic book in clinical medicine' is now ready for the medical students of our country and abroad.

It is my strong belief that bedside medicine (patient-oriented medicine) still holds effective in the present era of high-tech medicine, and this is why, I have attempted to write this monograph dealing with common clinical problems along with some fundamental information which a medical student should know at the end of his/her clinical training. In this rapidly changing global scenario, even with availability of sophisticated gadgets, modern technology and advanced investigations, clinical examination is the quicker and more cost-effective way in arriving at a logical diagnosis. I strongly believe that clinical medicine will never die even in the era of modern technology. The 'storytelling style' of the book narrates step-by-step details of history, analysis of symptoms, clinical methods, clinical pearls, history of medicine, relevance of clinical findings, differential diagnosis, details of investigations and logical management in a lucid language. The present edition deals with different must-know areas in clinical medicine in a student-friendly way. This book will teach both the science and arts of clinical medicine from the fundamentals to the most advanced level.

During my long tenure as a teacher for more than three decades, I feel that the skills needed for a comprehensive and competent clinical examination can only be mastered at the bedside by repeated clinical practice. The book emphasizes the basic approach to clinical medicine, and its problem-solving attitude helps the students prepare for the medicine practical (even in theoretical) at final MBBS, MD, DNB and MRCP level, and also in their professional life in future. This quick-reference ready-reckoner is full of valuable tips from beginning to the end. As clinical methods are scattered throughout the book, the students are **advised to follow the 'Contents' and 'Index' for easy reading**. It is advisable to set a 'mind map' of the chapters, as the students progress from first to last page. In many places, 'history of medicine' has been focused for the relevant topic under discussion. Now try to enjoy the world of clinical medicine.

This present edition contains 100 model long, short and spot cases, 416 photographs (elaborating clinical methods in details along with real-life pictures of patients), 51 tables, many drawings, flowcharts and innumerable questions with their logical answers. I have tried my best to avoid any ambiguity in the text. The book remains an invaluable resource for MBBS students, house officers, postgraduates studying MD, DNB, MRCP curricula, and junior teachers preparing for clinical teaching sessions. I feel really happy as the book is nicely accepted by academicians, students, teachers and leading physicians from different corners of the country and abroad. Healthy suggestions and constructive criticisms from the readers will always be appreciated by the author and received with gratitude.

I have immense pleasure in placing on record my appreciation for Mr Satish Kumar Jain (Chairman and Managing Director) and Mr Varun Jain (Director) of CBS Publishers and Distributors (CBSPD), New Delhi for publishing and distributing the book in India and abroad with great care. Mr SK Verma of CBSPD (VP, Marketing & Distributions) needs special mention who has guided me in every step of this long journey. Mr YN Arjuna (Senior Vice-President, Publishing, Editorial and Publicity) helped me by his constant input and encouragement, which have had a significant impact on the final texture of the text. I am also thankful to my wife Bijoya, son Dr Abhishek and daughter Ushasi, who have assisted me by their constant encouragement and support, and I remain indebted for their tolerance, patience and understanding during the preparation of the book.

Arup Kumar Kundu

arup2158@gmail.com
arup_kundu@hotmail.com

Preface to the First Edition

This is not a text book of medicine. This book is based on bedside clinics on hundred 'model cases' oriented to **oral and practical examinations** with special stress on clinical methods. I hope this book will be very much helpful to students of clinical medicine both undergraduate and postgraduate.

First, I wish to express my deep sense of gratitude to my parents and family members, whose constant encouragement has enabled me to complete this book.

Next, I take the opportunity to extend my heartfelt reverence and fathomless gratitude to all my respected teachers. I feel, I should make a special mention of the names of Prof P Sen MD (Cal), FRCP (Edin), FICA (USA), Prof S Sen FRCP (Edin), FICA (USA), Prof PC Das MD (Cal), FICA (USA), FCCP (USA); and Prof AK Kundu MD (Cal).

This book would never have been completed without the help of my wife Mrs Bijoya Kundu. I am greatly indebted to her.

I owe deep sense of gratitude to Prof SK Paul MO (Cal), without his constant encouragement, active guidance and blessings, this book would never have seen the light of the day.

I am very much grateful to Mr Bimal Dhur of Academic Publishers, whose advice has been of great help to me.

I am thankful to Mr Robin Chatterjee and Ms Lopamudra Paul for meticulously typing out the manuscript. I also heartily acknowledge Mr Kaustuv Paul of Crest Publishers who has taken immense pain in publishing this book.

I also express my thanks to all the staff of 'Abhinaba Mudrani' who have helped me in every step to complete the book.

In conclusion, I would like to admit that only few names appear in this acknowledgement, many too much unsung, have significantly contributed to and enhanced the quality of this book. To all, I am deeply obligated.

Arup Kumar Kundu

Perspectives

In 1816, Rene-Theophile-Hyacinthe Laennec invented the stethoscope — the single instrument that came to symbolise the bedside physician and the tool used by the clinicians for almost last two centuries.

The term patient is derived from the Latin word 'patiens', or 'to suffer'. A 'patient' is one who feels sick physically or mentally, and consults doctor for relief of his ailments. In clinical medicine, patients hold the key position. Naturally, it is the task of the physician that he should do the needful for the recovery of the patient. The target of medical practice is to relieve sufferings.

To relieve the sufferings of the patients, a doctor should ascertain at first, the nature of illness from which the patient is suffering from. In other words, the doctor has to diagnose the existing disease. Physical diagnosis makes the bridge between the study of disease and the management of illness. Clinical diagnosis is an artistic science, based on three kinds of medical information:

i. Communication with the patient (i.e. the history taking),
ii. Physical examination, and
iii. Investigations.

Clinical medicine deals with the first two parts of diagnosis, i.e. 'clinical examination' of a patient consists of history taking as well as physical examination. These are the most important parts and it starts as soon as the patient comes to the doctor. At no point can **history taking** (medical events that have already taken place) be considered as 'wastage' of time; in most of the cases, the diagnosis can be made with history alone. History taking is an art, which a doctor should learn over years by repeated practice. A physician should be an attentive listener and be friendly to the patient. Regarding history taking, it is my advice to the students of clinical medicine that they should try to disprove Ben Berston's comment, who told 'A funny thing happens to medical students on their way to becoming physicians; they forget how to hold a conversation'. An appropriate history guides the patient's management in a proper direction. While examining the patient, an experienced doctor not only 'sees' but also 'uses all of his senses' and gradually develops the keen 'power of observation' which is known as 'clinical eye' or 'clinical acumen'. These insights cannot be acquired in a short-cut way and there is no rule of thumb in it. To learn this, one has to go to the bedside of the patients for years together, to make keen observations, to examine them thoroughly and sympathetically, and to try to 'associate' different observations and findings. Gradually the person develops the inherent 'knowledge of correlation' with the help of clinical eye. This is why, Hippocrates commented, 'A great part, I believe, of the art of medicine is the ability to observe. Leave nothing, combine contradictory observations and allow yourself enough time'. *An experienced clinician not only hears but listens, not only sees but observes, and not only touches but feels.* One, who has sharp clinical eye, becomes successful in life in the long run.

Traditionally, the process of **physical examination** (clinical state at that given time) is divided into four parts like looking (inspection), feeling (palpation), tapping (percussion), and listening (auscultation). From our student days we have learned to determine 'where is the lesion' as well as 'what is the lesion' derived by physical examination to arrive at a definitive diagnosis; this is also true to the students of this generation too. It should be realised that inspection/palpation/percussion/and especially auscultation are skills acquired over years of training. We know that our professional progenitors relied more on power of smelling (sweetish musty odour of hepatic coma) and tasting as well (the sweetness of urine in diabetes mellitus), but these facts have lost their importance in today's modern medicine. A sincere and meticulous physical examination combined with in-depth as well as sound knowledge of internal medicine will help the physician to determine the most probable cause/causes of the patient's present ailments. At the beginning, a student should have an open mind (observe, listen and create). It is wise to consider the patients as living pages of books, and instead of examining from 'head to feet', I should rather advise students to examine patients from 'head to toes'.

Another important part of clinical medicine is doctor-patient relationship. It has got immense value in ultimate recovery of the patient. By the way of 'conversation' and physical examination, one sympathetic doctor gains confidence and wins trust of the patient. This should never be neglected. Whenever the confidence of the patient is achieved, it becomes easier for the doctor to get his cooperation to examine the painful areas or even the diseased private parts of the body. In a non-cooperative patient, diagnosis may be much more difficult and delayed.

Investigations help the doctor confirm the diagnosis made by clinical examination. Of course, clinical diagnosis by physical examination has limitations. No doubt, in many cases one has to take the help of newer and sophisticated investigations to arrive at a definitive diagnosis. Recently, there is a boom in investigational facilities like polymerase chain reaction (PCR), ELISA (enzyme-linked immunosorbent assay) test, ultrasound, CT (computed tomography) scan, NMR (nuclear magnetic resonance) scan, PET (positron-emission tomography) scan, and SPECT (single-photon emission computed tomography) scan where the patient is being fragmented into systems, organs, tissues, cells or even the smallest DNA, and very often these facilities erode the confidence of the clinicians concerned. Nowadays, a large section of doctors feel that clinical examination is not at all essential and diagnosis can be made easily with the help of sophisticated investigations only. But this is not at all true. The laboratory should be used as an aid for confirmation of diagnosis and the final approach should be to 'treat the patient', not the laboratory reports. Try to prepare yourself with a patient-oriented mindset, rather than laboratory-oriented mindset. One confident doctor should never disregard his own clinical findings; moreover, newer investigations are often very costly and out of reach of most of the patients of a developing country like India. It seems we have reached an era of intellectual bankruptcy where the doctors ask for 'all investigations' than to ask for 'rational investigations'. A long time back, Alvan R. Feinstein remarked, 'Clinical judgement depends not on knowledge of causes, mechanisms or names of disease but on a knowledge of patients. The background of clinical judgement is clinical experience; the things that clinicians have learned at the bedside is the care of sick people'. I do think that clinical judgement and insight are inborn faculties which increase with experience.

In spite of these facts we cannot ignore the importance of 'chemical' diagnosis and contribution of physics in medicine, e.g. the discovery of X-ray by Wilhelm Roentgen or ECG (electrocardiogram) by Willem Einthoven. So question arises, will this computer and sophisticated newer technology replace the physician's task of performing physical examination? The answer is simply 'no'. The computer necessarily deals with the cold literal aspects of words, whereas the doctors are trained to search for hidden meanings. To the question, 'is your pain continuing at the present moment'? — the mechanical computer only records 'yes' even when the patient shows agony while responding. The doctor reads far more to the patient's response to 'yes'. Moreover, detailed questioning and physical examination frequently build the first emotional contact between the doctor and the patient. Can a computer be sympathetic to the patient regarding his illness? Or can a fascinating electronic gadget replace the excellence of Giant Clinicians like Battista Morgagni, Leopold Auenbrugger, Rudolf Virchow, RTH Laennec, Sir William Osler, Adolph Kussmaul and Joseph Jules Francois Felix Babinski? A human brain created the computer, and thus a slave can neither demonstrate physical signs of the disease in a patient nor can interpret the complexities encountered to have a definitive diagnosis. It has to be remembered that technology cannot be a substitute for clinical examination or the doctor-patient bond, which heals before any medicine. An internet cannot replace examination of patients at the bedside. So there is reason to believe that clinical medicine will ever persist as a basic diagnostic method and investigations will remain as 'complementary' to the clinician.

Medical knowledge is not masterable. Unlike physics or chemistry, medicine is not a pure science. Half of what is true today will be proven to be incorrect in the next five years, and unfortunately we do not know which half that is going to be. The question arises whether medicine is a science, or an art, or an art based on science? The scientists say that medicine is sometimes considered a science, and sometimes an art, and the object of medical science is to study disease. I think medicine is an art based on science; medicine is supposed to be a scientific study whether its practice is an art. However, I should say that medicine is a philosophy, the elicitation is the art and its interpretation is the science. Today, every senior doctor is shouting in every corner of this globe that the art of clinical medicine is dying in the present teaching set-up with high-tech gadgets. I also think that they are mostly true; today, doctors are more powerful but more deaf. Medical students are advised to revive the dying art of medicine and to be good artists with sufficient scientific knowledge.

It is worthwhile to mention here that lack of clinical skills may be called as 'hyposkillia'! The physicians with deficiency of clinical skills cannot take proper history, cannot perform physical examination, cannot manage the patient with proper assessment and reasoning, and posses poor communication skills. So, a proper training is essential in initial days of medical curriculum as today's medical students are the practicing physicians of future. At first, a student learns from his teacher and then 'experience' teaches him. The term 'doctor' came from the Latin word '*docere*', which means 'to teach'.

In the beginning of their clinical training, the students should also remember these golden words: '**there is no substitute for watchful eyes, alert ears, and tactful fingers in a logical mind**' as Hippocrates told 'eyes, ears, nose and palpating fingers are the gems of a physician, while intact brain is the necklace'.

Contents

Abbreviations

ABG	Arterial blood gas
AFB	Acid-fast bacillus
AGN	Acute glomerulonephritis
AIDS	Acquired immune deficiency syndrome
AI/AR	Aortic incompetence/regurgitation
AKI	Acute kidney injury
ALL	Acute lymphoblastic leukaemia
AMI	Acute myocardial infarction
AML	Acute myeloid leukaemia
ANA	Antinuclear antibody
ARDS	Acute respiratory distress syndrome
ARF	Acute renal failure
AS	Aortic stenosis
ASD	Atrial septal defect
ATD	Antituberculosis drugs
AVM	Arteriovenous malformation
BAL	Brochoalveolar lavage
BHP	Benign hypertrophy of prostate
BMI	Body mass index
BP	Blood pressure
BT	Bleeding time
°C	Degree Celsius
CAD	Coronary artery disease
CCF	Congestive cardiac failure
C/F	Clinical features
CKD	Chronic kidney disease
CLD	Chronic liver disease
CLL	Chronic lymphocytic leukaemia
CML	Chronic myeloid leukaemia
CMV	Cytomegalovirus
CNS	Central nervous system
C/o	Complains of
COPD	Chronic obstructive pulmonary disease
CP angle	Cerebello-pontine angle
CPR	Cardiopulmonary resuscitation
CRF	Chronic renal failure
CRP	C-reactive protein
CT	Clotting or coagulation time
CT scan	Computed tomography scan
CVA	Cerebrovascular accidents
CVP	Central venous pressure
CVS	Cardiovascular system
CXR	Chest X-ray
D/D	Differential diagnosis
DIC	Disseminated intravascular coagulation
DKA	Diabetic ketoacidosis
DVT	Deep vein thrombosis
ECG	Electrocardiogram
EF	Ejection fraction
EPS	Extrapyramidal system
ESR	Erythrocyte sedimentation rate
ESRD	End-stage renal disease
°F	Degree Fahrenheit
FEV1	Forced expiratory volume in one second
FNAC	Fine needle aspiration cytology
FUO	Fever of unknown origin
GBS	Guillain-Barré syndrome
GERD	Gastroesophageal reflux disease
GFR	Glomerular filtration rate
GH	Growth hormone
GTT	Glucose tolerance test
Hb	Haemoglobin
HBV	Hepatitis B virus
HCV	Hepatitis C virus
HD	Hodgkin's disease
HIV	Human immunodeficiency virus
HLA	Human leucocyte antigen
HOCM	Hypertrophic obstructive cardiomyopathy
H/o	History of
HSP	Henoch-Schönlein purpura
IBD	Inflammatory bowel disease
IBS	Irritable bowel syndrome
ICP	Intracranial pressure
ICS	Intercostal space
ICU	Intensive care unit
IE	Infective endocarditis
IHD	Ischaemic heart disease
IHSS	Idiopathic hypertrophic subaortic stenosis
IIT	Increased intracranial tension
ILD	Interstitial lung disease
IM	Intramuscular
INR	International normalised ratio
IV	Intravenous
IVC	Inferior vena cava
JIA	Juvenile idiopathic arthritis
JVP	Jugular venous pressure
LA/RA	Left atrium/right atrium
LAF	Left atrial failure
LAH	Left atrial hypertrophy
LFT	Liver function test
LMN	Lower motor neurone
LV/RV	Left ventricle/right ventricle
LVF	Left ventricular failure
LVH	Left ventricular hypertrophy
MCL	Midclavicular line
MCTD	Mixed connective tissue disease
MDR	Multi-drug resistance
MI/MR	Mitral incompetence/regurgitation
MND	Motor neurone disease
MS	Mitral stenosis
NAD	No abnormality detected
NHL	Non-Hodgkin's lymphoma
NPH	Normal pressure hydrocephalus
NSAIDs	Non-steroidal anti-inflammatory drugs
OC pills	Oral contraceptive pills
PAH	Pulmonary arterial hypertension
PA view	Postero-anterior view
PCR	Polymerase chain reaction

PDA	Patent ductus arteriosus
PFT	Pulmonary function test
PND	Paroxysmal nocturnal dyspnoea
PPI	Proton-pump inhibitor
PSS	Progressive systemic sclerosis
PUO	Pyrexia of unknown origin
RA	Rheumatoid arthritis
RAH	Right atrial hypertrophy
R/E	Routine examination
RHD	Rheumatic heart disease
RNTCP	Revised National Tuberculosis Control Programme
RTI	Respiratory tract infections
RVF	Right ventricular failure
RVH	Right ventricular hypertrophy
SBE	Subacute bacterial endocarditis
SLE	Systemic lupus erythematosus
SOL	Space-occupying lesion
SPA	Spondyloarthropathy
STD	Sexually transmitted diseases
SVC	Superior vena cava
TB	Tuberculosis
TC/DC	Total count/differential count
TI/TS	Tricuspid incompetence/stenosis
TIA	Transient ischaemic attack
UMN	Upper motor neurone
USG	Ultrasonography
UTI	Urinary tract infection
VATS	Video-assisted thoracoscopic surgery
VPB	Ventricular premature beat
VSD	Ventricular septal defect
WHO	World Health Organisation
WNL	Within normal limit

Chapter 1

Long Cases

"Medicine is not only a science; it is also an art. It does not consist of compounding pills and plasters; it deals with the very process of life, which must be understood before they may be guided."
—**Paracelsus** (1493–1541), an alchemist, physician, astrologer and general occultist

Scheme of History Writing

Introduction

The first and foremost part of consultation is talking with the patient (to gather maximum possible information) while communication plays the pivotal role to the clinical examination. Most of the art of medicine lies in 'communication'. History taking remains the essence of medical practice. History taking is an immensely skilled technique, which requires a lot of practice; it helps to build up a rapport with the patient, which ultimately gives rise to a strong doctor-patient relationship. Clinical skills and bedside manners are acquired continuously during the lifetime by repeated practice and experience. Knowledge and experience are required to learn 'bedside clinical medicine', which are gained from clinical teachers and patients.

Clinical methods are the skills in clinical practice a doctor achieves during examining a patient, which are acquired in his lifetime by a combination of study and experience. A good *clinical eye* is essential to be a good clinician. Primary (first) impression is formed as soon as the patient enters the consultation room—the way the patient walks in the clinic, the way he/she interacts during conversation, change of body language during consultation, and the non-verbal communication (e.g. rubbing the centre of chest to describe heartburn; catch in breath, flushing, restlessness or change in eye contacts are signs of 'stress') may provide wealth of information and can give vital clinical clues. It is essential to understand the patient as a whole person. The consultation room environment should be comfortable, cool, well-ventilated, well-lighted and with a pleasant surroundings; the waiting area and the clinic-staffs should be patient-friendly and sensitive. Try to make the seating arrangement between the doctor and the patient in such a way, so that the patient remains in the centre of attention; try to pull up a chair at the bedside and sit at the patient's level to see and examine the patient comfortably while maintaining a good 'eye contact'.

The physician should be polite, cordial, humble and respectful to the patient, and professional in dress, behaviour and attitude. A doctor should be gentle and confident in his communication which help in gaining the faith of the patient. Always try to maintain and respect the patient's privacy (e.g. examining in a side room or by pulling the curtains at the bedside) and dignity. It is better to avoid phone calls and other jobs during history taking and examination. Allow the patient to tell their story in their own words without unnecessary interruption and as such an active listening in an open mind helps the physician to gather lot of information. A patient and sympathetic listening can provide a 'therapeutic catharsis' for the patient; it establishes a good doctor-patient relationship which may reduce the suffering of the patient and instil confidence in the treating doctor (Epictetus, the Greek philosopher). Smiling at the patient from time to time will encourage him/her to talk. Personal attention and a caring attitude also build a good doctor-patient relationship. After sympathetic listening with patience, the unnecessary part of the history may be discarded.

- An accurate history is the first step in determining the aetiology of patient's illness (~75%), and as such one may be able to make a diagnosis based on the history alone. Physical examination adds ~10%, while routine investigations (blood, urine, X-ray, etc.) add another 10% to the yield of diagnosis; hopefully, 5% patients may need special investigations (USG, CT scan, endoscopy) to reach the final diagnosis. So, most of the diagnosis can be made on the basis of history alone, while investigations are supplementary to the clinical diagnosis. This is why Sir William Osler once told 'if you listen carefully to the patients, they will tell you the diagnosis'.

Offer a greeting to your patient and try to make an introduction (ask the patient's name while reciprocate by saying that "I'm Dr. X"); often a shake hand gives a good start. Speak clearly and audibly using simple language avoiding medical titles and jargons. Always maintain a pace during history taking which is comfortable for the patient and to try to be on the patient's level in all respect. Assess the patient's mood, anger, frustration, anxiety and apprehension arising out of the disease itself. Do not be biased, rather show empathy and patience while recognising the emotion of the patient; be an attentive listener and behave friendly. Interview the patient in a soft tone so that the disease discussed remains confidential from others. Be sensitive and tolerant to patient's religious belief. The physician should be careful so that his/her personal beliefs do not prejudice the patients' care by any means. Ask for an *interpreter* while facing problem in communication due to difference in conversation language. If the patient is very ill or mentally confused, ask for a *third party* to collect information. Full concentration is paid to the patient and the barriers of communications (difficulty in hearing/vision, dysphasic/aphasic patient, emotionally disordered, i.e. angry or abusive patient) may be overcome by information obtained from a *relative.* Try to find out why the patient has come with an *accompanying person/persons.* Ask the patient how he/she reached the clinic; is it by car or ambulance or by walking, which may focus on severity/depth of the problem. Some patients are intelligent and deliver clear, concise, chronologically correct history while majority talk irrelevantly, and few patients are garrulous (i.e. talks a huge amount without describing the proper information) who may have to be interrupt appropriately; literacy and intellectual level of the patient are two important factors for a good history taking.

Remember, a patient may be male or female, young or elderly, educated or illiterate, silent or talkative, depressed or irritated or miserably distressed.

Many of the patient's symptoms are subjective (pain, migraine, gaseous distension of abdomen or angina pectoris) with absent physical signs. These facts are to be judged by the physician's experience. A 'pain scale' from 1 to 10 may be helpful to assess the severity of pain where 1 is very mild pain, whereas 10 is the severest pain the patient can imagine. A simple facial rash may be barely noticeable by an aged patient while it may be devastating for a professional actor; always try to interpret the 'severity of symptoms' by how they interact with their life. The skills of history taking can be obtained and maintained satisfactorily only by practice.

Many a time, *'direct'* or *'leading questions'* may prove relevant; these questions are direct and very specific with answer remaining between 'yes' or 'no' (e.g. in a patient presenting with sudden onset acute pain and swelling at the base of great toe may be asked by 'have you consumed alcohol last night?' and if the answer is 'yes', then the probability of gout increases). Sometimes the negative answer is equally important like the positive answer (a retrosternal chest pain which is not increased after exertion and not relieved by rest/nitrates is less likely to be angina pectoris). Sensitively explore the highly-sensitive matters like substance abuse, marital disharmony, sexual disorders or mental illness at the fag end of history taking. Ask the patient not to use pseudo-medical terms (heart attack/black-out/fits/sciatica/allergy/stroke/arthritis/pleurisy), rather instruct him/her to explain it because misinterpretation of medical terms is common amongst common people. Remember, in case of females, there might be some triggering influence of menstruation on migraine or pregnancy on heart failure, which are to be evaluated in those perspectives. Show a thankful attitude before concluding a conversation.

Always examine female patients in presence of a female attendant. Before starting the clinical examination, always take permission of the patient and explain briefly what you are going to do; if needed, examine the intimate/private parts at the last part of your examination and it is a must to seek permission sensitively for this purpose.

A provisional diagnosis could be built-up based mainly on history and clinical examination supplemented by appropriately ordered routine and special investigations.

It is useful to start with a 'structure of history' or 'scheme for history taking' with plan of physical examination protocol in mind.

Scheme (Format or Proforma) for History Taking

A. Particulars (biodata) of the patient Bed No. ....

1. Name
2. Age
3. Sex ('Gender' is a better terminology)
4. Race/religion
5. Occupation
6. Address
7. Date and time of admission
8. Date and time of examination

B. The history or history proper

1. Chief (presenting) complaints
2. History of (H/o) present illness
3. Past history
4. Family history
5. Personal and social history
6. Treatment history
7. Psychiatric history
8. Menstrual and obstetric history in women

C. Physical examination

I. General survey:

1. Appearance: Whether looks normal, ill, very ill, distressed, or moribund?
2. Level of consciousness: Whether alert, oriented and cooperative (e.g. obeying commands)
3. Apparent age (corroborative or not): Down syndrome, thalassaemia and a pituitary dwarf

look younger, and in progeria, precocious puberty or chronic exposure to sunlight the patient looks older than his/her chronological age

4. Decubitus (position of the patient in bed)—vide page 422
5. Build or built (skeletal framework): Average/ dwarf/tall stature (vide page 323)
6. Nutrition (nourishment of the body): Average/ undernutrition/obese. Try to determine the body mass index (BMI), i.e. weight (kg)/height (m^2)—vide page 327
7. Facies (facial appearance; vide page 319)
8. Pallor or anaemia (mild, moderate, severe): Probably 'pallor' is a better terminology
9. Cyanosis (central or peripheral type)
10. Jaundice (mild, moderate, severe/deep)
11. Neck artery (carotid arteries)
12. Neck vein (jugular venous engorgement, pressure and pulsation)
13. Lymph nodes (neck, axilla, epitrochlear, inguinal and popliteal groups)
14. Thyroid gland
15. Clubbing
16. Koilonychia
17. Pulse (with all the points; see the chapter on 'Pulse')
18. Respiration (rate, rhythm, type, depth and breathing pattern)
19. Temperature (record oral temperature)
20. Blood pressure (BP): Preferably record both in supine (compulsory) and standing position as this may detect postural hypotension (e.g. diabetes mellitus). Measurements both in right and left arms are sometimes necessary (e.g. supravalvular aortic stenosis); lower limb BP in selective cases (e.g. coarctation of aorta and aortic incompetence).
21. Oedema
22. Skin (hyperpigmentation, hypopigmentation, rash in face, scratch mark, ulcer), hairs (including scalp to see alopecia; hirsutism), and nails
23. Height and weight, arm-span, upper segment-lower segment ratio (anthropometry)
24. Any obvious deformity (of skull, spine, limbs, or swelling of abdomen) or outstanding feature (e.g. static tremor in parkinsonism)
25. Handedness (right, left, or ambidextrous) with level of intelligence (average, low, high)
26. Others: Examination of breasts (page 211), hydration status (page 329) and bony tenderness

II. Systemic examination:

1. Cardiovascular system (CVS)
2. Respiratory system
3. Gastrointestinal system (GI system)/alimentary system and hepatobiliary system
4. Nervous system
5. Genitourinary system
6. Lymphoreticular system
7. Locomotor system

D. Summary of the case (construct two paragraphs. First paragraph: Short history in two or three sentences, and second paragraph: Clinical examination findings in brief with major abnormalities in two or three sentences. Add positive plus important negative points in summary)

E. Provisional diagnosis (P/D) or working diagnosis: Most possible diagnosis considering the history and clinical examination

F. Differential diagnoses (D/D): Consider other possibilities in this setting

G. Relevant investigations (optional): Rational investigations in an aim to reach a final diagnosis.

- In the history sheet, one may add 'points in favour of diagnosis', after the provisional diagnosis.
- In the systemic examination, one should write 'all the systems', e.g. in a patient with pneumonia—first the respiratory system is dealt with in details and then the other systems are considered in brief.
- If the patient has IV drip, Ryle's tube, IV cannula, urinary catheter or chest drain, etc. mention it.
- Always try to stand on the right side of the patient during examination.
- Never forget to examine thyroid gland, breast (with permission) and spine in a patient.

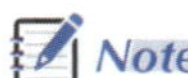
Note

Oncology, geriatric and psychiatric assessment are not within the purview of this boo

Facts to be known before Approaching to Diagnosis

- There is no substitute for careful history taking and an intelligent clinical examination. Excessive dependency on investigations can be harmful for the patient though investigations add to proper clinical diagnosis (only supplementary).
- Only reading books will not help to learn the skill of interrogating (i.e. symptoms) and examining (i.e. signs), which are mostly taught by the teachers in the hospital indoors or outdoors. Every patient is different and their reaction to a disease is also different, while no machine can analyse such a difference—try to learn this.
- 'Symptom' is a subjective evidence of physical disturbance observed by the patient, e.g. pain, headache, loose motion, etc. while 'sign' is an objective evidence of disease or physical disturbance noticed by the physician, e.g. tendemess, elevated blood pressure, detection of murmur in heart, etc. So, *symptom is what the patient says and sign is what the physician observes*. Thus, before examining a part of the body of a patient, the physician gets some idea of probable diagnosis on the basis of history (i.e. symptoms) which is corroborated by clinical

examination (i.e. signs) resulting in a 'clinical diagnosis' for the patient's ailments.

- 'Differential diagnoses (D/D)' are different diseases which share similar symptoms and signs, e.g. D/D of acute appendicitis is Meckel's diverticulitis. Provisional diagnosis is the most possible temporary diagnosis (may be changed in future) after clinical examination in the absence of complete information (e.g. investigations). 'Final diagnosis' or 'definitive diagnosis' is made after getting the results of investigations like blood or urine examination, or biopsy of a lymph node, etc.
- Importance of name: Identity, good doctor-patient relationship when called by name during conversation, and many a time it reflects the religion and the country where the patient lives.
- Rationality of mentioning age: A diagnostic clue comes in hand if one knows that some diseases are common in younger age (congenital disorders, acute rheumatic fever), while some are common in middle age (rheumatoid arthritis) and old age (malignancies, degenerative disorders, osteoporosis, parkinsonism).
- Regarding sex (gender): Systemic lupus erythematosus (SLE), thyroid and gallbladder disorders are more common in females, while gout and carcinoma of the lung are more prevalent in males. X-linked diseases (e.g. haemophilia) exclusively affect males.
- How religion helps in diagnosis? e.g. β-thalassaemia is common in Punjabi and Sindhi caste in India, while carcinoma of the penis is rarely seen in Muslims (due to circumcission of penile foreskin). Moreover diet, culture and spiritual belief (Fig. 1.1) are different from religion to religion which may increase the risk of acquiring a disease; consanguinity (i.e. marriage among relatives) are common in Muslim communities, and in some other religion and race (so, congenital disorders and autosomal recessive disorders are prevalent among them).

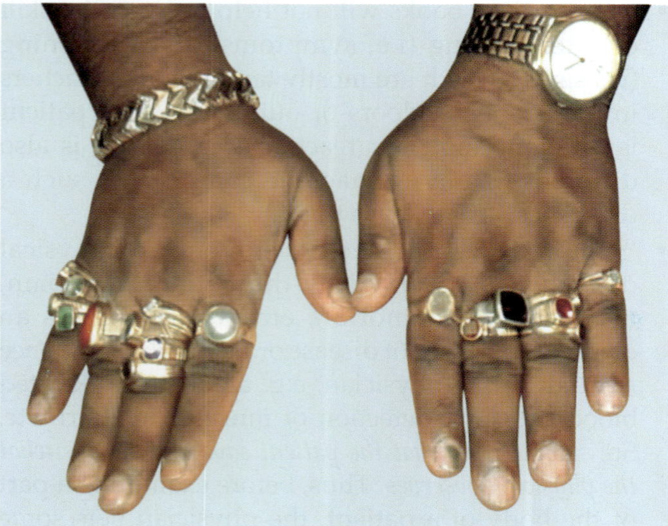

Fig. 1.1: 'Social or religious taboo'—putting multiple rings or metallic bracelet in hands to cure a disease

- Importance of occupation: Some particular type of occupation predisposes some specific diseases by change in pattern of lifestyle or exposing the person to toxic substances or injuries. People working in coal mines are in risk of development of coal-worker's pneumoconiosis while development of varicose veins is common in persons with prolonged standing like in security guards, tram drivers or traffic police.
- How address helps in diagnosis?: It is known that some diseases are common in a particular geographical area like arsenic toxicity in Taiwan, Eastern India and Bangladesh, while filaria is prevalent in Odisha state of India. Moreover, complete postal address is essential for follow-up patients and should be kept in hospital records.
- Do not hurt your patient physically or mentally. Be an empathetic listener and always try to build-up a healthy doctor-patient relationship. Try to learn how an 'informed consent' is taken from a patient or his/her relatives (i.e. getting written permission before conducting a 'procedure' like pleural aspiration in pleural effusion or lumbar puncture in a suspected patient of meningitis). As a trainee one cannot divulge the prognosis (i.e. outcome of a disease) but with maturity one student has to learn the skill to 'breaking a bad news' to the patient or his/her relatives clearly and sensitively (e.g. to parents of a child who is suffering from leukaemia). One student should have some idea about 'medical negligence' which is nothing but deviation from 'code of ethics' which binds the doctor to certain modes of conduct. Try to develop your 'communication skills' wholeheartedly by repeated practice.

History Taking

1. Chief (Presenting) Complaints

The patent may have many symptoms but a decision should be taken which symptom or symptoms led the patient to present in the clinic. Allow the patient to tell his/her complaints. It is better to ask him at the beginning by "Tell me what is your main problem" or "what is the most bothering problem for which you are here?" Major complaints give a clue to the organ or system involved, and guides the physician about the systems to be examined. If the patient gives a direct diagnosis (e.g. allergy), ask him/her to elaborate the symptoms and do not accept the diagnosis before confirmation; try to clarify precisely the vague symptoms like 'feeling very bad' or 'my head is jamming' or 'feeling tired while walking'. Help of relatives, accompanying persons or interpreter (described earlier) may be taken if there is any difficulty felt by the patient to narrate proper history. It is preferable to record patient's own words while avoiding medical terminologies e.g. instead of 'haemoptysis', mention coughing out of blood, and convulsions should be noted instead of 'epilepsy', while 'dyspnoea' should be replaced by difficulty in breathing.

Record the presenting symptoms with duration (from longest to shortest duration) in chronological order of their appearance in the patient's own language, avoiding technical terms. The chronological order of appearance of symptoms not necessarily matches with severity.

For example, if a patient of mitral stenosis (MS) diagnosed 10 years back is admitted/presented in the hospital on the previous day with cerebral embolism (cerebrovascular accident or CVA), the chief complaints in order will be: 1) Exertional breathlessness from time to time for last 10 years; 2) Chest pain, fatigability and pedal swelling (oedema) for last 3 years; and 3) Weakness of one side (e.g. left side) of the body for 1 day. However, the first system to be examined is nervous system for which the patient was admitted in the hospital (next the CVS is to be examined). So, it is to be realised that proper history taking is immensely skilled and fascinating.

2. History of Present Illness

It is the brief description of patient's illness from onset to till date. Elaborate the individual chief complaint in a logical manner in the light of:

a. It is the expansion of each chief complaint in relation to their mode of onset (acute/subacute/insidious), progress (progressive/regressive/static/with exacerbations and remissions), and duration. Progress during stay in the hospital should be enquired into (i.e. sequence of events). Aggravating and relieving factors relating to chief complaints may be asked for.
b. Use patient's own words and avoid scientific or medical terms as far as possible (joint pain is preferable term than arthritis).
c. Positive, plus important negative symptoms (absence of either paralysis in neurological disorder or breathlessness in cardiovascular diseases are negative points) should be recorded.
d. Preferably do not put leading questions (i.e. questions suggesting their own answers which may decrease the reliability of any information) but many a time direct relevant question makes an essential component of sensitive history taking.
e. Pain (site, radiation, character, periodicity, severity, aggravating or relieving factors, associated symptoms) and fever (range, axillary or oral, types i.e. intermittent/continued/remittent, chill and rigor, diurnal vanation, sweating, associated symptoms like headache/malaise, how relieved) should be described in details. Pain and fever are two most important symptoms which compel the patient to attend a doctor.
f. Record relevant associated symptoms (e.g. preceding visual disturbance in migraine, drenching sweat in hypoglycaemic coma, palpitations in association with angina pain).
g. Investigations and treatment received so far along with response.
h. Introductory questions: Time and date of appearance of first symptom/were you all right before this episode/have you suffered from similar illness in the past/what were you doing when the symptoms appeared/whether the symptoms interfered with normal activities or sleep/have you consulted a physician before/are you better or worse now/what else you want to say?
i. Generalities (basic general symptoms): Appetite, loss of weight, fatigue, sleep, bladder and bowel.

3. Past History

Ask about previous illness, operations, accidents or admissions to hospital in the past. Keeping the patient's chief complaints in mind, ask relevant past illness from the following events:

- Rheumatic fever (e.g. in valvular heart disease).
- Tuberculosis (e.g. in pleural effusion).
- Malaria (e.g. in recurrent pyrexia).
- Kala-azar (e.g. in a case of enlarged spleen).
- Jaundice (e.g. in cirrhosis of liver).
- Epilepsy (e.g. patient presenting with convulsions).
- Systemic hypertension (e.g. in a case of CVA).
- Diabetes mellitus (e.g. in a case of foot ulcer).
- Ischemic heart disease (IHD)/dyslipidaemia/thyroid disorder.
- STD (sexually transmitted diseases like gonorrhoea, syphilis, AIDS, etc.).
- Operations, trauma, injury, accidents, or procedures like catheterisation, bronchoscopy, biopsy.
- Fever, cough, atopy or allergy, haematemesis, melaena, bleeding per rectum, breathlessness, arthritis.
- **'H/o contact'** with persons suffering from tuberculosis or any contagious disease.
- **'H/o exposure (sexual)'** to STD.
- Any illness which demanded 'blood transfusion' (e.g. thalassaemia, any operation or accidents).
- Past hospital admissions (ask for reason behind).
- H/o travel (abroad or disease-prone areas) may give clue to malaria, dengue, tropical sprue, etc.
- Childhood illness, e.g. measles, mumps, rubella, chickenpox, whooping cough, poliomyelitis; birth history (asphyxiated or not), H/o any injury, umbilical sepsis, meningitis, immunisations and vaccinations history from the parents.
- H/o similar complaint, other major medical or psychiatric illness in the past.

- Few clinicians prefer to mention hypertension and diabetes within personal history.
- Read different chapters for relevant past history to be asked in specific system/cases.
- Never comment like 'past history nothing significant', rather say 'the patient had no history suggestive of tuberculosis, jaundice......and rheumatic fever.'

4. Family History

In a true sense, this includes 'first-degree relatives', i.e. parents, children and siblings though in a broader sense all near 'blood-relatives' like parents, brothers, sisters, uncles (paternal or maternal), nephew or niece may be considered. In a broader sense, 'second-degree relatives' are grandparents, uncle, aunt, nephew-niece, while the 'third-degree relatives' are cousin brothers/sisters, great grandparents, etc.

a. Ask whether any family member has had a similar illness? Or, are there any illness that run in your family (i.e. heredofamilial diseases having major genetic trends), e.g. thalassaemia, haemophilia, schizophrenia, Huntington's disease, breast carcinoma? Remember, mother's brother (i.e. maternal uncle) or sister's son may be affected in X-linked diseases like haemophilia.
b. Diseases of multifactorial aetiology that have familial aggregation (i.e. not a single gene disorder) should also be enquired like systemic hypertension, diabetes mellitus, IHD, bronchial asthma, dyslipidaemia, eczema, migraine, epilepsy, carcinoma (e.g. colon) or thyroid disorders.
c. Family history is important in hereditary (mentioned above), and communicable diseases (mumps, measles, chickenpox, scabies, tuberculosis) due to unavoidable H/o contact within family members.
d. Common 'environmental factors' such as poverty, smoking (active or passive), unbalanced diet are aetiology of many diseases, e.g. there are lots of deleterious effects of passive smoking in a woman who is having a heavy-smoker husband.
e. H/o consanguineous marriage (i.e. marriage among relatives) within the family should be recorded (autosomal recessive disorder, e.g. homocystinuria may result from consanguineous marriage). Is there any H/o adoption within the family?
f. Age and cause of death of first-degree relatives, if any, should be noted.
g. Lastly, the 'pedigree chart' representing three generatiouns (symbols used in construction of a family showing the pattern of inheritance should be plotted on a diagram) may be drawn.

Genetically transmitted diseases are:

- Autosomal dominant: There is vertical transmission, i.e. H/o similar type of illness in either of the parents/ grandparents. The examples are polycystic kidney disease, myotonic dystrophy or Huntington's disease.
- Autosomal recessive: There is horizontal transmission, i.e. similar illness is absent in the parents (the patient may be heterozygous). The examples are cystic fibrosis, sickle cell anaemia or phenylketonuria.
- X-linked recessive: There is oblique transmission. Common examples are haemophilia, colour blindness, etc. Read also page 469.

5. Personal and Social History

This includes H/o the patient, spouse and children only. At this juncture, try to find out more about the patient as a person while the questions should be asked in a sensitive and conversational way than as a routine one. Personal details and lifestyle of the patient should be noted carefully:

a. Marital status with number of children. Ask for the health of spouse and children.
b. Level of education obtained (gives an indirect idea of social status).
c. *Occupation* (working place and type of work immensely influence health. Nature and environment of job are important, i.e. a sedentary/desk job may initiate weight gain, whereas a laborious job may precipitate musculoskeletal ailments; a prolonged computer-associated job may initiate a back pain, or exposure to dust/chemicals/fumes may be complicated by pulmonary diseases; exposure to asbestos, silica or lead in the industrial work, working in coal mines or high altitude, or overstress in working place should be recorded). Ask about both present and past jobs. Any H/o unemployment?
d. Income (asked indirectly in a decent way) and social (socioeconomic) status: For example, the patient is a government service holder and comes from a middle class family. Socioeconomic status in India is measured by education, occupation and family income in "Kuppuswamy's socioeconomic status scale". But practically, patients are divided into three broad classes, i.e. upper, middle and lower. The diseases prevalent in lower class are tuberculosis, undernutrition, scabies, etc. while diabetes, hypertension, obesity and sedentary lifestyle are more common in upper socioeconomic status.
e. Dietary habit (for diagnosis of avitaminosis, malnutrition or obesity): Ether vegetarian or non-vegetarian, or takes mixed Indian diet. Enquire about frequency, time and variety of meals along with snacking habit. Is there any H/o dietary restrictions (e.g. avoidance of milk in irritable bowel syndrome or lactase deficiency)? Remember, vegetarian people may suffer from pernicious anaemia, or non-iodised salt consumption may develop into hypothyroidism and low-fibre diet (e.g. mutton) may produce constipation.
f. *Addiction* (tea, coffee, betel nut, smoking, alcoholism, or H/o '*substance abuse*', e.g. chewing or smoking tobacco or cannabis, alcohol consumption, LSD, cocaine, heroin, opium, tranquillisers, 'recreational drugs' such as Ecstasy, or any other illicit drug consumption): Try to estimate the amount of consumption of tobacco or alcohol. In female patients, ask about addiction sensitively.
g. Lifestyle: Whether performing exercise or regular morning walk? Enquire about the activities on weekdays and on weekends. Sleep, appetite, bowel and bladder habit, and weight gain/loss may be asked here (may be included in H/o of present

illness). Hobbies/pastimes/leisures (e.g. source of entertainment—attending club every alterate evening with unrestricted consumption of alcohol) and habits like having a pet are definitely important in specific cases (hydatid disease in those who keeps dog, and psittacosis pneumonia who keeps birds). Foreign travel (e.g. traveller's diarrhoea in persons coming from developed to developing country; *air travel* may pose problems like earache/middle ear problems/jet lag, and deep vein thrombosis; H/o accommodation while travelling, activities like water sports and sexual contacts, and travel vaccination), domestic and marital relationship, sexual history (the most sensitive part of history taking, e.g. impotence may imbibe psychosomatic disorders; ask for number of contacts, homosexual or bisexual partners, polygamy, contacts with prostitutes) should be taken into account.

Whether the patient is living alone, with family, or living alone with friend/relatives residing nearby (social history) should be recorded; income, office environment, family relationship, dependents at home are other components of social history taking.

h. *High risk behaviour*, e.g. IV drug abuse, multiple unprotected sexual exposure, homosexuality, etc. are important in hepatitis B or C infection, AIDS and SBE (subacute bacterial endocarditis). 'Needle sharing' gives rise to hepatitis B, C and HIV infection, right-sided infective endocarditis, abscess/cellulitis, and thrombophlebitis. Ask for H/o contraception. Always protect the patient's modesty.

i. Ethnic background is important in many diseases, e.g. thalassaemia and sickle cell disease.

- **Tobacco smoking** enquiry: Smoker (how long smoked, types like cigarette/bidi/cigar/pipe/hooka, and how much smoked [i.e. number of cigarettes] versus non-smoker [enquire about 'passive smoking']; estimate 'pack year' (see page 242) to assess the tobacco-related health hazards. Tobacco can also be chewed or taken as snuff. Cigar and pipe smokers inhale less smoke than cigarette/bidi smokers (thus, the former smokers have higher risk of oral, laryngeal and oesophageal carcinoma; other tobacco-related risks are relatively less). Ask the tobacco-chewer about the frequency, brand and quantity (they may suffer from severe submucosal fibrosis of the oral cavity).

  Major tobacco-related diseases are: Cardiovascular system/CVS (IHD, peripheral vascular disease, Buerger's disease), respiratory system (laryngeal carcinoma, chronic bronchitis, emphysema, bronchogenic carcinoma), gastrointestinal (GI) system (peptic ulcer, oral and oesophageal carcinoma), central nervous system/CNS (cerebrovascular accidents or CVA, addictions, tobacco amblyopia), haematological (AML), obstetrical (small babies) and genitourinary system (erectile dysfunction, renal cell carcinoma and carcinoma of urinary bladder).
- **Alcohol consumption:** Enquire about type of drink (beer, wine, whisky, gin, vodka), frequency, quantity and duration of drinking habit. In a 'social drinker', try to find out what it exactly means. Approximately one standard glass of wine, one peg (i.e. 60 mL) of spirits (whisky, gin, vodka), or half-pint of beer make *1 unit of alcohol*; a large peg contains 60 mL of beverage while a small peg has a capacity of 30 mL. The safe limit for men is 21 units/week (i.e. 168 g of ethanol) and that for women, it is 14 units/week (i.e. 112 g of ethanol). Consumption above these limits is hazardous drinking, which may lead to different alcohol-related disorders.

  Major alcohol-related disorders are: Hepatobiliary system (alcoholic hepatitis, cirrhosis of liver), GI system (oesophagitis, acute gastritis, peptic ulcer, pancreatitis), nervous system (cortical atrophy, cerebellar degeneration, tremor, seizures, delirium tremens, Wernicke's encephalopathy, dementia, Korsakoff's psychosis, peripheral neuropathy, proximal myopathy), CVS (hypertension, cardiomyopathy) and genitourinary system (erectile dysfunction, infertility).

Clinical Wisdom

Try to comment on 'substance abuse' in every case history, whether present or absent.

6. Treatment History

Both present and past treatment history are important to arrive at a diagnosis. Note:

a. Treatment received so far, for the present illness.
b. Any H/o allergy or reactions (e.g. drugs like sulphonamides or penicillins, animal hair, pollen, food material, metal may act like allergens).
c. H/o blood transfusion: Date, indication, frequency, amount and type (e.g. whole blood, plasma, packed cell, platelets, etc.).
d. Prolonged use of oral contraceptives (may precipitate CVA), penicillamine (used in Wilson's disease, which may develop into nephrotic syndrome) or vitamin C (may produce oxalate stone in urinary tract).
e. Intake of non-steroidal anti-inflammatory drug (NSAID) may give rise to acute gastritis, haematemesis or melaena, NSAID-induced asthma, and renal toxicity.
f. Regular use of oral contraceptives, vitamins, laxatives, sedatives or herbal remedies.
g. Any surgical intervention or H/o accidents in significant past should be asked for. Previous illness or operations may have a direct bearing on the present health; ask for pacemaker implantation, valve replacement, knee replacement, cochlear implantation or radium in the cervix, etc.
h. Immunisation (tetanus, hepatitis B, pneumococcal, influenza or herpes zoster vaccine).
i. Self-medication, if any.

7. Psychiatric History

A structured enquiry regarding psychiatric history is important. Observe the 'mood' of the patient, i.e. whether anxiety, depression, euphoria, irritability, confusion, obsession, mania, neurosis, bipolar disorder, phobia, altered perceptions and depersonalisation are present or not. Childhood, growing-up, interpersonal relationships, schooling, substance abuse, marital and sexual history are of immense important. Peptic ulcer, bronchial asthma, irritable bowel syndrome (IBS) are examples of *psychosomatic disorders*.

Common 'functional disorders' (where physical examination and investigations fail to reveal an underlying organic cause; many a time they are stress-induced) are chronic fatigue syndrome, chronic back pain, IBS, fibromyalgia and conversion disorder (previous 'hysteria').

8. Menstrual and Obstetric History

These history include the following:

a. Menarche (first occurence of menstruation, averaging 13 years).
b. Duration of menstruation (i.e. period or menses).
c. Quantity of blood loss (usually assessed by number of pads consumed or passage of clots).
d. Dysmenorrhoea, amenorrhoea, menorrhagia or other menstrual irregularities.
e. Date of last menstrual period (LMP). Remember, expected date of delivery (EDD) of a pregnant lady is calculated by EDD = First day of LMP +9 month and 7 days).
f. Menopause, post-menopausal bleeding, hormone replacement therapy (HRT) in post-menopausal women.
g. Obstetric history:
   - Number of pregnancies.
   - Outcome of pregnancies; H/o abortions, or carried to term; live birth (male/female).
   - Complications during pregnancy (e.g. toxaemia, gestational diabetes mellitus).
   - Mode of delivery (vaginal, forceps, Caesarean section).
   - Last childbirth.

- 'Gravida' means the number of times a female has been pregnant while 'Para' or 'Parity' means number of pregnancies which have crossed beyond the period of viability of foetus (i.e. 28 weeks).

Tips for Presenting a Long Case (A Model Answer)

Mr. XY, a 72 years-old retired executive from city of Mumbai, who is hypertensive, non-diabetic, smoker but non-alcoholic, was admitted in the medicine ward of this tertiary care hospital at 2 am of midnight with the chief complaints of....... for one month, ... for 1 day, and .... for 2 hours. He was apparently normal one month back, when he suddently noticed respiratory distress on exertion.

Now add H/o present illness, relevant past history, family history, personal history, social history and treatment history with definite positive, along with important negative points. If you listen to the history carefully, in most of the cases you will get a lead to diagnosis (Δ is shorthand symbol for diagnosis).

Start with general survey, followed by systemic examination (first examine the specific system getting clue from the history itself, and then examine the other systems sequentially). Tell the findings on general survey and the specific system examined (both positive and negative points); clinical findings on other systems should be mentioned, and if other system/systems do not record any finding, you may tell that 'nervous system reveals no abnormality' or 'other systems are within normal limit (WNL)'.

If it is possible to arrive at a provisional diagnosis, then tell that **'My diagnosis in this patient is**..........', or if there is no idea about provisional diagnosis, then tell in this way 'With this history and clinical findings, I can give some differential diagnoses/or it is a case of generalised lymphadenopathy/or it is a case of hepatosplenomegaly'.

SECTION 1: CARDIOVASCULAR SYSTEM (CVS)

The symptoms of CVS are mentioned below:

1. Chest pain (angina pectoris, acute myocardial infarction or AMI, pericardial pain, aortic dissection).
2. Breathlessness (dyspnoea, orthopnoea, paroxysmal nocturnal dyspnoea).
3. Palpitations.
4. Cough and expectoration.
5. Haemoptysis (expectoration of blood, or bloody sputum; seen in mitral stenosis).
6. Dizziness and syncope (aortic stenosis, hypotension, arrhythmia), black-out.
7. Convulsions or past H/o neurodeficit (e.g. mitral stenosis with atrial fibrillation having big left atrial clot gives rise to CVA).
8. Tiredness or fatigue (aortic stenosis, β-blocker therapy; exertional fatigue in heart failure).
9. Swelling of feet (peripheral oedema) or facial puffiness.
10. Intermittent claudication or limb pain.
11. Squatting or cyanotic spells (e.g. cyanotic congenital heart diseases).
12. Visual disturbance (retinal haemorrhage or embolism).
13. GI symptoms like anorexia, nausea, vomiting [digitalis toxicity or protracted congestive cardiac failure (CCF)], pain abdomen (mesenteric embolism, tender hepatomegaly in CCF, inferior wall AMI).
14. Renal symptoms like oliguria, nocturia (in CCF).
15. Hoarseness of voice or dysphagia (left atrial enlargement due to mitral valve disease, or aortic aneurysm).
16. Fever (SBE, pericarditis, rheumatic activity or rheumatic fever, AMI, deep vein thrombosis, atrial myxoma, Dressler's syndrome).
17. Fleeting joint pain, fever with sore throat, subcutaneous nodules for rheumatic heart diseases.
18. General symptoms—Appetite, loss of weight (cardiac cachexia) or gain in weight (due to oedema), sleep, bladder and bowel.

- No. 1, 2, 3, 6, 8 and 9 are cardinal symptoms in cardiology.

Scheme of Examination (Proforma)

A. Pulse

1. Rate
2. Rhythm
3. Volume
4. Condition of the arterial wall
5. Comparison between two radial pulses
6. Radio-femoral delay
7. Any special character
8. Other peripheral pulses

B. Blood Pressure (BP)

C. Examination of Neck Veins

1. Engorged or not
2. If engorged,
   i. Pressure
   ii. Pulsation: Present or not
   iii. Hepato-jugular reflux: Present or not

- In general survey, especially look for signs of: a) rheumatic fever and b) infective endocarditis.

D. Examination of the Heart

I. Inspection:

a. Inside the precordium,
   i. Shape: Presence of any deformity or bulging
   ii. Pulsation: Apical impulse; diffuse pulsation over precordium (*see* pages 41–42)
   iii. Engorged superficial veins: Present or not (*see* page 431)
   iv. Polythelia (accessory nipple): Often indicates underlying congenital heart disease, cardiomyopathy, etc. (Fig. 1.2)
   v. Any scar mark (especially for previous cardiac operation, pacemaker), sinuses

b. Outside (beyond) the precordium—Any pulsation present in (*see* pages 41–42),
   i. Aortic area
   ii. Pulmonary area
   iii. Parasternal areas (right and left)
   iv. Epigastrium
   v. Suprasternal area
   vi. Supraclavicular area
   vii. Carotid pulsation
   viii. Locomotor brachialis
   ix. Back: Especially at the inferior angle of scapula in coarctation of aorta (Suzman's sign)

c. Inspection of the BACK for scoliosis, kyphosis, gibbus, drooping of the shoulder, winging of the scapula; examine the skin for any sinus, ulcer, venous or arterial prominence, scar mark, etc.

- Look for midline sternotomy scar (Fig. 1.3A) for coronary artery by-pass surgery or prosthetic valve replacement, left submammary scar for mitral valvotomy (Fig. 1.3B), and left infraclavicular scar for implantation of pacemaker. A mark of needle prick with cotton swab over precordium indicates pericardiocentesis.

II. Palpation (Fig. 1.4):

a. Mitral area:
   1. Apex beat: (i) Site, and (ii) Character
   2. Palpable heart sound (M_1)
   3. Thrill

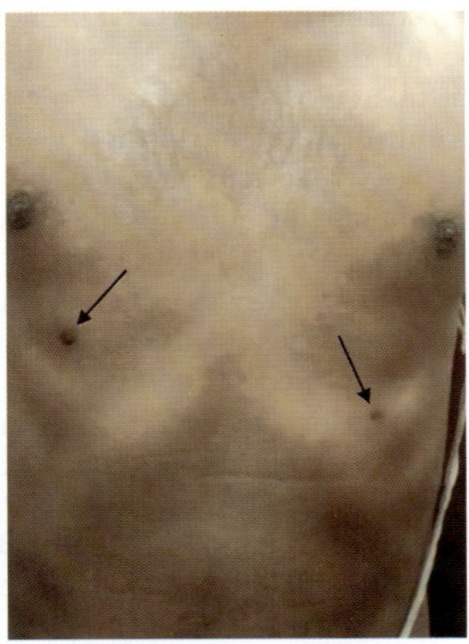

Fig. 1.2: **Accessory nipples,** which are present along mammary ridges and are often associated with congenital cardiac anomalies

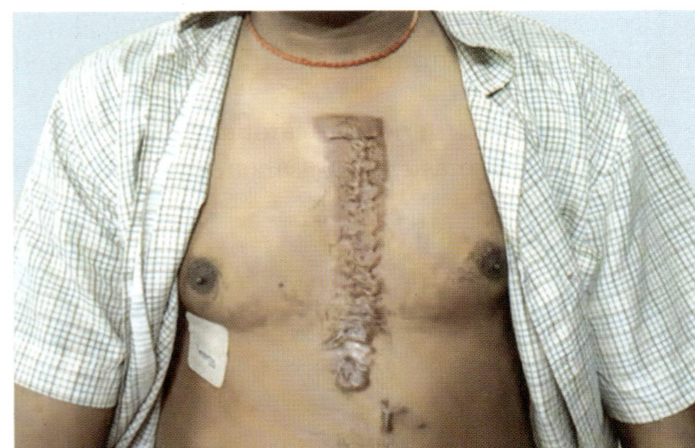

Fig. 1.3A: Keloid formation in midline **vertical** sternotomy **scar** done for **valve replacement**

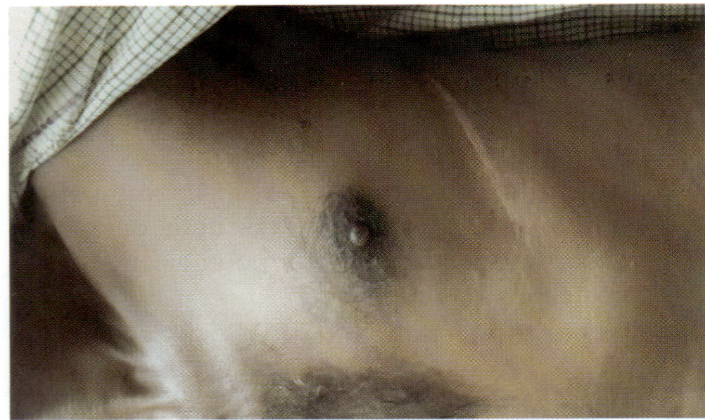

Fig. 1.3B: Left submammary **scar for mitral valvotomy**

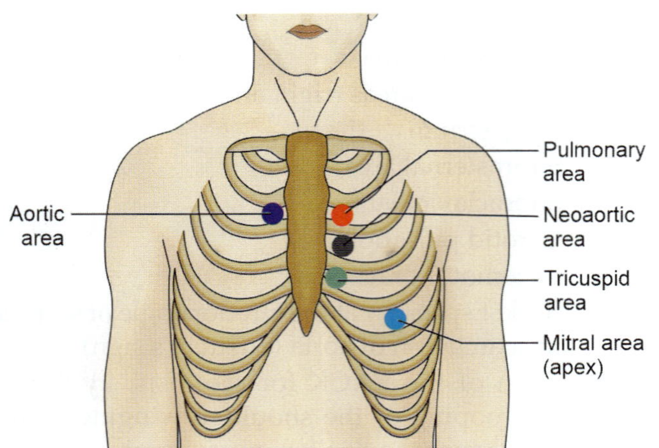

Fig. 1.4: Different **landmark areas of heart**

b. Pulmonary area:
   1. Pulsation
   2. Palpable heart sound (P_2)
   3. Thrill
c. Aortic area:
   1. Pulsation
   2. Palpable heart sound (A_2)
   3. Thrill
d. Tricuspid area:
   1. Left parasternal heave (page 410)
   2. Palpable heart sound (T_1)
   3. Thrill
e. Neoaortic area: For any thrill or pulsation
f. Direction of venous blood flow (in engorged superficial veins)
g. Thrill in carotid arteries (i.e. carotid shudder)
h. Epigastric or suprasternal pulsation, or any pulsation over the back
i. Palpable pericardial rub
j. Tracheal tug

- *See* pages 411–412 for different areas of heart, page 31 for thrill, pages 409–410 for palpation of heart sounds and parasternal heave.

III. Percussion: Not done routinely as it has limited value in today's clinical medicine (*see* pages 410–411).

IV. Auscultation:

a. Cardiac rate
b. Rhythm
c. Mitral area:
   1. Heart sounds (S_1 or S_2)
   2. Murmurs (in detail; pages 412–413)
   3. Adventitious sounds: S_3 or S_4, opening snap, ejection click, splitting of heart sounds, pericardial rub or knock, tumour plop, non-ejection click, prosthetic valve sounds
d. Pulmonary area: As in mitral area
e. Aortic area: As in mitral area
f. Tricuspid area: As in mitral area
g. Auscultation over neoaortic area
h. Auscultation over carotid arteries for bruit (after holding the breath), axilla and back
i. Venous hum at root of the neck (e.g. severe anaemia).

- It is better to write 'audible' in case of heart sounds which are not produced in that area. Thus, in pulmonary hypertension, S_2 (P_2) is loud but S_1 is audible in pulmonary area.
- Before doing any clinical procedure or manoeuvre (e.g. palpation of apex beat) always take permission of the patient and explain briefly what you are going to do.
- Before delivering the diagnosis, always think of some common disease by the 'law of probability'; if you give the provisional diagnosis of a rare disease, you are rarely correct. Remember the dictum: Uncommon presentations of common diseases are more common than common presentations of uncommon diseases.

MITRAL STENOSIS — CASE 1

Q. What is your diagnosis?

Give the provisional diagnosis (P/D).

It is a case of mitral stenosis (MS) of rheumatic origin without any evidence of congestive cardiac failure (CCF) or pulmonary hypertension, and the patient is in sinus rhythm at present.

Q. What is your case?

One should describe the summary (or salient features) without mentioning the P/D directly, e.g. Puja Devi, a 28 years female presented with gradually increasing breathlessness for last 10 months, and cough with haemoptysis for last 1 month. The breathlessness was gradually progressive, exertional, non-seasonal and NYHA (New York Heart Association) grade II in severity. Cough was not associated with rise of temperature. She had no H/o chest pain, swelling of legs, syncope, squatting (to exclude cyanotic congenital heart diseases), pain in legs during walking or any neurodeficit. She complained of occasional palpitations with mild exertion. Two weeks back, she experienced acute respiratory distress at middle of night due to paroxysmal nocturnal dyspnoea (PND). She was neither hypertensive nor diabetic; there was neither any H/o contact with tuberculosis nor any H/o exposure. She had an uneventful H/o childbirth, 4 years back. She gave definite H/o rheumatic fever in her childhood which affected mainly the big joints like knee, ankle and elbow following an attack of sore throat. The arthritis was fleeting in nature and was not associated with any skin lesion or chorea. She took inj. benzathine penicillin for few years but stopped suddenly.

The patient is alert, oriented, cooperative, and comfortable in bed. On examination, there is no anaemia; pulse is 76/minute, low volume, regular with all the peripheral pulses palpable equally; BP is 100/70 mm of Hg in supine position and the neck veins are neither engorged nor pulsatile. There is no deformity of precordium (precordial bulging indicates early onset and longer duration cardiac diseases). On palpation,

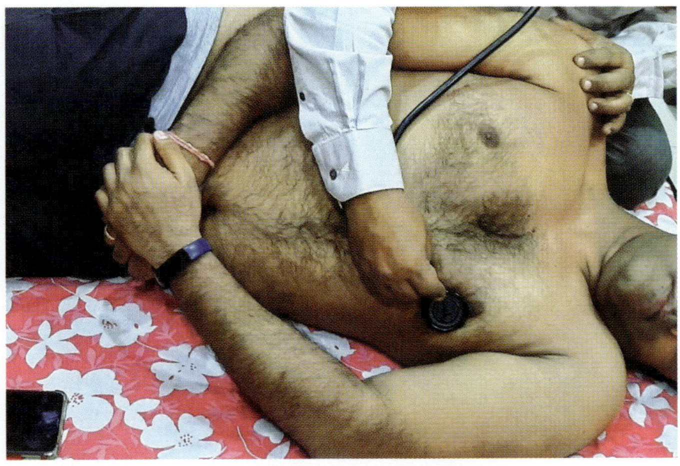

Fig.1.5: Auscultation of mitral area (especially for MS): Use bell while patient is in left lateral position

the apex beat is present in left 5th intercostal space (ICS) 1/2" inside the left midclavicular line (MCL) and is tapping in character (i.e. S_1 is palpable). A diastolic thrill is palpable in the mitral area which is best felt in left lateral position and in full expiration, and there is absence of left parasternal heave. On auscultation of the mitral area the 1st heart sound (S_1) is short, sharp, accentuated (i.e. loud), and the 2nd heart sound (S_2) is audible. Opening snap (OS) is heard medial to mitral area, just after S_2. There is a low-pitched mid-diastolic rumbling murmur with presystolic accentuation of grade IV intensity in the mitral area without any radiation (use the term 'radiation' or 'direction of selective propagation' but it is better to avoid the term conduction of murmur; see page 413 for explanation). The **murmur is best audible** at cardiac apex with the bell of stethoscope (placed lightly), in left lateral position (this position accentuates low-frequency sounds, increases the heart rate and transvascular flow), at the height of expiration and after doing mild exercise (Fig. 1.5). There is absence of split, click, rub, or murmur over other areas. Examination of the respiratory system revealed no abnormality (no adventitious sound, no hydrothorax, etc.), and there is absence of hepatosplenomegaly or ascites.

- Features of right ventricular hypertrophy (RVH) and pulmonary hypertension are absent here.
- Past H/o rheumatic fever, hypertension, diabetes mellitus, tuberculosis are important in all CVS cases (Table 1.1).
- A big summary is elaborated here for the sake of better understanding of the case history of MS.

Q. Give the summary of the case:

Give the short case history from the question discussed above.

Q. Provisional diagnosis in valvular heart diseases (standard format):

1. Anatomical: Mitral, tricuspid, aortic, pulmonary.
2. Structural abnormality: Stenosis, regurgitation (i.e. incompetence).
3. Aetiological: Rheumatic, congenital.
4. Complications: Pulmonary hypertension, CCF, subacute bacterial endocarditis (SBE), etc.
5. Rhythm: Sinus rhythm or dysrhythmia (e.g. irregularly irregular rhythm due to atrial fibrillation).

Clinical Wisdom

Some clinicians prefer to add NYHA classification in the provisional diagnosis (*see* page 26).

- Heart diseases may be congenital or acquired (e.g. rheumatic, ischaemic, cardiomyopathy, etc.)

Q. Why it is a case of mitral stenosis?

It is a case of mitral stenosis because of the following:

A. Symptoms (from the history):

a. Breathlessness or effort intolerance for last 10 months.
b. Cough with haemoptysis from time to time for last 1 month.
c. Attacks of paroxysmal nocturnal dyspnoea 2 weeks back.
d. Past H/o rheumatic fever (tell about the symptoms).

B. Signs:

a. Pulse: 76/minute, *low volume, regular*, no radio-radial or radio-femoral delay, all the peripheral pulses are palpable, neither any abnormality in the arterial wall nor there is any special character.
b. BP: Low (or normal)
c. Apex beat: Normal in position and tapping (due to accentuated S_1) in character. There is presence of diastolic thrill, best palpable in left lateral position and at the height of expiration. S_1 is palpable.
d. Auscultation (of the mitral area):
   S_1: Short, sharp and accentuated (loud and snapping S_1 is a very important clinical clue)
   S_2: Normal
   S_3 or S_4: Not audible at present
   Opening snap: Audible, just after S_2
   Murmur: Describe the classical murmur (as described in summary)
   Other areas: No murmur

- **Add features of pulmonary hypertension, if present.**
- Auscultatory cadence of murmur and heart sounds of MS seem to be as follows: ***ffout*** (presystolic murmur ending in loud S_1)–***ta*** (S_2)–***ta*** (opening snap)–***rrrou*** (mid-diastolic murmur).
- 'Usually' the apical impulse in an established MS is diffuse and formed by right ventricle. There is a diastolic thrill at apex, best palpable at left lateral position. There is sustained left parasternal heave as a result of RVH from pulmonary hypertension. The pulse becomes irregular in the presence of atrial fibrillation.

Q. If no past H/o rheumatic fever present:

Rheumatic fever is the commonest aetiology of MS and it is true in other valvular heart diseases. Forty percent

Table 1.1: Importance of past and family history in CVS

Past history	Family history
1. Rheumatic fever	1. Hypertension
2. Cyanotic spells with H/o squatting	2. Congenital heart disease
3. Recurrent respiratory tract infection	3. Rheumatic heart disease
4. Any murmur or cardiac lesion detected at school	4. Ischaemic heart disease (IHD) or cardiomyopathy
5. Hypertension, diabetes mellitus, IHD	5. Obesity, diabetes, dyslipidaemia
6. Thyrotoxicosis	6. Sudden (cardiac) death

- Examination of thyroid gland is a must in cardiovascular system work-up.

(40%) patients of MS do not give definite H/o rheumatic fever, still one should consider rheumatic fever as the probable aetiology. In that case it is better to say in P/D as 'a case of MS probably of rheumatic origin'.

Q. Queries in personal history:

H/o smoking, tobacco chewing, alcohol intake, IV drug addictions, sedentary lifestyle and diet (e.g. excess of salt and fat intake) are specially enquired for.

Q. How to diagnose congenital/early-onset cardiac disease?

1. History with ailments since birth/childhood with special reference to squatting.
2. Bulged precordium.
3. Clubbing with cyanosis plus polycythemia.
4. May be associated with dwarfism.

Q. What is 'precordium'?

It is the anterior chest wall which overlies the heart. In health, it is slightly convex and is associated with a smooth contour. The different deformities are:

a. Bulging: Early onset and longer duration cardiac diseases (e.g. congenital heart diseases or childhood-acquired valvular diseases), pericardial effusion, scoliosis, different chest deformities (*see* page 415), mediastinal tumours, left-sided pleural effusion.
b. Flattening: Fibrosis or collapse of the left lung, congenital deformity of chest, adherent pericarditis.

Clinical Wisdom

Systolic retraction of the lower part of precordium is sometimes seen in adherent pericarditis, and when seen in back of chest at 11th and 12th rib level with narrowing of intercostal space, it is known as **Broadbent's sign**.

Q. What is mitral facies?

It is the pinkish purple patches on cheeks. As low cardiac output in MS produces vasoconstriction, peripheral cyanosis is often seen in lips, tip of the nose and cheeks. Occasionally along with these, malar flush is seen due to vasodilatation (vascular stasis) in malar area. These features constitute 'mitral facies' which is appreciated in fair skin persons, and is **rarely seen in India**.

Q. Causes of malar flush:

1. High altitude.
2. Myxoedema.
3. Mitral stenosis.
4. Cushing's syndrome.
5. Thyrotoxicosis.
6. Chronic alcoholism.
7. Polycythemia.
8. Carcinoid syndrome.
9. Menopausal syndrome.
10. Pheochromocytoma.

Q. How loud S_1 in MS can be explained?

Due to persistent diastolic gradient across the mitral valve, the valve cusps remain wide open throughout the diastole and as soon as the ventricular systole starts, the widely opened mitral valve cusps close rapidly giving rise to loud S_1 (think of the sound produced when a door is closed from a short distance or from widely opened position, and it is obvious that closing the door from a long distance will produce more sound).

Q. Factors influencing the intensity of S_1 (Table 1.2):

Phonocardiographically four heart sounds (S_1, S_2, S_3, and S_4) are recorded but clinically two heart sounds (S_1 and S_2) are audible in most of the patients. The S_1 is best audible in the mitral area, while the S_2 is best audible in the aortic and the pulmonary area. The factors influencing S_1 are:

1. Position of valve cusps (mitral or tricuspid) at the onset of ventricular systole:
   a. Wide open valve cusps: MS or TS, hyperdynamic circulatory states (all produce loud S_1).
   b. Valve cusps remaining close to each other or cannot close completely (e.g. MI or TI): The S_1 becomes muffled, e.g. in myocarditis, myocardial infarction, heart failure, MI or TI.
2. PR interval (in ECG): S_1 is loud if PR interval is short, and S_1 becomes muffled if PR interval is prolonged.
3. Pliability of the valve cusps, e.g. calcification results in loss of pliability, and the heart sound becomes muffled or faint.
4. Ventricular muscle mass (booming S_1 is heard in patients with systemic hypertension leading to LVH).

Table 1.2: Variations in intensity of S_1

Loud S_1	Soft, distant or muffled S_1
1. Mitral stenosis, tricuspid stenosis	1. Mitral incompetence, tricuspid imcompetence
2. Sinus tachycardia due to any cause	2. Prolonged PR interval (e.g. 1° heart block), bradycardias
3. Hyperkinetic circulation, e.g. severe anaemia, pyrexia, exercise, pregnancy, thyrotoxicosis, Paget's disease, beriberi	3. Right or left ventricular dysfunction, AMI
4. Short PR interval, e.g. tachycardia, nodal rhythm, W-P-W syndrome	4. Calcified mitral/tricuspid valve
5. A loud S_1 is heard intermittently in complete heart block (cannon sound)	5. Obesity, emphysema, thick chest wall, pericardial effusion, constrictive pericarditis
6. Normally in children	6. Peripheral circulatory failure, shock, heart failure
Varying intersity of S_1	**Splitting of S_1**
1. Atrial fibrillation	1. Wide splitting—complete RBBS, left ventricular pacing, Ebstein's anomaly
2. Ventricular tachycardia	2. Reversed splitting—complete LBBB, right ventricular pacing, severe MS, left atrial myxoma
3. Complete heart block (cannon sound)	
4. Multiple extrasystoles	

- Wide split—when T_1 closes late to M_1, reversed split—M_1 comes later than T_1.

5. Heart rate: In tachycardia, S_1 tends to be loud as a result of short PR interval.
6. Intervening media between heart (valve cusps) and the stethoscope, e.g. emphysema, pericardial effusion or obesity diminishes the intensity of S_1.

- Normally the S_1 is dull and prolonged (lubb in 'lubb-dupp'), and is best audible at the apex. S_1 indicates the beginning of ventricular systole and is produced due to closure of atrioventricular valves. It has two components: mitral (M_1) and tricuspid (T_1); in health, M_1 comes earlier than T_1 and M_1–T_1 interval is 0.02 second. It is loudest at apex.
- S_1 coincides with carotid pulsation, while S_2 comes before or after the carotid pulsation. During auscultation of heart sounds in different areas, always palpate right carotid artery with the left thumb.

Q. Muffled S_1 in MS:

The S_1 is short, sharp and accentuated in MS. Muffled S_1 is found when MS is associated with:

1. Mitral incompetence (MI) or severe aortic incompetence (AI).
2. Mitral valve calcification.
3. Active rheumatic carditis (due to prolonged PR interval).
4. Digitalis overdose (due to prolonged PR interval).
5. Acute myocardial infarction.
6. Left atrial failure (LAF).
7. Atrial fibrillation (produces varying intensity of S_1).
8. Marked clockwise rotation of heart due to gross right ventricular hypertrophy (RVH) and consequently right ventricle is forming the apex.
9. Emphysema, severe obesity, thick chest wall (transmission of S_1 is hampered).

Q. Comment on apex beat in MS:

Usually the apex is in normal position. If the apex goes outward, think of RVH (from pulmonary hypertension) and if it is downward plus outward, think of LVH (i.e. search for associated MI, AI, AS, systemic hypertension). Normally, the apex is tapping (palpable S_1) in character though it may be diffuse (due to RVH). LVH is not a feature of isolated MS.

Q. How do you clinically assess the 'severity' of MS?

Features of severe MS at the bedside are:

1. Narrow S_2–OS gap (the smaller the gap, the more severe is the MS), and
2. Longer duration of mid-diastolic murmur

Clinical Wisdom

Remember, it is the duration and not the intensity of murmur, which assesses the severity of MS. Other signs of severity are—symptomatic patient, low volume pulse, RVH and pulmonary hypertension in ECG, and cardiomegaly (LA enlargement and/or RVH) in chest X-ray.

Q. Recognition of pliable mitral valve cusps:

1. Short, sharp, accentuated S_1, and
2. Presence of opening snap.

If the valve cusps are non-pliable (i.e. in calcification), S_1 will be muffled and the opening snap will not be heard.

Q. Why the murmur is mid-diastolic in MS and why there is presystolic accentuation?

The interval between closing of the aortic valve (S_2) and opening of the mitral valve is known as 'isovolumetric relaxation' period. Diastolic murmur of MS is heard as soon as the blood flows from the left atrium to left ventricle after opening of the mitral valve (i.e. in the mid-diastole). There is no blood flow in the isovolumetric relaxation period and this is why the murmur of MS is mid-diastolic, not early diastolic.

The last part of ventricular diastole (last rapid filling phase) actually coincides with atrial systole. Atrial systole increases the blood flow across the stenotic valve and thus, there is accentuation of the diastolic murmur (presystolic accentuation).

Q. Absent presystolic accentuation in MS:

The presystolic accentuation is absent in (only mid-diastolic rumble persists): 1. Artrial fibrillation, 2. Left atrial failure, and 3. Big left atrial thrombus.

Q. Why the MS murmur is localised without any radiation?

MS murmur is produced at mitral valve while blood is flowing from LA (lies posterior to LV) to LV (lies anterior to LA). As the flow of blood is in postero-anterior direction towards the apex, the murmur is localised without any radiation.

Q. What is an opening snap (mitral)?

A. Opening snap is produced due to billowing down of the closed mitral valve cusps at the onset of ventricular diastole (i.e. mitral valve will open just now but has not opened yet). It is:
   a. Sharp and high-pitched; heard immediately after S_2
   b. Best heard with the diaphragm of stethoscope
   c. Best heard after expiration with the patient in standing position
   d. Loudest in between the apex beat and the left sternal border
   e. Present in early diastole (at the end of isovolumetric relaxation period)
   f. It may be the loudest sound in the cardiac cycle. It was first described by Potain

B. It indicates:
   a. MS is organic
   b. Valve cusps are pliable (i.e. not calcified)
   c. Significant MS
   d. High left atrioventricular pressure gradient
   e. Severe AI, gross MI, gross pulmonary hypertension, atrial fibrillation, left atrial failure or SBE (subacute bacterial endocarditis) is absent
   f. Diminishing S_2–OS gap indicates increasing tightening of stenosis (severe MS)
   g. MS is readily amenable to surgery.

- Opening snap is also audible in tricuspid stenosis, ASD, VSD, PDA, posterior cuspal type of MI.
- OS should be differentiated from S_3 (*see* page 45) and splitting of S_2. To differentiate OS from splitting of S_2, ask the patient to stand. As standing reduces the venous return, the S_2-OS gap increases and A_2-P_2 gap of S_2, decreases on assuming standing position (dynamic auscultation).

Q. Aetiology of MS:

MS is 'almost always' or invariably of **rheumatic** in origin. Rarely the congenital form ('parachute' mitral valve—all chordae are inserted into a single left ventricular papillary muscle) may produce MS or very rarely it may arise from severe mitral annular calcification with extension onto the leaflets, carcinoid syndrome, collagen vascular disease (SLE), endomyocardial fibrosis or mucopolysaccharidosis. Organic MS results from shortening of chordae tendineae and fusion of commissures.

- **In clinical practice it is said that the commonest aetiology of MS is rheumatic. The second is rheumatic and the third is also rheumatic.**
- Rheumatic MS is much more common in females.

Q. Pathological types of MS:

1. Button hole, 2. Fish mouth, and 3. Funnel type.

- *Mitral valve apparatus* is composed of: 1. Valve leaflets, 2. Valve annulus, 3. Chordae tendineae, 4. Papillary muscles, and 5. Myocardium (the papillary muscles are attached here).

Q. Common symptoms of MS:

Dyspnoea (exertional), orthopnoea, paroxysmal nocturnal dyspnoea (PND), palpitations, syncope, fatigability, haemoptysis, recurrent bronchitis, cough, chest pain, right hypochondrial pain (tender hepatomegaly), oedema, and symptoms related to complications.

- Symptoms are due to:
  1. Symptoms due to low cardiac output: Fatigability, syncope.
  2. Symptoms due to left atrial failure (i.e. pulmonary congestion): Dyspnoea, orthopnoea, PND, cough, haemoptysis, recurrent bronchitis.
  3. Symptoms due to RVF: Swelling of legs (oedema), pain in right hypochondrium.
  4. Symptoms due to arrhythmia: Palpitations.
- Chest pain in MS is due to 1) RVH, 2) coincidental coronary atherosclerosis, or 3) coronary embolism.

Q. Lutembacher's syndrome:

Atrial septal defect (ASD) plus MS (of rheumatic origin).

Q. Changes noticeable when atrial fibrillation develops in MS:

1. Ventricular rate (heart rate) is about 100–140/minute.
2. **Irregularly irregular pulse with varying volume, and a pulse deficit >10.**
3. Varying intensity of S_1 (classical loudness of S_1 is lost); opening snap is not heard.
4. Absent a-wave in the neck veins or JVP.
5. **Presystolic accentuation of the diastolic murmur disappears as atria contracts in an uncoordinated**

and ineffective manner; only mid-diastolic rumble persists. It should be remembered that presystolic accentuation in MS is present, if the patient is in sinus rhythm.

6. Congestive cardiac failure may precipitate and embolic manifestations may appear (CVA, intermittent claudication, pain abdomen, etc).

- *Aetiology of atrial fibrillation* is rheumatic (commonly MS), ischaemic, hypertensive, thyrotoxicosis, cardiomyopathy, myocarditis, pericarditis, idiopathic or 'lone' atrial fibrillation (in elderly persons without any demonstrable cardio-pulmonary disease), following cardiothoracic surgery, congenital (especially ASD) and sinoatrial disease. Always rule out mitral valve lesion, thyrotoxicosis and hypertension in a case of atrial fibrillation.
- In atrial fibrillation, the atria usually fire impulses at a rate of 350–600/minute while the ventricles respond at irregular interval of 100–140/minute, and the pulse rate is usually 100–120/minute with pulse deficit.

Q. Changes occurring after left atrial failure in MS producing pulmonary oedema:

1. S_1 becomes muffled.
2. Opening snap is not heard.
3. Presystolic component of the murmur disappears, and
4. Presence of bilateral basal crepitations (fine).

Q. Which chamber of heart fails first in MS?

The left atrium. Chamber involvement in MS: LA → RV → RA.

Q. Which ventricle fails first in MS?

The right ventricle **(left ventricle does not fail in MS as mitral valve lies proximal to it)**.

- In the presence of left ventricular hypertrophy or failure in MS, think of associated valvular diseases like MI, AI, AS, systemic hypertension, ischaemic heart disease, or cardiomyopathy.

Q. What is tight or severe MS?

Normal cross-sectional area of mitral valve orifice is 4–6 cm^2 (average 5 cm^2). Grading of MS in relation to dimension of mitral valve orifice is: Minimal >2.5 cm^2, mild—1.6–2.5 cm^2, moderate—1–1.5 cm^2, and severe (tight/critical) <1 cm^2.

Q. What is juvenile mitral stenosis?

This type of MS is usually found in Indian sub-continent. In this situation, MS develops early in contrast to the western world, where the patients usually experience disability in the 4th decade. The criteria for diagnosis are:

1. Occurs below 18 years of age.
2. Pin-point mitral valve.
3. Atrial fibrillation is rare.
4. Valve calcification is uncommon.
5. Needs immediate operation.
6. Common in South-East Asia.

Q. Haemoptysis in MS—explanation:

The possible underlying mechanisms are:

1. Pulmonary apoplexy: Due to rupture of thin-walled, dilated bronchial veins or pulmonary veins (frank haemoptysis) resulting from sudden rise in LA pressure.
2. Winter bronchitis (chronic bronchitis): Blood-streaked mucoid sputum.
3. Acute pulmonary oedema: Profuse, pinkish, frothy sputum is produced due to rupture of capillaries into the alveoli.
4. Pulmonary infarction: Frank haemoptysis.
5. Overdose of anticoagulant therapy (rare): Often required to treat embolic manifestation in MS.
6. Pulmonary haemosiderosis: Rare.

Q. Unconsciousness and syncope in MS:

- Unconsciousness: Due to CVA (i.e. cerebral embolism) especially in MS with atrial fibrillation, leading to hemiplegia.
- Syncope: Usually due to low cardiac output (e.g. severe pulmonary hypertension, ball valve thrombus, cerebral embolism, atrial fibrillation with rapid ventricular rate).

Q. Most significant finding in your case:

The mid-diastolic rumbling murmur (due to turbulent blood flow through the narrowed mitral valve).

Q. What is damped MS?

In course of time, development of pulmonary hypertension diminishes the cardiac output (throttle effect) and results in temporary symptom-free period (period of illusion). Often the mid-diastolic murmur is not audible and thus known as silent MS.

- The diastolic murmur of MS may be absent in severe stenosis (due to low flow across mitral valve).

Q. When the classical signs of MS are absent?

1. Damped or silent MS.
2. In marked clockwise rotation of right heart: Diastolic murmur may not be audible.
3. Presystolic accentuation is absent in atrial fibrillation.
4. Loud S_1 is absent in mitral valve calcification.

Q. What is intermittent claudication?

This is a cramp-like pain, tightness and numbness (due to ischaemia) felt commonly in calves, thighs or buttocks on walking a certain distance, and characteristically relieved by taking rest. The 'claudication' (Latin meaning 'to limp') suggests peripheral vascular disease and the most important risk factor is smoking.

The common causes are:

1. Atheroma, severe atherosclerosis **(Fig. 1.6)** or embolism of lower limb arteries; Leriche's syndrome (saddle-shaped thrombosis at bifurcation of aorta, i.e.

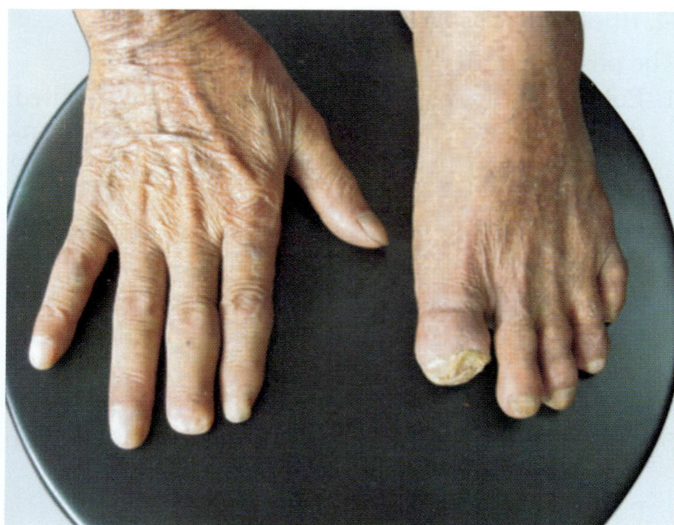

Fig. 1.6: Loss of pulp tissue in right middle finger and left great toe in **severe atherosclerosis**. The patient had H/o intermittent claudication

claudication of thigh and leg muscles, absent femoral pulses, cold-clammy-pale and cyanotic legs, with impotence) is an example of atherosclerothrombotic disease.

2. Buerger's disease (thromboangiitis obliterans; young heavy-smoker males).
3. Coarctation of aorta.
4. Arteritis.
5. Lumbar canal stenosis (patient often stoops forward during walking to reduce symptoms. If he continues to walk, paraesthesia in feet and even foot drop may develop): Pseudoclaudication.
6. Venous claudication (bursting pain on walking, previous H/o DVT), and
7. Over-exertion.

Palpation of peripheral pulses in legs, i.e. arteria dorsals pedis shows diminution in the volume of pulse in 1, 2, 3 and 4; in 5, 6 and 7, peripheral pulses remain normal but in 5, ankle jerk may be diminished or absent.

- **Vascular claudication** (No. 1, 2, 3, 4): Cold legs, pallor, hair loss, toenail atrophy and feeble pulse are common. Common risk factors are diabetes, smoking, hypertension and hypercholesterolaemia.
- **Neurogenic claudication** (No. 5 or cauda equina compression): Paraesthesia, limb weakness, diminished ankle jerk with normal pulse.

Q. Differential diagnosis (D/D) of mitral diastolic murmur:

1. Carey Coombs murmur: It is the soft mid-diastolic murmur of active rheumatic valvulitis (with nodules forming on the mitral valve leaflets), which is localised to the apex. The murmur varies in intensity from day to day and usually disappears after the acute attack. There is absence of loud S_1, opening snap and diastolic thrill. Oedema of the mitral valve cusps produce obstruction and gives rise to diastolic murmur. Other features of acute rheumatic fever (e.g. fever, arthritis, high ESR) may be present.
2. Austin flint murmur: It is a functional low-pitched, mid-diastolic rumbling murmur produced in a patient with severe AI. When the aortic regurgitant jet of blood impinges on the anterior mitral leaflet (thereby stenosing the mitral orifice relatively), a murmur (actually the murmur is due to both antegrade flow of blood from left atrium and regurgitant jet from AI) is audible with the features like:
   a. Mid-diastolic murmur with absence of presystolic component; heard in the mitral area.
   b. No diastolic thrill.
   c. S_1 is not loud.
   d. Absense of opening snap.
   e. Commonly found in syphilitic AI.
   f. Isometric hand-grip increases the murmur.
   g. Presence of AI murmur in the aortic area with features of LVH, plus
   h. Peripheral signs of AI (read the section on 'Aortic incompetence').
3. Functional mid-diastolic murmur: It is found in increased left-to-right shunt in ventricular septal defect (VSD), atrial septal defect (ASD), or patent ductus arteriosus (PDA). Increased flow through the normal mitral valve, as in VSD/ASD/PDA and severe MI, gives rise to a short mid-diastolic murmur. There is absence of diastolic thrill, opening snap and presystolic accentuation but S_3 may be present.
4. Left atrial myxoma: Myxoma is a benign tumour of the atrium, which may be sessile or pedunculated:
   a. Alteration of physical signs (murmur) with change of posture, H/o postural syncope.
   b. Tumour 'plop': A sound heard in late diastole as the pedunculated tumour comes to a halt.
   c. Constitutional symptoms like fever, weight loss, anaemia, arthralgia, rash, clubbing; high ESR.
   d. Embolic episodes.
   e. 2-D echocardiography is diagnostic.
5. Tricuspid stenosis: Mid-diastolic murmur with presystolic accentuation which is loudest at lower left sternal edge. Murmur increases at the height of inspiration. Features of RVH are never present.
6. Ball valve thrombus: The thrombus usually floats in the left atrium and obstructs the mitral orifice in diastole producing functional MS. Echocardiography is essential for final diagnosis.
7. Conducted murmur of AI: Early diastolic, soft blowing, no thrill, no opening snap. Peripheral signs of AI are present.
8. Cortriatriatum: A correctable rare malformation of heart where an abnormal fibromuscular diaphragm separates the left atrium into two chambers. Echocardiography and cardiac catheterisation are diagnostic.

9. Infective endocarditis with large vegetations obstructing mitral orifice: Stigmata of infective endocarditis (e.g. clubbing, splenomegaly) are present.
10. Rytand's murmur: Found in complete heart block.

- Nearest D/D of MS are left atrial myxoma and ball valve thrombus in the left atrium.

Q. Describe the classical attack of paroxysmal nocturnal dyspnoea (PND) (Fig. 1.7):

It is the sudden and dramatic development of acute dyspnoea occurring in the early hours of night, i.e. nearly 30 minutes to 2 hours after retiring to bed. The patient is awakened from sleep with a feeling of apprehension, intense suffocation and choking sensation. He sits upright gasping in the bed with the legs hanging by the side of the bed (to reduce left atrial pressure by gravitational pooling) or rushes to an open window in the hope that cool fresh air will relieve him. Dyspnoea (air hunger) progresses with profuse sweating. These are accompanied by a dry, repetitive cough which is due to **'acute interstitial oedema'** (fluid collection in interstitial tissue) resulting from pulmonary venous hypertension, when there is no collection of fluid within the alveoli. The attack may subside spontaneously within 30 minutes but often progresses to **'acute pulmonary oedema'** which may end fatally. The cough becomes productive with profuse, watery, pinkish and frothy sputum due to acute pulmonary oedema (collection of excess fluid within the alveoli making the lungs rigid with resulting dyspnoea).

PND signifies the earliest symptom of acute left-sided heart failure (due to LAF or LVF). Acute dyspnoea with wheeze and repetitive productive cough are features of **'cardiac asthma'**. Actually 'cardiac asthma' is closely related to PND and is characterised by wheezing due to bronchospasm which is most prominent at night. Acute pulmonary oedema is the severe form of cardiac asthma due to marked increase in pulmonary capillary pressure leading to alveolar oedema.

PND may be confused with nocturnal episodes of bronchial asthma (as it causes wheeze) which should be differentiated with care (*see* page 99). MS is probably the commonest cause of PND.

Clinical examination at the time of an attack of PND reveals:

a. Severe dyspnoea and orthopnoea; tachypnoea associated with air hunger and recruitment of accessory muscles.
b. Anxious and pale (ashen-grey pallor) patient with profuse sweating; cold, clammy extremities.
c. Central cyanosis.
d. Pulse: Tachycardia, feeble pulse.
e. BP: May be high (as hypertension is the commonest cause of PND). Hypotension is a poor prognostic sign.
f. JVP: Raised.

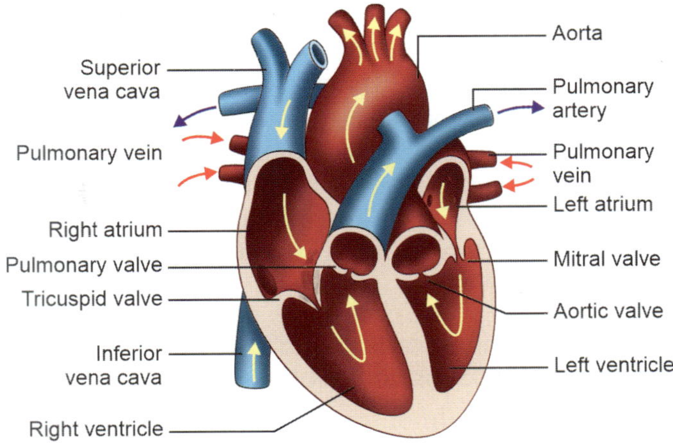

Fig. 1.7: Cardiac chambers, valves and great vessles

g. Heart: S_3 gallop rhythm; signs of underlying heart disease.
h. Lungs: Vesicular breath sound with prolonged expiration; bubbling crepitations +++ (predominantly basal), and scattered rhonchi is present.

- Acute pulmonary oedema is the phenomenon of 'cough, cough, cough—spit, spit, spit'.
- **So, causes of LAF and LVF are the basic causes for paroxysmal nocturnal dyspnoea or acute pulmonary oedema** (or cardiac asthma). PND is a symptom of decompensation of the left heart.
- 'Left side' of the heart encompasses the functional unit of left atrium, left ventricle, mitral valve and aortic valve, and 'right side' of the heart is used for the term encompassing right atrium, right ventricle, tricuspid valve and pulmonary valve.
- In recumbency, the rapid increase in venous return leads to pulmonary congestion and the left-sided chambers cannot cope up with this increased inflow in MS. Breathlessness in PND is due to inappropriate awareness of respiratory tract and firing of 'J' receptors at the alveolo-capillary junction in lung.
- LAF is left atrial failure and LVF is left ventricular failure. Dyspnoea, PND, orthopnoea and acute pulmonary oedema are progressive grades of symptoms of acute left-sided heart failure.

Clinical Wisdom

D/D of PND are nocturnal asthma, obstructive sleep apnoea and panic attacks.

Q. Why dyspnoea occurs in MS?

It is known that abnormally elevated LA-LV pressure gradient is the haemodynamic hallmark of MS. The events in MS go like this: ↑LA pressure →↑pulmonary venous pressure →↑pulmonary capillary wedge pressure → ↓ compliance of lung → dyspnoea (exertional). Ultimately, pulmonary arterial hypertension develops → RVH → right ventricular failure.

Q. Protective mechanisms to prevent pulmonary oedema in MS:

As the disease progresses to chronic mitral stenosis, there is development of:

1. High pulmonary vascular resistance (pulmonary hypertension).

2. Capillary-alveolar-interstitial barrier (obliterative change in pulmonary vascular bed), and
3. Broncho-pulmonary venous shunts.

Thus, it is clear that a recent onset MS patient may die of LAF (acute pulmonary oedema), and an old or chronic patient dies of RVF (from pulmonary hypertension). An old case of MS usually does not suffer from PND because of the development of protective mechanisms mentioned above.

Q. Causes of 'non-cardiogenic' pulmonary oedema (termed as 'ARDS' or acute lung injury):

Vide page 99. Pulmonary oedema is of two types: cardiogenic and non-cardiogenic. Non-cardiogenic pulmonary oedema is a clinical syndrome which leads to rapidly progressing respiratory distress, severe respiratory insufficiency and ultimately multi-organ failure. The causes of non-cardiogenic type are:

1. Diffuse pulmonary infections (viral, bacterial, fungal, *Pneumocystis jirovecii*).
2. Inhalation of toxins and irritants (phosgene, chlorine, smoke, ozone, high concentration of O_2).
3. Aspiration of vomitus, water (near drowning), acid/alkali poisoning, kerosine poisoning.
4. Narcotic (heroin, morphine, methadone, dextro-propoxyphene) and non-narcotic (nitrofurantoin) overdose/ effects.
5. Severe sepsis, gram-negative septicaemia, shock, major trauma, uraemia.
6. Acute haemorrhagic pancreatitis, *plasmodium falciparum* malaria, amniotic fluid/fat/air embolism, fulminant hepatic failure, insecticide poisoning, snake bite, high altitude, eclampsia.
7. Miscellaneous: Cardio-pulmonary bypass, major blood transfusion reaction, anaphylaxis (bee, wasp, snake venom, crab), major burns, head injury, chest trauma, high-altitude pulmonary oedema, SLE, DIC, lymphangitis carcinomatosa.

- In severe cases of pulmonary oedema, pink and frothy sputum comes out through the nose. **Remember, pneumonia (exudate) is not pulmonary oedema (transudate)**.
- 'Cardiogenic' pulmonary oedema (described in page 17): Results from left-sided heart failure (LAF/LVF), acute myocardial infarction, cardiac dysrhythmias, acute pulmonary thromboembolism.
- Right heart catheterisation by Swan-Ganz catheter allows differentiation of two types. **Cardiogenic:** Engorged neck veins, ↑CVP (central venous pressure) and ↑PCWP (pulmonary capillary wedge pressure) and **non-cardiogenic:** Normal left-sided atiral or ventricular pressure, neck viens are not engorged, and with normal CVP and PCWP.

Q. Why the dyspnoea is usually nocturnal in MS?

Probable theories are:

1. Venous return increases in recumbency.
2. Mobilisation of oedema fluid from extravascular to intravascular compartment on lying.
3. Adrenergic drive is reduced during sleep.
4. Heart rate increases during rapid eye movement (REM) sleep.
5. Reduction of vital capacity in supine position.
6. Elevation of left atrial pressure and fall in PaO_2 during sleep.

Q. Complications of MS:

1. Left atrial enlargement, acute left atrial failure and acute pulmonary oedema.
2. Pulmonary hypertension.
3. Right ventricular failure (RVF/CCF).
4. Atrial fibrillation (AF; most common), atrial flutter, ventricular or atrial premature beats.
5. Embolic manifestations (20%) due to AF (from dislodged clots formed in the LA):
   a. Cerebral arteries: 60% (cerebral infarction leading to hemiplegia)
   b. Peripheral arteries: 30% (e.g. aorta—Leriche's syndrome)
   c. Visceral arteries (renal, pulmonary, mesenteric, coronary): 10%
6. Haemoptysis.
7. Infective endocarditis: Very rare (more common in milder form of MS than in severe form); endocarditis is common in 'regurgitation' than in 'stenosis'.
8. Recurrent broncho-pulmonary infections due to chronic venous congestion in lung.
9. Complications due to giant left atrium (LA):
   a. Hoarseness of voice: Due to compression of left recurrent laryngeal nerve by enlarged LA (Ortner's syndrome); very rare.
   b. Dysphagia: Due to oesophageal compression.
   c. Clot present in a giant LA may give rise to embolic manifestations even in sinus rhythm.
   d. Rarely, collapse of the lung occurs due to pressure over left bronchus.
10. Jaundice, cardiac cirrhosis (in long-standing CCF).
11. Sudden death may be caused by ball valve thrombus where the LA outlet is blocked by large pedunculated thrombus.
12. Cardiac cachexia, stunted growth in juvenile variety, pulmonary haemosiderosis.

- Complications not related to severity of MS are atrial fibrillation, embolic manifestations and SBE.

Q. How do you like to investigate a case of MS?

A. Chest X-ray (PA view):
   a. Slight increase in transverse diameter of heart (due to RVH).
   b. '**Mitralisation**' of heart means straightening of the left border of heart and is due to (from above downwards):
      1. Aortic knuckle: Small (due to low cardiac output).

2. Convexity due to dilated pulmonary artery (due to pulmonary hypertension).
3. Left atrial appendages: Becomes prominent and produces a convexity.
4. Left border of left ventricle: No change.

c. Double contour of the right border of heart or double-density sign (shadow within shadow): The outer and upper border is due to LA, and the inner and lower border is due to RA enlargement.
d. Evidence of 'pulmonary hypertension': Dilated pulmonary arteries at hilum with peripheral pruning (i.e. peripherally pulmonary arteries taper sharply).
e. Dilatation of upper lobe pulmonary veins is known as upper lobe diversion (earliest X-ray feature of pulmonary venous hypertension). There may be hydrothorax.
f. Fan-shaped opacity ("Bat's-wing" appearance) from parahilar region to periphery indicates pulmonary oedema.
g. Kerley's B lines: Fine, dense horizontal lines at the base of the lung (in the region of costophrenic angles) due to distension of interlobular septa and lymphatics, with oedema.
h. Mitral valve calcification: Best seen in fluoroscopy or echocardiography.
i. Elevation of left upper lobe bronchus which becomes horizontal and producing wide carinal angle—splaying of carina (due to LA enlargement).
j. Multiple small opacities from secondary pulmonary haemosiderosis (subjects who had multiple haemoptysis may show haemosiderin deposits in the lungs) and parenchymal ossification: Rare.

B. Chest X-ray (RAO view): Right anterior oblique (RAO) view with barium-filled oesophagus is done. Oesophagus is pushed or curved backward (sickling of oesophagus) by the enlarged LA.

C. Chest X-ray (lateral view): Obliteration of retrosternal air space in left lateral view with slight increase in transverse diameter of heart (PA view) indicates RVH. 'Upturned' apex (in PA view) may result in boot-shaped configuration due to RVH. Pulmonary congestion or oedema, or mitral valve calcification may be evident.

D. Electrocardiography (ECG): In early stages, the ECG may be normal:
a. LA enlargement: Wide and notched P-wave (P-mitrale).
b. RVH.
c. 'f' waves replacing P-waves, if atrial fibrillation develops.

E. Blood examination (for active rheumatic carditis):
a. Total and differential count (TC and DC).
b. ESR.
c. ASO titre.

- All are raised in the presence of active rheumatic carditis.

F. Echocardiography (M-mode and 2-D): To see chamber enlargement, left atrial thrombus, valve pathology, valve movement, mitral orifice, etc. (in MS there are thickened immobile cusps, reduced valve area, LA enlargement and reduced rate of diastolic filling of LV). It is the most informative investigation.

G. Cardiac catheterisation: To determine the haemodynamic status of the patient (degree of stenosis, pressure measurement, oxygen saturation in blood samples). The pressure gradient between LA and LV is determined.

H. Doppler study: To know the functional status, speed and direction of blood flow in the heart chambers; to record pressure gradient across mitral valve and pulmonary artery systolic pressure.

- **Echocardiography confirms the diagnosis of valvular heart diseases.**

Q. Rationality of nervous system examination in MS, i.e. in CVS cases:

1. Hemiplegia or monoplegia may occur in a patient with MS (commonly with atrial fibrillation).
2. Sydenham's chorea.
3. Fundoscopy: Roth spot, hypertensive retinopathy.

Q. Rationality of respiratory system examination in MS, i.e. in CVS cases:

1. Respiration (tachypnoea, orthopnoea), haemoptysis, hoarseness of voice (rare).
2. Hydrothorax (from CCF).
3. Basal crepitations (from LVF) and diffuse rhonchi (from pulmonary oedema).

Q. Rationality of GI system examination in MS, i.e. in CVS cases:

1. Liver: Soft and tender liver with mild enlargement (may be pulsatile rarely) due to CCF.
2. Spleen: In the presence of SBE, spleen may be palpable.
3. Ascites may develop from CCF.
4. Mesenteric embolism, dysphagia (rare).

Q. Rationality of skeletal system examination in cardiac disorders:

1. Build:
   a. Tall: Marfan's syndrome (MI or AI).
   b. Stunted growth: Turner's syndrome (coarctation of aorta).
2. Kyphoscoliosis (shifting of apex beat, deformity of precordium).
3. Polydactyly or syndactyly (congenital heart disease).
4. Cubitus valgus (Turner's syndrome may be associated with coarctation of aorta).
5. Fingerisation of thumb with upper limb dysplasia (Holt-Oram syndrome with ASD).
6. Rheumatoid arthritis or ankylosing spondylitis (MI or AI), rheumatic arthritis (carditis).

- Heart diseases may be congenital or acquired. The external features for **congenital heart diseases** are cyanosis, clubbing, polycythemia, webbing of neck, hypertelorism, syndactyly, arachnodactyly, low set ears, cryptorchidism, etc. In **acquired heart diseases**, search for stigmata of rheumatic fever (arthritis, subcutaneous nodules, fever, etc.), infective endocarditis (anaemia, fever, petechiae, clubbing, splenomegaly, Osler's node, etc.) and coronary heart diseases (xanthelasma, arcus senilis, obesity, nicotine staining, ear lobe creases, etc.).

Q. Important points in general survey of CVS:

1. **Decubitus:** May be propped-up; orthopnoea.
2. Build: Dwarfism in cyanotic congenital heart diseases, tall in Marfan's syndrome.
3. Nutrition: Cardiac cachexia in severe chronic heart failure.
4. Facies: Mitral facies, central cyanosis, corneal 'arcus', xanthelasma, ear lobe pulsation in high jugular venous pressure (JVP).
5. **Anaemia:** Present in SBE (remember, anaemia can aggravate all heart diseases), Plethora (i.e. polycythemia) is important in cyanotic congenital heart diseases.
6. **Cyanosis:** Cyanotic congenital heart diseases, acute pulmonary oedema.
7. **Clubbing:** Cyanotic congenital heart disease, SBE, Eisenmenger's syndrome.
8. **Pulse:** Very important clue to diagnosis in different cardiovascular disorders.
9. **BP:** Must be seen in all patients; of immense value in diagnosis.
10. Respiration: Tachypnoea, orthopnoea, hyperventilation.
11. Temperature: Elevated in SBE, tuberculous pericarditis, rheumatic fever.
12. **Oedema:** CCF, constrictive pericarditis, pericardial effusion, tricuspid valve disease.
13. **Neck veins:** Reflecte central venous pressure; found in RVF (CCF).
14. Thyroid One should search for thyrotoxic features in all CVS disorders.
15. Jaundice: Rare; due to congestive hepatomegaly from CCF, or cardiac cirrhosis.
16. Skin: Osler's node, patechial haemorrhages, xanthelasma, rheumatic subcutaneous nodules.
17. Skeletal: Kyphoscoliosis, cubitus valgus, polydactyly.

Q. Treatment of MS:

Mild MS may need no treatment. The different modalities of treatment in moderate to severe MS are:

a. Drugs (medical treatment).
b. Percutaneous mitral balloon valvuloplasty (treatment of choice).
c. Valvotomy or commissurotomy: Closed and open (closed type is preferred). Open valvotomy needs open heart surgery with cardio-pulmonary by-pass.
d. Mitral valve reconstruction including annuloplasty.
e. Valve replacement or prosthesis (Starr-Edwards ball valve or Bjork-Shiley disc valve).

Q. Criteria for mitral valvuloplasty:

1. Significant symptomatic MS.
2. Pure MS (may have trivial MI).
3. Left atrium is free of clots.
4. MS with pregnancy.
5. Valve and sub-valvular apparatus are free of calcification.

Q. Indications of valvotomy:

1. Progressive symptomatic deterioration inspite of medical treatment.
2. MS with complications (as mentioned earlier), e.g. haemoptysis or pulmonary hypertension.
3. Asymptomatic patients with a single attack of thromboembolic manifestation.
4. MS with pregnancy where previous pregnancy was symptomatic.
5. Mitral valve orifice <1 cm^2.

Q. Contraindications of closed valvotomy:

1. MS with significant MI.
2. MS with left atrial thrombus.
3. Valvular calcification.
4. Presence of active rheumatic carditis.
5. Extremely tight stenosis.
6. Mitral valve distorted by previous operation (i.e. restenosis cases).

Actually, these are indications for open valvotomy.

Clinical Wisdom

Complications of surgery are development of MI, thromboembolism and restenosis. Approximately 30% patients develop restenosis at 10 years after mitral valvotomy. Loud S_1 and OS persist after mitral valve prosthesis.

Q. Treatment done in MS with MI:

Mitral valve replacement (prosthesis), Mechanical prosthesis like Starr-Edwards valve or Bjork-Shiley valve, or porcine bioprosthesis may be used. Prosthesis is done in grossly damaged valve and sub-valvular structures, and in presence of MI. Artificial valves may work for more than 20 years.

Q. Medical treatment in MS:

1. Treatment of CCF by restriction of physical activity, bed rest with proper 'back-rest', salt-restricted diet, diuretics, β-blockers, ACE inhibitors and digoxin (available as 0.25 mg tablet).
2. Antibiotic prophylaxis against infective endocarditis is advised though it is uncommon in pure MS (see the section on 'Aortic stenosis'). Secondary prevention of acute rheumatic fever is done.

3. Anticoagulation in the presence of atrial fibrillation or big left atrial clot to reduce the risk of systemic embolism. Anticoagulation (with warfarin), and aspirin/clopidogrel are required in cerebral embolism.
4. Treatment of atrial fibrillation with digoxin, β-blockers or rate-limiting calcium channel blockers, DC cardioversion, or oral anticoagulation (singly or in combination).
5. Management of complications like haemoptysis, acute pulmonary oedema, recurrent respiratory tract infections is done accordingly.

Q. MS with pregnancy: outline of management:

Rheumatic heart disease accounts for 90% of all cardiac diseases in pregnancy. Of these, MS is the commonest lesion. The principles of management are:

1. Schedule treatment of MS.

Clinical Wisdom

Functional degradation (e.g. patient deteriorates from grade I to grade II NYHA classification) occurs in pregnancy due to increase in cardiac output.

2. Increased bed rest. Oxygen inhalation, if necessary.
3. Adequate nutrition and correction of anaemia; low salt diet.
4. Digoxin may be needed though ACE inhibitors are contraindicated. Warfarin is to be avoided in 1st trimester. Prophylaxis for rheumatic fever should be continued.
5. Therapeutic abortion: In selected cases, e.g. with H/o repeated heart failure before conception, controlled heart failure in 1st trimester.
6. Mitral valvuloplasty: In symptomatic tight MS, in mid-trimester. The patients are usually symptomatic in second trimester, when the blood volume increases significantly.
7. Ideally all other cases should go into labour with scrupulous monitoring and not allowing the patient to strain in 2nd stage of labour.
8. Caesarean section may be performed, where indicated.
9. Patients are advised to restrict the number of children to one or two.

Q. Metallic mitral valve prosthesis in MS—auscultatory findings:

1. A metallic sound is audible in mitral area which coincides with S_1
2. Normal S_2
3. A metallic opening snap

Prosthetic valves are of two types:

- Metallic valve (produces clicking sound): Starr-Edwards, Bjork-Shiley, St. Judes valve.
- Tissue valve or biological valve (human—homograft; porcine or bovine—xenograft: does not produce clicking sound): Carpentier-Edwards, lonescu-Shiley, Hancock porcine valve.

Q. Complications of prosthetic valve:

Thromboembolism (needs life-long anticoagulation), infective endocarditis, valve failure/leaking/obstruction by thrombosis or calcification/perforation/rupture, microangiopathic haemolytic anaemia, bleeding (e.g. upper GI bleeding) due to anticoagulants.

Clinical Wisdom

One should not use abbreviations like MS, MI, PH, BP, etc.; use the full term, e.g. mitral stenosis, mitral incompetence, pulmonary hypertension, blood pressure respectively. In this book, abbreviations are used just to avoid repetition of long words. One should search for signs of active rheumatic carditis in all valvular heart diseases. Before stating the P/D as MS, one must be sure that there are no other valvular lesion like AI, MI or AS. If MS is associated with pulmonary hypertension, some changes develop in the palpatory and auscultatory findings—carefully search for them, often they are missed (read the section on 'Mitral incompetence' for the features of pulmonary hypertension).

MITRAL INCOMPETENCE — CASE 2

Q. What is your diagnosis?

This is a case of organic mitral incompetence (regurgitation or insufficiency) of rheumatic origin with features of congestive cardiac failure and pulmonary hypertension, and the patient is in sinus rhythm at present.

Q. What is your case?

Build up the summary. The symptoms are almost similar to that of MS. Symptomatology consists of exertional dyspnoea, orthopnoea, PND, fatigue, recurrent respiratory tract infections, palpitations, oedema feet due to CCF, and features of pulmonary hypertension or SBE (fever, embolic episodes, etc.)

Palpitations in MI are due to:

1. LVH, and/or
2. Atrial fibrillation (palpitations in MS are due to RVH or atrial fibrillation).

Q. Why it is a case of mitral incompetence (MI)?

It is a case of MI because of the presence of:

A. Symptoms (from the history):

a. Exertional dyspnoea for last 8 months, and
b. Palpitations for last 6 months.
(Plus past H/o rheumatic fever)

B. Signs:

a. Decubitus: Propped-up.
b. Pulse: Rate is 110/minute; otherwise normal arterial pulse (sometimes, the pulse is jerky or of good volume); describe all the points.
c. JVP: Engorged and pulsatile (CCF).
d. Oedema: Bipedal and pitting in nature (CCF).
e. Precordium: Bulged.
f. Epigastric pulsation: Present (RVH).

g. Apex: Present in left 7th ICS, ½" outside the left MCL (LVH); hyperdynamic in character; a systolic thrill is present in apical area which is best palpable in left lateral position and at the height of expiration.

h. Left parasternal heave: Present (RVH).

i. Palpation of pulmonary area: Diastolic shock (palpable P_2) present. There is neither any pulsation nor any thrill.

j. Auscultation:

   i. Mitral area:

   S_1: Soft

   S_2: Audible (with loud P_2)

   S_3 or S_4: Not audible at present; RVS_3 may be audible in CCF

   There is a high-pitched, soft blowing pansystolic murmur of Grade IV intensity which is best audible with the diaphragm of stethoscope, in left lateral position of the patient and at the height of expiration. The murmur is radiated towards the left axilla and inferior angle of left scapula **(hallmark of diagnosis).**

   ii. Pulmonary area: Ejection systolic murmur (different from pansystolic murmur at apex) with loud P_2.

   iii. Other areas: WNL, i.e. S_1 and S_2 are audible, and there is no murmur, split, click or rub.

[k.GI tract:

   i. Liver: Mild (enlargement), soft and tender hepatomegaly (CCF).

   ii. Spleen: Not palpable.

   iii. Ascites: Absent.

l. Respiratory system:

   i. Breath sound: Vesicular, rhonchi: Occasionally present, crepitations: Nil.

   ii. Hydrothorax: Not present.

m.Nervous system: Within normal limit (WNL)].

- Actually, these are features of MI with pulmonary hypertension and CCF.
- 'Rocking motion over the precordium' in each cardiac cycle in MI may be due to retraction of the left ventricle as well as expansion of the left atrium during systole.

Q. Different types of heart failure:

Heart (cardiac) failure is a condition where the heart can not function as a pump and is not able to maintain an adequate cardiac output for the needs of the body. It is usually classified as:

a. Left-sided or right-sided failure (*see* below).

b. High output or low output failure (*see* page 48).

c. Systolic cardiac failure (i.e. impaired systolic function with reduced cardiac output, e.g. IHD) or diastolic cardiac failure (i.e. impaired diastolic function with reduced ventricular filling, e.g. hypertension; the ejection fraction remains normal).

d. Acute heart failure (i.e. from mitral or aortic valvular disease) or chronic heart failure (i.e. from CAD or cardiomyopathy).

e. Forward failure (i.e. pumping of blood into arterial system is inadequate) or backward failure (i.e. filling of ventricles is inadequate resulting in elevated pressure in atria and venous system).

Q. Clinical features of LVH:

In LVH, apex goes down and outwards.

Q. Clinical features of RVH:

1. Apex goes outwards.
2. Left parasternal heave.
3. Epigastric pulsation.

- That is to say, right ventricular pulsations are seen in left parasternal and epigastric region.
- Cardiac apex remains down and outwards in combined LVH+ RVH.

Q. Cardinal signs of LVF (left heart failure/left-sided failure):

Three cardinal signs are:

1. Gallop rhythm (addition of S_3 or S_4, along with S_1 and S_2 produces **'triple rhythm'**. Triple rhythm with sinus tachycardia is known as **gallop rhythm**—so called because of its resemblance with the cadence produced by galloping of horses). So, *gallop rhythm indicates that the patient is in heart failure.*
2. Fine crepitations at both lung bases (i.e. basal crepitations).
3. Pulsus alternans.

- Sometimes, there are associated Cheyne-Stokes breathing, tachypnoea, central cyanosis, LVH and signs of underlying disease. The patient usually C/O exertional breathlessness (including orthopnoea and PND), nocturia, fatigue and mental confusion. Remember, pulmonary oedema is a feature of left-sided heart failure.
- **Gallop** is of two types:
  1. Quadruple gallop: Four distinct heart sounds due to audibility of S_3 and S_4 separately, and
  2. Summation gallop: The extra sound is produced as a result of superimposition of S_3 on S_4 (i.e. three audible sounds in one cardiac cycle).
- Ventricular galop (protodiastolic gallop) S_1, S_2, S_3; atrial gallop (presystolic gallop) S_1, S_2, S_4.

Q. Cardinal signs of RVF (right heart failure/right-sided failure/CCF):

Three cardinal signs are:

1. Engorged and pulsatile neck veins (Fig. 1.8).
2. Mildly enlarged, soft, tender liver.
3. Dependent bipedal oedema (pitting) (Fig. 1.9); or sacral oedema.

- Sometimes, there are associated cardiomegaly, peripheral cyanosis, pulsatile liver (rare), pansystolic murmur of TI and

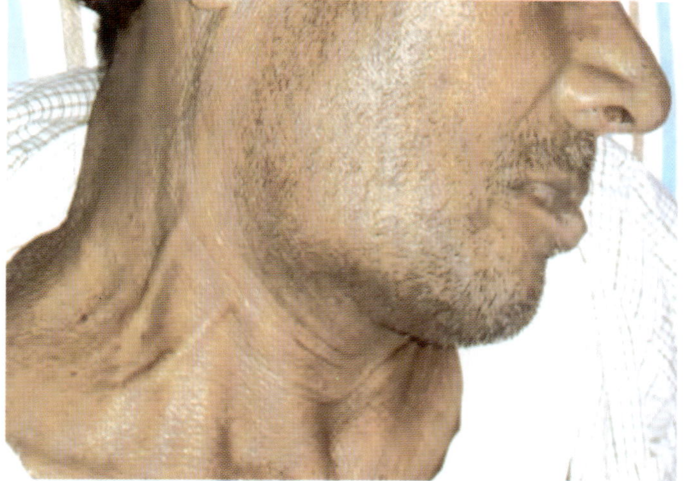

Fig. 1.8: **Engorgement** of both external and internal **jugular veins** in a patient with congestive cardiac failure

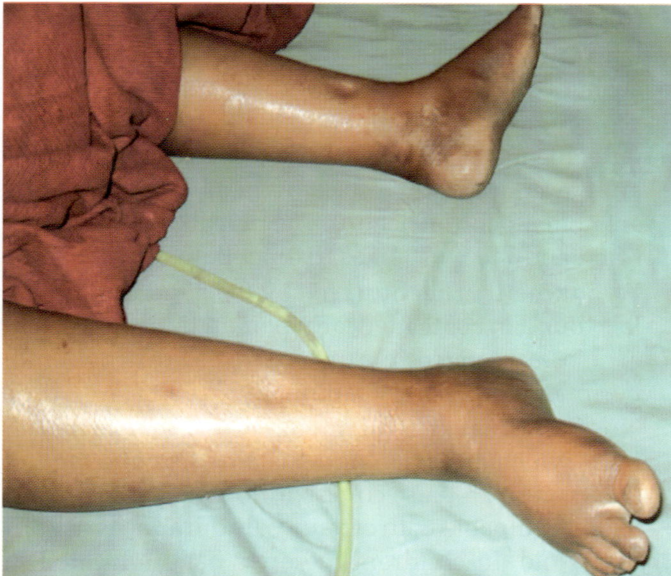

Fig. 1.9: Bilateral pitting pedal **oedema** in congestive cardiac failure

right ventricular gallop rhythm. The patient C/o weakness and fatigue, breathlessness, cough, oedema, nocturia, oliguria, GI tract disturbances (e.g. anorexia, nausea, vomiting, right hypochondriac pain due to stretching of hepatic capsule) and swelling of abdomen (ascites); there may be hydrothorax (commonly right-sided, may be bilateral) or jaundice (due to hepatic congestion). Cardiac cachexia (due to ↑ tumour necrosis factor, ↑basal metabolic rate, anorexia, nausea, vomiting) is not uncommon.

- Brain natriuretic peptide (BNP) is secreted primarily by the ventricles and an elevated level of BNP is used in the diagnosis of heart failure.

Q. Precipitating causes of cardiac failure in a patient of valvular heart disease:

- Severe anaemia, pregnancy, respiratory tract infections.
- Tachyarrhythmias, infective endocarditis, pulmonary thromboembolism, thyrotoxicosis.
- Ongoing rheumatic activity, unaccustomed exertion.

Q. What is apex beat?

It is the lowermost and outermost part of the precordium where a DEFINITE (most important, and not necessarily the maximum) thrust can be felt.

When the same cardiac pulsation is seen, it is called **apical impulse**. 'Cardiac impulse' is a better terminology than apical impulse because any 'pulsation seen' over the precordium may not correspond with the apex beat detected by palpation. If the apical impulse is not visible in supine position of the patient (best visible from the right side of the patient by a tangential view), the patient is turned to left lateral position when the apical impulse may be visible somewhere near the left anterior axillary line. Causes of non-visibility of apical impulse are same as causes of non-palpable apex (*see* below).

Clinical Wisdom

Be sensitive of the feelings of female patients while examining precordium.

Q. What is the significence of apex beat?

It is an important parameter by which one can assess the enlargement of heart (in the absence of push-pull effect of lung) and the activity of myocardium.

Q. How to localise the apex beat of the heart?

1. The patient should lie flat or supine. Place your whole flat of right palm over the precordium (always stand on the right side of the patient). Try to localise the definite thrust (not necessarily the maximum) with outstretched fingers (Fig. 1.10). If a definite thrust is palpable, confirm it by pulp of index or middle finger, and locate it by counting the ribs (Fig. 1.11); also look, how far it is from the left midclavicular line (inside or outside).
2. If the apex beat is not palpable in dorsal decubitus position, ask the patient to sit and lean forward. Again try to locate it by your outstretched fingers.

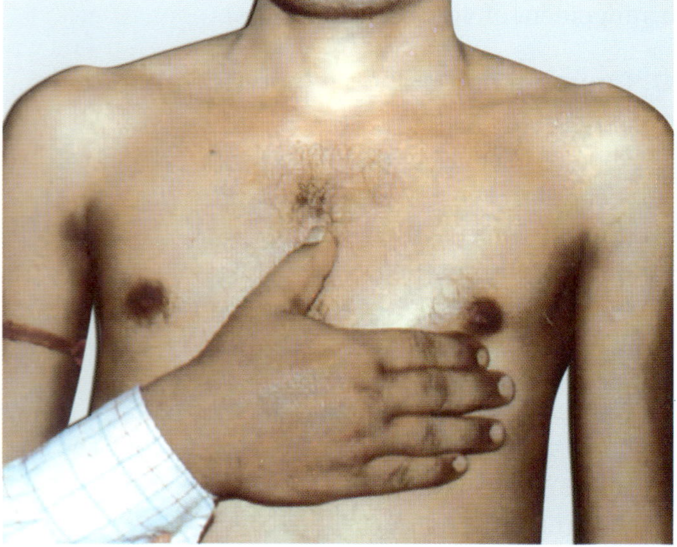

Fig. 1.10: **Palpation of cardiac impulse** with flat palm (supine position)

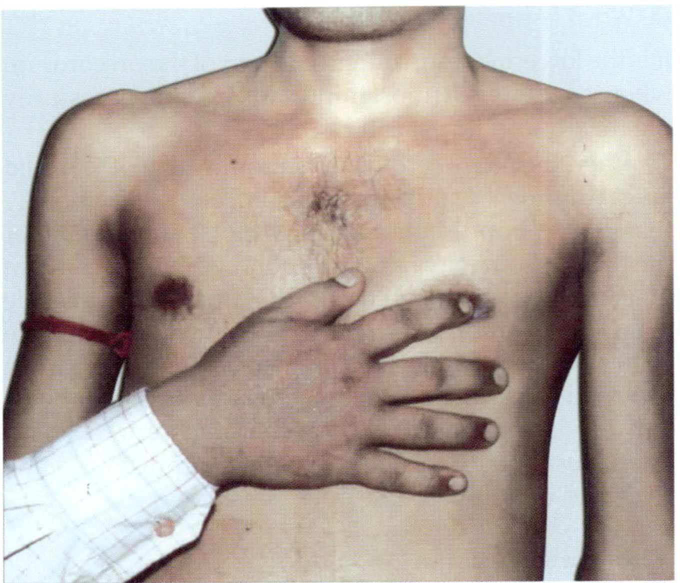

Fig. 1.11: **Localizing apex beat** with the finger tips (supine position)

3. If the apex is not palpable even in sitting position, place your right palm over the right side of the chest (to detect the presence of dextrocardia or dextroversion).
4. If still not palpable: Say that 'the apex could not be localised properly'.

- Remember, the heart has some mobility within the chest and thus never turn the patient to left lateral position for localisation of the apex beat (in left lateral position, apex shifts about 1–2 cm towards the left). **Normal position of the apex beat is in the left 5th ICS, ½" inside the left MCL (adult).**

Q. In palpating the apex, why the finger is lifted in systole when the ventricle is contracting?

This is due to the complex rotatory movement of the heart in systole (vortex-like movement), one manifestation of which is the forward movement of apex (the rotatory movement is due to the complex spiral arrangement of ventricular muscles).

Q. Causes of non-palpable (non-visible) apex:

1. Apex lying behind a rib.
2. Obesity or thick chest wall.
3. Pendular breast in elderly female.
4. Emphysema (COPD).
5. Pleural effusion (left).
6. Pneumothorax (left).
7. Constrictive pericarditis.
8. Pericardial effusion.
9. Acute myocardial infarction.
10. Deformity of the chest (gross kyphoscoliosis).
11. Thickened pleura (left).
12. Heart failure.
13. Shock.
14. Heart may be somewhere else (dextrocardia).

Q. Commonest cause of displaced apex:

Deformity of thoracic cage, usually scoliosis. So, never forget to inspect the back in any CVS case.

Q. Describe different characters of the apex beat:

The normal apex beat is early systolic outward thrust located at a point not more than 2–3 cm in diameter.

The different types are:

1. **Hyperdynamic** (volume overload apex): It means 'forceful and ill sustained' impulse found in conditions with diastolic overload of the left ventricle like MI, AI, VSD, PDA, high output states, etc. As there is no obstruction to the blood pumped from the left ventricle, the apex remains ill sustained.
2. **Heaving** (pressure overload apex): It is a 'forceful and well sustained' impulse found in conditions with systolic overload of the left ventricle like AS, systemic hypertension, coarctation of aorta, obstructive cardiomyopathy, etc. As there is some obstruction in left ventricular outflow tract, the apex becomes well sustained.
3. **Tapping:** When the accentuated first heart sound is palpable in MS or tachycardia due to any cause, it is known as tapping apex beat (remember, heart sounds are not palpable in health). The palpating finger is not lifted and the S_1 is felt as distinct palpable shock.
4. **Hypokinetic:** The thrust felt by the hand is minimal. It is found in acute myocardial infarction, pericardial effusion, constrictive pericarditis, myxoedema, peripheral circulatory failure.
5. **Normal:** Situated in the left 5th ICS, ½" inside the left MCL which is a brief, non-sustained, gentle tap not exceeding a 25-paisa coin size, not much forceful but usually palpable with certainty. Its duration is <1/3rd of systole. In children, the apex beat is located in the left 4th ICS and in lean-tail persons, it is usually present in the left 6th ICS.

- There may be double kicking apex beat in IHSS (idiopathic hypertrophic subaortic stenosis or hypertrophic cardiomyopathy) and ventricular aneurysm. Retractile apex is seen in severe tricuspid incompetence. Diffuse apical Impulse (>3 cm in diameter) is characteristic of LV aneurysm or LV dilatation. See-saw apex beat is found in ventricular aneurysm.
- Regarding the **character of the apex beat**, some clinicians prefer the terms 'right ventricular (RV)' or 'left ventricular (LV)' type. In **LV type** the apex goes downwards and outwards as well as there is a larger impulse (usually more than a 25-paisa coin), and the impulse is maximal at the apex; if there is a left parasternal impulse, it is asynchronous with the apex beat. Whereas in **RV type**, the apex is rotated outwards as well as there is production of left parasternal heave, and both are synchronous; in RV type, the cardiac impulse is maximal over the lower left sternal border.
- While **palpating for pulsations**, e.g. apex beat or any local pulsation—use the pulp of the fingers, for thrills—use the base of the fingers, and for parasternal lift or heave—use ulnar border of the hand or heal of the palm (i.e. thenar and hypothenar eminences) (**Fig. 1.12**).

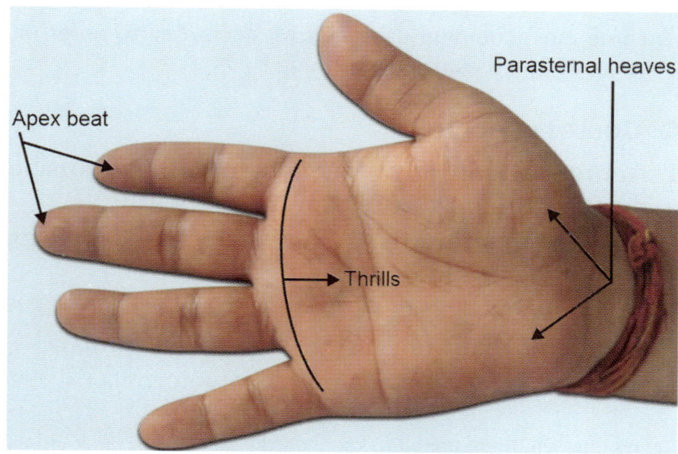

Fig. 1.12: **Palpating for pulsations** by hand

Q. Different positions of heart:

- Levocardia: Cardiac apex on left side of chest (situs solitus).
- Dextrocardia: Cardiac apex on right side of chest.
- Mesocardia: Cardiac apex over the centre of chest.
- Dextracardia with situs inversus (heart *per se* does not show any abnormality).
- Isolated dextrocardia: Dextrocardia without situs inversus; almost always have cardiac malformations.
- Isolated levocardia: Cardiac apex on left side with viscera rotated (partial or totally) to opposite side.
- Dextroversion: Always acquired; cardiac apex is on right side due to extracardiac causes like left-sided pleural effusion/pneumothorax, or right-sided fibrosis/collapse of lung (i.e. push-pull effects). Remember, trachea is moved to the right side too.

❍ 'Situs inversus' is the rotation of abdominal/thoracic organs to opposite side, either totally (totalis) or partially (partialis).

Q. Clinical features of pulmonary hypertension:

Normal pulmonary artery pressure is 25/10 mm of Hg. Pulmonary hypertension is said to be present when mean pulmonary artery pressure is >25 mm of Hg at rest or >30 mm of Hg during exercise.

A. Symptoms (from the history):

1. Breathlessness (often severe; exertional).
2. Easy fatigability.
3. Dizziness.
4. Syncope (due to low fixed stroke volume).
5. Chest pain (angina pectoris).
6. Cough (rare), palpitations, haemoptysis.

B. Signs:

1. Pulse: Low volume (due to reduced cardiac output).
2. Neck veins: a-wave is prominent; prominent v-wave in functional tricuspid incompetence.
3. Central cyanosis In right-to-left shunt, lung diseases (COPD, interstitial lung disease).
4. a. **Inspection:**
   i. Precordial bulge; visible pulmonary artery pulsation in left 2nd ICS.
   ii. Epigastric pulsation.

   b. **Palpation:**
   i. Apex goes outwards.
   ii. P_2: Diastolic shock, i.e. P_2 is palpable.
   iii. Left parasternal heave.
   iv. Pulsation of pulmonary artery may be felt in upper left parasternal areas.

   c. **Percussion:** Left 2nd ICS may be dull on percussion.

   d. **Auscultation (pulmonary area):** The **classical sequence of events** are:
   i. S_1: Audible.
   ii. Pulmonary ejection click.
   iii. Ejection systolic murmur (due to relative obstruction at pulmonary orifice).
   iv. Close splitting of S_2 with loud P_2.
   v. Graham Steell murmur: A high-pitched early diastolic decrescendo murmur due to functional pulmonary incompetence (pulmonary annulus dilatation).
   vi. Right-sided S_3 (right ventricular gallop): Heard at the lower left sternal border.

Among these features, the ejection systolic murmur with palpable as well as audible loud P_2 are commonly found. Remember: (i) Epigastric pulsation, (ii) Left parasternal heave, and (iii) Outward apex are features of RVH. RVH is usually present in a case of pulmonary hypertension of some duration.

- [Chest X-ray: Bulging right and left pulmonary arteries at hilum, peripheral pruning of large pulmonary arteries (i.e. a pruned tree appearance → enlarged proximal branches of pulmonary arteries with rapid tapering), enlargement of RV and RA of heart.
- ECG: RV strain or hypertrophy, and RA enlargement.
- Echocardiography (most useful): RV enlargement with paradoxical motion of interventricular septum. It estimates the pulmonary artery systolic pressure, left ventricular function and valvular disease.
- Pulmonary function test, lung scan, right heart catheterisation and pulmonary angiography in appropriate cases.]

❍ For demonstration of 'Signs' anywhere in clinical medicine, always start from general survey.

❍ Unless otherwise mentioned, pulmonary hypertension means pulmonary arterial hypertension. As soon as pulmonary hypertension develops from valvular heart disease, it protects the patient from pulmonary oedema.

Q. Causes of pulmonary hypertension:

Pulmonary hypertension is basically of two types: Primary pulmonary hypertension (No. 6 below) and secondary pulmonary hypertension (No. 1–7, except No. 6). The causes are:

1. Passive: From left-sided heart diseases like MS, MI, AI, AS.
2. Hyperkinetic (left-to-right shunt): ASD, VSD, PDA.
3. Vasoconstrictive (hypoxic): Chronic cor pulmonale, interstitial lung disease, high altitude.
4. Obstructive: Pulmonary thromboembolism (acute cor pulmonale).
5. Obliterative: SLE, systemic sclerosis, polyarteritis nodosa.
6. Neurohumoral or idiopathic: Primary pulmonary arterial hypertension (common in females in 3rd and 4th decades).
7. Miscellaneous: Sleep apnoea, Pickwickian syndrome, drugs like aminorex fumarate, porto-pulmonary hypertension, sarcoidosis, etc.

Q. Gradation of dyspnoea (cardiac):

Functional gradation of heart disease by New York Heart Association: '**NYHA classification**':

Class I: No limitation of activities with ordinary physical work (activity), i.e. asymptomatic though the patient is suffering from organic heart disease (there is no class 0). There is shortness of breath on unaccustomed exertion.

Class II: No limitation under resting condition but symptoms appear on ordinary activity.

Class III: Limitation of activities on mild exertion or less than ordinary physical activity.

Class IV: Limitation of activities at rest, restricting the person to bed or chair.

- Remember, this functional classification refers not only to dyspnoea but to symptoms like fatigue, palpitations, angina pectoris, etc. This is actually a *classification of cardiac disability*. Dyspnoea due to cardiovascular diseases should always be quantified by this classification.

Q. Aetiology of MI (chronic):

1. **Rheumatic** (commonest).
2. Functional: Associated with LVH (due to dilatation of mitral ring) as found in systemic hypertension, aortic valvular diseases (AS, AI), IHD, myocarditis, cardiomyopathy or acute rheumatic carditis.
3. Mitral valve prolapse syndrome (MVPS).
4. Dysfunction of papillary muscle or chordae tendineae (due to IHD, i.e. ischaemic heart disease).
5. Acute myocardial infarction (due to rupture of papillary muscle).
6. Traumatic: During mitral valvotomy (iatrogenic).
7. Infective endocarditis (due to perforation of mitral valve leaflet or chordae tendineae).
8. Collagen vascular diseases: Marfan's syndrome, SLE (Libman-Sacks endocarditis), rheumatoid arthritis, ankylosing spondylitis, Ehlers-Danlos syndrome, pseudoxanthoma elasticum, etc.
9. Dilated cardiomyopathy.
10. Congenital.

- Three most common causes of MI according to order of frequency are rheumatic, MVPS and IHD.

Q. Causes of acute MI:

1. Acute myocardial infarction (papillary muscle dysfunction/rupture of chordae tendineae).
2. Infective endocarditis (rupture of mitral valve cusps or chordae tendineae).
3. Trauma in the chest.
4. Acute rheumatic fever (due to mitral valvulitis).
5. Cardiac surgery (during mitral valvotorny).

- In acute MI, there are sinus tachycardia, a-wave in neck veins and short systolic murmur radiating to base.

Q. What is mitral valve prolapse syndrome (MVPS)?

The other names of this disease are systolic click-murmur syndrome, Barlow's syndrome, billowing mitral leaflet syndrome, or floppy mitral valve. There is excessive mitral leaflet tissue which is commonly involved with myxomatous degeneration. MVPS is frequently associated with Marfan's syndrome, Ehlers-Danlos syndrome and osteogenesis imperfecta. It is common in young females. The patient is usually asymptomatic or may present with palpitations or chest pain. A mid- or late systolic click (due to prolapse of the mitral valve) with high-pitched late systolic murmur (due to MI), best heard at the apex, is the classical auscultatory finding. 2-D echocardiography confirms the diagnosis. Treatment is done by reassurance, propranolol for chest pain and arrhythmia, antibiotic prophylaxis for SBE, antiplatelets (e.g. aspirin) for prevention of transient ischaemic attacks (TIA), and valve replacement by prosthesis for permanent remedy. Prognosis, as a whole, is good.

Q. What is seagull murmur?

If a patient develops SBE over MI, the character of MI murmur changes with a musical quality called seagull murmur. Here the ruptured chordae tendineae acts as the string of the musical instrument. Seagull murmur is also known as 'cooing dove murmur'. This type of musical murmur is also found in acute myocardial infarction (due to papillary muscle dysfunction), syphilitic AI and rarely in acute rheumatic fever.

Q. Can MI produce apical mid-diastolic murmur?

Yes. The increased flow through the valve in diastole may produce a low-pitched mid-diastolic rumbling murmur (functional MS), often with a S_3.

Q. Radiation of murmur if posterior mitral leaflet is affected:

In *posterior mitral leaflet* affection, pansystolic murmur of MI radiates to the anterior precordium and up to the pulmonary area (base of the heart). In a classical case of MI with radiation of murmur towards the left axilla and inferior angle of left scapula, the pathology remains in the *anterior mitral leaflet* (blood goes from LV to LA, i.e. anterior to posterior direction). Rheumatic MI predominantly affects anterior mitral leaflet.

Q. What is 'bruit"?

When the murmurs occur at the site of arterial stenosis, they are traditionally called bruits, e.g. renal artery bruit in renal artery stenosis. A short systolic bruit is produced in 50% or less obstruction, continuous bruit in 75% or more obstruction, and there is no bruit in 100% obstruction.

Q. Differential diagnosis (D/D) of your case:

The undermentioned conditions give rise to systolic murmur near apical area.

1. Functional murmur: Usually soft, not pansystolic, does not radiate to the axilla and without any thrill. No alteration with change of posture and respiration. Any condition which results in dilatation of left ventricle may give rise to functional MI.
2. VSD: History starts from early childhood. Rough, pansystolic murmur, best audible over the lower left parasternal area with radiation to right chest. Very often associated with systolic thrill.
3. Conducted murmur of aortic stenosis: Harsh, mid-systolic murmur.
4. Tricuspid incompetence (TI): Murmur best audible over the tricuspid area with positive **Carvallo's sign** (increase in intensity of murmur with inspiration), not conducted to the axilla, and may be associated with features of CCF (in functional TI, search for tender-pulsatile liver and engorged-pulsatile neck vein with prominent c-v complex).
5. Papillary muscle dysfunction.

Q. Definition of pansystolic or holosystolic murmur:

They start immediately with the S_1 and continue through to the S_2 (pansystolic). They always have a uniform intensity and thus known as holosystolic.

Q. Why the murmur of MI is pansystolic?

As soon as the LV pressure exceeds LA pressure, i.e. *just after the* S_1, the regurgitant jet of blood goes from LV to LA, and *continues to and through the* S_2 until the LA pressure exceeds LV pressure. This is why the murmur of MI is pansystolic in nature.

Q. How to describe the 'intensity' or 'grading' of a murmur?

The intensity of murmurs are divided into SIX GRADES **(Levine's grading system).** Grade I is a very faint murmur heard on careful auscultation, and grade VI murmur may be heard without a stethoscope and with the head just away from the chest (loudest).

If the murmur is associated with thrill, the grading is IV or IV+ (i.e. it may be grade IV, V or VI). Thrill is absent in grade I, II, and III. Though systolic murmurs are classified into six grades, diastolic murmurs are only graded up to IV.

Grade I: Very faint or soft (can be heard only in quiet surroundings)
Grade II: Soft
Grade III: Moderately loud
Grade IV: Loud with presence of thrill
Grade V: Very loud with associated thrill; still heard with the stethoscope lightly touching the chest
Grade VI: Extremely loud and still heard with the stethoscope off the chest, with associated thrill.

Q. How to assess the 'severity' of MI clinically?

Severe MI is assessed at the bedside by:

1. Presence of apical mid-diastolic flow murmur.
2. Left ventricular (apical) S_3.
3. Degree of LVH, and
4. Presence of systolic thrill with a loud murmur over the apical area.

Q. Surface marking of mitral valve:

It is obliquely placed behind the left 4th costal cartilage and the adjacent part of the sternum.

Q. What is mitral area?

It corresponds with the apex of the heart. Normally in an adult, the apex is situated in the left 5th ICS, 1/2" inside the left MCL. Suppose, in a patient the apex beat is palpable in the left 6th ICS, 1/2" outside the MCL (in LVH)—this (apical) area will be the mitral area of the patient. So mitral area is a mobile area according to the position of the apex or apical area, i.e. it is not a fixed area. Tricuspid, aortic and pulmonary areas are always fixed in their location. See page 411 for other details.

Different areas of heart (e.g. mitral, aortic, pulmonary or tricuspid area) do not correspond to surface markings of respective heart valve but denote areas where cardiac events in these four valves are best appreciated.

Q. When the patient is turned to left side while examining the CVS?

1. To note the 'character' of apex beat (Fig. 1.13).
2. For better palpation of the diastolic thrill (MS), and
3. For better auscultation of the diastolic murmur (MS).

- It is also said that in a case of MI, palpation of the systolic thrill and auscultation of the systolic murmur are better appreciated in left lateral position. Never turn the patient to the left to localise the site of apex beat.

Q. Palpate the mitral area:

Following four points are to be noted:

a. Site of apex beat.
b. Character of apex beat.
c. Palpable heart sound (M_1).
d. Any thrill.

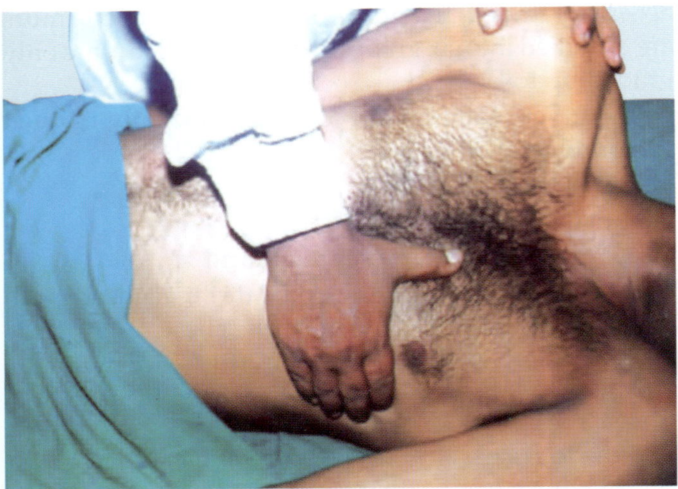

Fig. 1.13: Palpating **apex beat for character** (left lateral position)

Steps:

1. First locate the apex by proper clinical method described in page 23.
2. Then note the character of the apex beat: Turn the patient to left lateral position.
3. Next, one should confirm whether any palpable heart sound is present or not.
4. Lastly, feel for any thrill (one should put his left thumb over the right carotid): If there is any difficulty, turn the patient to left lateral position and try to palpate the thrill in a better way at the height of expiration.

Q. Complications of MI:

1. Acute LVF.
2. Infective endocarditis (more common than MS).
3. CCF.
4. Arrhythmias:
   i. Ventricular ectopics.
   ii. Atrial fibrillation (with embolic manifestations).
5. Giant left atrium may produce:
   i. Pressure symptoms: Dysphagia, hoarseness of voice.
   ii. Atrial fibrillation.
   iii. Left atrial thrombus and systemic embolisation (less common than MS).
6. Recurrent respiratory tract infections.

Q. How do you like to investigate a case of MI?

a. Chest X-ray (PA view): There is cardiomegaly due to:
   1. LVH.
   2. LAH (giant left atrium).
   3. Signs of pulmonary venous hypertension (in acute MI).
   4. RVH.

b. Curved barium-filled cesophagus pushed by enlarged LA in RAO view of chest X-ray.

c. ECG: The ECG may be normal in early stages. Following abnormalities are commonly seen:
   1. LAH (in most of the chronic cases).
   2. LVH (50% cases).
   3. Biventricular hypertrophy (25% cases).
   4. Atrial fibrillation.

d. Blood for (to detect active rheumatic carditis):
   1. TC and DC.
   2. ESR.
   3. ASO titre.

- All are raised with active rheumatic carditis.

e. Echocardiography (giant or aneurysmal left atrium may be seen): Done for confirmation with severity assessment.

f. Doppler study (it quantifies the regurgitation).

g. Cardiac catheterisation with left ventriculography.

Q. Treatment of MI:

1. Medical treatment: As in MS. MI of moderate severity can be managed medically. For the case described at the outset, digitalis and diuretic should be given to treat CCF; penicillin prophylaxis against SBE is a must. Digitalis and anticoagulants are added, if AF is present. Vasodilators (nitrates, ACE inhibitors) can reduce the regurgitant flow and may be helpful in severe cases.
2. Surgical treatment: Implantation of prosthesis (mitral valve replacement) is done under open heart surgery; sometimes, repair by mitral annuloplasty or valvuloplasty is done.

Q. Features of Digitalis Toxicity:

1. Non-cardiac: Anorexia, nausea, vomiting [due to direct stimulation of chemoreceptor trigger zone (CTZ) at medulla], and diarrhoea; these are the earliest signs of toxicity.
2. Cardiac:
   i. Premature ventricular beats (bigeminy and multiform).
   ii. Varying degree of AV block (bradycardia).
   iii. Paroxysmal atrial tachycardia with blook.
   iv. Ventricular tachycardia.
   v. Bidirectional tachycardia.
   vi. Sinus arrest.
   vii. Ventricular fibrillation.
3. Chronic toxicity:
   i. Weight loss.
   ii. Cachexia.
   iii. Gynaecomastia.
   iv. Xanthopsia (yellow vision).
   v. Agitation, psychosis, delirium.
   vi. Headache.

- Digitalis toxicity is managed by withholding digoxin, withdrawal of diuretic (hypokalaemia increases digitalis toxicity), giving potassium, administration of lignocaine or phenytoin to combat ventricular arrhythmias, and repeated application of anti-digoxin antibody (Fab fragments).
- **Blue vision (cyanopsia) is sildenafil-Induced, yellow vision is digitalis-induced, while red vision is found in polycythemia vera.**

Q. What is cadiac output, cardiac index and ejection fraction?

a. Cardiac output = Stroke volume (output per ventricle per beat) × heart rate.
   Normal: 5-6 litre/minute
b. Cardiac index = Cardiac output/minute/square meter of body surface.
   Normal: 3.3 litre/minute/m^2
c. Ejection fraction (EF)

$$= \frac{\text{End-diastolic volume} - \text{End-systolic volume}}{\text{End-diastolic volume}}$$

   Normal: 55–80%
   Left ventricular dysfunction (EF-related): Mild (40–50%), moderate (30–40%), severe (<30%).

Q. Why history of drug intake is important in cardiology?

1. Drugs can aggravate a disease (β-blockers in heart block, thyroxine in angina, amlodipine in oedema, salbutamol in palpitations, α-blockers in postural hypotension, steroids in systemic hypertension).
2. Drugs can mask a disease (antihypertensives in systemic hypertension, diuretics in MS).
3. Drugs can modify a disease (oral contraceptive pills in systemic hypertension).
4. Drugs can cure a disease or alter physical sign (diuretics abolish the gallop rhythm in heart failure).
5. Drugs can induce a disease (β-blockers in hyperlipidaemia, alcohol in cardiomyopathy).

Clinical Wisdom

Diastolic thrill in MS is a very frequent clinical sign, but systolic thrill in MI is rather uncommon.

AORTIC STENOSIS — CASE 3

Q. What is your diagnosis?

This is a case of valvular aortic stenosis (AS) of rheumatic origin without congestive cardiac failure and the patient is in sinus rhythm at present.

Q. What is your case?

Build up the summary. The chief presenting symptoms in AS are exertional dyspnoea, anginal pain, syncope and features related to LVF. All the symptoms are usually 'exertional'.

a. Dyspnoea is primarily due to elevation of the pulmonary capillary pressure and pulmonary oedema; later on PND may occur. Severe AS may exist for many years without producing any clinical disability.
b. Anginal pain is due to low aortic blood pressure and low cardiac output. Increased O_2 demand due to increased muscle mass (LVH) is also important. Thus, coronary blood flow cannot be maintained while on exertion.
c. Syncope or black-out may be due to low and fixed cardiac output, LVF, low BP or transient atrioventricular block (all causing cerebral hypoperfusion). Sometimes, the patient complains of light-headedness, faintness or giddiness.

- *Dyspnoea, angina pectoris and syncope are three cardinal symptoms of AS.* Many patients remain asymptomatic. Sometimes, a patient may be brought in the hospital emergency with 'sudden cardiac death'.

Q. Why do you say aortic stenosis?

It is a case of AS because of the presence of:

A. Symptoms (from the history):

a. Pain in the chest for 1 year.
b. Exertional dyspnoea for 9 months.
c. Occasional black-out for last 2 months. (plus past H/o rheumatic fever).

B. Signs:

a. Pulse: 72/minute, low volume, regular, no radio-radial and radio-femoral delay, arterial wall is not thickened, all the peripheral pulses are palpable and of 'anacrotic' in type (also called pulsus parvus et tardus). *'Carotid shudder'*, i.e. a systolic thrill in the carotid artery is felt.
b. BP: Low systolic BP (say, 95/80 mm of Hg) with low pulse pressure (in supine position).
c. Apex beat: In normal position (i.e. left 5th ICS, 1/2" inside the left MCL) and heaving in character (though there is LVH, apex is usually not shifted because AS causes concentric hypertrophy). There is no palpable heart sound, no thrill in the apical area.
d. Palpation of the aortic area: Systolic thrill felt. Best felt in full expiration with the patient sitting and leaning forward. The thrill is radiated along the carotid artery (carotid shudder).
e. Auscultation of the aortic area:
   S_1: Audible
   S_2 (A_2): Muffled (soft)
   S_3 or S_4: Not audible at present
   Ejection click (just after S_1): Present
   After the ejection click, a harsh midsystolic ejection murmur of grade V with direction of selective propagation towards the carotids is heard. The murmur is best audible in full expiration with the patient sitting and leaning forward, and with the diaphragm of stethoscope (Fig. 1.14) (occasionally the murmur of AS is transmitted to the mitral area and is known as *Gallavardin's phenomenon*).
f. Auscultation of other areas of heart and lung: Within normal limit. No adventitious sound heard.

[g. Examination of respiratory system, GI tract and nervous system revealed no abnormality.]

- The murmur of AS is known as saw-like murmur or crescendo-decrescendo murmur (never say 'diamond shaped' murmur as this is the phonocardiographic pattern of AS murmur).

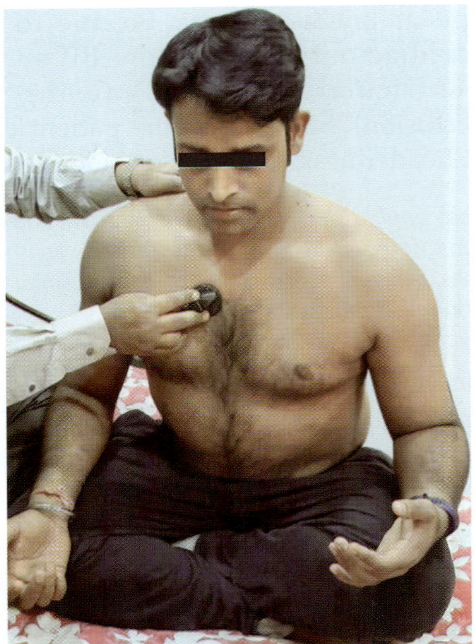

Fig. 1.14: Auscultation of aortic area: Use diaphragm while patient is sitting and leaning forward

- Add features of pulmonary hypertension, if present.
- The normal aortic valve averages 3–4 cm^2. If it is ≤1.0 cm^2 or having a mean pressure gradient >40 mm of Hg (normally, no gradient), the stenosis is critical.
- The pulse is not only small in volume but is slow in rising to a peak (plateau pulse).

Q. Why the murmur of AS is midsystolic?

The pressure gradient between the left ventricle and aorta is greatest in the middle of systole, and this is why the murmur of AS is midsystolic.

Q. Significance of ejection click:

Valve opening is normally silent. Ejection click is a sharp and high-pitched clicking sound heard immediately after the first heart sound due to sudden opening of the aortic or pulmonary valve (semilunar valves), and are best audible in aortic (in aortic stenosis) and pulmonary (in pulmonary stenosis) area respectively. **Its presence indicates that the stenosis is at the 'valvular' level and the stenosis (aortic stenosis or pulmonary stenosis) is of milder degree.** Pulmonary ejection click in pulmonary stenosis becomes less audible (soft) in inspiration, in contrast to all other right-sided events.

Aortic ejection click: AS, aortic aneurysm, systemic hypertension.

Pulmonary ejection click: PS, pulmonary hypertension.

Example of **'non-ejection click'** is mitral valve prolapse syndrome (MVPS).

Q. Aetiology of AS:

1. **Rheumatic** (it should be remembered that isolated rheumatic AS is rare; usually it is associated with MS, AI or MI: So, try to find them out. Aortic valve is the second most frequently affected valve in rheumatic fever after mitral valve).
2. Congenital (commonly bicuspid aortic valve): Young adult patients.
3. Calcific degeneration of the aortic valve (old age leading to aortic sclerosis): Vide page 46.
4. Associated with familial hypercholesterolaemia, mucopolysaccharidosis.
5. Functional: In severe AI, thyrotoxicosis, severe anaemia, etc.

- Calcific valvular disease is the commonest cause of AS.

Q. Types of aortic stenosis:

a. Valvular (involves valve cusps): Examples are described above in 'Aetiology of AS'.
b. Supravalvular (rare; constriction at the first part of aorta): May be associated with Elfin facies, mental retardation, hypercalcaemia.
c. Subvalvular (narrowing at outflow tract of left ventricle; special variety is IHSS): Idiopathic hypertrophic subaortic stenosis.

- Elfin facies: Broad forehead, pointed chin, cupid's bow-like upper lip, upturned nose, hypertelorism and low set ears (seen in supravalvular AS and when associated with mental retardation and hypercalcaemia, it is known as William's syndrome).

Q. Causes of RVH:

1. Pulmonary hypertension (especially MS and other left-sided valvular diseases, COPD).
2. Pulmonary stenosis.
3. Tricuspid incompetence.
4. ASD and VSD with initial left-to-right shunt.
5. Fallot's tetralogy.
6. Cardiomyopathy.
7. Hyperdynamic circulation.

Q. What are the causes and types of LVH?

LVH is of two types: Concentric and eccentric.

A. **Concentric** (muscle mass increases at the cost of left ventricular cavity, i.e. left ventricle is more hypertrophied than dilated due to pressure overload—so the apex is not shifted much). The examples are basically left ventricular outflow tract obstruction, and are:
   1. AS.
   2. Systemic hypertension.
   3. IHSS.
   4. Coarctation of aorta.

B. **Eccentric** (left ventricle is more dilated than increase in its muscle mass and is due to volume overload—so the apex goes down and outwards). The examples are:
   1. Systemic hypertension.
   2. MI or AI.
   3. Ischaemic heart disease (IHD).
   4. Severe anaemia (hyperdynamic circulation).

5. Thyrotoxicosis.
6. Cardiomyopathy (dilated).
7. VSD.
8. PDA.

- **Combined A + B are the causes of LVH.**
- Hypertrophy of ventricle is commonly due to pressure overload (e.g. systemic hypertension), and dilatation is the result of volume overload (e.g. AI, MI).

Q. Causes of right atrial hypertrophy (RAH):

1. Tricuspid stenosis.
2. Tricuspid incompetence.
3. Pulmonary hypertension.
4. RVH of some duration (e.g. MS, COPD).
5. Pulmonary thromboembolism.
6. ASD, Ebstein's anomaly.

Q. Causes of left atrial hypertrophy (LAH):

1. MS.
2. MI (giant left atrium may be seen).
3. LVH of some duration.
4. Left atrial myxoma, VSD, PDA.

Q. Causes of biventricular hypertrophy (LVH + RVH):

1. Cardiomyopathy (dilated).
2. Ventricular septal defect.
3. Myocarditis.
4. Ishaemic heart disease.
5. Systemic as well as pulmonary hypertension.
6. Hyperkinetic circulation (e.g. in severe anaemia).

Q. Meaning of a thrill:

This is palpable low-frequency vibrations with the sensation like 'purring of a cat', and is always associated with heart murmur. It is synonymous with 'palpable murmur'. A thrill is always described by its site and timing.

Q. How to determine the timing of a thrill?

Palpate the thrill with the whole flat of the right palm (mainly by the base of the fingers). While palpating for a thrill, always put your left thumb over the right carotid artery at the level of the upper border of thyroid cartilage to confirm the timing. If the thrill is synchronous with carotid pulsation, it is systolic in timing and if it appears before (or after) carotid pulsation, it is diastolic thrill. Many clinicians adjust the timing of a thrill with the apex beat instead of carotid pulsation.

Always remember:

a. In mitral or apical area: Diastolic thrill is very common.
b. In all other areas (base of the heart and tricuspid area): Systolic thrill is more common.
c. In pulmonary area: Thrill may be continuous or systolo-diastolic, e.g. PDA.

Clinical Wisdom

It is seen that thrill is usually present in stenotic lesions and generally absent in regurgitant lesions of the heart. The presence of a thrill, most of the time, indicate that the murmur is organic.

- Sudden appearance of thrill usually indicates SBE or failure of prosthetic valve.
- Austin Flint murmur and Carey Coombs murmur do not have thrills.

Q. Thrill in different areas of the heart:

A. Mitral area:

a. *Systolic:*
   1. MI (commonest).
   2. VSD.
   3. ASD (ostium primum type)
b. *Diastolic:*
   1. MS (commonest).
   2. Left atrial myxoma (very rare).

B. Aortic area: Congenital or acquired AS (thrill in aortic area is almost exclusively systolic). Rarely, there is diastolic thrill of acute, severe AI.

C. Pulmonary area: Usualy it is systolic thrill:

1. Pulmonary stenosis.
2. ASD
3. High VSD.
4. Fallot's tetralogy.
5. PDA (sometimes, continuous thrill).

- Graham Steell murmur is usually not associated with diastolic thrill.

D. Tricuspid area: Usually it is systolic thrill:

1. VSD.
2. Tricuspid incompetence.
3. ASD (ostium primum).
4. Pulmonary stenosis (infundibular type).

Q. Causes of systolic murmur in base of the heart:

A. Aortic area:

1. Aortic stenosis (AS).
2. Systemic hypertension.
3. Coarctation of aorta.
4. Functional (from AI).
5. Aortic sclerosis (old age).
6. Aneurysm of aorta.

B. Pulmonary area:

1. Pulmonary hypertension.
2. Pulmonary stenosis (PS).
3. Hyperkinetic circulatory states.
4. ASD.
5. Fallot's tetralogy.
6. Innocent murmur.

Q. Classify 'organic' murmurs (Fig. 1.15):

A. Systolic (murmur between S_1 and S_2):

1. Ejection systolic or mid-systolic: Starts after the S_1 and ends before the S_2. Examples are AS, PS and ASD.
2. Pansystolic: Starts immediately with the S_1 and continues through to the S_2, and typically they are of uniform intensity (holosystolic), e.g. MI, TI and VSD.
3. Late systolic, e.g. MVPS, IHSS, papillary muscle dysfunction.

B. Diastolic (murmur between S_2 and S_1):

1. Early diastolic: AI and pulmonary incompetence (Graham Steell murmur).
2. Mid-diastolic: MS, TS, Austin Flint murmur, Carey Coombs murmur, and flow murmur in ASD, VSD or PDA.
3. Presystolic or late diastolic: MS, TS, atrial myxoma.

C. Continuous (murmur begins is systole and ends in diastole through S_2):

1. PDA.
2. Ruptured sinus of Valsalva.
3. Pulmonary arteriovenous fistula.
4. Aortopulmonary window.
5. Coronary arteriovenous fistula.
6. Coarctation of aorta (rare).

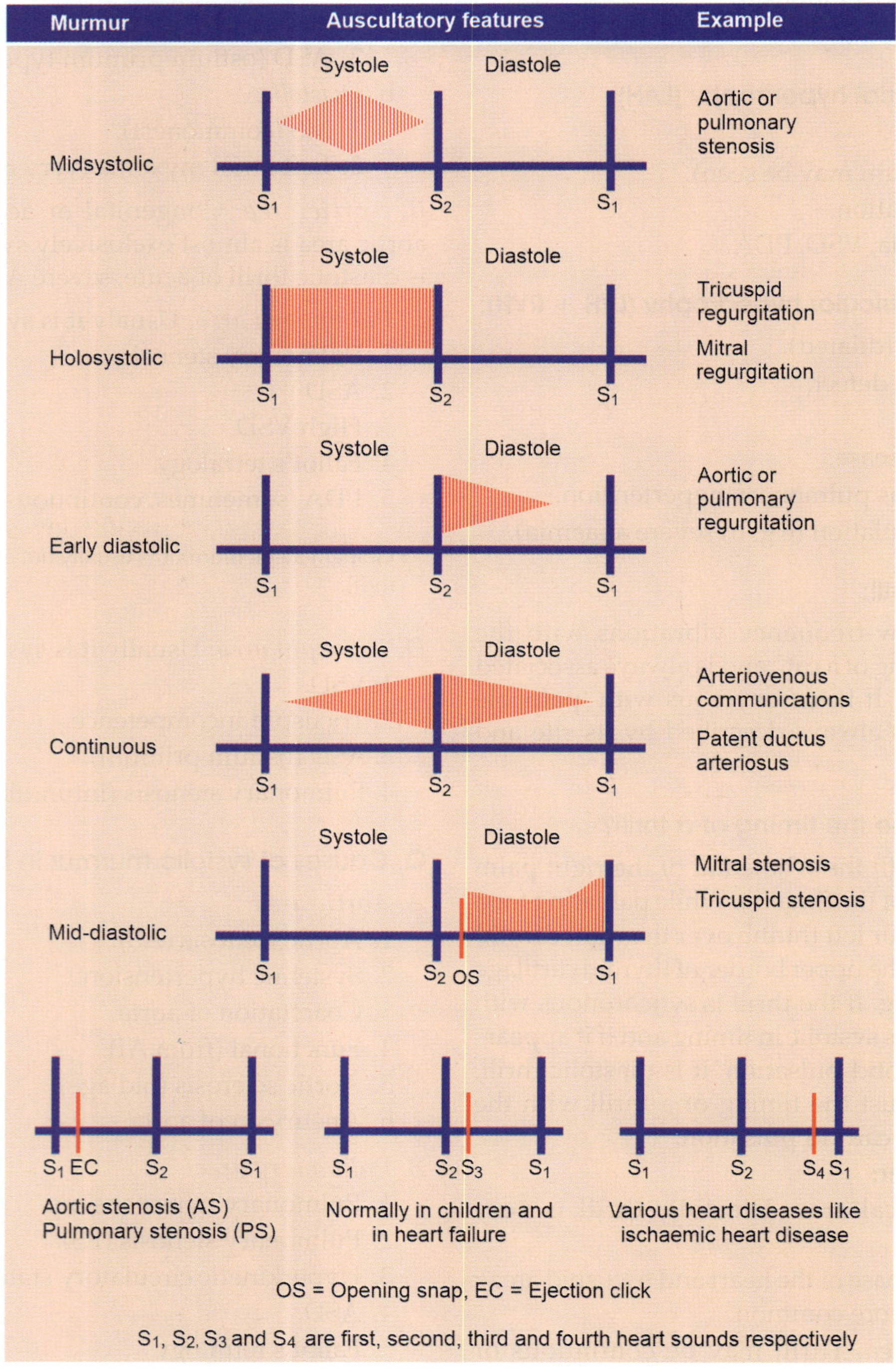

Fig. 1.15: Different murmurs and sounds in heart diseases

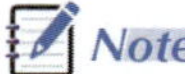 Note

Read more details of 'murmur' from page 412.

Q. Innocent murmur:

These are commonly found in **children** (Still's murmur) and usually disappear as the child grows older. Here, the heart with its valves are absolutely normal. Possible mechanisms are:

a. Hyperkinetic circulatory states in children due to increased heart rate, and
b. Increased resistance of the pulmonary vascular bed in children.

The characteristics are:

1. Usually systolic, soft (up to grade II) and musical, low-pitched vibration; localised.
2. No thrill.
3. Best heard over the lower left sternal border.
4. Heard best in supine position and may disappear in upright position; often the murmur is heard after exercise, crying or fever. Best heard with the bell of stethoscope.
5. Associated with normal heart sounds, chest X-ray and ECG.

Q. Haemic murmur:

Sometimes, an ejection systolic murmur is heard in the pulmonary and the aortic area when the person suffers from severe anaemia (so called haemic). The possible mechanisms are:

a. Increased flow of blood through the pulmonary artery, and
b. Dilatation of the pulmonary artery.

These mechanisms also play their part in other hyperkinetic circulatory states like pregnancy, thyrotoxicosis, high fever, etc. Often severe anaemia produces mitral systolic murmur due to ring (mitral) dilatation. This type of murmur disappears after correction of the primary disease. They are never associated with abnormality in ECG. Sometimes, a systolic thrill is associated with haemic murmur.

Q. Functional murmur:

In functional murmur, there is no organic heart disease present at the site of production of murmur and is produced only due to increased flow of blood.

The common examples are:

1. Systolic murmur in the pulmonary area in a case of ASD.
2. Early diastolic Graham Steell murmur of pulmonary hypertension (functional pulmonary incompetence).
3. Functional systolic murmur in aortic area (functional AS) in a case of severe AI.
4. Apical mid-diastolic murmur in a case of severe AI (Austin Flint murmur).

Characteristics:

1. Usually systolic, may be diastolic.
2. Intensity of murmur: Not very loud.
3. Commonly without a thrill (remember, presence of thrill does not exclude functional murmur).
4. Not distributed to a wide area (more or less, localised).
5. Does not change much with change of posture.
6. Does not produce cardiomegaly (haemodynamically insignificant).
7. Murmur disappears after correction of the increased flow.

Q. Flow murmur:

These are flow-related soft, ejection murmur heard over pulmonary area due to altered physiological states like severe anaemia, thyrotoxicosis, pyrexia, etc.

Q. Changing murmur:

These are the murmurs which change their character or intensity from time to time, e.g.

1. Infective endocarditis,
2. Atrial myxomas, and
3. Atrial ball valve thrombus.

Q. How to assess the 'severity' of AS clinically?

Severe AS is assessed at the bedside by the presence of:

1. H/o effort dyspnoea, effort angina and/or effort syncope.
2. Low volume pulse with a slowly rising plateau (e.g. delayed carotid upstroke).
3. Systolic decapitation of BP (low systolic pressure due to low and fixed cardiac output; in a patient with isolated AS, systolic BP never goes above 150 mm of Hg).
4. Soft S_2.
5. Paradoxical splitting of S_2: The splitting happens to occur only during expiration.
6. Presence of S_4.
7. Systolic thrill and heaving apex beat.
8. Harsh, loud and long murmur with late systolic peaking.

Q. Describe second heart sound (S_2):

Normally the S_2 is short and high-pitched (dupp in 'lubb-dupp'). It indicates the beginning of ventricular diastole and is produced due to closure of aortic (A_2) and pulmonary (P_2) valves. S_2 has two components: Aortic (A_2) and pulmonary (P_2); A_2 is best audible in aortic area and P_2 is in pulmonary area; A_2 comes earlier than P_2.

Q. Splitting of S_2 (Table 1.3)?

In health, there is a gap of 0.03 second between A_2 and P_2. Splitting of A_2–P_2 becomes wider in inspiration, where as splitting of A_2–P_2 is narrowed in expiration. Normal physiological splitting of S_2 is audible in children and young adults in inspiration. Splitting of S_2 is of three types:

1. Physiological: When the splitting is present only during inspiration, it is physiological splitting. Here A_2 occurs earlier than P_2.
2. Reversed (paradoxical): Splitting occurs only during expiration. Here pulmonary valve closes earlier than aortic valve.
3. Pathological: Splitting of S_2 is audible both in inspiration and expiration.

Table 1.3: Different types of splitting of S_2

A. Wide and fixed (i.e. no change with respiration) splitting: 1. Atrial septal defect (hallmark of ASD) 2. CCF (severe right heart failure) 3. Massive pulmonary thromboembolism 4. Total anomalous pulmonary venous connection (TAPVC) 5. Right ventricular pacing
B. Wide and variable splitting: 1. RBBB (right bundle branch block) 2. Pulmonary stenosis 3. Left ventricular pacing 4. Ventricular septal defect (VSD)
C. Reversed (paradoxical) splitting: 1. Severe aortic stenosis 2. LBBB (left bundle branch block) 3. Systemic hypertension 4. Severe left ventricular dysfunction

Q. Single S_2:

1. Severe AS (with absent A_2), aortic atresia (absence of aortic valve).
2. Severe PS (with absent P_2), pulmonary atresia (absence of pulmonary valve).
3. Fallot's tetralogy (absent P_2).

Q. Causes of loud S_2:

a. Loud P_2: Pulmonary hypertension, pulmonary artery dilatation.
b. Loud A_2: Systemic hypertension, dilated aorta, aneurysm of aorta, hyperkinetic circulatory states.

Q. Causes of soft S_2:

Soft A_2: AS, AI
Soft P_2: PS

- Palpable S_2 (either P_2 or A_2) is known as **diastolic shock** or **diastolic knock.**
- Loud (both) P_2 and A_2 may be found in patient with thin chest wall, and combined pulmonary hypertension plus systemic hypertension.

Q. Murmur of bicuspid aortic valve:

Usually the AS-murmur is heard but sometimes, AI-murmur is also present. The AI-murmur is haemodynamically insignificant and in bicuspid aortic valve, features of AS is always greater than AI.

Q. Who invented the stethoscope?

The French physician R.T.H. Laennec (1816) invented the stethoscope. His idea of listening heart sounds by a roll of thick paper landed in modern stethoscope with the passage of time.

Q. Diagnosis of acute rheumatic fever:

It is done by revised **JONES CRITERIA**, updated in 1992 (after Dr. T. Duckett Jones).

A. Major manifestations:
1. Carditis
2. Polyarthritis
3. Chorea
4. Erythema marginatum
5. Subcutaneous nodules

B. Minor manifestations:
1. Fever
2. Arthralgia
3. Previous rheumatic fever
4. High ESR or positive C-reactive protein (CRP)
5. Leucocytosis
6. Increased PR interval on ECG

The presence of:
a. Two or more major manifestations, or
b. One major + 2 or more minor manifestations strongly suggest rheumatic fever **with**

One supporting evidence of preceding streptococcal infection such as:
a. H/o recent scarlet fever (i.e. a good clinical history).
b. Positive throat culture for group A *Streptococcus*.
c. Increased ASO (antistreptolysin O) titre or titre of other streptococcal antibodies.

- Do not forget to take the H/o sore throat, 2–4 weeks prior to the onset of acute rheumatic fever. Evidence of recent streptococcal infection (within 45 days) is particularly valuable if only one major manifestation is present.
- Acute rheumatic fever occurs in children aged 5–15 years, and develops as a delayed sequel to pharyngeal infection caused by group A beta-haemolytic streptococci, i.e. *Streptococcus pyogenes* (type 5 most commonly causes rheumatic fever; other rheumatogenic M-serotypes are 1, 3, 6, 14, 18, 19, 24, 27 and 29). Streptococcal skin infection never produces rheumatic fever.
- The WHO (2002–2003) criteria for the diagnosis of rheumatic fever is a minor variation of revised Jones criteria but AHA-revised Jones criteria (2015) is a bit different (AHA is American Heart Association).

Q. Bedside diagnosis of 'acute rheumatic carditis':

This is a '**pancarditis**' developing from acute rheumatic fever involving endocardium, myocardium and pericardium to varying degree. The clinical features are:

A. Pericarditis:
1. Pericardial rub (usually C/o chest pain).
2. Pericardial effusion (rare and always mild).

B. Myocarditis:
1. Relative tachycardia (pulse rate rises by >10/ minute with per degree (°F) rise of temperature).

2. 'Tic-tac' quality of heart sounds (due to tachycardia and mimic foetal heart sounds).
3. S_1: Muffled or soft (reflected as prolonged PR interval in ECG).
4. S_3: Gallop rhythm due to heart failure.
5. Congestive heart failure.
6. Heart size: Enlarged (apex goes down and outwards due to cardiac dilatation). It is a very important bedside clinical sign.
7. Conduction defects: Dropped beat in pulse due to heart block.
8. Arrhythmias may occur.

C. Endocarditis:

1. The appearance of:
   a. Soft systolic murmur due to mitral incompetence.
   b. Soft early diastolic murmur in the aortic area due to acute involvement of the aortic valve (murmur of AI).
   c. Carey Coombs murmur: Due to mitral valvulitis (temporarily producing MS as a result of oedema of the mitral valve cusps), or
2. Change in the character of existing organic heart murmurs.

- Rheumatic subcutaneous nodules are almost always associated with active carditis.
- An accelerated heart beat during rest or sleep makes the clinician suspicious of carditis.

Q. Appearance of murmur in rheumatic valvulitis (carditis) from acute rheumatic fever:

In order of sequence, they are:

1. MI murmur.
2. AI murmur.
3. Carey Coombs murmur (mimicking MS).

Q. Investigations done in acute rheumatic fever:

A. Blood:
   1. Anaemia, polymorphonuclear leucocytosis, raised ESR.
   2. Raised ASO titre (>200 Todd units in adult and >333 Todd units in children).
   3. Raised C-reactive protein (CRP) and other acute phase reactants (e.g. serum complements)
   4. Other streptococcal antibodies: Antihyaluronidase (AH), anti-streptokinase (ASK), anti-streptozyme (ASTZ), and anti-DNase B (antideoxyribonuclease B). Nowadays, anti-DNase B and ASO titre are preferred for diagnosis.
   5. Positive throat swabs culture for Group A streptococci in 25–40% cases.

B. ECG (evidence of carditis):
   1. Sinus tachycardia.
   2. Prolonged PR interval.
   3. 2° heart block (rare).
   4. Features of pericarditis.
   5. T wave inversion.
   6. Reduction in QRS voltage.

C. Chest X-ray: Cardiomegaly, pulmonary congestion or evidences of heart failure.

D. Echocardiography: Cardiac dilatation with valve abnormalities (in case of carditis).

Q. Latent period from rheumatic fever to organic valvular heart disease:

In temperate climates, this gap is usually 15 years. In India, organic disease (mainly MS) develops much earlier (latent period may be as short as 1–2 years), and frequently causes serious symptoms before the age of 20 years. This happens to be due to repeated attacks of severe carditis in India.

Q. Characteristics of rheumatic arthritis:

1. Most common in children (5–15 years); commonest 'major' manifestation (75%).
2. Big joints are involved (knee, ankle, hip, elbow; knee, most commonly); but no joint is immune to the inflammatory process. Small joints of hand and feet may be affected as seen in rheumatoid arthritis. Joint involvement is usually asymmetrical. Involved joints are red, hot, swollen, painful and tender.
3. Typically it is **fleeting or migratory in nature** (i.e. as the inflammation of one joint is subsided, others tend to become affected); the affection of joints in rheumatoid arthritis is 'additive' (one above other) in nature.
4. Spine, sternoclavicular and temporo-mandibular joints are rarely affected (affected more in rheumatoid arthritis).
5. Recovery is complete (rare in rheumatoid arthritis).
6. Usually there is no residual deformity (rarely, recurrent attacks of arthritis may lead to minor deformities of the hand at MCP joints—Jaccoud's arthritis). Deformity is very common in rheumatoid arthritis.
7. Muscle spasm and muscular wasting are not common (common in rheumatoid arthritis).
8. No radiological abnormality (rheumatoid arthritis have characteristic erosive X-ray features).

- **Arthritis** means inflammation of the joint, i.e. pain plus swelling of the joint. **Arthralgia** means subjective presence of joint pain only (no inflammation, no swelling). *Acute rheumatic fever bites the heart and licks the joint in children, whereas it bites the joints and licks the heart in adults.*
- Post-streptococcal reactive arthritis (PSRA) rarely occurs after group A streptococcal pharyngitis without other major criteria of rheumatic fever. There may be symmetrical small joint involvement, which is usually 'additive'.

Q. 'Signs of activity' in acute rheumatic fever:

1. Fever.
2. Tachycardia.
3. Clinical evidence of carditis.
4. Leucocytosis with high ESR.

Q. Active rheumatic carditis with low ESR—reason behind:

The patient is in heart failure (remember, acute rheumatic fever is always associated with high ESR).

Q. Causes of high ESR:

1. All acute infections (e.g. tuberculosis).
2. Severe anaemia.
3. Pregnancy.
4. Old age.
5. Collagen vascular diseases (e.g. SLE).
6. Malignancy.
7. Multiple myeloma (stormy ESR).
8. Vasculitis.
9. Acute rheumatic carditis.
10. Temporal arteritis.

- ESR is the rate at which erythrocytes migrate through the plasma, and its alterations point towards presence as well as intensity of an inflammatory process. **Very high ESR** is seen in multiple myeloma, temporal arteritis and advanced tuberculosis.
- Normal ESR in men is 0–15 mm/hr and in women it is 0–20 mm/hr. ESR reflects changes in plasma proteins. Some clinicians use ESR as 'sickness index'.

Q. Causes of very low ESR:

1. Polycythemia (COPD, Fallot's tetralogy).
2. Congestive cardiac failure.
3. Congenital fibrinogen deficiency.
4. Sickle cell anaemia.
5. Hereditary spherocytosis.
6. Macrophage activation syndrome (MAS).

- Low ESR is due to diminished plasma protein or abnormal red cells making rouleaux formation impossible.

Q. What are acute phase reactants?

These are a class of liver-produced proteins, which rise in response to cytokines synthesised in tissue injury, e.g. in inflammation. Common phase reactors are fibrinogen, haptoglobulin, ferritin, α_1-antitrypsin, serum amyloid-A protein (SAP), mannose-binding protein, C_3 complement, ceruloplasmin, C-reactive protein (CRP), hepcidin, procalcitonin and orosomucoid. In clinical practice, estimation of C-reactive protein is commonly done. These proteins are responsible for rise in the ESR and thus ESR is an indirect measure of acute phase response. Phase reactors serve as markers for 'disease activity'.

- 'Negative' acute phase reactors are albumin, transferrin and fetuin (i.e. their serum level is diminished in acute inflammation).
  1. ESR ↑ with CRP normal: Old age, anaemia, multiple myeloma, pregnancy and SLE.
  2. CRP ↑ with ESR normal: Early phase of inflammation (as CRP increases within 6 hours of inflammation).

Q. Differential diagnosis (D/D) of your case:

It is a patient of valvular AS (due to the presence of ejection click and soft A_2). The D/D are:

1. Subvalvular aortic stenosis: Characterised by,
   a. Early diastolic murmur of AI (common).
   b. No ejection click.
   c. In IHSS variety: Double kicking apex beat and pulsus bisferiens may be present.
   d. The murmur does not radiate to carotids.
   e. No poststenotic dilatation.
   f. Heart size tends to be larger.
2. Supravalvular aortic stenosis: Characterised by:
   a. Right radial pulse better felt than left; systolic BP of right arm >left arm (Coanda effect) and is known as anisosphygmia.
   b. No ejection click.
   c. Systolic thrill and murmur transmitted to carotids (thrill is more conspicuous than other types).
   d. May be associated with mental retardation, Elfin facies, squint, infantile hypercalcaemia.
   e. A_2: Normal/accentuated.
   f. No poststenotic dilatation.

 *Note*

Also consider other *causes of systolic murmur in the aortic area* (pages 31 and 33).

Q. Complications of AS:

1. Acute LVF (rapidly progressive).
2. Right-sided heart failure (CCF).
3. Infective endocarditis.
4. Tachy- and bradyarrhythmias.
5. Precipitation of angina pectoris or syncope.
6. Sudden death due to complete heart block (as a result of extension of aortic valve calcification to AV node) or ventricular fibrillation.

- Bleeding per rectum resulting from angiodysplasia of colon may be associated with valvular AS.

Q. How do you like to investigate a case of AS?

1. X-ray chest (PA view):
   a. Normal sized heart due to concentric hypertrophy of left ventricle or LVH.
   b. Poststenotic dilatation of ascending aorta.
   c. Calcification of aortic valve (in left anterior oblique view or on fluoroscopy).
2. Fluoroscopy: Aortic valve calcification is seen.
3. ECG:
   a. LVH.
   b. LAH.
   c. First degree heart block.
   d. LBBB, complete heart block (when aortic valve calcification extends into conducting system).

4. Blood for (to detect active rheumatic carditis):
   a. TC and DC
   b. ESR
   c. ASO titre
   } All are increased in active carditis
5. Echocardiography shows calcified aortic valve, LVH; Doppler estimate of gradient, etc.
6. Cardiac catheterisation: To identify associated coronary artery disease or to assess the gradient across the aortic valve.
7. Coronary angiogram: To rule out co-existing IHD in patients of AS with angina pectoris.

Q. How will you like to treat this case?

By. 1. Medical management: As in MS. Treatment of angina, atrial fibrillation and LVH should be done carefully. β-blockers and strenuous exercise should preferably be avoided.
2. Asymptomatic AS: Review regularly for development of angina, syncope or heart failure.
3. In childhood, adolescence or pregnancy: Valvotomy; adults and elderly: Valvuloplasty.
4. For calcific AS: Aortic valve replacement (prosthesis)

Q. Describe the classical pain of angina pectoris:

First description of typical angina pectoris was given by William Heberden in 1770.

Characteristics:

1. Commonly retrosternal; sometimes, felt in left side of the midline.
2. Constricting, pressing or squeezing in nature; along with a sense of chocking. Often described as 'like a band around the chest'.
3. Radiation: Both upper extremities (left> right), shoulders, lower jaw, neck, back, rarely to the upper abdomen. Radiation to the ulnar aspect of the left arm is characteristic.
4. Exertional commonly. It increases with emotion, exposure to cold or walking uphill after a heavy meal.
5. Duration is usullally 2–5 minutes; seldom lasts for more than 20 minutes.
6. Relieved by rest, or after taking sublingual nitrates or nitroglycerin.
7. Usually associated with palpitations and diaphoresis.

Clinical Wisdom

A chest pain present in the left inframammary region is usally not due to IHD. The pain of **myocardial infarction** is also retrosternal, more severe, lasts longer than 30 minutes, persists at rest, and very often associated with breathlessness, nausea, vomiting, diaphoresis, pallor and collapse. There is tachycardia with feeble pulse, hypotension (↓ BP), muffled heart sounds with gallop (CVS) and basal crepitations in lungs. If the anginal pain occurs at rest ('rest pain') think of acute myocardial infarction, unstable angina, vasospastic angina (Prinzmetal's angina) and emotion-induced angina.

The diagnosis of ischaemic chest pain depends on history and different investigations [rest ECG, cardiac enzymes study (CK-MB, troponin T, troponin I), stress testing (treadmill test or TMT), thallium stress test, Holter monitoring, echocardiography and Doppler study, and the most specific coronary angiography].

Q. Syncope, fainting or black-out—definition and aetiology:

Definition: Syncope is sudden and transient loss of consciousness with inability to stand upright as a result of impairment of cerebral blood flow (i.e. postural collapse). The aetiology are:

1. Simple syncope, i.e. due to vasovagal phenomenon (in an unpleasant sight, micturition syncope, cough syncope, carotid sinus syncope or acute severe pain due to any cause).
2. Cardiovascular (complete heart block, AS, IHSS, sick sinus syndrome, hypersensitive carotid sinus syncope, prolonged QT syndrome, acute pulmonary thromboembolism, Eisenmenger's syndrome, other brady- or tachyarrhythmias, massive AMI, left atrial ball valve thrombus or myxoma).
3. Metabolic or drug-induced (hypoglycaemia, hypocalcaemia, alcohol intoxication; methyl dopa, prazocin, vasodilators or diuretics-induced postural hypotension).
4. Postural hypotension (in patients receiving antihypertensives and vasodilator drugs).
5. Nervous system disorders (vertebro-basilar insufficiency, diabetic autonomic neuropathy, GB syndrome, familial dysautonomia, glossopharyngeal neuralgia).
6. Others: Hyperventilation and hysterical fainting, breath-holding (children), internal bleeding, unknown causes.

- Exertional syncope is classical in aortic stenosis. In pre-syncope, the patient feels dizzy with loss of postural tone but with preserved consciousness. Common causes of syncope are vasovagal attack, Stokes-Adams syndrome (complete heart block), postural hypotension, micturition syncope and carotid sinus syncope.
- **Dizziness:** A sensation of light headedness or faintness.
- **Vertigo (or giddiness):** A sense of loss of balance and unsteadiness with a feeling of rotation of environment or body.
- **Drop attack:** Sudden unexpected episodes of lower limb weakness with a fall in the ground where awareness is preserved. It is common in middle-aged women, and presumably of brainstem in origin.

Q. D/D of syncope with episodic weakness/fainting:

Hyperventilation syndrome, hypoglycaemia, acute blood loss (hypovolaemia), vertigo, transient ischaemic attack, severe anaemia, etc.

Q. Describe the 'black-out' in this patient:

1. Present for last 2 months.
2. Persists for few seconds.
3. Almost always exertional.
4. No H/o trauma.

5. Absence of convulsions.
6. Repeated attacks.
7. Preceded by light-headedness.
8. Always in upright posture.

Q. How to take the H/o dyspnoea in a patient?

Following points should be noted carefully in each patient of respiratory distress **(Table 1.4)**:

1. Onset—acute or gradual? Does it occur at rest?
2. Paroxysmal or exertional? How much exertion is needed? Is it proportional to exertion?
3. Any H/o PND, or orthopnoea, or platypnoea, or trepopnoea?
4. Seasonal variation present or not?
5. Associated with wheezing or not? Any cough with expectoration?
6. Grading of dyspnoea (NYHA classification for cardiac causes and MMRC scale for respiratory causes).
7. Whether associated with pain chest (pneumothorax), shock (myocardial infarction), fever (consolidation), angina (AMI)?
8. Time of appearance: Early night (cardiac asthma), early morning (bronchial asthma).
9. Progressive or not?
10. How releived? by drugs/rest/change of smoky environment/squatting/change of posture/by expectoration of tenacious sputum, or by inhaler or nebuliser?
11. Does the patient smoke? If yes, number of cigarettes smoked per day.

Q. Enumerate the different causes of dyspnoea:

The major causes of dyspnoea are due to cardio-respiratory abnormalities:

1. Respiratory: Bronchial asthma, COPD, airways obstruction, lobar consolidation and broncho-pneumonia, spontaneous pneumothorax, pleural effusion, pulmonary thromboembolism, pulmonary oedema, bronchogenic carcinoma, fibrosing alveolitis (ILD), pulmonary infections (pneumonias).
2. Cardiovascular: Acute left ventricular failure (e.g. AMI, valvular heart disease), SVC syndrome, cyanotic congenital heart diseases, pericardial effusion and cardiac tamponade, constrictive pericarditis, rapid cardiac arrhythmias, IHD, cardiomyopathy.
3. Metabolic: Diabetic ketoacidosis, uraemia, high fever.
4. Neurological: Depression of respiratory centre from motor neurone disease, GB syndrome, bulbar poliomyelitis, syringobulbia; raised intracranial tension, diaphragmatic or respiratory muscle paralysis, myasthenia gravis.
5. Mechanical: Huge ascites.
6. Psychogenic: Hysterical hyperventilation, anxiety neurosis.
7. Physiological: High altitude, exercise, hyperpyrexia, obesity, severe anaemia.

- Common causes: Bronchial asthma, COPD, cardiogenic and non-cardiogenic pulmonary oedema, interstitial lung disease (ILD) and severe anaemia.
- Commonly missed causes: Severe anaemia, pulmonary hypertension and diaphragmatic palsy.

Q. Dyspnoea where chest is clear on auscultation:

1. Pulmonary thromboembolism.
2. Metabolic acidosis.
3. Severe anaemia.
4. Hyperventilation (e.g. hysterical).
5. CNS causes (i.e. respiratory centre abnormality).
6. Diaphragmatic palsy.

- 'Silent chest' in acute severe asthma in an important cause.

Q. Management of acute rheumatic fever in a nutshell:

1. Bed rest: Especially for fever, arthritis, arthralgia, carditis and heart failure.
2. High calorie, salt restricted diet.
3. Chorea: Reassurance, sedatives like clonazepam or chlorpromazine, and in severe cases haloperidol, sodium valproate or carbamazepine is used.

Table 1.4: Differentiation between dyspnoea of pulmonary and cardiac origin

Dyspnoea due to pulmonary aetiology	Dyspnoea due to cardiac aetiology
1. Wheezing or stridor	1. PND and orthopnoea
2. Cough with expectoration precedes dyspnoea	2. Dyspnoea precedes cough with expectoration
3. Pleuritic chest pain	3. Associated angina, syncope, palpitations; hypertension
4. Pyrexia	4. Rapid progression of symptoms
5. Cyanosis (++ or +++)	5. Little or no cyanosis (+)
6. Seasonal variation	6. Erect posture or squatting may relieve
7. Progression over many years	7. Oedema is an important sign
8. Response to oxygen and bronchodilators	8. Response to diuretics and digoxin
9. Absence of obvious cardiac disease	9. Physical signs of cardiac disease

4. Symptomatic treatment:
   a. Arthritis, arthralgia, fever: Aspirin (acetylsalicylic acid) in a dose of 80–100 mg/kg/day in children and 4–8 g/day in adults in 4–5 divided doses is started, and continued for 2 weeks. If symptoms subside, a lower dose of 60–70 mg/kg/day (in children) is continued for a further 2–4 weeks. Other NSAIDs like naproxen at a dose of 10–20 mg/kg/day gives good symptomatic response.
   b. Patient without carditis: Aspirin is preferred.
   c. Patient with carditis but without heart failure: Aspirin ± glucocorticoid (role of corticosteroids are doubtful in carditis but majority of cardiologists believe that they help in rapid resolution of heart failure). Prednisolone 1–2 mg/kg/day (maximum of 80 mg) is given orally for a period of 2 weeks and then tapered off over next 2 weeks.
   d. Patient with carditis and heart failure: Majority opine that corticosteroid is mandatory over and above aspirin.
   e. Antibiotics: Single injection of 1.2 million units of benzathine penicillin, IM (after proper skin test) is given to eradicate group A streptococcal infection, if present. Oral penicillin (penicillin V) 500 mg twice daily (250 mg twice daily for children ≤27 kg), orally for 10 days, or erythromycin 40 mg/kg/day, orally may be used for 10 days (in patient allergic to penicillin).
5. Secondary prevention of acute rheumatic fever: The mainstay of controlling rheumatic heart disease is secondary prevention. The dose of inj. benzathine penicillin is 1.2 million units, IM (after proper skin test) given at 4 weekly interval (in endemic areas and high-risk cases, the interval is 2–3 weekly); dose of penicillin in children (≤27 kg) is 0.6 million units. Instead oral penicillin V may be used 250 mg twice daily or oral erythromycin 250 mg twice daily (in penicillin allergy). Controversies exist regarding duration of therapy and the guideline is:
   a. Rheumatic fever without proven carditis: 5 years after the last attack or until the age of 21 years, whichever is longer.
   b. Rheumatic fever with carditis but having no residual valve damage: 10 years after the last attack or 21 years of age, whichever is longer.
   c. Rheumatic fever with carditis along with residual heart disease: 10 years after the last episode or until the age of 40, whichever is longer. Few clinicians prefer to give penicillin lifelong in this situation.
   d. If valvular surgery is done: Penicillin prophylaxis is continued lifelong.

- Salicylate toxicity is pain abdomen, acute gastric erosion, nausea, vomiting and tinnitus; aspirin increases the risk of Reye's syndrome in children. Rheumatic recurrences are less likely with increasing age. Prophylaxis against infective endocarditis is also needed in valve damage.

AORTIC INCOMPETENCE — CASE 4

Q. What is your diagnosis?

This is a case of valvular aortic incompetence (regurgitation or insufficiency) of rheumatic origin without congestive cardiac failure and the patient is in sinus rhythm at present.

Q. What is your case?

Try to build up the summary. Aortic incompetence (AI) remains asymptomatic for years or decades. Main symptoms of aortic incompetence are:
1. Palpitations.
2. Awareness of the heart beat, especially when lying on the left side; pulsatile or throbbing sensation.
3. Chest pain (angina pectoris, or due to pounding of heart against chest wall).
4. Dyspnoea (exertional).
5. Features of LVF or CCF (orthopnoea, PND, oedema, etc).

Q. Peripheral signs of AI (chronic):

Start from hands and go to the neck, head and then downwards to the legs systematically in search of peripheral signs. **Peripheral signs are produced as a result of 'wide pulse pressure'.** They are:
1. Visible capillary pulsation (Quincke's sign) at nail-beds or lip, i.e. blanching and quick refill:
   a. When light pressure is applied to the tip of fingers or nails, there is alternate flushing and pallor of the nail-bed, or
   b. When a glass slide is pressed on the everted lower lip, it produces alternate redness and blanching.
2. Prominent digital artery pulsation: Hold the flexed fingers of the patient with your fingers in flexed position to feel the pulsation.
3. High volume collapsing pulse or Corrigan's pulse (water-hammer pulse).
4. **Locomotor brachialis** (Fig. 1.16): Look at the medial side of lower arm (with semiflexed elbow) for 'tortuous and highly pulsatile' brachial artery. Tortuosity is the most important component of locomotor brachialis and thus, it is commonly found in arteriosclerosis (old age).

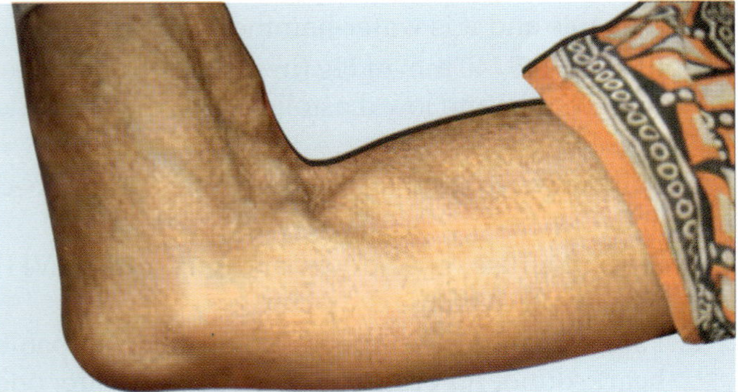

Fig. 1.16: **Locomotor brachialis** seen in a patient of thrombotic stroke

5. Blood pressure: Wide pulse pressure with high systolic BP and low diastolic BP (even Korotkoff sounds may continue upto 0 mm of Hg). Pulse pressure is usually >60 mm of Hg.
6. **Corrigan's sign:** Dancing carotids in neck.
7. de Musset's sign (named after a French poet): To and fro head-nodding synchronous with each carotid pulsation or heart beat (systolic extension of neck).
8. Visible pulsation in the suprasternal (jugular) notch.
9. 'Pistol shot' sound or Traube's sign: Booming sound produced after pressing the stethoscope over femoral artery.
10. Systolic murmur on compression of the femoral artery *proximally*.
11. Duroziez's murmur: Diastolic murmur on compression of the femoral artery *distally*.
12. **Hill's sign:** Increase in the femoral artery systolic BP >20 mm of Hg above the brachial artery systolic BP. In health, the systolic difference between two extremities remains within 20 mm of Hg. In severe AI, the difference is >60 mm of Hg. It is very important and specific sign of AI.

- **Pulsations in different areas in AI** are named after different clinicians. Pulsations in uvula, liver and enlarged spleen are respectively known as Muller's sign, Rosenbach's sign and Gerhardt's sign. Changes in pupil size with each cardiac systole is known as Landolfi's sign. Alternate flushing and blanching of forehead is known as Lighthouse sign, and pulsation of retinal artery is Becker's sign. Bozzolo sign is pulsatile nasal mucosa while Dennison sign reflects pulsatile cervix. *Duroziez's sign* is the combination of No. 10 and 11, and are appreciable after adjusting the pressure of chest piece of stethoscope over the femoral artery.

Q. Why do you say aortic incompetence?

It is a case of AI because there are presence of:

A. Symptoms (from the history): Palpitations, throbbing sensation all over the body, chest pain, dyspnoea for last 2 years. Past H/o rheumatic fever is also present.

B. Signs:

a. Pulse: 80/minute, regular, high volume, neither there is any inequality nor any delay, arterial wall is not thickened, all the peripheral pulses are 'nicely' palpable and it is water-hammer in type.
b. BP: Say, 145/40 mm of Hg (in supine position), i.e. high systolic and low diastolic BP. So, there is wide pulse pressure.
c. **All the peripheral signs are present** (described above).
d. Apex: Diffuse, goes down and outwards (LVH) with hyperdynamic character.
e. Palpation of the aortic area: No thrill, no palpable heart sound, no pulsation [though very rare, one may get a diastolic thrill (5%) in aortic area or in lower left sternal border].
f. Ausculation of the aortic area:
   S_1: Audible
   S_2 (A_2): Muffled (soft)
   S_3 or S_4: Not audible at present
   Murmur—High-pitched, soft blowing, early diastolic decrescendo murmur of grade III which is best audible in sitting and leaning forward position, in full expiration and with the diaphragm of stethoscope. The murmur is radiated towards the apex and is best heard at neoaortic area (left 3rd ICS).

- Occasionally, the murmur may radiate up to left axilla due to higher position of apex, and is known as *Cole-Cecil murmur*. Sometimes, S_3 may be heard.

g. Other areas of heart and lungs: Within normal limit.

- Add features of pulmonary hypertension, if present. Always examine the neck for thyroid enlargement in a patient with wide pulse pressure.

[h. Examination of respiratory system, GI tract and nervous system revealed no abnormality].

- AI remains asymptomatic for years after years, but once decompensated, patients start deteriorating rapidly.

Clinical Wisdom

In AI, search for the stigmata of Marfan's syndrome, ankylosing spondylitis or rheumatoid arthritis.

Q. Different types of murmur found in AI:

1. Classical early diastolic, soft blowing, high-pitched murmur in the aortic or neoaortic area.
2. Ejection systolic murmur of functional AS in the aortic or neoaortic area.
3. Austin Flint murmur: Mid-diastolic rumbling murmur (flow murmur) in the mitral area.

Q. How to assess the 'severity' of AI clinically?

Bedside assessment of severe AI is done by:

1. Presence of marked peripheral signs (i.e. wide pulse pressure).
2. Hill's sign of more than 60 mm of Hg (difference in systolic BP between lower and upper extremity 20–40 mm of Hg: Mild AI, 40–60 mm of Hg: Moderate AI, and >60 mm of Hg: Severe AI). Hill's sign is due to the phenomenon of recruitment of impulses.
3. Long duration of early diastolic decrescendo murmur.
4. Presence of Austin Flint murmur.
5. Pulsus bisferiens (read the section on 'Water-hammer pulse').
6. S_1: Soft S_2.

Q. Aetiology of chronic AI:

1. **Rheumatic** (80%).
2. Traumatic.
3. Infective endocarditis.

4. Bicuspid aortic valve.
5. Atherosclerotic.
6. Cystic medial necrosis.
7. Marfan's syndrome (look for tall stature).
8. Ankylosing spondylitis (look for stooped posture).
9. Rheumatoid arthritis (look for deformed fingers)
10. Reiter's syndrome (i.e. reactive arthritis).
11. Dissecting aneurysm of aorta.
12. Syphilitic (H/o exposure should be taken).

- First 4 causes are due to 'valve involvement' and others produce AI by 'ring dilatation' due to aortic root disease.

Q. Causes of acute AI:

Peripheral signs are absent in acutely developing AI. Acute AI develops from:
1. SBE.
2. Trauma to the chest.
3. Dissection of aorta.
4. Acute rheumatic fever (carditis or valvulitis).
5. Prosthetic valve dysfunction.

Q. Clinical features of 'acute AI':

1. Acutely ill and symptomatic (breathlessness, chest pain) patient.
2. 100% patients have acute left heart failure. It is a medical emergency and should be tackled duly.
3. Peripheral signs are absent (normal or low pulse pressure).
4. No cardiomegaly.
5. Diastolic thrill is present in majority of patients.
6. S_1: Soft to absent.
7. Short, soft, early diastolic murmur.

Q. AI with normal or low pulse pressure:

Normally AI patients have wide pulse pressure. The causes of low pulse pressure are:
1. Acutely developing AI (see above).
2. Associated with AS or tight MS.
3. AI with CCF.
4. AI associated with systemic hypertension.

Q. Is there any systolic murmur present in the aortic area in your case?

No, occasionally a harsh systolic murmur of 'functional' AS of grade II to V may be heard in the aortic area. This murmur may be transmitted towards carotids. This is caused by increased flow across the aortic valve and does not necessarily indicate an organic AS (for the difference between organic and functional AS, read the section on 'Aortic stenosis and aortic incompetence').

Q. Features of rheumatic AI:

1. Age: Young age group.
2. H/o rheumatic fever present in majority of patients.
3. Involvement of other valves: May be present.
4. Diastolic thrill: Usually absent.
5. A_2: May be diminished (soft) or absent.
6. Murmur: Best audible in left 3rd ICS (neoaortic area), blowing in character.
7. Peripheral signs: Present.

Q. Features of syphilitic AI (rarely seen nowadays):

1. Age: Older age group (>40 years).
2. H/o exposure to syphilis: Present.
3. Usually isolated lesion. Anginal pain is more common.
4. Diastolic thrill: May be present (commoner than rheumatic).
5. Right parasternal heave: Very often present.
6. A_2: Usually loud (tambour quality).
7. Murmur: Best audible along right sternal border (right 3rd ICS); ringing, cooing or musical.
8. Peripheral signs: More marked than rheumatic AI.
9. Austin Flint murmur: May be present.

- If the early diastolic murmur of AI is best audible along right sternal border, it suggest syphilis, Marfan's syndrome, dissecting aortic aneurysm or ankylosing spondylitis, and is due to dilatation of ascending aorta.
- In atherosclerotic AI, the A_2 is ringing in quality.

Q. Causes of pulsation at different areas:

A. Carotid pulsation:
1. Exertion, emotion and excitement.
2. Aortic incompetence (Corrigan's sign).
3. Hyperkinetic circulatory states like severe anaemia, thyrotoxicosis, pyrexia, pregnancy, etc.
4. Atherosclerosis.
5. Aortic aneurysm.
6. Kinked carotid artery (right > left).

B. Suprasternal (jugular) notch pulsation:
1. Hyperkinetic circulatory states like severe anaemia, thyrotoxicosis, pyrexia, pregnancy, etc.
2. Aortic incompetence.
3. Coarctation of aorta.
4. Unfolding of the arch of aorta (old age; commonly in patient with systemic hypertension).
5. Aneurysm of the arch of aorta.
6. High arch of aorta (congenital).
7. Abnormal thyroidea ima artery.

C. Pulsation over the pulmonary area:
1. Children (physiological).
2. Pulmonary hypertension (severe).
3. ASD.
4. PDA.
5. VSD.
6. Idiopathic dilatation of pulmonary artery.

D. Pulsation over the aortic area:
1. Dilatation of the ascending aorta due to aneurysm.
2. Chronic aortic incompetence.

E. Left parasternal pulsation:

1. RVH (due to any cause).
2. LAH (rare).
3. ASD (left parasternal lift).
4. Aortic aneurysm.

F. Right parastemal pulsation:

1. Dextrocardia.
2. Dextroversion (due to extracardiac cause, i.e. cause in lung, pleura, thoracic cage).
3. Aneurysm of the ascending aorta.
4. Right atrial hypertrophy due to any cause.

G. Epigastric pulsation (Fig. 1.17):

1. Excitement, especially in a thin person (normal aortic pulsation; physiological).
2. Right ventricular hypertrophy (RVH).
3. Transmission of aortic pulsation by any growth present in front of aorta like gastric carcinoma (pulsation disappears after adopting knee-elbow position)—i.e. transmitted pulsation.
4. Aneurysm of the abdominal aorta (expansile pulsation).
5. Transmitted hepatic pulsation in tricuspid incompetence.

H. Pulsation at the back:

1. Coarctation of aorta *(Suzman's sign).*
2. Pulmonary arteriovenous fistula.

I. Intercostal pulsation: Absent in health; present in ventricular aneurysm (RV or LV).

J. Juxta-apical: Ventricular aneurysm.

K. Apical: Normally in health, LVH or RVH.

- The epigastric pulsation is felt with the tip of the index finger inserted upwards and obliquely under the xiphoid process **(Fig. 1.17)**, or it is often better seen after tangential application of light.
- Parasternal pulsation is common in hyperdynamic circulation (e.g. pregnancy) and thin chest wall.

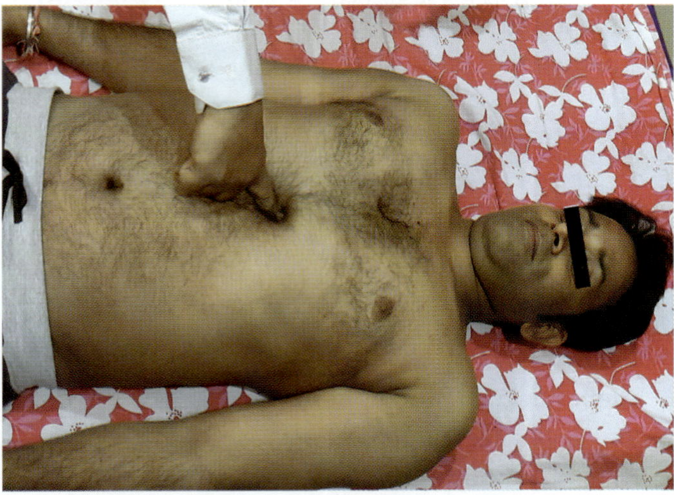

Fig. 1.17: Examination of **epigastric pulsation**

Q. Importance of joint involvement in CVS:

1. Acute rheumatic arthritis.
2. Rheumatoid arthritis, ankylosing spondylitis may be associated with AI or MI.
3. Arthralgia may be seen in valvular heart diseases complicated by SBE.

Q. Why the murmur of AI is early diastolic?

The leaking back of blood from the aorta to the left ventricle is greatest in early part of diastole for obvious reason (as pressure in the aorta is more than that of the left ventricle in early diastole). In the mid-diastole, no leak is possible as the pressure in the aorta and the left ventricle becomes equal.

Q. Differential diagnosis (D/D) of your case?

1. PDA, coronary arteriovenous fistula, ruptured sinus of Valsalva: Considered for wide pulse pressure; they produce continuous murmur.
2. Graham Steell murmur (rare): Considered for early diastolic murmur in pulmonary area; features of pulmonary hypertension are present without any peripheral sign of AI.

Q. Complications of AI:

1. Acute LVF.
2. Infective endocarditis.
3. Congestive cardiac failure.
4. Arrhythmias.
5. Heart block.
6. Angina pectoris (especially nocturnal).

- Angina is due to low diastolic BP compromising coronary artery perfusion pressure, and marked LVH.

Q. How do you like to investigate a case of AI?

1. X-ray chest (PA view):
   a. Cardiomegaly (LVH): A large heart is also known as Cor bovinum or bovine heart.
   b. Aortic root dilatation (prominent aortic knuckle).
   c. Aortic valve calcification (raises the possibility of concomitant AS).
2. ECG:
   a. LVH.
   b. Conduction defects.
3. Blood for (to detect active rheumatic carditis):
   a. TC and DC.
   b. ESR.
   c. ASO titre, and
   d. VDRL and Kahn test (for syphilis); ANF, rheumatoid factor, CRP to exclude connective tissue diseases.
4. Echocardiography (M-mode and 2-D): Diagnosis, assessing severity and possible cause of lesion.
5. Cardiac catheterisation: To assess for coronary artery disease in patients requiring surgery.
6. Colour doppler study: Most sensitive for detecting mild AI and pressure gradient in AI.

Q. How will you treat this case?

1. Medical management: As in MS; underlying cause, e.g. infective endocarditis or syphilitic aortitis needs to be treated. Chronic AI with significant volume overload needs vasodilator therapy with hydralazine, nitrates or ACE inhibitors.
2. Surgical: Aortic valve replacement (prosthesis), or aortic valve repair by valvuloplasty or annuloplasty; ideal time of operation is selected after haemodynamic or echocardiographic evidence of left ventricular dysfunction but before the development of significant symptoms.

Clinical Wisdom

Diastolic thrill in the aortic area is rare in AI. If really a diastolic thrill is present, it is better to think of syphilitic origin, ruptured sinus of Valsalve, or AI developed from dissecting aneurysm.

Q. What is 'base of the heart'?

'Base of the heart' includes aortic and pulmonary area. For better understanding, *see* page 409.

Q. Common causes of palpitations:

Palpitations are "abnormal unpleasant awareness of one's own heartbeat". Palpitations may be transient or persistent. Patients describe it as racing heart or pounding heart.

A. Cardiac:

1. AI, MI, TI, MS.
2. ASD, VSD, PDA.
3. Paroxysmal atrial tachycardia.
4. Atrial fibrillation.
5. Ventricular ectopics.
6. Bradyarrhythmias.

B. Non-cardiac:

1. Hyperkinetic circulatory states like severe anaemia, thyrotoxicosis, arteriovenous shunt, anxiety, unaccustomed exertion, pyrexia, Paget's disease.
2. Drug-induced, e.g. sympathomimetics (e.g. salbutamol, vasodilators (e.g. nifedipine), atropine.
3. Non-organic diseases, e.g. excessive smoking, exercise, anxiety states, cardiac neurosis, hysteria.
4. Miscellaneous: Hypoglycaemia, pheochromocytoma, menopause.

Clinical Wisdom

All valvular heart diseases described so far are chronic rheumatic heart diseases (RHD).

MITRAL STENOSIS AND MITRAL INCOMPETENCE: CASE 5

Q. What is your diagnosis?

This is a case of organic mitral incompetence (regurgitation or insufficiency) and mitral stenosis of rheumatic origin with pulmonary hypertension but without any evidence of congestive cardiac failure or arrhythmia at present (start with the dominant lesion).

Clinical Wisdom

Never use the term 'double mitral' lesion or MS with MI (abbreviations) in the examination. A combined lesion is difficult to be diagnosed correctly by an undergraduate student. But if one is meticulous and to the point in the clinical examination, it is not very difficult to diagnose the lesion. In a patient with MS and MI, both may be organic or the MS may be functional, if present with gross MI. When both are organic lesions, it is the duty of a student to determine the predominant (haemodynamically significant) one.

Q. Palpatory findings in the apical area in this patient:

1. Site of the apex beat is in left 6th ICS, 1/2" outside the left MCL (LVH due to MI).
2. Character: Hyperdynamic (due to MI).
3. Palpable S_1: Absent.
4. Thrill: Systolic thrill, best felt in left lateral position with full expiration.

   Here, all the features point towards predominant MI.

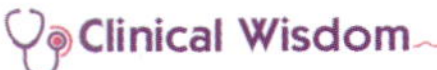

Clinical Wisdom

Remember, diastolic thrill in MS is more common than systolic thrill in MI (in the mitral area).

If MS is the predominant lesion, the findings in the apical area would be:

1. Site: Left 5th ICS, 1/2" outside the left MCL (RVH).
2. Character: Tapping.
3. Palpable S_1: Present.
4. Thrill: Diastolic thrill, best felt in left lateral position with full expiration.

Q. Is pulmonary hypertension present here?

Yes. In a combined lesion of MS and MI, pulmonary hypertension is usually present though it depends mainly on the duration of the disease.

- MS>MI → commonly dyspnoea on exertion → orthopnoea → PND → haemoptysis; palpitations in AF.
- MI>MS → commonly palpitations → dyspnoea on exertion → orthopnoea → PND.

Q. What are the evidences of MI present here?

Read the differentiation **(Table 1.5)** carefully and give your answer accordingly.

Q. Why this is MI murmur, not TI?

Describe the classical MI murmur. It is best heard over the mitral area with typical radiation (i.e. towards the left axilla and inferior angle of left scapula), which increases with expiration. The TI murmur is best heard in lower left parasternal area, localised and increases with inspiration **(Carvallo's sign)**.

Table 1.5: Determination of dominant lesion in combined MS and MI

Features	MS>MI	MI>MS
A. Symptoms:		
Haemoptysis, H/o PND, systemic embolisation, palpitations, CCF, pulmonary congestion, chest pain	+++	+
B. Signs:		
1. Pulse	Low volume, features of atrial fibrillation are more common	Within normal limit (not low volume); may be 'collapsing'
2. BP	Low systolic BP	Within normal limit
3. Apex	Already described	Already described
4. Left parasternal heave	+++	+
5. S_1	Short, sharp and accentuated (snapping)	Soft or muffled
6. Opening snap	**Usual and the lesion is organic**	OS is absent in a dominant MI
7. S_3	Absent	**Present; presence of S_3 signifies dominant and gross MI**
8. Diastolic murmur	Classical murmur of MS	Short mid-diastolic flow murmur without presystolic accentuation (due to functional MS)
9. Systolic murmur	Pansystolic blowing murmur of MI without radiation	Classical pansystolic murmur of MI with radiation
C. Investigations:		
1. Chest X-ray (PA view)	LAH + RVH	LVH + LAH
2. ECG	See the section on 'MS' (LVH is not present)	See the section on 'MI' (LVH is usually present)
3. Echocardiography	Final diagnosis with certainty (thick, immobile cusps with diminished rate of diastolic filling)	Final diagnosis with certainty (LA enlargement with hyperdynamic LV)

Q. Conditions associated with S_3 (third heart sound):

S_3 signifies diastolic overload of the ventricles. It occurs during the first rapid filling phase of cardiac cycle (in ventricular diastole). LV S_3 signifies LVF, while RV S_3 indicates RVF. It is a ventricular distension sound and the clinical associations are:

1. Healthy young adults (<40 years) and children, pregnancy, athletes.
2. Heart failure (LVF or RVF).
3. Chronic MI, TI, AI.
4. Hyperkinetic circulation like severe anaemia, thyrotoxicosis, etc.
5. ASD, VSD or PDA; dilated cardiomyopathy.

Q. Conditions associated with S_4 (fourth heart sound):

It signifies systolic overload of the ventricles. It occurs during the last rapid filling phase of cardiac cycle (in ventricular diastole) which also coincides with the atrial systole. Presence of S_4 is always pathological. It is an atrial contraction sound and the clinical associations are:

1. Ischaemic heart disease, especially acute myocardial infarction.
2. Aortic stenosis.
3. Systemic hypertension.
4. Rarely, in normal individuals (above 60 years).
5. Hypertrophic cardiomyopathy.

Q. How to auscultate for S_3 or S_4?

S_3 or S_4 is best heard at the **apex** with the **bell** of stethoscope placed lightly. Sometimes, they are best heard with the patient turned to **left lateral** position; often they are better felt than heard. They are low-pitched sounds.

Left-sided S_3 (LVF) is best audible at the apex during expiration while the right-sided S_3 (RVF) is best heard at the lower left sternal border during inspiration.

- Multiple heart sounds are characteristic of Ebstein's anomaly—Split S_1, split S_2, opening snap and S_4.

Q. Can you accentuate gallop sounds?

Elevate both lower limbs at 60° → maintain the position for 30 seconds → cardiac output ↑→ accentuation of gallop sounds. In this way a latent S_3 can be made audible. Isometric handgrip also accentuate gallop.

Q. How and where the "bell" of stethoscope is used?

During the use of the bell, it should be placed very lightly over the skin. More pressure will tighten the skin and smother the low-frequency sounds. It is made for listening low-pitched sounds (80–150 Hz) like:

1. Murmur of MS and TS.
2. S_3 or S_4.
3. Foetal heart sounds.
4. Venous hum.

Clinical Wisdom

'Diaphragm' of stethoscope is used for high-frequency sounds (>300 Hz) like S_1, S_2, all murmurs except MS and TS, opening snap, pericardial knock, etc. Bruits are better picked up by bell.

Q. What is dynamic auscultation (Table 1.6)?

Circulatory dynamics can be altered by application of certain body manoeuvres (respiration, isometric

Table 1.6: Dynamic manoeuvres in differentiation of murmurs

Manoeuvres	Increased	Decreased
1. Isometric handgrip (↑ afterload)	AI, MI, VSD	HOCM, MVPS
2. Valsalva monoevure (↓ venous return)	HOCM, MVPS	All organic murmurs except HOCM and MVPS
3. Squatting (↑ venous return and ↑ peripheral resistance)	AS, AI, MI, MS	HOCM, MVPS
4. Standing (↓ venous return)	HOCM, MVPS	AS, MI
5. Both leg raising (↑ venous return)	All right-sided murmur	HOCM, MVPS
6. Inspiration (↑ venous return)	All right-sided murmur	Pulmonary ejection click
7. Expiration (↑ cardiac output of left heart)	All left-sided murmur	—
8. Amyl nitrite (↓ arterial pressure and ↑ cardiac output)	HOCM, AS, MVPS	AI, MI

- HOCM (hypertrophic obstructive cardiomyopathy), MVPS (mitral valve prolapse syndrome).

handgrip, Valsalva manoeuvre, leg raising, etc.) and administering certain vasoactive substances (amyl nitrite, phenylephrine), and auscultation of these events in the CVS is known as dynamic auscultation.

Q. Cardinal points to diagnose dominant lesion (MS + MI):

1. History.
2. Pulse.
3. Apex (LVH or RVH, hyperdynamic or tapping).
4. S_1 (loud or muffled).
5. S_3 (S_3 signifies significant MI).
6. Opening snap (always signifies dominant MS).
7. Mid-diastolic rumbling murmur with presystolic accentuation signifies predominant MS; only short mid-diastolic murmur points towards a dominant MI.

Q. D/D of opening snap (Table 1.7):

1. Splitting of S_2.
2. S_3, and
3. Pericardial knock.

Q. Mitral diastolic murmur: Organic or functional?

Functional MS (from gross MI) will have the following features:

1. Pulse: Normal volume.
2. Diastolic thrill in mitral area: Absent; rather a systolic thrill of MI may be present.
3. S_1: Not very loud.
4. Presystolic accentuation (of the murmur) is absent.
5. Opening snap—absent; rather S_3 is heard due to significant MI.
6. Features of LVH.

Q. What is the aetiology of your case?

Rheumatic; an organic MS with MI is virtually always from chronic rheumatic heart disease (RHD).

Q. How will you manage this case?

1. Prophylaxis against rheumatic recurrence.
2. Mitral valve replacement in severe cases (prosthesis).
3. Treatment of complications:
   a. Heart failure.
   b. SBE.
   c. Atrial fibrillation.
   d. Embolic manifestations.

AORTIC STENOSIS AND AORTIC INCOMPETENCE: CASE 6

Q. What is your diagnosis?

This is a case of organic aortic incompetence (regurgitation or insufficiency) and aortic stenosis of rheumatic origin without any evidence of congestive cardiac failure and the patient is in sinus rhythm at present (start with the dominant lesion).

Table 1.7: Differentiation between opening snap and S_3

Features	Opening snap	S_3 (LV)
1. Where found	MS	Heart failure or chronic MI
2. Best audible	At lower left parasternal region; with the diaphragm of stethoscope on standing	At apex; with the bell of stethoscope in left lateral position
3. Pitch	High-pitched	Low-pitched
4. Palpability	Not palpable	May be palpable
5. Timing	0.04–0.12 seconds after A_2 (early part of diastole)	0.14–0.16 seconds after A_2 (mid-diastole)
6. Effect of standing	S_2–OS gap widens	S_2–S_3 gap unchanged
7. After treating heart failure	OS becomes louder	S_3 vanishes

Clinical Wisdom

Do not use the term 'double aortic' lesion or AS with AI (abbreviations) in the examination. Often a functional systolic murmur is heard in a patient with severe AI. Thus, one has to determine whether the AS is organic or functional. Lastly, in a combined AS with AI, dominant lesion (haemodynamically significant) should be diagnosed. It is worthwhile to remember that combined AS with AI is usually of rheumatic in origin.

Q. Cardinal points to diagnose dominant lesion (AS + AI) (Table 1.8):

1. History: Angina and syncope are seen more in AS. Palpitations and dyspnoea are common in AI.
2. Pulse.
3. BP.
4. Apex.
5. S_3 or S_4.
6. Ejection click.
7. Peripheral signs of AI (best indicator of severity of AI lesion).

Q. Aortic stenosis murmur: Organic or functional?

1. History: Patients with organic AS will give H/o angina and/or syncope.
2. Pulse: Low volume, often anacrotic in nature (in organic AS).
3. BP: Systolic decapitation of BP in organic lesion.
4. Apex: Heaving in organic lesion.
5. Systolic thrill in aortic area: Present in organic lesion (very rarely, functional AS may give rise to systolic thrill).
6. Ejection click: Always in favour of valvular (organic) AS.

- In a functional AS, peripheral signs of AI will be very prominent like presence of water-hammer pulse, dancing carotids, etc. Thus in a functional AS, pulse is of high volume.

Q. Expected BP in patients where AS>AI and AI>AS:

If AS>AI—the approximate BP will be 90/65 mm of Hg and if AI > AS—the approximate BP will be 130/20 mm of Hg. So, measurement of BP should be done carefully in all CVS patients.

Q. What is aortic sclerosis murmur?

In aged persons suffering from atherosclerosis with or without hypertension, there is fibrosis, thickening and calcification of bases of the aortic valve cusps. These may give rise to harsh, ejection systolic murmur up to grade IV in some cases. Differentiate aortic sclerosis from aortic stenosis by:

a. No H/o syncope, angina or heart failure.
b. Normal pulse volume.
c. Absence of thrill.
d. No shifting of apex beat.
e. Normal A_2.

Table 1.8: Determination of dominant lesion in combined AS and AI

Features	AS>AI	AI > AS
A. Symptoms:		
1. Effort angina, dysponea on effort, effort syncope, black-out, etc.	+++	+ (chest pain, dyspnoea may occur)
2. Palpitations, throbbing	+ (palpitations)	+++
B. Signs:		
1. Pulse	Low volume. Pulsus bisferiens (tidal > percussion wave)	High volume collapsing pulse; pulsus bisferiens (percussion > tidal wave)
2. BP	Low systolic BP. Pulse pressure is low	Wide pulse pressure due to high systolic and low diastolic BP
3. Peripheral signs of AI	±	+++
4. Apex	Heaving, apex may be in normal position	Hyperdynamic, down and outwards (LVH)
5. Thrill	Always systolic; palpated on aortic area and on carotids	a. Rarely present; systolic thrill due to functional AS b. Very rarely diastolic thrill may be palpable along the left sternal border
6. S_3	Absent	May be present
7. S_4	May be present	Absent
8. Ejection click	Present in mild-to-moderate AS	Rare; sometimes present in severe AI
9. Diastolic murmur	Very short duration AI murmur	Classical mumur of AI
10. Systolic murmur	Classical murmur of AS	Functional midsystolic ejection murmur may be audible
C. Investigations:		
1. Chest X-ray (PA view)	Read the section on 'AS'	Read the section on 'AI'
2. ECG	Read the section on 'AS'	Read the section on 'AI'
3. Echocardiography	Final diagnosis with certainty	Final diagnosis with certainty

f. Localised (aortic area) murmur.
g. Often by the features of atherosclerosis like thick peripheral arteries, kinked carotids, locomotor brachialis, suprasternal pulsation, xanthelasma (deposition of lipids) (Fig. 1.18) around the eyes. Occasionally, the calcification becomes excessive and thus, produces severe aortic valve obstruction. This is known as 'calcific aortic stenosis' (*see* aetiology of 'AS' in page 30).

- Aortic sclerosis and mitral valve prolapse syndrome (MVPS) are haemodynamically stable cardiac lesions.

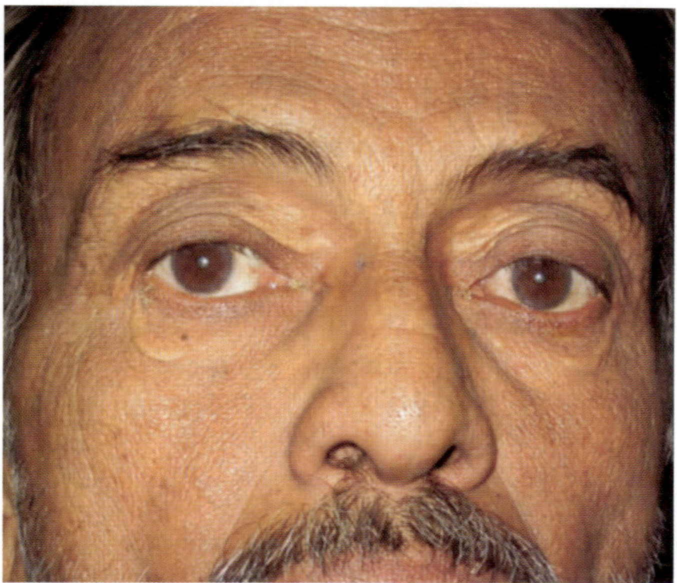

Fig. 1.18: **Xanthelasma** (soft, yellowish, plaque-like lesion) around the eyes and cataract are seen in a patient with ischaemic heart disease; xanthelasma is regarded as a physical sign of underlying hyperlipidaemia

Q. What is the possible aetiology of your case?

Rheumatic. Sometimes, the bicuspid aortic valve (congenital) produces features of combined AS and AI though the AI lesion is insignificant (always AS>AI). Bicuspid aortic valve is the most common congenital malformation of the heart though it may go undetected in early life.

Q. Signs of aortic arch aneurysm:

Aneurysm of aorta is an abnormal dilatation of aorta involving all three layers of aortic wall. The features are:

1. Swelling in the anterior chest wall.
2. Pulsation in the upper part of anterior chest wall.
3. Suprasternal pulsation.
4. Difference between right and left radial pulses (radio-radial delay) and blood pressure.
5. Left 2nd ICS is dull on percussion.
6. Loud tambour like A_2; ejection click.
7. Systolic murmur in the aortic area.
8. **'Tracheal tug'** (Fig. 1.19): It is the downward pull of trachea synchronous with each cardiac systole.

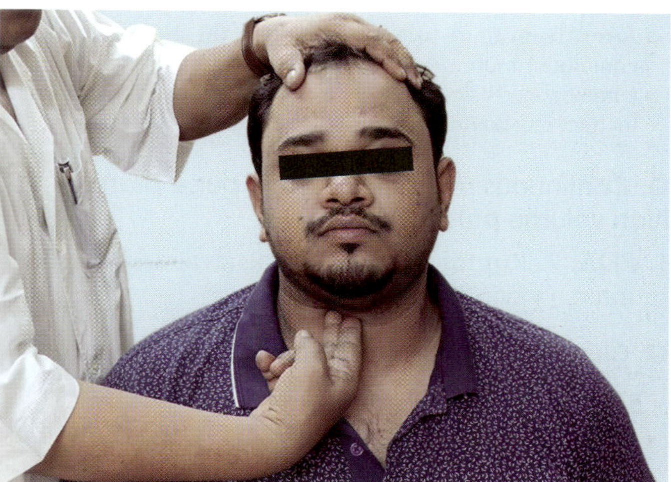

Fig. 1.19: Eliciting **tracheal tug**

Stand behind the erect (upright) patient. Raise the chin, slightly stretch the neck backwards, and apply upward pressure on the trachea with two fingers placed on the lower border of cricoid cartilage. A downward traction is felt on the trachea (*Oliver's sign*). This sign is also seen in COPD patients when the downward tracheal pull is felt on each inspiration (*Campbell's sign*).

Q. Differential diagnosis (D/D) of your case:

Actually, a patient with AS and AI having systolic and diastolic murmur in the aortic area mimic 'continuous murmur'. The common causes of **continuous murmur** (begins in systole and extends through second heart sound into part or whole of diastole) are:

1. Patent ductus arteriosus (PDA, 'Train in the tunnel' murmur, machinery murmur, Gibson's murmur): Commonly found in female patients with water-hammer pulse and continuous murmur with late systolic accentuation, best audible in left infraclavicular area and lett 2nd ICS. Thrill may be systolic or systolo-diastolic.
2. Ruptured sinus of Valsalva: Dramatic onset of chest pain with continuous murmur along the left sternal border.
3. Coronary arteriovenous fistula: Along left sternal edge, superficial, harsh.
4. Pulmonary arteriovenous fistula: Along left 2nd ICS.
5. Aortopulmonary window: Along left 3rd ICS.
6. Rarely, in coarctation of aorta (better auscultated at the back).
7. Mammary souffle (in pregnancy): Best heard over the mammary area, and 2nd to 4th ICS.
8. Venous hum at root of the neck (Devil's murmur): Actually it is a D/D of continuous murmur.
9. VSD with AI, AS with AI, and MS with MI mimic continuous murmur.
10. Anomalous origin of left coronary artery from pulmonary artery.
11. After Blalock-Taussig shunt operation done in Fallot's tetralogy: In upper sternal area.

- Arteriovenous fistula anywhere in the body produces continuous murmur.
- Lutembacher's syndrome, branch pulmonary artery stenosis, thyrotoxicosis and Paget's disease are other causes.

Q. Continuous murmur with high pulse pressure (i.e. high volume pulse):

1. PDA, 2. Ruptured sinus of Valsalva, and 3. Aorto-pulmonary window.

Q. Clues to diagnose multivalvular lesions:

It needs experience but one may follow this format:

1. Mild or moderate AI is frequently missed. Carefully listen to the aortic and then the neoaortic area (Erb's point) in sitting posture of the patient, in full expiration and with the diaphragm of stethoscope, in the search of an early diastolic murmur. For confirmation, measure the BP to record the pulse pressure.
2. Short mid-diastolic murmur of MS is often missed. Thus, it is a dictum to listen the mitral area with the bell of stethoscope, in left lateral position and with full expiration. For corroboration, carefully auscultate for loudness of S_1.
3. Murmur of insignificant MS may be pronounced after little exercise, if the condition of the patient permits (e.g. in the absence of heart failure).
4. Carefully palpate the brachial and carotid arteries. Actually, the commonest cause of pulsus bisferiens is combined lesion of AS and AI. If you get pulsus bisferiens in your patient, you are sure about the presence of two valvular heart diseases (rarely, it is seen in isolated AI).

Q. Causes of LVF (or pulmonary oedema):

1. Systemic hypertension.
2. IHD, i.e. acute myocardial infarction.
3. AI, AS, MI.
4. Cardiomyopathy.
5. Coarctation of aorta.
6. Myocarditis.
7. Severe anaemia.
8. VSD, PDA.
9. Rapid and excess fluid infusion or blood transfusion.

Q. Causes of RVF (CCF):

1. Secondary to left-sided heart failure (LVF/LAF).
2. COPD.
3. Pulmonary hypertension due to any cause.
4. ASD, VSD or PDA.
5. Pulmonary stenosis or incompetence.
6. Pulmonary thromboembolism.
7. Cardiomyopathy.
8. Myocarditis.
9. Right ventricular myocardial infarction.
10. Tricuspid incompetence.

Q. Causes of LAF:

1. Mitral stenosis.
2. Left atrial myxoma.
3. Ball valve thrombus in the left atrium.
4. Mitral atresia (rare).

Q. Causes or RAF:

1. Tricuspid stenosis.
2. Secondary to RVF.
3. Right atrial myxoma (very rare).

- **Bernheim effect:** It is the RV pressure change resulting from LVH without developing pulmonary hypertension. Actually, interventricular septum hypertrophies from LVH (the septum bulges within RV) and produces obstruction to right ventricular outflow (i.e. decreased RV compliance) and thus, manifests as prominent a-wave in the neck vein without developing RVH or RVF, while lungs are clear on auscultation. This is also observed in HOCM.
- Commonest cause of RVF is LVF.

Q. Causes of biventricular failure:

1. RVF following chronic left-sided heart failure.
2. Hyperkinetic circulation, e.g. severe anaemia, thyrotoxicosis, arteriovenous shunts.
3. Ischaemic heart disease (e.g. AMI).
4. Myocarditis: Viral, rheumatic, diphtheritic, etc.
5. Dilated cardiomyopathy.
6. Patients with systemic hypertension and pulmonary hypertension (commonly from COPD).
7. Multiple valvular heart disease.

Q. High output and low output heart failure:

A. High output failure: There is no lesion in the heart and the cardiac output is higher than normal. The causes are:
   1. Thyrotoxicosis.
   2. Severe anaemia.
   3. Arteriovenous fistula.
   4. Pregnancy.
   5. Chronic cor pulmonale.
   6. Cirrhosis of liver.
   7. Paget's disease.
   8. Beriberi.

B. Low output failure: Commonly there is a lesion in the heart and the cardiac output is lower than normal. The causes are:
   1. MS, MI, AS, AI.
   2. Ischaemic heart disease (IHD).
   3. Myocarditis.
   4. Cardiomyopathies.
   5. Systemic hypertension.
   6. VSD, PDA, ASD.
   7. Infective endocarditis.
   8. Pericardial effusion.

Q. Causes of sudden cardiac (heart) failure:

1. Acute myocardial infarction.
2. Malignant or accelerated hypertension.
3. Dissection of aorta.
4. Massive pulmonary thromboembolism.
5. Arrhythmias (e.g. ventricular fibrillation).
6. Circulatory overload (fluid infusion or blood transfusion, severe anaemia).
7. Myocarditis.
8. Valvular heart diseases.
9. Subacute bacterial endocarditis.

Q. Accelerated and malignant hypertension:

A. Accelerated hypertension: Significant recent and rapid increase in BP level associated with evidence of vascular damage on fundoscopic examination but **without papilloedema**.

B. Malignant hypertension: Severe accelerated hypertension with diastolic BP> 140 mm of Hg with haemorrhage, exudate and **papilloedema** found on fundoscopic examination, and is often associated with one or more of the following:
   a. Rapidly deteriorating renal function (oliguria).
   b. Cardiac decompensation (acute LVF).
   c. Central nervous system manifestations, e.g. hypertensive encephalopathy (severe headache, vomiting, convulsions, coma).

It is papilloedema, and not the diastolic BP—which is important here. This rare complication of hypertension is associated with accelerated microvascular damage with fibrinoid necrosis, and intravascular thrombosis. If untreated, death may occur due to complications.

Q. Management of multivalvular heart diseases:

Treatment for complications like CCF, embolic manifestations, and prophylaxis aginst SBE and rheumatic fever is done.

1. Mild to moderate: Follow-up. Severe AS with AI is managed by aortic valve replacement (prothesis).
2. MS with AI: First the AI is dealt with and next the MS. If MS is operated before AI, there will be left ventricular overload (blood coming from LA and aorta both) and ultimately LVF occurs. Actually, in practice both the operations are done simultaneously.
3. MS with AS: MS protects the heart from failure. First deal with AS and then MS.

INFECTIVE ENDOCARDITIS — CASE 7

Q. What is your diagnosis?

This is a patient of rheumatic mitral incompetence (MI) complicated by subacute bacterial endocarditis (SBE) and without any heart failure or dysrhythmia at present.

Q. Reasons behind your diagnosis:

A. Symptoms (from the history): Fever with chills present persistently with diaphoresis, arthralgia, lassitude, anorexia, pain in the loin, etc; over and above dyspnoea, fatigue, chest discomfort and palpitations due to MI.

B. Signs:

1. Anaemia: Severe, with a peculiar pallor (cafe-au-lait pallor).
2. Temperature (oral): Elevated (101°F) with chill and rigor; toxic look.
3. Clubbing: Present (may be painful).
4. Pulse: Tachycardia, regular in rhythm (describe all points).
5. Petechiae, Osler's node and splinter haemorrhage: Present.
6. Pansystolic murmur (due to pre-existent MI) with a musical quality—'Seagull murmur'. There may be change in the pre-existent murmur or appearance of a new diastolic murmur.
7. Mild, tender splenomegaly (30–40%) with occasional splenic rub.
8. Renal angle is tender.
9. Arthralgia or arthritis.
10. Ophthalmoscopy: Roth spots in <5% cases.

Q. Hands in SBE (Fig. 1.20):

Meticulous hand examination at the bedside often gives a clue to diagnosis of SBE.

1. Clubbing (10%). It takes 3–6 weeks to develop.
2. Pallor (due to anaemia).
3. Osler's node (15%): Painful and tender papule about the size of pinhead to pea, and is seen in the *pulp of fingers*, toes and palms (due to septic embolism or arteritis). The nodes usually last for 1–5 days.
4. Splinter haemorrhage (10%, also known as Horder's line): Linear longitudinal haemorrhage under the nail (other causes of splinter haemorrhage are trauma, trichinosis, leukaemia, scurvy, psoriasis, rheumatoid arthritis, systemic vasculitis).
5. Janeway's spot: Large, non-tender maculopapular lesion in *palms* (and soles).
6. Temperature: Elevated.
7. Petechiae (40–50%) may be found in dorsum of hands.
8. Infarction or gangrene of the fingers due to embolism rarely.
9. Nail-fold thrombi (due to embolisation).
10. Painful finger tips, loss of pulses (embolic manifestation).

- 3, 4, 5, 7, Roth spots, nephritis and positive rheumatoid factor are immunological phenomenon.
- Features of septic embolisation: 3, 4, 5, 7–10, painful splenomegaly, CNS and renal manifestations.
- Though initially thought to be an exclusive manifestation of SBE, Roth spots are also non-specific sign of blood dyscrasias (e.g. acute leukaemias) and anaemia (e.g. aplastic anaemia).

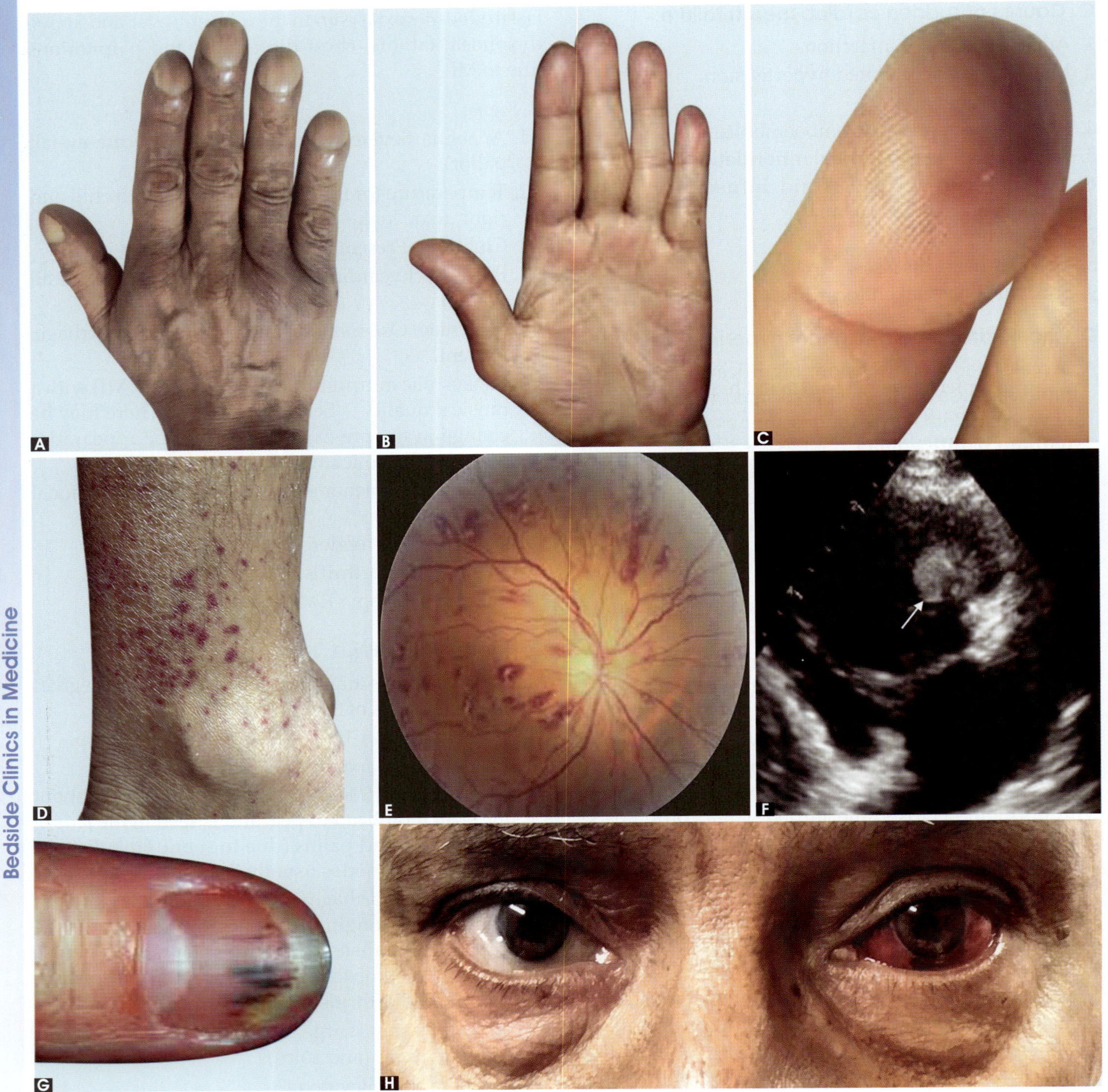

Fig. 1.20: Different stigmata **(or signs) of infective endocarditis**: A. Clubbing; B. Janeway's lesions; C. Osler's node; D. Petechial rashes; E. Roth spots; F. Vegetation seen in echocardiography; G. Splinter haemorrhage; H. Subconjunctival haemorrhage

Q. D/D you like to consider in your patient (SBE-mimickers):

The features like unexplained fever, cardiac murmur and embolic phenomenon may be present in:

1. Acute rheumatic fever.
2. Atrial myxoma (left).
3. Marantic endocarditis.
4. Systemic lupus erythematosus.
5. Anticardiolipin antibody syndrome.
6. Different (selective) causes of PUO.

Q. The clinical findings in different systems in SBE:

Virtually all the systems are affected in SBE like:

1. General: Pyrexia, pallor, malaise, anorexia, diaphoresis, weight loss.
2. CVS: Breathlessness, pain chest, palpitations, tachycardia, changing of pre-existent murmur or appearance of new murmur, CCF and conduction defects.
3. Kidneys: Haematuria (due to autoimmune nephritis or renal infarction), glomerulonephritis, loin pain due to embolic renal infarction, tender renal angle.

4. Lungs: Haemoptysis, chest pain, pleural rub (embolic infarction of lung).
5. Nervous system: Headache, meningitis, embolic stroke, convulsions, intracranial haemorrhage due to ruptured mycotic aneurysm, encephalopathy.
6. Blood vessels: Cold periphery due to loss of pulses as a result of embolisation.
7. Skin and mucous membrane: Petechiae, purpura, subungual haemorrhage.
8. Hands: Described above.
9. Eyes (Fig. 1.20): Red eyes, sudden blindness, subconjunctival haemorrhage, Roth spots.
10. Haematopoietic: Fatigability, anaemia, leucocytosis, thrombocytopenia, ↑ ESR and ↑ CRP.
11. Spleen: Splenomegaly, pain in left hypochondrium, splenic rub (due to splenic infarction).
12. Bowel: Pain abdomen, mesenteric artery embolism, bowel infarction.

- Read modified Duke criteria for the clinical diagnosis and NICE (National Institute for Health and Care Excellence) guidelines for prophylaxis of infective endocarditis from any standard textbook.

Q. How to establish the diagnosis of SBE?

1. Blood:
   a. Anaemia (normocytic-normochromic).
   b. Leucocytosis (neutrophilia).
   c. Thrombocytopenia.
   d. Raised ESR and high C-reactive protein (CRP).
   e. Blood biochemistry: Urea, creatinine, bilirubin and alkaline phosphatase levels may be elevated.
   f. Immunoglobulins and complements: ↑ Serum immunoglobulins, ↑ circulating immune complexes and ↓ complement levels are characteristic.
   g. Repeated blood culture (typical organism for infective endocarditis are diagnosed from either of two seperate blood cultures drawn 12 hours apart which detect bacteraemia in 90% culture-positive cases; or detected from all of 3, or majority of 4 or more seperate blood cultures done, with the first and last blood cultures obtained at least 1 hour apart. Blood is drawn under aseptic technique from different venepuncture sites; both aerobic and anaerobic, and rarely fungal cultures are done). At least 10–20 mL blood is taken at a time which is not related to height of temperature. An indwelling IV line should not be used for collection of blood. *Streptococcus viridans is the commonest pathogen in SBE. Positive blood culture gives the definite diagnosis of SBE*. Presumptive antibiotic therapy should be started immediately after obtaining the blood culture samples.
2. Urine:
   a. Microscopic haematuria (frank haematuria is rare).
   b. Mild proteinuria.
3. Chest X-ray: Cardiac failure, cardiomegaly.
4. Electrocardiography (ECG): Sinus tachycardia, prolonged PR interval, AV block (if septum is involved).
5. Echocardiography (2-D): To assess valve damage, identification of vegetations (small/sessile polypoidal), progress of vegetations, and abscess detection:
   a. Demonstration of parent disease (e.g. MI here) with chamber dilatation.
   b. Detection of vegetations (>2 mm by transthoracic echo and <2 mm by transoesophageal echo).
6. Bone marrow culture and serological study for *Candida, Histoplasma* and *Brucella* may be helpful in culture-negative cases.

- Positive past H/o recent dental extraction, genitourinary instrumentation or IV drug abuse is important in diagnosis of SBE.
- **'Vegetations'** (the basic lesions in SBE) are solid mass made up of platelet, fibrin and organism, and grow at the site of endothelial damage in endocardium or valve, which may ultimately give rise to embolism.

Q. Features in the nervous system (in SBE):

They are due to embolism or mycotic aneurysm. The features are:

1. Toxic psychosis, meningitis, metastatic brain abscess.
2. Convulsions, hemiplegia, intracranial haemorrhage due to haemorrhagic infarcts, subarachnoid haemorrhage (mycotic aneurysm), coma.
3. Roth spots: Yellowish, elliptical, *flame-shaped haemorrhage with a pale centre* present in the retina and is found in ophthalmoscopy. This is due to deposition of circulating immune complex (other causes of Roth spots are aplastic anaemia, leukaemia, scurvy, dysproteinaemia and HIV retinopathy).

Clinical Wisdom

Fundoscopy is essential in CVS for SBE (Roth spots), systemic hypertension (retinal haemorrhage, papilloedema), SVC syndrome (papilloedema) and AI (pulsation of retinal artery).

Q. Right-sided endocarditis:

Right-sided endocarditis has some specific characteristics like:

1. *Commonest organism is Staphylococcus aureus.*
2. Affects mainly the tricuspid valve and rarely the pulmonary valve.
3. Common in drug addicts or patients receiving central venous catheters.
4. Prognosis is relatively better.
5. Systemic embolisation is rare though pulmonary infection and infarction are not uncommon.
6. Clinical features: Cough, pleurisy, chest pain, haemoptysis and recurrent pulmonary lesions.

- Cardiac signs may be absent in right-sided endocarditis.

Q. Clinical spectrum of infective endocarditis:

It is of two types: acute and subacute.

1. Acute bacterial endocarditis: See below (next question).
2. Subacute bacterial endocarditis (SBE): Caused by less virulent organisms with an indolent course. Cardiac damage occurs slowly, and rarely metastasize unless complicated by a major embolic event. Organisms are *Streptococcus viridans* (commonest), staphylococci, HACEK organisms (*Haemophilus species*, *Actinobacillus* or *Aggregatibacter*, *Cardiobacterium*, *Eikenella* and *Kingella* species), fungi (*Candida*) or *Rickettsia*. SBE affects a patient who is suffering from either rheumatic heart disease or congenital heart disease, or has undergone some sort of cardiac surgery (e.g. valvotomy, prosthesis).

Q. Acute bacterial endocarditis:

1. Often involves the normal heart with a rapidly progressive course (SBE invariably involves damaged heart), and is caused by highly virulent and invasive organisms.
2. Right-sided involvement (tricuspid valve) is common; pneumonia may be present.
3. *Clubbing is not a feature.*
4. Common in IV drug abusers.
5. Source of CVS involvement is often evident, i.e. there may be preceding staphylococcal abscess or pneumococcal meningitis. *Staphylococcus aureus is the commonest pathogen.*
6. Cardiac and renal failure develop rapidly.
7. Rapid onset with fulminant course, damages cardiac structures very rapidly and haematogenously metastasize in extracardiac sites.

Q. Causes of culture-negative SBE:

This accounts for 5–10% of cases and they are:

1. Partially treated patients.
2. Fungal, yeast infection, anaerobic organism or Q fever (needs special culture).
3. Intermittent bacteraemia.
4. L-form (cell-wall deficient form) of organism, fastidious organism (e.g. H. parainfluenzae).
5. **Marantic endocarditis** (non-bacterial thrombotic endocarditis, usually in elderly dying patients with advanced carcinomatosis; reported to occur in AIDS patients too).
6. Libman-Sacks endocarditis (non-bacterial verrucous endocarditis in SLE).
7. Right-sided endocarditis.

- 5 and 6 are examples of non-infective endocarditis.

Q. Complications of SBE:

Heart failure, rupture of chordae tendineae, aortic incompetence (i.e. destruction of valve), embolic manifestations (in brain, kidney or spleen), mycotic aneurysm at bifurcation of cerebral arteries, aortic root abscess (leads to complete heart block), myocardial abscess, lung abscess (from right-sided endocarditis), osteomyelitis and vasculitis-like features.

Q. Poor prognosis in SBE:

1. Prosthetic valve, fungal or gram-negative endocarditis.
2. Culture-negative endocarditis.
3. Presence of congestive cardiac failure.
4. Involvement of multiple valves.
5. Polymicrobial bacteraemia.
6. Large vegetations.
7. Mycotic aneurysm.
8. Immunocompromised host.
9. Aged patient.

Q. Cardinal features of SBE for 'bedside' diagnosis:

1. Fever (persistent or swinging), toxic look.
2. Pallor.
3. Clubbing.
4. Mild splenomegaly.
5. Microscopic haematuria, and
6. Embolic manifestations.

- As soon as SBE is diagnosed, it should be managed very promptly. The life of the patient is in danger if there is delay in the diagnosis and initiation of treatment. **So, it is a rule to examine all CVS patients for anaemia, pyrexia, clubbing and splenomegaly.**

Q. SBE with absence of fever:

1. CCF.
2. Uraemia.
3. Fungal endocarditis.
4. Severe sepsis.
5. Prior antibiotic therapy.
6. Elderly patients.

Q. Predisposing factors for infective endocarditis:

a. Acute: IV drug abuse, previous cardiac surgery, alcoholics.
b. Subacute: Rheumatic and congenital heart diseases, prosthetic valve, dental extraction, tonsillectomy, minor surgery (e.g. circumcision), IV catheter, instrumentation like catheterisation, cystoscopy, GI endoscopy or bronchoscopy.

Q. Cardiac diseases predisposing SBE:

1. Mitral and aortic valve diseases (mainly regurgitant diseases, as regurgitant jet damages the endocardium and predisposes a bed for seeding of the micro-organism) i.e. MI, mitral valve prolapse, AI commonly, MS, AS rarely.
2. VSD, PDA, bicuspid aortic valve, Fallot's tetralogy, rarely ASD.

3. Prosthetic heart valves, indwelling catheters.
4. Prior cardiac surgery (valvotomy, valve replacement).

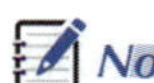

Note

Read the management of CCF, LVF, atrial fibrillation, rheumatic fever and SBE from standard textbooks.

SECTION 2: RESPIRATORY SYSTEM

The cardinal symptoms of respiratory system are:

1. Cough.
2. Expectoration or sputum production.
3. Haemoptysis (expectoration or spitting out blood, or bloody sputum).
4. Chest pain (pleural pain).
5. Breathlessness.
6. Wheezing or stridor (audible sounds).

Other symptoms are:

7. Hoarseness of voice.
8. Heaviness in the chest.
9. Fever (pulmonary tuberculosis, lung abscess, pleurisy, pneumonia, empyema thoracis).
10. Swelling of feet, e.g. oedema (in chronic cor pulmonale).
11. Epistaxis (nosebleeds), symptoms related to upper respiratory tract/ear/nose/throat (e.g. sinusitis, rhinitis, running nose, sneezing, ear infection or discharge, sore throat), or painful swallowing (e.g. septic tonsillitis).
12. Syncope (e.g. cough syncope), bone pain (hypertrophic osteoarthropathy or rib pain in bronchogenic carcinoma), snoring (may indicate obstructed breathing which may lead to obstructive sleep apnoea) or altered mentation (respiratory failure). Enquire for smoking-related symptoms.
13. General symptoms: Appetite, loss of weight (pulmonary tuberculosis or bronchogenic carcinoma), fatigue, sleep, bladder and bowel.

- *Upper respiratory tract* extends from external nares to the junction of larynx with trachea (i.e. up to lower border of cricoid cartilage), and includes nasal cavity, nasopharynx, sinuses, oropharynx and larynx. *Lower respiratory tract* includes trachea, lobar bronchus, segmental bronchi, generations of tracheo-bronchial tree and alveolar air sacs (**Fig. 1.21**).

Scheme of Examination (Proforma)

A. Upper Respiratory Tract (URT)

1. Nose (congestion, discharge, crusting, hypertrophied turbinate, bleeding spots and polyp) and nasal septum (deviation); nostrils and alae nasi (nasal flare e.g. in respiratory distress).
2. Mouth breathing (e.g. adenoids) or purse-lip respiration (e.g. COPD).
3. Air sinuses are tested for tenderness (maxillary sinus—press over the malar prominence by thumb; frontal sinus—press over the medial side of supraorbital ridge by thumb, or ask the patient to sit and lean forward, and ask for any heaviness over forehead; ethmoidal sinus—press by thumb against the medial wall of the orbit).
4. Pharynx [throat, gum, teeth (caries tooth), palate, cheeks, tongue, posterior pharyngeal wall, post-nasal drip], nasopharynx, tonsils with oral hygiene; halitosis present or not.
5. Larynx: Could not be examined (examined by direct and indirect laryngoscopy).

- The purpose of examination of URT is to determine whether it is healthy/unhealthy, or favouring aspiration or not. Remember, nose is the gateway to the lungs.

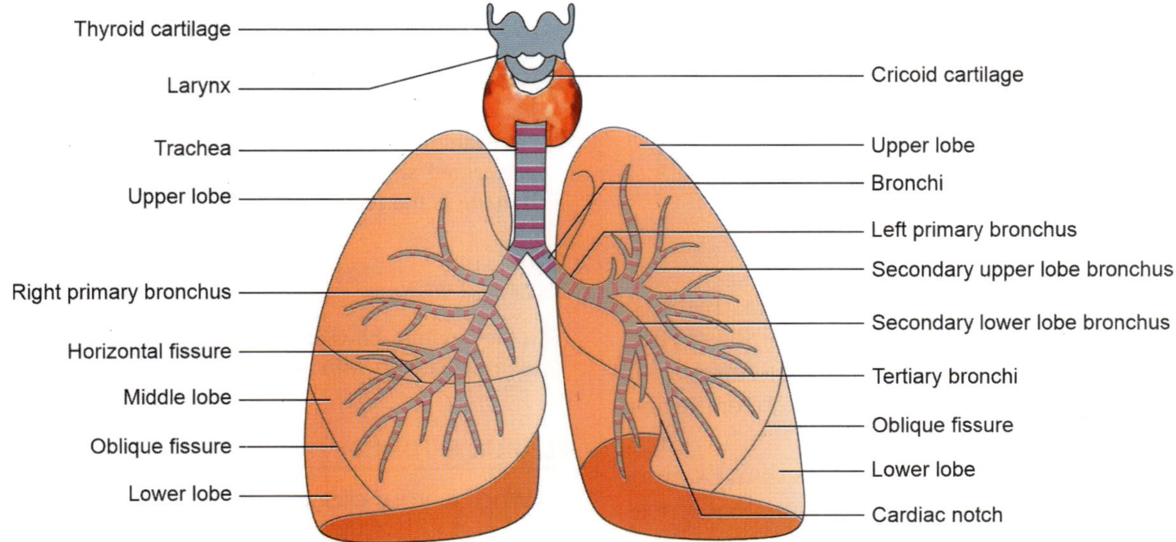

Fig. 1.21: Schematic representation of the **airways, fissures and lobes of the lungs**

B. Examination of the Chest (Lower Respiratory Tract)

I. Inspection (also vide pages 415–418):

1. Shape of the chest.
2. Movement of the chest.
3. Apical impulse (stand on the right side of the patient and look tangentially over precordium).
4. Respiration: Rate, rhythm, type, depth and breathing pattern(vide page 418).
5. Venous prominence (inspect the veins in standing or sitting position after coughing).
6. Fullness or depression:
   i. Unilateral or bilateral
   ii. Localised or generalised.
7. Supraclavicular and infraclavicular fossae; crowding of ribs.
8. Whether both the nipples are at the same level or not.
9. Whether accessory muscles of respiration are working or not.
10. Wheezing or stridor (audible sounds).
11. Intercostal suction.
12. Skin (front and back): Gynaecomastia (from bronchogenic carcinoma), pigmentation, sinus (e.g. from empyema, cold abscess or systemic fungal infection), scars (axillary scar for pneumonectomy or pneumothorax draining), ulcer, herpes zoster, puncture mark, any swelling (e.g. cold abscess or metastatic nodule), visible pulsations, breasts, parietal oedema (e.g. amoebic liver abscess, empyema thoracis, or lymphoedema), shiny skin over empyema thoracis, blue markings for radiotherapy over sternum, etc.
13. *Back* (also vide page 59): Spine should be examined in details. Scoliosis, kyphosis, drooping of the shoulder, winging of the scapula, gibbus, position of inferior angle of both scapulae, symmetry of interscapular areas (spino-scapular distance), ankylosing spondylitis, 'straight back', and arterial or venous prominence. Also observe the skin condition (e.g. sinus) over back.

- Any deformity after thoracic operation, e.g. thoracoplasty, should be carefully looked for.
- Trail's sign (or sternomastoid sign) is a finding on inspection (vide page 73).

II. Palpation:

1. Surface temperature.
2. Tenderness (rib tenderness in trauma, fracture or secondary metastasis; costochondral junction tenderness in Tietze's syndrome; muscle tenderness in myositis; intercostal tenderness or punch tenderness in liver abscess or empyema thoracis).
3. Corroboration of the findings of inspection: Examine the chest asymmetry, spinal deformity and tenderness, direction of venous flow (vide page 431), details of any swelling present, parietal oedema, etc.
4. Position of the trachea and the apex beat (i.e. position of the mediastinum).
5. Movement of the chest (always measure the expansion of the chest by a tape in full inspiration and in full expiration).
6. Vocal fremitus (vide page 71).
7. Any other palpatory findings, i.e. 'palpable accompaniments' (vide page 71) like friction fremitus, rhonchial fremitus, palpable coarse crepitations, subcutaneous emphysema, palpable pericardial rub.

- Some clinicians prefer to add 'cricosternal distance' in palpation (vide page 95).

III. Percussion (for the format, vide page 80):

	Right	Left
a. Conventional percussion	–	–
b. Shifting dullness	–	–
c. Coin percussion	–	–

d. Hepatic and cardiac dullness: Lost or not (both are lost in emphysema); delineate the upper border of hepatic dullness along the right MCL. Cardiac dullness is not done routinely.

e. Traube's space and tidal percussion (may be included).

IV. Auscultation:	Right	Left
a. Breath sounds (vesicular, bronchial and bronchovesicular)	–	–
b. Vocal resonance (diminished or increased; whispering pectoriloquy, aegophony)	–	–
c. Adventitious sounds or added sounds (rhonchi, crepitations and pleural rub)	–	–
[d. Miscellaneous (succussion splash, post-tussive suction, coin sound, pneumothorax click, tinkling crepitations, etc.)]	–	–

- It is better to auscultate all over the chest without leaving any space unexamined.
- Never forget to examine the **upper respiratory tract** and the **back** in respiratory system.
- **No examination of the respiratory system, however carefully performed, should be considered entirely satisfactory or final, if made in the recumbent position.**

Clinical Wisdom

See the 'sputum-bowl' and mention the specific abnormality present in patients with respiratory system.

PLEURAL EFFUSION — CASE 8

Q. What is your diagnosis?

This is a case of left-sided massive pleural effusion, probably of tuberculous in origin.

Q. Why do you say so?

This is a case of pleural effusion (excess quantity of fluid collected within pleural cavity) because there are presence of:

A. Symptoms (from the history):

a. Evening rise of temperature for last 1 month.
b. Dry cough with left-sided chest pain for 20 days.
c. Heaviness on left side of chest for 15 days.
d. Respiratory distress for last 2 days.

B. Signs:

1. General survey:

a. Decubitus: Prefers to lie on left lateral decubitus. The patient is not comfortable in bed.
b. Respitration: 28/min, abdomino-thoracic in type and the rhythm is regular. There is less movement on left side of chest. Accessory muscles of respiration are working.
c. Lymph nodes: Not palpable (rarely, few matted non-tender or slightly tender cervical lymph nodes may be palpable in tuberculosis).
d. Anaemia: Mild.
e. Pulse: 90/min, regular, mention other points.
f. Temperature: 100.8°F (oral) at present.
g. Emaciation: Present.
h. Nicotine staining of the fingers (e.g. pleural effusion developing from bronchogenic carcinoma): Absent.

2. Inspection:

a. Upper respiratoy tract is within normal limit.
b. Increased respiratory rate of 28/min. Accessory muscles of respiration are working.
c. Fullness of intercostal spaces on left side of chest. Diminished movement of chest on left side.
d. Apical impulse could not be visualised.
e. Absence of intercostal suction.

3. Palpation:

a. Diminshed movement on left side of chest and the expansion is 1½″ as measured by the tape.
b. *Trachea is shifted to the right side* and apex beat could not be localised (i.e. impalpable)—[If apex beat can be localised in a left-sided pleural effusion, it will be situated somewhere near the sternum, i.e. towards the right side].
c. Vocal fremitus is diminished on left side.
d. Absence of tenderness over chest.
e. Friction fremitus: Absent.
f. Normal palpatory findings on right chest.

4. Percussion: Stony dullness on the whole of left side of chest which does not alter with change of posture, i.e. shifting dullness is absent. Traube's space is dull on percussion. Tenderness is absent while percussing the chest. Normal resonant note on right side of chest.

5. Auscultation:

a. Diminshed vesicular breath sound on left side (or absent breath sound). Normal vesicular breath sound on right side.
b. Vocal resonance: Diminished on left side; normal vocal resonance on right side.
c. Adventitious sounds: Crepitations, rhonchi or pleural rub is absent on both sides of chest.

- Sometimes, there is tubular breath sound, bronchophony and whispering pectoriloquy (with increased vocal fremitus), and aegophony present at the upper border of moderate pleural effusion.
- **Vocal fremitus, percussion and auscultation are carried out in the following way:**
  1. Anterior chest: Along MCL or midclavicular line [supraclavicular (apex), infraclavicular, mammary and inframammary area]. Remember, apex of the lung is percussed from back.
  2. Lateral chest: Along MAL or midaxillary line (axillary and infra-axillary area).
  3. Back:
     i. Upper part: Suprascapular area,
     ii. Middle part: Interscapular area,
     iii. Lower part: Infrascapular area (along scapular line)
- The stony dullness of 'right'-sided pleural effusion is continuous with liver dullness while in 'left'-sided pleural effusion, the dullness is continuous with cardiac dullness with loss of Traube's space tympanicity.
- A small pleural effusion on the right or left side may be detectable only by tidal percussion.

Q. What is your case?

Build up the summary from the symptoms and signs, and try to say systematically as described above.

Q. Why it is not a case of pneumothorax?

Presence of stony dullness on percussion rules out pneumothorax (pneumothorax is tympanitic on percussion) and establishes the diagnosis of pleural effusion.

Q. Why it is not a case of hydropneumothorax ?

There is absence of shifting dullness, succussion splash, and classical horizontal fluid level.

Q. Provisional diagnosis in respiratory system diseases (standard format):

1. Anatomical: Lung (left/right/bilateral) and/or pleural disease.
2. Pathological: Fibrosis/collapse/consolidation/pleural effusion/restrictive lung disease.
3. Aetiological: Tuberculosis, malignancy, occupational, traumatic, smoking-induced.
4. Complications (optional): Cor pulmonale/respiratory failure.

Q. Important points in general survey of respiratory system:

1. **Decubitus:** May be propped-up; orthopnoea.
2. Nutrition: Emaciation in tuberculosis, bronchogenic carcinoma, diabetes mellitus and AIDS (DM and AIDS are often associated with pulmonary tuberculosis).

3. Facies: Moon face due to SVC syndrome; sarcoidosis (lupus pernio).
4. Anaemia: Tuberculosis, bronchogenic carcinoma, massive haemoptysis.
5. Jaundice: Bronchogenic carcinoma metastasizing in liver, antituberculosis drug-induced hepatitis, disseminated tuberculosis, pulmonary thrombo-embolism.
6. **Cyanosis:** Acute severe asthma, tension pneumothorax, lobar pneumonia, etc.
7. **Clubbing:** Bronchogenic carcinoma, bronchiectasis, lung abscess, empyema thoracis, etc.
8. Pulse: Pulsus paradoxus in acute severe asthma.
9. **Lymph nodes:** Especially the supraclavicular glands (tuberculous), scalene nodes (bronchogenic carcinoma), Virchow's gland (bronchogenic carcinoma) and glands in the posterior triangle of neck.
10. **Respiration:** Tachypnoea, orthopnoea, hyperpnoea, etc.
11. Temperature: For any infective aetiology like tuberculosis, lung abscess, pneumonia, etc.
12. Oedema: From chronic cor pulmonale.
13. Eye: Horner's syndrome (bronchogenic carcinoma), subconjunctival haemorrhage (chronic cough, SVC syndrome), chemosis of conjunctiva (SVC syndrome), polycythemia (COPD), phlyctenular keratoconjunctivitis (primary tuberculosis), uveitis in ankylosing spondylitis and episcleritis in rheumatoid arthritis, choroidal tubercles in retina (miliary tuberculosis), colour blindness (ethambutol toxicity), ptosis in myasthenia gravis, and papilloedema (COPD and SVC syndrome).
14. Hands: Nicotine staining, clubbing, cyanosis, wasting of the small muscles of one hand (thoracic inlet syndrome), warm and moist hand (type II respiratory failure) and flapping tremor.
15. Skin: Erythema nodosum, scars and sinuses in neck, scrofuloderma (tuberculous lymphadenitis with extension in skin), blue radiotherapy mark with India ink over the chest (for treatment of SVC syndrome).
16. Any obvious deformity: Gibbus (due to caries spine), kyphoscoliosis, different chest deformities.

- Examination of **eye in clinical medicine**—search for exophthalmos, enophthalmos, periorbital oedema, ptosis, squint, xanthelasma, nystagmus, cataract (e.g. steroid use) and pupillary abnormalities (e.g. miosis and mydriasis).

Q. What is pleural effusion?

Collection of serous fluid within the pleural cavity (in-between visceral and parietal layers of pleura) is *pleural effusion*. Only when the character of the fluid is transudate, it is known as *hydrothorax*.

Actually, the collection of fluid (resulting from increased hydrostatic pressure or decreased plasma oncotic pressure) occuring with a 'normal pleura' is ultrafiltration of plasma (transudate) in **hydrothorax**; it is usually bilateral. While the effusion due to 'pleural diseases' more nearly resemble plasma (exudate) which results from increased capillary permeability in **pleural effusion**, and is commonly unilateral but may be bilateral.

Q. Causes of pleural effusion:

A. Exudative (pleural effusion):

a. Pneumonia (bacterial and viral): Possibly the commonest cause worldwide.
b. Tuberculosis (possibly the commonest cause in India).
c. Bronchogenic carcinoma.
d. Pulmonary infarction (may be transudative in character).
e. Collagen vascular diseases like SLE (as a part of polyserositis), rheumatoid arthritis.
f. Pleural mesothelioma.
g. Lymphoma and leukaemias (haemothorax).
h. Meigs' syndrome (many authorities believe it to be transudative in nature).
i. Acute pancreatitis, subphrenic abscess, ruptured amoebic liver abscess, oesophageal perforation.
j. Asbestosis-associated pleural effusion (benign).
k. Uraemia, septicaemia, bleeding disorders.
l. Post-myocardial infarction syndrome (rare).
m. Chylous pleural effusion.
n. Yellow nail syndrome (rare; effusion due to lymphoedema).
o. Drug-induced (*see* below).
p. Familial Mediterranean fever (rare).

B. Transudative (hydrothorax):

a. Congestive cardiac failure (CCF).
b. Nephrotic syndrome.
c. Cirrhosis of liver.
d. Hypoproteinaemia (malnutrition) with severe anaemia.
e. Constrictive pericarditis, pericardial effusion.
f. Myxoedema.
g. SVC syndrome.
h. Peritoneal dialysis.

a, b, c, and d, under (A) are most common causes of pleural effusion.

- Major types of pleural effusion are: transudative (serous), exudative (straw-coloured), empyema (purulent), haemorrhagic (bloody) and chylous (milky) effusion.
- **'Polyserositis'** is inflammation of several membranes (i.e. pleura, peritoneum, pericardium) at the same time, and is commonly due to collagen vascular diseases (e.g. SLE), tuberculosis or septicaemia.

Q. How to diagnose hydrothorax?

1. Affection is usually bilateral.
2. Presence of anasarca.

3. Evidence of CCF, cirrhosis of liver, nephrotic syndrome, or severe anaemia with malnutrition.
4. Absence of signs of inflammation (i.e. no H/o fever, local tenderness, etc.).
5. Transudative nature of pleural fluid on aspiration.

In patients with hydrothorax, always look for collection of fluid in other serous sacs. So, one should be careful in detecting oedema, pericardial effusion, ascites, hydrocele, etc. in a case of hydrothorax.

Q. Haemorrhagic pleural effusion (haemothorax):

1. Neoplasm: Primary or secondary, pleural mesothelioma.
2. Chest trauma (during paracentesis or placement of central line; post-thoracic surgery).
3. Tuberculous effusion.
4. Bleeding diathesis.
5. Lymphoma and leukaemias.
6. Anticoagulant therapy.
7. Pulmonary infarction.
8. Acute haemorrhagic pancreatitis.
9. Asbestos-ralated pleural effusion.

- Pleural effusion resulting from mesothelioma usually does not shift the mediastinum as mesothelioma encases the lung on the affected side and is commonly related to asbestos exposure.
- In haemothorax, pleural fluid heamatocrit is greater than 50% of peripheral blood heamatocrit. If the fluid is kept on standing in a test tube, clot formation is complete in traumatic aspiration while the clot is incomplete in haemothorax.

Q. Chylous (milky) pleural effusion:

It results from leakage of chyle (thoracic duct lymph) into the pleural space and is due to:

1. Trauma (e.g. thoracic surgery).
2. Tuberculosis.
3. Malignancy.
4. Lymphoma.
5. Filariasis.
6. Myxoedema (gold paint effusion).
7. Congenital absence of thoracic duct.
8. Yellow nail syndrome.

Q. Bilateral pleural effusion:

1. Rheumatoid arthritis.
2. SLE.
3. Lymphoma and leukaemias.
4. Bilateral tuberculous effusion (rare).
5. Pulmonary infarction.
6. Multiple pleural metastases, septicaemia.

- Remember, hydrothorax is usually bilateral.

Q. Predominent right-sided pleural collection:

1. Rupture of amoebic liver abscess into pleural cavity.
2. Cirrhosis of liver.
3. Congestive cardiac failure.
4. Meigs' syndrome (fibroma of the ovary with ascites and pleural effusion).
5. Right-sided subphrenic abscess.

Q. Predominant left-sided pleural collection:

1. Acute pancreatitis.
2. Oesophageal rupture (Boerhaave's syndrome).
3. Dressler's syndrome (post-myocardial infarction syndrome with fever and chest pain).
4. Left-sided subphrenic abscess.
5. Aortic dissection.

Q. Recurrent pleural effusion (reappearance after thoracentesis):

1. Bronchogenic carcinoma.
2. Pulmonary tuberculosis.
3. Congestive cardiac failure.
4. Collagen vascular diseases.
5. Pleural mesothelioma.
6. Lymphoma.

Q. Acutely developing pleural effusion:

1. Trauma to the chest wall.
2. Pulmonary infarction.
3. Acute pancreatitis.
4. Rupture of amoebic liver abscess, oesophageal rupture or aortic dissection.

Q. Drug-induced pleural disease and/or pleural effusion (pleural fluid is eosinophilic):

1. Nitrofurantoin.
2. Methysergide.
3. Amiodarone.
4. Dantrolene sodium.
5. Bromocriptine.
6. Procarbazine.

- Drug-induced lupus (i.e. hydralazine or procainamide-induced) may give rise to pleural effusion.

Q. Causes of empyema thoracis (purulent effusion):

Collection of pus within the pleural cavity is known as empyema thoracis. The causes are:

1. Rupture of tuberculous cavity or post-pneumonic (bacterial).
2. Secondary infection of haemothorax or pleural effusion.
3. Rupture of subphrenic abscess or perforation of oesophagus.
4. Rupture of lung abscess (mostly staphylococcal—thin walled and multiple); bronchiectasis.
5. Septicaemia or pyaemia.
6. Traumatic (penetrating wounds of chest, after chest aspiration or liver biopsy).

Q. Bedside diagnosis of empyema thoracis (purulent effusion):

1. Patient looks toxic and prostrated; loss of weight.
2. Hectic rise of temperature with rigors and sweating.
3. Tachycardia as well as tachypnoea.
4. Development of clubbing.
5. Intercostal tenderness (patient winces with pain on application of pressure) as well as fullness.
6. Skin is red, oedematous and glossy overlying empyema.
7. *Plus*, signs of pleural effusion.
8. Rarely, a swelling in the chest wall is seen which gives impulse on coughing—**'empyema necessitans'** (i.e. pus collected under the skin of the chest wall due to rupture of purulent material from the pleural cavity, which communicates with the empyema thoracis).

Q. What is meant by 'stony dullness' on percussion over pleural effusion?

1. Extreme form of dull note elicited by percussion, *plus*
2. Feeling of increased resistance by the percussing finger.

Q. Bronchial breath sound above the fluid level in pleural effusion—mechanism behind:

It is said that air conducted through the relaxed or collapsed lung (compression collapse) produces tubular breath sound (so, there are bronchial breath sound, bronchophony and whispering pectoriloquy). Pleural effusion produces compression collapse and conductivity of the sound through collapsed (airless) lung is increased if the bronchus remains patent.

Q. Classical findings at the upper border of moderate pleural effusion:

1. Actually there is horizontal upper border of fluid level. Ellis's S-shaped curve, so called a classical finding of pleural effusion (i.e. highest level of dullness is in axilla in comparison to anterior and posterior wall, and thus assuming the shape of the letter 'S') is not demonstrated clinically. It is said that the upper border of fluid level sweeps towards the axilla due to capillary suction, and the highest point of fluid in axilla is just a radiological observation.
2. Skodaic resonance (after Czech physician Joseph Skoda) on percussion: It is observed just above the upper border of moderate effusion and the note (hyperresonant) mimics the percussion over an empty wooden box (boxy note). It is due to compensatory emphysema.
3. Bronchial breath sound (tubular): May be audible and is due to relaxed lung.
4. Pleural rub, rarely.
5. Aegophony.

- Remember, fluid is a good conductor of sound though the breath sound is diminished vesicular or absent over pleural effusion because of the fact that the sounds have to travel first through air in the alveoli and then through the fluid (i.e. change of media). In massive pleural effusion, when there is no air in lung parenchyma (i.e. compression collapse), the tracheal sounds traverse directly through the fluid resulting in bronchial breath sound (rarely found).

Q. In health, who keeps the trachea in the midline?

The equally negative intrapleural pressure on both sides.

Q. Is it possible to have trachea shifted towards the side of pleural effusion?

It is possible in a case of pleural effusion (malignant) developing from ipsilateral bronchogenic carcinoma. If we go through the basic physiology, it is very easy to understand.

A. In absorption collapse (due to endobronchial growth, i.e. bronchogenic carcinoma or foreign body impaction):
   1. Bronchus: Not patent (obstructed),
   2. Intrapleural pressure: Remains negative, and
   3. Trachea: Shifted to the same side. It is the more negative intrapleural pressure which draws the trachea to same side.

B. In compression collapse (due to pleural effusion, pneumothorax or hydropneumothorax):
   1. Bronchus: Patent,
   2. Intrapleural pressure: Positive, and
   3. Trachea: Pushed to the opposite side due to positive intrapleural pressure.

Now, if we deal with a case of bronchogenic carcinoma with **malignant pleural effusion**, the tussle between (A) and (B) will determine the position of trachea. If (B) plays more, trachea will go to the opposite side and if (A) plays more, **trachea will be shifted towards the same side.** If (A) and (B) play equally, trachea will remain in the midline.

So, if the pulling effect on trachea by absorption collapse (i.e. bronchogenic carcinoma) overcomes the pushing effect on trachea by compression collapse (i.e. pleural effusion), trachea remains on the same side of effusion. **Remember, a pleural effusion commonly shifts the trachea to the opposite side.**

Q. Red flag signs in pleural effusion:

1. Trachea shifted to the side of effusion.
2. Rapid and recurrent collection of fluid.
3. Developing into empyema thoracis.

Q. Pleural effusion present but trachea remains in the midline:

The possibilities are:

1. Mild pleural effusion (only the apical impulse is shifted to opposite side).
2. Malignant pleural effusion secondary to bronchogenic carcinoma (as described above).

3. Loculated or encysted pleural effusion (both the apical impulse and trachea may not shift).
4. Bilateral pleural effusion (if the amount of collection is more or less equal bilaterally).
5. Pleural effusion associated with mesothelioma of pleura.
6. Coincidental association of pleural effusion with ipsilateral apical fibrosis.

Q. Observation on inspection of 'back' in respiratory system:

Inspection of back (in respiratory system or CVS) **is always done in standing position** (if the condition of the patient permits) to avoid undue obliquity. Go to the back of the patient and look for:

1. Kyphosis (look from sides in profile).
2. Scoliosis (may be responsible for mediastinal shifting).
3. Drooping of the shoulder (signifies apical fibrosis or collapse, or trapezius paralysis).
4. Winging of the scapula (long thoracic nerve palsy or spinal deformity: Prominent medial border of scapula on the affected side is seen).
5. Whether the inferior angle of scapula on both sides are at the same level or not.
6. Interscapular area (spino-scapular distance): Compare between two sides of chest.
7. Intercostal suction.
8. Gibbus (Fig. 1.22) (acute angulation in the spine due to collapsed vertebra which is commonly developing from caries spine, and sometimes as a result of metastasis, or trauma).
9. Ankylosing spondylitis (stiff and immobile spine): May produce restrictive lung disease.
10. Loss of normal thoracic kyphosis or straight back present, or not.

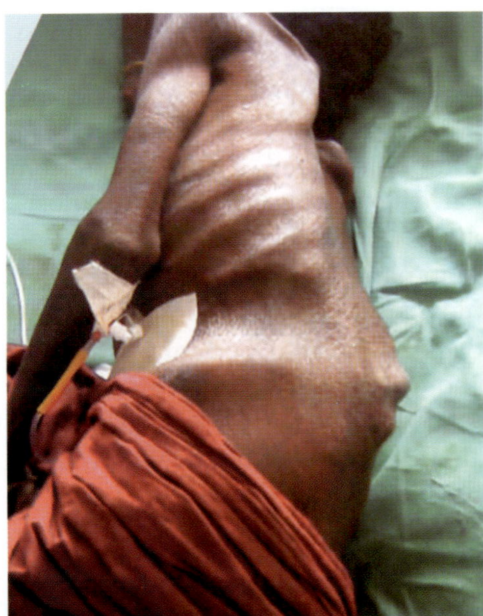

Fig. 1.22: **Gibbus**–acute angulation of vertebra; here it is due to metastasis from lung

11. Crowding of ribs (both in the front as well as the back).
12. Skin condition: Scar, sinus (e.g. tuberculosis), herpes zoster, local oedema, venous prominence, arterial pulsation (Suzman's sign), pigmentation, deformity after thoracic operation, e.g. thoracoplasty, etc.
13. Movement: Whether both the sides are moving simultaneously and symmetrically, or not.

Q. Importance of past history in pleural effusion:

Any H/o:

1. Fever, cough, chest pain, heaviness in chest, respiratory distress (as the case discussed).
2. Tuberculosis (or H/o contact).
3. Asbestosis (mining, textile workers, pipe fitters or shipbuilder): So, take occupational history.
4. Diabetes mellitus (prone to develop pulmonary tuberculosis).
5. Smoking (for malignant pleural effusion).
6. Skin rash, joint pain or swelling, neck swelling (lymphadenopathy): For collagen vascular diseases, lymphoma, etc.
7. Swelling all over the body (anasarca with hydrothorax).
8. Haemoptysis (tuberculosis, bronchogenic carcinoma, etc).
9. Trauma (to the chest wall).
10. Similar type of illness in significant past (recurrence) or in the family (e.g. tuberculosis).

Q. Differential diagnosis (D/D) of your case:

A. Pneumonic consolidation:

1. Acute onset with high fever, rusty sputum and chest pain.
2. Pulse respiration = 2:1 or 3:1 (normal ratio is 4:1); there is tachypnoea.
3. Trachea and apex beat: **Normal** in position (i.e. no shifting).
4. Percussion: **'Woody dullness'**.
5. Auscultation: Tubular breath sound, bronchophony, whispering pectoriloquy, aegophony, crepitations and pleural rub may be present.

B. Thickened pleura:

1. Long history.
2. Crowding of ribs with drooping of the shoulder. Depression of intercostal spaces with reduced movement on the affected side.
3. Trachea and apex beat may be shifted towards the diseased side (in fibrothorax).
4. Dull note on percussion but **never stony dull**.
5. Diminished vesicular breath sound with diminished vocal resonance. Bronchial breath sound is never heard. Pleural rub may or may not be present.
6. Commonly an end result of tuberculosis, empyema thoracis, asbestosis or haemothorax.

- Often known as **fibrothorax** (diffuse pleural thickening when the entire lung is surrounded by fibrotic pleura) and its clinical findings depend on degree of pleural thickening. There is blunting of costophrenic angle with tenting of diaphragm in chest X-ray.

C. Fibrosis or collapse (absorption) of the lung:

1. Crowding or ribs, drooping of the shoulder and retraction of intercostal spaces; flat chest.
2. **Apex beat and trachea are shifted towards the affected side.**
3. Impaired resonance on percussion; never stony dull.
4. Diminished vesicular breath sound with occasional crepitations (collapse with patent bronchus gives rise to bronchial breath sound).

D. Empyema thoracis: Already described.

E. Bronchogenic carcinoma:

1. H/o cough, haemoptysis, chest pain and emaciation in an aged patient; chronic smoker.
2. Superior mediastinal syndrome.
3. Cervical adenopathy (scalene group especially); clubbing.
4. **Usually no shifting of mediastinum** unless complicated by pleural effusion.
5. Localised rhonchi or crepitations.

F. Pericardial effusion: Considered only in left-sided pleural effusion.

1. Trachea is in normal position (i.e. no mediastinal shift).
2. Tympanicity on Traube's space percussion: Retained (lost in left-sided pleural effusion).
3. JVP: Engorged and may be pulsatile. Kussmaul's sign may be present.
4. Pulsus paradoxus.
5. Apex beat (if possible to localise) is medial to outer border of cardiac dullness.
6. Muffled heart sounds.

G. Subphrenic abscess:

1. H/o recent abdominal operation or appendicitis, etc.
2. Fever (hectic) with chill and rigor; pain in upper abdomen.
3. Rigidity in upper abdomen.
4. Absence of stony dullness in chest (on percussion).

[*H. Liver abscess—considered only in right-sided pleural effusion:*

1. H/o intestinal amoebiasis may or may not be present.
2. Patient looks toxic; fever with chill; shiny skin over the right lower chest.
3. Severe upper abdominal pain with right-sided intercostal tenderness present.
4. Upper border of liver dullness goes upwards].

- No. (A), (B), (C), (D), (G), (H) and pleural effusion cause dullness on percussion at lung base.

Q. Further confirmation of your diagnosis:

1. Chest X-ray: PA and lateral view, PLUS.
2. Aspiration of pleural fluid (absolute proof).

Q. Other findings on percussion in pleural effusion:

1. Area of dullness (triangular) on percussion against the vertebral column at the base of opposite lung (Grocco's triangle): Probably due to shift of posterior mediastinum to the opposite side pushed by effusion.
2. Loss of tympanicity of Traube's space (in left-sided pleural effusion).
3. Tidal percussion at the base of lung posteriorly may detect right- or left-sided small pleural effusion.

Q. Why there is dyspnoea in pleural effusion?

Dyspnoea occurs if there is,

1. Massive collection and/or
2. Rapid collection.

Pleural effusion produces (compression) collapse of the lung with shifting of the mediastinum to opposite side which leads to reduction in the vital capacity.

Q. Examination of CVS in respiratory diseases:

Search for dilated superficial veins over chest wall as well as engorged, non-pulsatile neck vein (SVC syndrome), pericardial effusion (as a complication of anasarca), and signs of RVH and RVF (chronic cor pulmonale). Special emphasis is given on features of pulmonary hypertension, if there is any.

Q. Examination of GI system and genitourinary system in respiratory diseases:

1. Halitosis (e.g. lung abscess).
2. Jaundice: ATD-induced hepatitis, disseminated tuberculosis, bronchogenic carcinoma metastasising in liver.
3. Hepatosplenomegaly: Liver or spleen may be palpable due to the push effect of massive pleural effusion commonly, rather than the cause of pleural effusion. Liver may be soft and tender in chronic cor pulmonale (liver of CCF). Splenomegaly is common in lymphoma, miliary tuberculosis, SLE and amyloidosis.
4. Ascites: In patients with hydrothorax (e.g. CCF), or disseminated tuberculosis.
5. Hydrocele or scrotal oedema: In patients with hydrothorax.
6. Abdominal lump: Pre- and paraaortic lymph nodes are palpable in lymphoma (which may produce pleural effusion or SVC syndrome).
7. Hernial sites: Should be examined as protracted cough is common in COPD.
8. Genitourinary system: Hydrothorax from nephrotic syndrome and uraemic lung from CRF may be present.

Q. Examination of nervous system in respiratory diseases:

1. Neck rigidity/stiffness: If present, goes in favour of tuberculous meningitis or meningism due to pneumonia.
2. Higher function may be altered in SVC syndrome or respiratory failure.
3. Features of respiratory failure in a case of myasthenia gravis.

- Horner's syndrome (bronchogenic carcinoma), myasthenic syndrome (Lambert-Eaton syndrome) and peripheral neuropathy may develop from respiratory illness; the last two are non-metastatic complications of bronchogenic carcinoma.

Q. Lymphadenopathy in a case of pleural effusion:

1. Tuberculosis (especially in the posterior triangle of neck, supraclavicular fossa, axilla).
2. Lymphoma (generalised lymphadenopathy).
3. Bronchogenic carcinoma (scalene node, Virchow's gland).
4. Acute leukaemias (cervical, axillary).
5. SLE (generalised lymphadenopathy).
6. AIDS (generalised lymphadenopathy).

Splenomegaly with pleural effusion is common in lymphoma, miliary tuberculosis, acute leukaemias, collagen vascular diseases (e.g. SLE) and cirrhosis of liver (hydrothorax, right-sided)

Q. What is 'phantom tumour'?

Occasionally, effusion (transudate) forms between the lobes of lung (interiobar effusion) and produces a rounded opacity in chest X-ray, which mimics a solitary pulmonary nodule or mass lesion (sharply marginated with bi-convex appearance). It is confirmed by USG or CT scan. The mass usually disappears with the resolution of effusion and this is why they are known as phantom tumour. Phantom tumour may be seen in congestive cardiac failure, which 'vanishes' after diuretic therapy (does not require pleural tapping).

Q. Subpulmonic effusion and its diagnosis:

Here the effusion collects underneath the lung and the chest X-ray (PA view) gives an impression of elevated hemidiaphragm. To confirm the diagnosis, a chest X-ray in LATERAL DECUBITUS position (affected side down) is taken which shows the pleural fluid layering out along the lateral chest wall. It is confused with subphrenic abscess.

Clinically, the left-sided subpulmonic effusion is diagnosed by loss of Traube's space tympanicity and the right-sided effusion is suspected in abnormal tidal percussion on right side.

Q. How massive pleural effusion is diagnosed clinically?

In massive pleural effusion, the dullness (on percussion) extends up to the 2nd ICS or above. Radiologically, it produces dense opacification of hemithorax with mediastinal shift. Usually pleural effusion is designated as mild (<500 mL), moderate (500–1500 mL) and massive (>1500 mL) according to the collected amount of fluid. Massive effusion commonly results from malignancy, CCF, tuberculosis, cirrhosis of liver and trauma.

Q. Points in favour of tuberculous aetiology in your patient:

The points in favour are:

1. Presence of anorexia, night sweats, malaise and loss of weight for last 2 months.
2. H/o evening rise of temperature and cough for approximately 1 month.
3. H/o contact.
4. Emaciation.

Tuberculous effusion is thought to be due primarily to a hypersensitivity reaction to tuberculous protein. Other hypersensitivity reactions of tuberculosis are erythema nodosum and phlyctenular keratoconjunctivitis.

Q. Complications of pleural effusion:

1. Thickened pleura.
2. Empyema thoracis.
3. Collapse (compression) of the lung followed by fibrosis later on.
4. Spread of infection (tuberculosis) to pericardium or peritoneum.
5. Cardio-respiratory embarrassment as a result of massive pleural effusion.
6. Acute pulmonary oedema (rare): As a complication of rapid pleural aspiration.
7. Hydropneumothorax (iatrogenic): May develop after pleural aspiration.

Q. How do you like to investigate a case of pleural effusion?

1. Blood: TC, DC, ESR, sugar (PP), serum amylase, any abnormal cell (high ESR and mild lymphocytosis are in favour of tuberculous aetiology; leucocytosis in pneumonia).
2. Chest X-ray (PA view):
   a. Triangular homogeneous opacity with a curved upper border which is concave medially and upwards, and extends upto axilla.
   b. Obliteration of costophrenic angle (earliest site of fluid collection).
   c. Massive effusion produces unilateral homogeneous opacity.
   d. Displacement of mediastinum to the opposite side.
   e. *Lateral view* is done to differentiate it from lobar consolidation.

- Encysted pleural effusion may not obliterate the costophrenic angle.

- 'Lateral decubitus film': Suspected subpulmonic effusion or 'small' pleural effusion.
- Repetition of chest X-ray should be done in all cases after therapeutic paracentesis thoracis.
- A wider than normal interlobar fissure is seen in interlobar effusion.

Clinical Wisdom

Approximately, 20% patients of tuberculous effusion may have co-existing lung diseases.

3. Aspiration of pleural fluid (thoracentesis or pleural tapping): For diagnostic purpose, at least 50 mL fluid should be aspirated. It helps by:
   a. Confirmation of diagnosis of pleural effusion.
   b. Examination of the nature of fluid: Transudate or exudate [physical character (clear in hydrothorax, straw-coloured in tuberculosis, red in haemorrhagic effusion, milky white in chylous, anchovy sauce-like from ruptured amoebic liver abscess and purulent in empyema thoracis), biochemical (protein and sugar; ↑LDH in exudate, ↑adenosine deaminase activity in tuberculosis), and cytological (RBC, WBC, malignant cells) examination] **(Table 1.9)**.
   c. Smear examination: Gram's stain, Ziehl-Neelsen stain, Leishman's stain for microfilaria or special stains for detection of malignant cells.
   d. Culture of the aspirated fluid (bacteriological, including culture of *M. tuberculosis* in Lowenstein-Jensen media). Bactec system of culture technique gives result within 7 days in favour of tuberculous effusion. Culture of pleural fluid for pyogenic bacteria is also done.
   A chest X-ray should be repeated after aspiration of pleural fluid to see the pulmonary parenchyma, especially in a suspected case of bronchogenic carcinoma. Sometimes, ultrasonography (USG) is done to differentiate an encysted pleural effusion from pleural tumour or pleural thickening, and to localise effusion before aspiration or pleural biopsy.
   e. ELISA (IgG or IgM) test of pleural fluid: Not very helpful.
   f. Special tests: Pleural fluid adenosine deaminase activity (↑ in tuberculosis), high levels of soluble interleukin-2 (IL-2) receptors and interferon-gamma (IFN-γ) in tuberculosis, and PCR study (polymerase chain reaction) to detect organisms including tubercle bacilli.

Table 1.9: Differentiation between transudate and exudate

Tests	Transudate	Exudate
(A) Routine:		
1. Appearance	Clear or light yellow. No froth on shaking	Straw-coloured, cloudy, purulent, milky, haemorrhagic. Froth formation on shaking
2. Protein	<3.0 g/100 mL	>3.0 g/100 mL
3. LDH	Low (<200 IU/L)	High (>200 IU/L)
4. Pleural fluid LDH	<2/3rd of normal upper limit of serum LDH	>2/3rd of normal upper limit of serum LDH
5. Pleural fluid LDH/serum LDH ratio	<0.6	>0.6
6. Plueral fluid protein/serum protein ratio	<0.5	>0.5
(B) Cytology:		
7. RBC	<10000/mm^3	>100000/mm^3
8. WBC	<1000/mm^3	>1000/mm^3 (>50% lymphocytes in tuberculosis and neoplasm; >50% polymorphs in acute infections)
9. Mesothelial or malignant cells	Not found	May be seen in neoplasm
(C) Special:		
10. pH	>7.3	<7.3
11. Specific gravity	<1.016	>1.016
12. Glucose	Same as blood concentration	Low in infections and neoplasm (very low in rheumatoid arthritis)
13. Amylase	–	High in pancreatitis, oesophageal rupture and neoplasm
14. Microbiology	Negative	Positive

- No. 4, 5 and 6 are known as **Light's criteria** in pleural effusion (to differentiate transudate from exudate).
- Some clinicians opine that **SFAG** [serum-fluid albumin gradient (i.e. 'serum albumin' minus 'fluid albumin')] value may determine the nature of the fluid, i.e. SFAG >1.2 g/dL is transudate, while <1.2 g/dL is exudate.
- The same calculation may be done by 'serum protein' minus 'fluid protein' and if >3.1 g/dL, it is transudate and if <3.1 g/dL, it is exudative in nature.

Cartridge-based nucleic acid amplification test (CB-NAAT) is known as GeneXpert test, which is helpful in early diagnosis of tuberculosis (usually done from sputum).

4. Sputum examination [it is done for 2 consecutive days (as per RNTCP) for AFB]:
   a. For demonstration of AFB (surest test for tuberculosis): Rarely positive.
   b. To diagnose the aetiology of pneumonia (if effusion develops from pneumonia).
   c. For malignant cells (exfoliative cytology).
5. Mantoux test (not much informative):
   a. Positive in cases of tuberculosis.
   b. May be negative in lymphoma.
6. Fine needle aspiration cytology (FNAC) or excision biopsy of lymph nodes (axillary, cervical or scalene node): May give a clue to the aetiology.
7. Imaging: Ultrasonography (especially in ICU setting or to diagnose encysted pleural effusion), CT scan or MRI scan detects fluid as small as 50 mL, and may be done if facilities are available.
8. Pleural biopsy (by Abram's, Cope's or trucut needle): Especially in malignancy or tuberculosis.
9. Serological tests like rheumatoid factor, antinuclear factor, complement level, etc.
10. Bronchoscopy and biopsy of the lung (in a suspected case of bronchogenic carcinoma).
11. Thoracoscopy and biopsy (pleura is inspected after inducing an artificial pneumothorax).

- Pleural fluid adenosine deaminase (ADA) activity: 40–60 U/L is borderline activity and >60 U/L is high activity in favour of tuberculosis.
- Pleural fluid NT (N-terminal)-proBNP>1500 pg/mL is diagnostic of effusion due to CCF.

Q. Minimal collection of pleural fluid for clinical detection:

At least 500 mL of fluid is necessary for clinical detection (minimally 300 mL fluid is required for radiological detection by-X-ray). Normal amount of pleural fluild in health is 5–15 mL.

For clinical or radiological detection of mediastinal shift, 1.5 litre of pleural fluid is required.

Q. Possible causes of malignant pleural effusion:

1. Bronchogenic carcinoma (commonest).
2. Metastatic carcinoma (often from breast or thyroid).
3. Pleural mesothelioma.
4. Lymphoma.
5. Acute leukaemias.

- These are the causes of rapid and repeated accumulation of pleural fluid.

Q. Indications of paracentesis thoracis (thoracentesis):

1. Diagnostic: For physical character, biochemical, cytological and bacteriological study of pleural fluid to come to a definite diagnosis. At least, 50 mL fluid should be aspirated.
2. Therapeutic: If there is:
   i. Respiratory distress.
   ii. Massive collection.
   iii. Rapid collection of fluid.
   iv. Bilateral pleural effusion.
   v. Intrapleural introduction of drugs for pleurodesis.
   vi. Suspected secondary infection of effusion.

   Fluid should be aspirated slowly and as much as possible until it is harmful for the patient. Few clinicians advocate not to aspirate more than 1 litre of pleural fluid on the first occasion because of the risk of developing acute pulmonary oedema. The area of maximum dullness on percussion (usually in the mid-axillary line) should be the appropriate site for aspiration of fluid. Nowadays, USG-guided pleural aspiration is preferred.

   The **'triangle of safety'** (by British Thoracic Society) for putting chest drain to evacuate air or fluid is bounded by: anterior—lateral border of pectoralis major, posterior—lateral border of latissimus dorsi, inferior—the 5th ICS, and apex—axilla. There is less chance of injury to internal organs, if air or fluid in pleural cavity is extracted by this route.

Q. Complications of pleural aspiration or pleural tapping (thoracentesis):

It is always done under strict aseptic condition with slow withdrawal of fluid. The complications are:

1. Pleural shock.
2. Empyema thoracis or haemothorax.
3. Hydropneumothorax or haemopneumothorax.
4. Acute pulmonary oedema (non-cardiogenic; unilateral)—If fluid is removed very quickly.
5. Air embolism.
6. Cardio-respiratory embarrassment with circulatory collapse.
7. Subcutaneous emphysema.

Q. How to clinically suspect a malignant effusion?

Clinical: Elderly, smoker, cachectic patient with nicotine stain and clubbing, palpable scalene or Virchow's lymph node which are hard and fixed.

Pleural fluid: Rapid and repeated collection of haemorrhagic fluid. In chest X-ray, a convex bulge may be seen above the concave fluid level and the trachea may be shifted to the side of pleural effusion.

Q. Special characteristics of tuberculous effusion:

1. It is possibly the commonest cause of plueral effusion in India and is usually associated with primary tuberculosis. It is commonly unilateral and rarely bilateral.

2. Straw-coloured or amber-coloured; EXUDATE in character (see below).
3. >50% lymphocytes with paucity of eosinophils.
4. Cobweb coagulum formed in pleural fluid.
5. pH is towards the acidic side.
6. Adenosine deaminase activity (ADA) in the fluid is elevated (>40 U/L) with elevated level of interferon-gamma (IFN-γ >140 pg/mL), presence of mycobacterial DNA (detected by PCR).
7. Paucity of AFB in pleural fluid. Yield:
   a. Pleural fluid: AFB is found in 6–8% cases.
   b. Ultracentrifused fluid: AFB is detected in 25–30% cases.
   c. Pleural biopsy: AFB is detected in 80% cases.
8. Pleural fluid culture for *M. tuberculosis* is 45% sensitive.

- **'QuantiFERON-TB Gold test'** is a test which defects latent as well as active tuberculous disease. The test measures a component of cell-mediated immune reactivity to *M. tuberculosis* and is based on quantification of IFN-γ released from sensitized lymphocytes. The test requires a blood sample and the result is available within 24 hours (logistically convenient). It is not affected by prior BCG vaccination. This test is also known as 'interferon-gamma release assays (IGRAs)'.

Q. How to assess the movement of the chest by palpation?

One has to assess whether both sides of the chest are moving simultaneously and symmetrically, or not. This is conventionally done at 3 places:

A. Front:

Place both palms firmly laterally on the lower rib cage in such a way that the thumbs touch each other in the middle anteriorly with a fold of skin in between the thumbs. Place the palms on the chest wall at the end of expiration. Now note the separation of the thumbs and feel over the palms with inspiration. Usually this is done *at the level just below the nipples ('lower' anterior chest)* (Fig. 1.23). Lower chest movement is known as **'bucket-handle' movement** (mainly lateral movement).

Normal expansion of the chest in an adult is at least 5 cm (5–8 cm normally), and expansion of 2 cm or less is abnormal. In severe emphysema and ankylosing spondylitis, it is found to be 1 cm or less.

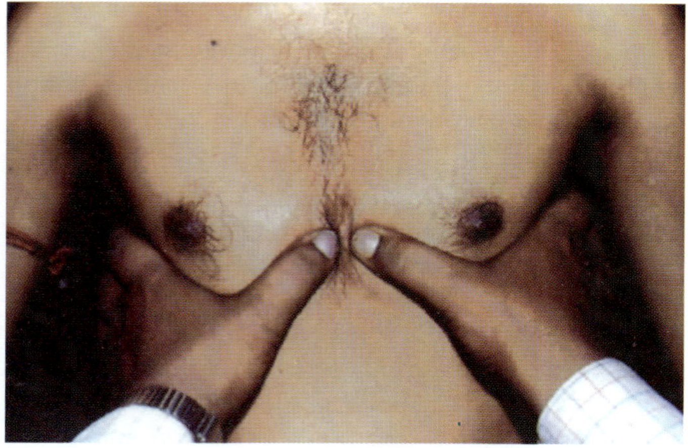
Fig. 1.23: Examining movement **of the chest (lower anterior** part)

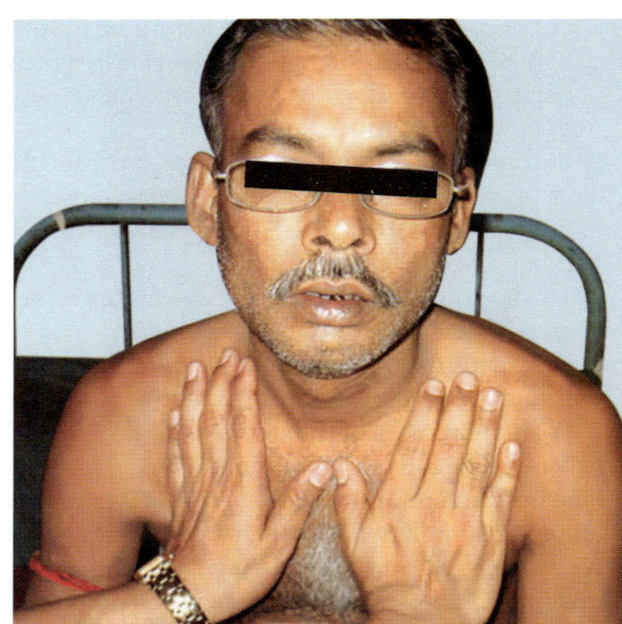
Fig. 1.24: Examining **movement of the chest (upper anterior** part)

Clinical Wisdom

According to many clinicians, the respiratory movement of the 'upper' anterior chest is determined by placing both palms side by side with thumbs touching the midline (terminal part of other fingers will fall over clavicles). Now, note the elevation or lifting of palms, and not the speration of thumbs to assess the movement of the 'upper' anterior chest (Fig. 1.24). Upper chest movement is known as **'pump-handle' movement** (mainly upward movement).

B. Back:

a. At the interscapular region: Place the palms firmly vertically side by side. Note the elevation or lifting of palms with inspiration.
b. At the infrascapular region (at the level of T_{10}) (Fig. 1.25): Same manoeuvre, as done in the 'lower' anterior part of the chest. Note the separation of thumbs with inspiration.
c. *Apex* (Fig. 1.26): Patient will sit, and standing behind the patient place two paims on the shoulder (over the clavicle) in such a way that thumbs touch each other in the nape of the neck at the level of the vertebra prominens (C_7). Note the feeling of upward movement of trapezius or lifting of palms with inspiration (not the separation of the thumbs). The movement of the apex may be examined from the front in a patient who is unable to sit (patient will lie down and palms will be placed over the clavicles from the front).

After the clinical assessment of movement of the chest, always measure the expansion (in the lower part of anterior chest wall and infrascapular region at back) with a measuring tape. Take the measurement both in inspiration and expiration (Fig. 1.27A and B).

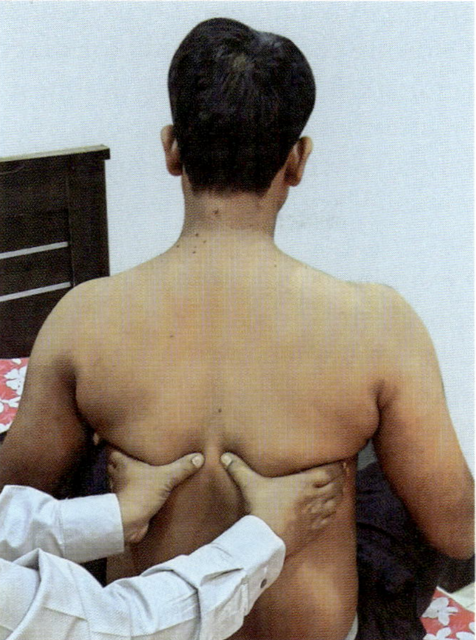

Fig. 1.25: Examining **movement of the chest (lower posterior part)**

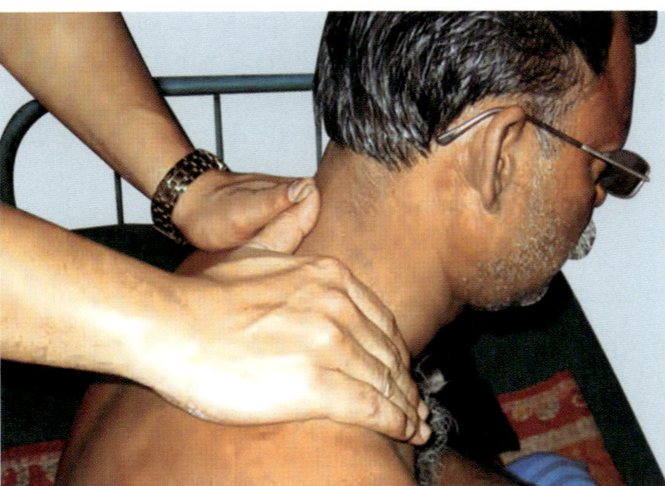

Fig. 1.26: Examining **movement of the chest** from back (**apical** area)

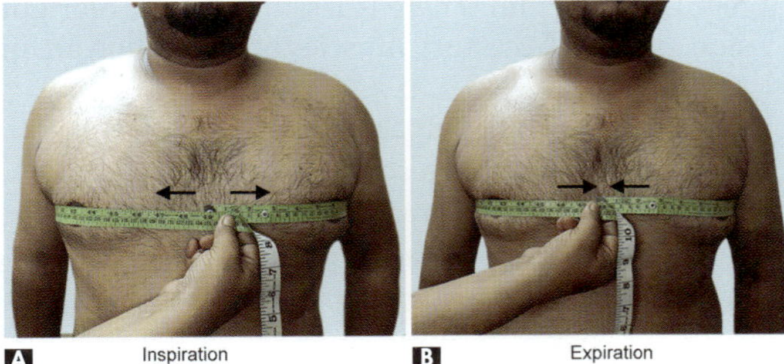

Fig. 1.27A and B: Measuring **expansion of chest:** (A) in inspiration and (B) in expiration

- The side with diminished expansion is likely to be the pathological side.
- Upper and middle lobe expansion is best assessed from the front while lower lobe expansion is measured from the back.

Q. Restriction of chest movement:

In health, both the sides of the chest move simultaneously and symmetrically without any bulging or indrawing.

Restriction of chest movement occurs in:

A. Unilateral:

1. Pleurisy.
2. Chest trauma*.
3. Pleural effusion.
4. Pneumothorax.
5. Hydropneumothorax.
6. Collapse of the lung.
7. Fibrosis of the lung.
8. Thickened pleura.
9. Consolidation of the lung.
10. Empyema thoracis.

B. Bilateral:

1. Emphysema.
2. Diffuse interstitial fibrosis.
3. Hydrothorax (bilateral).
4. Ankylosing spondylitis.
5. Sometimes in bronchial asthma.
6. Weak inspiratory muscles, e.g. myasthenia gravis, respiratory paralysis (e.g. GB syndrome).
7. Any extensive bilateral disease.
8. Obesity (i.e. hypoventilation syndrome).

*Due to severe chest pain, fractured ribs, flail segment following trauma or previous thoracoplasty.

Q. What do you mean by 'expansion' of the chest?

Expansion and movement of the chest are not interchangeable terms, e.g. in emphysema, chest may move but there is little expansion. 'Expansion' is the difference between inspiration and expiration, and is commonly measured by a tape (Fig. 1.27A and B).

Q. Why there is aegophony above the level of effusion?

It is due to interceptions of the relaxed lung as well as the fluid level, with the low-pitched component of the sound (i.e. there is change in lung acoustics).

Q. Why the upper margin of fluid goes towards axilla in chest X-ray?

This is a radiological illusion. A horizontal section of hemithorax at the level of the upper margin of fluid shows that there is same amount of fluid present anteriorly, posteriorly and laterally. But it is a fact that X-ray beam traverse more fluid laterally than they do centrally because of the peculiar shape of hemithorax. So we see the curved upper margin going towards axilla in X-ray picture.

Some clinicians opine that it is due to capillary suction between two pleural layers, which draws the fluid up.

Q. How will you manage a case of pleural effusion?

1. Rest in bed with good nutritious diet.
2. NSAID: To relieve chest pain.
3. Aspiration of pleural fluid, if there is respiratory distress or rapid collection.

4. 'Chest physiotherapy' should be encouraged to help in the expansion of lower chest (e.g. clapping on the chest wall by cupped hand).
5. According to aetiology:
   a. Tuberculous:
      i. Antituberculosis chemotherapy.
      ii. Sometimes, corticosteroid is added to prevent pleural adhesion and fibrosis (20–40 mg daily for 6–12 weeks with gradual tapering).
   b. Malignancy:
      i. Repeated aspiration of pleural fluid.
      ii. Pleurodesis (obliteration of the pleural space by adhesion) is done by tetracycline, bleomycin, mustine hydrochloride, talcom powder, *Corynebacterium parvum*, etc.
      Alternatively, thoracotomy with pleurectomy or pleural abrasion may be tried.
      iii. Treatment of bronchogenic carcinoma or lymphoma is done accordingly.
   c. Hydrothorax: Specific treatment of CCF or cirrhosis of liver is done.

Q. Management of empyema thoracis:

Diagnosis of empyema is made by clinical features, radiology (similar to pleural effusion) and aspiration of pus by a wide-bore needle through an intercostal space over the area of maximum dullness. Then bacteriological examination of pus is done accordingly.

A. Treatment of non-tuberculous empyema:

a. Acute:

i. Intercostal tube drainage through water-seal drainage system.
ii. Proper antibiotic therapy after sensitivity test (arbitrary use may produce resistance).
iii. It pus is very thick, rib resection and clearing of empyema cavity are done; a wide-bore tube helps in prolonged drainage.

b. Chronic: It is the domain of thoracic surgeon.

i. Resection of empyema sac in toto (if the underlying lung is healthy).
ii. Thoracotomy and decortication of pleura (in patients with thickened pleura). Decortication means stripping of the whole of thickened visceral pleura.

B. Treatment of tuberculous empyema:

a. Antituberculosis chemotherapy.
b. Repeated drainage of pus through a wide-bore needle or tube-drainage.
c. Rarely, surgery is necessary.

Conclusion

1. Always look for puncture mark, benzene stain or cotton seal in the lower chest (indication of pleural aspiration).
2. Shifting of mediastinum to the opposite side, stony dullness on percussion, and diminished (or absent) vesicular breath sound and vocal resonance on the affected side are **cardinal points for diagnosis**.
3. Examine for shifting dullness in the chest to exclude hydropneumothorax in all cases of pleural effusion.
4. Never forget to write measurement of the chest in two phases, i.e. both in full inspiration and in full expiration
5. Always examine the upper respiratory tract (nose, nasal septum, air sinuses, pharynx) at the beginning of clinical examination of respiratory system.
6. **Do not forget to examine the breast, testes and spine in a patient of pleural effusion.**

PNEUMOTHORAX — CASE 9

Q. What is your diagnosis?

It is a case of right-sided spontaneous pneumothorax of closed type, probably of tuberculous aetiology.

Q. Why do you say so?

It is a case of pneumothorax (presence of air within pleural cavity) because there are presence of:

A. Symptoms (from the history):

a. Rise of temperature with dry cough for last 2 months,
b. Pain in the right chest for 1 day, and
c. Respiratory distress for 1 day.

- Breathlessness and pain chest started suddenly.

B. Signs:

1. General survey:

a. Decubitus: Propped-up position at present. The patient prefers to lie on right lateral decubitus and becomes breathless on left lateral decubitus; not comfortable in bed.
b. Respiration: 30/min, abdomino-thoracic in type and regular in rhythm. There is less movement on right side of chest. Accessory muscles of respiration are in action.
c. Lymph nodes: Not palpable.
d. Cyanosis: Absent at present.
e. Pulse: 84/minute and regular; mention other points.
f. Temperature: 100°F (oral) at present.

2. Inspection:

a. Upper respiratory tract is within normal limit.
b. Increased respiratory rate of 30/min.
c. Intercostal spaces are full on right side.
d. No intercostal suction; accessory muscles of respiration are working at present.
e. Diminished movement on right side of chest.
f. Apical impulse is seen on left side of the chest, below the left nipple and placed more outward than normal.

3. Palpation:

a. Diminished movement on right chest. Expansion of chest is $1\frac{1}{2}$", as measured by the tape.

b. *Trachea is shifted towards left side. Apex beat is palpable at left 5th ICS, 1″ outside the left MCL.*
c. Vocal fremitus is diminished (or absent) on right chest. Normal vocal fremitus on left side.
d. Absence of local tenderness all over in the chest.

4. Percussion:

a. Tympanitic note on all over the right chest.
b. Obliteration (reduction) of liver dullness, and the upper border of dullness is present on right 6th ICS in the right MCL.
c. Shifting dullness: Absent.
d. Normal resonant note on percussion over left side of the chest.

5. Auscultation:

a. Breath sound is diminished vesicular (or absent) on right chest.
b. Vocal resonance is diminished (or absent) on right chest.
c. Adventitious sounds: Neither rhonchi nor crepitations are heard. Pleural rub is absent.
d. Coin sound: Present on right chest.

Auscultatory findings on the left side of chest are normal.

- Pyrexia may be absent in pneumothorax; sudden onset of unilateral pleuritic *chest pain and dyspnoea are two chief complaints*.
- The chest in pneumothorax is known as 'tympanicity with silence' (i.e. tympanitic note on percussion with diminished or absent breath sound).
- A small pneumothorax may be asymptomatic without any abnormal physical sign in chest.

Q. What is your case?

Build up the summary from the symptoms and signs, and say systematically as mentioned above.

Q. Describe the dyspnoea (H/o present illiness) in your patient:

The dyspnoea is due to collapse (compression) of the lung. It is:

1. Acute (sudden) in onset which compelled the patient to attend hospital immediately.
2. Sense of something being torn inside the chest, at the beginning of symptoms.
3. Not associated with wheezing (may be associated with wheezing in a COPD patient).
4. Dyspnoea at rest.
5. Not relieved by drugs, rest, squatting, etc. minimally relieved by adopting sitting posture or by right lateral decubitus position.
6. Associated with stabbing chest pain.
7. Non-progressive.
8. No H/o PND.
9. Not associated with 'shock and collapse' at the onset.
10. Cough aggravated the breathlessness.

- For gradation of 'respiratory' dyspnoea i.e. MMRC dyspnoea scale, see page 192.

Q. Describe the chest pain (H/o present illness) in your patient:

1. It is sharp, and stabbing or tearing in nature; acute in onset and excruciating.
2. Present on the right side of chest.
3. Increases by coughing, laughing, sneezing, jolting and deep inspiration.
4. Associated with dry cough.
5. The patient is forced to take shallow breathing and suppression of coughing.
6. Not relieved by any drug or by any other measure, forced the patient to attend hospital.
7. Without any radiation (i.e. localised).
8. In all respect, it is a **pleuritic pain**.

Q. Importance of past history in pneumothorax:

1. Respiratory distress (COPD may be an aetiology of pneumothorax).
2. Tuberculosis.
3. Haemoptysis.
4. Trauma.
5. Prolonged recumbency with calf pain (indicates pulmonary thromboembolism: As D/D of dyspnoea of sudden onset).
6. Similar episode (recurrent pneumothorax) in the past.
7. Chest pain (IHD): Indicates acute myocardial infarction (D/D of dyspnoea and pain chest).
8. Systemic hypertension (LVF may be a D/D of acute onset dyspnoea).
9. Chronic smoking.

Q. Other possible auscultatory findings in pneumothorax:

1. Amphonic breath sound may be heard on the affected side (open type).
2. **Pneumothorax click:** Sharp clicking sound synchronous with the heart beat may be heard in left-sided 'shallow' or small pneumothorax.
3. Hamman's sign (in case of pneumomediastinum): Read the section on 'Pericardial rub'.

Q. How to examine for subcutaneous emphysema?

It is the presence of air in the subcutaneous soft tissue and is also known as **'surgical emphysema'** (older term). When one gives light pressure after placing the fingers fanwise on the affected area, a peculiar spongy or crackling sensation (crepitus) is obtained. If a stethoscope is placed and pressed there, crepitations-like sound is heard. It may extend from face to the foot resulting in diffuse swelling of the part. The clinical associations are:

1. **Pneumothorax** (after intercostal tube drainage) or severe bronchial asthma (air may track into mediastinum resulting in mediastinal emphysema).

2. Rib fracture which penetrates the lung, i.e. penetrating injury to the chest wall.
3. Fracture of paranasal air sinus.
4. Rupture of the oesophagus.
5. Laryngeal perforation (accidental).
6. Gas gangrene.

- Always search for subcutaneous emphysema in a case of pneumothorax having tube drainage.

Q. Types of pneumothorax:

1. *Artificial:* Artificially done to control tuberculosis by inducing collapse of the lung (not used nowadays because of availability of antituberculosis drugs) or to differentiate radiologically among the lesion in pleura, lung and chest wall (diagnostic purpose).
2. *Traumatic:* Chest trauma (stab injury), thoracic surgery, after pleural or lung biopsy, CVP recording through subclavian vein, fractured ribs, pericardiocentesis, bronchoscopy.
3. *Spontaneous:*
   a. Closed [mild (<20% of radiographic volume in chest X-ray), moderate (20–50%) and large (>50%) variety]: Usually develops due to rupture of emphysematous bulla or from rupture of subpleural tuberculous focus. The communication between pleura and lung closes by fibrin clot, and usually does not reopen. Trapped air is slowly reabsorbed and collapsed lung reexpands in 2–4 weeks. Dyspnoea is not very severe and infection of pleural space does not occur. Pneumothorax is small though there may be presence of mediastinal shift.
   b. Open: There is development of free communication between pleural space and bronchus (*broncho-pleural fistula*). Air goes in and out of the pleural space with inspiration and expiration respectively. Expansion of collapsed lung is hampered and infection of the pleural space is a common complication (pyopneumothorax). Open type usually originates from the tuberculous cavity, lung abscess or apical subpleural bleb. Amphoric breath sound may be auscultated. The patient is dyspnoeic and there is presence of mediastinal shift. Penetrating wound of the chest also produces open type of pneumothorax. Pyrexia is common.
   c. Tension (valvular): The pleuro-pulmonary communication acts as a check-valve which allows air to enter into the pleural cavity during inspiration, coughing, sneezing and straining but prevents escape of air during expiration. Very large amount of air may be trapped within the pleural cavity in this way. Dyspnoea is very severe and progressive with cyanosis, and mediastinal shift is obvious (thus, there is shock and collapse). Central cyanosis is present. **It is a medical emergency** and the patient should be tackled immediately to treat respiratory failure.

- **Clinical classification of pneumothorax:** Closed type, open type and tension type.

Q. Pneumothorax in relation to atmospheric pressure:

1. Closed type: Intrapleural pressure < Atmospheric pressure.
2. Open type: Intrapleural pressure = Atmospheric pressure.
3. Tension type: Intrapleural pressure > Several times of atmospheric pressure.

Q. What is normal intrapleural pressure?

Normal intrapleural pressure is –2.5 to –6 mm of Hg. It is the negative intrapleural pressure, i.e. –2.5 mm of Hg, (subatmospheric) which keeps the lungs in apposition with the chest wall (at the end of expiration). At the height of inspiration, it becomes more negative, i.e. –6 mm of Hg.

Q. Recent classification of spontaneous pneumothorax:

Spontaneous pneumothorax is one where air develops within the pleural space without antecedent trauma to the thorax. It is basically of two types:

A. **'Primary'** spontaneous pneumothorax:
   a. Without underlying known lung disease,
   b. Usually due to rupture of apical subpleural blebs of 1–2 cm in diameter,
   c. In tall, thin individuals between 20–40 years of age, and
   d. Usually in smokers; may have positive family history. Approximately 50% have recurrence.

B. **'Secondary'** spontaneous pneumothorax:
   a. With underlying lung disease (different aetiology are mentioned below),
   b. Usually from COPD and active cavitary pulmonary tuberculosis,
   c. Most common in older persons, and
   d. More dangerous than primary variety because of underlying lung disease.

- Source of air in pneumothorax is from lung, mediastinum or outside of body (i.e. atmosphere).

Q. Aetiology of pneumothorax:

1. Rupture of an apical subpleural bleb or bulla (usually in young patients).
2. Rupture of a subpleural tuberculous focus or tuberculous cavity.
3. Rupture of the pulmonary end of pleuro-pulmonary adhesion.
4. Rupture of subpleural emphysematous bullae (usually in elderly).
5. Staphylococcal lung abscess.
6. Penetrating or non-penetrating trauma (e.g. pleural biopsy, thoracentesis) to the chest.
7. Bronchogenic carcinoma.

8. Pulmonary infarction.
9. Rupture of 'Honeycomb lung' (bronchiectasis, scleroderma, histiocytosis X disease, tuberous sclerosis).
10. Bronchial asthma.
11. Whooping cough.
12. Cystic fibrosis.
13. Rupture of oesophageal carcinoma.
14. Rupture of a tension cyst in lung.
15. Artificial pneumothorax.
16. Pneumoconiosis.
17. Catamenial pneumothorax: Rare disorder in women over 25–30 years, occuring within 48 hours of onset of menstruation; probably due to intrapleural endometriosis; recurrent and usually right-sided, treated by OC pills to suppress ovulation, or by danazole, surgical explorations and pleurodesis. Haemoptysis may also associated with.
18. Caisson's disease (decompression sickness).
19. ARDS (especially, under mechanical ventilation), AIDS.
20. Mechanical ventilation.

- 1, 2, 3 and 4 are principle causes of pneumothorax. Aetiology No. 1 is usually congenital and probably the commonest cause worldwide. No. 1 is primary variety while rest are secondary.

Q. Causes of recurrent (more than twice) spontaneous pneumothorax:

1. Patients with emphysematous bulla or apical subpleural bleb.
2. Cystic fibrosis.
3. Rupture of bronchogenic carcinoma or oesophageal carcinoma.
4. Patient with lung cysts.
5. Catamenial pneumothorax.
6. Honeycomb lung.
7. AIDS.
8. Ehlers-Danlos syndrome, Marfan's syndrome, α_1-antitrypsin deficiency, lymphangioleiomyomatosis.

Q. Causes of bronchopleural fistula:

1. Tuberculous cavity.
2. Lung abscess.
3. Necrotising pneumonia.
4. Following lung resection.
5. Chest trauma.
6. Barotrauma.
7. Empyema thoracis.
8. Chemo- or radiotherapy for lung cancer.

- Bronchopleural fistula is often used synonymously with open pneumothorax.

Q. Percussion note over normal lung:

Lung is resonant on percussion while abdomen is tympanitic. When the air in a cavity of sufficient size is set into vibration, the character of the sound becomes tympanitic, e.g. in the case of percussion over stomach. On the other side, the lung alveoli are small pockets of air seperated by numerous septa which dampen down the sound from tympanitic to resonant note.

Q. Differentiation between different characters (quantitative) of percussion note:

It is described below from higher to lower note (pitch and loudness) of resonance:

A. Resonant note:

1. Tympanitic (abdomen, pneumothorax)
2. Hyperresonant (emphysema)
3. Resonant (normal lung field)
4. Impaired resonance (thickened pleura)

B. Dull note:

5. Woody dullness (consolidation of the lung)
6. Stony dullness (pleural effusion)

- Qualitative types of percussion note: coin sound over pneumothorax or cracked-pot sound over a cavity.

Q. Tympanitic note (a drum-like resonance) on percussion:

1. Pneumothorax.
2. Superficial, big, empty cavity.
3. Over a large emphysematous bulla.
4. Subpleural lung cyst.
5. Sliding hiatal hernia (left side only).
6. Over Traube's space (i.e. fundus of stomach).

- Remember, tympanitic note is elicited on percussion over any hollow viscus.

Q. Hyperresonant note (slightly increased normal resonance on percussion):

1. Emphysema.
2. Occasionally over lung cyst.

- Hyperresonance or tympanitic note is more difficult to detect than the dullness.

Q. Impaired note (slightly diminished normal resonance) on percussion:

1. Thickened pleura.
2. Fibrosis of the lung.
3. Collapse of the lung.
4. Over pulmonary neoplasm.
5. Early pleural effusion.
6. Consolidation of the lung (early).

- No. 1–6 may produce dull note too.

Q. Dull note (an impaired note of greater degree) on percussion:

1. Consolidation (**woody dullness**; an older terminology).
2. Pleural effusion, empyema thoracis and over 'hydro' part of hydropneumothorax **(stony dullness)**.

Q. Causes of acute chest pain:

1. Ischaemic heart disease (IHD), i.e. angina pectoris or acute myocardial infarction.
2. Acute dry pleurisy due to any cause (e.g. tuberculosis, pneumonia).
3. Spontaneous pneumothorax.
4. Diffuse oesophageal spasm (may be food-related), gastroesophageal reflux disease (GERD).
5. Acute pulmonary thromboembolism.
6. Musculoskeletal pain: Rib fracture (trauma, cough), secondary deposits in rib (malignancy, multiple myeloma), osteomalacia, osteoporosis producing fracture, osteomyelitis, costochondritis (Tietze's syndrome; symptoms become worse with sneezing, coughing and movement of the chest), abscess or furuncle on the chest wall, myositis, fibrositis, intercostal myalgia (Bornholm disease—intercostal muscle involvement by Coxsackie B virus infection), thrombophlebitis of anterior thoracic vein (Mondor's disease), arthritis of shoulder joint or spine, intercostal neuralgias.
7. Acute dry pericarditis.
8. Acute tracheobronchitis, mediastinitis.
9. Aortic stenosis, hypertrophic cardiomyopathy.
10. Dissecting aneurysm.
11. Herpes zoster on the chest wall.
12. Anxiety states/psychogenic (cardiac neurosis).
13. Iatrogenic: From procedures like thoracentesis, thoracoscopy or chest tube insertion.
14. *Abdominal disorders*, e.g. hiatal hernia, acute cholecystitis, acute pancreatitis, perforated peptic ulcer, ruptured amoebic liver abscess, subphrenic abscess, splenic flexure syndrome.

- Local **tenderness** is found in 6 and 11; 2 and 7 may produce tenderness.

Q. Enumerate the causes of 'retrosternal' chest pain:

1. Ischaemic heart disease (angina or AMI).
2. Oesophagitis or diffuse oesophageal spasm, hiatal hernia.
3. Acute dry pericarditis.
4. Acute mediastinitis.
5. Diaphragmatic hernia.
6. Mediastinal tumour or mediastinal emphysema.
7. Aneurysm of the aorta.
8. Dissecting aneurysm.
9. Tracheitis.
10. Psychogenic.

- Causes of chest pain remain within a) Retrosternal (central), b) Peripheral (non-central, e.g. causes of pleurisy), and c) Musculoskeletal pain (non-central). Pain originating from lung, pleura or chest wall is peripheral and pain due to centrally situated structures like heart, mediastinum, aorta, trachea or oesophagus is central (retrosternal).

- **Precordial catch:** Sudden, momentary stabbing pain at cardiac apex experienced by normal subjects; physiological and does not indicate organic heart disease.
- Sharp stabbing left 'submammary pain' associated with anxiety is known as cardiac neurosis or Da Costa's syndrome. In contrast, a patient of AMI (organic coronary artery disease) often describes the chest pain by putting a clenched fist over the sternum **(Levine's sign)**.

Q. Dyspnoea of acute or sudden onset:

1. Cardiac asthma (cardiogenic pulmonary oedema).
2. Acute severe asthma (status asthmaticus).
3. Acute exacerbation of chronic obstructive pulmonary disease (COPD), or acute viral/bacterial bronchitis.
4. Acute laryngeal obstruction (child—foreign body, diphtheria, acute epiglottitis, oedema of glottis; adult—foreign body like dentures, loose teeth, tetany, mucus plugs, oedema of glottis, etc.).
5. Spontaneous pneumothorax (tension type).
6. Anaphylaxis (oedema of glottis).
7. Acute pulmonary thromboembolism.
8. Rapidly accumulating massive pleural effusion.
9. Diabetic ketoacidosis.
10. Lobar pneumonia (severe).
11. Cardiac tamponade.
12. ARDS.
13. Hysterical hyperventilation (dyspnoea is more at rest than on exertion), claustrophobia.

- 1–7, 12 and 13 are very important causes in day-to-day practice. Acute obstruction of upper airway with food, followed by sudden collapse is known as 'Cafe coronary syndrome'.
- **Classification of dyspnoea according to time course of onset:**
  a. In seconds: 4, 5, 6 and 7
  b. In hours: 1, 2, 9, 10, 11 and 13
  c. In days: 3, 8 and 12
  d. In weeks to months: Severe anaemia, pleural effusion, COPD, weakness of respiratory muscles, e.g. myasthenia gravis.
- Dyspnoea in respiratory diseases are basically due to ventilatory defect (pneumonia, COPD), diffusion defect (ILD) and perfusion defect (acute pulmonary thromboembolism).

Q. Chest pain with dyspnoea (elaborated in page 74):

1. Spontaneous pneumothorax.
2. Acute myocardial infarction.
3. Trauma to the chest wall.
4. Acute pulmonary thromboembolism.
5. Dissection of aorta.
6. Acute dry pleurisy (especially from consolidation).
7. Psychogenic.

- Usually (No. 5) develops from Marfan's syndrome, hypertension, coarctaion of aorta and pregnancy.

Q. Chest pain with circulatory collapse (shock) or syncope:

1. Acute myocardial infarction.
2. Tension pneumothorax.

3. Acute pulmonary thromboembolism.
4. Dissection of aorta.
5. Cardiac tamponade.
6. Pneumomediastinum.
7. Acute pancreatitis.
8. Upper gastro-intestinal bleeding.

Q. Different types of fremitus over chest:

Fremitus is synonymous with 'palpable vibrations'. The different types are:

1. Vocal fremitus.
2. Friction fremitus (palpable pleural rub).
3. Rhonchial fremitus (palpable rhonchi; rhonchi are better felt than crepitations).
4. Tactile fremitus:
   a. Palpable coarse crepitations,
   b. Palpable subcutaneous emphysema,
   c. Palpable pericardial rub.

- Except the vocal fremitus, others are sometimes called as **'palpable accompaniments'**.
- **Vocal fremitus** is the palpation of laryngeal vibrations on the chest wall when the patient speaks some words repeatedly in a constant tone and voice (e.g. 'one, one, one', or 'ninety-nine, ninety-nine, ninety-nine'). Place the palm of the hand (thenar and hypothenar eminences) or the ulnar border of right hand over the intercostal spaces on the chest, comparing the corresponding areas on both sides **(Fig. 1.28)**. Always use the same hand for examining both the sides (use right hand). Avoid the area of cardiac dullness on left side and place the hand a bit laterally. Start from above downwards in the front, sides and back of the chest. For changes (diminished or increased) in vocal fremitus, see page 88, as causes for changes in vocal fremitus are exactly the same as that of vocal resonance. Nowadays, vocal fremitus is losing its importance.

Q. How cough is analysed at the bedside?

Cough is a violent expiratory blast which occurs against a partially closed glottis. It is the most important protective reflex of the respiratory tract. A cough can be a conscious, voluntary act or an uncontrollable, involuntary reflex. Clinical approach to cough is done by:

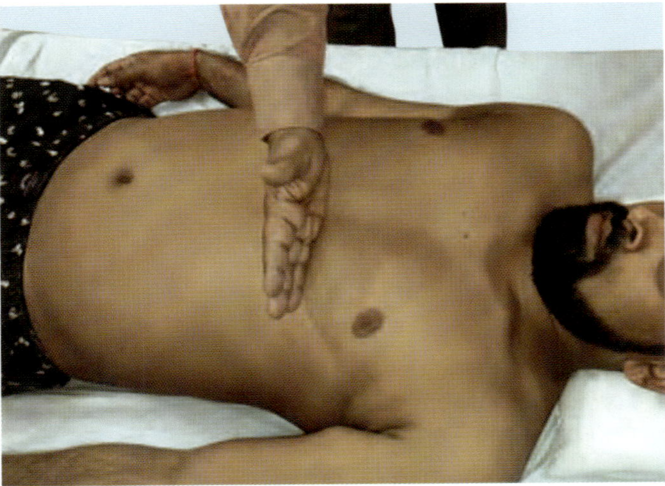

Fig. 1.28: Demonstrating **vocal fremitus**

1. Duration (days/months/years); acute <3 weeks, subacute (3–8 weeks), chronic >8 weeks.
2. Variability (daytime/nocturnal/morning, and seasonal or postural variation).
3. Precipitating or triggering factors (dust/fumes/pollen/cold air, lying down → gastroesophageal reflux disease or CCF) and relieving factors (e.g. cough suppressants).
4. Sputum analysis (*see* below), i.e. character of cough.
5. Types (dry/wet/bovine—see below).
6. Haemoptysis: Present or not.
7. Associated symptoms (post-nasal drip, gastro-esophageal reflux disease or occult asthma—these are common causes of long-standing, undiagnosed cough); wheezing? seasonal?
8. Chest pain (pleuritis) or breathlessness (COPD): Present or not.
9. H/o drug intake: ACE inhibitor, β-blocker, NSAID.
10. Presence of pre-existing disease, e.g. allergic rhinitis, bronchial asthma.

Q. Types of cough:

Analysis of cough to reach its origin is a major task of clinicians.

1. Dry (non-productive): Acute dry pleurisy, acute tracheobronchitis, interstitial lung disease (ILD).
2. Wet (productive): Bronchiectasis, lung abscess, resolution stage of lobar pneumonia.
3. Hacking (pharyngeal cough): Heavy smokers, chronic pharyngitis.
4. Whooping: In whooping cough, there is rapid succession of dry coughs which gather speed gradually and end in a deep inspiration during which the characteristic 'whoop' (noise) is heard.
5. Brassy (with a metallic sound): In carcinoma of larynx or tracheal compression.
6. Bovine (laryngeal cough): In recurrent layngeal nerve palsy, which is commonly due to bronchogenic carcinoma (the explosive nature of cough is lost); or in respiratory muscle paralysis.
7. Spluttering cough: In tracheo-oesophageal fistula (cough during swallowing).
8. Barking: Harsh and loud cough; found in epiglottitis, whooping cough and hysteria.
9. Nocturnal: Chronic bronchitis, LVF, tropical eosinophilia, post-nasal drip, aspiration.
10. Morning: Smokers, chronic bronchitis, bronchiectasis.
11. 'Croupy' cough: Laryngitis, especially in children.
12. Foetid cough: In bronchiectasis and lung abscess, there is foul smelling expectoration.
13. Paroxysmal cough: Chronic bronchitis, whooping cough, foreign body inhalation and aspiration.
14. Nagging cough: Post-nasal drip, GERD, cough-variant asthma, ACE inhibitor-induced.
15. Recurrent cough since childhood: Cystic fibrosis, childhood asthma, congenital heart disease, cystic disease of lung, hypogammaglobulinaemia.

16. Long duration cough: Pulmonary tuberculosis, bronchial asthma, ILD, COPD, bronchogenic carcinoma.
17. Cough with postural variation (postural cough): Bronchiectasis, lung abscess, gastroesophageal reflux disease (GERD), bronchopleural fistula.

- Stimulation of parietal pleura (e.g. during aspiration of pleural effusion or pleural biopsy) may induce cough.

18. Otogenic: Reflex dry cough from vagal stimulation by impacted wax or foreign body in auditory canal.

- Different causes of cough lie in respiratory (pharyngeal and laryngeal, tracheobronchial, lungs and pleural), cardiovascular, mediastinal or psychogenic illness. Reflex aetiology of cough is liver abscess or subphrenic abscess.
- Acute (URT infection, pneumonia, common cold), subacute (bronchial asthma) and chronic (COPD, bronchiectasis, pulmonary tuberculosis, smokers) cough—classified according to duration of cough. Cough is alarming when associated with haemoptysis, dyspnoea, chest pain, pyrexia or loss of weight.

Q. Profuse purulent sputum:

1. Bronchiectasis.
2. Lung abscess.
3. Sometimes, chronic bronchitis.
4. Empyema throacis ruptured into bronchus.
5. Tuberculous cavity.
6. Cystic fibrosis, resolving pneumonia.

- 1, 2 and 4 are causes of **profuse and offensive sputum.** Infection with anaerobic organisms and necrotising pneumonia also produce offensive sputum.
- Normal amount of tracheobronchial secretion in health is <100 mL/day. **Profuse sputum** (bronchorrhoea) means approximately a 'teacupful' (>100 mL) of sputum production per day, while a 'teaspoonful' expectoration per day is designated as **small sputum.**

Q. How sputum (expectoration or 'phlegm') is analysed clinically ?

1. Amount (profuse or scanty).
2. Character (serous, mucoid, purulent, mucopurulent).
3. Colour (yellow or green in bacterial infection, black in pneumoconiosis, rusty in lobar pneumonia, pinkish in LVF and anchovy-sauce in ruptured amoebic liver abscess into lung).
4. Odour or taste (offensive or not).
5. Mixed with blood (haemoptysis) or not.
6. Sputum production influenced by change of posture (e.g. bronchiectasis, lung abscess) or there is any diurnal variation (e.g. morning sputum production in bronchiectasis).

Q. How to palpate the trachea?

Normal position of trachea in a healthy person is **central** or slight deviation to the right side. The upper 4–5 cm of trachea, which lies in between cricoid cartilage and jugular notch, can be felt in the neck.

Steps (Fig. 1.29A):

1. Trachea should be palpated in standing (most preferable) or sitting position with arms placed symmetrically on two sides and chin held in the midline. Be gentle and explain what you are going to do. The patient may slightly flex his neck to relax the sternomastoids. **Trachea should not be examined in lying down position** unless the patient is very ill.
2. One may fix the head of the patient with his left hand. Standing in front of the patient (patient looking directly forward), place the right index finger on the cricoid cartilage (trachea starts from lower border of cricoid) and slide it down over the tracheal rings up to the suprasternal notch.
3. Now slide the index finger in the space between the sternomastoid muscle and trachea on both sides (never poke the finger, otherwise the patient may start coughing). **The space is narrowed and feels more resistant on palpation with deviation of trachea to that side.**

- It is better to have the patient's and examiner's head at the same level by proper adjustment (while sitting). Always exclude goitre (by inspection only) before palpating the trachea.

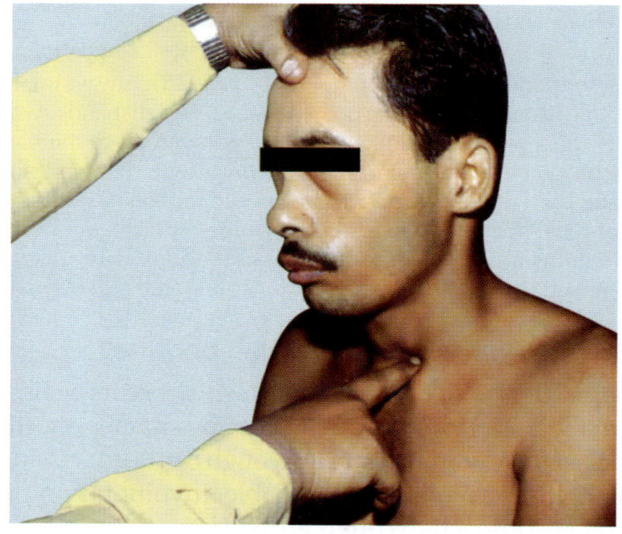

Fig. 1.29A: Palpation of the trachea in sitting posture

Q. Shifting of trachea and apex beat:

A. To same side (pull effect):

1. Fibrosis of the lung.
2. Collapse of the lung (absorption collapse).
3. Grossly thickened pleura.
4. Pneumonectomy.

B. To opposite side (push effect):

1. Pleural effusion.
2. Pneumothorax.
3. Hydropneumothorax.
4. Empyema thoracis.
5. Pyopneumothorax.
6. Haemothorax, haemopneumothorax.

- **Tracheal shifting is absent** in consolidation, emphysema, bronchial asthma, interstitial lung disease, bronchitis, bronchiectasis and lung abscess.
- **'Mediastinal shifting'** *means shifting of trachea (superior mediastinum) PLUS shifting of apex beat (interior mediastinum).* Trachea is commonly shifted in diseases of the upper part of chest (like shifting of trachea to same side in apical fibrosis or collapse) and predominantly apex beat is shifted in involvement of the lower part of chest (like shifting of the apex beat to opposite side in mild-to-moderate pleural effusion though a massive pleural effusion shifts the trachea too).
- Remember, mediastinum may be shifted in scoliosis.
- To summarise, **causes of displacement of apex beat** are LVH, RVH, mediastinal shift (pleuro-pulmonary diseases), thoracic deformity (e.g. scoliosis) and dextrocardia.

Q. How to differentiate dextrocardia from dextroversion?

In dextrocardia (congenital), heart is present in right hemithorax with apex pointing to the right while trachea remains central in position. In dextroversion due to extracardiac causes (e.g. left-sided pleural effusion or pneumothorax, or right-sided fibrosis or collapse of the lung), both trachea and apex beat will be shifted to the right.

To differentiate dextrocardia from dextroversion, always palpate the trachea.

Q. What is sternomastoid sign?

It is the undue prominence of lower part of sternomastoid muscle due to deviation of trachea to that side. This is also known as **Trail's sign**. It is a finding on inspection (Fig. 1.29B).

Q. Shifting of trachea without any lung pathology:

1. Severe scoliosis, straight back syndrome.
2. Enlarged lymph nodes on one side of neck.
3. Huge enlargement of one lobe of thyroid gland.
4. Aneurysm of the arch of aorta.
5. Any superior mediastinal growth (e.g. lymphoma).

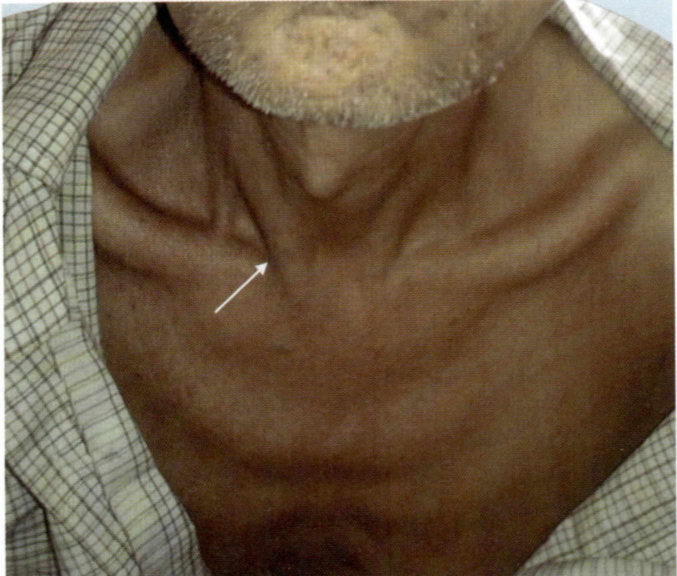

Fig. 1.29B: **Trail's sign.** The right sternomastoid seems prominent with deviation of trachea to the right side

Q. Elicitation of "coin sound":

It is classically found in pneumothorax (and rarely, in the 'pneumo' part of hydropneumothorax). Coin sound is mostly found in a **tense pneumothorax** (elicited by coin percussion) and is also known as bell sound, bell tympany, bruit-de-airain or 'distal anvil sound'. The bell-like sound resembles the sound of 'hammer on an anvil'. The clinical examination goes like this:

1. The observer stands at the back. A metallic coin (one rupee coin preferably) is placed over the upper part of front of the affected chest and is percussed with a similar type of coin when the observer listens at the back (just diametrically opposite to the point of percussion) with the diaphragm of stethoscope. A high-pitched tympanitic bell-like metallic sound (ringing sound) is heard in a patient with tense pneumothorax. It is necessary to compare the sound with the healthy side (which produces a dull thud as the normal lung does not transmit the ringing metallic sound distinctly). The patient helps here by fixing one coin in the anterior chest wall with his left hand and also by beating it with another coin with his right hand (Fig. 1.30A), Or
2. An alternative method: the patient fixes the diaphragm of observer's stethoscope over the anterior chest wall (observer stands at the back of the patient and throws the stethoscope over the patient's shoulder) while the observer himself puts a coin in the back and strikes it with the second coin. In these methods, one coin is acting as pleximeter finger while the other is serving the purpose of percussing finger (Fig. 1.30B).

- A lax or 'shallow' pneumothorax (left side) may give rise to **pneumothorax click**.

Q. D/D you will consider in this case:

A. **Causes of unilateral tympanitic or hyperresonant note with diminished breath sound:**

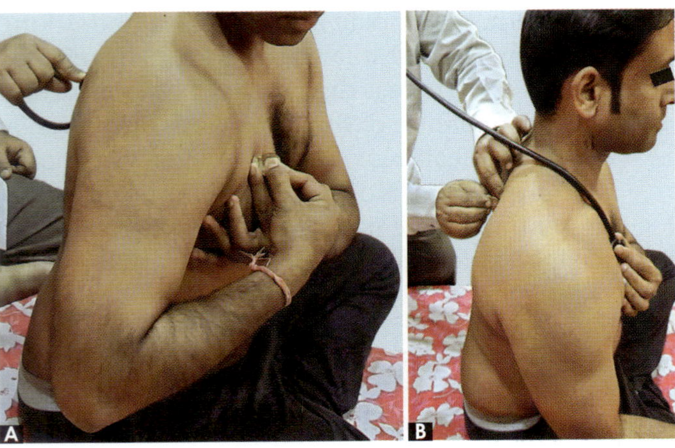

Fig. 1.30: A. Eliciting **coin sound**; B. Eliciting coin sound (alternative method)

1. Large emphysematous bulla: Symptoms of chronic bronchitis may be present. Large subpleural bulla (appear as avascular radiolucent areas with thin curvilinear wall in X-ray) may resemble pneumothorax.
2. Lung cyst: May be difficult to distinguish from pneumothorax (in contrast to pneumothorax, there is neither mediastinal shifting nor any collapsed lung at hilum in case of lung cyst).
3. Superficial, big, empty cavity (connected with a patent bronchus):
   a. Cavernous breath sound.
   b. Post-tussive suction.
   c. Post-tussive crepitations.
   d. Cracked-pot sound on percussion.

[4. Sliding hiatal hernia: May have chest pain, dysphagia, heart burn, respiratory distress due to nocturnal regurgitation. The whole chest is not tympanitic. Breath sound is not totally absent in the *left side of chest*.]

B. **Causes of chest pain with dyspnoea:**

1. Acute myocardial infarction: Occurs in middle aged or aged persons, retrosternal chest pain with radiation to left hand, drenching sweat and shock. Breathlessness with signs of heart failure may be found.
2. Acute pulmonary thromboembolism: Sudden onset of pain chest with dyspnoea, haemoptysis and circulatory collpase are present. Tachycardia, low BP, elevated JVP, RVgallop rhythm, loud P_2 are not uncommon. Normal resonant note on percussion over the chest with paucity of signs on auscultation. H/o prolonged recumbency or signs of deep vein thrombosis (DVT) in legs may be noted.
3. Trauma to the chest: H/o trauma, 'point of tenderness' may be detected. Normal resonant note on percussion. Typical findings of pneumothorax are lacking.
4. Acute dry pleurisy: Dyspnoea is not so common but chest pain is present. Pleural rub is audible and no sign of pneumothorax can be detected.
5. Dissection of aorta: Abrupt onset of tearing retrosternal chest pain and dyspnoea (mimicking acute myocardial infarction) with pain referred to the back. There is discrepancy between carotid pulses, difference of BP in two arms, arrhythmia, shock and features of acutely developing aortic incompetence. No sign of pneumothorax is present. The patient is commonly hypertensive or having Marfan's syndrome or in the third trimester of pregnancy.
6. Massive collapse of the lung: H/o aspiration of foreign body may be present. Mediastinal shifting is towards the side of collapse. Impaired resonance note is revealed on percussion over affected lung. Breath sound is diminished vesicular or absent (as bronchus is obstructed by foreign body).

Q. Complications of pneumothorax:

1. Hydropneumothorax.
2. Pyopneumothorax.
3. Empyema thoracis.
4. Haemopneumothorax.
5. Thickened pleura.
6. Circularoty collapse; acute respiratory failure.
7. Atelectasis of lung.
8. Surgical emphysema and pneumomediastinum.

Q. How do you like to investigate this case?

1. Chest X-ray (PA view): Done in **erect posture**. Sometimes, the X-ray is taken **after full expiration,** especially in a small pneumothorax. The radiological features are:
   a. Increased radiolucency on right side of the chest with absence of bronchovascular markings in that area.
   b. Collapsed right lung is seen as a homogeneous opacity with sharp outline (present paracardiac or paravertebrally).
   c. Shifting of mediastinum towards the left side.
   d. The left lung is showing mottled opacity in the apical area (signs of pulmonary tuberculosis): May be normal.
   e. Costophrenic angles are clear.

- Chest X-ray may reveal as little as 50 mL of air in pneumothorax. In supine X-ray chest, most of the air in pneumothorax acumulates in subpulmonic location.
- Remember, in large lung cyst or large bulla (mimics pneumothorax in chest X-ray) there is no mediastinal shifting.

2. CT scan of chest (most acurate imaging modality): To distinguish from bulla.
3. Blood: TC, DC, ESR (increased lymphocytes with high ESR point towards tuberculosis).
4. Mantoux test: Positive in tuberculous aetiology.
5. Sputum for AFB for consecutive 2 days (RNTCP) along with culture for *M. tuberculosis*.
6. Lung function tests: FEV_1, FVC, PEFR, etc. (to detect underlying emphysema, COPD, etc).

Q. Management of pneumothorax:

1. Small pneumothorax (less symptoms): The air gets absorbed spontaneously within few days and no treatment is required. The patients with underlying lung disease (COPD) cannot tolerate even a small pneumothorax and in that case air must be removed. Small pneumothorax needs close observation with serial radiographic monitoring.
2. Large pneumothorax or tension pneumothorax: O_2 inhalation at 8–10 litres/minute with propped-up position. A self-retaining catheter is inserted into the pleural cavity (in sitting position) *in the 2nd ICS along the MCL (preferable)*, or in the 4th or 5th ICS behind the anterior axillary fold (more comfortable for the

patient and cosmetic for a female patient though not used routinely). The tube is now connected to a water-seal drainage system. If no bubbling of air within the bottle is seen for 24 hours, or the patient is relieved of dyspnoea, or the chest X-ray shows complete re-expansion of lung, the tube is removed. The whole process takes approximately 3–4 days.

3. Recurrent spontaneous pneumothorax: Chemical pleurodesis is done by intrapleural instillation of kaolin, talcom powder, minocycline, 50% glucose solution, iodised oil, etc. Alternatively, parietal pleurectomy or pleural abrasion may be tried. Smoking should be stopped.
4. Antituberculosis chemotherapy, whenever indicated. Sometimes, antibiotics are used to prevent secondary infection; antibiotics are always used in open type.
5. Surgery:
   a. Thoracoscopy and cauterisation of the breach in the pleura, or excision of the bulla.
   b. VATS with pleurectomy and pleural abrasion (in recurrent type when pleurodesis fails).
   c. Decortication and closure of bronchopleural fistula, lobectomy or thoracoplasty.

- Surgery is usually required for open type (cauterisation of the opening, or open thoracotomy and direct closure of fistula). Open thoracotomy is needed in failure of the lung to re-expand after 5–7 days, or bilateral pneumothorax, or recurrent pneumothorax. VATS is video-assisted thoracic surgery.
- The rate of reabsorption of air is about 1.25% of the total radiographic volume per day and thus, a 50% pneumothorax (occupying 50% of hemithorax) will take 40 days to resolve totally.
- **Points to be remembered:** Small pneumothorax with <20% collapse of the lung needs no active treatment, while pneumothorax with >33% collapse of the lung and tension pneumothorax need urgent treatment.

Q. Immediate management of tension pneumothorax:

It is an acute medical emergency and if not managed immediately, death may occur.

a. O_2 inhalalation and propped-up position.
b. Do not wait for the chest X-ray, and immediately insert a wide-bore needle (16 G, BD needle) into the pleural space through the 2nd ICS at MCL (in sitting position). If large amount of gas escapes from the needle (with an audible hissing sound), the diagnosis is confirmed and the patient gets relieved. The needle should be left in place until an intercostal tube drainage with water-seal drainage system can be arranged at the earliest opportunity. If the tension penumothorax is dealt in this way, circulatory collapse (cardio-respiratory embarrassment) can be prevented. If hydropneumothorax is developed, a seperate drain is introduced at a lower level to drain the fluid.
c. Treatment of shock, haemodynamic instability (e.g. tachycardia, hypotension) and circulatory collapse, if present (tension pneumothorax → mediastinal shift plus severe hypoxaemia → diminished venous return → inadequate cardiac output) is done accordingly.

Q. Water-seal drainage: Whether working properly or not?

The tube coming out from the pleural cavity should be placed under water. Exit-tube (for air) will always remain above the water level in the bottle. Look for bubbling of air in the water. The whole channel is patent and working if:

1. During each expiration or coughing, more bubbling occurs, and
2. During inspiration, water column ascends within the tube, which remains under water.

- The bottle should be kept below the level of thorax. If the water-seal drainage is required to continue for more than a week, the tube should be removed (always remove after clamping it) and a new tube is attached (the then may change the site of insertion in the chest).

Follow-up—look for bubbling of air in the water present in the bottle, blockage of the tube by kinking or clot, tube malposition, and retrograde flow back into the chest.

Q. Reasons behind failure of the lung to re-expand in due time:

1. The lung is trapped, or
2. A major bronchus is obstructed, or
3. Presence of bronchopleural fistula, or
4. Water-seal drainage is not working properly.

Q. Will you advise any respiratory exercise?

Yes. The patient is advised to inflate incentive spirometer, air pillows, balloons or football bladder, which will help in expansion of the collapsed lung. Before discharge from hospital, the patient is advised not to smoke, and must stop to fly or dive for 3 months.

Q. Basic treatment strategy in pneumothorax:

1. Closed type: Observation, water-seal drainage if necessary
2. Open type: Water-seal drainage system, treat hydropneumothorax or pyopneumothorax. Consult thoracic surgeon. Treat with proper antibiotic.
3. Tension type: Always tackle this medical emergency by water-seal drainage system.

Clinical Wisdom

PLUS, Antituberculosis chemotherpy, if indicated.

Q. Pneumothorax is seen in X-ray plate: will you treat ?

Presence of any one of the following is an indication to initiate treatment.

1. Dyspnoea.
2. Cyanosis.

3. Gross mediastinal shifting.
4. Pneumothorax occupying >50% of hemithorax.
5. With underlying lung disease (e.g. COPD).
6. Circulatory collapse.

Immediate treatment by intercostal tube drainage with underwater seal is necessary.

Q. Describe the antituberculosis drug (ATD) treatment:

It is the standard practice for patients with pulmonary and lymph node disease:

A. Short course chemotherapy **for 9 months** with three drugs regimen:
   1. Rifampicin: 450 mg/day, if <50 kg and aged; 600 mg/day, if >50 kg.
   2. INH (isoniazid): 300 mg/day.
   3. Ethambutol: 25 mg/kg/day or
      Pyrazinamide: 20–35 mg/kg/day (maximum 2.5 g) or
      Inj. streptomycin (IM): 1 g/day, if >45 kg; and 0.75 g/day, if <45 kg.
      'Initial phase' for 2 months with 1+2+3, and 'Continuation phase' for 7 months with 1+2.

B. Short course chemotherapy **for 6 months** with four drugs regimen (standard regimen):
   1. Rifampicin: 450 mg/day, if <50 kg and aged; 600 mg/day, if >50 kg.
   2. INH (isoniazid): 300 mg/day.
   3. Ethambutol: 25 mg/kg/day.
   4. Pyrazinamide: 20–35 mg/kg/day (maximum 2.5 g).

'Initial phase' for 2 months with 1 + 2 + 3 + 4, and 'Continuation phase' for 4 months with 1 + 2.

Clinical Wisdom

If ethambutol has to be continued after 2 months for any reason (like rifampicin toxicity, etc.), the dose will be 15 mg/kg/day. Bone tuberculosis should be treated for 9 months while tuberculous meningitis should receive treatment for 1 year. All the drugs should be taken in empty stomach and in single daily dose. Pyridoxine 10 mg/day is added to prevent peripheral neuropathy induced by INH.

Q. Corticosteroids in tuberculosis:

As steroids reduce inflammation and limit tissue damage, steroids are now recommended in patients with tuberculous affection of the following though opinion differs from clinician to clinician:

1. Pleural effusion (some cases).
2. Pericardial disease.
3. Meningeal disease (reduces adhesions) or CNS tuberculosis.
4. Endobronchial disease (especially in children).
5. Extensive pulmonary disease.
6. Genitourinary tuberculosis.
7. Ophthalmic disease.
8. Hypersensitivity antituberculosis drug reactions.
9. Laryngeal or adrenal tuberculosis (Addison's disease).
10. Phlyctenular keratoconjunctivitis.

Steroids should always be given under cover of antituberculosis chemotherapy. If corticosteroid is given alone, tuberculosis will spread all over the body.

Q. Common side effects of antituberculosis drugs (ATD):

ATDs are known for their varieties of adverse effects like:

- Rifampicin: Nausea, vomiting, red-orange urine, flu syndrome, hepatitis, vasculitis, thrombocytopenia.
- INH: Peripheral neuropathy, hepatitis, lack of mental concentration, psychosis, convulsions.
- Ethambutol: Optic neuritis, arthralgia, hypersensitivity (rare).
- Pyrazinamide: Hepatitis, anorexia, nausea, vomiting, gout, fever, rash.
- Streptomycin: Giddiness, loss of renal function, deafness.
- PAS: Nausea, vomiting, goitre, blood dyscrasia, hypothyroid, hepatic damage.
- Thiacetazone: Exfoliative dermatitis, gastrointestinal reactions, hepatitis.
- Cycloserine: Depression, psychosis, headache, somnolence, convulsions.
- Ethionamide or prothionamide: Nausea, jaundice, neuropathy, metallic taste in mouth.
- Kanamycin, amikacin, capreomycin, viomycin: Giddiness, loss of renal function, deafness.

- *First five drugs are 'first-line drugs' and others are 'second-line drugs'*. First four drugs are first-line essential drugs while streptomycin, rifabutin and rifapentine are first-line supplemental drugs.
- PAS is para-amino salicylic acid, and INH is isoniazid.
- Other drugs are: Rifabutin, rifapentine, bedaquiline, quinolones (ciprofixoacin, levofloxacin, sparfloxacin), macrolides (clarithromycin, azithromycin), amikacin, phenazines (clofazimine), linezolid, co-amoxyclav, different immunomodulators (cytokine immunotherapy).
- Rifampicin, streptomycin, INH and pyrazinamide are bactericidal drugs. Rifabutin and rifapentine are rifampicin-related ATDs. Newer ATDs are delamanid, pretomanid and sutezolid.

Q. What is DOTS?

Directly Observed Treatment Short-course (DOTS) chemotherapy is the backbone of Revised National Tuberculosis Control Programme (RNTCP) in India. It is the administration of potent antituberculosis regimens to a patient having tuberculosis, in an intermittent manner, under direct supervision. As poor adherence to therapy is responsible for prolonged illness, relapse and resistance, supervised therapy 3 times per week definitely improves compliance. For DOTS, the patients are divided into 3 categories (I, II and III). Nowadays, DOTS-plus strategy is adopted where prevalence of MDR-tuberculosis is high. Read DOTS in details from any standard textbook. From 2019, concept of category I, II and III are not followed.

In developing country like India, multi-drug resistance tuberculosis (MDR-TB) and extensively drug-resistant tuberculosis (XDR-TB) are very high. Tuberculosis is now a notifiable disease in India.

Clinical Wisdom

RNTCP was renamed as 'National Tuberculosis Elimination Programme (NTEP)' on 1st January of 2020 with a target to eliminate tuberculosis by 2025. The four strategic pillars to eliminate tuberculosis are 'Detect-Treat-Prevent-Build (DTPB)'. DOTS is an integral part of NTEP.

Q. Prognosis of pneumothorax:

It depends on:

1. Type of pneumothorax (closed, open or tension).
2. Amount of air present (indicates mediastinal shifting).
3. Underlying disease (emphysema, COPD).

It is important to remember that a small pneumothorax in an aged patient with COPD is more dangerous than a large pneumothorax in a young individual.

Conclusion

1. Always look for puncture mark, benzene stain or cotton seal in the upper chest (anteriorly or axilla). If a tube or catheter is seen with water-seal drainage system, the diagnosis of pneumothorax is obvious (sometimes, a hydropneumothorax may be present with water-seal drainage).
2. Shifting of mediastinum to the opposite side, diminished or absent breath sound with tympanitic note on percussion on the affected side are **cardinal points for diagnosis** (there is loss of liver dullness in right-sided pneumothorax and loss of cardiac dullness in left-sided pneumothorax).
3. Search for shifting dullness in the chest to exclude hydropneumothorax in all cases of pneumothorax.
4. Remember, breath sound may be absent in both pneumothorax and pleural effusion, and in that case percussion note is the only guide (pneumothorax—tympanitic, pleural effusion—stony dullness) for diagnosis. Never forget that bronchial breath sound may be audible at the upper border of moderate pleural effusion as well as in case of open pneumothorax (bronchopleural fistula).

HYDROPNEUMOTHORAX — CASE 10

Q. What is your diagnosis?

This is a patient of right-sided hydropneumothorax, probably of tuberculous in origin.

- Hydropneumothorax is collection of both fluid (lower part) and air (upper part) in the pleural cavity.

Q. What are the cardinal features of hydropneumothorax ?

The hallmark of diagnosis in hydropneumothorax are 3 'S':

1. Shifting dullness,
2. Succussion splash, and
3. Straight (horizontal) fluid level (upper limit of dullness is horizontal).

Q. Is there any other feature present?

1. In a sitting patient, the percussion note over air-containing upper part is tympanitic, and fluid-containing lower part is stony dull.
2. Tinkling sounds or metallic crepitations (especially after coughing) heard by stethoscope in upper chest—due to shifting of drops of fluid falling on main bulk of fluid.
3. Positive coin sound in upper chest (rare).

Q. Why do you say hydropneumothorax?

One of the common aetiology of hydropneumothorax in the day-to-day practice is secondary infection of an open type of pneumothorax, or sympathetic collection of fluid in closed or tension pneumothorax. Thus, the patient will have **symptoms** like:

a. Dyspnoea.
b. Pain chest.
c. Splashing sound during jolting.
d. Cough.
e. Heaviness in the chest.
f. Pyrexia.

The physical **signs** in hydropneumothorax are more or less similar to pneumothorax. While eliciting the signs mentioned above, one should be careful about (to differentiate from pleural effusion):

A. During percussion:

i. There is horizontal fluid level (so called Ellis's S-shaped curve in pleural effusion, if any), and
ii. Shifting dullness (absent in pleural effusion).

B. During auscultation, one should search for:

i. Amphoric breath sound (bronchial breathing): As bronchopleural fistula is a common cause of hydropneumothorax (pleural effusion rarely may have bronchial breath sound),
ii. Succussion splash (absent in pleural effusion).
iii. Tinkling sounds (absent in pleural effusion), and
iv. Positive coin sound in upper chest (absent in pleural effusion).

So, describe the symptomatology and signs with special reference to above points to prove the rationality of your diagnosis.

Q. Aetiology of hydropneumothorax:

1. Rupture of a subpleural tuberculous focus or cavity (commonest cause).

2. Rupture of subpleural lung abscess (staphylococcal): Bronchopleural fistula.
3. Chest injury (penetrating).
4. Acute pulmonary infarction.
5. Following cardiac surgery.
6. Cystic disease of the lung.
7. During aspiration of fluid in pleural effusion (Iatrogenic).
8. Secondary infection of pneumothorax, especially after water-seal drainge.
9. Pneumonia, COPD, malignancy.

- No. 2 produces pyopneumothorax (pus and air), and No. 3 haemopneumothorax (blood and air).

Q. How shifting dullness is elicited?

Due to the presence of free fluid and air within the pleural cavity, dullness (fluid) shifts from one place to other within chest with the change of posture of the patient (similar mechanism as ascites). The clinical method is:

1. In **sitting position** of the patient, percussion is done in the conventional method in *anterior chest wall* along the MCL. In hydropneumothorax, the lower part of the affected chest will be stony dull and the upper part tympanitic.
2. Now the percussion is done in **lying down position** when the fluid gravitates in the dependent part and the air comes in front. Percussion along the MCL in anterior chest wall in lying down position will elicit tympanitic resonance all over the anterior chest. So, the lower part of anterior chest which was dull on percussion in sitting position becomes tympanitic in lying down position, i.e. dullness shifts.
3. The same procedure can be done along midaxillary line (MAL) in the *lateral chest wall* in sitting position, and then the patient is asked to lie down in lateral decubitus position (with healthy side downwards) for repetitions of percussion (findings are same as 1 and 2 above).

- Alternative method: Few clinicians follow this manoeuvre. First, percussion of the *back* is done in sitting position of the patient (while the lower part will be stony dull and upper part tympanitic) and the patient is then instructed to bend forward in the same sitting position. Percussing again in the back, after few seconds, will reveal tympanitic note over whole of the back of the patient as fluid goes more anteriorly by forward bending.

Q. Demonstrate succussion splash (Hippocratic succussion) in chest:

By the method of percussion, the upper border of dullness is detected in the lateral chest wall along the MAL, in sitting position of the patient. Now the diaphragm of stethoscope is placed on the air-fluid level and the patient is shaken from side to side vigorously. A splashing sound (like splashing sound of intact coconut) is audible with every jerk. Sometimes, the sound can be heard without the help of stethoscope (unaided ear, i.e. ear placed over the chest wall and the patient is shaken from side to side). The stethoscope may also be placed in the anterior or posterior chest wall at the air-fluid level to demonstrate succussion splash. The splash is absent if the fluid is thick or loculated. Succussion splash in the chest is always pathological and is found in:

1. Hydropneumothorax, pyopneumothorax or haemopneumothorax.
2. Herniation of stomach in the thorax.
3. Rarely, over a large cavity in the lung partially filled with exudate.

Q. How to elicit the horizontal fluid level?

This is classically found in hydropneumothorax. In sitting position of the patient, percussion is done from above downwards in the front (along MCL), lateral chest wall (along MAL) and back (along scapular line) in the conventional method. During percussion from above downwards, a point of dullness is reached in the front, lateral chest wall and back where markings are given by the skin pencil. Now, these three points are joined transversely and a horizontal line is drawn encircling the affected chest wall. This is the upper horizontal border of fluid level.

Clinical Wisdom

Ellis's S-shaped curve in pleural effusion does not exist today. Actually, it is a radiological observation (highest level of fluid in axilla). Previously the lesson was that the highest level of dullness (elicited by percussion) is present in axilla (so called Ellis's S-shaped curve) though it is not true. The upper limit of fluid in pleural effusion is also horizontal like hydropneumothorax but it is not easily demonstrable.

In hydropneumothorax, the difference in the note of percussion (from above downwards, it is tympanitic to stony dullness) is very distinct and clear cut in comparison to pleural effusion (from above downwards, it is resonant note to stony dullness). So the term 'horizontal fluid level' is classically used in hydropneumothorax.

Q. What is midclavicular line (MCL), midaxillary line (MAL) and scapular line?

One should be acquainted with the surface marking of these lines to examine the respiratory system properly.

- MCL: It is a vertical line drawn from the centre of the clavicle, i.e. *above*, the line is passing midway between the middle of the suprasternal (jugular) notch and the acromion process; the *lower* point is the midinguinal point (midpoint between anterior superior iliac spine and symphysis pubis).
- MAL: It is a vertical line drawn from axilla, which is midpoint between anterior and posterior axillary folds.
- Scapular line: It is a vertical line passing through the inferior angle of scapula.

Clinical Wisdom

In respiratory system, percussion and auscultation are done along these lines.

Q. From which ICS, the axilla starts?

The 4th intercostal space (ICS).

Q. Surface marking of 'root or hilum of the lung':

It is the space in-between the spine and vertebral border of scapula at the level of T_5, T_6 and T_7 vertebrae on both sides. In health, bronchovesicular breath sound is audible here.

Q. Purpose of percussion in clinical practice:

It is done to note the resonance or dullness of an organ, and also to know the:

1. Content (state of underlying tissue, i.e. whether solid organ, fluid or gas is present),
2. Contour (topographical percussion), and
3. Depth (usually by percussion, we get an idea upto a depth of 2 inches).

- Percussion indirectly diagnoses **tenderness over chest** (e.g. empyema thoracis, liver abscess, rib fracture, secondary deposits in ribs, osteomyelitis, costochondritis and Bornholm disease).
- A lesion of <2 cm diameter does not produce any change in the percussion note.

Q. Purpose of percussion over chest:

1. Conventional or general percussion.
2. Liver or cardiac dullness.
3. Coin percussion.
4. Shifting dullness.
5. Tidal percussion, and
6. Traube's space percussion.

Q. Three cardinal rules of percussion:

1. Percuss from resonant to dull area, or more resonant to less resonant area.
2. Pleximeter finger should be placed parallel to the border of the organ to be percussed and the line of percussion should be perpendicular to that arbitrary border.
3. Heavy percussion for deeply placed viscera (e.g. upper border of liver) and light percussion for superficial viscera (e.g. lower border of liver or lung).

- The art of respiratory medicine remains in performing 'percussion'.
- The method of percussion was first described by Leopold Auenbrugger (1722–1809) when he was a medical student. He (son of a wine-seller) acquired this art from his father, who used to percuss over the barrels of wine to know its fullness.

Q. How far can you go during conventional percussion in the chest?

In the MCL, MAL and scapular line, the **lower border of lung extends** upto 6th rib, 8th rib and 10th rib respectively. The **lower limit of pleura is present** two-spaces downwards than the lung (along those lines), i.e. at 8th rib, 10th rib and 12th rib, respectively. These are true in a patient with quiet respiration.

So, conventionally (as per anatomy is concerned) one should percuss:

1. Along MCL: Up to 7th ICS (the space just above the lower limit of pleura).
2. Along MAL: Up to 8th ICS (upper border of spleen lies at 9th rib).
3. Along scapular line: Up to 11th ICS (the space just above the lower limit of pleura).

Q. Basic principles for conventional percussion over the chest:

The art of percussion can be learnt only by experience and it goes like:

1. The dorsal aspect of middle phalanx of the middle finger of left hand **(the pleximeter finger)** is kept firmly over the chest wall without any airspace in-between (i.e. over intercostal spaces) and is struck suddenly with the tip of the middle finger of right hand **(the percussing or plexor finger)** perpendicularly (with "hammer effect")—mediate percussion. The entire movement is delivered from the right wrist joint (a loose swinging movement), and not from the elbow. Strike once or twice on the pleximeter finger (avoid repeated heavy striking). The other fingers of the left hand should not touch the chest wall.
2. **Ask the patient to sit.** Direct percussion is done over bones and indirect percussion for other areas. First percuss the clavicle (direct percussion) and then the anterior chest wall along MCL. *The first palpable interspace in anterior chest wall is 2nd ICS.* Keep the hands hanging by the side while percussing the **anterior chest wall along MCL.** During percussion of **axilla along MAL,** patient's hands are kept over the back of his head. While **percussing the back,** cross the patient's hands over the opposite knees or shoulders when the patient bends forward (this position wide aparts the scapulae), and percuss in a bat's-wing or fish-bone pattern. Lastly, **percuss the apex of the lung from the back** of the patient keeping the patient's hands hanging by the sides (read Kronig's isthmus from page 82). The front of the chest is more resonant on percussion than the back due to lesser bulk of musculature.
3. Always percuss from above downwards and compare the note on the identical site on the opposite side of chest. All the areas should preferably be percussed in sitting position of the patient.

- While percussing the left side of anterior chest wall, always follow the left MCL (do not deviate laterally, because the most outer border of cardiac dullness lies 1/2 inch inside the left MCL). One may start percussion from apparently healthy side, or the right side of the chest (if it is not possible to detect the diseased side from history). Use light percussion for anterior chest and heavy percussion for posterior chest wall (as thick muscles are there at the back). Percussion is done over ICS and thus never percuss over ribs.

- On the left side, while percussing the anterior chest wall from above downwards, there is a transition from resonant note of lung to tympanitic note of stomach, while on the right side lung resonance changes over to liver dullness. It is wise to hear as well as feel the purcussion.
- Sternum is percussed directly (like clavicular percussion) to assess mediastinum (page 410).

Clinical Wisdom

The art of percussion should be learned by relentless practice at the bedside. The students are advised to percuss over a hollow cupboard (hyperresonant), wooden piece (dull), and then over a solid brick wall (stony dullness) to get confidence.

Q. Format of percussion over the chest (Fig. 1.31A and B):

A. Anterior chest wall—Along MCL:

1. Over the clavicle (direct percussion)
2. Infraclavicular area (clavicle to 3rd rib)
3. Mammary area (3rd to 6th rib)
4. Inframammary area (6th rib to 7th ICS, or lower costal margin)

Both the sides of the chest should be percussed with special reference to:

Right side	*Left side*
• Conventional percussion	• Conventional percussion
• Shifting dullness	• Shifting dullness
• Liver dullness	• Cardiac dullness
• Coin percussion	• Coin percussion
• –	• Traube's space percussion

B. Lateral chest wall (right and left side)—Along MAL:

1. Axillary area (4th ICS to 6th rib)
2. Infra-axillary area (6th rib to 8th ICS, or lower costal margin)

C. Posterior chest wall (right and left side):

1. Suprascapular (above the spine of scapula): Percussion is done from medial to lateral side keeping pleximeter finger vertically parallel to spine over suprascapular area.
2. Interscapular (between the medial border of scapula and spine → T_2 to T_7 vertebrae → in a 'fish-bone pattern' percussion from above downwards keeping pleximeter finger obliquely).
3. Infrascapular (below the inferior angle of scapula → T_7 to T_{11} vertebrae: *Along scapular line* from above downwards keeping pleximeter finger obliquely).

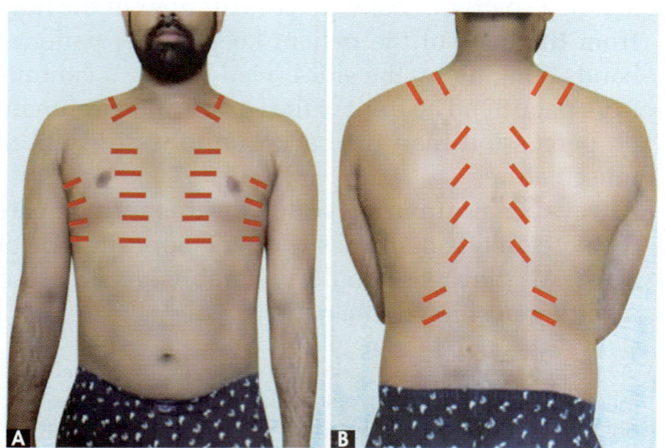

Fig. 1.31A and B: Areas of **percussion over chest**—front and sides (axillae) (A) back of chest (B)

D. Apical (or supraclavicular area): Always done from the back (read "Kronig's isthmus")—Right and left side.

Q. How to count the ribs and ICS in clinical practice?

First place the right index finger in the suprasternal (jugular) notch and then go downwards till the **sternal angle** (angle of Louis) is felt as a transverse bony ridge (junction of the body of the sternum and manubrium sterni). If the finger is moved sideways, it will touch the 2nd ribs. Now count the ribs with ICS from above downwards.

Posteriorly, the ribs and ICS are counted from below upwards (difficulty faced in a muscular body or in an obese patient). If the arms rest by the side of the body, the inferior angle of scapula lies at the level of T_7 vertebra (or the 7th rib)—this may be of some help in counting ribs or ICS in the back.

- **Angle of Louis** or sternal angle corresponds with the disc space between T_4 and T_5 vertebrae posteriorly, and anteriorly it is the landmark for tracheal bifurcation. It also corresponds to the upper border of right atrium and thus regarded as a 'reference point' to measure the jugular venous pressure (JVP).

Q. Traube's semilunar space and its importance (Fig. 1.32):

This is a triangular space or semilunar topographic area in the left lower chest anteriorly which is bounded by:

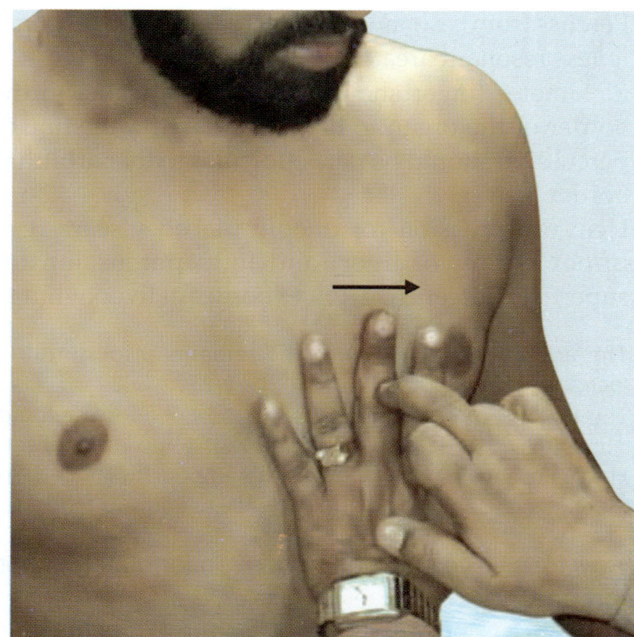

Fig. 1.32: Percussion of **Traube's space**

Laterally: Left midaxillary line.
Above: Left dome of diaphragm and left lung, i.e. the left-sided 6th rib.
Below: Left lower costal margin.

Detection: The triangle is percussed in a supine (or sitting) patient with left arm abducted during normal breathing, across one or more level from its medial to lateral margin, i.e. from xiphisternum to left midaxillary line across 6th and 7th intercostal space keeping the pleximeter finger parallel to lett sternal border **(Barkun's method)**.

Importance: Normally the space is tympanitic on percussion as **it contains the fundus of stomach**. The tympanicity of Traube's space (after Ludwig Traube) is lost in:

a. Carcinoma involving the fundus of stomach or full stomach.
b. Left-sided pleural effusion.
c. Enlarged left lobe of liver.
d. Massively enlarged spleen or ruptured spleen.
e. Situs inversus totalis (Traube's space is present on the right side).
f. Achalasia cardia (often the fundal gas is absent).

- Traube's space is shifted upwards in fibrosis or collapse of the left lower lobe of lung, and left-sided diaphragmatic palsy. Traube's space tympanicity is retained in pericardial effusion.
- Percussion of the Traube's space is a useful screening test for splenomegaly (specificity of 75%).

Q. Upper border of liver dullness—Clinical detection and possibilities of shifting:

To delineate the upper border of liver dullness, perouss the anterior chest wall along right MCL from above downwards. Normally the **upper border of liver dullness is present in right 5th ICS at MCL.** It is:

A. Lowered or obliterated:

1. Emphysema.
2. Pneumothorax (right-sided).
3. Perforation of abdominal hollow viscus, e.g. perforation of peptic ulcer.
4. Chilaiditi's syndrome (interposition of colon between liver and diaphragm: An anatomical variation).
5. Cirrhosis of liver (liver becomes shrunken).
6. Visceroptosis of liver (i.e. downward displacement of abdominal viscera).
7. After laparotomy or laparoscopy (pneumoperitoneum induced by CO_2).

B. Elevated:

1. Amoebic or pyogenic liver abscess.
2. Subdiaphragmatic abscess (right).
3. Diaphragmatic palsy (right).
4. Pleural effusion (right).
5. Basal pneumonia (right).
6. Increased intra-abdominal tension due to ascites or pregnancy.

- *The upper border of liver dullness is present in right 7th and 9th ICS when percussed along midaxillary and scapular line respectively.*
- The upper border of liver dulluess can not be delineated in right-sided pleural effusion.

Q. Where do you beat in clavicular percussion?

Traditionally it is a **direct percussion** (clavicle acts as pleximeter finger) done by right middle finger,

i. Over the most prominent part of clavicle, or
ii. Over the medial 1/3 rd of the clavicle.

During percussion, stretch the overlying skin downwards with the left thumb so that the percussing finger does not slip over the clavicle. It is a light percussion. Few clinicians advise to place pleximeter finger over clavicle to reduce pain while percussing.

Q. What is tidal percussion (Fig. 1.33)?

In health, while percussing during delineating the 'lower border of lung', there is difference in resonance by one space in full inspiration. It happens to be due to the downward movement of diaphragm and tidal percussion demonstrates diaphragmatic movement. Today, in the era of imaging facilities, this crude method has little practical value and is only of historical interest. The clinical method goes like this:

The patient will sit with hands crossed over the knees or shoulders. First **percuss the lower back** along the scapular line at the end of forced expiration and then percuss the same place at the height of full inspiration. Note the increase in resonance by one space after full inspiration. The clinical importance lies in:

1. Paradoxical resonance, i.e. there is dull note on inspiration and resonant note on expiration due to paradoxical movement of diaphragm in 'diaphragmatic palsy'.

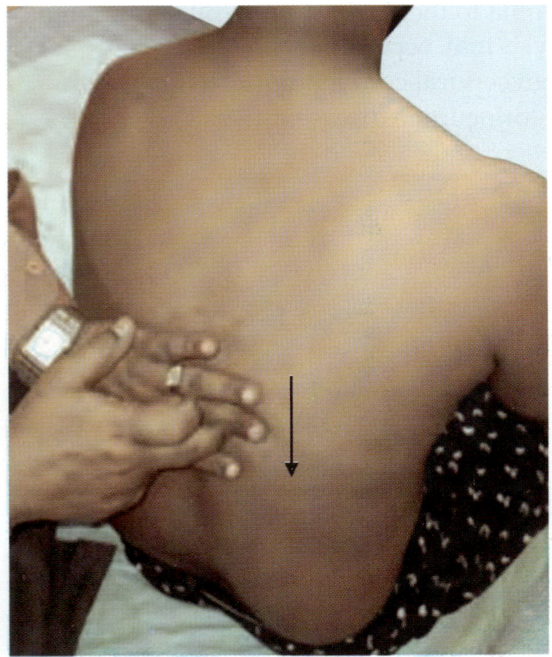
Fig. 1.33: Method for **tidal percussion**

2. Dullness which does not change on inspiration or expiration indicates basal pneumonia, basal pleurisy (or pleural effusion) or subdiaphragmatic abscess.

Q. What is Kronig's isthmus?

It is a small area (a band of resonance of 5–6 cm width, connecting the lung resonance on the anterior and posterior chest on each side) in the apex of the lung (supraclavicular area) which is bounded:

Medially: By neck muscles, and laterally: By the ipsilateral shoulder joint,

Anteriorly: By the clavicle, and posteriorly: By the trapezius muscle.

Kronig's isthmus is elicited by percussion over the apex of the lung (**percussion done from the back** of the patient), where the note is normally resonant. The area becomes dull on percussion in the presence of apical tuberculosis, Pancoast's tumour or apical pneumonia. *The pleximeter finger should be placed over the supraclavicular fossa, across the anterior border of trapezius, perpendicular to the clavicle* (Fig. 1.34).

- The apices of lungs rise about 2–3 cm above the clavicle on both sides.

Q. What is percussion myokymia?

In some chronic wasting diseases, e.g. pulmonary tuberculosis, if a light tap is applied over the chest (on the sternum or near the sternum), it may produce transient twitching of pectoral muscles for few seconds as a result of undue irritability. This phenomenon is also known as 'myotatic irritability'.

Q. Diagnosis of diaphragmatic palsy:

Unilateral paralysis is more common than bilateral paralysis. Unilateral paralysis commonly results from tumour (bronchogenic carcinoma), birth injury, surgery or trauma to the mediastinum. Bilateral phrenic nerve paralysis may occur due to:

a. High cervical cord injury (C_3 to C_5).
b. Motor neurone disease.
c. Poliomyelitis.
d. Demyelinating disease.
e. Polyneuropathies (e.g. GB syndrome).
f. Bilateral involvement by mediastinal lesions.

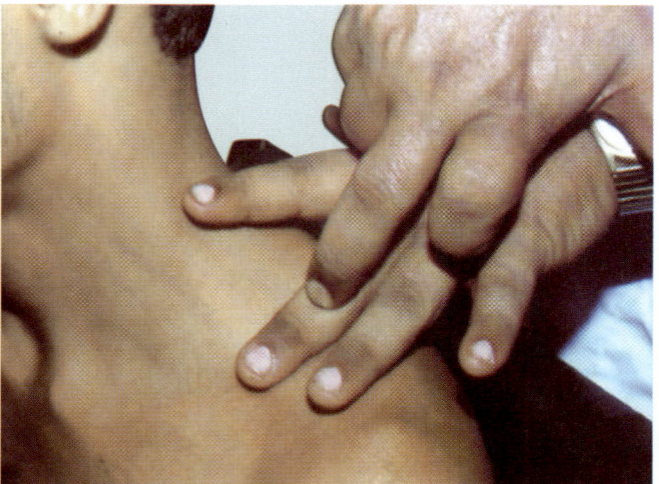

Fig. 1.34: **Percussion of the left apex** of lung from behind

Diaphragmatic palsy is diagnosed by:

1. Dyspnoea in supine posture.
2. Abdominal movement is less in comparison to thoracic movement.
3. As a whole the respiratory excursions in chest are diminished.
4. Tachypnoea may be present with intercostal suction.
5. **Paradoxical respiration:** Depression of abdomen with inspiration, and bulging with expiration. It is best observed in unilateral palsy and is known as 'see-saw movement' of abdomen.
6. Tidal percussion (see above).
7. Counting sign: Majority of healthy individuals can count up to 20 and beyond in one breath. Here the patient can not count aloud up to 10 in one breath (sometimes, it is seen that COPD patients can not count up to 20 in one breath; often it is observed that patient of myasthenia gravis starts counting normally but the voice becomes unintelligible after crossing 10).
8. Litten's sign: Absence of indrawing of subcostal margin during inspiration.
9. Elevated hemidiaphragm in chest X-ray, which is confirmed by fluoroscopy.
10. **Sniff test** (diagnostic on fluoroscopy): When the patient is asked to sniff, there is upward motion of the affected hemidiaphragm (the unaffected diaphragm descends). Sniff test can also be confirmed by USG.

- Patient with diaphragmatic palsy will have difficulty in sniffing—a rough test for assessing the integrity of diaphragm. Bilateral diaphragmatic palsy is a cause of sleep apnoea. Treatment is done by diaphragmatic pacing or nighttime assisted ventilation.
- Paradoxical inward movement of abdomen during inspiration (Hoover's sign) is a common feature in severe COPD.

Q. Put your hand over lower lobe of left lung:

Place your hand in the lower part of back of the chest on left side. Actually when seen **from behind,** mainly the lower lobes are seen while a small area near the apex is occupied by the upper lobes. When seen **from front**, the upper and middle lobes on the right, and the upper lobe on the left side occupy the most. When seen **from sides** (axillary region), parts of all the lobes are accessible.

Q. Absent shifting dullness in hydropneumothorax: is it possible?

Shifting dullness is absent in loculated or encysted variety of hydropneumothorax. A patient with small air and large fluid, or large air and small fluid may not have shifting dullness.

Q. Diagnosis of pyopneumothorax developed from hydropneumothorax:

1. Patient will be toxic and prostrated; loss of weight.
2. Hectic rise of temperature with rigors and sweating.
3. Tachycardia as well as tachypnoea.
4. Intercostal tenderness with fullness, and tenderness on percussion (patient winces with pain).
5. Skin is red, oedematous and glossy over lower part of affected chest.
6. Development of clubbing, *plus*
7. Signs of hydropneumothorax.

Q. D/D you will consider in your case:

1. Pyopneumothorax.
2. Pleural effusion.
3. Herniation of stomach in the thorax.
4. A large lung abscess partially filled with exudate.

Q. Clinical differentiation between pleural effusion and hydropneumothorax:

Theoretically there may be many differences but basic bedside dissimilarities are:

Pleural effusion:

1. Percussion note above the fluid level: Skodaic resonance.
2. Shifting dullness: Absent.
3. Coin sound in upper chest: Absent.
4. Succussion splash: Absent.
5. Classical horizontal fluid level: Present but difficult to demonstrate on percussion.
6. Breath sound and vocal resonance: Commonly diminished vesicular breath sound with diminshed vocal resonance is audible though bronchial (tubular) breath sound, bronchophony, aegophony and whispering pectoriloquy may be heard at the upper border of moderate effusion.

Hydropneumothorax:

1. Percussion note above the fluid level: Tympanitic.
2. Shifting dullness: Present.
3. Coin sound in upper chest: May be present.
4. Succussion splash: Present.
5. Horizontal fluid level on percussion: Easily demonstrated.
6. Diminished vesicular breath sound with diminished vocal resonance at the upper border of fluid level. There may be bronchial (amphoric) breath sound in bronchopleural fistula.

Q. How do you like to investigate this case?

The investigations will be done in the line of both pleural effusion and pneumothorax already described but the X-ray features will be different in hydropneumothorax.

Chest X-ray (PA view) in **erect posture** shows:

1. Horizontal fluid level on right chest.
2. Increased radiolucency above the horizontal level which is lacking in lung markings ('pneumo' component) and a homogeneous opacity below the horizontal level ('hydro' component).
3. Shifting of trachea and cardiac shadow towards the left side.
4. The left lung shows wooly opacities in apex (i.e. apical tuberculosis).

It is worthwhile to remember that in erect posture, the fluid remains below and the air above. The collapsed lung is usually hidden within the fluid and is not visible in X-ray (rarely, collapsed lung is visible paravertebrally).

Blood (R/E), sputum examination and Mantoux test are done routinely.

Q. How will you manage a patient of hydropneumothorax ?

1. Intercostal tube drainage through water-seal drainage system is applied as done in pneumothorax. The catheter is introduced in the *dependent part* in such a way that fluid can come out through the tube (special tube with multiple perforations like 'Romodrain') and the air is absorbed or expelled in due course of time.
2. Antituberculosis chemotherapy.
3. Proper antibiotics (in case of pyopneumothorax).
4. Surgery in resistant cases with pyo-or haemo-pneumothorax.

CONSOLIDATION OF THE LUNG — CASE 11

Q. What is your diagnosis?

This is a case of consolidation of the lower lobe of left lung.

Q. Why do you say so?

This patient is suffering from consolidation because there are presence of

A. Symptoms (from the history):

a. High fever with chill and rigor, sweating, fatigue and headache for last 5 days.
b. Harassing dry cough for 3 days.
c. Pain on the left side of chest, and dyspnoea for 2 days.

B. Signs:

1. *General survey:*
   a. Patient looks toxic and ill, but conscious and co-operative at present.
   b. Decubitus: Propped-up at 45°.
   c. Cyanosis: Absent at present.
   d. Respiration: 30/min, regular and predominantly abdomino-thoracic in type.
   e. Pulse: 90/min, regular (describe other paints in pulse).
   f. Pulse: Respiration: 3:1 (in health, it is 4:1).
   g. Herpes labialis: Present on left side; tonsils–WNL.
   h. Temperature (oral): 100°F at present.
   i. Neck stiffness: Absent (to diagnose meningism).

2. *Inspection:*
   a. Upper respiratory tract reveals no abnormality.
   b. Absence of intercostal suction but accessory muscles of respiration are working.
   c. Absence of fullness or flattening of chest wall in both the sides.
   d. Apical impulse: Seen below the left nipple, approximately 3" lateral to midline.
   e. Diminished movement on left side of chest, mainly the lower part of back and lateral aspect.
3. *Palpation:*
   a. Restricted movement on left side of chest.
   b. *Trachea and apex beat are normal in position (i.e. no mediastinal shifting).*
   c. Vocal fremitus: Increased on left side (lower part of lateral aspect and back mainly).
   d. Friction fremitus: Present in lower part of back, on the left chest (with local tenderness).
4. *Percussion:* Woody dullness on left side of chest (lower part), mainly at the back and lateral aspect. The outline of woody dullness is irregular and limited.
5. *Auscultation:* All the positive findings are present mainly on the left base (left infrascapular region).
   a. Tubular breath sound (high-pitched bronchial).
   b. Increased vocal resonance: Bronchophony and whispering pectoriloquy.
   c. Aegophony.
   d. Pleural rub.
   e. Absence of rhonchi and crepitations (as lung is solidified and liquefaction is yet to start).

- The right lung seems to be normal clinically. Characteristic rusty sputum may not be found.
- The surface marking of the dullness in consolidation and collapse follows the distribution of affected lobe which is not seen in pleural effusion. Features of acute dry pelurisy is present here.
- The involvement of lung in acute bronchopneumonia is usually patchy, bilateral and more widespread in lower lobes.

Q. Why do you say consolidation of the lower lobe?

The signs are predominantly present in the back and at basal region.

Q. Pathological "stages of pneumonia" with auscultatory findings:

There are four stages in the natural course of illness in pneumonia:

a. Stage of hyperaemia or congestion: Diminished vesicular breath sound with fine crepitations (indux crepitations)—24–48 hours.
b. Stage of 'Red Hepatisation' (2–4 days) }*
c. Stage of 'Grey Hepatisation' (4–8 days) }*
   *Classical features of consolidation described above.
d. Stage of resolution: Breath sound is vesicular or rarely bronchovesicular in type. Coarse crepitations are heard (redux crepitations): >8 days (usually 2–3 weeks).

- Respiratory symptoms and signs in consolidation are often absent in elderly, alcoholic, immunocompromised or neutropenic patients.

Q. Classification of pneumonia:

Pneumonia or 'consolidation' (synonym: pneumonitis) is defined as acute inflammation or exudative solidification of the lung parenchyma. Pneumonias are classified in a number of ways like:

a. Main classification (classification by aetiology):
   1. 'Primary' pneumonia [*Streptococcus pneumoniae* (most common), *Staphylococcus aureus, Haemophilus influenzae, Klebsiella pneumoniae,* etc.]—usually community-acquired (in normal healthy individuals).
   2. 'Secondary' pneumonia (occurs when the host is weakened):
      i. Acute bronchopneumonia, acute lobular or hypostatic pneumonia.
      ii. Benign aspiration pneumonia.
      iii. Suppurative or necrotising pneumonia (lung abscess): Commonly by *Staphylococcus aureus* and *Klebsiella pneumoniae*.
      iv. Hospital-acquired pneumonia (nosocomial).
      v. In immunocompromised host (*Pneumocystis jirovecii* infection in AIDS).

- Lung abscess may be a part of 'primary' pneumonia.

b. Empiricist's classification (most commonly used; classification by mode of acquiring):
   1. Community-acquired pneumonia (CAP) (*Streptococcus pneumoniae, Haemophilus influenzae*).
   2. Hospital-acquired pneumonia (nosocomial): Mainly by aerobic gram-ve bacilli, anaerobes.
   3. Pneumonia in immunocompromised host: *Pseudomonas aeruginosa, Pneumocystis jirovecii.*
c. Anatomical classification:
   1. Lobar (homogeneous consolidation of one or more lobes of lung).
   2. Lobular (bronchopneumonia, if bilateral).
   3. Segmental (benign aspiration pneumonia).
d. Aetiological classification:
   1. Infective: Bacterial, viral, rickettsial, yeast and fungi, protozoa (*Pneumocystis jirovecii*).
   2. Chemical agents: Irritant gases, aspiration of vomitus, kerosine oil, etc. (kerosine oil produces 'lipoid pneumonia').
   3. Physical agents: Irradiation.
   4. Hypersensitivity reaction: SLE, Stevens-Johnson syndrome, Loeffler's syndrome.
e. Radiological classification (classification by site):
   1. Alveolar or air space pneumonia (pneumococcal mainly): Air bronchogram in chest X-ray.
   2. Bronchopneumonia (*Haemophilus influenzae*, etc.): Atelectasis is seen in chest X-ray.

3. Interstitial pneumonia (virus, *Mycoplasma*, etc.): Reticular or reticulonodular pattern in chest X-ray.

f. Behaviorist's classification:
   1. Easy, and
   2. Difficult: non-resolving.

- Nowadays, ventilator-associated pneumonia (VAP) with MDR and non-MDR pathogens pose problem in treatment (MDR = multi-drug resistance). VAP is a subtype of hospital-acquired pneumonia (HAP).

Q. Characteristics of viral pneumonia:

The commonly responsible viruses are influenza, parainfluenza, varicella, measles and respiratory syncytial virus (RSV). A novel coronavirus is responsible for severe acute respiratory syndrome (SARS) pneumonia.

1. Constitutional symptoms like anorexia, headache, myalgia, malaise are predominant. Fever and toxaemia usually precede respiratory symptoms.
2. Cough may be absent initially and sputum is mucoid in nature.
3. Haemoptysis, pleuritic chest pain and pleural effusion are rare.
4. **Spleen may be palpable** in the first week; tachypnoea may be absent.
5. **Paucity of physical signs** in chest but may develop later and seldom gross.
6. WBC count is usually normal.
7. Chest X-ray: Usually does not correspond to lobes or segments, which is typical of consolidation. Reticular or reticulonodular patterns may be seen.
8. Usually self-limiting; there may be failure of rapid resolution or response with antibiotics.

Q. Absence of physical signs of consolidation in lobar pneumonia: is it possible?

Yes. The possibilities are:

1. Deep-seated consolidation.
2. Associated pleural effusion or empyema thoracis.
3. When the bronchus is not patent (exudate fills the bronchus along with the alveoli)—as seen in 'massive pneumonia' caused by *Klebsiella pneumoniae* (Friedlander's pneumonia).

- Sometimes in hypostatic pneumonia, the classical signs of consolidation are lacking.

Q. What is massive consolidation?

It is the consolidation involving more than one lobe.

Q. Appearance of physical signs of consolidation:

The physical signs usually appear within 2 days, and usually disappear within 2 weeks.

Q. Appearance of radiological signs of consolidation:

Opacity in X-ray appears within 12–18 hours of the onset of illness. Radiological opacity usually disappears within 4 weeks.

Q. How to suspect development of effusion with pneumonia?

Development of effusion with pneumonia is known as 'synpneumonic' pleural effusion. When the effusion appears after resolution of pneumonia, it is called 'postpneumonic' pleural effusion. Together, they are known as 'parapneumonic effusion'. These terms are going to be obsolete nowadays.

Persistence of fever, stony dullness on percussion and shifting of mediastinum to the opposite side make the clinician suspicious about the development of pleural effusion. Radiology (obliteration of costophrenic angle in chest X-ray) further supports the diagnosis. These are simple exudative effusions.

Q. Causes of 'delayed resolution' of pneumonia:

Delayed resolution means when the physical signs persist for >2 weeks and the radiological features persist for >4 weeks after proper antimicrobial treatment. The possibilities are:

1. Inappropriate chemotherapy like incomplete treatment, suboptimal dose, wrong choice of antibiotics, drug resistance, irregular intake of drugs.
2. Complicated by pleural effusion, suppurative pneumonia or empyema thoracis.
3. Decreased host resistance (immunocompromised patient) like diabetes mellitus, chronic alcoholism, agranulocytosis, lymphoma, leukaemia, multiple myeloma, IV drug abusers, post-splenectomy, renal failure, corticosteroid or radiation therapy, chemotherapy, hypogammaglobulinaemia, AIDS, etc; elderly and debilitated patient.
4. Tuberculous pneumonia (needs specific anti-tuberculosis chemotherapy).
5. Partial obstruction of bronchus by a foreign body like dentures in the elderly or *bronchogenic carcinoma* (common in clinical practice).
6. Fungal or atypical pneumonia.
7. Pneumonia resulting from connective tissue diseases (e.g. SLE), pulmonary infarction, etc.
8. Recurrent aspiration in achalasia cardia or GERD.
9. Alternate diagnosis, e.g. pulmonary haemorrhage, pulmonary thromboembolic disease.

- **Common causes of 'non-resolution' of pneumonia** are inappropriate chemotherapy, bronchogenic carcinoma, aspiration of foreign body, diabetes mellitus (or immunocompromised host) or pneumonia caused by virulent organism (e.g. staphylococcal pneumonia).

Q. Possible causes of recurrent pneumonia:

Chronic bronchitis, SLE, multiple myeloma, diabetes, AIDS, recurrent aspiration in achalasia cardia or pharyngeal pouch or scleroderma, bronchiectasis, bronchial obstruction or bronchogenic carcinoma, cystic fibrosis, ciliary dyskinesia, hypogammaglobulinaemia, sequestration of the lung or foreign body aspiration.

Q. Is it possible to have shifting of trachea to the same side in pneumonia?

In pneumonia, trachea remains in the midline. Rarely, there may be same-sided shifting of trachea in massive pneumonia producing 'collapse-consolidation' (may be from bronchogenic carcinoma).

Q. Predisposing factors to pneumonia:

1. Cigarette smoking (strongest independent risk factor).
2. Upper respiratory tract viral infection, followed by *Streptococcus pneumoniae* infection.
3. Excess of alcohol.
4. Immunosuppression (diabetes mellitus, AIDS, corticosteroid therapy, chemotherapy).
5. IV drug abusers.
6. Bronchial obstruction (malignancy), bronchiectasis, aspiration from oesophageal obstructions.
7. Old age.
8. Severe liver disease, uraemia, COPD, postoperative (especially, abdominal operation).

- Sources of infection are from: Inhalation, aspiration, direct spread (e.g. intubation), haematogenous or from nearby focus of infection (contiguous spread).

Q. When will you advise hospitalisation in a patient of pneumonia ?

Hospitalisation is advised in:

1. Elderly patients (over 65 years of age) and with,
2. Severe dyspnoea with hypoxia (tachypnoea with respiratory rate >30/min).
3. Central cyanosis.
4. Fall of systolic BP (<90 mm of Hg) and diastolic BP (<65 mm of Hg).
5. Empyema, meningism, meningitis.
6. Altered mental status, delirium.
7. Shock.
8. Underlying serious cardio-pulmonary diseases, diabetes mellitus, uraemia.
9. Hypoxia (PaO_2 <60 mm of Hg), leucopenia (<4000/mm^3) or leucocytosis (>20000/mm^3, e.g. in empyema), high blood urea, or culture +ve pneumonia.

- The patient is referred to ITU (Intensive Therapeutic Unit) in No. 6, 7, 8, 9 and severe acidosis.
- Read the 'CURB-65 scoring' for pneumonia severity score from any standard textbook.

Q. What are the accessory muscles of respiration?

Normal muscles of respiration are intercostals (external and internal) and diaphragm. Accessory muscles are not required for respiration in health; they are required to assist breathing in respiratory embarrassment (e.g. acute severe asthma, COPD), and may therefore be active and prominent. They are:

1. Alae nasi (nasal flare).
2. Sternomastoid.
3. Scalenii.
4. Latissimus dorsi.
5. Trapezius.
6. Pectoralis major.
7. Serratus anterior.
8. Abdominal muscles (e.g. rectus abdominis).

Q. Common causes of 'intercostal suction':

Normally intercostal spaces expand and draw-out with inspiration. Intercostal suction is the drawing-in of the intercostal spaces with inspiration (prognostically worse) and is commonly seen in:

1. Foreign body within larynx or trachea.
2. Diphtheria.
3. Oedema of the glottis (in anaphylaxis).
4. COPD.
5. Bronchiolitis (in infants and children).
6. Bilateral diaphragmatic palsy.

- Intercostal suction is produced as a result of positive atmospheric pressure pressing the lower intercostal spaces in the face of increased negative intrathoracic pressure due to failure of air entry in respiratory tract from airway obstruction.

Q. What are the D/D you will consider in your case?

A. Pleural effusion:
   a. Gradual onset.
   b. Dry cough may be present; patient does not look toxic.
   c. **Mediastinal shifting to opposite side, stony dullness on percussion.**
   d. Diminished vesicular breath sound or absent breath sound with diminished or absent vocal resonance. Usually there is no added sound.

B. Collapse of the lung:
   a. Cause is detected from the history, e.g. aspiration, trauma, postoperative events, etc.
   b. Patient does not look toxic.
   c. **Mediastinal shift is towards the affected side**; flattening of chest and aggregation of ribs.
   d. Impaired resonance on percussion.

C. Bronchogenic carcinoma:
   a. Age is higher, male, smoker commonly
   b. Clubbing (even with HPOA).
   c. Cervical lymphadenopathy (hard).
   d. Emaciation.
   e. **Usually no shifting of mediastinum unless complicated by pleural effusion.**
   f. Localised crepitations over the mass. Features of SVC syndrome may be evident.

D. Pulmonary tuberculosis:
   a. Gradual onset of weight loss, anorexia, evening rise of temperature, night sweats.
   b. Physical signs are mainly present in apical region, if there are any.

c. Absence of high rise of temperature or rigor; longer history than pneumonia.
d. Classical signs of consolidation are absent.

E. Pulmonary infarction (thromboembolism):
a. Sudden onset of chest pain with dyspnoea.
b. Pyrexia is usually less.
c. There may be evidence of DVT in legs (Fig. 1.35).
d. Cough is not troublesome.
e. Patient is not toxic
f. Heamoptysis is much more common.

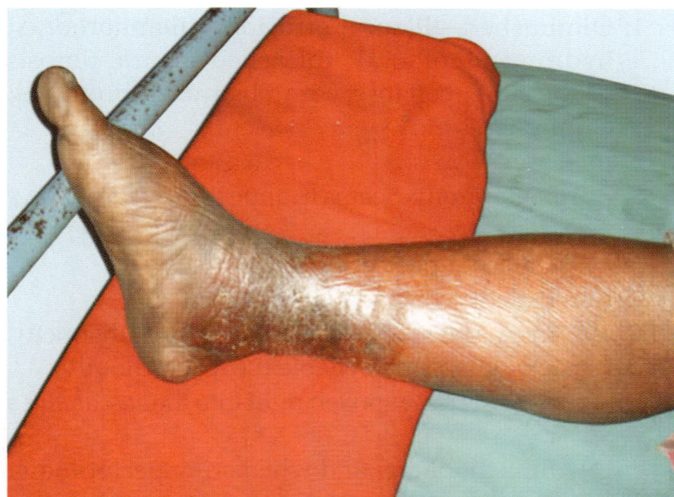

Fig. 1.35: **Deep venous thrombosis (DVT)** of calf muscles (with some eczematous changes in lower part of leg)

Q. Causes of haemoptysis (Table 1.10):

Coughing out of blood ranges from blood-streaking of sputum to frank blood.

A. Pulmonary:

1. Bronchitis (acute and chronic).
2. Plumonary tuberculosis.
3. Bronchiectasis.
4. Lung abscess.
5. Bronchogenic carcinoma.
6. Pneumonia (particularly, *Klebsiella*).
7. Pulmonary thromboembolism.
8. Lupus pneumonitis (i.e. from SLE).
9. Foreign body in bronchus or lung.

B. Cardiovascular:

10. Mitral stenosis (severe).
11. Acute left ventricular failure.
12. Primary pulmonary hypertension.
13. Eisenmenger's syndrome.

C. Coagulation disorder:

14. Haemorrhagic diathesis (leukaemia, haemophilia).
15. Anticoagulant therapy.

D. Miscellaneous:

16. Vasculitis (Wegener's granulomatosis).
17. Arteriovenous malformations.
18. Trauma (e.g. penetrating lung injury).
19. Aspergilloma ('fungus ball').
20. Goodpasture's syndrome.
21. After bronchoscopy/lung biopsy.
22. Systemic hypertension.
23. Pulmonary haemosiderosis.
24. Hydatid disease of the lung.
25. Idiopathic.

- No. 1, 2, 3, 5, 6, 10 are common causes of heamoptysis. *Worldwide, chronic bronchitis is possibly the commonest cause of haemoptysis*. **Recurrent haemoptysis** is commonly due to chronic bronchitis, bronchiectasis, bronchogenic carcinoma and pulmonary thromboembolism. Sources other than lower respiratory tract like nasopharyngeal bleeding or laryngeal carcinoma may be a cause of haemoptysis.
- Spurious haemoptysis: Bleeding from upper respiratory tract or oral cavity.
- Pseudohaemoptysis: Infection with Serratia marcescens, which produces a red pigment.

Q. What is massive haemoptysis?

Variably defined as 'coughing out of blood' in excess of 600 mL/24 hours is 'massive' one and potentially lethal and life-threatening due to combined effect of blood loss (haemodynamic decompromise) as well as asphyxia. Severe haemoptysis is >200 mL/24 hours.

Table 1.10: Bedside differentiation between haemoptysis and haematemesis

Features	Haemoptysis	Haematemesis
1. Definition	Coughing out of blood	Vomiting out of blood
2. Symptoms	Symptoms of pulmonary and CVS diseases	Symptoms of upper GI tract diseases
3. Content and colour	Blood is mixed with sputum, bright red in colour and 'frothy' from admixture of air	Blood is mixed with food particles, may be coffee-ground in colour
4. Premonitory symptoms	Premonitory symptoms like cough, salty sensation or tickling sensation in throat	Nausea, vomiting, retching, fainting, abdominal discomfort, perspiration
5. Melaena	Melaena does not occur (very very rarely may occur, if blood is ingested)	Usually followed by melaena on the next day
6. Amount	Relatively less; shock is rare	Huge in amount; patient may be in impending shock
7. Taste	Saline taste	Bitter taste
8. Reaction	Alkaline (blue litmus remains unchanged); pH normal like blood	Acidic (blue litmus turns red); pH is acidic

Q. Special signs in a 'cavity' within the lung:

Pulmonary cavity is an area of liquefaction necrosis within the lung (may remain empty or filled with secretion) and is usually communicating with a patent bronchus. The signs are:

1. Post-tussive crepitations (crepitations evoked by coughing due to dislodgement of thick cavitary fluid).
2. Post-tussive suction (high-pitched sucking sound audible during the phases of long inspiration following a bout of cough): Hallmark sign of a thin-walled superficial, compressible cavity connected with a patent bronchus.
3. Cracked-pot sound by percussion over (a tympanitic note) empty communicating cavity (mimics the sound produced by percussion over a broken earthenware vessel).

Q. Findings over a superficial, big, empty cavity connected with a patent bronchus:

Common signs are described below. Physical signs are absent in deep-seated cavity.

1. Slight reduction in chest movement on affected side.
2. Absence of mediastinal displacement.
3. Increased vocal fremitus.
4. Percussion: Hyperresonant or tympanitic note when filled with air (empty), impaired note when filled with exudate.
5. Cavernous breath sound (low-pitched bronchial) with bronchophony and whispering pectoriloquy.
6. Coarse crepitations (especially when filled with exudate); may be post-tussive.

Q. Common causes of pulmonary cavity:

1. Pulmonary tuberculosis (commonest), anaerobic infection in lung (lung abscess).
2. Lung abscess.
3. Necrotic degeneration of bronchogenic carcinoma (i.e. cavitating lung cancer).
4. Bronchiectasis.
5. Pseudocavity in large emphysematous bulla or lung cyst.
6. Wegener's granulomatosis, rheumatoid arthritis, pulmonary infarction, fungal cavity.

Q. Vocal resonance (voice sounds) and its classification:

A. Definition: This is the auscultation of laryngeal vibrations transmitted to the chest wall and nothing but the auscultatory homologue of vocal fremitus, or the resonance in the chest of sounds made by the voice.

B. Method of elicitation:

1. The patient will pronounce repeatedly syllables like 'one, one, one' or 'ninety-nine, ninety-nine, ninety-nine'.
2. The patient will speak in a constant tone and voice (the depth and intensity of voice remaining the same); the voice should be clear.
3. Both sides of the chest are auscultated area by area, **comparing with the corresponding site on the other side.** Auscultation starts from above downwards in the front, sides and back of the chest.
4. It is better to start from the apparently healthy side. Do not auscultate over clavicle, sternum and scapula.

C. Classification:

I. Quantitative change:

1. Diminished—Pleural effusion, pneumothorax, hydropneumothorax, thickened pleura, fibrosis of the lung, collapse with obstructed bronchus, emphysema, etc.
2. Increased—
   i. **Bronchophony:** Seems to appear from the *earpiece of stethoscope*.
   ii. **Whispering pectoriloquy:**
      a. Patient whispers.
      b. Increased sound is heard clearly or distinctly, i.e. syllable by syllable (i.e. pectoriloquy).
      c. It seems to be spoken right into the *auscultator's ear*.

      Bronchophony and whispering pectoriloquy are classically heard over consolidation. It is also heard in collapse with patent bronchus, over a superficial empty cavity, sometimes above the level of pleural effusion, and in an open pneumothorax.

II. Qualitative change:

Aegophony: This is a qualitative change in vocal resonance with nasal intonation mimicking the bleating of a goat. It is classically found over consolidation and sometimes, above the level of pleural effusion. Though the speech remains intelligible, the removal of low-pitched elements of the sound explains the nasal bleating quality of aegophony (i.e. there is selective transmission of high-pitched components of the sound).

- The mechanism of production of quantitative increase in vocal resonance and that of bronchial breath sound is same, and naturally both are present in a single patient.

Q. What is normal vocal resonance?

1. The sound seems to be produced at the *chest piece of stethoscope*,
2. Heard as indistinct rumble, and
3. Individual syllables are indistinguishable.

Q. What is bronchopneumonia?

It is the diffuse, widespread and patchy alveolar consolidation associated with bronchial and bronchiolar inflammation, usually affecting both the lower lobes. The children (as a complication of measles or whooping cough) and elderly (as a complication of influenza or bronchitis) persons are most vulnerable.

Q. Complications of pneumonia:

A. Pulmonary:

1. Delayed resolution.
2. Lung abscess or cavitation.
3. Pleural effusion.
4. Empyema thoracis.
5. Parapneumonic effusion.
6. Organising pneumonia.
7. Pyopneumothorax.
8. Pneumatocele.
9. Fibrosis of the lung, rarely.
10. Respiratory failure.

B. Neurological:

1. Mental confusion (psychosis).
2. Meningism.
3. Meningitis (rare).
4. Cerebral abscess.

C. CVS:

1. Myocarditis.
2. Endocarditis.
3. Pericarditis.
4. Peripheral circulatory failure.

D. GI tract: Meteorism (distended tense abdomen due to gaseous accumulation), hepatitis.

E. Musculoskeletal: Septic arthritis.

F. Septicaemia, herpes labialis, thrombophlebitis, uraemia, ARDS, multiorgan failure.

- Pneumatocele: Multiple thin-walled cyst-like lesions in staphylococcal pneumonia.

Q. What is atypical pneumonia?

These are a group of pneumonia which do not behave like lobar pneumococcal pneumonia **(typical pneumonia)** and do not respond to penicillin. This type of 'atypical' pneumonia is not severe and is caused by *Chlamydia psittaci* (psittacosis), *Coxiella burnetii* (Q fever), *Legionella pneumophila* and *Mycoplasma pneumoniae*. Predominent features are dry cough, constitutional symptoms (and as such more than respiratory symptoms), abnormality in chest X-ray inspite of lack of physical signs in chest.

Q. How will you investigate pneumonia?

1. Blood examination: TC, DC and ESR. TC shows polymorphonuclear leucocytosis. Persistence of leucocytosis signifies lung abscess or empyema formation, and absence of leucocytosis carries a bad prognosis (atypical pneumonia). Toxic granulation within the neutrophils indicates bacterial pneumonia. ESR tends to be high. HIV testing is done in selected cases.
2. Sputum examination:
   i. For identification of organism (with aerobic and anaerobic culture), and
   ii. Detection of sensitivity to antibiotics.

   Always an attempt should be made to establish a microbiological diagnosis, if possible. Administration of nebulised hypertonic saline often helps in expectoration. Many a time false-positive results come out (non-pathogenic organism from oropharynx). In our country, sputum should always be examined for identification of AFB. So, smear examination of sputum by both Gram and Ziehl-Neelsen stains, and culture and sensitivity test of sputum should be done.
3. X-ray chest (PA and lateral view): This is helpful for confirmation of diagnosis. Homogeneous opacity with air bronchogram is seen involving segments, part of a lobe or lobes of lung. Rarely, reticular patterns may be seen (viral, *Mycoplasma pneumoniae*). Pleural effusion or empyema may be present. Follow-up X-ray after 7–10 days is important to assess the response to therapy and for diagnosis of development of any complication.

   Sites of lung involvement in pneumonia are as follows: Right lung is involved more because of its continuity with the trachea; apical area is affected more in tuberculosis or *Klebsiella pneumoniae* infection; basal segments of lower lobes in standing or sitting-up position, and posterior segment of upper lobes and superior segment of lower lobes are mostly affected in a recumbent patient.
4. Blood culture: This is done in severe pneumonia (in hospitalised patients), especially when the sputum examination is negative. PCR tests are available for a number of pathogens.
5. Serological tests: For the diagnosis of *Mycoplasma pneumoniae, Coxiella burnetii, Legionella pneumophila* or viral infections; a four-fold rise in antibody titre repeated after 10 days suggests a recent infection. Pneumococcal antigen can be detected in pneumococcal pneumonia.
6. Biomarkers: Acute phase reactants like CRP and procalcitonin are elevated in the presence of inflammatory response, especially to bacterial pathogens. Detection of galactomannan antigen test in serum or BAL helps in diagnosis of *Aspergillus fumigatus*-induced pneumonia.
7. Nose and throat swabs: May be cultured for viruses or examined under electron microscope.
8. Pleural fluid: If there is formation of parapneumonic effusion, the fluid may be aspirated for microbiological examination.
9. Pulmonary function test (PFT), pulse oximetry and arterial blood gas (ABG) analysis: Usually hypoxia with hypocarbia is seen (type I respiratory failure). It is done in the management of seriously ill patients in anticipation of assisted ventilation.
10. CT scan of thorax, if an obstructing tumour in suspected.
11. Bronchoalveolar lavage (BAL) or transtracheal aspiration for microscopic examination and culture.

12. Bronchoscopy: May be done when there is evidence of an obstructing tumour or foreign body.
13. Lung biopsy (transthoracic, CT-guided or videoscopy assisted): Rarely needed. Sometimes, open lung biopsy is done in patients who are immunocompromised, e.g. *Pneumocystis jirovecii* infection in AIDS.

Q. Line of management of pneumonia:

1. *General:* Rest in bed, good nutritious diet (high calorie with plenty of fluids).
2. *Specific:* Antibiotics; usually given after sputum examination. If sputum is unobtainable or unhelpful, start with erythromycin 500 mg QDS, orally, or amoxycillin 500 mg TDS, orally. In hospital-acquired pneumonia and pneumonia in immunocompromised host, a third-generation cephalosporin should be started.
3. *Symptomatic (hospitalisation, wherever indicated):*
   a. O_2 inhalation in high concentration to all hypoxaemic patients.
   b. Cough suppression by methadone, pholcodine, etc. in harassing non-productive cough; otherwise, expectoration should be encouraged.
   c. Hydrocortisone for peripheral circulatory failure.
   d. IV fluid infusion for dehydration and hypotension.
   e. Warmth, counterirritants and analgesics (e.g. paracetamol or NSAIDs) for pleural pain. Opiates may be used with extreme caution in poor respiratory function.
   f. Inj. diazepam (use cautiously) for delirium.
   g. Assisted ventilation in respiratory failure.
   h. Postural drainage and chest physiotherapy in cases of suppurative pneumonia.
   i. Thromboprophylaxis: Low-molecular weight heparin (LMWH) with elastic stockings in legs to prevent DVT, if admitted for >12 hours.
4. *Prevention:* Pneumococcal vaccine taken for once in lifetime and is advised for adults >65 years, and in asthma, COPD, diabetes, uraemia, chronic liver disease, alcoholics, immunocompromised and asplenic individuals. Influenza vaccine is recommended to those who are at high risk of mortality from pneumonia (taken every year).

Conclusion

Mediastinum (trachea and apex beat) is not shifted in consolidation. Fever (may have chill and rigor), cough (initially dry and painful, later on productive), haemoptysis (rusty sputum or frank haemoptysis), gross anorexia, headache and bodyache, pleuritic chest pain, tachypnoea and herpes labialis with features of consolidation (typical pneumonia) are common mode of presentations.

The **hallmarks of diagnosis** are:

1. Absence of mediastinal shifting.
2. (Woody) dullness on percussion on the affected side.
3. Tubular breath sound, bronchophony and whispering pectoriloquy with aegophony on the affected side.

BRONCHIAL ASTHMA — CASE 12

Q. What is your diagnosis?

It is a case of bronchial asthma with recent acute paroxysmal attack.

Q. Why do you say so?

This patient is suffering from bronchial asthma because of the presence of:

A. Symptoms (from the history):

1. Cough with mucoid expectoration for last 2 years.
2. Respiratory distress for 2 years with acute exacerbation for last 3 days.

   [**H/o present illness:** Describe dyspnoea, fever, cough, chest pain, H/o oedema, seasonal variation, etc. if any; C/o wheezing and chest tightness during coughing. H/o exacerbation of cough/wheezing at night and after exercise, and improvement with bronchodilator (inhaler) therapy.

   Past history: Chronic exposure to dust and smokes. H/o repeated cough and cold in the childhood. Recurrent attacks of rhinorrhoea and angioneurotic oedema present. There is no H/o PND. He was admitted in hospital once in the past with same ailments.

   Personal history: Smoker (15 cigarettes/day for last 14 years) and bus driver by profession. Reported to have normal BP.

   Family history: Maternal uncles suffer from same type of respiratory distress].

- Family history regarding bronchial asthma, hay fever and eczema are important in respiratory system. Occupational history, e.g. exposure to coal mines, asbestos, silica dust, or H/o exposure to cotton dust, pollen, perthenium, feather, or pets (i.e. pigeon, parrot) should always be taken into account. In personal history, H/o allergy and atopy should be asked for. Drugs like β-blockers or aspirin can induce bronchoconstriction. For bronchiectasis, ask for H/o measles, influenza or whooping cough in childhood.
- 'Triggering factors' of asthma are childhood viral pulmonary infections, different allergens (e.g. pollen, dust-containing mite, cotton, etc.), exercise, cold air, emotional stress, exposure to pets, indoor pollution, cigarette smoke, aspirin/β-blockers, occupational dust and GERD.

B. Signs:

1. *General survey:*
   a. Decubitus: Propped-up at 45°. The patient is in respiratory distress but is conscious and oriented.
   b. Cyanosis: Absent at present.
   c. Neck veins: Within normal limit (neither engorged nor pulsatile).
   d. Polycythemia: Absent (present in patients with COPD).
   e. Respiration: 28/min, regular and without purse-lip respiration.

f. Temperature: 101°F (oral) at present.
g. Pulse: 92/min, regular, without any special character (describe all other points).
h. Flapping tremor: Absent (i.e. to exclude respiratory failure).

2. *Inspection:*
   a. Accessory muscles of respiration are working.
   b. Wheezing: Present
   c. Upper respiratory tract: Hypertrophied inferior turbinate; no nasal polyp seen.
   d. Indrawing of suprasternal and supraclavicular fossae without any intercostal suction.
   e. Shape of the chest: Normal.
   f. Respiration: 28/min, regular in rhythm and predominantly thoraco-abdominal in type.

❍ Severe bronchial asthma persisting from childhood may have 'pigeon chest'.

3. *Palpation:*
   a. Apex beat: Cannot be localised properly (due to overinflation of the lung).
   b. Trachea: In the midline (central). Tracheal tug: Absent.
   c. Movement: Both the sides are moving simultaneously and symmetrically, and the expansion of chest is 2″ (measured by the tape).
   d. Vocal fremitus: Symmetrically reduced all over the chest (bilaterally and uniformly).
   e. Rhonchial fremitus: Present.
4. *Percussion:*
   a. Resonant (or hyperresonant due to overinflation) note all over the chest (bilaterally and uniformly).
   b. Liver dullness: Present at right 5th ICS at right MCL.
   c. Cardiac dullness: Within normal limit.
5. *Auscultation:*
   a. Vesicular breath sound with prolonged expiration present all over the chest.
   b. Vocal resonance: Diminished uniformly all over the chest.
   c. Adventitious sounds:
      i. *Sibilant (high-pitched), polyphonic biphasic rhonchi (more marked on expiration) scattered all over the chest.*
      ii. Coarse crepitations at the lung bases.
      iii. Absence of pleural rub.

❍ With the history, symptoms and signs, bronchial asthma is basically a clinical diagnosis.

Q. Describe the 'breathlessness' (dyspnoea) in your patient (Table 1.11):

1. Acute respiratory distress for last 3 days though he is suffering from mild to moderate breathlessness from time to time for last 2 years. He is a chronic smoker.
2. This attack is paroxysmal, and is probably precipitated by respiratory tract infections.
3. Exertional at present. MMRC scale?
4. H/o seasonal variations (increased in winters).
5. Associated with wheezing.
6. Associated with cough and there is production of mucoid expectoration.
7. No H/o pain chest.
8. No H/o PND.
9. The disease was stationary for last 2 years (non-progressive).
10. Breathlessness used to relieve by inhaled drugs (bronchodilators) and taking rest.

Q. What do you mean by wheezing and stridor?

A. Wheezing:

1. High-pitched musical sound heard from a distance (especially heard by bed-partner at night).
2. *Better heard in expiratory phase.*
3. Indicates small airways obstruction.
4. Usually associated with rhonchi in the chest.

Clinical associations:

a. Bronchial asthma (most classical).
b. Chronic bronchitis (or COPD).
c. Tropical eosinophilia.
d. Cardiac asthma.
e. Carcinoid syndrome.
f. Endobronchial disease (neoplasm).
g. GERD with aspiration.
h. Toxic gas inhalation.

Table 1.11: Modified Medical Research Council (MMRC) dyspnoea scale

Grade	Degree of breathlessness related to activities
0	Breathessness only on strenuous exercise
1	Short of breath when hurrying on level ground or walking up a slight hill
2	Walks slower than persons of same age on the level because of breathlessness
3	Stops for breath after walking about 100 yards or after a few minutes on level ground
4	Too breathless to leave the house, or breathless while dressing, undressing or washing

❍ Actually, try to assess the severity by asking to what extent the lifestyle is affected. MMRC dyspnoea scale determines the gradation of **respiratory dyspnoea**. NYHA classification is for **cardiac dyspnoea**.

Clinical Wisdom

Bronchial asthma is associated with reversible wheezing whereas COPD with irreversible one.

B. Stridor:

1. Low-pitched crowing or croaking sound (loud) heard from a distance.
2. *Better heard in inspiratory phase.*
3. Indicates partial larger airways obstruction like larynx, trachea and major bronchus.
4. Very common in children.
5. *Laryngeal stridor is a medical emergency* and urgent respiratory support may be required.

Clinical associations:

a. Foreign body inhalation in larynx or trachea.
b. Laryngeal oedema (angio-oedema from anaphylaxis).
c. Laryngeal diphtheria, whooping cough.
d. Vocal cord palsy due to *recurrent laryngeal nerve paralysis* (other features of recurrent laryngeal nerve paralysis are bovine cough and hoarseness of voice).
e. Croup (acute laryngotracheobronchitis).
f. Acute epiglottitis.
g. Paratracheal and subcarinal lymph nodes pressing over main bronchi (e.g. bronchogenic carcinoma).
h. Laryngismus stridulus in tetany.
i. Rapidly progressive laryngomalacia, papilloma of larynx.
j. Subglottic involvement from Wegener's granulomatosis.

Clinical Wisdom

Stertor: Noisy breathing due to partial barrier in air passages at naso-oropharyngeal level; at laryngeal level–**stridor**, tracheal level–**rattling noise**, and small airways (bronchial) level–**wheezing**.

Q. Classify respiratory disorders:

a. Obstructive ventilatory defect: Bronchial asthma, COPD, bronchiectasis, cystic fibrosis; FEV_1 is grossly ↓, VC↓ or normal, and FEV_1/VC↓.
b. Restrictive ventilatory defect: Pleural diseases, interstitial lung disease, alveolar diseases, neuromuscular disorders (myasthenia gravis, GB syndrome), thoracic cage abnormalities (severe kyphoscoliosis, ankylosing spondylitis, obesity); FEV_1 is slightly ↓, VC ↓↓, and FEV_1/VC normal or ↑.
c. Obstructive + restrictive ventilatory defect: Bronchiectasis, sarcoidosis, hypersensitivity pneumonitis.

Q. What is 'bronchial asthma'?

It is a chronic inflammatory disorder of the airways where the tracheobronchial tree shows increased responsiveness to multiplicity of intrinsic and extrinsic stimuli, producing 'reversible' airflow obstruction (due to muscle spasm, mucosal oedema and viscid secretion), and are characterised by paroxysm of dyspnoea, cough, tightness of chest and wheezing. Classically bronchial asthma has three characteristics like airflow limitation, airway hyperresponsiveness and bronchial inflammation. Bronchial asthma is of two types:

1. Episodic asthma (definite external cause is present): Early onset, extrinisic or atopic, and
2. Persistent or chronic form (no causative agent found): Late onset, intrinsic or non-atopic types.

Q. What is 'acute severe asthma'?

This condition was previously known as **'status asthmaticus'**. It is a severe airway obstruction where paroxysm of acute asthmatic attacks occur (i.e. exacerbation of asthma) without any remission in between and is not controlled by conventional bronchodilators within 24 hours. Remission is usually attained by the use of corticosteroid and sometimes, by respiratory assistance. This is a life-threatening attack of bronchial asthma and should be treated urgently. The clinical features are:

1. Severe dyspnoea (orthopnoea) with wheezing, tachypnoea, restlessness.
2. Active accessory muscles of respiration.
3. Unproductive cough in the presence of profuse bronchial secretions.
4. Profuse sweating.
5. Central cyanosis.
6. Tachycardia.
7. Pulsus paradoxus.
8. Inability to complete a sentence in one breath.
9. Diminished breath sound with minimal or absence of high-pitched polyphonic rhonchi: 'Silent chest' (airflow may be insufficient to produce rhonchi, and is a grave sign).
10. PEFR (peak expiratory flow rate) is <50% of predicted or patient's best.

- Drug-induced asthma: Asthma precipitated by certain drugs like β-blockers, aspirin or NSAID.
- Cough-variant asthma: Here the main symptom is dry cough instead of classic dyspnoea or wheezing.

Q. What are exercise-induced asthma and nocturnal asthma?

a. Exercise-induced asthma:

- Induced by exercise (the dry and/or cold air is the main trigger).
- There is increased execution of respiratory tract.
- Due to degranulation of mast cells.

b. Nocturnal asthma: There is overnight fall of FEV_1 of >20% due to airway cooling, low plasma cortisol at night, increase in vagal tone and decrease in catecholamines at night.

Q. How to assess the severity of bronchial asthma at the bedside?

Clinical parameters of life-threatening asthma are:

1. Exhaustion and unable to complete a sentence in one breath; inability to lie supine.
2. Confusion and diminished level of consciousness. Feeble respiratory effort.
3. Pluse rate > 120/min.
4. Pulsus paradoxus.
5. Central cyanosis.
6. Silent chest (ominous sign) on auscultation.
7. Hypotension.
8. Coma.
9. Unrecordable PEFR.
10. Arterial blood gas (ABG) analysis:
    - Normal or high $PaCO_2$ >5–6 KPa (37.5–45 mm of Hg) even with O_2 therapy.
    - Severe hypoxaemia, pO_2 <8 KPa (60 mm of Hg).
    - Low pH <7.2 or high H^+ concentration.

❍ It is said that tachypnoea and apparent distress may be misleading. In life-threatening asthma, there may be bradycardia and arrhythmia. No. 1, 2, 5, 8, 9 and 10 warrant assisted ventilation.

Q. What is chronic obstructive pulmonary disease (COPD)?

According to new definition as per GOLD 2023, it is a heterogeneous lung condition where there is chronic, persistent, often progressive obstruction to airflow (major site being the small airways) due to chronic bronchitis, emphysema, and chronic bronchiolitis (small airway disease). The airflow limitation is progressive and 'not fully reversible'. Often it is known as chronic obstructive lung disease (COLD) or chronic obstructive airway disease (COAD). The nearest D/D is chronic severe bronchial asthma.

COPD may be associated with number of co-morbidities, e.g. IHD, hypertension, diabetes, heart failure or malignancy, suggesting that COPD may be a part of generalised systemic inflammatory process. Systemic features of COPD are muscle wasting, weight loss and osteoporosis due to increased level of TNF-α in circulation.

❍ GOLD is Global Initiative for Chronic Obstructive Lung Disease.

Q. Risk factors for development of COPD (i.e. aetio-pathogenesis):

1. Environmental pollution, occupational exposure to organic and inorganic dust/chemical agents, indoor air pollution (e.g. fuel used for cooking and heating).
2. Cigarette smoking.
3. Genetic predisposition (e.g. α_1-antitrypsin gene, MMP-12 gene).
4. Infection.
5. Ageing, low birth weight and bronchial hyper-responsiveness.

Q. What are the alterations in breathing?

1. Dyspnoea: Abnormally uncomfortable subjective awareness of breathing. Dyspnoea is a subjective symptom and related to undue consciousness for the increased respiratory effort ('dys' means 'difficult, painful', and 'pnoia' means 'breathing').
2. Orthopnoea: Breathlessness in recumbent (lying down) position and is of such a degree as to make the patient sit upright for relief. The patient may sleep in a chair or uses some extra pillows at night (often quantified by number of pillows, e.g. 'two-pillow orthopnoea'). There is less efficient lung movement in lying down position, and sitting gives relief to the patient by helping in descent of liver with free diaphragmatic movement as well as diminishing the venous return in a failing heart.
3. Trepopnoea: Breathlessness only in left or right lateral decubitus position, most often in patients with heart disease (CCF); may be found in pleural effusion or pneumothorax while lying in lateral decubitus position with healthy side downwards.
4. Tachypnoea or polypnoea: Increased rate of respiration, e.g. >20/min is tachypnoea (normal respiratory rate in an adult is 14–18 breaths/min). Very high respiratory rate is observed in lobar pneumonia. Many a time, it is the only clue to shortness of breath or presence of respiratory disease.
5. Bradypnoea: Abnormaly low respiratory rate (e.g. <10/min) with slow breathing, commonly due to opium or morphine poisoning, increased intracranial tension, myxoedema coma, carbon dioxide narcosis, hypothermia, alkalosis, cardiac arrest, head injury, or respiratory centre abnormality.
6. Hyperventilation: Increased depth of respiration (ventilation in excess of metabolic needs).
7. Hyperpnoea: Increase in rate and depth of respiration (increased ventilation due to increased metabolic needs).
8. Platypnoea or orthodeoxia: Breathlessness only on assuming upright position, i.e. just opposite to orthopnoea. Though rare, it happens to be due to some cardiac diseases (e.g. left atrial myxoma or left atrial ball valve thrombus), massive pulmonary thromboembolism, pulmonary arteriovenous fistula, hepato-pulmonary syndrome or in selective paralysis of intercostal muscles.
9. Sighing respiration: It is functional in nature, and occurs mostly in young females and children. It is a shallow nervous breathing with intermittent deep inspiration punctuated by frequent sighs. It is found in the presence of relatives or parents, and never occurs during sleep or when the patient is unmindful; if associated with 'hyperventilation syndrome', the patient may complain of giddiness,

black-out, tingling of extremities, circumoral numbness, palpitations, and chest wall tightness with local tenderness elicited all over the chest. Restlessness, anxiety and panic attacks are common. Features of tetany (e.g. carpopedal spasm) may be manifested in some cases. Tachypnoea and occasionally tachycardia may be present. This type of hyperventilation returns to normal during sleep, and often associated with underlying anxiety or depression.

10. Cheyne-Stokes respiration: This is a form of periodic respiration where periods of apnoea (cessation of breathing for at least 10 seconds or more) rhythmically alternate with periods of hyperpnoea, each phase lasting for about 30 seconds, and the whole cycle is usually completed in less than 2 minutes. The rate and depth of respiration increase to a maximum (hyperpnoea), and then decrease when breathing virtually ceases (apnoea). The hypercapnoea (as a result of apnoea) stimulates brainstem centres resulting in hyperventilation drive, which washes out CO_2 resulting in depression of respiratory centre leading to apnoea. It is commonly seen in:
    a. Healthy infants, adults during deep sleep, in high altitude (physiological).
    b. Severe cardiac failure (acute LVF).
    c. Uraemia.
    d. Narcotic poisoning (opium, barbiturates).
    e. Increased intracranial tension (e.g. stroke involving the brainstem).
    f. Metabolic encephalopathy.
    g. Severe cardio-pulmonary embarrassment.
11. Kussmaul's breathing: Vide infra.
12. Stertorous breathing: Breathing with rattling noise in throat (i.e. fall-back of tongue, pharyngeal secretions), often seen in deep coma, deep sleep or in dying patients, is known as stertorous breathing.
13. Cogwheel breathing: An interrupted type of breathing pattern, seen particularly in nervous/anxious/weeping individuals.
14. Gasping respiration: Dying patients often take few deep, irregular and intermittent inspirations mimicking a 'fish out of water', is known as 'gasping' respiration. It is the terminal respiratory pattern of lower brainstem damage.
15. Apneustic breathing (lesion in lower pons): Deep, gasping inspiration with a pause of 2–3 seconds after full inspiration.
16. Ataxic respiration (lesion in medulla): Rhythm is chaotic, varying in rate and depth.
17. Paradoxical respiration: Diaphragmatic palsy, high spinal cord lesions.
18. Purse-lip respiration: Vide page 97.

- Major receptors in lung are: Stretch receptors, irritant receptors and juxtacapillary (J) receptors.

Q. Common causes of orthopnoea, tachypnoea, hyperpnoea and hyperventilation:

A. Orthopnoea:
1. CCF.
2. LVF.
3. Bronchial asthma.
4. COPD or interstitial lung disease (ILD).
5. Massive pleural effusion.
6. Pericardial effusion (cardiac tamponade).
7. Huge ascites.
8. Bilateral diaphragmatic palsy.

B. Tachypnoea:
1. Nervousness, exertion, anxiety.
2. Fever.
3. Acute lobar pneumonia, asthma.
4. LVF.
5. COPD (hypoxia).
6. Shock, ARDS; chest injury.
7. Acidosis (metabolic).
8. Hysteria.

C. Hyperpnoea:
1. Severe exertion, e.g. 100 or 200 meter race.
2. Metabolic acidosis (Kussmaul's breathing).
3. High altitude.
4. Severe aneamia.
5. Hysteria (panic attacks).

D. Hyperventilation:
1. Hysteria.
2. Pain anywhere in the body, fever, anoxia.
3. Anxiety neurosis.
4. Salicylate overdose.
5. Metabolic acidosis.

- **Bendopnoea:** This recently reported (introduced in 2014) novel symptom is defined as shortness of breath within 30 seconds while bending forward (e.g. bending over to tie a shoe), and is seen in heart failure.

Q. What is Kussmaul's breathing (air hunger)?

Deep sighing, rapid breathing at a regular rate and with a hissing sound (i.e. there is hyperpnoea with increased rate and depth of respiration) is known as Kussmaul's breathing. It (panting for breath) is commonly seen in metabolic acidosis and is also known as 'acidotic breathing'. The causes are:

1. Ketoacidosis (diabetes, alcoholic).
2. Uraemia.
3. Lactic acidosis.
4. Sometimes in hepatic coma.

Q. Features of upper airway obstruction (e.g. laryngeal oedema):

1. Restlessness with hyperactive accessory muscles of respiration.
2. Dyspnoea and even orthopnoea.

3. Cough (croupy cough in diphtheria).
4. Stridor.
5. Central cyanosis.
6. Intercostal suction.
7. Signs of exhaustion.

Q. Bedside diagnosis of advanced airflow obstruction (COPD or bronchial asthma):

1. Dyspnoea and even orthopnoea (sometimes with purse-lip breathing).
2. Hyperactive accessory muscles of respiration.
3. Reduction in the length of trachea palpable above the suprasternal notch (cricosternal distance).
4. Tracheal tug (tracheal descent during inspiration; if the **cricosternal distance**, i.e. the distance between suprasternal notch and the inferior border of cricoid cartilage is reduced to less than 3 finger breadths, it indicates hyperinflation of the lungs (e.g. COPD). Normally, the cricosternal distance is approximately 3–4 finger breadths)—also known as Campbell's sign. Vide also page 47.
5. Inspiratory excavation of the suprasternal and supraclavicular fossae.
6. Expiratory filling of neck veins.
7. Central cyanosis.
8. Intercostal suction.
9. Relative increase in antero-posterior diameter of the chest.
10. Wheezing.

- Characteristic 'tripod' position (patient sits with knee bending and flexed head placed in between knees) and Hoover's sign (paradoxical inward movement of rib cage with each inspiration) may be seen in advanced COPD.
- Facies in COPD: Anxious look with bluish discolouration of tip of the nose, lips and ear lobules with purse-lip respiration.

Q. How to assess 'respiratory depression' (e.g. opium poisoning) at the bedside?

1. Features of hypoxia (vide page 100).
2. Presence of central cyanosis.
3. Shallow respiration (expansion of the chest will be less).
4. Decreased respiratory rate (bradypnoea).
5. Diminished air entry in lungs (diagnosed by auscultation).

- **Hypoventilation** is regular, rhythmic and shallow breathing (may be due to brainstem defects, alveolar disorder, chest wall defects or massive obesity).

Q. Breath sound over compensatory emphysema:

Usually it is harsh vesicular. Compensatory emphysema is usually unilateral.

Q. Bedside diagnosis of emphysema (Table 1.12):

1. Asthenic body build with short and thick neck.
2. Barrel-shaped chest.
3. Purse-lip respiration (i.e. prolonged expiration through pursed lips).
4. Non-localisation of the apex beat.
5. Diminished chest expansion.
6. Diminished vocal fremitus.
7. Hyperresonant note on percussion bilaterally.
8. Loss of both liver and cardiac dullness.
9. Breath sound will be diminished vesicular with prolonged expiration.
10. Diminished vocal resonance.
11. Usually rhonchi and crepitations are absent. Sometimes, there is wheezy rhonchi.
12. Heart sounds: Distant (muffled).
13. Liver and spleen may be palpable due to descent of diaphragm.

- Added to these 13 points, there are features of 'advanced airflow obstruction' (question above).
- **Emphysema** is the permanent overinflation of air spaces in lung distal to terminal bronchioles as well as destruction of alveolar septae. Emphysema is of four types: centriacinar (more common), panacinar (less common), paraseptal, and scar or irregular. The most common cause is smoking.

Q. Adventitious sounds—Classification of crepitations:

Crepitations are discontinuous (<20 millisecond in duration), non-musical, bubbling or crackling (wet) sound produced by the passage of air through exudate-filled bronchi, bronchioles, alveoli, big cavity, or due to sudden snapping open of the relatively stiff alveoli at inspiration. The crepitations have a gurgling quality.

Table 1.12: Bedside differentiation of chronic bronchitis and emphysema

Features	Predominant chronic bronchitis	Predominant emphysema
Breathlessness	Mild-to-moderate	Severe
Cough	Develops before dyspnoea	Develop after dyspnoea
Cyanosis	More	Less
Oedema	Present	Absent
Sputum production	Profuse	Scanty
Respiratory tract infections	More common	Less common
Cor pulmonale	Common	Late and often terminal

A. Fine crepitations (end-inspiratory): Soft, high-pitched and <10 millisecond in duration, and is produced due to presence of exudate in the alveoli. The causes are:

1. LVF (at lung bases).
2. Fibrosis of the lung.
3. Indux crepitations of pneumonia (i.e. early stage of consolidation).
4. Fibrosing alveolitis or ILD **(velcro crepitations)**: See below for its mechanism of production.

- Velcro crepitations—sound resembles as if two strips of adhered velcro tapes are being seperated.

B. Coarse crepitations (biphasic): Louder, low-pitched and <20 millisecond in duration, and is produced due to presence of exudate in the bronchi, bronchioles, alveoli or big cavities. The causes are:

1. Acute bronchopneumonia.
2. Bronchiectasis or chronic bronchitis.
3. Lung abscess or pulmonary cavity.
4. Redux crepitations of pneumonia (i.e. resolution stage of consolidation).
5. Cystic diseases of lung.
6. Pulmonary oedema (often called 'death rattle' when occurs as a terminal event).

- Fine crepitations are known as crackling rales, while coarse crepitations as bubbling rales.

Q. Recent classification of crepitations:

The older term for crepitations is 'rales' and the new terminology for crepitations is '**crackles**'. Commonly, crepitations are described by the undermentioned **two points**:

1. To note their timing in relation to respiratory cycle, and
2. Whether they are affected by coughing or not. Crepitations heard in fibrosing alveolitis are due to sudden snapping open of the relatively stiff alveoli at the end of inspiration, and are uninfluenced by coughing. Crepitations in the presence of secretions is confirmed by the observation that they either disappear temporarily or reduce in number after coughing.

- Crepitations of LVF are often silenced by bending forward.

Q. What is post-tussive crepitations?

These are crepitations heard after coughing and may be diagnostic of superficial tuberculous cavity, early pneumonia or lung abscess.

Q. Types of crepitations in relation to phases of respiration:

a. Inspiratory:

1. Early: Chronic bronchitis, bronchiolitis.
2. Mid: Bronchiectasis, pneumonia.
3. Late: Fibrosing alveolitis, pulmonary oedema, lung abscess, cavity within the lung.

b. Expiratory: Severe airway obstruction, e.g. bronchial asthma.

c. Biphasic (both inspiratory and expiratory): Bronchiectasis, pulmonary oedema ('death rattle').

Q. Causes of bilateral basal crepitations:

1. LVF.
2. Bronchiectasis
3. Fibrosing alveolitis.

Q. D/D of 'crackling sound' over chest:

1. Crepitations.
2. Pleural rub.
3. Subcutaneous emphysema.
4. Rib fracture.
5. Gas gangrene.
6. Auscultation over hairy skin.
7. Pressing stethoscope in an uneven chest (over prominent ribs).

Q. Adventitious sounds—Classification of rhonchi?

Rhonchi are continuous (>250 millisecond in duration), uninterrupted musical (dry), whistling sound produced in the narrowed bronchi or bronchioles as a result of muscle spasm, collection of viscid secretion, mucosal oedema or narrowing by an endobronchial growth.

A. Old classification:

1. High-pitched rhonchi which are produced in smaller bronchi or bronchioles, and of squeaky quality is known as 'SIBILANT' rhonchi (end-inspiratory or early-expiratory): Found in bronchial asthma.
2. Low-pitched rhonchi which are produced in larger bronchi, and of snoring quality is known as 'SONOROUS' rhonchi (biphasic): Found in endobronchial growth affecting a large bronchus.

B. Recent classification:

1. ***Monophonic rhonchi:*** May be inspiratory or expratory or both, and may change in intensity with change of posture. It is produced due to narrowing of a single bronchus by tumour, mucus accumulation or foreign body (i.e. localised obstruction), which produces a single musical note.
2. ***Polyphonic rhonchi:*** Particularly heard in expiration and are characteristically found in diffuse airflow obstruction, e.g. bronchial asthma, chronic bronchitis or COPD. They denote dynamic compression of bronchi. This is the most common type of rhonchi where the musical sound (rhonchi) contains several notes of different pitch, and results from oscillation of many large bronchi at a time.

- It is preferable to call rhonchi as **wheezes** (new terminology).

Q. Common causes of rhonchi:

1. Bronchial asthma, COPD.
2. Wheezy bronchitis.

3. Cardiac asthma (LVF).
4. Tropical pulmonary eosinophilia.
5. Laryngeal oedema, foreign body or tumour obstructing bronchus (fixed monophonic).

Q. What is chronic cor pulmonale?

It is a condition where there is right ventricular hypertrophy with or without right ventricular failure resulting from diseases affecting the structure (i.e. lung parenchyma and vasculature) and/or function of the lung. This is also known as 'pulmonary heart disease' or heart disease secondary to disease of the lung.

a. *Disorders of lung parenchyma:* **COPD (commonest cause)**, bronchial asthma, pneumoconiosis, fibrosing alveolitis, scleroderma, etc.
b. *Diseases of pulmonary vessels:* Primary pulmonary hypertension, recurrent pulmonary thromboembolism, polyarteritis nodosa, etc.
c. *Disorders affecting movements of thoracic cage (i.e. affecting the function of the lung):* Severe kyphoscoliosis, ankylosing spondylitis, neuromuscular disorder like poliomyelitis, thoracoplasty, Pickwickian syndrome (hypoventilation with extreme obesity, may have obstructive sleep apnoea), etc.

Q. What is acute cor pulmonale?

It is synonymous with acute pulmonary thromboembolism where **right ventricle dilates with or without its failure**. As a result, acute pulmonary hypertension develops from massive pulmonary thromboembolism.

Q. Bedside features of chronic cor pulmonale:

a. Symptoms: Cough, expectoration, breathlessness (may not be relieved by sitting up), atypical chest pain, weakness, pedal swelling, excessive day time somnolence.
b. General survey:
    1. Orthopnoea or a stooping forward position in bed: Tachypnoea; purse-lip respiration.
    2. Central cyanosis.
    3. Pulse: Tachycardia, may be water-hammer in character; regular (mention all other points).
    4. Face: Dusky and plethoric (due to polycythemia).
    5. Hands: Warm and blue, may have flapping tremor.
    6. Neck veins: Engorged and pulsatile (RVF).
    7. Oedema: Bipedal pitting oedema (RVF).
    8. Engorged veins may be seen in the forehead.
    9. Nicotine staining of the finger (as commonly a smoker).
c. Inspection:
    1. Hyperactive accessory muscles of respiration with intercostal suction.
    2. Barrel-shaped chest with features of emphysema.
    3. Epigastric pulsation (RVH) (Fig. 1.17).
d. Palpation:
    1. Tracheal tug may be evident.
    2. Apical impulse may not be localised due to emphysema (outward apex—RVH).
    3. Palpable P_2 (diastolic shock)
    4. Left parasternal heave (RVH).
    5. Liver: Enlarged, soft and tender (RVF).
e. Percussion: Hyperresonant note all over the chest with loss of hepatic and cardiac dullness.
f. Auscultation:
    1. Diminished vesicular breath sound with prolonged expiration.
    2. Occasional rhonchi with or without coarse crepitations.
    3 Vocal resonance: Diminished all over the chest uniformly.
    4. Loud P_2.
    5. Right ventricular gallop (RVF) may be audible.
    6. Pansystolic murmur of TI is audible in high pulmonary artery pressure.

Actually, it is a mixture of signs of emphysema PLUS signs of pulmonary hypertension. Emphysema overshadows all the inspectory and palpatory signs in the chest, and one has to depend on **epigastric pulsation (RVH), engorged and pulsatile neck vein (RVF), and loud P_2 (due to pulmonary hypertension)** to diagnose a case of chronic cor pulmonale.

Q. Why a COPD patient purses the lips (Fig. 1.36)?

Pursing of lips during expiration helps the patient to maintain high intrabronchial pressure (i.e. to keep high end-expiratory pressure) above that within the surrounding alveoli (alveoli are overinflated or air-trapped in COPD) and thus prevents the collapse of bronchial walls by overinflated alveoli.

Q. Who is a 'blue bloater'?

In COPD patients with 'predominant chronic bronchitis', there is severe hypoxia with hypercapnia, pulmonary hypertension and RVF from the very early stage though

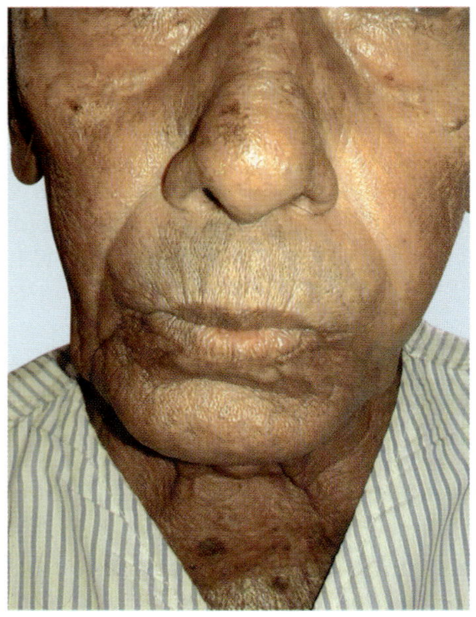

Fig. 1.36: **Purse-lip respiration** in COPD

the ventilatory capacity is well preserved. They suffer from cyanosis (blue), oedema (bloated) and thus known as blue bloaters. Cough with sputum production is the main feature while dyspnoea is less common. There is repeated episodes of RVF and respiratory failure.

Q. Who is a 'pink puffer'?

In COPD patients with 'predominant emphysema', there is gross impairment of ventilatory capacity and as a result they usually suffer from severe disabling exertional dyspnoea. They are not cyanosed at rest (so, pink) because the arterial O_2 is sufficient to saturate haemoglobin and usually try to blow off the excess CO_2 (puffer). They maintain a near-normal PaO_2 and $PaCO_2$. The occurance of RVF and respiratory failure are late and often terminal. The patient is usually lean and thin.

Q. Complications of COPD:

1. Recurrent pulmonary infections (very common).
2. Chronic cor pulmonale.
3. Spontaneous pneumothorax (due to rupture of emphysematous bulla).
4. Right ventricular failure (often a part and parcel of chronic cor pulmonale).
5. Type II respiratory failure.
6. Increased incidence of peptic ulcer.
7. Complications of chronic cough (*see* below).
8. Systemic symptoms: Decrease in muscle mass (sarcopenia), loss of weight, osteoporosis.

Q. What are the D/D you will entertain in your case?

1. Chronic bronchitis **(Table 1.12)**:
   a. Often a smoker, commonly male, usually overweight.
   b. Family history is absent.
   c. It is *defined as* chronic cough with expectoration on most days for at least 3 months in a year, for 2 or more consecutive years.
   d. Symptom-free childhood.
   e. Episodes of frequent respiratory tract infections.
   f. Copious mucoid sputum.
   g. Wheeze and rhonchi+.

- Chronic bronchitis is associated with chronic cough with expectoration (phlegm). A patient of *chronic bronchitis with acute exacerbation* presents with pyrexia, and persistent or recurrent mucopurulent sputum production.

2. Tropical eosinophilia:
   a. Nocturnal cough; breathlessness in a young patient.
   b. H/o urticaria, worm infestation.
   c. Absolute eosinophil count >3000/mm^3.
   d. High level of filarial antibody.
   e. Miliary mottlings in the chest X-ray.
3. Allergic aspergillosis:
   a. Episodic cough, wheezing and dyspnoea.
   b. Migratory densities in chest X-ray.
   c. Sputumn contains Aspergillus fumigatus.
   d. High eosinophil count in blood.
4. Cardiac asthma: Described in the section on 'Mitral stenosis' and **Table 1.13**.
5. Acute bronchopneumonia:
   a. No family history.
   b. Extremes of ages.
   c. Patient will be toxic.
   d. Fever; bilateral patchy involvement affecting mainly the lower lobes.
   e. Recently developing dyspnoea.

- D/D of **'acute severe asthma'** in clinical practice are acute LVF, acute exacerbation of COPD, ARDS, bronchiolitis and tension pneumothorax.
- **Recurrent bronchospasm** is classically seen in bronchial asthma, recurrent pulmonary thromboembolism, tropical eosinophilia, carcinoid syndrome (tumour), acute exacerbation of chronic bronchitis/emphysema,and cardiac asthma (acute LVF).

Q. Complications of bronchial asthma:

1. Acute severe asthma.
2. Recurrent bronchitis and pneumonia (from infections).
3. Atelectasis (collapse) of the lung or bronchiectasis (from mucous plugs).
4. Emphysema.
5. Pneumothorax (spontaneous).
6. *Complications of cough* like chest and abdominal wall soreness, exhaustion, headache, severe vomiting, rib fracture (especially in elderly with osteoporosis or multiple myeloma), cough syncope, spontaneous pneumothorax, subconjunctival haemorrhage, frenal ulcer, urinary incontinence; prolapse of rectum, hernia or uterus.
7. Chronic cor pulmonale and respiratory failure (in late stage).

Q. What is respiratory failure (Table 1.14)?

It is a condition which is characterised by abnormality in blood gases (PaO_2 <60 mm of Hg and/or $PaCO_2$ >50 mm of Hg). The normal arterial blood gases are no longer maintained and the lung function is inadequate for the metabolic needs of the individual. It is of four types (mainly types I and II):

1. Type I: Low PaO_2 with normal or low $PaCO_2$; also known as hypoxaemic respiratory failure. It is found in pulmonary oedema (acute LVF), pneumonia, ARDS (acute lung injury), bronchial asthma, fibrosing alveolitis, pulmonary thromboembolism, pneumothorax, hysterical hyperventilation.
2. Type II: High $PaCO_2$ with low PaO_2; also known as hypercarbic failure or 'ventilatory failure'. It is found in chronic bronchitis, emphysema, acute exacerbation of asthma or COPD, gross kyphoscoliosis, ankylosing spondylitis, trauma, neuromuscular disorders like

Table 1.13: Bedside differentiation between bronchial and cardiac asthma

Features	Bronchial asthma	Cardiac asthma (e.g. LVF)
1. Present history	Longer duration of breathlessness	Shorter duration of breathlessness
2. Past history	Allergy, rhinitis and atopy; past H/o similar attacks	No H/o allergy may have H/o IHD, hypertension or valvular heart disease
3. Family history	Often positive	Negative
4. Onset	Late night or early morning*	Early hours of night or midnight*
5. Age	Any age, usually young	Usually elderly
6. Clinical features	a. Scanty, mucold and tenacious expectoration b. Dyspnoea and distress + c. Signs > symptoms d. Wheeze +++ e. Cyanosis + + f. Perspiration: Less common g. Pulsus paradoxus h. BP: Usually normal i. Apex beat: Normal character j. There may be obliteration of liver and cardiac dullness k. RVH: May be present l. Heart sounds are muffled m. Rhonchi +++, crepitations + n. May have 'silent chest' o. Usually relieved by bronchodilators	a. Profuse, pinkish and frothy expectoration b. Dyspnoea and distress +++ c. Symptoms > signs d. Wheeze + e. Cyanosis + f. Perspiration: Common g. Pulsus alternans h. BP: May be hypertensive** i. Apex beat: Heaving or tapping j. Cardiac dullness may be increased due to LVH k. LVH: May be present l. Gallop rhythm present m. Rhonchi +, crepitations + + + n. Breath sound is not altered o. Usually relieved by sitting-up posture or diureties

*Bronchial asthma: Bronchospasm due to 'morning dipping' as a result of circadian changes of cortisol and catacholamines level. Cardiac asthma: Venous return increases after lying down.
**As hypertension is the commonest cause of cardiac asthma.

Table 1.14: Features of respiratory failure at the bedside

Features due to hypoxia	Features due to hypercapnoea
1. Restlessness, tachypnoea	1. Headache (bifrontal or occipital)
2. Impaired judgement	2. Reduced psychomotor activity
3. Mental confusion	3. Drowsiness, confusion or even coma
4. Depression of consciousness level	4. Flapping tremor (asterixis)
5. Central cyanosis	5. Water-hammer pulse and capillary pulsation
6. Tachycardia, systemic hypotension	6. Flushed and warm extremities (e.g., hands)
7. Cardiac arrhythmias	7. High blood pressure
8. Damage to organs like liver and kidney	8. Muscle twitching (fasciculation)
9. Convulsions	9. Papilloedema
10. Coma	10. Chemosis of the conjunctiva

Hypoxic features are more prominent in type I failure. It was previously known as 'alcoholic type' as the patient becomes restless. Severe hypoxia may lead to bradycardia and systemic hypertension.

Features of hypercapnoea are more pronounced in type II failure. It was previously known as 'anaesthetic type' as the patient becomes drowsy. Majority of hypercapnoic features are due to cerebral and peripheral vasodilatation. The spectrum is also known as hypercapnoic encephalopathy or **carbon dioxide narcosis.**

- Features of **hypocapnoea** are: hyperventilation, dizziness, circumoral paraesthesia.

myasthenia gravis, polyneuritis, poliomyelitis; depression of respiratory centre by narcotics or anaesthetics; end-stage of type I failure.

- Type III: From lung atelectasis (perioperative) and
- Type IV: From hypoperfusion of respiratory muscles, e.g. shock.
- So, respiratory failure results from disorders of lung, chest wall, diaphragm, neuromuscular structures and CNS. **Commonest cause of respiratory failure is chronic bronchitis.**

Q. Bedside assessment of pulmonary function:

1. Tachypnoea.
2. Central cyanosis.
3. Rising pulse rate.
4. Inability to speak.
5. Progressive exhaustion.
6. Altered sensorium.
7. Profuse sweating.

8. Pulsus paradoxus.
9. Inability to blow out a match at 6" distance.
10. Asynchronous respiration (i.e. in respiratory muscle fatigue).
11. Silent chest.

If present, immediately check the arterial blood gas and start mechanical ventilation accordingly.

Q. What is ARDS?

ARDS is a non-specific reaction of the lungs to a wide variety of insults, and by far the commonest one is sepsis. Previously called adult respiratory distress syndrome (ARDS) is nowadays known as acute respiratory distress syndrome or 'acute lung injury' (ALI). This is a severe form of type I respiratory failure caused by non-cardiogenic pulmonary oedema, or it is an acute hypoxaemic respiratory failure following a systemic or pulmonary insult without having any evidence of cardiac failure. Acute lung injury is a less severe disorder which can evolve into ARDS at any point of time. ARDS is a serious disorder which is characterised by damage of alveolar epithelium as well as pulmonary capillary endothelium, where the alveoli become flooded with protein rich oedema fluid. The salient features are tachypnoea followed by dyspnoea, central cyanosis and crepitations throughout both lung fields; chest X-ray reveals diffuse, bilateral, interstitial and alveolar infiltrates ('fluffy' shadow).

ARDS is also characterised by normal pulmonary capillary wedge pressure (≤18 mm of Hg) and a PaO_2/F_iO_2 (inspiratory O_2 fraction) ratio <200 mm of Hg; in ALI, there is normal pulmonary capillary wedge pressure (≤18 mm of Hg) and a PaO_2/F_iO_2 ratio is between 200 and 300 mm of Hg. In new 'Berlin definition' of 2012, there is no category called ALI. Read the causes of non-cardiogenic pulmonary oedema from the section on 'Mitral Stenosis'.

Q. How do you like to investigate bronchial asthma?

1. Peripheral blood film: May show eosinophilia. Polymorphonuclear leucocytosis occurs in the presence of respiratory tract infections.
2. Sputum examination: Reveals,
   a. Eosinophils,
   b. Charcot-Leyden crystals (rhomboid crystals derived from eosinophils),
   c. Laennec's pearls,
   d. Curschmann's spiral (mucus casts of small airways),
   e. Dettrich's plugs, and
   f. Bronchial casts.
3. Chest X-ray: May be normal or shows overinflation of lungs (due to emphysema). Rarely, there may be segmental or lobar collapse due to obstruction of bronchus by tenacious mucus. *In worsening dyspnoea, always rule out the presence of pneumothorax or consolidation.* HRCT scan of thorax helps to exclude other diseases.
4. Arterial blood gas (ABG) analysis: In between the paroxysms, there is low PaO_2 with normal or low $PaCO_2$. But in acute severe asthma, there is low PaO_2 with high $PaCO_2$.
5. Lung or pulmonary function tests (PFT) (spirometry):
   a. FEV_1.
   b. FEV_1/FVC.
   c. PEFR.

   The effects are seen before and after application of bronchodilator drugs (most useful initial investigation). These values are low in bronchial asthma. There is marked diurnal variation in PEFR (no diurnal variation in chronic bronchitis or emphysema) and the value is lowest in the morning (early morning dipping).
6. ECG (to exclude RVH in cor pulmonale) and echocardiography (in disproportionate dyspnoea).
7. Skin hypersensitivity tests: Done by 'prick method'. It may identify the allergen in an atopic individual (wheal and flare reaction after intradermal injection of common allergens).
8. Serum IgE: Elevated serum IgE level supports atopy.

Q. What will be the outline of management of bronchial asthma?

1. Rest in bed in propped-up position with most O_2 inhalation at the rate of 4–6 litres/ minute.
2. Salbutamol or terbutaline: By IM or IV route in a dose of 250–500 µg, or inj. aminophylline with a loading dose of 5.0 mg/kg of body weight by slow IV infusion over 20 minutes and maintenance dose of 0.5 mg/kg/hour, given as a continuous IV infusion (in acute case). Nebulised salbutamol (5 mg) or terbutaline (10 mg), driven via oxygen is better than aminophylline to tackle acute situations. Tablet salbutamol (2 mg), terbutaline (2.5 mg) or theophylline (100 mg) may be given three times daily, or doxophylline 400 mg twice daily, in between the attacks. Long-acting β_2-stimulants like salmeterol or formeteral or bambuteral are now used routinely as inhaler or spacer. Levosalbutamol inhalation produces less tachycardia compared to salbutamol.
3. Corticosteroids: Hydrocortisone hemisuccinate 200 mg IV may be given in acute severe asthma as a loading dose, followed several hours later by an infusion regulated to deliver 3 mg/kg every 6 hours. Nowadays corticosteroid (beclomethasone, budesonide or fluticasone as inhaler, or oral prednisolone) is also used in between the attacks.
4. Sodium chromoglycate inhalation 20 mg, four times daily in between the attacks; recently nedocromil sodium is used as 4 mg, 2–4 times daily.
5. Ipratropium bromide (anticholinergic) inhalation two puffs of 20 µg each four times daily, or tablet ketotifen (antihistaminic) 1 mg twice daily may be given in between the attacks.

6. Leucotriene antagonist, montelukast (10 mg, orally, once daily) or zafirlukast (20 mg, orally, BD) may be used to provide control of mild-to-moderate persistent asthma.
7. Sedatives, tranquillisers or narcotics should preferably be avoided.
8. Treatment of pulmonary infection with proper antibiotics. Expectorants or mucolytics (bromhexine, acetylcysteine) may be used.
9. Desensitisation or immunotherapy by repeated subcutaneous injections of gradually increasing dose of extracts of allergen/allergens may be tried (doubtful value).
10. Recent development: Omalizumab (recombinant humanized monoclonal antibody which modulates IgE-associated inflammation), mepolizumab, and benralizumab in corticosteroid-resistant severe asthma. Bronchial thermoplasty is a novel technique (by radiofrequency waves).

- Acute severe asthma needs special management. Read the step-up and step-down drug treatment of bronchial asthma from any standard textbook.
- One can read Global Initiative for Asthma (GINA) guidelines for its control.

Q. Management of acute exacerbation of COPD (i.e. type II respiratory failure):

This condition is managed by oxygen (continuous low concentration O_2 by Venturi mask), nebulised bronchodilator (e.g. salbutamol) with an anticholinergic (ipratropium), prednisolone (orally, 30–40 mg/day) or hydrocortisone (IV route), antibiotics (in suspected chest infections), diuretics (in oedema), chest physiotherapy (rescue from respiratory secretions), and respiratory support by non-invasive ventilation like BiPAP (Bi-level Positive Airway Pressure), if necessary.

Q. Side effects of pure (100%) oxygen therapy:

1. Cough and bronchial irritation as it is both irritant and toxic; drying of secretions.
2. 'Carbon dioxide narcosis' occurs when high O_2 concentration is given to patients with respiratory failure who thrives on 'hypoxic drive', e.g. in COPD patients **(Table 1.15)**.

Table 1.15: Oxygen cascade in human body and atmosphere

Different levels	Partial pressure of oxygen (pO_2 in mm of Hg)
Atmosphere	160
Inspired air	150
Alveolus	104
Artery	95
Vein	40
Tissue level	<40 (average 23)
Expired air	120

3. Retrolental fibroplasia (blindness) and broncho-pulmonary dysplasia: In premature infants.
4. Pulmonary oedema and ARDS.
5. Consolidation of the lung.
6. Absorption collapse (in low ventilation/perfusion zones).
7. Respiratory depression.

- Newborn and infants are more susceptible to effects of pure O_2 than older children and adults.
- Indications of **hyperbaric O_2 therapy** are poisoning (CO, cyanide), decompression sickness, gas gangrene, air embolism, thermal burns and mediastinal emphysema.
- Common therapeutic **'indications of O_2 therapy'** are acute exacerbation of bronchial asthma, COPD, acute pulmonary oedema, ARDS, respiratory paralysis and severe anaemia.

Conclusion

The **hallmark of diagnosis** of bronchial asthma is sibilant, polyphonic rhonchi (mainly expiratory) present all over the chest.

SECTION 3: GASTROINTESTINAL AND HEPATOBILIARY SYSTEM

The cardinal symptoms of GI system are enlisted below:

1. Anorexia (loss of appetite), dyspepsia, indigestion; dysgeusia, pica.
2. Dysphagia, odynophagia (painful swallowing); toothache, bleeding gum, dentures.
3. Nausea, vomiting, retching, eructation, hiccough (singultus).
4. Heartburn (pyrosis, i.e. a hot, burning retrosternal discomfort and pain in the neck, e.g. GERD), water brash (salivary hypersecretion with sudden filling of mouth with watery fluid, common in normal individuals after heavy meals) and regurgitation (effortless appearance of gastric contents in mouth), which is common in GERD; feeling of lump in the throat (globus hystericus).
5. Jaundice, yellow urine, pruritus.
6. Pain abdomen (e.g. a. Colicky: Intestinal, biliaryand ureteric, b. Inflammatory: Peritonitis, IBD, c. Ischaemic: Mesenteric angina, renal infarction, d. Metabolic: Diabetic ketoacidosis, e. Haematological: Sickle cell crisis, f. Referred: AMI, caries spine).
7. Haematemesis.
8. Melaena.
9. Haematochezia.
10. Bleeding per rectum.
11. Alteration in bowel habit.
12. Stool (colour, odour, frequency): Diarrhoea or constipation, mucus in stool, worms in stool.
13. Swelling in the abdomen, distension of the abdomen (e.g. ascites) or mass in the abdomen.

14. Wind or flatulence (belching or flatus).
15. Loss of weight (unexplained and unintentional weight loss >3 kg in previous 6 months is 'significant').
16. Pedal oedema; features of malnutrition (e.g. vitamin deficiency).
17. Oliguria (e.g. hepato-renal syndrome from cirrhosis of liver).
18. Neuropsychiatric manifestations (inversion of sleep rhythm, drowsiness from hepatic pre-coma).
19. Fever (intestinal tuberculosis, lymphoma, amoebic liver abscess, infective diarrhoea, ulcerative colitis, subphrenic abscess, spontaneous bacterial peritonitis).
20. General symptoms: Fatigue, bladder symptoms, etc.

- **Dyspepsia** is the summation of a variety of GI symptoms, e.g. anorexia, early satiety plus flatulance. It is the medical term for indigestion and is usually of 3 types: reflux-like, ulcer-like and dysmotility-like dyspepsia.
- Difficulty in defecation with straining (dyschezia), and upleasant feeling of incomplete evacuation with a constant desire for defecation (tenesmus) fall within 'alteration in bowel habit'; **tenesmus** is due to bacillary dysentery, acute proctitis, carcinoma of the rectum and impacted feces.
- Do not forget to take the H/o hernia or haemorrhoids. Other minor symptoms are halitosis, dry mouth, ulcers in mouth (e.g. aphthous ulcer) or pain in the oral cavity.
- Aproximately 200–2000 mL of flatus (wind) is normally passed per day. Too much flatus production is commonly due to aerophagia (air ingestion or swallowed air), malabsorption or lactase deficiency.
- The GI tract measures 8 metre in length extending from stomodium (mouth) to proctodium (anus).

Clinical Wisdom

Terminology associated with alimentary system:
- Appetite: Pleasurable desire to eat.
- Hunger: Unpleasant sensation produced as a result of empty stomach as well as peristaltic contraction.
- Satiety: A sensation of satisfaction after taking food.
- Sitophobia: Fear of eating (e.g. in oropharyngeal dysphagia, pulmonary aspiration of food occurs during swallowing).
- Phagophobia: Fear of swallowing (e.g. in rabies, tatanus and hysteria).
- Nausea: Feeling or desire to vomit.
- Retching: Laboured and rhythmic contraction of respiratory and abdominal muscles preceding vomiting.
- Dysgeusia: Altered taste sensation. Bad taste in mouth is due to poor oral hygiene, chronic sinusitis or tonsillar infection, advanced carcinoma of stomach or oesophagus, drug-induced and psychogenic.

Scheme of Examination (Proforma)

A. Upper GI Tract

1. Lips.
2. Teeth.
3. Gum.
4. Cheeks (buccal mucosa).
5. Tongue.
6. Fauces and tonsils.
7. Palate (with movement of soft palate).
8. Floor of the mouth.
9. Breath (halitosis or foul smell).
10. Oropharynx.

A torch, a tongue depressor and a pair of gloves are necessary for examination of oral cavity. It is not possible to examine the oesophagus at the bedside; ask the patient for dysphagia, odynophagia, heart burn, or give the patient a glass of water or biscuits, and ask him to swallow. Oesophageal disorder is analysed by barium swallow, upper GI endoscopy, and motility study by manometry and isotope Tc^{99} taken with solid or liquid food.

B. Examination of the Abdomen

I. Inspection:

1. Shape of the abdomen.
2. Flanks: Full or not (ascites makes the flanks "full").
3. Venous prominence (examine in sitting or standing position while asking the patient to cough).
4. Umbilicus:
   i. Position of the umbilicus and the slit:
      a. Whether inverted or everted.
      b. Whether situated midway between xiphisternum and symphysis pubis, or not.
      c. Whether the slit is circular, transverse or vertical.
   ii. Venous prominence around the umbilicus (caput medusae from portal hypertension).
   iii. Hernia (umbilical hernia may contain omentum, bowel or fluid): Look for the expansile impulse on coughing in standing position of the patient.
   iv. Granuloma, adenoma (raspberry tumour), endometriosis (looks raw and red).
   v. Nodules around the umbilicus (e.g. metastatic nodule from intra-abdominal malignancy).
   vi. Bluish discolouration around the umbilicus (Cullen's sign from haemoperitoneum) or Grey Turner's sign (discolouration of skin in the abdominal flanks due to haemoperitoneum).
   vii. Omphalolith (inspissated desquamated epithelium with other debris): Especially in the elderly.
   viii. Sinus (malignant or tuberculous peritonitis, Crohn's disease, patent urachus).
5. Condition of the skin: Ulcer, striae, pigmentation, scar and puncture mark, sinus, stoma (ileostomy, colostomy), fistula (Crohn's disease), keloid.
6. Any localised swelling or visible mass.
7. Movement of the abdomen:
   i. Respiratory movement (whether all quadrants of the abdomen is moving with respiration or not).
   ii. Pulsations.
   iii. Peristalsis.

8. Hernial sites like:
   i. Inguinal ii. Femoral
   iii. Umbilical iv. Epigastric, or
   v. Incisional hernia (look for midline and oblique incision marks over abdomen).
9. Hair (secondary sexual hair: Loss of pubic hair, virilism, etc).
10. Groin and genitalia (maintaining patient's dignity).

- During inspection of the abdomen, extend the legs of the patient.
- Ask the patient to stand and note the presence of impulse on coughing on the hernial swellings.
- For **observation of respiratory movements, pulsations and peristalsis**: Squat down by the side of the bed to have a tangential inspection, or shine a light tangentially across the patient's abdomen. Movements of the abdomen: In health, abdomen bulges during inspiration and retracts during expiration. Paradoxical abdominal movement is seen in diaphragmatic palsy, and abdominal movements are absent in peritonitis. For pulsation and peristalsis, read pages 259 and 429, respectively.
- Finally, inspect the posterior abdominal wall (back)—skin, spine, any swelling, etc.

II. Palpation:

a. Superficial:
   1. Surface temperature.
   2. Tenderness or hyperaesthesia.
   3. Parietal oedema.
   4. Consistency or feel (normal elastic feel, or muscle guard or rigidity).
   5. Localised lump.
   6. Divarication of recti (if any) detected by rising test.
   7. Direction of blood flow in prominent abdominal wall veins.
   8. Pulsation (transmitted or expansile).
   9. Fluid thrill with girth of the abdomen at the level of umbilicus.
   10. Cough impulse at hernial orifices.

- Measure the girth of the abdomen at the level of umbilicus with the help of a tape.
- Divarication of recti: Widely seperated two rectus abdominis muscles (e.g. post-surgery and lax abdomen).

b. Deep:
   1. Liver (in details).
   2. Spleen (in details).
   3. Gallbladder (in details).
   4. Kidneys (in details).
   5. Colon.
   6. Palpation of the testes (it is a must).
   7. Any other lump or mass in the abdomen.
   8. Deep tender spots: McBurney's point, gall-bladder point, epigastric point, renal angle, etc.
   9. Rebound tenderness.
   10. Dipping method in ascites.
   11. Examination of hernia and its orifices, and external genitalia (for examination of hernia, ask the patient to stand and cough with turning the head to other side). Palpate both groins.
   12. The aorta, paraaortic glands and common femoral vessels.
   13. Urinary bladder.

- **Rebound tenderness** (Blumberg's sign): First give firm pressure over the abdomen, and then 'suddenly' take off the hands. The patient complains of severe pain in the abodmen if the sign is positive. This is positive in peritonitis (basically inflammation of parietal peritoneum) from any cause, including acute appendicitis.
- For deep palpation, conventionally palpate with the dominant hand. In any obese, muscular or poorly relaxed patient, the left hand is placed over the right hand **(i.e. using both hands)** to exert more pressure during palpation. Dipping method is adopted in the presence of ascites. The *abdominal aorta* is palpated by placing both hands vertically with extended fingers (eight fingers of both hands except thumbs), which are held side by side, and the palpation is carried a little above and to the left of umbilicus **(Fig. 1.37)**.
- Palpate both iliac fossae for thickened and tender colon (e.g. colitis), and pelvic colon for fecal mass (i.e. *scybala*, which pits on pressure).
- **Groin** should be carefully examined for inguinal lymph nodes, hernia and femoral pulsation.
- Enquire about pain in the abdomen and it is preferable to examine the painful part at the last.

III. Percussion:

1. General note of the abdomen (tympanitic note in health is elicited by 'light' percussion).
2. Upper border of liver (and splenic) dullness.
3. Percussion of Traube's space.
4. Band of colonic resonance over a kidney lump.
5. Shifting dullness.
6. Urinary bladder: Full or empty.

IV. Auscultation:

1. Peristalsis (bowel sounds).
2. Hepatic/splenic rub.

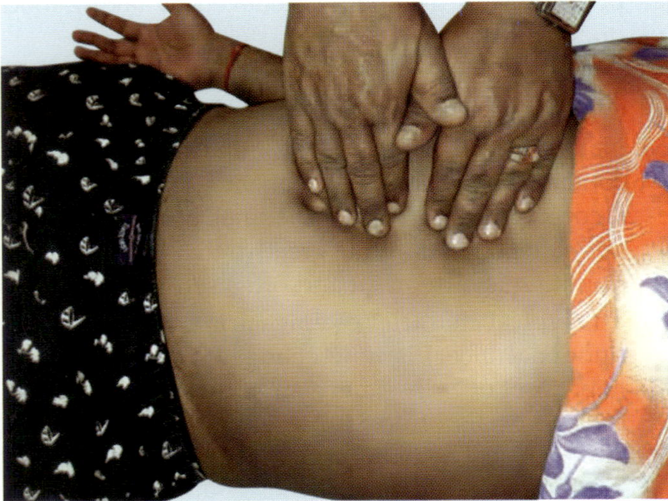

Fig. 1.37: Palpation of **abdominal aorta**

3. Venous hum.
4. Bruit (e.g. hepatic bruit, renal artery bruit, bruit of aneurysm of the aorta).
5. Ausculto-percussion and succussion splash (in pyloric stenosis).
6. Foetal heart sounds (in pregnancy).

C. Per rectal examination (optional)

- **Examine '3S'** such as spine (for metastasis), scrotum (for testicular tumour) and supraclavicular fossa (Virchow's gland for abdominal malignancy).
- Abdominal examination is never completed without examining external genitalia and performing rectal examination. It is important to examine the anus too. Per rectal examination is important in females to note fullness of pouch of Douglas by ovarian cyst, fluid collection or malignant deposits. **Per vaginal examination** is often helpful to diagnose the nature of an abdominal mass.

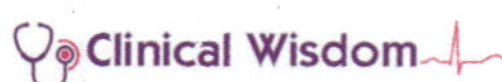

Red flag signs in gastroenterology: Persistent vomiting, profound anorexia, protracted jaundice, progressive weight loss, GI bleeding, dysphagia, prolonged pyrexia, progressive anaemia, palpable hard mass, alteration in bowel habit (rule out malignancy of colon) and chronic diarrhoea.

PYLORIC STENOSIS — CASE 13

Q. What is your diagnosis?

This is a patient of pyloric stenosis possibly developed from chronic duodenal ulcer.

Q. Reasons behind your diagnosis:

This is a case of pyloric stenosis because:

1. The patient is giving a long history of duodenal ulcer. Previously the pain was present in epigastrium, appeared in empty stomach (or there was H/o hunger pain; appeared 90 minutes to 3 hours after a meal) with history of heartburn, water brash, nocturnal pain (between midnight and 3 AM) and pointing sign. The pain is relieved by taking food or antacid.
2. Distension of the upper part of abdomen with foul smelling gaseous eructation and belching.
3. Nausea as well as *projectile vomiting* is present which contains food taken by the patient 1–2 days back and is copious in amount, and the smell of the vomitus is very offensive. Vomiting greatly relieves the patient. Vomiting is infrequent and often self-induced.
4. The typical character of epigastric pain (of chronic duodenal ulcer) is now changed and instead the new onset of early satiety, and a sense of epigastric fullness or discomfort is present. The periodicity of pain is lost. The pain has lost its relationship with food in the last few months.
5. Rapid loss of weight and increasing constipation.
6. Features of tetany is present (alkalosis caused by vomiting; rarely seen). Signs of dehydration +.
7. **A diffuse swelling** is present in the upper abdomen.
8. **Visible peristalsis** from left to right hypochondrium is seen (see the section on 'Visible peristalsis').
9. **Succussion splash** is heard (splashing sound heard on shaking the patient's abdomen).
10. **Ausculto-percussion** over the abdomen reveals gastric distension.

- A lump in the upper abdomen may be felt in carcinoma of the pylorus presenting as gastric outlet obstruction.
- 'Early morning vomiting' is characteristic of pregnancy, raised intracranial pressure, anxiety disorder, chronic alcoholism and uraemia.
- Psychogenic vomiting is frequent, of small volume and usually with a noisy sound.

Q. What is your case?

Build up the summary from the history and physical findings.

Q. Aetiology of 'gastric outlet obstruction':

1. Chronic duodenal ulcer.
2. Carcinoma of the stomach (antrum).
3. Oedema of the pylorus.
4. Congenital hypertrophic pyloric stenosis.
5. Adult hypertrophic pyloric stenosis.
6. Hypertrophic gastritis, rarely.
7. Gastroparesis (e.g. from diabetes mellitus).
8. Bezoars (trichobezoars or phytobezoars).
9. Gastric lymphoma or Crohn's disease.
10. Compression by pancreatic carcinoma.

- Chronic duodenal ulcer → duodenal cicatrisation → fibrotic stricutre → pyloric stenosis.
- Gastric outlet obstruction may be prepyloric, pyloric or duodenal.

Q. Common differential diagnosis you will consider in your case:

1. Carcinoma of the antrum:
   a. Age will be higher.
   b. History is short.
   c. Classical presentation of gastric carcinoma (vide infra).
   d. Rarely, epigastric pain relieved with food.
2. Adult hypertrophic pyloric stenosis:
   a. No past H/o peptic ulcer disease.
   b. Other features are like classical pyloric stenosis.
3. Intestinal obstruction:
   a. Peristalsis will be periumbilical.
   b. Abdomen will be tympanitic.
   c. Obstipation (absolute constipation, i.e. no passage of feces and flatus).
   d. Bowel sounds gradually diminish.

4. Primary carcinoma of liver (predominantly involving the left lobe):
   a. History is short.
   b. Jaundice (rare).
   c. Vomitus is not offensive.
   d. Neither peristalsis seen nor any succussion splash heard.
   e. Hard, tender, nodular liver; emaciation.

Q. Common physical signs in gastric carcinoma:

1. Tender mass in the epigastrium (hard lump).
2. **Anaemia**.
3. **Asthenia** (cachexia).
4. Vomiting (often coffee-ground coloured), haematemesis and/or melaena.
5. Jaundice (due to hepatic metastasis).
6. Liver: Enlarged, tender, hard with nodular surface and sharp margin; hepatic rub may be present due to metastasis.
7. Palpable Virchow's gland (palpable hard and fixed lymph nodes in between two heads of left sternomastoid muscle—*Troisier's sign*).
8. Metastatic nodules around the umbilicus (Sister Marie Joseph's nodule).
9. Ascites (due to malignant peritonitis).
10. Visible gastric peristalsis (vide page 429).
11. Succussion splash (due to gastric outlet obstruction).
12. Krukenberg's tumour (due to metastasis in the ovary): Detected by P/V examination.
13. Blumer's shelf (shelf-like mass in the prerectal pouch): Detected by P/R examination.
14. Rarely, there may be dermatological features like acanthosis nigricans, dermatomyositis, migratory thrombophlebitis (Trousseau's sign), etc.

- Sister Marie was nursing superintendant of St. Mary's Hospital, Rochester, USA.

Clinical Wisdom

Examination of neck glands, jaundice, anaemia, ascites are important in a patient suffering from gastric outlet obstruction. **Anorexia** is a very important symptom in gastric carcinoma (i.e. '3A'—anorexia, asthenia and anaemia). The tympanicity of Traube's space percussion is often lost.

Q. How to elicit succussion splash (Hippocratic succussion) in abdomen?

This is the characteristic splashing sound heard in pyloric obstruction when gastric contents (meal or drink) are retained for more than 4 hours in the stomach. The sign is elicited by shaking the patient from side to side and simultaneously listening the splashing sound (reflects the presence of gas and fluid in an obstructed organ) by placing the diaphragm of stethoscope over the distended area in the epigastruim. The splash is often realised by palpation (by placing hands over epigastrium) and heard without the help of stethoscope. This splashing sound may be normally present after taking a large amount of water.

Q. How to elicit ausculto-percussion?

This method helps to *delineate the enlarged stomach* in cases of pyloric stenosis and sometimes in acute dilatation of the stomach. Put the diaphragm of stethoscope over the epigastrium and scratch the upper part of the abdomen by finger or a pen/pencil in a centrifugal fashion downwards and sideways. Note the sudden change in character of the sound and mark individual points (the sudden change in sound) with a skin pencil. The pencil marks are joined to get the outline of distended stomach, which generally crosses the umblicus in a patient with pyloric stenosis. This method is called 'ausculto-scratching'. In the classical method of ausculto-percussion, a doctor percusses the stomach centrifugally (in the direction away from the stethoscope) while the other doctor listens the sudden changes in character of the sound putting the stethoscope over the epigastrium. This manoeuvre lost its importance due to upper GI endoscopy.

Q. Medical causes of peptic ulcer:

1. Cirrhosis of liver.
2. COPD.
3. Hyperparathyroidism.
4. Polycythemia vera.
5. Cushing's syndrome.
6. Chronic renal failure.
7. Systemic mastocytosis.
8. NSAID or corticosteroid therapy.

Q. How will you confirm your diagnosis in a case of gastric outlet obstruction?

1. Typical history with physical findings.
2. Analysis of gastric contents (fractional test meal):
   a. Volume of gastric aspiration will be >200 mL after overnight fasting.
   b. The colour of the juice is coffee-ground (in gastric carcinoma).
   c. Bile is absent in all the samples.
   d. Aspirate is offensive and contains food residue (classical pyloric stenosis).
   e. Pentagastrin-fast achlorhydria virtually diagnoses gastric malignancy.
3. Barium meal X-ray of stomach and duodenum:
   a. Grossly dilated stomach with excessive fasting contents.
   b. Lesion at or near the pylorus.
   c. **Failure of the stomach to evacuate the meal even after 6 hours (characteristic)**.
4. Upper GI endoscopy: Diagnostic and a standard practice now.
   a. Can identify the obstruction and its degree.

b. Old food material may be seen.
c. May identify carcinoma in the antrum (biopsy may be taken).

5. USG of the abdomen: To see the origin of epigastric fullness, hepatic metastases from gastric carcinoma.
6. FNAC (fine needle aspiration cytology) or excision biopsy of a palpable cervical lymph node (may diagnose carcinoma of stomach causing gastric outlet obstruction).
7. Liver biopsy may be done (to diagnose metastases from gastric carcinoma).
8. Blood biochemistry: Persistent vomiting may give rise to hypokalaemia, hypochloraemia and metabolic alkalosis. Hyponatraemia and high blood urea level may be present.

- Coffee-ground colour vomitus (e.g. in gastric carcinoma) is due to coversion of haemoglobin to acid haematin by gastric acid and it indicates bleeding in the stomach.

Q. How are you going to manage your case of pyloric stenosis?

1. Repeated stomach wash or gastric decompression is done (at 2–4 hourly interval for 3–4 days) to remove all food debris.
2. Correction of dehydration, dyselectrolytaemia and metabolic alkalosis are done by:
   a. 5% dextrose and normal saline.
   b. Injection potassium chloride 80–100 mmol/day.
3. Proton pump inhibitors may reduce pyloric oedema or heal ulcer.
4. Gradually the patient is put on oral diet. At first liquid, then semisolid diet is started.
5. Elective surgery: Surgery is required in majority of patients in the long run. Vagotomy with gastrojejunostomy, or subtotal gastrectomy is done according to the choice of the surgeon. Endoscopic balloon dilatation of the obstructed outlet may be done instead of surgery.

Q. Late complications after gastric surgery:

1. Recurrent ulceration.
2. Afferent loop syndrome.
3. Dumping syndrome: Early and late.
4. Bile reflux gastropathy.
5. Postvagotomy diarrhoea.
6. Osteomalacia and osteoporosis.
7. Haematological complications: Iron deficiency and megaloblastic anaemia.
8. Maldigestion and malabsorption.
9. Small stomach syndrome.
10. Nutritional weight loss.
11. Adenocarcinoma of gastric stump.

Q. Describe the normal peristaltic sound:

'Bowel sounds' are produced by the movement of feces, fluid and flatus within the bowel lumen as a result of peristalsis. Place the stethoscope on one side of the abdominal wall and keep it there minimally for one minute until the bowel sounds are heard. Usually the stethoscope is placed just to the right of the umbilicus. Stethoscope should not be shifted from site to site. Normal bowel sounds are intermittent (at 5 or 10-second's interval) low- or medium-pitched gurgles mixed with occasional high-pitched tinkle (Fig. 1.38).

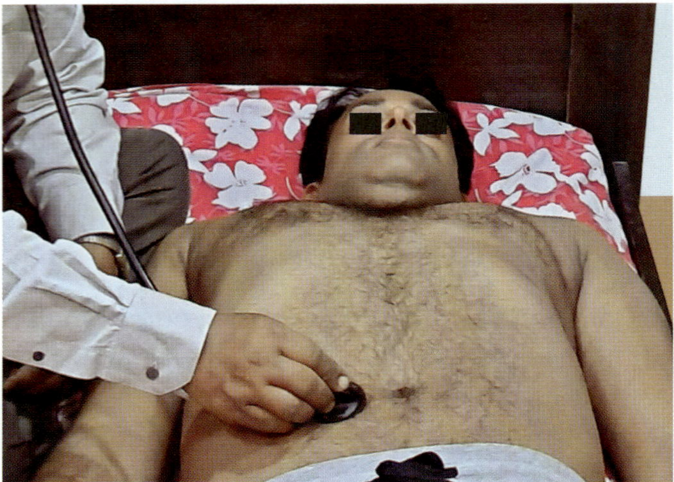

Fig. 1.38: Auscultation of **bowel sounds**

In mechanical **intestinal obstruction:** Frequent loud low-pitched gurgles (borborygmi) are heard, often interspersed with high-pitched tinkles occurring in a rhythmic pattern with peristalsis. As a whole, the peristaltic *sounds are exaggerated*. Bowel sounds are also exaggerated in diarrhoea, malabsorption and severe GI bleeding.

In **paralytic ileus and peritonitis:** Abdomen is *silent* (complete absence of bowel sounds over a 4-minute period).

While dealing with a patient related to gastrointestinal system, one should be careful in examining:

1. Anaemia.
2. Jaundice.
3. **Neck glands** (Virchow's gland especially).
4. Oedema (nutritional, malabsorption).
5. Ascites (cirrhosis, peritonitis).
6. Organomegaly in abdomen.
7. Hernial sites.
8. **Testes.**
9. **Spine (referred pain from caries spine)**, and
10. Rectum (per rectal examination).

ACUTE VIRAL HEPATITIS — CASE 14

Q. What is your diagnosis?

This is a case of acute viral hepatitis probably due to type B virus infection, the patient is in the icteric stage and without any sign of hepato-cellular failure at present.

Q. What is the reason behind your diagnosis?

This is a case of acute viral hepatitis because:
The patient suffered from high fever with mild chill

and rigor, aches and pain all over the body 8 days back, and these ailments persisted for next 5 days. Initially, it was associated with profound anorexia, nausea and vomiting. At the onset, he also had urticarial rashes and arthralgia. The colour of the urine was yellow from the very beginning, and the patient complained of yellowish discolouration of eyes for last 5 days. The patient is having slightly pale stool from day before yesterday. He also complained of dull-aching, non-colicky, non-radiating pain in the right hypochondrium. Neither he is suffering from generalised pruritus nor any bleeding diathesis at present.

There is no past H/o dental extractions, tattooing, acupuncture, blood taken (by unsterile syringe) for any investigational purpose within last 6 months or 'high risk behaviour' (all predispose to type B infection), Jaundice, biliary colic, drug intake (like OC pills, rifampicin, INH), amoebic dysentery or alcohol intake. There was H/o receiving blood transfusion 3 months back when he suffered from a serious street accident. No family member or persons in his locality is suffering from similar type of illness (vide Type A infection). Thus, the disease started acutely and is progressing gradually. For the last 8 days of illness, he is feeling extremely weak.

On examination, there is presence of moderate degree of jaundice; liver is enlarged 4 cm below the right costal margin at right MCL, soft, tender with rounded and regular margin; it has a smooth surface and there is absence of pulsation, rub or bruit. Spleen is just palpable, soft and non-tender. The gallbladder is not palpable and there is discomfort on percussion over the right lower chest. There is neither any free fluid in the abdomen nor any sign of hepato-cellular failure present. CVS, nervous system, respiratory system and genitourinary system are essentially within normal limit.

- Splenomegaly and cervical adenopathy are present in 10–20% cases of viral hepatitis.
- Look for needle track marks, tattoos and evidence of body piercing (for type B and C).

Q. Give the summary of the case:

Described above.

Q. 'Extrahepatic associations' of type B infection:

1. 'Serum sickness-like' syndrome manifested by arthralgia or arthritis (affecting small joints), fever, urticarial rash (present in this patient), angio-oedema and rarely haematuria or proteinuria.
2. Polyarteritis nodosa (systemic necrotising vasculitis).
3. Acute glomerulonephritis.
4. Polymyalgia rheumatica.
5. Essential mixed cryoglobulinaemia (arthritis with cutaneous vasculitis, commoner in hepatitis C).
6. Guillain-Barré syndrome.
7. Myocarditis.

- Porphyria cutanea tarda, essential mixed cryoglobulinaemia, leucocytoclastic vasculitis, arthritis, NHL, lichen planus and sicca syndrome are *extrahepatic clinical associations with hepatitis C.*

Q. Chief complaints of your patient:

1. Anorexia, nausea and vomiting for last 8 days.
2. Yellowish discolouration of urine for last 7 days.
3. Yellowish discolouration of eyes for last 5 days.
4. Fever for 5 days (initial 5 days of illness).
5. Pain in the right upper abdomen for last 3 days.

Q. Common symptoms of acute viral hepatitis:

1. Anorexia, nausea and vomiting.
2. Arthralgia, myalgia and headache.
3. Pharyngitis, cough and coryza.
4. Fatigue and malaise.
5. Dark urine.
6. Clay-coloured stool (cholestasis due to canalicular obstruction by swelling of hepatocytes).

Q. Probable causes of marked anorexia:

1. Acute viral hepatitis.
2. Tuberculosis (especially, pulmonary and gastro-intestinal).
3. Malignancies (especially, stomach and pancreas), lymphomas and leukaemias.
4. Chronic diseases like cirrhosis of liver, chronic renal failure, CCF, Addison's disease.
5. Drugs, e.g. chloroquine, quinine, digitalis, metronidazole, erythromycin.
6. Psychogenic: Depression, emotional upset, anorexia nervosa.
7. Chronic smoking, chronic alcoholism.

Q. Enumerate common causes of persistent (protracted) vomiting:

1. Acute viral hepatitis, acute gastritis, viral/bacterial infections of intestine, raised intracranial pressure (ICP), diabetic ketoacidosis, adrenal crisis, AMI (especially inferior wall), Ménière's disease, acute labyrinthitis, migraine, pyloric stenosis, renal failure (acute or chronic), psychogenic.
2. Surgical abdomen, e.g. acute pancreatitis or cholecystitis, peritonitis, intestinal obstruction.
3. Miscellaneous: Hyperemesis gravidarum, chronic alcoholism, drug-induced (e.g. digoxin), hypercalcaemia, motion sickness, corrosive poisoning, food poisoning.

Q. Different functional (psychosomatic or non-organic) disorders of GI tract:

Halitosis (bad breath) or bad taste, atypical chest pain (due to oesophageal motility disorder), functional dyspepsia (e.g. anorexia), globus hystericus, excessive belching or aerophagia, psychogenic vomiting, functional bloating or gaseous distension, rumination syndrome, irritable bowel syndrome, functional constipation and diarrhoea.

Q. Agents responsible for acute viral hepatitis:

1. Hepatitis A, B, C, D and E.
2. Yellow fever virus.
3. Epstein-Barr virus.
4. Cytomegalovirus.
5. Herpes simplex virus.
6. Coxsackie B virus.

- A and E viruses typically cause acute infections. The B, C and D viruses commonly cause both acute and chronic infections.
- Other infective causes of acute hepatitis are: Non-viral—Leptospira (Weil's syndrome), toxoplasma and coxiella; post-viral—Reye's syndrome in children (aspirin-induced).
- **'Acute hepatitis'** is due to acute viral hepatitis (see above) plus, drugs (e.g. rifampicin), poison (copper sulphate, mushroom), alcohol, Wilson's disease and autoimmune hepatitis.

Q. Features of different types of viral hepatitis (types A to E):

Type A:

1. Transmission: Faecal-oral route commonly (percutaneous and sexual route—uncommon).
2. Age: Children and young adults.
3. Seasonal influence: In winter and rainy seasons.
4. Incubation period: 15–45 days (mean 30 days).
5. Severity: Generally mild.
6. Chronicity: Never occurs.
7. Prognosis: Excellent.
8. Carrier state: Never occurs.
9. Australia antigen: Negative.
10. Peak ALT: 800–1000 IU/L.

Type B:

1. Transmission: Usually parenteral (also sexually transmitted). Perinatal transmission ++.
2. Age: Any age group may be affected (young adults, babies, toddlers).
3. Seasonal influence: Occurs round the year.
4. Incubation period: 30–180 days (mean 60–90 days).
5. Severity: Occasionally severe (<1% having fulminant hepatic failure).
6. Chronicity: Occurs in 1–10% (90% of neonates).
7. Prognosis: Not bad but worse with increasing age.
8. Carrier state: Occurs (0.1–30%).
9. Australia antigen (HB_SAg): Positive.
10. Peak ALT: 1000–1500 IU/L.

- Humans are the only source of infection. HB_SAb is protective.

Type C:

1. Transmission: Parenteral (sexual transmission uncommon).
2. Age: Any age may be affected (common in adults).
3. Seasonal influence: Occurs round the year.
4. Incubation period: 15–160 days (mean 50 days).
5. Severity: Moderate.
6. Chronicity: Commonly occurs (50%).
7. Prognosis: Not good, not bad (moderate).
8. Carrier state: Exists (0.5–1%).
9. Australia antigen: Negative.
10. Peak ALT: 300–800 IU/L.

- Accounts for more than 90% of post-transfusion hepatitis. Anti-HCV is not protective.

Type D (Delta virus):

1. Transmission: Commonly parenteral (also sexually transmitted). Perinatal transmission +.
2. Age: Any age (as type B virus).
3. Seasonal influence: Occurs round the year (as type B virus).
4. Incubation period: 30–180 days (mean 60–90 days).
5. Severity: Occasionally severe.
6. Chronicity: Commonly occurs.
7. Prognosis: Good in acute variety, poor in chronic variety.
8. Carrier state: Variable (10–20% in pregnant women).
9. Australia antigent: Positive (as there is 'coinfection' with or 'superinfection' on type B).
10. Peak ALT: 1000–1500 IU/L.

- Delta virus requires hepatitis B virus for replication, i.e. it has no independent existence.

Type E:

1. Transmission: Only by faecal-oral route.
2. Age: Young adults.
3. Seasonal influence: Commonly after monsoon and flood but sporadic, isolated cases occur.
4. Incubation period: 14–60 days (mean 40 days).
5. Severity: Usually mild.
6. Chronicity: None.
7. Prognosis: Good (mortality is very high in women in the last trimester of pregnancy).
8. Carrier state: Does not exist.
9. Australia antigen: Negative.
10. Peak ALT: 800–1000 IU/L.

- Faecal-oral route: Type A and E; Parenteral route: Type B, C, D; Chronicity: Type B, C, D.
- Hepatitis C is the commonest cause of post-transfusion hepatitis.
- Hepatitis A, B and C viruses are transmitted through saliva too.

Clinical Wisdom

Type A and type B hepatitis were previously known as infective hepatitis and serum hepatitis, respectively. Hepatitis C and hepatitis D were also known as non-A non-B hepatitis and delta virus hepatitis respectively.

Q. Risk factors for type B and type C hepatitis:

The risk factors are: IV drug abuse, blood transfusion, sharing contaminated syringe and needle, tattooing or acupuncture, promiscuous sex or male homosexuality, multiple sexual partners, foreign travel, chronic haemodialysis and organ transplantation. Sexual transmission is uncommon in type C hepatitis.

Q. Describe hepatitis G virus (HGV):

It is a RNA virus (hepatitis A, C, D, E and G are RNA virus, while hepatitis B virus is a DNA virus). HGV is transmitted through blood transfusion (risk factors are like HCV). It is the sixth heterotropic viral agent. Extensive investigations have failed to show that HGV plays a causal role in acute or chronic liver disease and thus, it does not seem to be a serious human pathogen. Hepatitis TT virus (transfusion-transmitted virus, a DNA virus) is also unlikely to be a significant cause of liver diseases.

Q. Type of jaundice in your case:

It is hepato-cellular jaundice.

Q. Complications of acute viral hepatitis:

1. 'Serum sickness-like' syndrome (described previously).
2. Fulminant hepatitis (massive hepatic necrosis): Leads to hepato-cellular failure, which is the most feared complication.
3. Cholestatic viral hepatitis (protracted obstructive jaundice): May persist upto 20 weeks.
4. Relapsing hepatitis (biochemical/clinical): Return of symptoms and signs of acute hepatitis during recovery phase.
5. Post-hepatitis syndrome (symptoms like malaise, anorexia, nausea or right hypochondriac pain persist though LFT remains more or less normal; common in anxious persons and reassurance is necessary).
6. Chronic carrier state.
7. Chronic hepatitis (lobular, persistent and active).
8. Cirrhosis of liver (postnecrotic variety).
9. Hepato-cellular carcinoma (hepatoma).
10. Rare: Pancreatitis, myocarditis, aplastic anaemia, peripheral neuropathy, atypical pneumonia, transverse myelitis, papular acrodermatitis in children, renal failure, polyarteritis nodosa.

Q. Stages of acute viral hepatitis:

There are three stages:

1. Prodromal stage.
2. Icteric stage (i.e. stage of clinical jaundice), and
3. Recovery stage.

Q. Clinical types of viral hepatitis:

1. Acute icteric hepatitis: Common type.
2. Anicteric hepatitis.
3. Fulminant hepatitis.
4. Relapsing hepatitis.
5. Cholestatic hepatitis.
6. Post-hepatitis syndrome.
7. Chronic hepatitis.

Q. What is anicteric hepatitis?

Here, jaundice is not clinically evident (only biochemical hyperbilirubinaemia up to 3 mg/dL), and the symptoms are few though the liver becomes enlarged and tender. It is a mild illness though there is bilirubinuria and elevation of aminotransferases. These patients usually suffer from chronic liver disease (e.g. chronic active hepatitis) later in life. The diagnosis is difficult and requires a high index of suspicion.

Q. Differential diagnosis you will consider in this case:

D/D of acute viral hepatitis at the bedside are:

1. Differentiate among the 5 types of viral hepatitis (the present case suffers from type B infection. There is H/o receiving blood transfusion, and presence of urticaria, arthralgia at the onset of the disease).
2. Hepatic amoebiasis or amoebic liver abscess:
   a. H/o amoebic dysentery may be present.
   b. Liver is enlarged and very tender.
   c. Intercostal tenderness (right) is present.
   d. Fever with chill and rigor, excessive sweating at night.
   e. Patient may look toxic.
   f. Jaundice, splenomegaly, marked anorexia are not very common features.
3. Alcoholic hepatitis:
   a. H/o chronic alcoholism.
   b. Stigmata of alcoholic liver disease (read the section on 'Cirrhosis of liver').
   c. Jaundice with enlarged, tender liver.
   d. Anorexia, weight loss.
4. Carcinoma of liver:
   a. Commonly affects middle aged or older persons.
   b. Progressive jaundice may be present (commonly in secondary malignancy of liver).
   c. Liver feels hard, tender and nodular.
   d. Anaemia, hard lymph nodes in neck and cachexia are prominent features.
   e. Fever and splenomegaly are usually absent.
   f. Ascites is not uncommon.
5. Drug-induced hepatitis:
   a. H/o intake of hepatotoxic drugs (rifampicin, INH, oral contraceptive pills).
   b. Malaise before onset of jaundice.
   c. Occasionally arthralgia, rash and fever are present.
   d. Liver is enlarged and may be tender.

- It is often very difficult to differentiate drug-induced hepatitis from acute viral hepatitis.

6. Haemolytic jaundice:
   a. Anaemia with mild jaundice.
   b. Freshly voided urine is acholuric (i.e. not yellow).
   c. Leg ulcers may be present.
   d. Typical facles may be revealed (vide 'Thalassaemia').
   e. Splenomegaly in almost all the cases.
   f. Non-tender liver, if at all palpable.
7. Congestive cardiac failure:
   a. Cardiomegaly with underlying heart disease.
   b. Features of CCF.
   c. Liver is enlarged, soft and tender.
   d. Clinical jaundice is not commonly seen (latent jaundice may be present).
8. Acute malaria:
   a. Fever with chill and rigor. Typical paroxysm with cold, hot and sweating stage.
   b. Anaemia.
   c. Anorexia and jaundice are not so common.
   d. Splenomegaly is more prominent than hepatomegaly.
9. Cirrhosis of liver:
   a. Long H/o dyspeptic symptoms.
   b. H/o GI bleeding.
   c. Signs of portal hypertension and hepato-cellular failure.
   d. Liver is enlarged but non-tender.
   e. Splenomegaly.
10. Chronic hepatitis (see below).
11. Yellow fever, Weil's disease, infectious mononucleosis, obstructive jaundice, etc.

Q. Enumerate the causes of 'prolonged jaundice':

Jaundice present for >6 months may be arbitrarily called as 'prolonged jaundice'. The causes are,

1. Cholestatic viral hepatitis.
2. Chronic hepatitis.
3. Carcinoma of liver (secondary variety commonly).
4. Cirrhosis of liver (especially, biliary cirrhosis).
5. Thalassaemia.
6. Drug-induced hepatitis (e.g. rifampicin, INH, chlorpromazine).
7. Extrahepatic biliary obstruction (e.g. stone, stricture, carcinoma of the head of pancreas).
8. Alcoholic hepatitis.
9. Wilson's disease.
10. Other causes like Gilbert's syndrome, primary biliary cirrhosis, hereditary spherocytosis, sickle cell anaemia, autoimmune haemolytic anaemia, sclerosing cholangitis, etc.

- 'Prolonged jaundice' may be given as a **long case**.

Q. Causes of enlarged and tender liver:

Read the section on 'Hepatosplenomegaly'.

Q. What is cholestatic viral hepatitis?

It is commonly associated with type A (more common) or type B infection. The jaundice gradually deepens (canalicular obstruction due to oedema of hepatocytes) and intense pruritus appears. Jaundice, hepatomegaly and LFT abnormalities may persist for many months but ultimately the recovery is complete (i.e. prognosis is good). It is often very difficult to differentiate this condition from surgical cholestasis (read the section on 'Jaundice').

Q. Give an outline of chronic hepatitis:

A. Definition:

It is a chronic inflammatory reaction in the liver present on clinical or other grounds (biochemical/serological) without improvement for 6 months or longer.

B. Aetiology:

1. Hepatitis B, C, and D.
2. Autoimmune hepatitis (itself a seperate entity).
3. Drugs (methyl dopa, INH, oxyphenisatin, ketoconazole, nitrofurantoin).
4. Wilson's disease, α_1-antitrypsin deficiency, alcoholic liver disease, non-alcoholic steatohepatitis (NASH) and ulcerative colitis.
5. Cryptogenic.

C. Types:

1. Chronic lobular hepatitis (milder form): Histology resembles unresolved acute viral hepatitis.
2. Chronic persistent hepatitis (milder form): The limiting plate between hepatocytes and portal zones is intact, and piecemeal necrosis is not seen. There is expansion of the portal zone by infiltration with mononuclear cells.
3. Chronic active hepatitis (severe form): There is erosion of limiting plate, presence of piecemeal necrosis, formation of 'rosette' and 'bridging necrosis'; prognosis of this disease is very bad, which can lead to cirrhosis and hepato-cellular failure.

- The above described 3 categories are not very helpful for prognostication. The new more informative classification of chronic hepatitis is based on 1. Aetiology, 2. Histological activity or grade (evidences of inflammation and necrosis), and 3. The stage (extent of fibrosis and reflects the level of progression of the disease).

D. Clinical features:

1. Fatigue, malaise, anorexia, fever.
2. Failure to recovery from acute hepatitis.
3. Jaundice (persistent or intermittent).
4. Hepatomegaly with or without splenomegaly.
5. Stigmata of chronic liver disease (CLD).
6. Signs of hepato-cellular failure.

E. Diagnosis:

1. High bilirubin level with very high aminotransferase levels; prolonged prothrombin time.

2. Antinuclear factor (ANF), anti-smooth muscle antibody may be present.
3. Hypoalbuminaemia with hyperglobulinaemia (autoimmune variety).
4. Detection of viral markers (antigen and antibody), e.g. HCV RNA and anti-HCV.
5. Copper kinetics: Serum copper and ceruloplasmin, urine copper estimation.
6. Elastography (fibroscan) is a non-invasive bedside investigation to measure hepatic fibrosis.
7. *Liver biopsy:* Diagnostic (described above in 'Types').

Clinical Wisdom

Commonest cause of 'acute hepatitis': Globally–HEV, in India–adults HEV and children HAV, and
'Chronic hepatitis': Globally–HCV, in India—HBV.

Q. Association of lymphadenopathy with jaundice:

1. Lymphoma.
2. Leukaemia (ALL).
3. Viral hepatitis (cervical and rarely epitrochlear).
4. Infectious mononucleosis.
5. Disseminated tuberculosis.
6. Disseminated carcinomatosis.

Q. How do you like to investigate a case of viral hepatitis?

1. Blood for TC, DC and ESR: Leucopenia (neutropenia with relative lymphocytosis). Blood picture becomes normal as jaundice appears. Atypical lymphocytes (virucytes) may be seen. ESR is high in pre-icteric phase and returns to normal with jaundice.
2. Liver function tests (LFTs):
   a. Serum bilirubin: High (in most instances the total bilirubin is equally divided between the conjugated and unconjugated fraction, or conjugated fraction is increased).
   b. SGOT (AST) and SGPT (ALT): Increased (normal value is 10–40 IU/L).
   c. Prothrombin time: If increased, indicates extensive hepato-cellular necrosis and a worse prognosis. **Prothrombin time is the best prognostic indicator of hepato-cellular failure.**
   d. Alkaline phosphatase: Slight increase (moderately increased in cholestatic hepatitis; normal value is 35–130 IU/L).
   e. Serum proteins: Mild elevation of gamma-globulin is common in acute viral hepatitis.
3. Urine and stool examination:
   a. Urobilinogen in urine appears in pre-icteric phase, disappears as jaundice is evident and reappears with recovery.
   b. Bilirubin appears in urine before clinical jaundice develops.
   c. Rarely proteinuria may be present.
   d. Stool: May reveal steatorrhoea.
4. Serological diagnosis:
   a. HB_SAg (Australia antigen) Positive in Type B (appears 6 weeks after infection and usually disappears by 3 months). IgM anti-HBc is diagnostic of acute HBV infection.
   b. Anti-HAV of IgM class: Positive in Type A variety.
   c. Anti-HCV (+ve after 6 weeks of infection); and HCV RNA: Positive in Type C variety.
   d. Anti-HDV and anti-HEV antibodies of IgM type are present in hepatitis D and E, respectively.
   e. Serology for cytomegalovirus or Epstein-Barr virus.
5. Blood glucose level may be low (due to vomiting, ↓ intake, poor hepatic glycogen).
6. Imaging: Ultrasonography (commonly used to differentiate other causes of jaundice) or CT scan of liver (USG is superior to CT scan).
7. Liver biopsy: Usually it is **not required to diagnose acute viral hepatitis.** It is important in differentiating cirrhosis, chronic hepatitis, drug-induced hepatitis from acute viral hepatitis.
8. Work-up to differentiate from cirrhosis of liver, alcoholic hepatitis (AST: ALT>2 and high gamma-glutamyl transpeptidase), autoimmune chronic active hepatitis (enzymes >10 times and gamma-globulin >2 times of normal), hepatic amoebiasis (positive indirect haemagglutination test, chest X-ray) should be done.

- Bad prognostic sign: Serum bilirubin >20 mg/dL, very high transaminases and prothrombin time increased by >3 seconds.

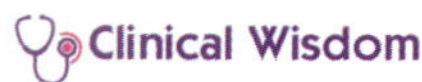

Clinical Wisdom

One should always search for K-F ring in the eyes in all cases of recurrent jaundice in young individuals (to exclude Wilson's disease producing cirrhosis of liver).

Q. Common clinical differences between type A and type B infection:

Characteristics of type A infection are:

1. Fever may be high, and may be >102°F.
2. Onset is very acute.
3. Cholestasis is more common.
4. Fulminant hepatitis is less common.
5. Less severity of illness with most patients making a complete recovery.
6. Post-hepatitis syndrome is more common.
7. No chronicity, no carrier state.
8. Simultaneous infection of other family members or persons in the same locality.
9. Serum sickness-like syndrome does not occur (very characteristic of type B).
10. Usually there is no past H/o blood transfusion, needle prick, etc.

Q. How to recognise that recovery has started in acute viral hepatitis?

1. Appetite returns.
2. Stool becomes normal coloured (from white or clay colour).
3. Urine and eyes become less yellowish.
4. Bilirubin and enzymes level return towards normal.

Q. Who is a 'carrier' of type B infection?

Persistence of HB_SAg for more than 6 months is known as 'carrier'.

- The annual spontaneous clearance rate of HB_SAg is 1–2%; in **incidental positivity for HB_SAg,** test for HB_eAg, HBV DNA and SGPT. Most of them are healthy carrier and do not develop progressive liver disease. But if surveillance shows positive HB_eAg and HBV DNA, it indicates ongoing infectivity; presence of IgG anti-HBc points towards chronicity. So, regular follow- up is mandatory with reassurance to the patient.

Q. How the ongoing infectivity and/or chronicity is diagnosed in type B infection?

a. Ongoing infectivity (viral replication) is diagnosed by the presence of HB_eAg and positive serum HBV DNA (by PCR technique).

b. Chronicity is diagnosed by the presence of positive serum IgG anti-HBc.

- In acute hepatitis B: HB_SAg and IgM anti-HBc are diagnostic.

Q. Discuss the post-exposure prophylaxis:

a. Hepatitis A: It is often necessary for household and institutional 'intimate' contacts, or travellers. Immune globulin (IG) is administered in a dose of 0.02 mL/kg of body weight by IM route as soon as possible. Hepatitis A vaccine (Havrix) should also be given (0.5 mL), IM, in 2 doses at 0, 6–12 months in 2–18 years age group; over 18 years, it is given (1 mL) by 2 injections in the same schedule of 0, 6–12 months.

b. Hepatitis B:
   - i. HBIG: 0.5 mL (neonates) or 0.06 mL/kg (adults) as single dose immediately by IM route, plus
   - ii. Hepatitis B vaccine (Engerix-B, hepavax): 3 doses (each of 1 mL) are given by IM route (always in deltoids) at 0, 1 and 6 months; accelerated schedule of 0, 1, 2, and 12 months are also approved (preferred). Booster dose is not considered routinely (protection appears to be excellent in normal schedule) except in immunocompromised and haemodialysis patients.

c. Hepatitis C or E: At present, vaccine against hepatitis C is not feasible though a vaccine against hepatitis E is successfully used in China.

d. Hepatitis D: No immunoprophylaxis; susceptible persons are given hepatitis B vaccine.

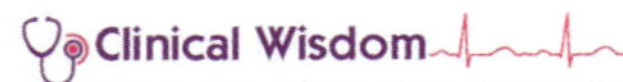

Pregnancy is not a contraindication to vaccination against hepatitis B. Vaccination against hepatitis B will give protection from delta virus infection too. HBIG may be repeated at 4 weeks.

Q. Indications for hepatitis B vaccination:

1. Surgical staffs, dental staffs and medical students.
2. Hospital and laboratory staffs in direct contact with blood.
3. Patients and staffs in haematology (e.g. haemophilia), oncology, and haemodialysis departments.
4. Mental subnormality (e.g. Down syndrome).
5. IV drug abusers.
6. Homosexually and bisexually active men, prostitutes; HIV infection or AIDS.
7. All newborns.
8. Babies born to HB_SAg +ve mother.
9. Accidental exposure to HB_SAg +ve blood.
10. Close family and sexual contacts of HB_SAg +ve carriers.

- 1 to 7 require pre-exposure prophylaxis (0, 1, 6-month's schedule), and 8 to 10 require post-exposure prophylaxis (accelerated). In post-exposure prophylaxis, HBIG should be given along with the vaccine.

Q. Who discovered Australia antigen?

In the year 1967, Baruch Samuel Blumberg, American physician and geneticist, discovered the hepatitis B surface antigen (HB_SAg) and was awarded Nobel prize in Medicine for his discovery in 1976.

Q. Diagnosis of hepatitis C virus infection:

1. Read the clinical characteristics mentioned earlier.
2. Serological test for HCV antibodies (anti-HCV) is usually positive after 6 weeks of infection.
3. Presence of HCV-RNA is detected by polymerase chain reaction (PCR), 1-2 weeks after infection.
4. Genotyping (6 major genotypes of hepatitis C) by restriction fragment length polymorphism (RFLP).

Q. How will you manage your case?

There is no specific treatment for acute viral hepatitis. Treatment is totally supportive.

1. Bed rest with bathroom privileges till jaundice persists. Restrict physical activity.
2. Diet: Low-fat, high carbohydrate, high-calorie diet (a diet containing 2000–3000 Kcal per day should be given). The food must be palatable. Plenty of fluids to drink.
3. Avoid close physical contacts in acute stage. Avoid alcohol and hepatotoxic drugs, and sharing comb/rajors. Regular surveillance on clinical parameters as well as liver function tests is done. Hospitalisation is usually not necessary. Reassurance, as recovery is the rule in majority.

4. Symptomatic treatment:
   a. Antiemetics: Domperidone, metoclopramide or ondansetron may be used.
   b. Sedatives: Should not be used. If the patient is very restless, oxazepam may be given.
   c. Vitamins: Parenteral injection of vitamin K, 10 mg by IM route may be given for consecutive 3 days if prothrombin time is high. Other vitamin supplements are not necessary.
   d. Severe vomiting with fluid loss: 10% dextrose drip may be given.
   e. Cholestyramine or UDCA (ursodeoxycholic acid) is advocated for intense pruritus from cholestasis.
5. Treatment of hepato-cellular failure (e.g. in fulminant hepatitis) may be done accordingly.

- Steroids should not be used in acute viral hepatitis. Keep the patient on minimal drugs.

Q. Patient of viral hepatitis becomes drowsy—significance:

Patient is going towards acute hepatic failure, i.e. hepatic pre-coma (encephalopathy).

CIRRHOSIS OF LIVER — CASE 15

Q. What is your diagnosis?

This is a case of decompensated chronic liver disease (CLD) probably macronodular cirrhosis of liver with features of portal hypertension and hepato-cellular failure following type B hepatitis, and the disease is progressing.

- Chronic liver disease (CLD) is defined as liver diseases persisting for 6 months or longer.

Q. Why do you say so?

This is a case of cirrhosis of liver because:

A. From the history:

a. Past H/o hepatitis B infection 12 years back.
b. Fatigue, weight loss, flatulent dyspepsia, anorexia and low grade fever for last 6 months.
c. Haematemesis, melaena, swelling of legs and progressive distension of abdomen for last 10 days.
d. Scanty micturition for last 5 days.
e. Drowsiness, inversion of sleep rhythm for last 2 days (say, if present).

B. Physical examination:

a. General survey

1. Malnutrition.
2. Anaemia: Moderate.
3. Jaundice: Mild.
4. Hepatic facies.
5. Oedema feet.
6. Obvious swelling of abdomen.
7. K-F ring in the eyes: Absent.
8. Flapping tremor: Absent.

b. Systemic examination

1. Abdomen:
   i. Venous prominences over abdomen, especially in the epigastrium with flow of blood away from the umbilicus.
   ii. Liver is 1 cm palpable, firm, non-tender with sharp and irregular margin; chiefly the left lobe is palpable (liver may not be palpable, especially in late stages, when it shrinks in size due to progressive hepatocyte destruction and accompanying fibrosis).
   iii. Moderate, non-tender splenomegaly (palpated by dipping method).
   iv. Ascites: Present, which is confirmed by shifting dullness.
2. Skin changes:
   i. Spider naevi.
   ii. Palmar erythema.
   iii. Diffuse pigmentation of skin.
   iv. White nails or leuconychia (due to hypo-albuminaemia).
   v. Scanty axillary and pubic hair. There is loss of male pattern of hair.
3. Gynaecomastia and bilateral testicular atrophy (soft and small testes; there is loss of testicular sensation too), [or atrophy of breast (females)].
4. Neurological changes: Nothing abnormal at present (say, if present).

Summary: This is a case of cirrhosis of liver because of:

- Long history.
- H/o jaundice, haematemesis, melaena and bipedal pitting oedema.
- Poor nutritional status, and
- Features of portal hypertension and hepato-cellular failure.

Clinical Wisdom

Measurement of BMI is not judicious in the presence of ascites and just mention the height and weight in such a case.

Q. What is your case?

Build up the summary.

Q. Importance of past history:

1. Jaundice (viral hepatitis).
2. Drugs (e.g. rifampicin, INH, OC pills; NSAID for melaena) or any herbal remedies taken.
3. Blood transfusion or transfusion of any blood products (viral hepatitis B or C); recent tattooing or acupuncture, drug abuse, needle sharing.
4. Alcohol consumption.
5. Tuberculosis (ascites due to tuberculous peritonitis).
6. Haematemesis or melaena (peptic ulcer, ruptured oesophageal varix, gastric malignancy).

7. Fever (tuberculosis, hepato-cellular failure, etc).
8. Haematochezia (lower GI malignancy, haemorrhoids).
9. Abnormal movements (chorea in Wilson's disease).

Q. Queries in personal and family history:

Vide pages 6–7 with special reference to alcohol intake. Dose of alcohol consumption, type of drink, daily/weekly pattern should be mentioned with duration. The patient in discussion, takes mixed Indian diet. Family history may be positive in Wilson's disease.

Q. Importance of family history in alimentary system:

- *Similar illness in the family:* Acute diarrhoea, food poisoning and acute viral hepatitis.
- *Genetic hepatic disorders:* Wilson's disease, haemochromatosis and α_1-antitrypsin deficiency.
- *Genetic intestinal disorders:* Familial polyposis coli, inflammatory bowel disease and carcinoma of colon.

Q. Features of portal hypertension:

1. Evidences of porto-systemic anastomosis (collateral circulation) at different sites (Fig. 1.39):
   a. Lower end of oesophagus: Rupture of 'oesophageal varix' produces haematemesis and melaena.
   b. Around the umbilicus: Caput medusae (classical caput medusae is rare); and also seen in the anterior abdominal wall, especially in the epigastrium.
   c. Rectum and anal canal: Haemorrhoids.
2. Splenomegaly (sine qua non and single most bedside cardinal finding), and
3. Ascites.

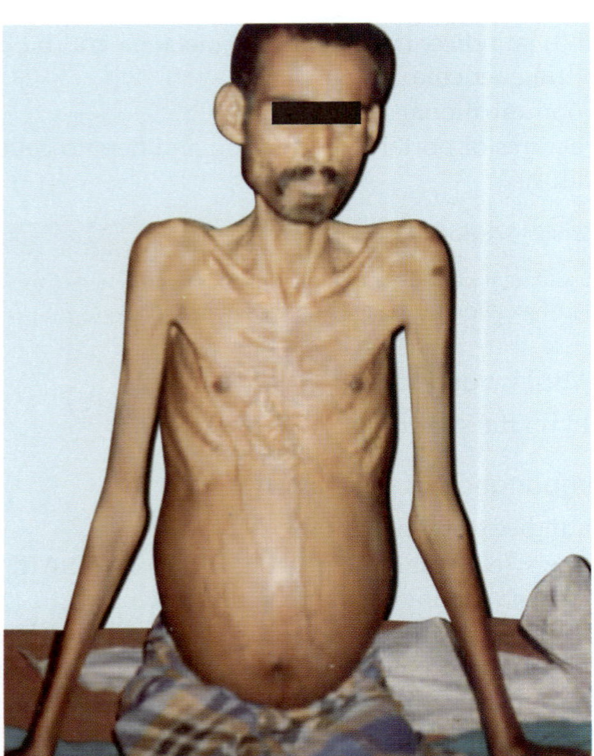

Fig. 1.39: **Portal hypertension.** Prominent and tortuous veins over the abdomen as well as ascites are present. The patient is grossly emaciated—a classical case of **cirrhosis of liver**

- It is often said that **fetor hepaticus** is a feature of portal hypertension (due to porto-systemic shunting of blood) but it should be remembered that underlying hepato-cellular failure must be present to have fetor. Portal hypertension is unlikely if splenic enlargement can not be demonstrated clinically or by radiographically.
- **Caput medusae:** Looks like Greek Goddess Medusae's hair after Minerva had turned it into snakes, i.e. snakes radiated from head (caput) of Medusae.

Q. Features of hepato-cellular failure:

1. General failure of health (loss of flesh).
2. Jaundice.
3. Skin changes (read the section on 'Palmar erythema' too):
   a. Spider naevi.
   b. Palmar erythema (liver palm).
   c. Diffuse pigmentation.
   d. White nails or leukonychia (due to hypoalbuminaemia).
   e. Clubbing (common in biliary cirrhosis).
   f. Loss of axilary and pubic hair (due to hyperoestrogenaemia); alopecia.
   g. 'Paper money' skin (usually on upper arms); white spots (arm and buttock).
   h. Dupuytren's contracture (especially in alcoholics).
4. Endocrine changes:
   a. Gynaecomastia (breast atrophy in females).
   b. Testicular atrophy (bilateral).
   c. Loss of axillary and pubic hair.
   d. Menstrual irregularities in females.

- Other endocrine features are loss of libido and impotence.

5. Bleeding manifestations: Petechiae, purpura and ecchymosis (chiefly due to hypoprothrombinaemia and sometimes due to low platelet count).
6. Fever (related to endotoxaemia with production of cytokines).
7. Fetor hepaticus (sweetish-faecal smell of the breath and urine due to methyl mercaptan and volatile dimethyl sulphide; the smell resembles that of dead mouse). Fetor hepaticus indicates severe hepatocellular failure with extensive collateral circulation (i.e. porto-systemic anastomosis).
8. Hepatic encephalopathy (potentially reversible neuropsychiatric complication—Disturbed consciousness with inversion of sleep rhythm, personality changes, intellectual deterioration, psychiatric abnormalities with asterixis): Personality changes, e.g. irritability and loss of family concern, and constructional apraxia, i.e. inability to reproduce simple diagrams with blocks are common.
9. Ascites and bipedal oedema.
10. Circulatory changes:
    A. Hyperkinetic circulation:
       a. Capillary pulsation.

b. Bounding pulse (high pulse pressure with low diastolic BP).
c. Tachycardia.
d. Hyperdynamic apex.
e. Ejection systolic murmur at the apex.

B. Central cyanosis and clubbing: Due to development of pulmonary arteriovenous shunts, which may lead to hypoxia (i.e. platypnoea).

- To diagnose a case of cirrhosis of liver, one should search for features of **both** portal hypertension and hepato-cellular failure. Pedal oedema (pitting) develops as a result of hypoproteinaemia, while additional factor is functional IVC obstruction due to ascites.
- A female distribution of body hair may be seen in male cirrhotics (e.g. less frequent shaving).
- Features accountable for both hepato-cellular failure and portal hypertension: ascites and fetor hepaticus (according to some hepatologists).
- **Testicular atrophy** is also noted in lepromatous leprosy, mumps, myotonic dystrophy and trauma to testis.

Q. Presence of ascites in cirrhosis of liver:

It indicates hepato-cellular failure with portal hypertension, i.e. it is decompensated cirrhosis with portal hypertension.

Q. Features of 'hyperoestrogenaemia' in hepato-cellular failure:

Diminished hepatic clearance of precursor androstenedione results in its peripheral conversion to oestrogen, and manifests as:

1. Spider naevi.
2. Palmar erythema.
3. Gynaecomastia (breast atrophy in females).
4. Bilateral testicular atrophy and infertility.
5. Loss of beard (H/o less shaving), axillary and pubic hair; alopecia.
6. Menstrual irregularities.
7. Loss of libido.

- Actually, **these are the stigmata of chronic liver disease (CLD).**

Q. Describe 'hepatic facies':

Hepatic facies is characteristic of chronic liver disease, e.g. cirrhosis of liver.

1. Shrunken eyes.
2. Hollowed temporal fossa.
3. Pinched-up nose with malar prominence.
4. Parched lips.
5. Muddy complexion of skin (blending of pallor, jaundice and melanosis).
6. Sallow and dry face.
7. Icteric tinge of conjunctiva.

Q. How to narrate a complete diagnosis in cirrhosis (standard format)?

a. **Aetiological:** Alcohol, type B hepatitis, toxins, Wilson's disease, NASH, etc.
b. **Morphological:** Micronodular, macronodular or mixed nodularity.
c. **Functional assessment (compensated or decompensated):**
   1. Portal hypertension.
   2. Hepato-cellular failure.
   3. Evolution: Progressing, regressing or stationary.

Q. Morphological classification of cirrhosis:

a. Micronodular (<3 mm in size): Alcoholism, malnutrition, old age, anaemia, haemochromatosis.
b. Macronodular (may be few centemeter in size): Post-HBV, post-HCV, Wilson's disease.
c. Mixed: Features both micro- and macronodular cirrhosis, e.g. biliary cirrhosis.

- Micronodular = Laennec's cirrhosis, and macronodular cirrhosis = postnecrotic or postviral.
- When regeneration is slow, micronodules are developed.

Q. Special stigmata of alcoholic cirrhosis:

1. Bilateral enlarged parotids.
2. Gynaecomastia.
3. Testicular atrophy with loss of body hair.
4. Wasting of muscle mass, and
5. Dupuytren's contracture.

- **Enlarged bilateral parotids** are seen in suppurative parotitis, mumps, cirrhosis of liver, Sjögren's syndrome, sarcoidosis, leukaemic or lymphomatous deposits, postoperative patients, IgG_4 disease, drug-induced (Iodides, guanethidine), parotid neoplasms, HIV infection, acromegaly or amyloidosis. **Unilateral parotid swelling** is common in early mumps, suppurative parotitis, obstruction of parotid duct, and leukaemic or lymphomatous deposits (Fig. 1.40).
- Damage of Leydig cells of testis occurs with high dose of alcohol, resulting in androgen deficiency.

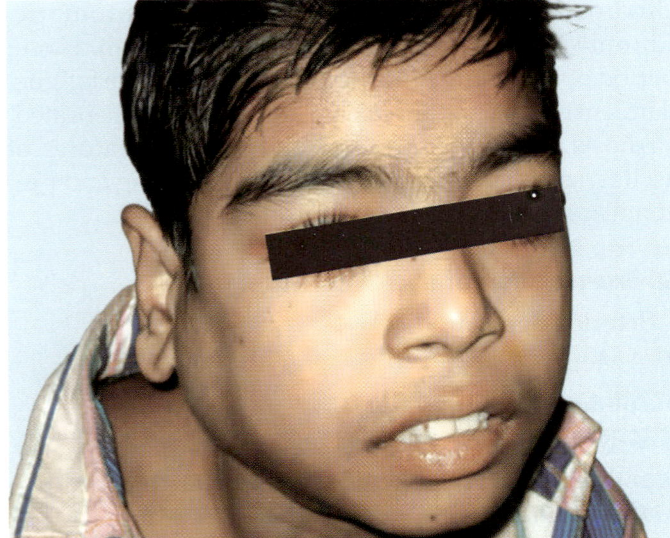

Fig. 1.40: **Parotid enlargement** by leukaemic deposits in right parotid gland in acute lymphoblastic leukaemia; pallor of the face cannot be overlooked

Q. 'Cirrhogenic' or danger dose of alcohol:

The danger dose of alcohol consumption is >80 g/day. Most alcoholic cirrhotics consume 160 g/day for at least 8 years. *A steady daily intake is more dangerous* than intermittent drinking.

Alcohol equivalents:

Whisky → 30 mL = 10 g
Country liquor → 45 mL = 10 g
Wine → 100 mL = 10 g
Beer → 250 mL = 10 g

- **Alcoholic liver disease** are fatty liver, alcoholic hepatitis and alcoholic cirrhosis. Hepato-cellular carcinoma is a complication, especially in men.

Q. Aetiology of cirrhosis of liver:

1. Alcoholic.
2. Biliary (primary or secondary).
3. Cryptogenic (when no aetiology can be determined, i.e. idiopathic).
4. Postnecrotic or postviral (HBV, HCV, HDV).
5. Cardiac or congestive.
6. Metabolic: Wilson's disease, haemochromatosis, glycogen storage disease, α_1-antitrypsin deficiency, galactosaemia, cystic fibrosis, tyrosinaemia.
7. Drugs: Methotrexate, amiodarone, methyl dopa, halothane.
8. Miscellaneous:
   i. Indian childhood cirrhosis.
   ii. Budd-Chiari syndrome.
   iii. Intestinal by-pass surgery.
   iv. Autoimmune hepatitis (lupoid).
   v. Non-alcoholic steatohepatitis (NASH).
   vi. Primary sclerosing cholangitis.

Q. Compensated and decompensated cirrhosis:

Cirrhosis can be symptomatic or asymptomatic. Chronic liver disease usually passes through a long period of minimum non-specific symptoms like fatigue, flatulent dyspepsia, anorexia—known as 'compensated' cirrhosis, and appearance of one or more features of ascites, jaundice, encephalopathy, GI bleeding and precoma are known as 'decompensated' cirrhosis.

Q. Examination of eye in cirrhosis:

1. Icteric tinge (jaundice).
2. Anaemia.
3. Bitot's spot.
4. K-F ring.
5. Subconjunctival haemorrhage (due to hypoprothrombinaemia).

- Always search for K-F ring in a patient with cirrhosis of liver, especially in younger cirrhotics.

Q. Common sites for varices in portal hypertension:

1. Lower end of oesophagus (commonest).
2. Gastric varices.
3. Colo-rectal.
4. Rarely, duodenal.

Q. Describe the 'liver' in cirrhosis (in a classical case):

The liver may not be palpable in the presence of ascites. Usually the liver is,

1. Palpable, 1 cm below the right costal margin at right MCL (often the left lobe is better palpable in the epigastrium) and moving with respiration. *The liver is enlarged in early cirrhosis, and may be shrunken and not palpable in advanced disease.*
2. **Firm in consistency.**
3. **Sharp and irregular margin.**
4. Surface is finely irregular (portal or Laennec's cirrhosis) or coarsely irregular (postnecrotic).
5. Non-tender.
6. Upper border of liver dullness may be lowered (in 6th or 7th ICS at right MCL).
7. No bruit.
8. No rub.
9. No pulsation.

- There is **moderate splenomegaly in cirrhosis**.

Q. Aetiology of portal hypertension:

A. Pre-sinusoidal:

a. Extrahepatic (**portal vein thrombosis**, or extrahepatic obstruction or EHO):
   1. Umbilical sepsis in neonates.
   2. Portal pyaemia.
   3. Exchange transfusion in neonates.
   4. Oral contraceptives, pregnancy.
   5. Abdominal trauma.
   6. Portal lymphadenopathy (lymphoma, metastasis).
   7. Hyperviscosity syndrome (myeloproliferative disorders).
   8. Malignancy of liver and pancreas.
   9. Protein C or S deficiency, antithrombin III deficiency, factor V Leiden.
   10. Secondary to cirrhosis of liver.
   11. Idiopathic.

- Extrahepatic portal vein obstruction (EHO) is the commonest cause of portal hypertension in children.

b. Intrahepatic:
   1. Schistosomiasis.
   2. Congenital hepatic fibrosis.
   3. Sarcoidosis.
   4. Lymphoma.
   5. Leukaemic infiltrations.
   6. Primary biliary cirrhosis.
   7. Arsenic, vinyl chloride and copper intoxication.
   8. Idiopathic portal hypertension.

B. Post-sinusoidal:

a. Intrahepatic (better known as 'intrahepatic parenchymal'):
   1. **Cirrhosis of liver (commonest cause of portal hypertension in adults)**.
   2. Acute alcoholic hepatitis.
   3. Hypervitaminosis A.
   4. Cytotoxic drugs.
   5. Veno-occlusive disease (by Jamaica bush tea containing toxic pyrrolizidine alkaloids).
   6. Partial nodular transformation of liver.
   7. Metastatic malignancy of liver.

b. Extrahepatic:
   1. **Budd-Chiari syndrome** (obstruction of hepatic veins commonly by thrombosis at any site from efferent vein of the lobule to the entry of the IVC into right atrium).
      i. Pregnancy.
      ii. Oral contraceptives.
      iii. Abdominal trauma.
      iv. Malignancy of liver, kidney, adrenal, testis, etc.
      v. Membranous obstruction of IVC (webs, diaphragms).
      vi. Hyperviscosity syndrome (myeloproliferative disorders, e.g. polycythemia).
      vii. Thrombophilic states (antiphospholipid syndrome, protein C or S deficiency).
      viii. Paroxysmal nocturnal haemoglobinuria.
      ix. Right atrial myxoma.
      x. Others: Vasculitis (Behcet's disease), liver abscess, sickle cell disease.
      xi. Idiopathic.
   2. Constrictive pericarditis.
   3. Severe right heart failure (rare).

- Actually, **sinusoidal causes of portal hypertension** are 1, 2, 3, 4 and 6 of (B)-a.
- Two rare causes of portal hypertension are tropical splenomegaly syndrome and haematological disorders with massive splenomegaly (increases hepatic blood flow).
- In **Budd-Chiari syndrome,** there may be added features of inferior vena caval obstruction (distended veins over flanks and back, plus gross pedal oedema) over and above portal hypertension and hepato-cellular failure. There is classical triad of abdominal pain, ascites and tender hepatomegaly. Abdominal Doppler ultrasound, CT, MRI and liver biopsy are helpful in diagnosis.

Q. Summary of aetiology of portal hypertension (Figs 1.39 and 1.41):

- Pre-hepatic: EHO, i.e. portal vein thrombosis and splenic vein thrombosis.
- Hepatic:
  a. Pre-sinusoidal: Non-cirrhotic portal fibrosis (e.g. schistosomiasis, arsenic toxicity).
  b. Sinusoidal: Cirrhosis of liver.
  c. Post-sinusoidal: Veno-occlusive disease.

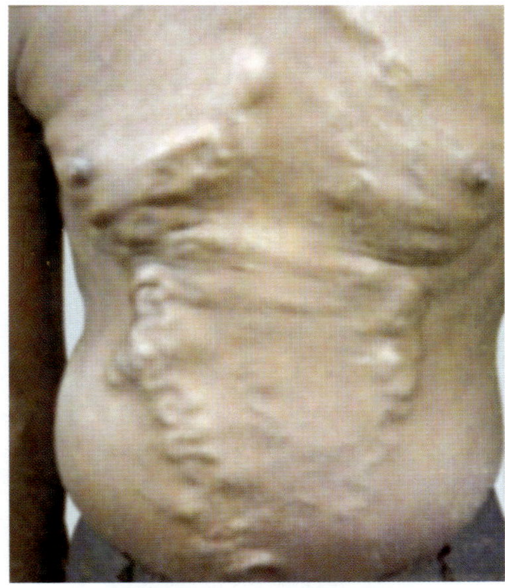

Fig. 1.41: Portal venous obstruction showing prominent collaterals. Venous hum is audible over the visible veins

- Post-hepatic: Budd-Chiari syndrome, IVC obstruction, constrictive pericarditis.

Q. What is non-cirrhotic portal fibrosis (NCPF)?

NCPF is an intrahepatic pre-sinusoidal cause of portal hypertension. The disease is characterised by moderate to massive splenomegaly with anaemia, 'preserved hepato-cellular function' and a benign prognosis in majority though in the late stages, nodular transformation may occur. Though recurrent haematemesis is common as a presenting feature, hepatic encephalopathy is uncommon. Ascites is unusual in NCPF. Endoscopy reveals oesophageal varices, splenoportalvenography (SPV) shows massive dilatation of portal and splenic veins with presence of collaterals; liver biopsy demonstrates varying degree of portal fibrosis with maintained lobular architecture. The possible aetiologies are:

1. Idiopathic portal hypertension (previously known as Banti's syndrome),
2. Schistosomiasis,
3. Congenital hepatic fibrosis,
4. Chronic arsenic ingestion (mainly through tube-well water; common in India and Bangladesh), and
5. Vinyl chloride, antiretroviral therapy: May be responsible.

The D/D of NCPF is tropical splenomegaly syndrome occuring in a patient of chronic malaria.

Q. Features of extrahepatic obstruction (EHO) (Fig. 1.42):

The patients present at an earlier age (causes mentioned in page 116) with episodes of haematemesis and/or melaena, not accompanied by hepatic decompensation. Stigmata of cirrhosis, jaundice, ascites and hepatic coma from bleeding are uncommon. **Liver is usually soft**, if at all palpable. There is massive splenomegaly with signs

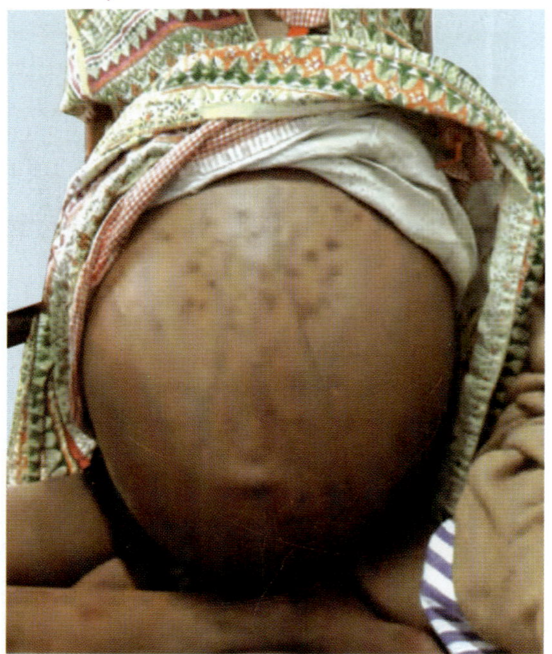

Fig. 1.42: Portal hypertension with huge ascites from extra-hepatic obstruction **(EHO)** with signs of counterirritation over abdomen

of portal hypertension. SPV demonstrates the collaterals and feeder vessels.

Clinical Wisdom

Splenomegaly in different types of portal hypertension are: 1. Cirrhosis: Moderate, 2. NCPF: Enlarged up to midline, 3. EHO: Massive (crossing umbilicus).

Q. What is NASH or NAFLD?

Diffuse accumulation of neutral fat (triglycerides) in hepatocytes may give rise to mild to moderate enlargement of liver, and is known as non-alcoholic steatohepatitis (NASH) or non-alcoholic fatty liver disease (NAFLD). 'Fatty liver' is divided into two types:

1. Macrovesicular (large fat droplets in hepatocytes): Alcohol, obesity, diabetes mellitus, starvation, drugs (steroid, oesotrogen, amiodarone), total parenteral nutrition, jejunoileal by-pass, Indian childhood cirrhosis.
2. Microvesicular: Reye's syndrome, acute fatty liver of pregnancy, drugs (tetracycline, valproate), toxins (yellow phosphorus).

Most patients are asymptomatic and may only complain of mild right hypochondriac discomfort. Hepatomegaly and mild elevation of aminotransferases are common. Fatty liver is reversible but if untreated, NAFLD can progress to NASH, with the subsequent development of cirrhosis (1%) and hepato-cellular carcinoma. Insulin resistance is present in virtually all patients of NASH/NAFLD, and NAFLD is now considered as hepatic component of metabolic syndrome. Elastography (fibroscan) is used to evaluate the degree of hepatic fibrosis. Ursodeoxycholic acid (UDCA), statins, vitamin E, metformin and pioglitazone are used empirically as pharmacotherapy of fatty liver; obeticholic acid is a promising drug. The patients are always encouraged to lose weight.

Clinical Wisdom

Metabolic dysfunction-associated fatty liver disease (MAFLD) and metabolic dysfunction-associated steatohepatitis (MASH) are the new terms suggested in 2020 targeting to replace NAFLD and NASH, related to systemic metabolic dysregulation.

Q. Pain abdomen in cirrhosis:

1. Tuberculous peritonitis.
2. Spontaneous bacterial peritonitis (SBP): Infection of ascitic fluid without any obvious primary source of infection.
3. Peptic ulcer (common in cirrhotics).
4. Chronic cholecystitis (1/3rd of cirrhotics have pigment gallstones).
5. Portal vein thrombosis.
6. Pancreatitis (common in alcoholic cirrhosis).
7. Cirrhosis turned into hepato-cellular carcinoma (hepatoma).
8. Zieve's syndrome (haemolysis, pain abdomen, hyperlipidaemia in an alcoholic patient).

Q. Fever in cirrhosis:

1. Tuberculous peritonitis.
2. Spontaneous bacterial peritonitis (SBP).
3. Hepato-cellular failure.
4. Transformation into hepatoma.
5. Associated chronic active hepatitis.
6. Tuberculosis (pulmonary or intestinal).
7. Other causes of fever like malaria, enteric fever, UTI, etc.

Q. Haematemesis and/or melaena in cirrhosis:

1. Ruptured oesophageal varices (commonest).
2. Peptic ulcer.
3. Portal hypertensive (congestive) gastropathy.
4. Gastric erosion (NSAID-induced).
5. Rupture of gastric varices.
6. Mallory-Weiss tear.
7. Bleeding tendency.
8. Ulcer due to sclerotherapy.

- In approximately 50% cases, the source of upper GI bleeding in cirrhosis is from peptic ulcer or portal hypertensive gastropathy.

Q. Definition of cirrhosis of liver:

Cirrhosis is a pathological term. It is the chronic and diffuse involvement of liver parenchyma of varied aetiology, which is clinically characterised by features of portal hypertension and hepato-cellular failure in varying combination, and pathologically by irreversible **necrosis**, extensive **fibrosis** as well as regenerative **nodule formation** in such a way that the normal architecture of liver is totally lost.

Q. Importance of examination of other systems in cirrhosis:

A. Respiratory system:
   a. Evidence of hydrothorax (commonly right-sided).
   b. Evidence of pulmonary tuberculosis (common in cirrhosis).
   c. Emphysema (in α_1-antitrypsin deficiency).

B. CVS: Evidence of circulatory changes, already mentioned in 'Features of hepato-cellular failure'.

C. Nervous system: Neuropsychiatric manifestations of hepato-cellular failure (hepatic encephalopathy) are described below (*see* page 121).

D. Genitourinary system:
   a. Facial puffiness due to renal failure (hepato-renal syndrome) with oliguria.
   b. Testicular atrophy and loss of pubic hair.

Q. Causes of haematemesis (*see* **Table 1.1**):

A. Common causes:

1. Chronic duodenal ulcer (commonest cause).
2. Erosive gastritis.
3. Variceal bleeding (ruptured oesophageal varices).
4. Chronic gastric ulcer.
5. Carcinoma of the stomach.
6. Mallory-Weiss syndrome.
7. Peptic oesophagitis.
8. Duodenal erosions.
9. Oesophageal carcinoma.
10. Portal hypertensive gastropathy.

B. Less common causes:

1. Leiomyoma and leiomyosarcoma of the stomach.
2. Lymphoma of the stomach.
3. Duodenal diverticula; hiatal hernia.
4. Blood dyscrasias (leukaemia, thrombocytopenia).
5. Anticoagulant therapy.
6. Rendu-Weber-Osler disease.
7. Pseudoxanthoma elasticum.
8. Uraemia.
9. Amyloidosis.
10. Vasculitis.
11. Arteriovenous malformations or Dieulafoy's lesion.
12. Corrosive ingestion (e.g. strong acid or strong alkali).
13. 'Spurious' haematemesis (e.g. swallowed nosebleed).
14. Aorto-duodenal fistula; haemobilia.
15. Watermelon stomach (gastric antral vascular ectasia, e.g. in scleroderma).
16. Idiopathic.

- All the above mentioned causes may produce **melaena**.
- Dieulafoy's lesion: Easily overlooked, small, superficial mucosal defect of stomach that involves an end artery which remains as large as its feeding artery → pressure erosion of the epithelium by the vessel → ultimately the vessel ruptures.

Q. Describe the characteristic features of melaena:

Melaena is 'altered blood in stool' with the following characteristics:

1. Black tarry stool (due to production of acid haematin); sticky too.
2. Offensive (acid haematin is altered by bacteria), and with a characteristic odour.
3. 'Semisolid' in consistency; often it is difficult to flush out.
4. Red-coloured fluid comes out from the stool after addition of water in it.
5. Usually associated with vertigo, dizziness or syncopal attack during defecation.

Approximately 60 mL of blood is required to produce a 'single black stool' and blood should remain at least 8 hours within the gut lumen to produce melaena. Haematemesis (vomiting out of blood) and melaena usually denote bleeding from the proximal gut **(proximal to the ligament of Treitz)** but bleeding from the lower gut may rarely produce melaena provided the gastrointestinal transit time is sufficiently prolonged. Occult blood test in stool may remain positive for 7 days even after the colour of stool becomes normal. Majority of patients with haematemesis usually have melaena; one event of bleed can give rise to 5–6 episodes of melaena. To produce clinical signs, the patient should bleed minimally 500 mL of blood from GI tract. Rarely, 'swallowed blood' may give rise to melaena (spurious), e.g. epistaxis.

Q. What is haematochezia?

It is the passage of bright red blood per rectum mixed with or without stool. It signifies bleeding from a source which is usually **distal to the ligament of Treitz**. The common examples of lower GI tract bleeding are haemorrhoids, anal fissure and fistula, trauma (foreign body), proctitis, ischaemic colitis, ulcerative colitis, diverticulitis, colo-rectal polyp, malignancy of colon and rectum, angiodysplasia of colon, arteriovenous malformations, blood dyscrasias, pseudomembranous colitis and 'gay bowel syndrome' in male homosexuals. Massive upper GI bleed may give rise to bright or dark red 'maroon' coloured stool, if there is hurried peristalsis or the transit time is reduced. Haematemesis, melaena and haematochezia are symptoms of acute GI bleeding.

Q. Causes of black stool:

1. Melaena.
2. Ingestion of iron (as a haematinic): Usually associated with 'hard' stool.
3. Ingestion of bismuth (in the treatment of chronic duodenal ulcer).
4. Intake of licorice, charcoal (orally used in treatment of poisoning) or black berries.

- No. 2, 3 and 4 stools are non-sticky, and often known as pseudomelaena.

Q. Blood in stool: What are the different forms?

1. Frank blood or haematochezia.
2. Altered blood or melaena.
3. Invisible blood or occult blood (detected chemically).

NSAID, hookworm infestation and colo-rectal cancer are common causes of occult blood in stool.

- **Obscure GI bleeding:** Where the cause of GI bleeding (haematemesis, melaena and haematochezia) is not found after proper and extensive investigations.

Q. Prerequisites for occult blood test (guaiac test) in stool:

Bleeding from GI tract may be intermittent and thus the test should be performed for several (usually three) consecutive days.

1. 3 days meat-free, high-fibre diet (to avoid false-positive result) is advocated.
2. Patient should not have been taking vitamin C (may result in false-negative test).
3. Intake of NSAID and iron should be stopped. The patient may avoid toothbrush for 3 days.

Q. Indications of blood transfusion in haematemesis and/or melaena:

Transfusion is required if,

1. Patient is in persistent shock.
2. There is H/o syncope.
3. Pulse rate is >100/minute.
4. Systolic BP is <100 mm of Hg.
5. Haemoglobin concentration is <10 g/dL.

Q. Definition of portal hypertension:

Portal vein is a 5.5–8 cm long vein formed by the union of superior mesenteric vein and splenic vein, behind the head of the pancreas at about the level of L_2 vertebra. Approximately, 2/3rd of hepatic blood flow and 1/2 of the O_2 supply to the liver are provided by the portal vein.

Normal pressure in the portal vein is 5–8 mm of Hg or 10–15 cm of saline. Portal hypertension is **defined** as sustained elevation of portal pressure >30 cm of saline (measured at surgery) or a direct percutaneous transhepatic portal vein pressure >12 mm of Hg.

Q. How oesophageal varices, caput medusae and haemorrhoids are formed in cirrhosis?

In cirrhosis, the porto-systemic anastomosis at different levels give rise to:

- **Oesophageal varices (at lower end of oesophagus):**
  a. Portal venous system: Left gastric vein, short gastric vein and posterior gastric veins communicate with,
  b. Caval venous system: Intercostal veins, diaphragmo-oesophageal vein and azygos minor vein.
- **Caput medusae (around umbilicus):**
  a. Portal venous system: Paraumbilical veins communicate with,
  b. Caval venous system: Superficial veins of the anterior abdominal wall.
- **Internal haemorrhoids (ano-rectal varices):**
  a. Portal venous system: Superior rectal vein communicates with,
  b. Caval venous system: Middle and inferior rectal veins.

Q. What is Child-Pugh classification in cirrhosis?

In cirrhosis, Child's grade is used to assess the hepato-cellular function. The determining 5 factors are: serum bilirubin, serum albumin, ascites, hepatic encephalopathy and prothrombin time. Every patient is assigned a class (A, B and C). Class A is 'prognostically' better and class C is the worst. Child-Pugh scoring system (scores 5–15 encompassing class A [5–6], B [7–9], C [10 or above]) are used to assess prognosis and is a reliable predictor of survival. A score ≥7 indicates cirrhosis with decompensation.

Q. 'Predictors' of bleeding from varices and variceal 'grading':

A. Best predictors of bleeding from varices are:
   1. Size of the varix (larger the size, the more likely it is to bleed).
   2. Presence of red signs (red colour correlates with the flow of blood through the varix), and
   3. Hepato-cellular function (hepatic failure promotes bleeding).

B. Grading of varices (endoscopic):
   1. Grade 1: The varices (slight protrusion above mucosa) can be depressed with insufflations.
   2. Grade 2: The varices occupying <50% of the lumen.
   3. Grade 3: The varices (occupying >50% of the lumen) are confluent around the circumference of the oesophagus.

- Red signs: 'Cherry-red spots' viewed on endoscopy suggest imminent rupture of varices.
- There are many classificaton (grading) of oesophageal varices. The Westaby classification (grading) is mentioned above.

Q. Anaemia in cirrhosis:

The possible explanations are:

1. Haematemesis and/or melaena: Blood loss.
2. Anorexia producing malnutrition: Nutritional.
3. Malabsorption.
4. Hypersplenism.
5. Haemolysis in alcoholic cirrhosis (with hyper-lipidaemia, it is known as Zieve's syndrome).

Q. Jaundice in cirhosis:

1. Impaired bilirubin metabolism, i.e. failure to excrete bilirubin (commonest).
2. Progressive hepatic injury.
3. Intrahepatic cholestasis.
4. Haemolysis (rare).
5. Viral hepatitis from blood transfusion (given to combat haematemesis or melaena).

Q. How to suspect that cirrhosis has transformed into hepatoma?

1. Rapid deterioration of general health.
2. Pain in right upper abdomen appears; fever may be there.
3. Rapidly developing huge ascites, not responding to conventional therapy.
4. Progressive hepatomegaly with hard and nodular liver.
5. Bruit may be audible (due to ↑ vascularity); rub is not uncommon.
6. Increase in serum alkaline phosphatase and α-fetoprotein.

Q. Features of hepatic encephalopathy (HE):

HE is a neuropsychiatric syndrome due to biochemical disturbance in performing function of brain. The stages are:

A. Stage of hepatic pre-coma:

a. Symptoms:
   i. Alteration in behaviour (may be restless or violent initially).
   ii. Impairment of memory and intellectual deterioration.
   iii. Inability to concentrate, apathy, slowness and brevity of response.
   iv. Disturbed consciousness and inversion of sleep rhythm (daytime sleep with arousal at night) with hypersomnia **(one of the early changes)**.
   v. Drowsiness, disorientation and confusion; features of cerebral oedema.
   vi. Changes in personality.
   vii. Slurred and monotonous speech.
   viii. Rarely, convulsions and myoclonus.

b. Signs:
   i. Higher functions: Disorientation in time, place and person; dysarthria.
   ii. Flapping tremor (asterixis); handwriting: Micrographia.
   iii. Constructional apraxia (elicited by positive Reitan trail-making test, drawing test).
   iv. Rigidity.
   v. Ankle clonus: May be present.
   vi. Plantar response: Flexor.
   vii. Gait: Ataxic.

B. Stage of hepatic coma:

a. Patient is in deep coma.
b. Flapping tremor: Absent.
c. Tone of muscles: Flaccid.
d. Jerks or deep reflexes: Absent.
e. Plantar response: Extensor.

- EEG (electroencephalogram) shows symmetric high voltage triphasic waves changing down to the delta ranges (slow activity) in hepatic encephalopathy.
- **'Minimal' hepatic encephalopathy** (i.e. early hepatocellular failure): Few patients are clinically normal but show significant impairment in their psychometric performance and electrophysiological variables including the EEG.
- **D/D of hepatic encephalopathy** (in the setting of alcoholic cirrhosis of liver) are hypoglycaemia, alcohol intoxication, delirium tremens, Wernicke's encephalopathy and subdural haematoma.

Q. Precipitating factors for hepatic encephalopathy in cirrhosis:

1. Upper gastrointestinal bleeding (from ruptured varices or peptic ulcer).
2. Excess protein in diet.
3. Overzealous use of diuretics (produces hypokalaemia → alkalosis; NH_3 cannot be converted into NH_4^+; so, hypokalaemia is very dangerous in cirrhotic patient).
4. Infection (sepsis); trauma.
5. Surgery (even operation on a small abscess): Produces fluid loss and electrolyte imbalance.
6. Paracentesis abdominis (volume >3–5 litres).
7. Sedatives, hypnotics; anaesthesia.
8. Electrolyte imbalance (hypokalaemia, hyponatraemia).
9. Acute alcoholic debauch.
10. Porto-systemic shunts made surgically or formed spontaneously (large shunts).
11. Constipation; vomiting, dehydration and diarrhoea (produces dyselectrolytaemia).
12. Uraemia.

Clinical Wisdom

Anaemia, hypoxia, hypoglycaemia and hypotension are also important precipitating factors.

Q. Aetiopathogenesis of hepatic encephalopathy:

The different hypothesis are:

1. Increase ammonia level in blood (most important): NH_3 combines with α-ketoglutaric acid in the Krebs' cycle and forms glutamic acid. So there is substrate deficiency in Krebs' cycle. NH_3 is the most readily identified toxin though it is not solely responsible for altered mental status.
2. Increase in short-chain fatty acids.
3. Rise in false neurotransmitters like octopamine.
4. Rise in methionine level.
5. Increased sensitivity of CNS neurones to gamma-aminobutyric acid (GABA), an inhibitory true neurotransmitter in the CNS.
6. Increased conversion of tryptophan to inhibitory neurotransmitter serotonin.
7. Ratio of aromatic amino acids (phenylalanine, tyrosine and tryptophan) to branched-chain amino acids (leucine, isoleucine and valine) is raised.

8. Excessive manganese deposition in the basal ganglia.
9. Increased circulating levels of endogenous benzodiazepines.
10. Different gut-derived neurotoxin (not removed by liver because of vascular shunting).

- Two general factors responsible for hepatic encephalopathy are liver failure and shunting of portal blood directly to the systemic circulation by-passing the liver.
- NH_3 (acts as a neurotoxin) also depresses cerebral blood flow and glucose metabolism.

Q. Define fulminant hepatic failure:

It is a clinical syndrome resulting from massive necrosis of liver cells with sudden and severe impairment of hepatic function (it is virtually a medical hepatectomy). The definition usually includes a time frame of 12 weeks from the onset of jaundice, in patients without pre-existing liver disease.

1. Fulminant: Hepatic failure develops within 2 weeks from the onset of jaundice.
2. Sub-fulminant: Hepatic failure develops between 2–12 weeks of the appearance of jaundice. Acute liver failure has been recently classified as,
   a. Acute (0–4 weeks)
      i. Hyperacute (0–7 days)
      ii. Acute (8 days–4 weeks)
   b. Subacute (29 days–12 weeks)
   c. Late-onset hepatic failure (8–24 weeks)

Q. Common causes of acute (fulminant) hepatic failure:

The causes vary from place to place, and they are:

1. Acute viral hepatitis (commonest).
2. Drug-induced (halothane, rifampicin-INH combination, paracetamol overdose).
3. Mushroom or copper sulphate poisoning.
4. Weil's disease.
5. Acute Budd-Chiari syndrome.
6. Shock and multiorgan failure.
7. Wilson's disease.
8. Acute fatty liver of pregnancy.
9. Reye's syndrome (patients <16 years and aspirin-induced).
10. Autoimmune hepatitis.
11. Eclampsia/HELLP syndrome (haemolysis + elevated liver enzymes + low platelets—a life-threating pregnancy-induced complications).

Clinical Wisdom

The clinical features are anorexia, fatigue, nausea/vomiting, jaundice, coagulopathy, distension of abdomen, hepatomegaly and ascites.

Q. D/D you like to consider in your case:

A. On aetiological basis:

a. Cryptogenic cirrhosis: This term is now used interchangeably with postnecrotic cirrhosis (the case described at the outset) but the terminology should be reserved for the patients where the aetiology is not known (10% of all cirrhotics). Clinical presentation in both the types are almost same. In many cases of cryptogenic cirrhosis, unrecognised NASH/NAFLD may play a role.
b. Alcoholic cirrhosis: Male preponderance, H/o intake of alcohol in cirrhogenic dose (commonly ≥one pint of alcohol taken daily for 8 years), jaundice is less persistent, mild ascites, alcoholic stigmata present, H/o pancreatitis and peptic ulcer; spleen is less commonly palpable.
c. Primary biliary cirrhosis: Commonly in middle-aged woman with persistent generalised pruritus, dark urine and pale stool, jaundice with scratch marks in skin, clubbing, pigmentation, xanthelasma and xanthomas, gradual development of ascites, oedema and hepato-cellular failure
d. Wilson's disease (hepatolenticular degeneration) (Fig. 1.43): Young patient with hepatosplenomegaly and K-F ring in cornea, neurological manifestations like chorea, slurred speech, drooling of saliva, dystonia, tremor are not uncommon. Positive family history may be obtained. The serum copper and ceruloplasmin are low though copper is accumulated in liver and brain; hepatic copper >250 µg/g of dry weight of liver is diagnostic (by liver biopsy). It is being treated by penicillamine, elemental zinc and trientine.
e. Indian childhood cirrhosis: Age group is 6 months to 5 years, onset around first year of life with progressive distension of abdomen, irritability, low

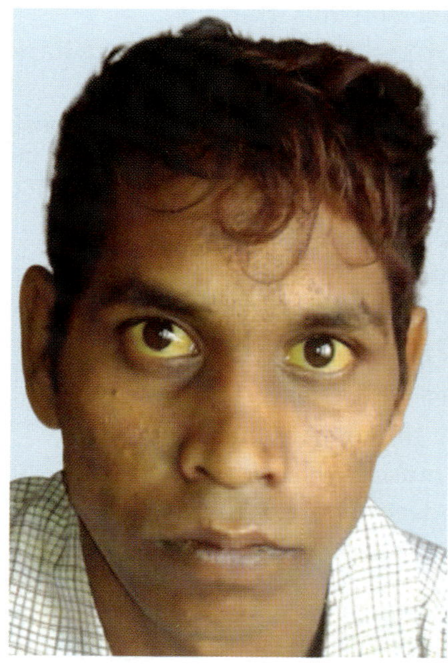

Fig. 1.43: Wilson's disease with jaundice and K-F ring in eyes

grade fever, firm liver with 'sharp leafy margin', splenomegaly with progressive hepato-cellular failure.

f. α_1-antitrypsin deficiency: Young age group, patient (PiZZ phenotype) usually suffers from respiratory distress due to emphysema or bronchiectasis along with chronic liver disease.

g. Secondary biliary cirrhosis: H/o previous surgery in biliary tract with H/o ascending cholangitis. There is presence of pain in the right hypochondrium. This type of cirrhosis results from partial or total obstruction of the CBD for more than one year. Other features are like that of primary biliary cirrhosis.

B. D/D done by:

a. Hepatomegaly.
b. Splenomegaly.
c. Ascites (never forget to make D/D with constrictive pericarditis).
d. Causes of haematemesis and melaena.
e. D/D of jaundice.

❍ Mention the D/D of your case according to the findings elicited and then apply your judgement. Cirrhosis of liver should be read along with the section on 'Ascites'.

Q. What is cardiac cirrhosis?

Prolonged passive venous congestion to liver from valvular heart disease, constrictive pericarditis or long-duration congestive cardiac failure may lead to cirrhotic changes in liver ('nutmeg liver' with alternating red and pale areas), and is known as cardiac cirrhosis. Clinical examination shows firm, non-tender and non-pulsatile hepatomegaly, features of right-sided heart failure, and stigmata of chronic encephalopathy with waxing and waning. This is a very rare cause of cirrhosis in clinical practice. Liver biopsy is diagnostic and the treatment aims at underlying heart disease.

Q. Can it be a case of carcinoma of liver?

No. Characteristics of carcinoma of liver are:

1. Cachexia, loss of weight, very rapid course.
2. Large, tender, grossly nodular, hard liver with bruit or hepatic rub.
3. **Absence of splenomegaly.**
4. Jaundice is of variable degree (secondary carcinoma of liver may be present with jaundice, hepatoma usually presents without jaundice).
5. Ascites (often tender) with pedal oedema.
6. Neck glands may be palpable.
7. Usually there is no porto-systemic venous collaterals.

Q. Differentiation between primary and secondary carcinoma of liver:

- **Primary (hepato-cellular carcinoma or hepatoma; 10%):** H/o hepatitis B or C infection, or cirrhosis of liver, or chonic arsenicosis, age 40–50 years, usually single nodule without umbilication, hepatic bruit present (due to ↑ vascularity), hepatic rub +, usually there is absence of jaundice with ↑α-fetoprotein. Alkaline phosphatase is elevated.
- **Secondary (90%):** H/o primary carcinoma in GI tract (stomach, colon), bronchus, breast or thyroid (primary source is not detected in 50%), aged patient with multiple nodules of variable size having umbilication (due to necrosis), hepatic bruit absent but rub ++, usually with obstructive jaundice along with ↑ levels of alkaline phosphatase and carcinoembryonic antigen (CEA) while α-fetoprotein is usually not high. Hepatic metastasis is common due to its dual blood supply (portal vein and hepatic artery).

❍ In both the situations, liver feels hard, irregular and tender (may or may not be tender).

Q. Nodular liver, jaundice, splenomegaly, ascites: can it be carcinome of liver?

In carcinoma of liver, there is absence of splenomegaly. Rarely, this case may be a primary hepato-cellular carcinoma (hepatoma) transformed from cirrhosis of liver. Presence of splenomegaly indicates the origin from cirrhosis of liver.

Q. Portal hypertension with massive splenomegaly:

Portal hypertension is usually associated with moderate splenomegaly. In massive splenomegaly, think of:

1. Extrahepatic obstruction (i.e. presinusoidal-extrahepatic causes).
2. Cirrhosis with hypersplenism.
3. Non-cirrhotic portal fibrosis (NCPF).
4. Rarely in tropical splenomegaly syndrome.

Q. Complications of cirrhosis:

1. Portal hypertension (variceal bleeding, congestive or portal gastropathy, hypersplenism, etc.).
2. Hepato-cellular failure and hepatic encephalopathy (acute on chronic and chronic).
3. Ascites and spontaneous bacterial peritonitis (SBP).
4. Hepato-renal syndrome (functional renal failure with normal tubular functions develop due to circulatory or haemodynamic changes): Occurs in 10% cases.
5. Acute and chronic pancreatitis.
6. Cholecystitis with pigment stone.
7. Peptic ulcer.
8. Septicaemia (gram-negative) and tuberculosis.
9. Portal vein thrombosis.
10. Hepato-cellular carcinoma (hepatoma) as a late complication.
11. Coagulopathy (factor deficiency, thrombocytopenia, fibrinolysis).
12. Hepato-pulmonary syndrome (HPS).
13. Porto-pulmonary hypertension.

14. Haematological complications (anaemia, haemolysis, neutropenia, thrombocytopenia).
15. Hepatic osteodystrophy or bone disorders (osteopenia, osteoporosis, osteomalacia).

- Cirrhotics may be hypoxaemic due to **hepato-pulmonary syndrome** (intrapulmonary shunting through direct arteriovenous communications → may be a result of NO overproduction), **porto-pulmonary hypertension** (pulmonary hypertension as a result of vasoconstriction and obliteration of pulmonary arterial system → leading to dyspnoea and fatigue), and hydrothorax. HPS is manifested by orthodeoxia (platypnoea), breathlessness, clubbing, central cyanosis and spider naevi.

Q. How do you suspect that spontaneous bacterial peritonitis (SBP) has developed?

SBP is suspected by appearance of fever, abdominal pain, increasing ascites not responding to diuretics, diminished bowel sounds and appearance of features of hepatic encephalopathy. The organisms (*E coli, Klebsiella,* enterococci) enter the peritoneum by haematogenous spread. Diagnostic aspiration should be performed immediately. It is an acute emergency and should be treated urgently with antibiotics (e.g. 3rd-generation cephalosporins). Norfloxacin 400 mg, BD-daily for 7 days is recommended for prevention.

Q. Sudden worsening (decompensation) of stable cirrhosis—reasons behind:

1. Consider the precipitating factors for hepatic encephalopathy, e.g. bleeding, hypokalaemia.
2. Development of spontaneous bacterial peritonitis or tuberculous peritonitis, or sepsis.
3. Transformation into hepatoma.
4. Formation of chylous ascites as a result of rupture of dilated abdominal lymphatics.
5. Portal vein thrombosis.
6. Development of renal or cardiac failure.

Q. Possible causes of death in cirrhosis:

1. Hepatic encephalopathy.
2. Cerebral oedema and ↑ICT.
3. Intercurrent infection (septicaemia).
4. Respiratory failure.
5. Coagulopathy.
6. Renal failure.
7. Hypoglycaemia, hypokalaemia.
8. Acid-base imbalance.

- Actually, these are the complications of fulminant hepato-cellular failure.

Q. Renal failure in cirrhosis:

Renal failure in a patient with hepato-cellular failure may be due to various factors, e.g.

1. Acute tubular necrosis precipitated by infection, haemorrhage or drugs (e.g. gentamicin),
2. If associated with primary kidney disease, or
3. Hepato-renal syndrome: When there is change in blood volume or shifting of fluid within the body compartment, this syndrome precipitates. The syndrome is due to increased pre-glomerular vascular resistance and thus the blood flow is diverted away from the renal cortex with resultant reduced GFR. *The kidneys are structurally normal but functionally abnormal.* There is progressive oliguria, ↑ in serum urea and creatinine with ↓ Na^+ and ↑K^+. The prognosis is poor.

Q. Investigations you like to perform in your case:

1. Blood examination-TC, DC, ESR, Hb%:
   a. Microcytic-hypochromic anaemia due to haematemesis and melaena.
   b. Pancytopenia may be seen in hypersplenism, macrocytic anaemia in alcoholics.
   c. ESR is increased in the presence of infection (like tuberculosis, SBP).
   d. Serum urea, creatinine, sugar and electrolytes (as a routine).
   e. Viral markers: HBV (HB_S Ag, HB_e Ag, IgG anti-HBc), HCV (anti-HCV).
2. Stool for occult blood test: May be positive.
3. Rectal examination (haemorrhoids are not palpable unless thrombosed) and proctoscopy for demonstration of internal haemorrhoids; slit-lamp examination of cornea for detection of K-F ring.
4. Chest X-ray: May show tuberculosis or hydrothorax.
5. Liver function tests:
   a. *Total protein is diminished with low albumin and high globulin.* **Albumin and globulin ratio is altered** (normal albumin level is 3.5–5.5 g/dL and that of globulin is 2–3.5 g/dL). ↓Albumin is due to impairment of hepatic protein synthesis whereas ↑ globulin results from non-specific stimulation of reticulo-endothelial system.
   b. Serum bilirubin: Normal or raised.
   c. SGOT and SGPT (AST and ALT): Mild elevation.
   d. Alkaline phosphatase: Slightly increased.
   e. Serum cholesterol: Low.
   f. Prothrombin time (PT): Increased and does not return to normal level with vitamin K therapy (it is a very important 'prognostic marker' of hepato-cellular damage. Normal prothrombin time is 12–16 seconds). Increased prothrombin time is a bad prognostic sign.
6. Serum autoantibodies: Antinuclear antibody, anti-smooth muscle antibody and anti-mitochondrial antibody may be present in varying percentage in autoimmune hepatitis, primary biliary cirrhosis and cryptogenic cirrhosis.
7. Serum immunoglobulins are increased, e.g. IgG in autoimmune hepatitis, IgA in alcoholic cirrhosis and IgM in primary biliary cirrhosis.
8. Barium swallow X-ray of oesophagus demonstrates 'worm-eaten appearance' or 'moth-eaten appearance'

(mutiple filling defects) at the lower part of oesophagus due to the presence of oesophageal varices. Sometimes, gastric varices may be seen by barium meal examination.

9. Endoscopy of upper GI tract: Shows oesophageal or gastric varices, peptic ulcer, or congestive gastropathy (looks beefy-red; mosaic pattern of red and yellow mucosa with petechial haemorrhage). It is a very important and reliable primary investigation for portal hypertension.
10. Straight X-ray of abdomen: Usually not informative. It may show increased hepatic and splenic size, or ground-glass opacity of ascites.
11. Examination of ascitic fluid: Transudate in nature if not complicated by tuberculosis or SBP. Serum-ascites albumin gradient (SAAG) is ≥1.1g/dL (indicates underlying portal hypertension).
12. USG (or, CT or MRI scan) of liver, spleen, portal vein (size), any collaterals, presence of thrombosis (in portal vein, splenic vein, hepatic vein, IVC), and for any free fluid in the abdomen—in cirrhosis of liver, there is heterogenous echo-pattern of liver (liver size <10 cm), splenic enlargement (>13 cm), presence of ascites and increase in diameter of portal vein (≥13 mm). **USG is superior to CT or MRI scan in diagnosing cirrhosis.**
13. **Liver biopsy (USG-guided): The gold standard test and confirms the diagnosis of cirrhosis of liver** (by Vim-Silverman, Menghini or 'Trucut' needle). Biopsy specimen can be especially stained for copper and iron.

Clinical Wisdom

Clinical suspicion of cirrhosis should be confirmed immediately by combination of laboratory and imaging tests, and finally by liver biopsy.

14. Percutaneous intrasplenic pressure measurement: Increased in portal hypertension.
15. Percutaneous transhepatic portal venography or splenoportalvenography (SPV): For the demonstration of site of obstruction and nature of collaterals. In SPV, the intrahepatic pattern in cirrhosis is known as 'tree in winter' appearance; 'cut off' sign is observed in NCPF.
16. Wedged hepatic venous pressure (normal 5–6 mm of Hg): Increased in cirrhosis of liver, i.e. >20 mm of Hg (never increased in NCPF).
17. Special investigations where facilities are available:
    a. Visualisation of portal venous system by Doppler ultrasound.
    b. Duplex Doppler ultrasonography for measurement of portal blood flow.
    c. Portal venography by digital subtraction angiography.
    d. Magnetic resonance angiography for portal vein.
18. Electroencephalogram (EEG): Triphasic waves are seen in fulminant hepatic failure.

- Serum copper and ceruloplasmin estimation may be done for detection of Wilson's disease, serum iron/TIBC/ferritin for haemochromatosis, and serum α_1-antitrypsin for aetiological diagnosis.

Q. Management of cirrhosis of liver:

1. Rest: Absolute bed rest in decompensated stage (reduction of physical activity reduces metabolic demands of liver and increases the renal perfusion).
2. Diet: Salt-free high protein diet (>1g/kg/day). Protein is restricted judiciously at the onset of hepatic encephalopathy.
3. Treatment of infection by proper antibiotics: SBP is treated by co-amoxyclav (amoxycillin 1 g, clavulinic acid 200 mg, IV, 8–12 hourly), or cefotaxime (1 g, IV, 12 hourly) plus gentamicin (60 mg, IV, 8 hourly), or piperacillin-tazobactam (4.5 g, IV, 6 hourly) for 5–7 days.
4. Treatment of variceal haemorrhage by:
    a. Blood transfusion.
    b. Vasopressin, terlipressin, octreotide or infusion of somatostatin.
    c. Sengstaken tube.
    d. Endoscopic sclerotherapy of varices or band ligation.
    e. Transjugular intrahepatic portosystemic stent shunting (TIPSS).
    f. Lastly, oesophageal transection (rarely used; poor outcome).
5. Treatment of hepatic encephalopathy by:
    a. Protein-restricted diet. Vegetable protein is less ammoniagenic, better tolerated and more laxative.
    b. Lactulose: 15–30 mL three times daily (dose is adjusted to ensure at least two to three semisolid stools per day). Lactitol may be used in lactulose-intolerant patients.
    c. Neomycin 4 g/day or metronidazole 200 mg, QDS, orally has now been replaced by rifaximin, 550 mg BD orally for 5–7 days.
    d. Enemata: Neutral phosphate, magnesium sulphate, mannitol—administer 8–12 hourly for 2–3 days.
    e. L-ornithine L-aspartate (LOLA) given parenterally or orally promotes hepatic removal along with detoxification of NH_3.
    f. Inj. Mannitol (20%): 100 mL, 8 hrly, IV in hepatic pre-coma.
    g. Maintenance of calorie, fluid and electrolytes. Supplement with zinc.
    h. Probiotics: Reduces intestinal NH_3 production.
6. Injection of vitamin K for coagulopathy—1 amp. (10 mg) of inj. vit. K, IM or IV daily for consecutive 3 days.
7. Judicious use of sedatives, if necessary: **Safe sedatives** in liver disease are oxazepam, temazepam,

chlormethiazole, phenobarbitone, etc. (morphine or paraldehyde are absolutely contraindicated).

8. Management of ascites by paracentesis, diuretics; control of oedema.
9. Control of aetiological factors:
   a. Abstinence from alcohol intake.
   b. Penicillamine in Wilson's disease.
   c. Phlebotomy or desferrioxamine in haemochromatosis.
10. Management of fulminant hepatic failure in an 'intensive care unit' with experienced management team.

- Over and above, inj. ranitidine 50 mg, IV, 6–8 hourly is given; dialysis is done for renal failure. Fresh frozen plasma is given if prothrombin time is >1.5 times more than normal.
- Safest analgesic in cirrhosis is paracetamol. Neomycin is available as 350 mg tablet and avoided in the presence of renal failure (not used nowadays).
- Gross protein restriction as first-line treatment is not recommended nowadays as it may lead to deteriorating nutritional state in already malnourished patients.
- **Prevention of recurrent variceal haemorrhage** is done by sclerotherapy, banding, TIPSS, propranolol and porto-systemic shunt surgery.

Q. How lactulose acts in hepatic encephalopathy?

Lactulose is a synthetic non-absorbable disaccharide. In the caecum, it is broken down into acetic acid and lactic acid, and thus the fecal pH drops. Its mechanism of action are:

1. Produces acidic diarrhoea (acts as an enema or bowel wash).
2. As intestinal pH is acidic, NH_3 absorption is less (NH_3 is converted into NH_4^+).
3. Promotes incorporation of N_2 within the intestinal bacteria.
4. The drop in fecal pH helps in the growth of lactose-fermenting organisms and suppresses the NH_3-forming bacteria (*Bacteroides*).
5. It may detoxify short-chain fatty acids.

- Nowadays, some clinicians use lactitol (approximately 30 g/day) instead of lactulose. Lactitol is available in powder form; it is less sweet, produces less flatulence and have a quicker action.

Q. Promising drugs in hepato-cellular failure:

a. Acute: Flumazenil (benzodiazepine receptor antagonist), IV branched-chain amino acid, levodopa, L-ornithine L-aspartate (LOLA), sodium benzoate, zinc, probiotics.
b. Chronic: Bromocriptine (dopamine agonist).

Q. Drugs causing reduction of portal hypertension:

1. Vasopressin.
2. Glypressin (terlipressin).
3. Somatostatin and octreotide.
4. Propranolol (commonly used for prevention of recurrent bleeding).
5. Clonidine.
6. Nitroglycerin.
7. Isosorbide mononitrate, and
8. Verapamil.

Q. Identification points for cirrhosis of liver:

1. Features of portal hypertension, and
2. Signs of hepato-cellular failure.

Always palpate the liver and spleen by 'dipping method' in the presence of ascites. *Splenomegaly is a very important bedside clinical finding to diagnose a case as cirrhosis of liver.* Never forget to examine for spider naevi, palmar erythema, gynaecomastia, scanty pubic hairs and testicular atrophy.

SECTION 4: NERVOUS SYSTEM

The cardinal symptoms of nervous system comprise of:

A. Higher functions:

1. Unconsciousness or alteration of consciousness, delirium, photophobia (↑sensitivity to light).
2. Loss of memory; illusion, delusion or hallucination; emotional disturbance.
3. Behavioural abnormality with speech defects.

B. Cranial nerves:

Cranial nerves	*Symptomatology*
I	Abnormal sensation of smell
II	Blurred vision, loss of vision, oscillopsia, flashes and floaters
III, IV, VI	Drooping of upper eyelid, diplopia, squint, head tilt
V	Difficulty in mastication, jaw deviation, loss of sensation over face
VII	Deviation of angle of the mouth, facial asymmetry, food accumulation at one side of mouth, epiphora, salivary dribbling, loss of taste sensation, lagophthalmos, difficulty in eye closure
VIII	Vertigo, deafness or difficulty in hearing, tinnitus, dizziness, loss of balance
IX, X	Speech difficulty or hoarseness of voice, nasal intonation of voice or nasal regurgitation of food or fluid, dysphagia, chocking
XI	Difficulty in movement of neck or shoulder, drooping of shoulder, fall-back of head
XII	Weak movement of tongue, wasting of the tongue, dysarthria, difficulty in chewing

C. Motor system:

1. Loss of power or weakness, or clumsiness of movements.
2. Wasting/thinning, or swelling (pseudohypertrophy) of limbs.

3. Fasciculation.
4. Flexor spasms.
5. Abnormal (involuntary) movements.
6. Pain in the muscles, or stiffness of muscles.
7. Heaviness in muscles.
8. Unsteady gait.

D. Sensory system:

1. Anaesthesia.
2. Paraesthesia.
3. Tingling or numbness.
4. Analgesia.
5. Hyperaesthesia, hypoaesthesia.
6. Root pain.
7. Girdle-like sensation.
8. Sensation of walking on cotton wool (e.g. tabes dorsalis).
9. Causalgia.
10. Trophic ulcer.
11. Ataxia of gait with diurnal variation.

E. Increased intracranial tension (IIT):

1. Headache.
2. Vomiting (projectile).
3. Convulsions.
4. Blurred vision.
5. Behavioural changes.
6. Coma.

F. Cerebellar system:

1. Swaying while walking (loss of balance), unsteadiness of gait or H/o tendency to fall (ataxia).
2. Weakness (as a result of hypotonia).
3. Difficulty in shaving, taking food to mouth and incoordination of speech.
4. Tremulousness (i.e. shaking) of hands while reaching for objects.

G. Autonomic nervous system (includes bladder and bowel function):

1. Retention of urine; feeling of sensation of bladder fullness.
2. Precipitancy, urgency, hesitancy, or urinary incontinence.
3. Burning micturition [(signifies UTI); H/o catheterisation].
4. Impotence (in males).
5. Diarrhoea (loose stools or rectal incontinence) or constipation.
6. Abnormal sweating (increased or diminished), palpitations, postural syncope.

- For other features of autonomic nervous system, read the section on 'Trophic changes'.

H. Miscellaneous:

1. Fever (meningitis, brain abscess).
2. Pain in the neck (meningitis, subarachnoid haemorrhage, cervical spondylosis).
3. H/o fall or seizures (epilepsy); H/o migraine: head or spinal injury; faintness (pre-syncope).
4. Sudden psychological changes like depression or euphoria, agitation, sleep disorder.
5. Discharge of pus from the ear (e.g. bacterial meningitis) (Fig. 1.44).
6. Bleeding tendency (e.g. thrombocytopenia) any H/o nose or ear bleed?
7. Rigidity, poverty of movement or frequent fall (e.g. parkinsonism).
8. Recurrent DVT (e.g. calf pain in antiphospholipid syndrome).
9. H/o birth injury or anoxic injury.
10. Any symptom related to vaccination.

- Regarding **loss of power in the motor system**, enquire about involvement of ↓↓

I. Upper limbs:
  a. Proximal (lifting of arm above the head, combing, placing an object on a high shelf).
  b. Distal (writing, sewing, typing, buttoning or objects falling off the hand).

II. Lower limbs:
  a. Proximal (climbing upstairs and going downstairs, squatting and getting up from squatting position, getting up from bathtub).
  b. Distal (slipper falling from the feet, i.e. difficulty in gripping).

III. Trunk muscles: Ask the patient to sit up from supine position (unable to roll on the bed or get up).

IV. Neck muscles: In bilateral sternomastoid weakness (e.g. myotonic dystrophy), head drops backwards;

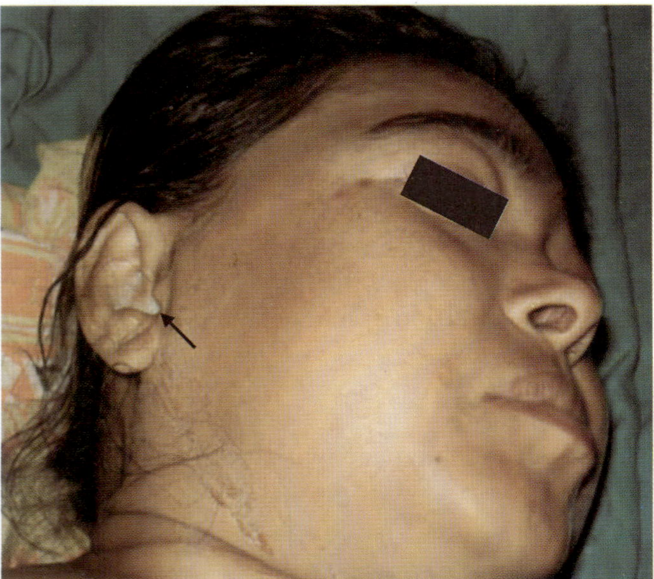

Fig. 1.44: A case of **meningitis** on the day of admission with **discharging right ear** (whitish pus seen)

while in neck extensor weakness (e.g. motor neurone disease), head drops forward (i.e. chin-on-chest).

Moreover, ask about the ability of standing (with or without support), walking (with or without support), running, etc. Predominant distal weakness is due to pyramidal tract involvement or peripheral neuropathy.

- Regarding **sensory abnormality**: Anaesthesia—loss of sensation, paraesthesia—tingling sensation (may be so intense as to be painful), analgesia—loss of pain sensation, hyperaesthesia—increased touch sensation, hyperalgesia—increased pain sensation to mildly painful stimuli, causalgia—burning, disagreeable sensation found in neuritis, allodynia—perception of pain evoked by non-painful stimulus, hyperpathia—perception of pain that spreads out and outlasts the stimulus in time (i.e. excessive response to pain).
- Regarding seizures or convulsious, enquire from relatives or eye-witness: onset and duration, frequency, precipitating factor, any aura, associated cognitive-motor-sensory deficit—if any, H/o tongue bite or urination, any automatism, post-ictal confusion, H/o head injury/seizure disorders in family/perinatal asphyxia or infection.

Q. 'Evolution' of symptoms in neurology (in history):

1. Sudden onset, rapidly evolving neurodeficit with variable recovery: Vascular, traumatic or demyelination.
2. Gradually progressive course over months (ICSOL, nutritional or toxin-induced) or over years (degenerative disorders).
3. Episodic weakness with full recovery: Epilepsy, migraine, periodic paralysis.
4. Temporary focal weakness: Transient ischaemic attack (TIA) and Todd's palsy (epilepsy).
5. Waxing and waning: Demyelinating (i.e. multiple sclerosis) or vascular malformations.
6. Sudden worsening of a slowly progressive illness: Haemorrhage within a ICSOL.

Scheme of Examination (Profoma)

A. Whether the patient is conscious, alert and co-operative

B. Higher functions:

1. Level of consciousness.
2. Appearance and behaviour.
3. Orientation with time, place and person.
4. Emotional state (euphoria, depression, hostile), i.e. the mood; sleep and dream.
5. Illusion, delusion or hallucination; thought (form and content).
6. Memory.
7. Intelligence.
8. **Speech** and language (with handedness).

C. Cranium and spine (bruit, deformities, short neck, kyphoscoliosis, etc.)

D. Signs of meningeal irritation (neck rigidity, Kernig's sign, Brudzinski's sign), straight leg raising (SLR) test and examination of carotid arteries

E. Cranial nerves:

1. Olfactory (I): Test the smell sensation with common bedside objects like soap, toothpaste, perfumes, etc.
2. Optic (II)
   i. Acuity of vision.
   ii. Field of vision.
   iii. Colour vision.
   iv. Ophthalmoscopy or fundoscopy (not essential in UG, mandatory in PG).
3. Oculomotor (III), trochlear (IV) and abducens (VI)
   i. Ptosis.
   ii. Squint.
   iii. Enophthalmos or exophthalmos.
   iv. Power of extraocular muscles: External ocular movements on follow and on command.
   v. Nystagmus.
   vi. Pupil: Size, shape, reaction (direct light reflex, consensual light reflex and accommodation reflex).
4. Trigeminal (V)
   i. Motor function (masseter, pterygoids and temporalis).
   ii. Sensory function (sensation over the face—touch, pain and temperature).
   iii. Corneal reflex: Right and left side.
   iv. Jaw jerk.
5. Facial (VII)
   i. Palpebral fissure, frowning, symmetry of blinking, eye closure, nasolabial folds, angle of the mouth, blowing, whistling, showing the teeth, epiphora, dribbling of saliva.
   ii. Power of individual facial muscle.
   iii. Upper half of face escaped or not.
   iv. Taste sensation of anterior 2/3rd of the tongue.
   v. Hyperacusis.
6. Vestibulocochlear (VIII)
   i. Hearing or auditory (or cochlear) function: Watch test, Rinne's test, Weber's test.
   ii. Vestibular function: Positional nystagmus (usually not done).
7. Glossopharyngeal (IX) and vagus (X)
   i. Soft palate: Movements (on saying '*Aaah*').
   ii. Pharyngeal or gag reflex.
   iii. Taste sensation of posterior 1/3rd of the tongue.
8. Accessory (spinal part) [XI]
   i. Power of sternomastoids.
   ii. Power of trapezius.
9. Hypoglossal (XII)
   i. Power of tongue muscles.
   ii. Deviation.
   iii. Atrophy (i.e. size, shape, wasting).
   iv. Fasciculation (or any abnormal movement).

F. Motor functions:

a. Nutrition (inspection and palpation of muscles): Attitude, atrophy or hypertrophy, etc.

	Right	Left
b. Tone		
i. Upper limb	–	–
ii. Lower limb	–	–
c. Power		
i. Upper limb	–	–
ii. Lower limb	–	–
d. Coordination		
i. Upper limb: (finger-nose test)	–	–
ii. Lower limb: (heel-shin test)	–	–
e. Involuntary movements		

G. Sensory functions:

a. Superficial or exteroceptive
   - i. Pain
   - ii. Touch
   - iii. Temperature (hot and cold): Usually not done; a rough assessment may be carried out at the bedside by using the metal of a tuning fork or metal part of stethoscope (cold perception) and by rubbing both palms (hot perception)–*see* page 486.

b. Deep or proprioceptive
   - i. Vibration sense
   - ii. Muscle sense
   - iii. Pressure sense
   - iv. Joint sense
   - v. Position sense

c. Cortical
   - i. One point (tactile) localisation
   - ii. Two point discrimination
   - iii. Stereognosis
   - iv. Graphaesthesia
   - v. Sensory extinction (perceptual rivalry).

- Is there a definite line of demarcation of sensory loss in the trunk?
- Both fine and crude touch sensations should be tested.
- Read details of sensory functions from page 485.

H. Reflexes:

	Right	Left
a. Superficial		
1. Abdominal		
i. Upper	–	–
ii. Middle	–	–
iii. Lower	–	–
2. Cremasteric	–	–
3. **Plantar response**	–	–

- Corneal, anal and gag reflex are superficial reflex.

	Right	Left
b. Deep		
1. Biceps jerk	–	–
2. Triceps jerk	–	–
3. Supinator jerk	–	–
4. Knee jerk	–	–
5. Ankle jerk	–	–
6. Clonus (ankle and patellar)	–	–

c. Visceral (sphincteric)
   1. Swallowing: The patient should be asked for dysphagia (with liquids, solids or both).
   2. Bladder: The patient is asked regarding bladder and urethral sensation, retention, incontinence, urgency, or difficulty in controlling or initiating micturition.
   3. Bowel: Whether facing any difficulty with defecation (constipation or incontinence).

d. Other reflexes
   1. Glabellar tap.
   2. Grasp reflex (on both sides).
   3. Palmo-mental reflex (on both sides).

I. Trophic changes

Bed sore, trophic ulcer, Charcot joint, changes in skin and hair.

J. Cerebellar functions: Titubation, scanning speech, pendular knee jerk, intention tremor, finger-nose test, dysdiadochokinesia, nystagmus and reeling gait.

K. Autonomic functions: Temperature regulation, postural hypotension, impotence, abnormal sweating, dry skin, palpitations, bladder dysfunction, nocturnal diarrhoea, Horner's syndrome, pupillary reactions, Valsalva manoeuvre, trophic changes.

L. Stance and gait (including Romberg's sign)

Clinical Wisdom

After examination of central nervous system (CNS), peripheral nervous system (PNS) should be examined—**Peripheral nerves are examined** for thickening, nodularity and tenderness. Commonly examined peripheral nerves are:

a. Great auricular nerve at neck
b. Ulnar nerve at elbow
c. Radial nerve at wrist
d. Common peroneal nerve at the neck of fibula
e. Posterior tibial nerve around medial malleolus
f. Sural nerve at the lateral part of ankle and foot

These nerves are commonly thickened in reference to leprosy. Read the causes of 'Thickened peripheral nerves' from the section on 'Leprosy'.

- In the general survey, mention about neurocutaneous markers (e.g. cafe-au-lait spots), stigmata of atherosclerosis or features of chronic alcoholism.

HEMIPLEGIA — CASE 16

Q. What is your diagnosis?

This is a case of left-sided complete hemiparesis (or hemiplegia) in the stage of recovery due to cerebral thrombosis probably involving the lenticulostriate branch of middle cerebral artery and the lesion is in the right internal capsule.

Q. Why do you say so?

This right-handed male patient aged 72 years was complaining of weakness of the left side of his body for last 10 days. At the onset when he was about to go to bathroom at about 5 am, he suddenly felt weak and could not move his left side. The episode was sudden in onset and the evolution of paralysis was completed within 6 hours. The patient complained of headache and vertigo at the beginning of the attack but neither he lost consciousness nor there was any H/o fall though there was some behavioural abnormalities present at that moment. He was suffering from mild speech difficulty (i.e. regarding fluency) and was immediately hospitalised. The patient also said that the weakness was marked in the left upper limb in comparison to left lower limb. There was no loss of bladder and bowel control. He had no H/o vomiting, convulsions, double vision, nasal regurgitation or nasal intonation but he complained of deviation of face to the right side during eating, speaking or attempted smiling. Though the disease started acutely, he was gradually improving in the hospital.

There was no H/o fever, head injury, palpitations, chest pain, breathlessness, previous neurodeficit of this type which recovered completely (e.g. TIA); no family H/o diabetes mellitus, hypertension or tuberculosis was obtained. There was no H/o contact with tuberculosis, no H/o exposure to STD (sexually transmitted diseases). He did not give any H/o diabetes mellitus; a non-smoker by habit. There was no H/o waxing and waning of his symptoms. For the last few days, he was on physiotherapy. He was a government service holder and came from a middle class family.

On examination, it shows that the patient is conscious, alert and cooperative. He is hypertensive but neither there is any valvular heart disease present nor there is presence of any bruit over the carotids. He is suffering from UMN paralysis of left upper and lower limbs including the paralysis of lower half of left face (i.e. UMN type of facial paralysis in the left), i.e. left-sided complete hemiparesis (or hemiplegia). The UMN paralysis of left side of the body is suggested by the presence of clasp-knife spasticity, loss of superficial reflexes, brisk tendon reflexes and presence of extensor plantar response. The neurological examination of right side of the body was essentially normal.

Q. What is your case?

Say the summary as above.

Q. Importance of 'past history' in hemiplegia:

1. Similar type of attacks or monoplegia in the past which recovered completely (indicates TIA).
2. Head injury (subdural haematoma).
3. Hypertension (TIA, cerebral thrombosis or haemorrhage, lacunar infarction).
4. Diabetes mellitus (often associated with hypertension and accelerates the atherosclerosis).
5. Rheumatic fever (valvular heart disease and cerebral embolism).
6. Epilepsy or convulsive disorder (Todd's palsy), or migraine (hemiplegic migraine).
7. Tuberculosis (tuberculoma, tuberculous arteritis or tuberculous meningitis).
8. Intake of oral contraceptives with duration (may predispose to strokes in females, if used for more than 5 years), anticoagulants or aspirin; any bleeding tendency.
9. Fever (meningitis, cerebral abscess, encephalitis, leukaemia or lymphoma).
10. H/o exposure to STD (neurosyphilis).
11. Dyspnoea or pain chest (mitral stenosis or recent acute myocardial infarction).
12. Intermittent claudication (atherosclerosis, arteritis).
13. Recent weight loss (tuberculosis).

- Pattern of seizure disorder (e.g. **epilepsy**): Prodromal phase—change of mood (aura), tonic phase—spasm of all muscles, unconsciousness and fall, clonic phase—jerks in limbs and trunk, tongue bite, and post-ictal phase—confusion, amnesia, headache and flaccidity.
- **Todd's palsy**: Following epileptiform convulsions there may be development of paralysis (commonly monoplegia, rarely hemiplegia) due to exhaustion of cerebral neurones, and is known as Todd's palsy. Todd's palsy usually recovers within 24 hours. TIA and hemiplegic migraine also recover within 24 hours.

Q. Importance of 'family history' in hemiplegia:

1. Hypertension.
2. Diabetes mellitus.
3. Similar illness among other members of the family, especially in young patients (cerebral diplegia, spinocerebellar degeneration, etc.).
4. Epilepsy or migraine.

Q. Importance of 'personal history' in hemiplegia:

Hypertension, diabetes, hyperlipidaemia, smoking, obesity and a strong family history of CVA. Bladder and bowel habit, loss of weight, H/o seizure disorder or tuberculosis, and occupational exposure are enquired.

Q. Chief complaints (clinical presentations) of your patient:

1. Weakness of the left side of body for last 10 days.
2. Deviation of the face to right side while eating or speaking, for last 10 days, and
3. Difficulty in speech for last 10 days.

Q. Enquiry regarding paralysis (in H/o present illness):

a. Date of onset: Note the specific date and time of onset of paralysis.

b. Mode of onset:

i. Sudden: Vascular, infective, traumatic and demyelinating.

ii. Gradual: Intracranial space-occupying lesion (ICSOL).

Clinical Wisdom

- Cerebral embolism: Develops in seconds (stormy).
- Cerebral thrombosis: Develops in minutes and hours.
- Cerebral haemorrhage: Very sudden in onset which relentlessly progress.
- Infective: Develops in hours and days.
- Demyelinating disease (multiple sclerosis): Develops in days and weeks.

c. Precipitating factors:

i. During sleep or soon after rising from bed: Cerebral thrombosis.

ii. During exertion, activity: Cerebral embolism.

iii. At the height of emotion: Cerebral haemorrhage.

iv. During activity, exertion or height of emotion: Subarachnoid haemorrhage.

v. Following fever: Cerebral abscess, encephalitis, meningitis.

vi. Following convulsions: Todd's palsy, cerebral haemorrhage or thrombosis.

d. Evolution of paralysis:

i. Paralysis extends over hours to days ('stroke in evolution').

ii. Paralysis is 'total' or maximal from the beginning **(completed stroke)**: Usually completed within 6 hours.

iii. Increase in a stepwise manner, i.e. repeated episodes of TIA leading to fully evolved stroke **('stuttering hemiplegia')**.

e. Progress of paralysis:

i. Improving, stationary or deteriorating (a complete recovery usually indicates cerebral embolism or demyelinating disease).

ii. Waxing and waning (means exacerbations and remissions): In demyelinating diseases.

f. Degree and duration of paralysis: Weakness or total loss of power, with duration.

g. Motor symptoms: See the symptomatology.

Q. Meaning of few terminologies in clinical neurology:

'Plegia' means complete or near complete paralysis, and **'paresis'** means weakness or partial paralysis.

1. Hemiplegia: Paralysis of one half of the body (especially of face, arm and leg), i.e. it is a facio-brachio-crural paralysis. The trunk is exempted due to bilateral innervation.
2. Hemiparesis: Weakness of one half of the body (especially of face, arm and leg).
3. Paraplegia: Paralysis of both the lower limbs (mostly due to spinal cord lesion).
4. Paraparesis: Weakness of both the lower limbs.
5. Diplegia: Bilateral hemiplegia of cortical origin where the lower limbs are more affected than the upper limbs (i.e. cerebral palsy).
6. Quadriplegia or tetraplegia: Paralysis of all the four limbs, and trunk (a feature of cervical cord disease).
7. Pentaplegia: Quadriplegia along with respiratory muscles paralysis (e.g. GB syndrome).
8. Monoplegia: Paralysis of one limb—
   i. Brachial monoplegia: Paralysis of one upper extremity.
   ii. Crural monoplegia: Paralysis of one lower extremity.
9. Crossed hemiplegia: Paralysis of ipsilateral cranial nerves (LMN type) with contralateral hemiplegia (a feature of brainstem disease).
10. Cruciate hemiplegia: Brachial monoplegia of one side with contralateral crural monoplegia.
11. Bi-brachial paralysis: Paralysis of both the upper extremities.
12. Bilateral (double) hemiplegia: Paralysis of all the four limbs, trunk, and total face.
13. Paraplegia with right brachial monoplegia: 3 limbs are involved (triplegia), i.e. paralysis of right upper limb and both the lower limbs.

- Hemiplegia and hemiparesis may be complete or incomplete (see page 135).

Q. Definition of upper motor neurone (UMN) and lower motor neurone (LMN) (Flowchart 1.1):

UMN: Pyramidal cells (generally the Betz cells of area 4) and their axons upto the cranial nerve nuclei, or anterior horn cells are called UMN (i.e. corticobulbar or corticonuclear, and corticospinal tracts respectively).

LMN: The anterior hom cells and its dendrite up to the motor end plate, and cranial nerve nuclei with the cranial nerves constitute the LMN. LMN is the final common pathway for all motor impulses, both voluntary and automatic.

- Motor unit: It is defined as the single alpha motor neurone and the muscle fibres it innervates.

Q. What are 'strokes'?

The term 'stroke' is used to identity all forms of cerebrovascular accidents (CVA). A stroke or CVA is defined as 'focal neurological deficit of abrupt onset due to a vascular lesion, lasting longer than 24 hours, and is manifested, either as brain infarction or haemorrhage'. Stroke is a better term than CVA.

Q. Diseases under CVA, i.e. types of CVA:

1. Cerebral thrombosis.
2. Cerebral embolism.
3. Cerebral haemorrhage.
4. Subarachnoid haemorrhage.

Flowchart 1.1: Compartmentalisation of nervous system (NS) disorders

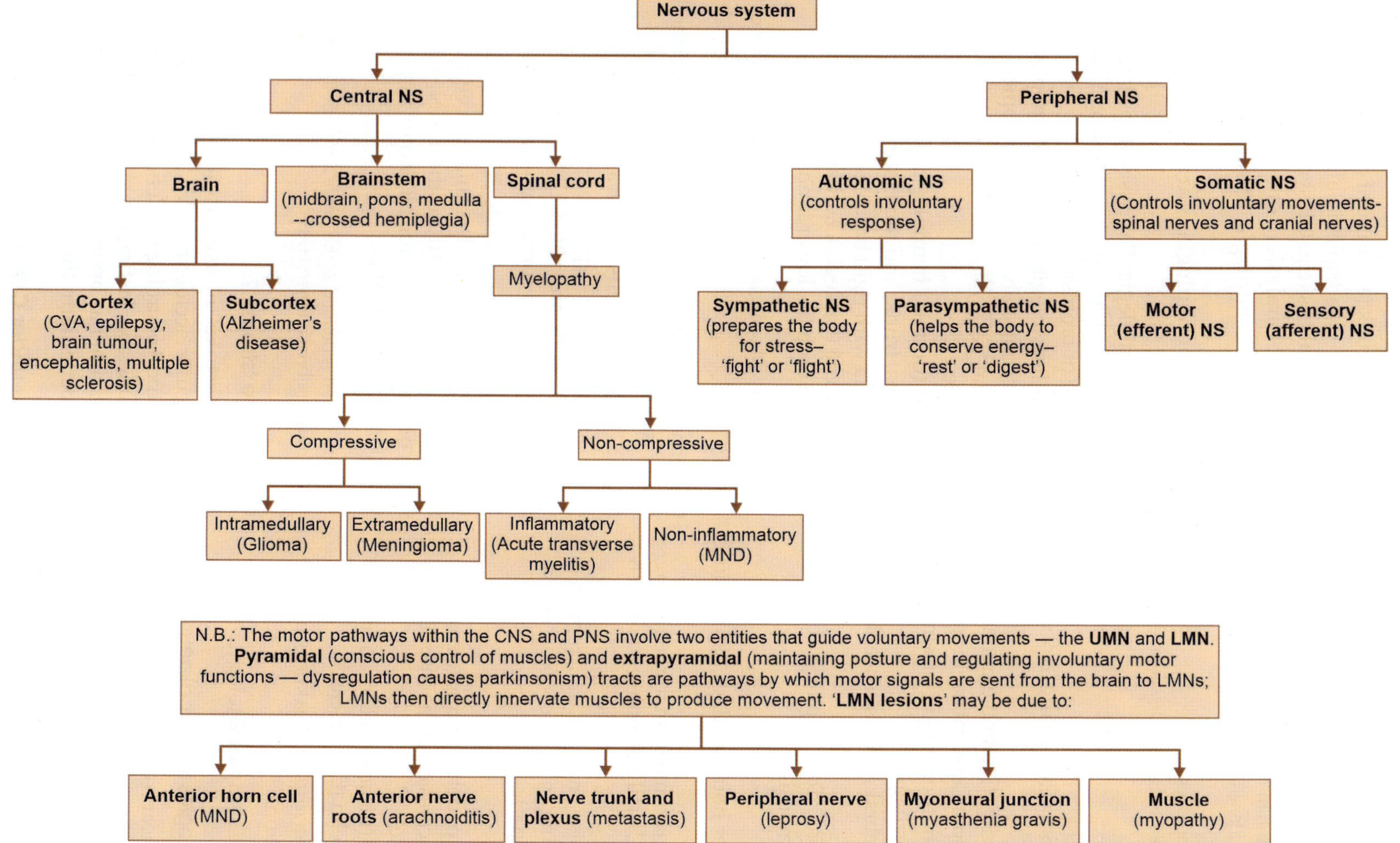

Note: The cranial nerves are considered components of PNS although I, II and V nerves are more accurately looked upon part of CNS. Spinal nerves are classified as part of PNS.

Table 1.16: Features of UMN and LMN palsy

UMN palsy	LMN palsy
1. Muscle groups or limbs are affected	1. Paralysis of individual muscle supplied by that segment or nerve
2. Paralysis of voluntary movements	2 Paralysis of muscles
3. Wasting is minimal and usually due to disuse atrophy	3. Atrophy and wasting are cardinal features
4. Clasp-knife spasticity (hypertonia)	4. Flaccidity (hypotonia)
5. Fasciculation is absent	5. Fasciculation may be present
6. Power is less affected than LMN type	6. Power is very much affected (may be Grade 0)
7. a. Superficial reflexes: Lost or diminished b. Deep reflexes or jerks: Brisk c. Clonus: May be present	7. a. Superficial reflexes: Lost or diminished b. Deep reflexes or jerks: Lost or diminished c. Clonus: Absent
8. Trophic changes in skin: Rare	8. Trophic changes in skin: Common
9. Plantar response: Extensor	**9. Plantar response: Flexor or no response**
10. Area of body involved: Large	10. Area of body involved: Small
11. Reaction of degeneration in the muscles: Absent	11. Reaction of degeneration in the muscles: Present

- Actually, there is no paralysis of muscles in UMN palsy (loss of dexterity) and it can be proved by the fact that the hemiplegic patient may run away from the room if the room suddenly catches fire (Table 1.16).
- In UMN lesion, symptoms occur early than the signs; and in LMN lesion, signs appear early than the symptoms.

5. Hypertensive encephalopathy.
6. Others (inobvious stroke): Multiple sclerosis, Todd's palsy, cerebellar haemorrhage or infarction, venous sinus thrombosis, subdural or epidural haematoma, cerebral metastasis, etc.

Clinical Wisdom

Gradual onset hemiplegia occurs due to:
1. Cerebral tumour.
2. Chronic subdural haematoma.
3. Cerebral abscess.
4. Meningitis and encephalitis.
5: AIDS (due to toxoplasmosis or primary CNS lymphoma).
6: General paralysis of insane (GPI).

- Stroke may be haemorrhagic (20%) or ischaemic (80%). Cerebral thrombosis and cerebral embolism result in cerebral ischaemia, and ultimately lead to **cerebral infarction**. Cerebral vasculitis (e.g. SLE) may also give rise to cerebral infarction. Cerebral infarction is the commonest cause of hemiplegia in the elderly. Cerebral infarction literally means death of brain tissue.
- **'Stroke mimickers'** are multiple sclerosis, hemiplegic migraine, cerebral tumour or abscess, and head injury.

Q. What is lacunar infarction?

It is the most common type of ischaemic stroke. These are small, deep infarcts developed as a result of atherothrombotic or lipohyalinotic occlusion of perforating or penetrating arteries (30–300 μm) within the brain substance. The 'lacuna' (cavity after healing of infarction) measures 2 mm to 2 cm in diameter. The major risk factor remains hypertension. Lacunes literally means 'lake' of fluid observed at autopsy. It may present as: 1) Pure motor hemiparesis, 2) Pure sensory stroke, 3) Ataxic hemiparesis, and 4) Clumsy hand, dysarthria syndrome. Pseudobulbar paisy may occur after multiple lacunar infarcts.

Q. Importance of examination of CVS in hemiplegia:

I. Method of examination:
  1. Pulse: Rate, rhythm (regular or irregular), volume, condition of the arterial wall (thickened or not), comparison with opposite side, radio-femoral delay (whether there is any delay present or not, especially when the patient gives H/o intermittent claudication) and any special character.
  2. Peripheral arterial pulses:
     i. **Carotids:** Kinking, diminished pulsation, or any bruit present over carotids or not (examination of neck is a must in a patient of CVA as carotid thrombus may be dislodged and cause cerebral thrombosis).
     ii. Brachial: Locomotor brachialis (a feature of arteriosclerosis) (*see* Fig. 1.16).
     iii. Femoral.
     iv. Arteria dorsalis pedis, and
     v. Any bruit over the eyeballs (for arteriovenous malformation).
  3. Blood pressure: High in cerebral haemorrhage and cerebral thrombosis (may be high in subarachnoid haemorrhage).
  4. Jugular veins.
  5. Apical impulse.
  6. Heart sounds.
  7. Murmur: Always search for a mitral diastolic murmur (for MS), especially in cerebral embolism.

II. Rheumatic heart disease (especially mitral stenosis): Cerebral embolism.

III. Hypertensive heart disease: TIA, lacunar infarction, cerebral thrombosis and haemorrhage.
IV. Ischaemic heart disease: Mural thrombus may dislodge.
V. Cyanotic congenital heart disease: May give rise to cerebral abscess, paradoxical embolism.
VI. Syphilitic heart disease: Tabes dorsalis and GPI (not seen nowadays).
VII. Subclavian steal syndrome: The patient complains of dizziness, diplopia, ataxia and/or collapse after use of one arm (no neurodeficit is produced but one should search for difference between pulse and BP in two upper limbs, and a bruit over the suprascapular area), resulting from stenosis of subclavian artery proximal to origin of vertebral artery. The syndrome results from stolen blood from the brain via the vertebral artery when the said arm is in use.

Clinical Wisdom

Carotid bruit, irregular pulse in atrial fibrillation and cardiac murmurs are of immense clinical importance in hemiplegia.

Q. Different sources in the heart for cerebral embolism:

The **sources of embolism** are:

1. Atrial fibrillation (from IHD, MS or MI): Left atrial thrombus may dislodge.
2. SBE (always search for mild splenomegaly).
3. Left atrial myxoma.
4. Right-to-left shunt in the heart (paradoxical embolism in Fallot's tetralogy).
5. Left ventricular thrombus or mural thrombus in recent acute myocardial infarction.
6. Left ventricular aneurysm.
7. Mitral valve prolapse.
8. Prosthetic heart valve.

Q. Special points in the physical examination in hemiplegia:

A. General survey:

a. The patient is conscious and cooperative.
b. Facies: Angle of the mouth is deviated to the right side on attempted talking.
c. Decubitus: Supine position in bed at present.
   i. Upper limb (left): Flexed, adducted and semipronated; lying helplessly.
   ii. Lower limb (left): Extended, adducted and plantiflexed, lying helplessly.
   iii. Right side (upper plus lower limbs): Within normal limit.
d. Neck veins: Neither engorged nor pulsatile.
e. Pulse: 70/min and regular, mention all the points; condition of the arterial wall may be thickened. Record the features of atherosclerosis (page 140), if there are any.
f. BP: It is compulsory to record the BP in all long cases; it is better to record BP on non-paralysed limb to avoid recording of low BP due to vasomotor paralysis on paralysed side; 185/100 mm of Hg in this patient.
g. Respiration: Record rate, rhythm, type, depth and breathing pattern.
h. Temperature: Record the axillary temperature (do not take oral temperature in facial palsy).
i. Oedema: May present on the paralysed side due to prolonged immobility (↓ venous and lymphatic flow) as well as affection of vasomotor nerves (reflex sympathetic dystrophy).
j. Any obvious deformity: Absent.

○ Mention all the points in general survey.

B. Nervous system:

a. The patient is conscious, alert, oriented and cooperative.
b. Higher functions including speech: Mention all the subheadings like level of consciousness, appearance and behaviour, memory, etc.—NAD (no abnormality detected) or WNL (within normal limit); a bit dysarthric (due to facial palsy) and unable to speak fluently; right-handed person.
c. Cranium and spine: Within normal limit.
d. Neck rigidity, Kernig's sign: Absent; carotids: Within normal limit.
e. Cranial nerves:
   i. VIIth cranial nerve: There is UMN type of paralysis on the left side of face as evidenced by,
      Epihora (left).
      Flattened nasolabial fold (left).
      Deviated angle of the mouth (right) while showing teeth.
      Weakness of buccinator, orbicularis oris, platysma (left).
      Upper face on left side (frontal belly of occipito-frontalis, corrugator superciliaris and upper part of orbicularis oculi) escaped paralysis.
   ii. Other cranial nerves: Fundoscopy for papilloedema. Mention the subheadings under the different cranial nerves: NAD.
f. Motor functions:

	Right	*Left*
i. Nutrition	Normal. No wasting seen	Normal, plus write down the attitude of left side from the 'Decubitus'. No wasting
ii. Tone	a. Upper limb: Normal	Clasp-knife spasticity in both the limbs.
	b. Lower limb: Normal	Flexor tone is increased more in upper limb and extensor tone is

(Contd...)

	Right	Left
		increased more in lower limb
iii. Power	a. Upper limb: Grade V	Grade III in both the limbs
	b. Lower limb: Grade V	
iv. Co-ordination	a. Upper limb: Normal	Could not be tested properly
	b. Lower limb: Normal	
v. Involuntary movements	None	None

g. Sensory functions:
- i. Superfical
- ii. Deep
- iii. Cortical

} NAD

❍ Mention the subheadings.

h. Reflexes:

	Right	Left
i. Superficial		
a. Abdominal		
x. Upper	Normal	Lost
y. Middle	Normal	Lost
z. Lower	Normal	Lost
b. Cremasteric	Normal	Lost
c. Plantar response	**Flexor**	**Extensor**
ii. Deep		
a. Biceps jerk	Normal	**Brisk**
b. Triceps jerk	Normal	**Brisk**
c. Supinator jerk	Normal	**Brisk**
d. Knee jerk	Normal	**Brisk**
e. Ankle jerk	Normal	**Brisk**
f. Clonus	Absent	Absent (say, if present)

iii. Visceral
- a. Swallowing
- b. Bladder
- c. Bowel

} within normal limit

iv. Other reflexes
- a. Glabellar tap — Normal
- b. Grasp reflex — Absent (absent bilaterally)
- c. Palmo-mental reflex — Absent (absent bilaterally)

i. Trophic changes: Absent.
j. Cerebellar functions: Within normal limit.
k. Autonomic functions: Normal.
l. Stance and gait: Classical hemiplegic gait. The patient walks by tilting the pelvis while the left leg is making 'circumduction'. Read the section on 'Abnormal gait'.

❍ Mention the jaw jerk under Vth cranial nerve.

C. CVS: See the answer of the question 'Importance of examination of CVS in hemiplegia' mentioned earlier (write the points from 1 to 7 under I).

D. Respiratory system:
- i. Shape of the chest
- ii. Movement of the chest
- iii. Trachea and apex beat

} within normal limit

- iv. Percussion: Normal resonant note on both sides.
- v. Breath sound: Vesicular.
- vi. Vocal resonance: Normal on both sides.
- vii. Adventitious sound: None.

E. GI tract and genitourinary system:
- i. Mouth, tongue, teeth, gum: NAD.
- ii. Shape of the abdomen WNL.
- iii. Umbilicus: Inverted.
- iv. Rigidity (abdominal): Absent.
- v. Hepatosplenomegaly: Not present.
- vi. Any lump felt: None.
- vii. Fluid thrill and shifting dullness: Absent. Percussion for bladder fullness done.
- viii. Auscultation: Normal peristaltic sound.
- ix. Genitalia: NAD.
- x. P/R examination: Not done.

F. Lymphoreticular system:
- i. Anaemia: Absent.
- ii. Lymphadenopathy: Absent.
- iii. Sternal tenderness: Absent.
- iv. Haemorrhagic spots: Absent.

Q. Clinical types of hemiplegia:

1. Complete hemiplegia (with UMN type VIIth nerve palsy in the side of hemiplegia).
2. Incomplete hemiplegia (hemiplegia without affection of VIIth cranial nerve).
3. Crossed hemiplegia (when the site of lesion is in the brainstem): Ipsilateral LMN type cranial nerve paralysis (i.e. at the side of brainstem lesion) with contralateral hemiplegia.

Q. Importance of headache, convulsions and coma (i.e. features of IIT) in strokes:

a. Headache
- i. Severe headache accompanying the paralysis: Subarachnoid haemorrhage (sudden onset of excruciating occipital headache), cerebral haemorrhage, hypertensive encephalopathy.
- ii. Headache preceding the paralysis for months: SOL (space-occupying lesion), subdural haematoma.
- iii. Mild headache: Cerebral thrombosis or embolism.

b. Convulsions
- i. Generalised convulsions preceding the paralysis: Todd's palsy (post-epileptic), hypertensive encephalopathy or SOL.
- ii. Focal or generalised convulsions occurring few months prior to paralysis: SOL.
- iii. Convulsions just prior to the paralysis may be seen in cerebral haemorrhage, thrombosis or embolism.

Convulsions do not occur in subarachnoid haemorrhage.

c. Unconsciousness

1. From the beginning: Commonly cerebral haemorrhage.
2. In cerebral thrombosis, cerebral embolism, subarachnoid haemorrhage or hypertensive encephalopathy: Usually the patients remain conscious but may be drowsy.

Q. What is projectile vomiting of increased intracranial tension (IIT)?

It is the sudden vomiting which is not preceded by nausea (common in children) and the vomitus is forcefully projected to a distance from the patient.

In food poisoning and pyloric stenosis, the patient may have projectile vomiting.

Q. Enquiry regarding the bladder and bowel symptoms in neurology:

Following questions are put to a hemiplegic or paraplegic patient,

1. Is there any increased frequency or urgency?
2. Do you feel burning sensation during micturition?
3. Is there any problem in initiation of micturition (hesitancy or precipitancy)?
4. Can you feel the urine passing?
5. Can you stop the flow of urine in the midstream at will?
6. Is there any dribbling of urine?
7. Is there any sense of bladder fullness?
8. Is there any associated rectal disorder (incontinence of stool, diarrhoea or constipation, etc.)? or any difficulty in anal sensation?
9. Is there any disorder of potency (in males)?
10. Have you ever catheterised in recent past?

Clinical Wisdom

1, 2, 3 and 10 are important in hemiplegia. In paraplegia, all the points are important.

Q. Type of bladder involvement in your patient:

The chief complaint of the patient is burning micturition at present (seen in many cases) as he was catheterised on admission (and as such now suffering from UTI). There is no loss of bladder control.

Q. Point out the signs of UMN lesion in your patient:

Demonstrate the points mentioned below:

1. VIIth cranial nerve: UMN palsy (as upper face on the left-side escaped paralysis).
2. Power: Loss of power.
3. Tone: Clasp-knife spasticity (hypertonia).
4. Reflexes:
   a. Abdominal: Lost.
   b. Jerks: Brisk.
5. Plantar response: Extensor.

- All the features are left-sided in this patient. Add clonus, if present.

Q. Why there is VIIth nerve palsy (UMN type) in hemiplegia?

The VIIth cranial nerve nuclei are divided into upper and lower part by an arbitrary horizontal line, and the upper part supplies muscles of upper face while the lower part supplies the lower face. **All cranial nerve nuclei are bilaterally supplied by pyramidal fibres (corticonuclear fibres) except the lower part of the VIIth cranial nerve nuclei which receive pyramidal fibres only from the opposite side.** So the lower face is easily affected (i.e. it means UMN type of VIIth nerve palsy) in a patient of hemiplegia.

Q. Trunk and abdominal muscles in hemiplegia:

These are not involved in classical hemiplegia (lesion at internal capsule) due to their bilateral representation at the cortex.

- Abdominal muscles (T_7–L_1): Do the 'rising test' and analyse **"Beevor's sign"** (**Fig. 1.45**) (*see* page 151).
- Intercostal muscles (T_1–T_{12}): During respiration, observe the movements of intercostals as well as the ribs.
- Extensors of spine (all segments of spinal nerve): Patient lies prone and tries to raise his shoulders from the bed against examiner's resistance. Back muscles (e.g. erector spinae) are seen to contract (**Fig. 1.46**).

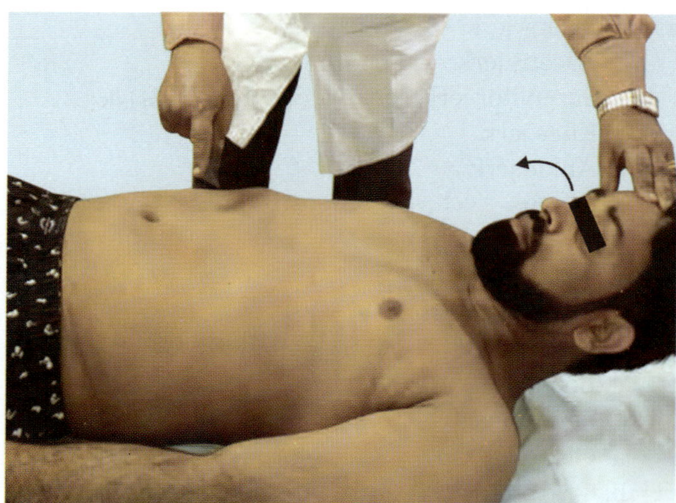

Fig. 1.45: Muscle power testing of **abdominal muscles**

Q. Different 'stages of hemiplegia' and their clinical diagnosis:

1. Stage of neural shock (for few hours to days, and may extend up to 2–3 weeks).
2. Stage of recovery.
3. Stage of residual paralysis.

- In neurological disorders, neural shock may be 'cerebral' (e.g. hemiplegia) or 'spinal' (e.g. acute transverse myelitis). The different stages of hemiplegia are:

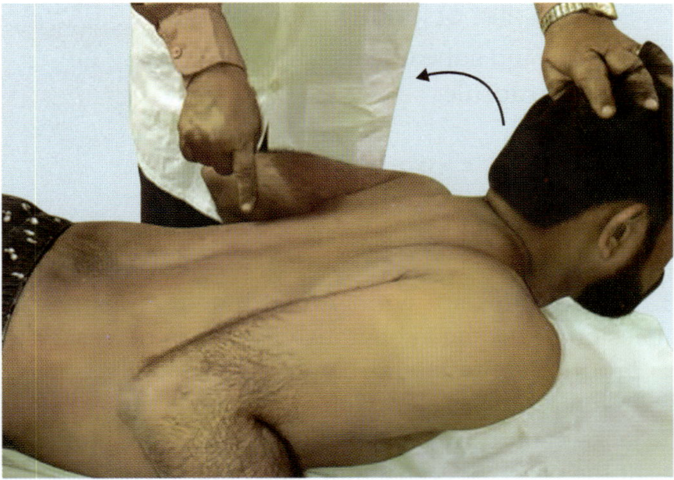

Fig. 1.46: Muscle power testing of **extensors of spine**

A. Stage of neural shock (a stage when all reflex activity is suppressed):
   i. Patient may be drowsy or in coma.
   ii. Aphasia.
   iii. Hypotonia of muscles or flaccidity with gross diminution of power.
   iv. Jerks are usually absent.
   v. Retention of urine and there may be spontaneous evacuation of feces.
   vi. Plantar response: No response or equivocal.

Neural shock stage may be prolonged with co-existing bed sore, UTI or malnutrition.

B. Stage of recovery: Recovery usually occurs in the following order:
   i. Face earliest.
   ii. Lower limb (first the extensors recover).
   iii. Upper limb (first the flexors recover).
   iv. Dorsiflexion of foot (minimally recovered).
   v. Finer movements of fingers (usually do not recover).

C. Stage of residual paralysis: Patient lives with some residual paralysis and walks in classical hemiplegic gait. During recovery of UMN lesion reflex recovers first, then comes tone and lastly power regains (proximal power recovers earlier than distal power). Plantar response may remain extensor on the affected side throughout life.

Q. Importance of examination of cranial nerves in hemiplegia:

It helps in localisation of the site of lesion. The olfactory and optic nerves are actually built up of central nervous tissue rather than peripheral nerves. The disposition of other cranial nerve nuclei in the brainstem are as follows:

a. Midbrain: IIIrd and IVth.
b. Pons: Vth, VIth, VIIth and VIIIth.
c. Medulla: IXth, Xth, XIth and XIIth.

Common examples of *'brainstem syndromes'* are:

1. Weber's syndrome: Paralysis of IIIrd crainal nerve of one side (LMN type) with contralateral hemiplegia (crossed hemiplegia): Lesion is at **midbrain**.
2. Millard-Gubler syndrome: Paralysis of VIth cranial nerve (LMN type) ± VIIth cranial nerve palsy (LMN type) with contralateral hemiplegia (crossed hemiplegia): Lesion is at **pons**.
3. Dejerine syndrome (medial medullary syndrome): Paralysis of XIIth cranial nerve of one side (LMN type) with contralateral hemiplegia (crossed hemiplegia): Lesion is at **medulla**.

- Crossed hemiplegia always indicates the lesion in the brainstem.
- Damage to brainstem recticular activating system may lead to coma.

Q. Importance of VIIth cranial nerve examination in hemiplegia:

It helps in localisation of the site of lesion in hemiplegia. For example:

a. UMN type of VIIth cranial nerve palsy in the side of hemiplegia (as this case is): Lesion is 'above' the pons (opposite side).
b. LMN type of VIIth cranial nerve palsy with contralateral hemiplegia, i.e. crossed hemiplegia (lesion is at VIIth cranial nerve nucleus): Lesion is 'at' pons on the side of VIIth nerve palsy.
c. No facial nerve involvement (incomplete hemiplegia): Lesion is 'below' the level of pons.

- *UMN type of VIIth cranial nerve palsy is always associated with same-sided hemiplegia while hemiplegia, if at all present with LMN type of VIIth cranial nerve palsy, is always crossed.*

Q. Eye position in hemiplegia:

a. Hemisphere lesion: Eyes deviated towards the side of lesion in cerebral hemisphere.
b. Pontine lesion: Eyes deviated to the paralysed side.
c. Putamen lesion: Loss of conjugate lateral gaze.
d. Thalamic lesion: Loss of upward gaze, down or skew deviation, lateral gaze palsies, unequal pupil.

Q. Functions of pyramidal and extrapyramidal system:

a. Pyramidal tract: Helps in volitional movements, especially the skillful movements (movement of fingers and hands, e.g. writing, sewing, buttoning, playing piano, etc.). It also integrates motor activity (i.e. when agonists contract, the antagonists are made to relax).
b. Extrapyramidal tract:
   i. Maintains muscle tone and posture.
   ii. Maintains emotional, automatic and associated movements (i.e. swinging of the hands during walking).
   iii. Checks abnormal involuntary movements.
   iv. Helps in integrated motor activity.

Q. Blood supply of the brain in a nutshell:

It is worthwhile to remember that carotid system (from two internal carotid arteries) and vertebrobasilar system (from two vertebral arteries) anastomose at the base of the skull to form 'circle of Willis'. The branches of cerebral arteries from 'circle of Willis' supply the brain.

a. Anterior cerebral artery (ACA): Supplies branches to frontal and parietal lobes, to part of internal capsule; *it also supplies the paracentral lobule*, i.e. the centre for movements of the lower limbs plus the centre for micturition and defecation.
b. Middle cerebral artery (MCA): Supplies the motor, sensory and speech areas.
c. Posterior cerebral artery (PCA): Supplies the visual cortex, brainstem, thalamus, occipital lobe and part of the temporal lobe; part of the posterior limb of the internal capsule.

Q. Blood supply of the internal capsule:

a. Anterior limb: Upper half—MCA (lenticulostriate branch), and lower half—ACA (Heubner's artery).
b. Posterior limb: Upper half—MCA, and lower half—anterior choroidal and posterior communicating artery.

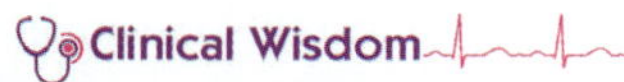

Pyramidal fibres take origin from Betz cells of cerebral cortex (motor area or area 4) and descend towards corona radiata. While descending from corona radiata, pyramidal tract occupies the anterior 2/3rd of the posterior limb of the internal capsule and genu. Anterior limb contains the fibres for the face while fibres for the tongue and mouth lies at the genu. Pyramidal fibres occupying the anterior 2/3rd of the posterior limb continue downwards and occupy the middle 3/5th of the peduncles of midbrain. Then the fibres descend through pons and medulla, and majority of the fibres cross to the opposite side to occupy the lateral column in the spinal cord.

- As pyramidal tract has contralateral supply, hemiplegia occurs contralateral to the side of lesion in brain.

Q. Features of anterior cerebral artery (ACA) involvement:

If it is blocked 'distal' to the anterior communicating artery, there is:

1. Hemiplegia and hemisensory loss of the opposite side of body where lower limbs are much more involved (crural dominance) than upper limbs (in hemiplegia due to blocked middle cerebral artery, the weakness is more marked in upper limbs, i.e. there is brachial dominance).
2. Face is not involved.
3. Urinary incontinence is very common.
4. Presence of mental symptoms (emotional disturbance)
5. Presence of 'released reflexes' (see page 437).

- If anterior cerebral artery is blocked 'proximal' to anterior communicating artery, there is development of complete hemiplegia (hemiplegia + face involvement) on the opposite side with or without aphasia.
- In Heubner's artery involvement (a perforating branch of anterior cerebral artery), opposite sided facio-brachial (face + hand) paralysis occurs.

Q. Possible sites of lesion in hemiplegia:

1. Cortical and subcortical.
2. Internal capsule.
3. Brainstem.
4. Spinal.

Q. Characteristics of each site of lesion:

a. Cortical:

1. As the fibres are widely distributed, an extensive lesion (outcome is obviously grave) is necessary to produce contralateral hemiplegia. Usually cortical lesion produces contralateral **monoplegia**.
2. Jacksonian convulsions and headache are common at the onset. Speech abnormality is present.
3. Flexors and extensors of both the upper and the lower limbs are equally involved, and so the involvement of tone of muscles.
4. There may be cortical type of sensory loss (e.g. astereognosis).

- Cortical function is assessed by convulsions, aphasia, apraxia and agnosia.

b. Subcortical (or at the level of corona radiata):

1. Subcortical lesion involves more fibres than the cortical lesion of equal size. Usually it produces contralateral **monoplegia** but hemiplegia on the opposite side may occur. There is absence of cortical signs like convulsions or dysphasia.
2. Involvement of adjacent thalamocortical fibres results in impairment of postural sensibility, tactile localisation and discrimination in the affected limbs.

c. Internal capsule:

1. It is the most common site of lesion in a CVA.
2. As the fibres are densely packed, a small lesion produces **complete hemiplegia** on the opposite side.
3. Hemianaesthesia and homonymous hemianopia occur as a result of damage to the sensory and the visual fibres respectively, which lie posterior to the pyramidal tract at internal capsule.
4. Global aphasia (in left-sided lesion) or apractagnosia (in right-sided lesion).
5. Flexor tone is increased in upper limb as the extensor tone in lower limb (in hemiplegic side). Classical position of the hemiplegic limbs:
   a. Upper limb: Flexed (elbow, wrist and fingers), adducted and semipronated.
   b. Lower limb: Extended, adducted and plantiflexed.
6. Cranial nerve involvement: Only UMN type of VIIth cranial nerve involvement on the side of paralysis, as discussed earlier.

- **Apractagnosia:** A type of agnosia marked by inability to use objects or perform skilled motor activities.

d. Brainstem:

1. Dizziness, vertigo and vomiting may be present.

2. Always **crossed hemiplegia**.
3. See the different brainstem syndromes discussed earlier and localise the site of lesion (vide page 137).
4. Gaze paralysis. Change in pupil is common, even Horner's syndrome may be seen.
5. Involvement of the cerebellum may be there.
6. If midbrain and medulla are involved: There will be quadriplegia, decerebrate rigidity, Cheyne-Stokes breathing or coma.

e. Spinal hemiplegia: Though rare, lesion lying below the medulla but above the C_5 spinal segment may produce **'ipsilateral' hemiplegia** (as the pyramidal fibres have already crossed in medulla) without any cranial nerve involvement (i.e. incomplete hemiplegia).

Q. Classical features of cerebral thrombosis, embolism, haemorrhage, etc.:

a. Cerebral thrombosis:
1. Middle aged or elderly; commonest cause of CVA.
2. Very often hypertensive and atherosclerotic.
3. Onset is less rapid than cerebral embolism or haemorrhage; usually with step-wise progression.
4. Mild headache and convulsions may occur. There may be transient loss of consciousness.
5. Often there is past history of TIA (single or multiple).
6. Occurs during sleep or soon after rising from bed.
7. Carotid bruit with diminished carotid pulsation highly supports cerebral thrombosis.

b. Cerebral embolism:
1. Commonly in young females.
2. Valvular heart disease or sources of embolism (discussed earlier) may be evident.
3. Pulse may be irregularly irregular (e.g. atrial fibrillation).
4. Develops in seconds (dramatic, stromy or 'bolt from the blue') during exertion, activity or any time; warning sign of TIA may be present.
5. Headache and convulsions are usually absent; there may be transient loss of consciousness.
6. Shifting hemiplegia may occur. Recovery may be very rapid.
7. Evidence of systemic embolisation may be present.

c. Cerebral haemorrhage:
1. Usually above the age of 40 years.
2. Develops acutely at the height of emotion or excitement. Develops over minutes and hours which progresses relentlessly.
3. Almost all are hypertensive.
4. Headache, recurrent vomiting or convulsions are present in most of the patients. Unconsciousness gradually progresses to deep coma. Early recovery is unusual.
5. Heart may show features of LVH.
6. Features of atherosclerosis may be present (as in thrombosis).
7. Conjugate deviation of eyes and Cheyne-Stokes breathing are common.
8. Very rarely, neck rigidity may be elicited.

- Lenticulostriate branch of MCA is (Charcot's artery of cerebral haemorrhage) commonly involved in hypertensive haemorrhage.
- Features of **pontine haemorrhage** are pin-point pupil, pyrexia and paralysis (3P).
- Common sites of **intracerebral haemorrhage** in order of frequency are: Basal ganglia, especially Putamen → thalamus → frontal or parietal lobes → pons (brainstem) → cerebellum. Bleeding in cortex is rare.

d. Subarachnoid haemorrhage:
1. Usually in young adults (also known as 'apoplexy of the young'). It may occur in older age group. Subarachnoid haemorrhage occurs as a result of rupture of berry aneurysm or arteriovenous malformations. It accounts for about 10% of strokes.
2. Bursting occipital headache (sudden and severe) commonly precedes (often called 'as the worst headache of my life'); usually does not give rise to convulsions but loss of consciousness (50%) may be present.
3. Occurs during activity or at the height of emotion.
4. Neck rigidity and Kernig's sign are present (cardinal signs at bedside).
5. Hemiplegia or aphasia is absent in most of the patients.
6. Fundoscopy may reveal subhyaloid haemorrhage.
7. Sometimes, there is paralysis of IIIrd, IVth, VIth cranial nerves, or monoplegia or hemiplegia (due to local pressure effect of berry aneurysm or vascular spasm).

E. Carotid hemiplegia:
1. Middle aged or elderly.
2. Very often hypertensive and atherosclerotic.
3. History of TIA is commonly found.
4. There may be H/o claudication of the jaw.
5. Kinking of the carotid artery, inequality of the pulse volume in two carotids or a bruit may be heard at the site of the block (i.e. examination of neck should be done in all CVA patients).
6. Ipsilateral visual disturbances (amaurosis fugax—transient mono-ocular blindness) and contralateral sensory-motor deficit.

- **Hypertensive encephalopathy** is an acute syndrome where severe hypertension is associated with nausea, vomiting, excruciating headache, transient abnormalities in speech or vision, convulsions, mental confusion and coma. Focal neurological signs are rarely seen but papilloedema is usually present. The symptom complex results from constriction of cerebral arterioles and cerebral oedema. Neurodeficit is fully correctable if acute hypertension is properly controlled.
- Following events are **common in hypertensive patients** like cerebral haemorrhage or thrombosis, TIA, carotid atheroma, lacunar infarction, subarachnoid haemorrhage and hypertensive encephalopathy.

Q. Features of 'atherosclerosis' (see Fig. 1.6)

Features of atherosclerosis should be assessed in a patient of stroke, especially of thrombotic variety.

1. Age of the patient is usually above 50 years.
2. There may be H/o symptoms like IHD, TIA, intermittent claudication or hypertension.
3. *Risk factors* like diabetes mellitus, smoking, hyperlipidaemia, central obesity may be present.
4. Condition of the arterial wall: Thickened (arteriosclerosis), feels like a cord and often tortuous (Monckeberg's medial sclerosis), and may be associated with:
   i. Locomotor brachialis (arteriosclerosis) (see Fig. 1.16).
   ii. Tortuous temporal arteries, and
   iii. Kinked carotids.
5. There may be presence of suprasternal pulsation.
6. Features of hyperlipidaemia like xanthelasma is seen around the eyes.
7. Often associated with corneal 'arcus' and diagonal ear lobe crease (surrogate marker).
8. Change of arterial and venous ratio, and arteriovenous nipping in ophthalmoscopy.
9. Chest X-ray may reveal unfolding of aorta or aortic calcification.

Clinical Wisdom

Carotid artery intima-media thickness, i.e. CIMT (carotid intima-media thickness) determined by a non-invasive procedure like high-resolution B-mode USG gives assessment of 'atherosclerosis', which corresponds with the severity of coronary atherosclerosis in a patient.

Q. Risk factors in CVA:

1. Systemic hypertension (most important).
2. Diabetes mellitus.
3. Hyperlipidaemia.
4. Smoking.
5. Cardiac diseases (valvular and ischaemic).
6. Obesity.
7. Severe carotid stenosis.
8. Oral contraceptive pills.
9. High alcohol consumption.
10. Hyperviscosity syndrome (polycythemia thrombocythemia, etc.), bleeding diathesis.
11. Trauma.
12. Strong family history of CVA (heredity).
13. Sleep apnoea.

- Increased age, male sex (except in extremes of ages) and hyperhomocysteinaemia are other risk factors.
- Major risk factors: 1–7, and 10; minor risk factors: 8, 9 and 11–13.

Q. Common causes of 'strokes in young' (<40 years of age):

A. Causes:

1. Cerebral embolism (from cardiac sources like rheumatic heart diseases; vide pages 133–134).
2. Subarachnoid haemorrhage (rupture of berry aneurysm or arteriovenous malformations).
3. Arteritis or vasculitis (tuberculosis, syphilis, Takayasu's disease, collagen vascular diseases).
4. Accelerated atherosclerosis (secondary hypertension, familial hypercholesterolaemia, hypertriglyceridaemia, diabetes mellitus, nephrotic syndrome, SLE).
5. Hyperviscosity syndrome (polycythemia, thrombocytosis).
6. Demyelinating disease (multiple sclerosis).
7. Intracranial neoplasm (primary or secondary).
8. Encephalitis, meningoencephalitis.
9. Head injury (trauma).
10. Anticoagulant therapy, ITP, or treatment with oral contraceptive pills.
11. Cerebral abscess (rule out cyanotic congenital heart disease, otitis media or AIDS), tuberculoma.
12. Hemiplegic migraine.
13. Procoagulant states, e.g. Protein C and S deficiency, antithrombin III deficiency, hyperhomocysteinaemia, activated protein C resistance, factor V Leiden mutation, prothrombin mutations, antiphospholipid syndrome (Hughes syndrome).
14. Venous sinus thrombosis: Especially in the setting of puerperium.
15. Cerebral malaria.
16. Drug abuse (e.g. amphetamine or cocaine).
17. Miscellaneous: Arterial dissection, prosthetic valve, post-cardiac surgery, sickle cell disease, thrombotic thrombocytopenic purpura (TTP).
18. Hysteria.

B. Special investigations in young patients:

a. Full blood count with platelet, ESR, VDRL test, sugar, urea; X-ray, ECG and echocardiography.
b. Antinuclear factor (ANF), antibodies to double-stranded DNA.
c. Anti-cardiolipin antibodies (antiphospholipid syndrome may be a cause of stroke in young patients), protein C and S, antithrombin III; coagulation screening (thrombocheck test).
d. Prothrombin time (PT), activated partial thromboplastin time (aPTT).
e. Lupus anticoagulant.
f. Lipid profile.

- Atherosclerosis, the chief cause of cerebral ischaemia in the aged is seen less commonly in young patients with stroke. The causes and evaluation of 'strokes in young' are a bit different from the aged population.

Q. Possible causes of thromboembolism:

a. Arterial: Systemic hypertension, infected or sterile emboli of cardiac or vascular origin, septicaemia, hyperhomocysteinaemia, thrombotic thrombocytopenic purpura, atrial myxoma, Takayasu's arteritis, polyarteritis nodosa, oral contraceptive pills.
b. Venous: Venous insufficiency/obstruction, prolonged immobility, nephrotic syndrome, antiphospholipid syndrome, oral contraceptive pills, *plus* the 'procoagulant states' for both the categories (described above).
c. Arterial plus venous: Antiphospholipid syndrome, oral contraceptive pills and polycythemia vera.

Q. Major side effects of prolonged use of oral contraceptive pills:

CVA (thromboembolic strokes), DVT, hypertension, cholestatic jaundice, obesity, impaired glucose tolerance and worsened lipid profile, increased incidence of AMI, depression and abnormal liver biochemistry.

- Recently, in OC pills, low dose oestrogens have been combined with newer progestational agents, which cause less deleterious effects on carbohydrate and lipid metabolism, coagulation profile, vascular apparatus and liver function.

Q. Causes of recurrent/transient hemiplegia:

1. Transient ischaemic attack (TIA).
2. Post-epileptic or Todd's palsy.
3. Hypertensive encephalopathy.
4. Hemiplegic migraine.
5. Multiple sclerosis.
6. Cerebral arteriovenous malformations.
7. Hysterical hemiplegia.

- 'Reversible neurodeficit' is common in 1, 2, 4 and 7.

Q. Mention few causes of monoplegia:

a. Brachial monoplegia (upper limb):

1. CVA (cortical or subcortical lesion).
2. Multiple sclerosis.
3. Encephalitis.
4. Poliomyelitis.
5. Mononeuropathy.
6. Brachial plexus lesion.
7. Motor neurone disease (MND).
8. Hysterical or psychogenic.

b. Crural monoplegia (lower limb):

1. Thrombosis of paracentral artery.
2. Granuloma affecting frontal lobe.
3. Multiple sclerosis.
4. Cauda equina lesion.
5. Sciatic nerve palsy.
6. Prolapsed intervertebral disc (PIVD).
6. Mononeuropathy.
8. Hysterical or psychogenic.

Q. Causes of hemiplegia:

1. Cerebrovascular accidents (page 131).
2. Strokes in young (page 140).
3. Gradual onset hemiplegia (page 133).
4. Recurrent and reversible hemiplegia (page 141)

Actually, these are sumtotal causes of hemiplegia.

Q. Can you prevent the first episode of stroke or CVA?

The answer is 'no' but one should try to focus on the following facts to prevent the first episode like control of BP, diabetes, dyslipidaemia, obesity (lifestyle modification), and stoppage of smoking and alcohol. Though controversial, few neurologists advise prophylactic aspirin (males >50 years and females >65 years). Control of atrial fibrillation by anticoagulants or antiplatelet drugs, treating all patient with high risk of embolism (e.g. SBE, MS, left atrial myxoma), avoidance of oral contraceptive pills or hormone replacement therapy may be judicious.

Q. Why do you consider cerebral thrombosis in this case?

1. As the onset was dramatic, I think the pathology is a 'vascular catastrophe'.
2. Though there is presence of hypertension, neither the patient gave any H/o vomiting and convulsions at onset nor he was unconscious. So, I am not thinking of cerebral haemorrhage in this case. As there is absence of neck rigidity, no H/o bursting occipital headache but there is presence of hemiplegia, I am not thinking of subarachnoid haemorrhage in this patient.
3. The CVS is within normal limit. The patient is not suffering from any valvular heart disease or atrial fibrillation. So, chance of cerebral embolism is less.
4. So, I say it is a case of CVA due to thrombosis which is the 'most common' cause of stroke in advanced age.

Q. Why do you say the site of lesion is in the internal capsule?

It is known that in a patient of hemiplegia if there is,

1. UMN type of VIIth nerve palsy to the side of hemiplegia: The lesion lies in the opposite internal capsule.
2. LMN type of VIIth nerve palsy with contralateral hemiplegia: The lesion lies in the brainstem (pons) opposite to hemiplegic site.
3. Hemiplegia without any cranial nerve involvement (known as spinal hemiplegia): The lesion lies in ipsilateral upper spinal cord (in between medulla to C_5 spinal segment).

As it is a case of left-sided complete hemiparesis, most likely the site of lesion is in the right internal capsule. It is the 'commonest site' of involvement in a patient with CVA, commonly involving the lenticulostriate branch of middle cerebral artery.

- Cortical and subcortical lesions usually produce monoplegia.

Q. 'Clinical' classification of stroke:

1. TIA (transient ischaemic attack): Abrupt neurological dysfunction (neurodeficit) due to cerebral ischaemia (without acute infarction) where symptoms last for <24 hours and the patient recovers completely.
2. Stroke in evolution (progressive stroke): The symptoms worsen gradually or in a step-wise pattern over hours or days. This is due to increasing size of infarction (usually due to gradual occlusion of a vessel by a thrombus), secondary haemorrhage or propagating cerebral oedema.
3. Completed stroke: The neurodeficit is complete from the beginning (usually within 6 hours) and persists for weeks and months, and often permanently.
4. Stuttering hemiplegia: Gradual stepwise development of neurodeficit by repeated episodes of TIA followed by fully evolved stroke.
5. Minor stroke: Usually the patient recovers within a week, without significant deficit.

[6. RIND (reversible ischaemic neurological deficit): Neurodeficit persists for >24 hours but recovers completely within 24–96 hours.

7. PNS (partial non-progressive stroke): Neurodeficit persists for >3 weeks but is either partial or terminates with minimal residual deficit.

6 and 7 are old terminologies, and are not preferred by neurologists nowadays.]

- Most neurologists still believe (recent view) that TIA is a stroke or may herald a stroke; the definition of TIA is unsatisfactory as clinical studies reveal that after 1 hour, ishaemic damage occurs. The arbitrary time of <24 hours is no longer used, as the end point is now tissue injury. TIA of (a) *carotid territory* manifests as transient contralateral weakness (monoparesis or hemiparesis), hemisensory loss, aphasia and transient ipsilateral mono-ocular blindness (amaurosis fugax) whereas, (b) *vertebro-basilar* TIA is manifested by vertigo, dysarthria, diplopia, vomiting, ataxia, dysphagia or sudden fall (drop attack). In TIA, the source of embolus may be clinically evidenced by carotid arterial bruit (i.e. stenosis), valvular heart disease/SBE, atrial fibrillation, recent acute myocardial infarction, or difference between BP of left and right arm.

Q. Classical signs of 'meningeal irritation':

1. *Neck rigidity (stiffness)* (Fig. 1.47):

a. In *supine position* of the patient, stand on the right side of the bed and place your left hand behind and below the patient's head; try to lift the head from the bed until the chin touches the chest and feel the resistance while flexing the head. Normally, the neck is supple and can be easily flexed passively. In the presence of neck rigidity, it is not possible to passively flex the neck fully. Neck rigidity occurs due to spasm of extensor neck muscles and in an attempt to do the test, the whole body may be raised up; head retraction represents an extreme form of neck rigidity. (Alternative method: by standing in front and right side of the patient, support the back of the head with both hands and

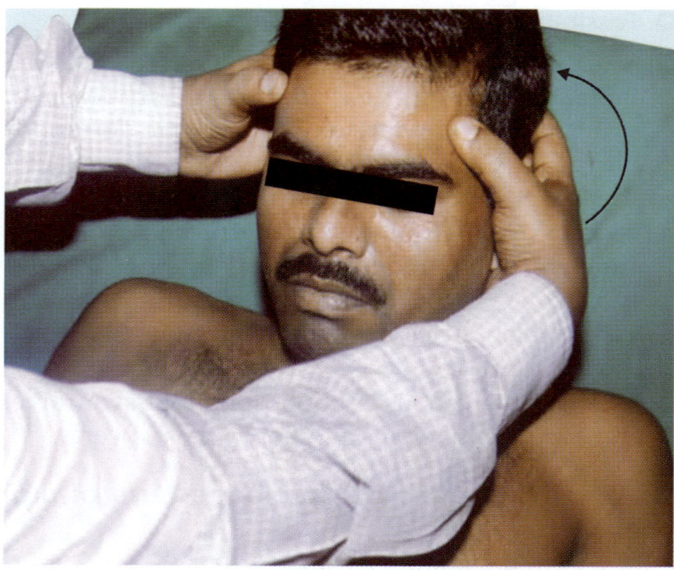

Fig. 1.47: Testing for **neck rigidity**

gently try to flex the neck so that the chin touches the chest). It is preferred to test for neck rigidity in supine position of the patient.

b. In *sitting position* of the patient (not a good method), ask him to touch the chin to the sternum (always with closed mouth).

Neck rigidity and Kernig's sign are present in:

i. Meningitis.
ii. Meningism.
iii. Subarachnoid haemorrhage.
iv. Meningoencephalitis.
v. Meningomyelitis.
vi. Tetanus, rabies, hysteria.
vii. Rarely in intracerebral haemorrhage.
viii. Spinal epidural abscess.
ix. Sometimes in posterior fossa tumour.
x. Cerebellar tonsillar herniation at foramen magnum.
xi. Retropharyngeal abscess.

- In clinical practice, No. 1, 2, and 3 are most important.

Clinical Wisdom

Sometimes, the **neck rigidity is absent** in deep coma, severe and terminal cases, or in infants. Passive resistance to head flexion may be present in cervical spondylosis (side-to-side movement is more restricted than antero-posterior movement), traumatic injury of cervical spine, Klippel-Feil anomaly or cerebral malaria. Neck stiffness may be felt in acute dystonia and parkinsonism.

2. *Kernig's sign* (Fig. 1.48): In supine position of the patient, flex his hip to 90° and then extend the knee to 90°. Now try to straighten the leg maintaining the hip in flexion. In the presence of meningeal irritation, it is impossible to straighten the leg because of the painful spasm of hamstring muscles (normally the leg can be easily straightened). *This sign is similarly positive in the conditions mentioned above.* Testing of neck rigidity is a more sensitive test of meningeal irritation than Kernig's sign.

3. Brudzinski's sign: It is a very helpful *sign of meningeal irritation in children.* It has two components:

a. Neck sign: Patient will lie supine with extended legs. Try to lift the head from the bed. There will be reflex flexion of the hip, or knee of one or both the limbs.
b. Leg sign: While passively flexing the thigh of any one limb, the other thigh or knee automatically becomes flexed.

- Kernig's and Brudzinski's sign are due to the presence of inflammatory exudate around nerve roots present in the lumbar theca, which results in muscle spasm. Brudzinski's sign is rare in adults.

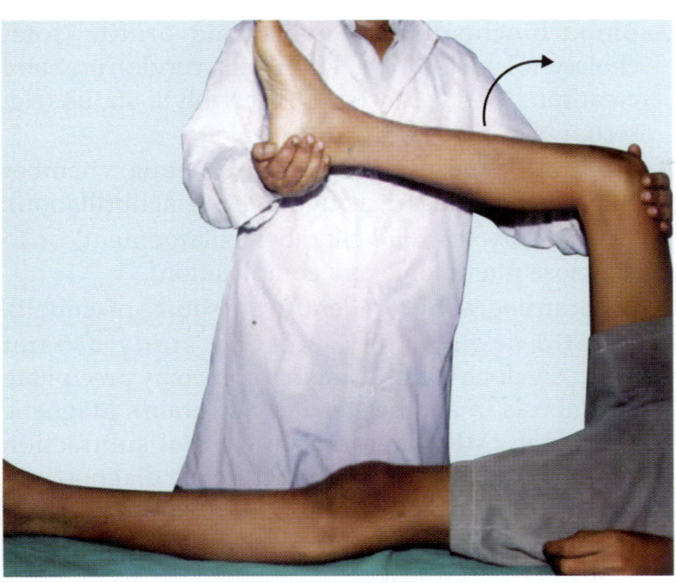

Fig. 1.48: Eliciting **Kernig's sign**

Q. How to differentiate meningism from meningitis?

Presence of neck rigidity and rise in CSF pressure are found in both the conditions but **meningitis** may have pain in the neck, positive Kernig's sign, turbid CSF and cellular changes in CSF. **Meningism** have no neck pain, less pronounced Kernig's sign, clear CSF with no cellular change.

Q. Diseases producing meningism in clinical practice:

1. Enteric fever.
2. Pneumonia (commonly atypical variety).
3. Empyema thoracis.
4. Diphtheria.
5. Acute pyogenic tonsillitis.
6. Viral encephalitis; or any viral infection.
7. Leukaemia, lymphoma, malignancy.
8. Weil's disease.

- *Meningism (meningeal irritation)* is usually due to some local or systemic infection but there is absence of any direct infection or inflammation of CNS.

Q. What is straight leg raising (SLR) test?

While the patient lies supine, try to elevate patient's 'extended' leg, keeping the hand behind the patient's heel. This movement (hip flexion) is possible up to 90° in a normal person. The test (SLR) is positive, i.e. restricted movement with pain is present in sciatica and prolapsed intervertebral disc (PIVD) due to stretching of nerve roots, while elevating patient's extended leg. Tight hamstring muscles often interfere with the test.

Lasegue's sign: Extension of the leg at knee, after flexing the thigh, will induce pain in PIVD. SLR and Lasegue's sign are tested in a patient with low back pain.

Q. Features of increased intracranial tension (IIT):

a. Symptoms:

1. Headache (intense deep-seated dull aching pain, worsened by exertion or change of posture, e.g. bending forward; headache may be severe on early morning hours or after coughing; holocranial headache).
2. Vomiting (sometimes, projectile, i.e. there is absence of nausea; unrelated to food).
3. Convulsions (usually generalised; focal due to SOL itself).
4. Altered consciousness to coma (retarded cerebration).
5. Drowsiness and mental deterioration may be present; visual problems like worsening of visual acuity and peripheral constriction of visual field.

b. Signs:

1. Pulse: Bradycardia; if the intracranial pressure continues to increase, the pulse becomes very rapid; there may be irregular pulse.
2. BP: There may be hypertension.
3. Respiration: Slow and deep respiration; later on it becomes rapid and shallow, and lastly Cheyne-Stokes breathing appears.
4. Papilloedema on fundoscopy; pupil: Unequal or abnormally reacting, may be fixed pupil.
5. **False localising signs** (signs which do not have localising value):
   i. Unilateral or bilateral, VIth or IIIrd nerve palsy.
   ii. Bilateral Babinski's sign.
   iii. Bilateral grasp reflex.
6. Bulged anterior fontanelle in infants.
7. A 'chronic IIT' may produce features of 'hypopituitarism', e.g. loss of body hairs, hypothyroidism hypoadrenalism, etc.

- **Examine:** Pulse, pressure, plantar response, papilloedema and paralysis, if any (5P).
- Bradycardia, systolic hypertension and irregular respiration are collectively known as **"Cushing's triad"** (due to cerebral herniation with brainstem compression necessitating urgent intervention).

c. Causes:

1. Cerebrovascular accidents (CVA).

2. Intracranial SOL (neoplasm, abscess, haematoma).
3. Meningitis, meningism, encephalitis.
4. **Benign intracranial hypertension** or pseudotumour cerebri (commonly from Addison's disease. corticosteroid withdrawal, COPD, overdose of vitamin A, hypoparathyroidism).
5. Circulatory block like aqueduct stenosis, 4th ventricle block in hydrocephalus.
6. Miscelaneous: Head injury, cerebral oedema, hypoxic encephalopathy, cortical venous sinus thrombosis.

d. Investigations:

1. X-ray of skull:
   i. Silver-beaten appearance (in children).
   ii. Sutural diastasis or separation (in children).
   iii. Erosion of posterior clinoid process.
   iv. Deepened sella turcica.
   v. Enlargement of internal auditory meatus.
2. CT or MRI scan: Diagnoses IIT (dilatation of ventricles and effacement of cisterns) with aetiology.

e. Treatment: It is done by propped-up position at 30°, IV mannitol (20%), glycerol (oral or IV), IV steroid (dexamethasone in vasogenic oedema surrounding a tumour or abscess, but not in CVA), furosemide (IV), rentention enema of magnesium sulphate, high-dose barbiturate therapy, or hyperventilation. Decompression surgery is indicated in significant IIT secondary to cerebral oedema.

- As a **false localising sign,** VIth cranial nerve is commonly involved because it has the longest intracranial course and thereby easily compressed at the bony prominences by IIT. Lumbar puncture is contraindicated in IIT with papilloedema because of the risk of development of 'cerebellar pressure cone syndrome' (sudden death due to compression of vital medullary centres as a result of descent of cerebellar tonsil).
- Features of **intracranial space-occupying lesion (ICSOL)** or mass lesion are: local effects (seizures), features of IIT, focal localising signs (uni- or bilateral VIth nerve palsy, ipsilateral hemiparesis, bilateral Babinski's sign), and others like mental changes or depression.

Q. What are the common causes of coma?

1. CVA (especially cerebral haemorrhage and massive cerebral infarction with oedema).
2. Encephalitis, meningitis, cerebral malaria, epilepsy, head injury, subdural or extradural haematoma, intracranial SOL, tentorial herniation.
3. Hypoglycaemia, diabetic ketoacidosis, renal failure, hepato-cellular failure, myxoedema coma, pituitary apoplexy, adrenal crisis, hyponatraemia.
4. Stokes-Adams syndrome, tight aortic stenosis, arrhythmias, respiratory failure (Type II).
5. Alcohol overdose, drug overdose, poisoning (barbiturate, opiate, organophosphorus), snake bite, hypothermia, heat stroke, severe sepsis.
6. Psychogenic.

Q. How do you like to investigate a case of hemiplegia?

1. **CT scan of the brain:** For proper initial evaluation, CT scan is mandatory to categorise the stroke into either ischaemic (thrombosis or embolism) or haemorrhagic origin. Cerebral haemorrhages (focal area of hyperdensity) are detected immediately whereas infarction (focal area of hypodensity) may take 48 hours or more to develop. CT scan helps to decide the line of management (e.g. regarding use of aspirin, anticoagulants or antiplatelet drugs). It also helps to diagnose the conditions which may simulate stroke, e.g. ICSOL, vascular malformation, etc. MRI scan may be done, though CT scan is preferred to MRI in acute stage.
2. Blood (routine examination): Hb%, TC, DC, platelet count, ESR.
3. Blood biochemistry: Sugar, lipid profile (total cholesterol, LDL, VLDL, HDL, triglyceride), urea and creatinine (renal functions), electrolyte status (e.g. serum Na^+, K^+).
4. ECG to diagnose myocardial ischaemia, chamber enlargement in heart, arrhythmia (atrial fibrillation).
5. Chest X-ray (cardiac chamber enlargement, or to diagnose pneumonia as a complication).
6. Echocardiography (to identify the source of emboli).
7. Carotid angiography and CSF study are not routinely done (carotid angiography may precipitate thrombosis in another territory of brain). Magnetic resonance (MR) angiography, digital subtraction angiography and lumbar puncture are diagnostic in subarachnoid haemorrhage.
8. Doppler flow studies in carotids (if facilities are available).

- Read the special investigations from 'Common causes of strokes in young' mentioned earlier (*see* page 140).

Q. What is the ideal line of management in hemiplegia?

After initial evaluation of neurological deficit, cardiovascular status, metabolic status (blood sugar, urea, creatinine and electrolytes) and haematological parameters (Hb%, coagulation profile) one may start management of hemiplegia with general supportive measures, anti-oedema management, and care of the co-morbid conditions.

1. Patient should lie in a railed cot. Insert Ryle's tube, put a self-retaining catheter and take care of the airway. Take care of the mouth (to prevent fungal infection), eyes and nutritional status. Nursing cares should be started by trained persons. O_2 therapy, if necessary (keep SpO_2 >94%).
2. Treat **cerebral oedema** by:
   a. 20% mannitol: 100 mL IV thrice daily (reduces cerebral oedema by osmotic diuresis). It is better to start 300 mL, IV rapidly as a bolus dose and then 100 mL, TDS, IV to be continued for 2–3 days.

b. Oral glycerol: 6 tsf thrice daily (usually taken with fruit juice).
c. Inj. furosemide: 40 mg IV stat, and as and when necessary.
d. Inj. dexamethasone (if not hypertensive): 4–6 mg, IM or IV, every 4–6 hourly may be tried in selected cases, e.g. chronic subdural haematoma (*contraindicated in CVA)*].

3. Treatment of diabetes mellitus, stress ulcer (by H_2RA or PPI), hypertension [maintain the BP at or just below 185/110 mm of Hg in cerebral infarction; and in cerebral haemorrhage, keep the BP a bit lower (i.e. 160/100 mm of Hg, or mean arterial pressure 130 mm of Hg) than the above reading; BP is gradually reduced over several days], hyperlipidaemia (atorvastatin 80 mg/day); avoid smoking; maintain fluid balance. Do not lower the BP much in acute stage because it will hamper the cerebral autoregulation, diminish the perfusion of ischaemic zones, and may exacerbate the size of infarction.
4. Antiplatelet drugs (in thrombosis): Aspirin (75–300 mg daily), clopidogrel (75 mg daily), or dipyridamole (50 mg thrice daily) or ticlopidine (250 mg twice daily) for long-term prophylaxis. Aspirin 300 mg daily should be started immediately as soon as the ischaemic stroke is confirmed, and reducing the dose to 75 mg daily after several days. Pentoxifylline, 400 mg, 8 hourly (haemorheology modifier, i.e. changes viscosity of blood) may be beneficial in cerebral infarction if used within 12 hours of onset of stroke (not accepted by all). Newer promising antiplatelet drugs are ticagrelor, triflusal and prasugrel. *Aspirin is strictly contraindicated in cerebral haemorrhage and very large infarction.*
5. Role of cerebral vasdodilators ('neuroprotective' agents) are contradictory (5% CO_2 with 95% O_2, cyclandelate, nicotinic acid, papaverine, aminophylline, etc.) due to steal phenomenon.
6. Treatment of atrial fibrillation (in embolism) and valvular heart disease is done accordingly.
7. Anticoagulant therapy may be given (heparin and warfarin) in an 'evolving stroke' if cerebral haemorrhage is ruled out by early CT scan. Anticoagulant therapy is not of value in the treatment of completed stroke. Anticoagulation is mandatory in cardiogenic embolic stroke.
8. Thrombolytic therapy (reperfusion therapy): Recombinant tissue plasminogen activator (r-TPA) may be beneficial if started within the first 3 hours of onset of an ischaemic stroke. Thrombotic stroke, if seen within 3 hours, may be treated with thrombolysis or heparin (without any contraindication like cerebral haemorrhage).
9. Surgery: Certain intracerebral haematomas are amenable to surgery (e.g. cerebellum); carotid endarterectomy is performed in carotid TIA. Surgery is done in subarachnoid haemorrhage.
10. Physiotherapy: Is done by an expert physiotherapist or physiatrist. **It should be started as soon as the patient recovers from the neural shock stage.** Change of posture in bed (2 hourly) must be done to avoid bed sores. *Physiotherapy is advised to prevent joint contractures and oedema of the limb, and to promote recovery of strength.* Compression stockings should be applied to paralysed leg to prevent deep vein thrombosis (DVT). Passive movement of the limb also prevents venous stasis and pulmonary embolism. Chest physiotherapy should be started to promote coughing out of expectorations. Manage swallowing difficulty.
11. Rehabilitation; speech and occupational therapy should be tried.

[12. Subarachnoid haemorrhage is managed by oral nimodipine 60 mg 6 times daily for 3 weeks to prevent vasospasm. Surgical clipping or coil occlusion of aneurysm afterwards in selected cases.]

- **Avoid** hypoxia, 5% dextrose infusion and corticosteroid in the treatment of CVA. Treat fever, dehydration and hyperglycaemia; haloperidol is given in severe restlessness.
- Antihypertensives used in ischaemic stroke are labetalol, enalaprilat, nicardipine, clevidipine or hydralazine.
- Always take care of bladder, bowel, back (bed sore), base of the lungs, and boost the morale (5B).

Clinical Wisdom

Mortality is approximately 20% in acute stroke. Poor prognostic signs are altered sensorium, old age, aphasia and brainstem signs. Recovery is variable and is usually incomplete. Recurrences are common.

PARAPLEGIA — CASE 17

Q. What is your diagnosis?

This is a case of spastic paraparesis (or paraplegia) in extension due to compressive myelopathy caused by caries spine and the lesion is at the level of T_{10} segment of the spinal cord.

- Previously known as Pott's paraplegia (i.e. paraplegia developing from spinal tuberculosis).

Q. Why do you say so?

This young male patient aged 32 years was complaining of severe weakness of both the lower limbs with loss of sensation for last one month. He also complained of anorexia, cough with evening rise of temperature for last 5 months. One month back, he noticed gradual weakness of the left leg which was followed by weakness of the right leg after 2 days. He also noticed numbness or loss of superficial sensations like touch, pain and temperature below the level of umbilicus for the same duration. The fever was intermittent in nature and was associated with night sweats. On repeated enquiry, he gave H/o *root pain*, i.e. sharp, constant, stabbing, electric shock-like pain which was distributed in the region below the umbilicus along with both the lower limbs. The pain used to aggravate by the change of posture, coughing, sneezing, jolting and movement of spine. He also complained of a special type of sensation, i.e. girdle-like sensation at the level of umbilicus. For the last 25 days, there was almost total and more or less, symmetrical paralysis of both the lower limbs; there was no H/o diurnal variation of weakness (vide myasthenia gravis). The patient did not complain of any involvement or weakness of the upper limbs. It seems that the disease started insidiously and was progressing gradually.

Initially, he was also suffering from hesitancy of micturition and was catheterised in the hospital on admission (he was admitted in the hospital 25 days back). He was unable to hold feces for the same duration (rectal incontinence). He specifically complained of bone pain at his back. Since his admission, there was no sign of recovery. The patient did not give any H/o flexor spasm.

There was no H/o headache, vomiting, convulsions, speech difficulty, facial weakness or any abnormal movements. No family H/o diabetes mellitus, hypertension or tuberculosis was found. There was no positive H/o exposure to STD, trauma to the spine or similar episodes in the past. He was not vaccinated in the recent past. He is neither diabetic nor hypertensive. On repeated enquiry, he gave H/o haemoptysis 3 months back which he ignored and did not attend any physician at that time.

On examination, it shows that the patient is conscious and cooperative. He is suffering from UMN paralysis of both the lower limbs. There is loss of superficial sensations below the umbilicus. A gibbus is seen at the level of 7th thoracic vertebra which is tender on palpation. The UMN paralysis of both the lower limbs is suggested by bilateral clasp-knife spasticity, brisk tendon reflexes, presence of clonus and extensor plantar response.

- **Paraplegia is basically of two types: spastic and flaccid.**

Q. What is your case?

Say the summary as above.

Q. Importance of 'past history' in paraplegia:

1. H/o tuberculosis.
2. H/o fever (tuberculosis, acute transverse myelitis, GB syndrome, lymphoma, leukaemia).
3. Primary chancre (exposure to STD).
4. Similar episodes in the past (may signify multiple sclerosis).
5. Spinal injury (produces compressive myelopathy).
6. Hypertension, diabetes mellitus as a routine.
7. H/o any lymphadenopathy (tuberculosis, lymphoma, malignancy) or vaccination (may precipitate acute transverse myelitis-like features).
8. Alcoholism or drugs like INH, vincristine (drug-induced peripheral neuropathy producing weakness of both lower limbs).
9. Pain in the spine (caries spine, metastasis in the spine).
10. Occupational history: H/o exposure to chemicals and toxins, weight lifting (e.g. PIVD).

Q. Importance of 'family history' in paraplegia:

1. Hypertension (as a routine).
2. Diabetes mellitus (as a routine).
3. H/o paraplegia in other members of the family (if present, may indicate hereditary spastic paraplegia, paraplegia with hereditary ataxia, or lathyrism).
4. Tuberculosis.

Q. Chief complaints (clinical presentations) of your patient:

1. Cough with evening rise of temperature for last 5 months.
2. Weakness of both the lower limbs for 1 month.
3. Loss of sensations of both the lower limbs for 1 month.
4. Hesitancy of micturition and loss of bowel control for 1 month.

Q. Enquiry regarding paralysis (in H/o present illness):

a. *Date of onset:* Note the specific date and time of onset of paralysis.
b. *Mode of onset:* Sudden (acute transverse myelitis, spinal injury, etc) or gradual (caries spine).
c. *Precipitaing factors:*
   i. Spinal injury.
   ii. Vaccination (commonly anti-rabies nervous tissue vaccine).
d. *Evolution of paralysis:* Whether both limbs are affected simultaneously or one after the other.
e. *Progress of paralysis:*
   i. Increasing in severity and extent: Cord compression.
   ii. Improving: Inflammatory, acute transverse myelitis or multiple sclerosis.
   iii. Static but progressing very slowly: Degenerative lesion (Friedreich's ataxia).
   iv. Waxing and waning: Multiple sclerosis.
f. *Degree and duration of paralysis:* Weakness or total loss of power, with duration.
g. *Motor symptoms:* See the symptomatology.

Q. Enquiry regarding sensory symptoms (in H/o present illness):

1. Loss of sensation (superficial and/or deep): Find out the upper border.
2. Girdle-like sensation or sense of constriction (find out the level).
3. Zone of hyperaesthesia (find out the level).

4. Root pain (ask for distribution and precipitating factors).
5. Sensation of pins and needles in the lower extremities (test for sensory functions).

Q. Cerebral paraplegia:

a. Causes: The lesion in paraplegia lies either in cerebral cortex, spinal cord, nerve roots, peripheral nerves, myoneural junction, or in muscles. Cerebral causes are extremely rare and always give rise to paraplegia in extension. The causes are:

1. Cerebral diplegia (Little's disease): Cortical cause of paraplegia.
2. Superior sagittal sinus thrombosis.
3. Parasagittal meningioma.
4. Thrombosis of unpaired anterior cerebral artery.
5. Hydrocephalus.
6. Bullet injury or trauma at paracentral lobule.

b. Features:

1. Extremely rare. H/o Jacksonian fits and cortical sensory loss present.
2. Spastic paraplegia in extension (may be flaccid in shock stage but never produces paraplegia in flexion).
3. Features of IIT may be present (headache, vomiting, convulsions). Bladder dysfunction is common.
4. Abnormalities in higher functions, speech difficulty, cranial nerve affection may be present.

Q. Causes of 'spastic' paraplegia (UMN type lesion):

a. Gradual onset

1. Cerebral causes: Cerebral diplegia, parasagittal meningioma, hydrocephalus.
2. Spinal causes:
   a. Compressive or transverse lesion in the spinal cord: Cord compression (*see* below).
   b. Non-compressive, or longitudinal lesion, or systemic diseases of the spinal cord:
      i. Motor neurone disease (MND), e.g. amyotrophic lateral sclerosis.
      ii. Multiple sclerosis, Devic's disease.
      iii. Friedreich's ataxia.
      iv. Subacute combined degeneration (i.e. from vitamin B_{12} deficiency).
      v. Lathyrism.
      vi. Syringomyelia.
      vii. Hereditary spastic paraplegia.
      viii. Tropical spastic paraplegia.
      ix. Paraneoplastic myelitis.
      x. Antiphospholipid antibody syndrome.
      xi. Radiation myelopathy.
      xii. Syphilitic meningomyelitis (rare).

b. Sudden onset

1. Cerebral causes: Thrombosis of unpaired anterior cerebral artery, superior sagittal sinus thrombosis, bullet injury at paracentral lobule.

Table 1.17: Differentiation between 'paraplegia in extension' and 'paraplegia in flexion'

Features	Paraplegia in extension	Paraplegia in flexion
1. Definition	1. Lower limbs take an extension attitude and the extensor muscles are spastic	1. Lower limbs take an attitude of flexion due to **'flexor spasms'** (even the heel may strike the back of thigh)
2. Pathology	2. Only pyramidal tracts are involved	2. Both pyramidal and extrapyramidal tracts (e.g. reticulospinal tract) are involved
3. Evolution	3. Early	3. Late
4. Clinical features		
a. Attitude	a. Hip extended and adducted, knee extended, and feet plantiflexed	a. Thigh and knee flexed, feet dorsiflexed. Adopts lateral decubitus posture in bed
b. Tone	b. Clasp-knife spasticity in extensor group of muscles	b. Tone is increased in flexor group of muscles
c. Jerks	c. Brisk	c. Present but diminished
d. Plantar response	d. **Extensor**	d. **Extensor but may be associated with flexor spasms**
e. Reflex evacuation of bladder and bowel	e. Absent	e. Present
f. Mass reflex	f. Absent	f. May be present

- **Spastic paraplegia is of two types: Paraplegia in extension and paraplegia in flexion** (Table 1.17).
- Thus, paraplegia in flexion is prognostically worse, and occurs in late stages of paraplegia or progressive lesion. Paraplegia in flexion is due to complete transection of spinal cord.
- **Mass reflex:** If the skin of the lower limbs or the lower abdominal wall is stimulated (below the level of lesion), there is reflex flexion of the lower trunk muscles and the lower limbs (i.e. flexor spasms), piloerection and penile erection, evacuation of the bladder, bowel and semen, and sweating. Mass reflex indicates severe spinal cord lesion. It is a reflex of spinal automatism. It indicates more severe spinal cord lesion.
- Flexor spasms may be severe in posterior column lesion (e.g. multiple sclerosis), in the presence of bed sores or urinary tract infection (as a result of constant stimulation of small unmyelinated nerve fibres) with cord lesion.

2. Spinal causes:
    a. Acute transverse myelitis.
    b. Injury to the spinal cord (fracture-dislocation or collapse of the vertebra).
    c. Thrombosis of anterior spinal artery (myelomalacia).
    d. Haematomyelia (from arteriovenous malformations, angiomas, or endarteritis).
    e. Post-vaccinal.
    f. Prolapsed intervertebral disc (PIVD).
    g. Spinal epidural abscess or haematoma.
    h. Radiation myelopathy.

- Compressive: 2 b), f) and g).
- Non-compressive: 2 a), c), d), e) and h).

Q. Causes of 'cord compression' (compressive aetiology in paraplegia):

I. Intramedullary (5%):

a. Glioma (astrocytoma).
b. Ependymoma.
c. Chordoma.
d. Syringomyelia, haematomyelia.

II. Extramedullary:

a. Intradural (15%)
  i. Meningioma.
  ii. Neurofibroma.
  iii. Patchy arachnoiditis (tuberculosis, syphilis sarcoidosis).
  iv. Arteriovenous malformations.
  v. Lipoma, dermoid, sarcoma.

b. Extradural (80%)
  i. Caries spine (Pott's paraplegia).
  ii. Myeloma, lymphomatous or metastatic deposits in the vertebra; osteomyelitis.
  iii. Patchy meningitis.
  iv. Prolapsed intervertebral disc (PIVD).
  v. Degenerative joint disease (spondylosis).
  vi. Fracture or dislocation of the vertebra (i.e. spinal injury), osteoporosis, Paget's disease.
  vii. Extramedullary haematopoiesis in thalassaemia.
  viii. Spinal epidural abscess or haematoma.
  ix. Extradural arteriovenous malformations.

- Cord compression produces paraplegia by: 1. Pressure effect, 2. Ischaemia (arterial), and 3. Congestion (venous).
- Intradural lesion (e.g. neurofibroma) gives a history of long duration while extradural lesion (e.g. malignancy) gives a short history.
- Spinal cord injury: Automobile accidents, gunshot or stab injury, sports injury or injury due to 'falls'.

Q. Causes of 'flaccid' paraplegia (LMN type lesion):

A. UMN lesion in shock stage, i.e. sudden onset spastic paraplegia in 'neural shock' stage, e.g. acute transverse myelitis, spinal injury.

B. Lesion involving anterior horn cells:
    a. Acute anterior poliomyelitis.
    b. Progressive musclular atrophy (variety of MND).
    c. Trauma.

C. Diseases affecting nerve roots: Tabes dorsalis, radiculitis, GB syndrome, malignancy.

D. Diseases affecting peripheral nerves:
    a. Acute infective polyneuropathy (GB syndrome).
    b. High cauda equina syndrome.
    c. Disease of peripheral nerves involving both the lower limbs.
    d. Lumbar plexus injury (e.g. psoas abscess or haematoma).

E. Diseases affecting myoneural junction:
    a. Myasthenia gravis, Lambert-Eaton syndrome, drugs like aminoglycosides or organophosphorus (OP) insecticides.
    b. Periodic paralysis due to hypo- or hyperkalaemia.

F. Diseases affecting muscles: Myopathy.

G. Hysterical or psychogenic paralysis.

- Note that *paraplegia may be developed due to lesion in cerebral cortex, spinal cord (compressive or non-compressive myelopathy), nerve roots, peripheral nerves, myoneural junction or muscles.* In clinical practice, we are more concerned with paraplegia due to lesions in the spinal cord (myelopathy).
- **Common causes of paraplegia** are: Trauma, tuberculosis, tumour, thrombosis (of anterior spinal artery) and transverse myelitis (5Ts).
- Common causes of flaccid paraplegia are GB syndrome and peripheral neuropathy.

Q. What is spinal (neural) shock?

It is a flaccid areflexic paralysis below the level of lesion in spinal cord after an acute insult (trauma, infarction or inflammation) to the cord. There may be urinary retention and constipation. Plantar response may be equivocal or 'no response'. Longer duration of shock suggests poor recovery. The common example is acute transverse myelitis.

Q. Classical features of acute transverse myelitis:

Though a common cause of non-compressive myelopathy (acute onset total transection of the cord), clinically somewhat **it behaves like compressive variety.**

1. Very often follows a viral illness (neurotropic virus) or post-vaccinal.
2. It behaves like flaccid paraplegia in neural shock stage. Onset is acute or subacute (evolve over several days to 2–3 weeks).
3. **Fever may be present before paralysis develops.**
4. **Bladder (retention of urine) and bowel (unable to pass stool) involvement are early.**
5. Though behaves like compressive variety, usually there is absence of root pain, spinal tenderness or spinal deformity. Back pain and progressive

paraparesis are presenting complaints. Girdle constriction at the level of lesion with zone of hyperaesthesia just above may be obtained. Mid-thoracic region is the most common site.

6. **Plantar response is extensor** and there is partial or complete sensory loss (all modalities), with a definite upper level (very important **point of difference with acute infective polyneuropathy** where these two features are, flexor and no demonstrable sensory loss respectively).
7. MRI scan is often required to exclude cord compression.
8. Majority (70%) recovers within 12 weeks.

- Plantar response may not be extensor, in the stage of neural shock.
- All the reflexes are usually lost below the level of lesion in the stage of neural shock (first 2–3 weeks). Thereafter, spasticity with brisk reflexes develop.
- **Causes of acute transverse myelopathy** are infections, trauma, multiple sclerosis, vasculitis (MCTD, SLE), nutritional, HIV, sarcoidosis, radiation, lightning injury, syphilis and anterior spinal artery occlusion (vascular).
- MRI of the spinal cord is done to rule out any alternate pathology (e.g. mass lesion). CSF pressure and cell count are usually normal but protein content is high.

Q. Features of acute infective polyneuropathy (Landry-Guillain-Barré syndrome):

1. There is an association with Epstein-Barr virus, measles, *Campylobacter jejuni* (causing diarrhoea), HIV, herpes zoster, cytomegalovirus, post-vaccinal and post-surgical events. The current hypothesis is in the favour of immunological reaction due to hypersensitivity, perhaps as a result of unidentified allergen directed against the myelin sheath of peripheral nerves. Truely speaking, *it is an acute post-infective polyradiculoneuropathy* (i.e. inflammatory demyelination involves spinal roots and peripheral nerves). Severe forms show secondary axonal degeneration. GB syndrome is usually monophasic and does not recur.
2. a. Common history of GB syndrome: Viral illness (e.g. respiratory catarrh) → after 2 weeks, sudden paralysis with sensory symptoms (paraesthesia) starts → paralysis progresses for 3 weeks and then stops → paralysis becomes static for 2 weeks → after 2 weeks recovery starts which is usually completed within 6 months → in incomplete recovery, residual disability persists.

   b. Incidence: In either sex; peak incidence is in between 20 and 50 years.
3. Monoplegia, paraplegia or quadriplegia **(proximal muscles are more affected)**. It is an acute (evolved over hours to days) **ascending LMN type of paralysis usually beginning in the legs.** Upper extremities may also be involved sequentially or at a time leading to quadriplegia. There may be bulbar palsy or respiratory muscle paralysis (i.e. breathing difficulty).
4. Bilateral VIIth (LMN type) cranial nerve palsy is not uncommon, though this is occasionally unilateral. Often papilloedema is noted (IInd).
5. **No sensory abnormalities demonstrated** (very characteristic) though sometimes the patients complain of distal paraesthesia.
6. Jerks are invariably absent (i.e. there is diffuse weakness with widespread loss of reflexes). Gross hypotonia is evident. **It is an areflexic, atonic ascending motor paralysis.**
7. Bladder and bowel are rarely involved.
8. **Plantar response: Flexor or no response.**
9. Autonomic disturbances (tachycardia, arrhythmia, postural hypotension/hypertension, pupillary abnormalities) are not uncommon.
10. Sensorium (consciousness): Clear throughout the disease process.
11. Albumino-cytological dissociation in CSF is characteristic.

- **There is subjective sensory symptoms (paraesthesia) without any objective sensory loss.**
- GB syndrome is also known as acute inflammatory demyelinating polyneuropathy (AIDP).
- Outcome: 1. Complete or near complete recovery 65%, 2. Residual disability 30%, and 3. Death 5% (respiratory paralysis or lung infection).

Clinical Wisdom

Georges Guillain (1876–1961) was professor of Medicine in paris, and JA Barré (1880–1967) was professor of neurology in Strasbourg, France.

Q. Features of 'atypical' GB syndrome (i.e. variants):

1. Distal muscle involvement.
2. Objective sensory impairment.
3. Papilloedema.
4. Descending paralysis.
5. Early bladder and bowel involvement.
6. Babinski's sign.
7. Glomerulonephritis.
8. Miller Fisher syndrome (ataxia, areflexia and external ophthalmoplegia) without significant limb weakness—a variant.
9. SIADH (syndrome of inappropriate ADH secretion).

Q. What is Brown-Sequard syndrome?

It is the hemisection of the spinal cord (e.g. bullet or stab injury, infarction of spinal cord, radiation myelopathy, intradural tumours or syringomyelia) and the features are:

1. ***Sensory:*** Loss of proprioception (joint, position, vibration sense) on the same side, and loss of pain and temperature sensations on the opposite side, 1–2 segment below the level of lesion.
2. ***Motor:*** Segmental LMN signs at the level of lesion; monoplegia of the lower limb or hemiplegia (UMN

lesion) on the same side may occur below the level of lesion (spastic paralysis).

3. *Reflexes:* Below the level of lesion, there are features of UMN lesion, i.e. superficial reflexes lost, brisk deep reflexes with extensor plantar response.

- There may be a band of hyperaesthesia on the same side just above the level of lesion.
- In lesion above T_1 level: Patient presents with Horner's sydrome.
- There is maximum motor loss on the same side and maximum sensory loss on the opposite side.

Q. Localisation of the level of lesion in a compressive myelopathy (Table 1.18):

Localisation of the level of compression in the spinal cord is done by:

1. Distribution of root pain: Ask for specific dermatomes involved (it is due to involvement of posterior nerve roots).
2. Upper border of sensory loss: Examine the patient from below upwards (i.e. from legs to thorax) for demonstration of upper border of sensory loss (due to affection of spinothalamic tract).
3. Girdle-like sensation or sense of constriction at the level of lesion (due to involvement of posterior column).
4. Zone of hyperaesthesia or hyperalgesia: This will localise the level of lesion one segment below, i.e. zone of hyperaesthesia is present just above the level of girdle-like sensation, and is due to compression of posterior nerve roots.
5. Analysis of abdominal reflex, i.e. if upper abdominal reflex is intact with loss of middle and lower one, the site of lesion is probably at T_{10} spinal segment.
6. Atrophy of the muscles in a segmental distribution (due to involvement of anterior horn cells).
7. Loss of deep reflexes, if the particular segment is involved. The reflexes will be brisk below the involved segment
8. Analysis of *Beevor's sign* (do the Babinski's 'rising test'. In paralysis of lower part of rectus abdominis, umbilicus moves upwards and in paralysis of upper part of rectus abdominis, umbilicus goes downwards): Beevor's sign detects the weakness of abdominal muscles.
9. Deformity (e.g. gibbus) or any swelling in the vertebra.
10. Tenderness in the vertebra.
11. The area of sweating may be of help (lack of sweating below the level) in localising the level of lesion.
12. The level can also be localised by X-ray of the spine, myelography, CT scan or MRI.

- The question of localisation of the level of lesion does not arise in non-compressive myelopathy.

Q. Determination of spinal segments in relation to vertebrae:

The spinal segments do not lie exactly under the overlying vertebra. The following formula determines the spinal segments related to a vertebral body.

1. For cervical vertebrae: Add 1.
2. For 1–6 thoracic vartebrae: Add 2.
3. For 7–9 thoracic vertebrae: Add 3.
4. The T_{10} arch overlies L_1 and L_2 segments.
5. The T_{11} arch overlies L_3 and L_4 segments.
6. The T_{12} arch overlies L_5 segment.
7. The L_1 arch overlies the sacral and coccygeal segments.

The first seven spinal nerves (C_{1-7}) come out above the corresponding vertebra while the C_8 spinal nerve comes out below the C_7 vertebra. Other spinal nerves exit below the respective vertebral body.

Clinical Wisdom

In the patient described at the outset, the T_7 vertebra is involved and thus, the spinal segment involved is T_{10} (by adding 3). Remember, in lower thoracic region the tip of a spinous process marks the vertebral body below.

- Altogether 31 pairs of spinal nerve roots emerge from the spinal cord. The segments in the cord are: cervical 8, thoracic 12, lumbar 5, sacral 5 and coccygeal 1. The lower end of spinal cord tapers to form **'conus medullaris'** at lower border of L_1 vertebra. The spinal roots below L_1 vertebra pass down in the spinal canal to emerge at their respective foramina, and thus form **'cauda equina'** (i.e. looks like horse's tail).

Q. Blood supply of spinal cord in a nutshell:

1. Aanterior spinal artery (1).
2. Posterior spinal arteries (2).
3. Small radicular arteries (31 pairs).
4. Intercostal artery, ascending and deep cervical arteries, vertebral artery, artery of Adamkiewicz (arises from a left posterior intercostal artery and some feeder arteries to join spinal arteries).

Q. Points to note in 'spine examination' in paraplegia:

I. 1. Kyphosis.
   2. Scoliosis.
   3. **Gibbus** (with paraspinal muscle spasm) (Fig. 1.22).
   4. Tenderness.
   5. Spina bifida.

II. Any scar (old trauma), tuft of hair over sacrum (spina bifida occulta), bed sore or sacral oedema.

Q. 'Paraplegia in extension' progressing to 'paraplegia in flexion': How to diagnose?

Spastic paraplegia may progress to paraplegia in flexion which is diagnosed by:

1. Appearance of flexor spasms.

Table 1.18: Differentiation between compressive and non-compressive myelopathy

Features	Compressive	Non-compressive
1. Bony deformity	+	–
2. Bony tenderness	+	–
3. Girdle-like sensation	+	–
4. Upper level of sensory loss	+	–
5. Zone of hyperaesthesia	+	–
6. Root pain	+	–
7. Onset and progress	Gradual	May be acute
8. Symmetry	Asymmetrical	Majority are symmetrical
9. Flexor spasms	Common	Usually absent
10. Pattern of neurodeficit	U-shaped*	Bilaterally symmetrical
11. Bladder and bowel involvement	Early	Usually late (early in acute transverse myelitis)
12. Classical example	Caries spine	Motor neurone disease

- No. 3, 4 and 5 are sometimes present in acute transverse myelitis.
- March of neurodeficit pattern*: U-shaped, i.e. first ipsilateral upper limb (UL), next ipsilateral lower limb (LL), next contralateral LL, and finally contralateral UL (Elsberg's phenomenon). In a slow cord compression the pyramidal tract is affected first, followed by the posterior column, and finally the spinothalamic tract.

2. Diminution of deep reflexes (jerks).
3. Diminution of ankle clonus in duration.

- In addition to pyramidal tract, there is involvement of extrapyramidal tracts like reticulospinal, rubrospinal, tectospinal or vestibulospinal tract in patients with paraplegia in flexion. It reflects significant cord damage with minimal chance of recovery (*see* **Table 1.17**).
- Pathophysiology: When the pyramidal tract alone is at jeopardy, the extrapyramidal system takes upper hand, resulting in increased tone of the antigravity muscles (i.e. paraplegia in extension). When the extrapyramidal system is at fault too, the spinal arc becomes dominant and there is relative increase in tone of the flexors (e.g. hamstrings) more than the extensors (i.e. development of paraplegia in flexion).

Q. Differentiation between intradural and extradural lesion of extramedullary pathology (Table 1.19):

- Intradural: Mode of onset is asymmetrical, root pain is more common, and spinal tenderness and deformity are –ve.
- Extradural: Respectively they are usually symmetrical, less common, and +ve.

Q. Abdominal reflex and its interpretations (Fig. 1.49):

It is a *polysynaptic nociceptive reflex*. The clinical method goes like this:

1. The patient lies supine and relaxed with exposed abdomen. The procedure is explained to him. Now the **stroke is given bilaterally in 3 places**–below the costal margins, at the level of the umbilicus and above the inguinal ligaments. Always compare right with the left side. Stroke is done lightly by a needle, a key or by the shaft of the hammer, on each side in turn.
2. **Stroke is given from outside to the centre on both the sides sequentially** (the dermatomes are criss-crossed at the midline and if the stroke starts from midline, eventually by chance, the opposite side may be stimulated). The hammer stick or orange stick should be placed at an acute angle with the abdominal skin and it should not caste any abrasion in the skin.
3. The normal reflex involves quick contraction of anterior abdominal musculature with movement of umbilicus in that direction. The reflex can be read by observing the movement of umbilicus (elevation, depression or lateral deviation), which is known as **Beevor's sign**. Root value: T_7–T_{12} (umbilicus at T_{10} level).

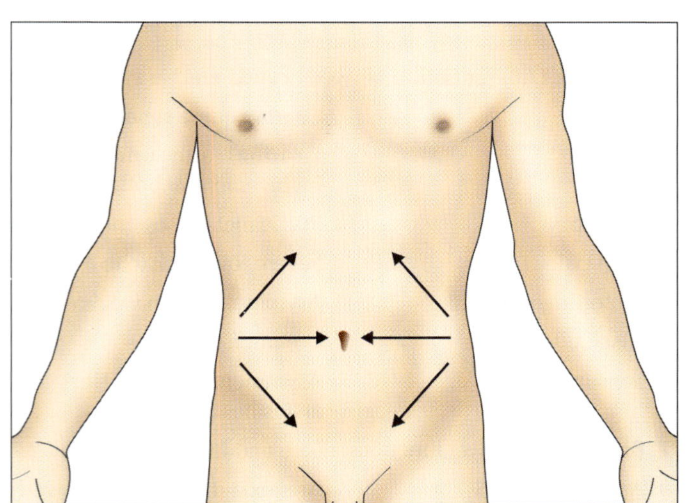

Fig. 1.49: Elicitation of **abdominal reflex**

Q. Loss of abdominal reflex:

a. Physiological:

i. Obesity.
ii. Lax abdominal wall.
iii. Multiparous woman.

Table 1.19: Discriminate between extramedullary (intradural) and intramedullary lesions

Features	Extramedullary	Intramedullary
1. Root pain	Early and common	Root pain is rare; burning in type and poorly localised
2. Sensory deficit	No dissociation of sensation; contralateral loss of pain and temperature with ipsilateral loss of proprioception	Dissociation of sensation common; spotty changes
3. Sacral sensation	Lost (early)	Sacral sparing
4. LMN involvement	Segmental	Marked with widespread atrophy; fasciculation seen
5. UMN Involvement	Early and prominent	Less pronounced; late feature
6. Reflexes	Brisk, early feature	Less brisk, late feature
7. Autonomic involvement (bladder and bowel)	Late	Early
8. Trophic changes	Usually not marked	Common
9. Vertebral tenderness	May be sensitive to local pressure	No bony tenderness in vertebrae
10. Changes in CSF (i.e. raised proteins)	Frequent	Rare

- Sacral sensation: In extramedullary lesion (e.g., cauda equina lesion) lower sacral sensations like S_{3-5} are impaired (i.e. **saddle anaesthesia**—loss of sensation restricted to buttocks, perineum and inner thighs), and in intramedullary lesion sensation is preserved in sacral dermatomes **(sacral sparing)**.

Table 1.20: Differentiation between cauda equine syndrome and conus medullaris lesion

Features	Cauda equina syndrome	Conus medullaris lesion
1. Onset	Gradual and unilateral (or asymmetrical involvement of both lower limbs)	Sudden and bilateral
2. Aetiology	PIVD, metastases, multiple myelomas	Intramedullary SOL (e.g. glioma)
3. Root pain	Severe low backache	Usually absent
4. Motor involvement	Asymmetric limb weakness	Muscle changes are not marked
5. Fasciculation	Common	Rare
6. Sensory loss	Asymmetric sensory loss (i.e. unilateral saddle anaesthesia)	Bilateral saddle anaesthesia (in late stage) or perianal sparing
7. Bladder and bowel functions	Late and less marked	Early and marked (flaccid bladder)
8. Anal reflex (S_2–S_4)	Areflexia it roots are involved	Anal reflex absent
9. Deep reflexes	Ankle and knee jerks are lost	Ankle and knee jerks are usually preserved
10. Trophic changes	Less	Early
11. Impotence	Less frequent	Frequent
12. Plantar response	Flexor or no response	Extensor (not always)

- Cauda equina lesion usually gives rise to LMN signs whereas conus medullaris lesion have UMN signs **(Table 1.20)**.

iv. Aged patient.
v. In the presence of ascites or pregnancy.
vi. Previous abdominal surgery.

b. Pathological:

i. LMN type of lesion affecting the corresponding reflex arc.
ii. Peripheral neuropathy.
iii. UMN type of lesion above the level of the reflex arc (hemiplegia or myelopathy).

- Abdominal reflex is lost early in multiple sclerosis, and retained long in MND and cerebral diplegia. In hemiplegia, the abdominal reflex is lost in the paralysed side only. Over-response occurs in anxiety and psychoneurosis. The reflex is absent in neonates and may disappear after repeated stimulation. Abdominal reflex (superficial reflex) is a local reflex arc modified by a 'cerebral arc', i.e. the pyramidal tract.

Clinical Wisdom

Beevor's sign can be elicited by 'rising test' too. When the umbilicus goes up it is called Beevor's sign while when it goes down, it is known as inverted Beevor's sign. Positive Beevor's sign (cephalad movement of umbilicus) is due to (a) dosral spinal cord pathology at D_{10} level, and (b) facio-scapulo-humeral muscular dystrophy.

Q. How cremasteric reflex is elicited?

Explain what you are going to do to your male patient. Scratch the medial side of upper thigh in a downward and inward direction (the patient lies supine with thigh remains abducted and externally rotated), and the response is brisk upward movement of ipsilateral scrotum and testicle due to contraction of cremasteric muscle. *Alternatively*, this reflex can be easily elicited by pressing over the sartorius in the lower third of Hunter's canal. The spinal segment responsible are L_1 and L_2. This reflex is lost in either UMN lesion or damage to $L_{1,2}$ spinal segments, or with hydrocele/hernia. It is also a *polysynaptic reflex*. Often it is very difficult to elicit this reflex in the elderly (easily elicited in children).

- **Different superficial reflexes are:** Corneal and conjunctival reflex (afferent Vth and efferent VIIth cranial nerve), gag reflex (afferent IXth and efferent Xth cranial nerve), abdominal reflex (T_7–T_{12}), cremasteric ($L_{1, 2}$), anal and bulbocavernosus reflex (S_2–S_4), and plantar reflex (S_1).
- **Anal reflex** (S_2–S_4): Gentle pricking or stroking of the skin on either side of the anus causes brisk contraction of the external anal sphincter which can be felt with a gloved finger at the anus. If the contraction of anal sphincter is perceived after stimulation of glans penis or clitoris, it is known as bulbocavernosus reflex (S_2–S_4).

Q. Special points in the physical examination in paraplegia:

A. General survey:

a. The patient is conscious and cooperative.
b. Decubitus: Lying helplessly without any movement of the lower limbs and with extension of all joints (lower limb). Upper limbs are within normal limit.
c. Lymph nodes: Not palpable (ref: tuberculosis, lymphoma, malignancy or HIV infection).
d. Pulse: 74/min and regular; mention all the points.
e. BP: It is compulsory to record the BP (in all long cases); 125/85 mm of Hg in the present case.
f. Respiration: 18/min, regular, abdominal in type (ref: respiratory depression in GB syndrome).
g. Pallor: Absent (may be present in vitamin B_{12} deficiency).
h. Temperature: Record the oral temperature (tuberculosis, acute transverse myelitis, UTI, etc.).
i. Oedema: Not present (may be present due to prolonged recumbency). Look for sacral oedema.
j. Skin: Absence of neurofibroma, cafe-au-lait spots or hypopigmented patches (e.g. leprosy).

- Mention all the points in general survey.

B. Nervous system:

a. The patient is conscious, alert, oriented and co-operative.
b. Higher functions: Mention all the subheadings—all are normal here; speech–normal.
c. Cranium and spine: Cranium is normal, presence of gibbus (T_7) with spinal tenderness.

- **One must examine the spine (gibbus, tendemess, or old surgical scar) in all patients with paraplegia.**

d. Neck rigidity, Kernig's sign: Absent; straight leg raising test: Negative.
e. Cranial nerves: No paralysis detected. Always search for optic atrophy (e.g. Friedreich's ataxia, multiple sclerosis) and VIIth nerve palsy (GB syndrome). Leukaemic or lymphomatous deposits may produce unilateral or bilateral VIIth nerve palsy (LMN type) with cord compression. Papilloedema may be found in GB syndrome. Mention the subheadings under different cranial nerves.
f. Motor functions: Both the upper limbs are within normal limit in all respect.
   i. Nutrition Helpless attitude of both the lower limbs; no atrophy at present.
   ii. Tone: Clasp-knite spasticity in both the lower limbs; extensor tone> flexor tone.
   iii. Power: Grade I in left leg and Grade II in right leg.
   iv. Coordination: Upper limbs: Normal. Lower limbs: Could not be tested.
   v. Involuntary movements: None present (search for fasciculation in the upper and lower limbs, e.g. MND). No flexor spasm seen.
g. Sensory functions: Both the upper limbs are normal.
   i. Superficial: Pain, touch and temperature.
   ii. Deep: Joint sense, position sense, muscle sense, pressure sense and vibration sense.
   iii. Cortical sensation: Point localisation, stereognosis.
   All are lost in both the lower limbs.

- **There is a definite line of demarcation of sensory loss at the level of umbilicus** (T_{10} dermatome). Below the level of umbilicus, there is no sensation present.

h. Reflexes:
   i. Superficial
      a. Abdominal:
         x. Upper: Present bilaterally (Beevor's sign +).
         y. Middle: Lost bilaterally.
         z. Lower: Lost bilaterally
      b. Cremasteric: Lost bilaterally
      c. **Plantar response: Extensor in both the lower limbs.**
   ii. Deep

	Right	*Left*
a. Biceps jerk	Normal	Normal
b. Triceps jerk	Normal	Normal
c. Supinator jerk	Normal	Normal
d. Knee jerk	Brisk	Brisk
e. Ankle jerk	Brisk	Brisk
f. ***Clonus (ankle and patellar)***	***Present***	***Present***

- Mention the jaw jerk under Vth cranial nerve.

Long Cases

iii. Visceral
   a. Swallowing: Normal at present.
   b. Bladder: Catheterised at present. A self-retaining catheter with continuous drainage into a urosac is seen.
   c. Bowel: Incontinence at present.
iv. Other reflexes: Glabellar tap, grasp reflex, palmo-mental reflex are WNL.

- Percuss the urinary bladder and confirm whether it is distended or not. Always see the colour of the urine present in the tube or urosac (chalky or turbid urine is seen in UTI, and orange coloured urine is a clue to intake of rifampicin).

i. Trophic changes: Bed sore present over sacrum **(must search for trophic changes in paraplegia)**.
j. Cerebellar functions: Normal (examinations involving lower limbs could not be performed).
k. Autonomic functions: Loss of sweating below the level of umbilicus.
l. Stance and gait: Could not be tested.

- **Sacrum should be examined in paraplegia** for the presence of oedema and/or bed sore.

C. Respiratory system: Search for:
i. Tuberculosis: Crepitations at the apex, consolidation or pleural effusion.
ii. Bronchogenic carcinoma: Mass or collapse, pleural effusion, SVC syndrome.
iii. Lymphoma: SVC syndrome or pleural effusion.

- Format of examination of 'Respiratory system' is similar to 'Hemiplegia'.

D. GI tract and genitourinary system: Palpate liver, spleen and examine for ascites (carcinoma, tuberculosis, lymphoma). Percuss for bladder fullness.

E. CVS: As in 'Hemiplegia'.

F. Lymphoreticular system: Examine for anaemia, sternal tenderness, haemorrhagic spots, lymphadenopathy, etc.

Clinical Wisdom

Special points in nervous system (may be added in history sheet): **Structures involved** in this patient—corticospinal tract, lateral spinothalamic tract, posterior column and T_{10} nerve roots (posterior).

Q. Grading of muscle power in neurology (by Medical Research Council Scale):

Grade 0: Complete paralysis (no visible muscle contraction).

Grade 1: A flicker of contraction only (visible or palpable) without any movement of joint.

Grade 2: Movements possible with gravity eliminated (i.e. side to side movement of a limb).

Grade 3: Movements possible against gravity but not against resistance offered by examiner.

Grade 4: Movements possible against gravity plus resistance but weaker than normal.

Grade 5: Normal power.

- Often, '+' or '–' 'symbols are used to improve the sensitivity of the grading.
- Weakness of small muscles of hands and feet does not require grading.

Q. How do you assess motor functions in neurology?

Motor system is assessed by these 5 points:
1. Nutrition or bulk of muscles (i.e. inspection and palpation of muscles).
2. Tone of muscles.
3. Power of muscles.
4. Coordination of movement.
5. Involuntary movements.

- Examination of *reflexes* and *gait* are additional points in motor function.

Q. Assessment of the nutrition of muscle:

Note the nutrition of muscles and observe the 'attitude' of the limb. It is assessed by:

a. Inspection:
i. Wasting or atrophy of muscles (e.g. convexity of deltoid or calf muscle is lost in wasting).
ii. Flattening of overlying skin or hollowness over the area.
iii. Prominent knuckles and other bony prominences.
iv. Prominent interosseous gutters (in hand and foot).
v. Prominent extensor/flexor tendons (in hand or foot).

Clinical Wisdom

Examine the big muscles like biceps, quadriceps, calves plus small muscles of the hands and feet. During inspection, other than *'attitude' of a limb*, one should look for atrophy, hypertrophy, fasciculation, contracture, deformity or flexor spasm.

b. Palpation: Normal muscle is elastic in feel. Atrophied muscles are small, soft and flabby on palpation.

c. Measurement: Measure the girth of the specific muscle by a tape from a fixed bony point and compare it with the identical point on the other side **(compulsory)**; usually the mid-muscle mass is measured. For the upper limb, the fixed bony point is the elbow (olecranon process) and for the lower limb, it is the tibial tuberosity (Fig. 1.50A and B). The difference in the circumference (comparing with the opposite side) will give objective evidence of wasting or hypertrophy. Remember, in a right-handed person the girth of right upper limb may be slightly more than that of left upper limb.

- **Muscles feel** doughy (rubbery) in pseudohypertrophic muscular dystrophy, semi-elastic in true hypertrophy, tender in myositis, hard and inelastic in polymyositis, firm in spasticity, and 'woody' in rhabdomyolysis.

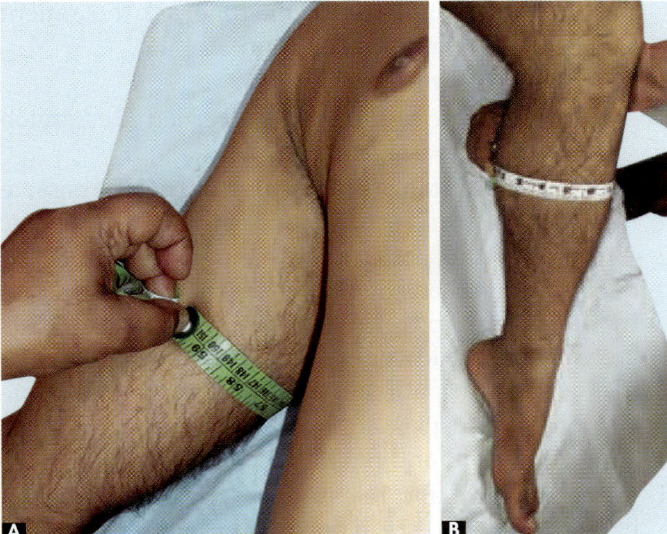

Fig. 1.50A and B: Measurement of **bulk of muscles** from a fixed point: (A) upper limb (from olecranon process); (B) lower limb (from tibial tuberosity)

- 'Atrophy' is defined as wasting or diminution in size of the muscle. If a patient have muscle atrophy in limbs, it is mandatory to measure the circumference of limbs for objective evidence (in long or short cases) (Table 1.21).

Q. Causes of hypo- and hypertonia:

Tone: It is defined as the resistance felt when a joint is moved passively through its range of movement, or it is the partially contracted condition of a muscle. Tone is of three types: normal (elastic type of resistance), hypotonia and hypertonia. Muscle tone is basically regulated by pyramidal and extrapyramidal pathways.

A. Hypotonia (diminished resistance to passive movements): The causes are:

1. LMN lesion due to any cause.
2. UMN lesion in shock stage.
3. Posterior column lesion (tabes dorsalis).
4. Chorea (the only extrapyramidal lesion with hypotonia).
5. Cerebellar lesion.
6. Myopathy (terminal stage).
7. Myasthenic crisis.
8. Polyneuropathy.
9. Down syndrome, rickets.
10. Deep sleep.
11. Drugs: Hypnotics, sedatives, muscle relaxants and anaesthetics.
12. Periodic paralysis, cataplexy, sleep paralysis.
13. Hypokalaemia or hypercalcaemia.
14. Emaciation.

- **LMN lesions** include anterior horn cell disease (poliomyelitis, syringomyelia, spinal muscular atrophy), anterior nerve root lesion or radiculopathy (arachnoiditis, radiculitis, GB syndrome, PIVD), nerve trunks and plexus lesion (metastasis, trauma), disorders of peripheral nerves (leprosy), diseases of myoneural junction (myasthenia gravis) and muscle disease (late stage of myopathy). Hypotonia is also known as **'FLACCIDITY'**.
- Hypotonia is usually associated with hyporeflexia, muscle wasting and weakness.
- **UMN lesions** include cortical, subcortical, brainstem and spinal cord lesion.

B. Hypertonia (increased resistance to passive movements): The causes are:

1. UMN lesion (clasp-knife spasticity).
2. Extrapyramidal lesion except chorea (lead pipe or cogwheel rigidity), e.g. parkinsonism.
3. Tetanus.
4. Hysterical hypertonia (resistance to passive movement increases in an irregular, jerky fashion in proportion to the effort applied by the examiner).
5. Sometimes in non-cooperative patients.
6. Tetany.
7. Myotonia during the contraction phase.
8. Strychnine poisoning.
9. Gegenhalten phenomenon (variable resistance found in catatonic states, e.g. encephalopathy, carbon monoxide poisoning, phenothiazine-induced; dementia): Classically a manifestation of frontal lobe disease where flexors and extensors are equally affected.
10. Decerebrate regidity (there is marked contraction of all extensor muscles in the body).
11. Catatonia (Fig. 1.51): A form of psychosis where the patient is hypomobile and mute, 'waxy flexibility' of the limbs.
12. Muscles around a painful joint.

- In health, tone is being inhibited by pyramidal tract (UMN), and vestibulospinal and reticulospinal tracts; thus hypertonia occurs in UMN, and extrapyramidal lesions.

Table 1.21: Differentiation between 'atrophy due to LMN lesion' and 'disuse atrophy'

Atrophy (LMN lesion)	Disuse atrophy (UMN lesion)
1. Usually atrophy occurs from distal to proximal muscles of a limb	1. Occurs in antigravity muscles of a limb (e.g., in hemiplegia)
2. Muscle power is very much reduced	2. Power loss is less than LMN lesion
3. Fasciculation may be evident	3. Fasciculation is never seen
4. Trophic changes may develop	4. Trophic changes are usually absent
5. Deep reflexes or jerks are lost or ↓	5. Deep reflexes or jerks may be brisk

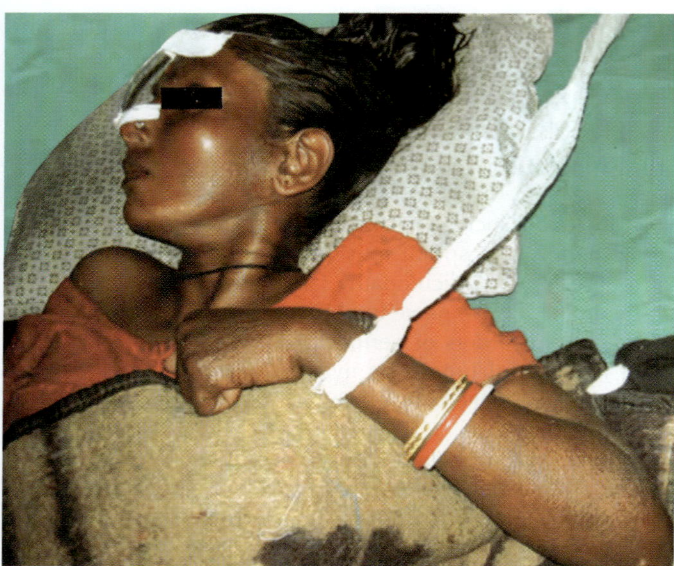

Fig. 1.51: Catatonic patient (hypertonia) holding a rigid posture for hours. It is the admixture of psychic and motor disturbance

- Hypertonia is of two types: **SPASTICITY** (pyramidal lesion) and **RIGIDITY** (extrapyramidal lesion). Spasticity is usually associated with brisk tendon reflex, clonus, Babinski's sign and classical pattern of weakness. Rigidity (e.g. parkinsonism) is frequently associated with bradykinesia, static tremor and postural abnormality. 'Reflex rigidity' is the muscle spasm in response to pain, e.g. neck rigidity in meningitis, board-like rigidity in peritonitis.
- Cooling increases and heat (warmth) decreases the tone.

Q. Features of hypotonia:

1. Unusual flexibility of joints leading to *increased* range of passive movement.
2. Inability to maintain sustained posture.
3. Muscles are soft and flabby, and smaller than normal.

In **hypertonia:** Muscles feel stiff and there is *diminished* range of passive movement.

Q. Clinical assessment of tone of muscles:

Tone may be **assessed at the bedside by the following methods**:

1. Classical method (Fig. 1.52A and B): By handling the limbs and moving them 'passively' at their various joints (to feel the resistance to passive movement)—

   Best method. While testing the tone, ask the patient to relax and be comfortable, and
   i. Expose the muscle fully.
   ii. Passively move the joint concerned (i.e. stretch the muscle passively).
   iii. Feel the resistance to stretching during the passive movement and see the contraction of the muscle.
2. Attitude of the patient: By seeing the attitude or decubitus, one can say that flexor tone has increased in the upper extremity and extensor tone has increased in the lower extremity on the affected side in a hemiplegic patient (i.e. in antigravity muscles).
3. Hypotonic muscles are smaller than normal, and abnormally soft and flabby on palpation.
4. When lifted up and released, a hypotonic limb falls like a log of wood (i.e. it behaves in such a way as the limb does not belong to the patient).
5. Ask the patient to outstretch the upper limbs and spread the fingers: Hypotonic limb may assume an abnormal posture, i.e. hyperextended at elbow, hyperpronated at forearm, flexed at wrist and hyperextended fingers at MCP joints is known as 'dinner-fork deformity'.

- Always compare with the opposite side while assessing tone.
- *Patient must be fully relaxed and comfortable* before assessing tone; patient's complete cooperation is essential to determine tone. If the patient fails to relex, divert his attention by conversing with him or ask him to count from 1 to 50. Examination of tone is difficult in neonates, a tense individual and in emotional states.

Q. Causes of cord compression at multiple levels:

1. Neurofibromatosis.
2. Patchy arachnoiditis.
3. Prolapsed intervertebral disc (PIVD).
4. Secondary deposits.
5. Cervical spondylosis.
6. Arteriovenous malformations.

Q. Causes of pure motor paraplegia:

1. Hereditary spastic paraplegia.
2. Lathyrism.

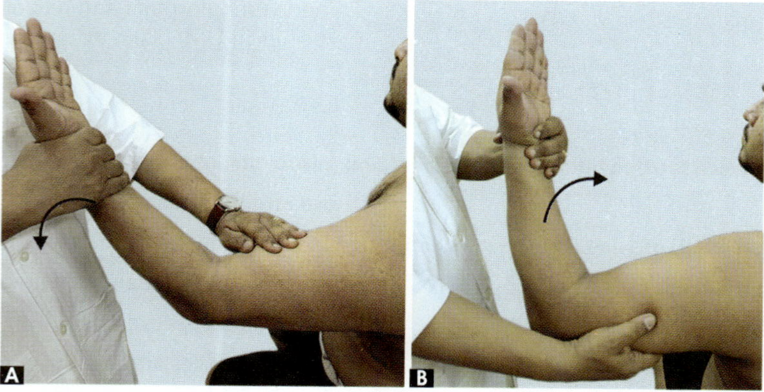

Fig. 1.52A and B: Elicitation of **tone:** Biceps (A) and triceps (B)

3. GB syndrome.
4. Amyotrophic lateral sclerosis (variety of MND).
5. Fluorosis.
6. Erb's spastic paraplegia (syphilitic).

Q. Recognition of minor weakness in a limb:

By early and easy fatigability.

Q. Sudden onset of 'generalised weakness' without loss of consciousness:

1. Transient ischaemic attack (TIA).
2. Hypoglycaemia (subjective weakness).
3. GB syndrome.
4. Acute transverse myelitis.
5. Acute anterior poliomyelitis.
6. Poisoning (botulinum).
7. Electrolyte imbalance ($\downarrow$K, $\uparrow Ca^{++}$, $\uparrow Mg^{++}$).
8. Snake bite (Elapidae group).
9. Myasthenic crisis.
10. Periodic paralysis ($\downarrow K^+$, $\uparrow K^+$, or thyrotoxic).
11. Sleep paralysis/cataplexy.
12. Hysterical.

- Patient with hypoglycaemia may go into coma, if not diagnosed in time.

Q. Possible aetiology of episodic paralysis:

1. Myasthenia gravis.
2. Hyperthyroidism.
3. Periodic paralysis ($\downarrow K^+$, $\uparrow K^+$, normokalaemic).
4. Botulinum poisoning.
5. Primary hyperaldosteronism.
6. GB syndrome.

Q. Possible causes of 'funny turns':

Episodes of lost or altered consciousness may be called as black-out, 'funny turns' or 'going dizzy'.
1. Hypoglycaemia.
2. Temporal lobe epilepsy.
3. Syncope.
4. Narcolepsy, cataplexy, sleep paralysis.
5. Hyperventilation and panic attacks.
6. Amnesic episodes.
7. Pseudoseizure (bizarre with vocalisation).
8. Basilar migraine.

Q. Spastic paraplegia with loss of deep reflexes:

Spastic paraplegia is associated with brisk jerks but jerks may be lost in:
1. Shock stage.
2. Sometimes seen in the presence of bed sore, urinary tract infection (UTI) or malnutrition: The reflex arc may be suppressed leading to loss of jerks.
3. Haematomyelia (sudden bleeding from a vascular malformation)/myelomalacia (thrombosis of a spinal artery with infarction).
4. Associated radiculitis.
5. INH therapy in caries spine causing peripheral neuropathy.
6. If contracture is developed in lower limbs.

- Bed sore, UTI or malnutrition may result in persistent flaccid paraplegia in UMN lesions.

Q. What are cranio-vertebral junction (CVJ) anomalies?

These are developmental anomalies around the cranio-vertebral junction, some of which may not produce any disability in life. They are **(congenital causes)**:
1. Platybasia (increase in the basal angle of the skull, usually asymptomatic).
2. Basilar invagination (elevation of floor of posterior fossa of the skull).
3. Atlanto-axial dislocation.
4. Occipitalisation of atlas.
5. Klippel-Feil anomaly (fusion of cervical vertebrae).
6. Arnold-Chiari malformation (medulla and cerebellum are extended downwards through foramen magnum).
7. Hypoplastic or separate odontoid process.

Acquired causes of cranio-vertebral anomaly are: trauma, rheumatoid arthritis or RA (atlanto-axial dislocation), ankylosing spondylitis, spinal metastasis, spinal tuberculosis, etc.

The usual **manifestations** of cranio-vertebral anomaly are:
1. Short neck, restricted cervical movements and low posterior hairline (Feil's triad).
2. *Spastic quadriparesis* of gradual onset; hypertonia, brisk jerks in all the limbs and Babinski's sign.
3. Wasting of the small muscles of hands.
4. Cerebellar signs and features of lower cranial nerve involvement.
5. Mirror-image movement, impaired position and vibration sense, etc.

Diagnosis is done by X-ray, CT or MRI scan of neck region, and is being treated by neck support (i.e. surgical stabilisation).

- **Low hairline** = hairline below C_4 vertebra.
- **Short neck** = Ratio of length of the body to length of the neck is >13: 1. Short neck in clinical medicine: Klippel-Feil anomaly, mucopolysaccharidosis, Turner's and Noonan's syndrome.

Q. Causes of quadriplegia or quadriparesis:

Weakness of all the four limbs can occur in the lesion from cortex to C_5 level of spinal cord:
1. Cerebral palsy.
2. Bilateral brainstem lesion (glioma).
3. Cranio-vertebral junction anomaly.
4. High cervical cord compression.
5. Cervical spondylosis (myelopathy).

6. Trauma to the neck.
7. Multiple sclerosis.
8. Acute anterior poliomyelitis.
9. Motor neurone disease.
10. GB syndrome.
11. Peripheral neuropathy.
12. Myopathy or polymyositis.
13. Myasthenia gravis (crisis).
14. Periodic paralysis.

Clinical Wisdom

Intermediate syndrome in OP poisoning and Elapidae snake bite (sudden onset) may give rise to quadriparesis.

Q. Features of 'high' cervical cord lesion:

High cervical cord lesion is seen in cranio-vertebral anomaly (e.g. RA), fracture-dislocation of upper cervical spine, haematomyelia, cervical spondylosis and cervical cord tumours. The common features are:

1. Horner's syndrome.
2. Features of injury to spinal accessory nerve (paralysis of sternomastoid and trapezius).
3. Features of injury to spinal tract of trigeminal nerve (i.e. analgesia and thermo-anaesthesia may be limited to ophthalmic and maxillary division in face).
4. Vertical nystagmus (down-beating).
5. Mirror-image movement (sometimes seen in Arnold-Chiari malformation).

- *Plus* there is quadriplegia.

Q. What is lathyrism?

It is a slowly evolving epidemic 'pure motor paraplegia' (spastic) due to consumption of *Khesari dal* or grass pea (lathyrus sativus, a drought-resistant pulse) for long period. Ultimately, the patients develop into disabling spastic paraplegia when they have to crawl on hands. Sensory function, bladder and bowel functions remain normal. It is common in UP, Bihar, Rajasthan and MP in India, and many persons either of the same family or of the same locality may be affected. The causative factor is a neurotoxin and is known as BOAA (Beta oxalyl amino alanine).

Q. What is arachnoiditis?

A non-specific term referring to inflammation of arachnoid, usually of unknown origin, which may result from tuberculosis, syphilis, sarcoidosis or a postoperative event (e.g. spinal surgery). Constant and severe bilateral asymmetric radicular limb pain is characteristic. Features of radiculopathy is pronounced than features of spinal long tracts involvement. Slight fever, features of root compression (e.g. areflexia) may be present. Lumbosacral region is commonly affected. Lumbar puncture may reveal partial or total spinal block. No satisfactory treatment is available.

Q. What is tropical spastic paraplegia?

It is the HTLV-I associated non-compressive myelopathy where the patient (commonly women) at her third to sixth decade of life complains of gradual onset of weakness of legs (paraparesis), muscle spasms, and is usually confined to wheel-chair within 10 years. Signs of UMN lesion are found in legs with variable sensory and bladder involvement. Usually the patient needs myelogram or MRI scan to exclude compressive myelopathy. Affected persons become seropositive for HTLV-L. Few patients show minor response to corticosteroid therapy. This is common in Japan, parts of South America and Western Africa.

Q. Possible causes of paraplegia with optic atrophy:

The second cranial nerve should always be examined in paraplegia. Optic atrophy is found in:

1. Hereditary: Friedreich's ataxia.
2. Demyelinating: Multiple sclerosis, Devic's disease.
3. Infections like tuberculosis, arachnoiditis, syphilis.
4. Subacute combined degeneration, pellagra.
5. Eale's disease (a rare ophthalmic disorder).
6. Subacute myelo-optic neuropathy (SMON), alcohol-induced.

- **Fundoscopy** in paraplegia: Caries spine (choroidal tubercles), GB syndrome (papilloedema) and acute transverse myelitis (optic neuritis).

Q. Recurrent attacks of 'myelitis' producing paraplegia:

SLE antiphospholipid antibody syndrome, Behcet's disease, MCTD, spinal AV malformations, neurosarcoid.

Q. Why do you say compressive myelopathy in this patient?

The features of **cord compression** are:

1. Usually of gradual onset but may be sudden.
2. Presence of root pain.
3. Symptoms start in one leg and then gradually involve the other leg. Both sensory and motor symptoms are present, and there is progressively increasing course of the disease.
4. *Asymmetrical signs and symptoms between two lower limbs are very suggestive.*
5. Spastic paraplegia with loss of superficial and deep sensation in varying degree and combination. There is presence of girdle-like sensation in the trunk with zone of hyperaesthesia above.
6. Bladder disturbance is common.
7. Deformity or tenderness in the spine goes in favour of cord compression.

All the above mentioned features are present in the patient discussed at outset.

Q. How caries spine causes paraplegia?

It is multifactorial and is due to:

1. Compression of the spinal cord by cold abscess (extradural): Commonest.

2. Tuberculous myelitis (involvement of the spinal cord from the bone).
3. Tuberculous endarteritis or thrombosis of the radicular artery: Responsible for the sudden onset of paraplegia or acute exacerbation of existing paraplegia.
4. Pachy meningitis or arachnoiditis.
5. Granulation tissue encircling the dura matter.
6. Compression by sequestrated bone (mechanical pressure).
7. Dislocation of vertebra: Rare.
8. Combination of multiple factors.

- **Caries spine should always be thought as the first cause of paraplegia in India, irrespective of age and sex of the patient.** *Mid-thoracic region is the commonly involved site.*

Q. Can it be a case of metastasis in the spine?

'Metastasis in the spine' is unlikely in this case as:

1. Age of the patient is only 32 years (though leukaemic and lymphomatous deposits in spine giving rise to paraplegia may be seen in the young).
2. Commonly there is sudden onset of paraplegia though gradual onset paraplegia may be seen.
3. No evidence of primary growth is found (like branchogenic carcinoma, gastric carcinoma, prostatic carcinoma). No lymphadenopathy is detected.
4. If allowed to do the X-ray of the spine, it would show that there is (caries spine) diminution of intervertebral space, collapse of the adjacent vertebrae and paravertebral cold abscess ('metastasis in the spine' shows destruction of the vertebra without any narrowing of the intervertebral disc space).

- Root pain is more common in malignancy than in caries spine. Tenderness and deformity of the spine are present in both though the tenderness is more common in malignancy. Metastasis causes paraplegia by (i) Compression by the deposits, and (ii) Collapse of the vertebra.

Q. Synopsis of bladder dysfunction in neurological diseases:

The conscious control of micturition has its centre within pre-frontal cortex. The urinary bladder receives neural supply from sympathetic (T_{11}–L_2 → The nerve of filling) and parasympathetic ($S_{2,3,4}$ → The nerve of evacuation) nerves. Bladder dysfunction arising out of neurological disorders is known as **neurogenic bladder**. Neurogenic bladder is divided into different types like:

A. *Uninhibited (cortical) bladder:* Found in frontal lobe tumours, CVA, parasagittal meningioma, hydrocephalus and dementia. There is urgency at low bladder volume (like a child below 2 years of age) with sudden uncontrolled evacuation of urine in inappropriate time and place. It is also known as 'mental incontinence' (loss of social control of micturition).

B. *Spinal bladder* (with or without autonomic dyssynergia):
   a. Incomplete lesion:
      i. Precipitancy: Due to involvement of inhibitory fibres, e.g. multiple sclerosis.
      ii. Hesitancy: Due to involvement of facilitatory fibres, e.g. incomplete cord compression.
   b. Complete lesion:
      i. Retention of urine with overflow incontinence: Commonly seen in 'neural shock stage' of acute transverse myelitis. Evacuation of the bladder is always incomplete.
      ii. **Automatic bladder (UMN bladder):** The evacuation is always complete. It is commonly seen when the 'neural shock stage' is over and evacuation occurs by local reflex arc. The bladder is small, spastic (hypertonic) and the patient complains of increased frequency, urgency and urge incontinence.
   c. Lesion in the local reflex arc:
      i. Sensory paralytic bladder (afferent fibres are affected): There is loss of awareness of fullness of bladder, e.g. tabes dorsalis, diabetes mellitus, multiple sclerosis. The patient feels difficulty in initiating micturition and in emptying the bladder. Large amount of urine collects in the bladder with a huge residual volume.
      ii. Motor paralytic bladder (efferent fibres are affected): Inability to initiate and continue micturition. It is commonly seen in pelvic neoplasm, trauma, polyradiculopathy, etc.
      iii. **Autonomous bladder (LMN bladder):** Commonly seen in cauda equina lesion, pelvic malignancy, spina bifida, etc. There is no sensation of bladder fullness but having continual dribbling (no voluntary control); it is a flaccid, atonic bladder. UTI is very common.

- Symptoms of neurogenic bladder are urgency, hesitancy, precipitancy, incontinence and retention of urine. Other causes of hesitancy and precipitancy in clinical practice are CVA, head injury, cerebral tumour, BHP, bladder neck obstruction, etc. Neurogenic bladder predisposes UTI; management requires assessment by urodynamic studies, proper catheterisation, drugs like oxybutynin (for detrusor spasticity) or terazocin (in failure of internal sphincter to relax), and surgery in some cases.
- **Urinary incontinence** (involuntary urinary leak) is of four types: *Urge* incontinence (uncontrolled passage of urine preceded by strong urge to void—due to overactivity of detrusor muscle; may have UTI or BHP), *stress* incontinence (urinary leak after stress, i.e. coughing, sneezing, and is commonly found in women after child birth), *overflow* incontinence (urinary leak due to chronic urinary retention), and *true* incontinence (voids urine at any time and at any position due to loss of sphincteric function, or 'continual incontinence' due to vesico-vaginal fistula).

Q. How do you like to investigate paraplegia?

1. Blood (R/E): Hb%, TC, DC, ESR; sugar, urea and creatinine.

2. Urine: Routine examination and culture-sensitivity test are done.
3. Mantoux test: Positive in tuberculosis and may be negative in lymphoma.
4. Chest X-ray: To exclude tuberculosis, bronchogenic carcinoma, lymphoma or metastasis.
5. **X-ray of the spine** (antero-posterior and lateral view): Helps in the diagnosis of caries spine, metastasis, fracture or dislocation of vertebra. It helps in detection of the site of spinal lesion.
6. Lymph node biopsy (if possible).
7. **MRI or CT scan** of spine, which helps to visualise the details of spinal cord, the coverings, spine and disc pathology. Myelogram is not done nowadays as MRI or CT scan is most preferable.
8. Lumbar puncture and CSF examination: Features of the Froin's loculation syndrome (below the level of cord compression) are:
   i. Low CSF pressure.
   ii. Xanthochromia.
   iii. Clot formation on standing.
   iv. High protein content.
   v. Positive Queckenstedt's test (i.e. no rise in CSF pressure following compression of the internal jugular vein).

   CSF examination may also be helpful in multiple sclerosis (oligoclonal bands), arachnoiditis and GB syndrome.
9. Miscellaneous: Muscle biopsy, muscle enzymes, EMG (demyelination in GB syndrome), blood for vitamin B_{12} estimation, VDRL and Kahn test, blood for HIV (these tests are done for non-compressive myelopathy), or albumino-cytological dissociation in GB syndrome. Serum prostate-specific antigen (PSA) for metastatic prostatic carcinoma and serum protein electrophoresis for multiple myeloma may be performed, if indicated.

- Froin's loculation syndrome usually results from spinal block as a result of spinal tumour.

Q. CSF features in GB syndrome:

1. Pressure: Normal.
2. May be xanthochromic.
3. Clots formation on standing.
4. High protein, normal sugar, and
5. No rise in cell count (i.e. albumino-cytological dissociation).

Q. Common causes of xanthochromia:

Yellowish discolouration of the CSF (xanthochromia) is due to:

1. Old subarachnoid haemorrhage (due to oxyhaemoglobin and bilirubin).
2. Guillain-Barré syndrome (due to high protein).
3. Acoustic neurofibroma (due to high protein).
4. Froin's loculation syndrome (spinal subarachnoid block and is due to high protein).
5. Deep jaundice (due to high bilirubin).
6. Massive old intracerebral bleed or haemorrhagic infarction (due to presence of old blood).

Q. Causes of albumino-cytological dissociation in CSF:

It means there is increased protein in CSF without any rise in cell count. The causes are:

1. Guillain-Barré syndrome.
2. Froin's loculation syndrome.
3. Acoustic neurofibroma.

Q. Complications of paraplegia:

1. Pressure sores (trophic changes).
2. Urinary tract infections.
3. Fecal impaction.
4. Contracture of limbs.
5. Deep vein thrombosis and pulmonary embolism.
6. Chronic renal failure.

Q. How do you like to manage paraplegia?

1. Adequate nutrition and fluid intake: In an adult, 3500 calories/day should be given. There is no need to put the patient on Ryle's tube. Arrange for an alarm bell at the bedside.

   The patient needs reassurance, physical and psychological support.
2. **Care of the bladder, bowel and trophic ulcers:**
   a. Bladder: Put a self-retaining catheter under aseptic technique, change the catheter regularly at 2–3 weeks' interval, bladder wash, to help in bladder control by application of clip to the drainage tube, R/E and C/S of urine—as and when necessary, antibiotics in UTI. Condom catheter may be used.
   b. Bowel: Treatment of constipation is done by adequate laxatives and at times manual evacuation may be necessary. Rectal incontinence is difficult to treat.
   c. Skin: Bed sores are formed due to loss of sensation and diminished blood supply. So the patient should be re-positioned every 2–4 hourly (change of posture) and the skin should be kept dry and clean. Specialised beds (air or water-cushioned bed), ripple mattresses, and soft bed coverings prevent development of bed sores. Trophic ulcers (if formed) are cleaned by hydrogen peroxide, and dressed by softa tulle. Aseptic care should always be taken. Plastic surgery: If necessary.
3. Muscle spasms and spasticity are treated by diazepam, baclofen (5 mg, thrice daily, orally), tizanidine (2 mg, thrice daily, orally) or botulinum toxin.
4. The underlying cause should be treated, e.g.
   a. In caries spine: Application of traction in early stage. Later on 'plaster jacket' is applied for

immobilisation. Antituberculosis chemotherapy is continued for at least 9 months to 1 year.

b. Treatment of carcinoma or lymphoma by radiotherapy and/or chemotherapy.

c. Acute transverse myelitis: High dose prednisolone (1 mg/kg/day) for two weeks with gradual tapering; high dose IV methyl prednisolone or plasma exchange may be very effective.

d. GB syndrome: Read the last question in section on 'Peripheral neuropathy'.

e. SLE, HIV infection, subacute combined degeneration should be treated accordingly.

5. Graded physiotherapy: Aim is to obtain the maximum development of all those muscles in which voluntary power remains as well as prevention of flexor contractures in the lower limbs. Passive movements are carried out in the lower limbs once or twice daily. Later on arrangement of wheel chair, walking calipers are done according to the necessity (rehabilitation). Breathing exercise should be done to prevent hypostatic pneumonia.
6. Surgery: Drainage of cold abscess, fusion of the verterbra, laminectomy for caries spine, skin grafting for bed sore are rarely needed. Rhizotomy is performed in severe unresponsive spasticity.

Clinical Wisdom

There is currently no cure for paraplegia. The treatment options available are physical therapy, medications and surgery.
It is the duty of the healthcare provider to assure the patient and to try to keep the moral of the patient high.

- **Acute transverse myelitis and GB syndrome are given as long cases.**

PERIPHERAL NEUROPATHY — CASE 18

Q. What is your diagnosis?

This is a case of peripheral neuropathy resulting from chronic alcoholism.

Q. How your patient presented himself?

The 52 years male patient presented in the hospital 2 weeks back with the chief complaints of:

1. Sensation of pins and needles (tingling and numbness) in the distal parts of the upper and lower limbs for last 6 months, with
2. Loss of power (or weakness) in all the four limbs for last 3 months which was more pronounced distally, and
3. Wasting (thinning) of the distal part of the limbs with pain in the limbs for last 1 month.

The onset of the disease was insidious and it was gradually progressive. The tingling sensation started distally and it was limited in the 'glove and stocking' distribution (feet earlier than hands). The weakness started in the distal part of all the four limbs on different dates. According to the patient, there was no weakness in the proximal muscles and the weakness was not related to repetitive use of muscles (vide myasthenia gravis). He complained of weakness in the grip and difficulty in holding objects. However, according to the patient, legs are weaker than hands; he gave H/o slippers falling from the feet. There was no H/o waxing and waning (vide multiple sclerosis). He had no H/o respiratory distress (vide GB syndrome). He is now facing difficulty in standing and walking while severity of all symptoms has increased over the last few weeks. The patient is not complaining of any bladder and bowel symptoms at present.

He did not suffer from haematemesis or melaena (due to alcoholism), headache, vomiting, convulsions, speech difficulty, diplopia, nasal regurgitation or intonation. There was neither any past H/o spinal trauma, fever, H/o contact with tuberculosis, H/o exposure to STD, white spots in the body (i.e. leprosy), vaccination in recent past, exposure to arsenicals or INH or vincristine, nor the patient was suffering from *diabetes mellitus*. The patient was taking alcohol in a dose of 60–90 mL of whisky, more or less, daily for last 16 years. There is no family history of such type of illness

- Preceding the 'glove and stocking' type of paraesthesia, there may be hyperaesthesia. The distal paraesthesia usually affects the feet first and then the hands are affected.

Q. Special points in the physical examination in peripheral neuropathy:

A. General survey:

a. The patient is conscious and cooperative.
b. Anaemia: Moderate.
c. Jaundice: Absent.
d. Decubitus: Dorsal decubitus at present, lying helplessly with bilateral foot drop.
e. Parotid glands: A bit swollen (due to chronic alcoholism).
f. Gynaecomastia: Absent.
g. Facies: A bit flushed and anxious (due to chronic alcoholism).
h. BP: 140/80 mm of Hg.
i. Skin: No white spots detected (vide leprosy).
j. All the limbs are lying helplessly with bilateral foot drop.
k. Ulnar and common peroneal nerves: Not thickened (vide leprosy).
l. Oedema: Nil.
m. Others: Dryness of skin, bruises, calluses, ulcers and skin colour changes in distal part of limbs.

- Mention all the points in general survey.

B. Nervous system:

a. The patient is conscious, alert, oriented and co-operative.

b. Higher functions: Normal; speech is not affected.
c. Cranium and spine: Within normal limit.
d. Neck rigidity, Kernig's sign: Absent; straight leg raising test: Negative.
e. Cranial nerves There is neither palatal palsy (diphtheria) nor VIIth nerve palsy (GB syndrome). Ophthalmoscopy: Not done (may reveal retinopathy in diabetes).
f. Motor functions:
   i. Attitude: Bilateral foot drop with paucity of spontaneous movements in the limbs.
   ii. Nutrition: Wasting of small muscles of the feet and hands. Wasting is seen in extensors of legs.
   iii. Tone: Diminished in all the limbs, especially in the distal muscles.
   iv. Power:
      Lower limbs: Proximal muscles are of grade V but extensors of legs are of grade II; flexor of legs are of grade III.
      Upper limbs: Proximal muscles are of grade V but the distal muscles are of grade IV.
      No involvement of trunk or respiratory muscles.
   v. Coordination:
      Upper limbs: Within normal limit.
      Lower limbs: Could not be tested.
   vi. Involuntary movements: Nil.
g. Sensory functions:
   1. Superficial: Pain, temperature and touch sensations are lost in the distal part of the limbs and it is rather bilaterally symmetrical involvement. Proximal sensations are relatively intact. No involvement of face and neck, and the sensory involvement is 'glove and stocking' in distribution (there is no 'definite' line of demarcation between normal and anaesthetic skin); patchy involvement.
   2. Deep:
      i. Vibration sense: Lost distally, impaired proximally.
      ii. Muscle sense: Calf muscles are tender on palpation and squeezing.
      iii. Position sense: Lost distally.
      iv. Joint sense: Lost distally.
   3. Cortical:
      i. One point localisation
      ii. Two point discrimination
      iii. Stereognosis
      iv. Graphaesthesia
      v. Sensory extinction
      } All are impaired

❍ In a patient of peripheral neuropathy, cortical sensations can not be tested properly.

h. Reflexes:

1. Superficial:	*Right*	*Left*
i. Abdominal	No response	No response
ii. Cremasteric	No response	No response
iii. Plantar response	**No response**	**No response**

2. Deep:	*Right*	*Left*
i. Biceps jerk	Normal	Normal
ii. Triceps jerk	Normal	Normal
iii. Supinator jerk	Diminished	Diminished
iv. Knee jerk	Diminished	Diminished
v. Ankle jerk	**Lost**	**Lost**
vi. Clonus	Absent	Absent

   3. Visceral:
      i. Swallowing
      ii. Bladder
      iii. Bowel
      } Within normal limit
   4. Other reflexes: Glabellar tap, grasp reflex and palmo-mental reflex revealed no abnormality.

❍ Plantar response is never extensor in peripheral neuropathy.

i. Trophic changes: A trophic ulcer is seen in the ball of the great toe of right foot; a large bed sore is seen over the sacrum. Charcot joint is not present.
j. Cerebellar functions: Normal.
k. Autonomic functions: Within normal limit (important in diabetes mellitus and GB syndrome).
l. Stance and gait: Could not be tested (there will be high-stepping gait if the patient could walk). Romberg's sign: Could not be tested.

C. GI tract and genitourinary system:

i. Angular stomatitis: Present.
ii. Glossitis: Present.
iii. Epigastrium: Tender on palpation.
iv. No venous prominence over abodomen.
v. Spleen: Not palpable.
vi. Liver: Mild enlargement, soft and tender.
vii. Ascites: Absent.
viii. Testes: Within normal limit.
ix. P/R examination: Not done.

❍ All the GI features are due to chronic alcoholism (vitamin and iron deficiency).

D. CVS:

i. Pulse and BP: Describe the pulse in details; BP is 140/80 mm of Hg (supine).
ii. Neck veins: Neither engorged nor pulsatile.
iii. Shape of the precordium: Within normal limit.
iv. Apex beat: Present in left 5th ICS, ½" inside the left MCL.
v. Pulsation in different areas: No pulsation seen.
vi. Palpation of different areas: No thrill, no pulsation felt, no plapable heart sound.
vii. Heart sounds: Within normal limit.
viii. Murmur: Absent.

E. Respiratory system:

i. Shape of the chest
ii. Movement of the chest
iii. Trachea and apex beat
} Within normal limit

iv. Percussion: Normal resonant note on both sides of the chest.
v. Breath sound: Vesicular.
vi. Vocal resonance: Normal on both sides.
vii. Adventitious sound: None.

F. Lymphoreticular system:

i. Anaemia: Moderate anaemia.
ii. Lymphadenopathy: Absent.
iii. Sternal tenderness: Absent.
iv. Haemorrhagic spots: Absent.

Q. Why do you say peripheral neuropathy?

Discuss the presenting symptoms plus important signs elicited. Give stress on power of muscles, details of sensory functions and trophic changes.

- Peripheral neuropathy will have LMN paralysis ± sensory abnormalities.

Q. Importance of 'past history' in peripheral neuropathy:

1. Diabetes mellitus, renal failure or leprosy.
2. H/o chronic alcohol intake.
3. Spinal trauma.
4. H/o contact with tuberculosis, vaccination in recent past, H/o exposure (HIV infection).
5. Exposure to drugs (INH, vincristine), solvents, pesticides or heavy metals.
6. Fever (areflexic paralysis in GB syndrome).

Q. Common causes of peripheral neuropathy:

A. Toxic:

1. Alcohol.
2. Pb, arsenic, Hg, TOCP poisoning.
3. Drugs: Vincristine, nitrofurantoin (NFT), INH (by causing pyridoxine deficiency).
4. Radiation.

B. Metabolic:

1. Diabetes mellitus.
2. Chronic renal failure (CRF).
3. Porphyria.
4. Hypothyroidism.
5. Amyloidosis.
6. Refsum's disease.

C. Infective or inflammatory:

1. Leprosy.
2. Diphtheria.
3. Landry-Guillain-Barré syndrome.
4. Viral hepatitis.
5. Enteric fever.
6. HIV infection.
7. Infectious mononucleosis.
8. Lyme disease.

D. Deficiency: Thiamine, nicotinic acid, pyridoxine, vitamin B_{12}, pantothanic acid, vitamin E and folate.

E. Connective tissue diseases:

1. SLE.
2. Rheumatoid arthritis.
3. Polyarteritis nodosa.
4. Cryoglobulinaemia.
5. Sjögren's syndrome.
6. Vasculitis.

F. Disseminated malignancy, paraneoplastic syndrome, lymphoma, multiple myeloma.

G. Hereditary or idiopathic (e.g. Charcot-Marie-Tooth disease).

- Pathogenesis of peripheral neuropathy is classified into two types: demyelinating and axonal. Acquired inflammatory demyelinating polyneuropathy falls into two major groups: acute form, i.e. GB syndrome (**AIDP**), and chronic forms, i.e. chronic inflammatory demyelinating polyneuropathy (**CIDP**; steroid-dependent).

Q. Enumerate neurological manifestation of alcohol abuse:

1. Features of alcohol inxication, and alcohol withdrawal (e.g. tremor).
2. Peripheral sensory-motor polyneuropathy.
3. Wernicke's encephalopathy (pyridoxine deficiency).
4. Korsakoff's psychosis (dementia).
5. Cerebellar degeneration (e.g. ataxia).
6. Optic atrophy, myopathy, rhabdomyolysis, central pontine myelinolysis.

Q. Six common causes of peripheral neuropathy in clinical practice:

1. Leprosy (commonest cause globally).
2. Diabetes mellitus.
3. GB syndrome.
4. Chronic renal failure (CRF).
5. Toxin-induced: alcohol or INH-induced.
6. Vitamin B_{12}, B_1, B_6, or nicotinic acid ↓.

Q. Classification of neuropathy by evolution:

- Acute (<4 weeks): GB syndrome, diphtheria, porphyria, malignancy, drugs (dapsone, TOCP, arsenic), thallium toxicity.
- Subacute (4–8 weeks): Alcoholic, nutritional, toxic (hexacarbon).
- Chronic (>8 weeks): Diabetes, CRF, CIDP, paraneoplastic.
- Long standing: Charcot-Marie-Tooth disease.
- Recurrent: Relapsing CIDP, porphyria, occupational toxic neuropathy, alcoholic, HIV/AIDS.

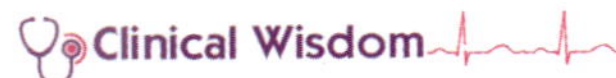

Small fibre neuropathy (neuropathy of symptoms): Muscle power and deep reflexes are less affected than the affection of pain and temperature sensations. The examples are diabetes, leprosy, alcoholism, sarcoidosis, HIV and paraneoplastic.

Large fibre neuropathy (neuropathy of signs): Significant motor disturbance and loss of deep reflexes with minimal sensory loss. There is loss of joint, position and vibration sense with sensory ataxia. Cisplatin neuropathy, pyridoxine neurotoxicity and Sjögren's syndrome are common examples.

Q. Sensations carried by long tracts:

a. The spinothalamic tract (lateral column) carries:

i. Pain.
ii. Temperature (hot and cold), and
iii. Crude touch (mainly goes through anterior spinothalamic tract).

- Lateral column also contains pyramidal tract (motor pathway).

b. The tract of Goll and Burdach (posterior column) carries:

i. Vibration sense
ii. Muscle sense
iii. Pressure sense
iv. Joint sense
v. Position sense

(i–v: Proprioception or deep sensation)

vi. Fine touch (well-localized touch), and
vii. Cortical sensations (assay parietal lobe functions)

- Testing of sensory functions are described in the section on 'Charcot joint'.
- Proprioceptive sensation goes through peripheral nerves, nerve roots, posterior column, medial lemniscus, thalamus, thalamoparietal fibres to sensory cortex (post-central gyrus of the parietal lobe, or area 3, 1 and 2 of Brodmann). Thus, proprioception is lost in lesions of those sites.

Q. Peripheral neuropathy with hypertension:

1. GB syndrome.
2. Polyarteritis nodosa.
3. Lead poisoning.
4. Chronic renal failure (CRF).
5. Porphyria (acute intermittent variety).
6. Amyloidosis.

Q. Predominantly motor neuropathy:

1. GB syndrome.
2. Porphyria.
3. Connective tissue diseases.
4. Diphtheria.
5. Paraneoplastic.
6. Infectious mononucleosis.
7. Lead poisoning.
8. HIV/AIDS.
9. Hereditary neuropathy.
10. Dapsone-induced.

- These are the causes of proximal motor weakness > distal motor weakness in peripheral neuropathy; also in **diabetic amyotrophy**, proximal muscles are predominantly affected.

Q. Predominantly sensory neuropathy:

1. Leprosy.
2. Drugs (vincristine, NFT, INH).
3. Diabetes mellitus.
4. Renal failure (initially).
5. Alcoholism.
6. Vitamin B_{12} and B_1 deficiency.
7. Hereditary sensory neuropathy.
8. HIV infection.
9. Paraneoplastic syndrome.
10. Thalidomide or cisplain toxicity.

Q. Peripheral neuropathy with cranial nerve involvement:

1. GB syndrome (VII).
2. Leprosy (VII).
3. Diabetes mellitus (III, IV, VI, VII).
4. Diphtheria (III, VI, IX, X).
5. Lyme disease (VII).
6. Sarcoidosis (VII).
7. Sjögren's syndrome (V).
8. Vitamin B_{12} deficiency (I, II).

Q. Painful peripheral neuropathy:

1. Diabetes mellitus.
2. Alcoholic polyneuropathy.
3. Carcinomatous neuropathy.
4. Vitamin B_1 and B_{12} deficiency.
5. Vasculitis.
6. Porphyria.
7. Uraemic neuropathy.
8. Arsenic-induced.
9. Amyloidosis.
10. Sjögren's syndrome.

Q. Drugs causing peripheral neuropathy:

1. INH.
2. Nitrofurantoin (NFT).
3. Vincristine.
4. Dapsone.
5. Thalidomide.
6. Cisplatin.
7. Suramin.
8. Amiodarone.
9. Pentamidine.
10. Pyridoxine (high dose).
11. Stavudine.
12. Paclitaxel.
13. Phenytoin.
14. Infliximab.

Q. Causes of mononeuritis multiplex:

It is the asymmetrical involvement of multiple non-contiguous peripheral nerves serially or at a time over days to years, and is usually due to arteritic involvement of vasa nervorum (i.e. multiple mononeuropathy). Diagnosis is done clinically and is supported by electrical studies (nerve conduction velocity). It gives a picture of distal symmetric neuropathy and is commonly found in:

1. Leprosy.
2. Diabetes mellitus.
3. Polyarteritis nodosa.
4. Sarcoidosis.
5. Rheumatoid arthritis.
6. Amyloidosis.
7. Vasculitis.
8. Trauma.
9. HIV and hepatitis C infection.
10. GB syndrome.
11. Paraneoplastic syndrome.
12. Cryoglobulinaemia.

The involvement is usually asymmetrical with predominant affection of the lower limbs.

Clinical Wisdom

- Neuropathy: Pathological process affecting a peripheral nerve or nerves.
- Peripheral neuropathy or polyneuropathy: A diffuse symmetrical disease process of peripheral nerves (peripheral means that the disorder is outside the CNS) involving the peripheral parts of body and gradually progressing proximally.
- Mononeuropathy: Focal involvement of a single nerve trunk (e.g. ulnar, radial or median nerve). This is commonly due to leprosy, diabetes, entrapment neuropathy, trauma or vascutitis.
- Mononeuritis multiplex: Already described above.
- Radiculopathy: A pathological process which affects the nerve roots.
- Neuronopathy: Affection of anterior horn cells.
- Plexopathy: Affection of plexus (brachial/lumbosacral).

Q. Which distal sensation is lost early in peripheral neuropathy?

Vibration sense is lost early in peripheral neuropathy (very common feature in diabetic neuropathy). Peripheral neuropathy follows the rule—'the longer the nerve fibre (i.e. axon length), the earlier is the involvement', and this is why the distal part of the body ('glove and stocking' distribution) is affected earliest and most (as distal part of the limbs are supplied by longer nerve fibres).

Q. How diphtheritic neuropathy presents?

1. Paralysis of the soft palate and posterior pharyngeal wall may occur very early (within 10 days).
2. Then paralysis of accommodation follows (difficulty in reading small letters).
3. Polyneuropathy usually develops 2–6 weeks after the onset of the disease. Weakness involves all the four limbs and descends from arms to legs.

- Among all cranial nerves the IIIrd, VIth, IXth and Xth nerves are commonly affected (in diphtheria).
- **Descending paralysis:** Botulism, myasthenia gravis, Elapidae snake bite, diphtheria and Miller Fisher syndrome.

  Ascending paralysis: GB syndrome, rabies, acute transverse myelitis, shellfish poisoning, periodic paralysis (hyperkalaemia and thyrotoxicosis) and tick palsy.

Q. Presentations of diabetic neuropathy:

1. Distal, symmetrical, sensory polyneuropathy (commonest).
2. Distal, symmetrical, mixed sensory-motor polyneuropathy: Mainly small fibre, mixed type or large fibre neuropathy.
3. Asymmetrical, proximal motor neuropathy (diabetic amyotrophy).
4. Asymmetric mononeuritis multiplex (painful).
5. Acute mononeuropathy (isolated, painless IIIrd, IVth and VIth cranial nerve palsy; affection of ulnar, median, femoral nerve rarely).
6. Radiculopathy (usually involves spinal nerves, over the chest wall or abdomen).
7. Autonomic neuropathy.

Q. Peripheral neuropathy with predominant upper limb involvement:

It is diphtheria, rabies and porphyria.

Q. Peripheral neuropathy with myelopathy:

SLE, paraneoplastic, Sjögren's syndrome, demyelination (e.g. AIDP).

Q. Peripheral neuropathy with significant autonomic involvement (autonomic neuropathy):

1. Diabetes mellitus (commonest).
2. GB syndrome.
3. Acute intermittent porphyria.
4. Peroneal muscular atrophy.
5. AIDS.
6. Amyloidosis.
7. Botulism.
8. Sjögren's syndrome.
9. Shy-Drager syndrome.
10. Riley-Day syndrome.

Q. Features of root lesion (radiculopathy):

a. **Anterior root:** Muscle atrophy and weakness in root distribution; rare.

b. **Posterior root:** Root pain, hyperalgesia and hyperaesthesia corresponding to the segments compressed. Different types of sensory abnormalities (e.g. hyperaesthesia) with an upper level which is usually a bit above the segmental level of the site of compression; commonly seen.

Table 1.22: Differentiation between myelopathy, neuropathy and myopathy

Features	Myelopathy	Neuropathy	Myopathy
1. Onset	1. Any age	1. Any age	1. Childhood
2. Tingling and numbness	2. Very rare	2. Present	2. Never occurs
3. Bladder and bowel involvement	3. Occurs	3. Usually absent	3. Never occurs
4. Atrophy and pseudo-hypertophy	4. Only atrophy	4. Only atrophy	4. Both present
5. Bilaterally symmetrical involvement	5. May be present	5. Initially asymmetrical	5. Present
6. Cranial nerve involvement	6. None	6. May be present (e.g., GB syndrome)	6. Never occurs
7. Girdle-like sensation	7. Present in compressive myelopathy and acute transverse myelitis	7. Absent	7. Never occurs
8. Sensory involvement	8. Upper border of sensory loss	8. Patchy	8. Never occurs
9. Motor Involvement	9. According to involvernent of myotome	9. Mainly distal	9. Predominantly proximal
10. Tone of muscles	10. Spasticity (except in shock stage)	10. Hypotonia (flaccidity)	10. Hypotonia (terminal stage)
11. Deep reflexes	11. Brisk (except in shock stage)	11. Lost or diminished	11. Usually normal
12. Plantar response	12. Extensor	12. Flexor or no response	12. Flexor
13. Confirmation	13. MRI, CT, myelography	13. Nerve conduction velocity (NCV)	13. Electromyography (EMG)

Q. What are the differential diagnosis of your case?

I. Aetiological differentiation:

a. Diabetes mellitus:
   1. H/o polyphagia, polydipsia and polyuria.
   2. H/o taking oral hypoglycaemic agents or insulin.
   3. Retinopathy invariably present in a case of diabetic neuropathy; there may be nephropathy.
   4. Susceptibility to infections and delayed wound healing.

b. Leprosy:
   1. Typical hypopigmented and anaesthetic skin lesion.
   2. Palpable peripheral nerves.
   3. Trophic changes.
   4. 'Leonine facies' may be present.

c. GB syndrome: Read the section on 'Paraplegia'.

d. Drug-induced.
   1. H/o prolonged intake of INH, NFT or vincristine.
   2. Predominantly sensory neuropathy.
   3. Presence of primary disease for which the drugs are taken, e.g. tuberculosis, leukaemia, etc.

e. Arsenical polyneuropathy:
   1. Early sensory symptoms; later on sensory-motor polyneuropathy.
   2. Rain-drop skin lesions with hyperkeratosis of palm and sole.
   3. People of known geographical area (different districts of West Bengal of India and Bangladesh) using deep tube-well water are predominantly affected.
   4. Mees' line in nail (white transverse banding of nails).
   5. Presence of anaemia with or without jaundice (due to hepatic involvement). There may be portal hypertension.
   6. Estimation of arsenic in hairs, nails, urine confirms the diagnosis.

II. Similarities in clinical features:

a. Tabes dorsalis:
   1. H/o exposure to STD at least 10 years back.
   2. Lightning pain; sensation of walking on cotton wool.
   3. Muscle sense is lost (calf muscles and even testicles are insensitive on squeezing—**Abadie's sign**).
   4. Loss of all modalities of posterior column sensations.
   5. Tabetic facies; Argyll Robertson pupil and optic atrophy may be seen.
   6. Romberg's sign is positive.

b. Subacute combined degeneration (SCD):
   1. Anaemia (± mild icterus).
   2. Glossitis; splenomegaly ±.
   3. Lhermitte's sign: Positive.
   4. Romberg's sign: Positive.
   5. Ankle jerk: Lost.
   6. Plantar response: Bilaterally extensor.

- **SCD** is the demyelination of pyramidal tract and posterior column of the spinal cord as a result of vitamin B_{12} deficiency. Distal paraesthesia, spastic weakness and difficulty in walking are common.

c. Myopathy (Table 1.22):
   1. History from childhood.
   2. No sensory loss.
   3. Predominantly proximal muscle weakness.
   4. Pseudohypertrophy plus atrophy.
   5. No bladder and bowel involvement.
   6. Plantar response: Flexor.

Q. What is TOCP neuropathy?

Triorthocresylphosphate (TOCP) poisoning is also known as 'ginger paralysis'—owing to the consumption of fluid extract of ginger which was used in the manufacture of bootleg alcohol and was adulterated with TOCP. Symptoms of TOCP polyneuropathy usually develop 10–20 days after the consumption of adulterated food (cooking oil) or drink, and produces bilateral wrist and foot drop with wasting of distal muscles of the limbs.

Q. Causes of foot drop (Fig. 1.53):

It is due to paralysis of the extensors of foot and peronei muscles. The common causes are:

1. Peripheral neuropathy (e.g. leprosy, diabetes mellitus).
2. Common peroneal nerve palsy (commonest cause of unilateral foot drop).
3. Prolapsed intervertebral disc (PIVD): Due to lesion in L_5 root.
4. Motor neurone disease (MND).
5. Sciatic nerve lesion
6. Peroneal muscular atrophy.
7. Vasculitis (e.g. polyarteritis nodosa).

- For 'wrist drop', read the section on 'Claw hand'.

Q. Altered muscle sense (or deep pain sensation):

Method: Muscles of calf or forearm are squeezed. Normally patient feels some discomfort.

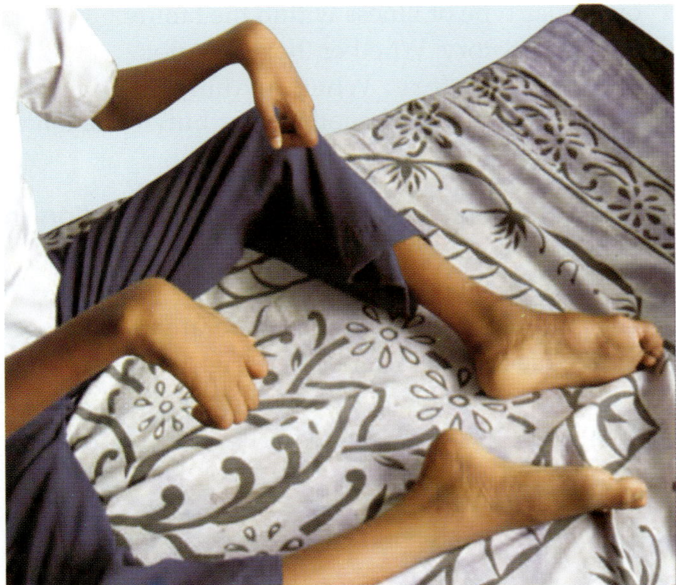

Fig. 1.53: Bilateral **wrist and foot drop** resulting from consumption of adulterated mustard oil

A. Diminished:
   1. Tabes dorsalis (Abadie's sign).
   2. Syringomyelia.
   3. Carcinomatous neuropathy.

B. Increased:
   1. Polyneuropathy.
   2. Myositis.
   3. Subacute combined degeneration.

- **Loss of testicular sensation** (it is the sickening sensation or pain felt in the abdomen on squeezing the testis) occurs in tabes dorsalis and diabetic autonomic neuropathy; a patient may complain testicular pain in vasculitis (e.g. polyarteritis nodosa). Inability to appreciate painful sensation on squeezing tendo-Achilles or calf muscles is known as **Abadie's sign** (found in tabes dorsalis).

Q. Investigations you like to perform in peripheral neuropathy:

1. Blood for R/E (peripheral smear for macrocytes in vitamin B_{12} or folic acid ↓), sugar, urea, creatinine, VDRL, Hb_SAg, autoantibodies (antinuclear factor or rheumatoid factor), serum folate and B_{12}, and thyroid and liver function tests.
2. **Nerve conduction velocity** or NCV (lowered in neuropathy but not in myelopathy or myopathy).
3. Nerve biopsy (usually sural nerve is selected at the ankle, especially in inflammatory pathology).
4. Electromyography or EMG (to differentiate neuropathy from myopathy and diseases of myoneural junction).
5. CSF (done in GB syndrome).
6. Miscellaneous: Slit-skin smear for leprosy, blood for ESR, protein electrophoresis for multiple myeloma, labial salivary gland biopsy for Sjögren's syndrome.

- 'Electrodiagnosis in neurology' is done by NCV and EMG. NCV shows features of demyelination, axonal or mixed injury; EMG reveals features of denervation.

Q. How do you like to manage your patient?

1. Complete abstinence from intake of alcohol.
2. Rest in bed.
3. Inj. vitamin B_1, B_6 and B_{12}: Twice weekly, deep IM, inj. methylcobalamin may be tried. For paraesthesia—Carbamazepine (300–1200 mg/day), aspirin (350–1200 mg/day) or amitriptyline (25–50 mg/day) may be given. For painful peripheral neuropathy pregabalin, tramadol, duloxetine, oxcarbazepine, gabapentin may be helpful.
4. Care of autonomic imbalance: Care of urinary bladder and controlling postural hypotension.
5. Physiotherapy and occupational rehabilitation in profound weakness.
6. Splinting of the foot (to manage foot drop); care of the foot ulcer and bed sore.
7. Empirical treatment with steroid is usually disappointing.

Q. Management of GB syndrome:

Treatment should be initiated as early as possible to get the maximum benefit.

1. Monitor the vital functions (patients may have autonomic instability), nutrition, DVT prophylaxis, and maintain airway, breathing and circulation.
2. High-dose intravenous immunoglobulin (IVIG) therapy (0.4 g/kg/day for 5 days or 2 g/kg over 2 days) may accelerate recovery if given at the earliest.
3. Plasma exchange: 200–250 mL plasma/kg in 5 sessions.
4. Physiotherapy (joint and chest).
5. Respiratory assistance in 'Respiratory Care Unit (RCU)' by intubation and positive pressure ventilation when the vital capacity falls below one litre. Good supportive care is given.
6. Corticosteroids or ACTH has shown no beneficial effects; it is better not to use them.
7. Occupational therapy and rehabilitation.

PARKINSONISM — CASE 19

Q. What is your diagnosis?

This is a patient of idiopathic parkinsonism.

- Dr James Parkinson, a physician from London, described the disease in 1817. Idiopathic perkinsonism is also known as 'shaking palsy'.

Q. How your patient presented himself?

This male patient aged 75 years presented himself with difficulty or paucity of movements (bradykinesia), tremor, and stiffness of limbs and joints (three cardinal symptoms of parkinsonism) for last 3 years. The difficulties started gradually and progressing slowly without any waxing and waning.

1. He is complaining of difficulty in initiation of movement. To start with, there is clumsiness of movement and now he is unable to perform day to day activities. He feels difficulty in getting up from sitting position, walking, doing finer activities like combing, eating or fastening buttons, and writing (the letters tend to be smaller and cramped at the end of a line—Micrographia).
2. Tremor is persisting for last 3 years which is mainly present in hands and occurs mostly at rest (static tremor). To start with, tremor was present in the left hand, followed by the right hand after 4 months. Recently the patient has noticed tremor of the legs, jaw and tongue. He has also complained of increasing tremor with emotional stress and diminution temporarily by willed movement (and diminution also during sleep as told him by family members).
3. Rigidity made him stiff and is responsible for his flexed attitude or 'stooped posture'. He knows from his relatives that his voice has turned into slow (dull) and monotonous type. Recently, he is feeling weakness of upper and lower extremities. He also complained of gait disturbance.

He was absolutely normal before 3 years. There is neither any H/o headache, vomiting, convulsions, diplopia, nasal intonation, nasal regurgitation nor there is any bladder and bowel disturbances. He has no complain regarding the sensory system. About the higher function, he is a bit depressed though there is no intellectual deterioration.

- *There is delay in initiation, slowness in expression and paucity in execution in parkinsonism.*
- Parkinsonism is known as akinesia-tremor-rigidity syndrome. **Postural instability,** the most disabling feature, is usually present in advanced disease contributing to falls and resulting injuries. Prevalence of the disease increases with age, especially over 70 years with a 1.5:1 male-female ratio.
- **Bradykinesia** is common in parkinsonism, myxoedema and depression.

Clinical Wisdom

Acronym 'TRAP' for parkinsonism—Tremor, rigidity, akinesia and postural instability.

Q. Importance of past, family, personal and treatment history:

A. Past history: H/o

a. Fever, convulsions, coma (indicates post-encephalitic variety; though there may be a long interval, usually parkinsonism develops during the subsequent 12 months).
b. Head injury (punch-drunk syndrome).
c. Exposure to STD (neurosyphilis).
d. Jaundice and chronic liver disease (Wilson's disease).
e. High BP (multiple infarction in brain).
f. CO or manganese intoxication.
g. Headache, vomiting and convulsions: Brain tumour.

B. Family history: H/o hypertension, diabetes mellitus or similar type of illness within the family.

C. Personal history: Whether 'boxer' or not.

D. Treatment history: Whether there is any H/o prolonged intake of phenothiazines, butyrophenones, tetrabenazine, etc.

Q. Special points in the physical examination in parkinsonism:

A. General survey:

a. The patient is conscious and cooperative.
b. Masked facies characterised by (Fig. 1.54A):
   i. Infrequent blinking with staring look (spontaneous ocular movements are lacking),
   ii. Loss of facial expression (looks blank and apathetic), and
   iii. Widened palpebral fissure.

- There may be associated titubation of head and drooling of saliva.

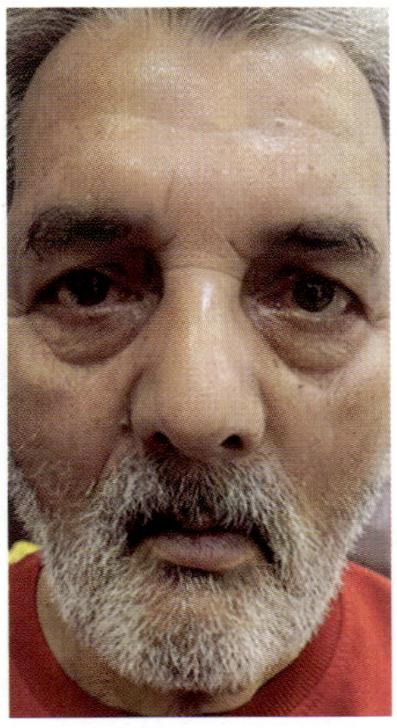

Fig. 1.54A: Mask facies in parkinsonism

c. Pulse: Write all the points. Condition of the arterial wall is normal (excludes atherosclerosis).
d. BP: 135/85 mm of Hg (excludes atherosclerotic variety).
e. Jaundice: Absent (for Wilson's disease).
f. Cornea: K-F ring is absent (for Wilson's disease).
g. Seborrhoea (greasy skin) and sialorrhoea: Absent (excludes post-encephalitic variety).
h. Outstanding features: Coarse and static tremor of hands; jaw tremor. Rate of eye blinking is reduced to <10/minute.
i. Posture: Flexed and stooped posture with impaired postural reflex.

❍ Mention all the points in general survey.

B. Nervous system:

a. Higher functions:
   i. The patient is conscious, alert, oriented and cooperative.
   ii. Normal intelligence and memory.
   iii. A bit depressed (dementia may develop in late stages).
b. Speech: Slow initiation, indistinct and **monotonous speech** without any fluctuation or modulations (bradylalia as well as hypophonia, and in advanced disease, speech is reduced to muttering). Palilalia (repetition of terminal words of own speech) in also present.
c. Cranium and spine: Within normal limit.
d. Neck rigidity and Kernig's sign: Absent.
e. Cranial nerves: Normal; Jaw jerk: Normal; oculogyric crisis: Absent.
f. Motor functions:
   i. Attitude: Flexed attitude in all the limbs with a stooped posture.
   ii. Nutrition: No wasting seen.
   iii. Tone: Increased in all the four limbs; flexor and extensor tone are equally increased; **rigidity** is mainly of lead pipe (plastic) in type. In the hands (i.e. at wrist joint), they are of cogwheel in type (due to static tremor).
   iv. Power: Grade IV in both upper and lower limbs.
   v. Coordination: Could not be tested properly.
   vi. Involuntary movements: Tremor is present. It is,
      1. **Static tremor** (or resting tremor) and does not increase at goal-point of an action.
      2. Coarse in type (4–6/second). It reduces on activity or holding something.
      3. More prominent in hands; bilateral and symmetrical.
      4. The patient can control the tremor temporarily by voluntary effort.
      5. There is predominantly contraction of flexor and extensors alternately with a prominent rotatory component between finger and thumb (pill-rolling, bread-cutting or drum-beating tremor); often changing to supination and pronation of forearm.
      6. Tremor is increased by emotion and disappears during sleep.
      7. Mostly present in the distal part of upper limb; and is also present in the jaw and tongue.
g. Sensory functions:
   i. Superficial
   ii. Deep
   iii. Cortical
   } NAD

❍ Mention the subheadings.

h. Reflexes:
   i. Superficial:
      1. Abdominal
      2. Cremasteric
      3. **Plantar response**
      } Within normal limit (bilaterally)
   ii. Deep:
      1. Biceps jerk
      2. Triceps jerk
      3. Supinator jerk
      4. Knee jerk
      5. Ankle jerk
      } Within normal limit (bilaterally)
      6. Clonus: Absent
   iii. Visceral:
      1. Swallowing
      2. Bladder
      3. Bowel
      } Within normal limit
   iv. Other reflexes:
      1. **Glabellar tap: Present**
      2. Grasp reflex: Absent (bilaterally).
      3. Palmo-mental reflex: Absent (bilaterally).
i. Trophic changes: Nil.
j. Cerebellar functions: Normal.
k. Autonomic functions: Within normal limit.

I. Stance and gait: There is **'festinant' gait**. The features are:
   i. Stance: Patient bends forward (universal flexion): Known as 'simian attitude'.
   ii. Difficulty in initiation of movement; the patient may freeze suddenly, i.e. glued to the floor.
   iii. Starts walking with rapid, short, shuffling steps as if the patient is trying to catch up his centre of gravity.
   iv. Paucity of automatic movements of both the upper limbs (i.e. less swinging movement of arms).
   v. Steps become more and more rapid with a tendency to run (festination) and the patient may ultimately fall like a telegraphic pole. The disease is characterised by loss of balance.
   vi. There is presence of propulsion (tendency to fall forward), retropulsion (walking backwards uninhibited, if pulled backwards) and lateropulsion (walking sideways better).
   vii. Impaired balance on turning (fractionated turn) and turns en block.
   viii. Difficult to stop suddenly, if pushed or pulled.
   ix. Can run faster than walking during emergency (kinesia paradoxa).

C. CVS: Within normal limit (search for the signs of atherosclerosis).

D. Respiratory system: Within normal limit.

E. GI tract and genitourinary system: Normal (search for hepatosplenomegaly due to Wilson's disease, especially in a young patient).

F. Lymphoreticular system: Within normal limit.

- Mention the subheadings in all the systems. Write plantar response as 'bilaterally flexor'.

Q. Chief complaints of your patient:

1. Difficulty of movements for 3 years.
2. Tremor in hands for 3 years.
3. Stiffness (rigidity) of muscles for 3 years, and
4. Postural instability for last 2 years.

Q. Causes of masked facies:

See the section on 'Scleroderma'.

Q. What is glabellar tap reflex (Myerson's sign) (Fig. 1.54B)?

In health, if a series of sharp finger tap (by index finger) is applied over the glabella (root of the nose), it evokes three or four blinks (bilateral closure of eyes) before the response is inhibited.

Precautions:

1. Tap should be light and done at a rate of 1/second up to 5 taps at a time.
2. Tap should be applied on standing behind the patient and the tapping finger is kept above the visual field (so that menace reflex does not play).

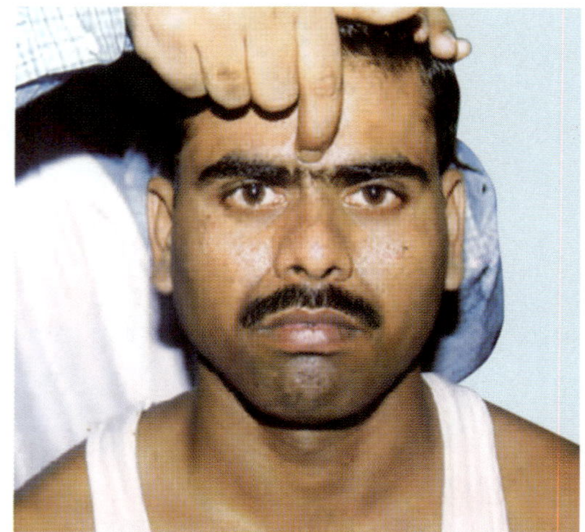

Fig. 1.54B: Eliciting **glabellar tap** standing behind the patient

3. Eyes should be kept open.

The afferent fibres are carried through Vth cranial nerve while the efferent fibres go through VIIth cranial nerve, and the centre for this reflex lies in pons.

Prolongation of glabellar tap (i.e. eyes continue blinking with each tap) response is seen in parkinsonism, diffuse cortical damage and senile dementia. This reflex tests the integrity of 'nigro-striatal pathway'.

Q. Differentiation between spasticity and rigidity:

Hypertonia is of two types: spasticity and rigidity.

A. Spasticity

1. Alaways in pyramidal tract (UMN) lesion. Spasticity takes some time to develop.
2. Tone is of clasp-knife in type [hypertonia is felt maximally at the beginning of passive movement when the limb is fairly flexed or extended, and the resistance is decreased (gives away) if the movement is continued]: Quick movement is better to elicit spasticity.
3. Hypertonia is marked in flexors of upper limbs and extensors of lower limbs, i.e. more in antigravity muscles. Power: Reduced.
4. Jerks or deep reflexes: Brisk; clonus may by present. Abdominal reflexes are lost.
5. Plantar response: Extensor
6. Involuntary movements are not seen,

- Clasp-knife spasticity is the lengthening and shortening reactions in muscles, originally described by Sherrington.

B. Rigidity

1. Seen in extrapyramidal lesions.
2. Tone is of lead pipe or cogwheel in type: Slow movement is better to elicit rigidity.
   a. Lead pipe: Uniform resistance present throughout the entire range of passive movement, and is mostly appreciated in legs and trunk; also known as plastic type rigidity.
   b. Cogwheel: Fluctuant resistance to passive movement due to presence of static tremor (as if a

lever is rubbing on the teeth of a cogwheel); best observed in wrist joint and neck.
3. Hypertonia is marked in both the limbs equally, i.e. flexors and extensors of all the four limbs are equally affected. Power: Normal.
4. Jerks or deep reflexes: Normal; clonus: Absent. Abdominal reflexes are preserved.
5. Plantar response: Flexor
6. Very often associated with involuntary movements (e.g. tremor).

- Causes of rigidity: Extrapyramidal lesions, decorticate rigidity, decerebrate rigidity, hysterical and reflex rigidity (i.e. neck rigidity in meningitis).

Q. Aetiology of parkinsonism (Table 1.23):

1. Idiopathic (Parkinson's disease or paralysis agitans): Usually occurs in middle aged or elderly.
2. Atherosclerotic (vascular or 'multi-infarct').
3. Post-encephalitic (von Economo's disease): Becoming increasingly rare.
4. Punch-drunk syndrome (or dementia pugilistica) in boxers (i.e. traumatic or repeated head injury).
5. Wilson's disease.
6. CO, CS_2, methyl-phenyl-tetrahydropyridine (MPTP, used for recreational purposes) and manganese dust intoxication.
7. Neurosyphilis, HIV-induced.
8. Drug-induced (reversible parkinsonism): Phenothiazines (chlorpromazine), butyrophenones (haloperidol), tetrabenazine, reserpine, metoclopramide.
9. Cerebral tumour (involving basal ganglia, rare).
10. Huntington's disease.
11. Normal pressure hydrocephalus (NPH).

Clinical Wisdom

1, 2 and 3 are the most common causes. According to some neurologists, vascular or atherosclerotic variety does not exist, and thus remains a topic of controversy. Paralysis agitans is a degenerative disorder.

- All Parkinson's disease suffer from parkinsonism but not all parkinsonism have Parkinson's disease. Post-encephalitic variety, drugs and Wilson's disease may develop into **parkinsonism in young age**.
- Parkinsonian disorders are classified into: a. Primary (i.e. Parkinson's disease: No. 1), b. secondary (No. 2–11) and c. parkinsonism-plus syndrome (*see* later).

Q. Components of extrapyramidal system:

1. Caudate nucleus.
2. Putamen.
3. Globus pallidus.
4. Red nucleus.
5. Substantia nigra.
6. Subthalamic nucleus of Luys.
7. Dentate nucleus (of cerebellum).
8. Reticular formation (of brainstem).

Q. Eye signs in parkinsonism:

1. Infrequent blinking, staring look (serpentine stare).
2. Impaired pursuit movement of eyeball.
3. Reflex blepharospasm (Myerson's sign).

Table 1.23: Differentiation between idiopathic and post-encephalitic parkinsonism

Features	Idiopathic	Post-encephalitic
1. Age	1. Elderly or late middle-aged	1. Relatively younger
2. Onset	2. Insidious	2. Sudden
3. Past history	3. Nothing particular	3. Gives history of encephalitis
4. Presentation complaint	4. Mainly tremor	4. Rigidity with impaired higher function
5. Higher function	5. Normal	5. Often mentally dull
6. Cranial nerves	6. Normal	6. *Oculogyric crisis* (sustained, involuntary upward conjugate deviation of eyeballs)
7. Rigidity	7. Usually of cogwheel in type	7. Lead pipe in type (due to absence of tremor)
8. Tremor	8. Most prominent feature, i.e. tremor > rigidity	8. Less prominent; rigidity is the main feature, i.e. rigidity > tremor
9. Reflexes	9. Normal	9. Jerks are brisk and *plantar response is extensor* due to involvement of pyramidal tract
10. Autonomic features	10. None	10. Flushing of skin, seborrhoea, sialorrhoea, behavioural disturbances, hiccoughs and orthostatic hypotension
11. L-dopa therapy	11. Good response	11. Poor response
12. Lewy body	12. Present	12. Absent

- **Oculogyric crisis** may be seen in drug-induced dyskinesia (e.g., metoclopramide-induced), petit mal epilepsy and post-encephalitic parkinsonism. The head may tilt backwards and body may take a posture of opisthotonus.

4. Oculogyric crisis (post-encephalitic).
5. Reversed Argyll Robertson pupil.
6. On gentle closing the eyes, there is fluttering of eyelids (blepharoclonus).
7. Hypometric saccades.

Q. Symptoms of extrapyramidal diseases:

A. Hyperkinesia (excessive involuntary movements):
   1. Tremor (static).
   2. Chorea.
   3. Athetosis.
   4. Hemiballismus.
   5. Myoclonus.
   6. Dyskinesia.
   7. Dystonia.
   8. Tics.

B. Hypokinesia or akinesia: Poverty and slowness of movement (e.g. parkinsonism).
C. Ataxia (postural disorder).
D. Rigidity.

- Hyperkinesia, hypokinesia and akinesia are collectively known as **'movement disorders'**.

Q. What are the stages of parkinsonism?

The Hoehn and Yahr scale for staging is:
Stage I: Unilateral involvement (so called hemi-parkinsonism).
Stage II: Bilateral involvement but no postural abnormality.
Stage III: Bilateral involvement with mild postural abnormality.
Stage IV: Stage 3 plus severe postural abnormality requiring substantial help.
Stage V: Severe, fully developed disease; patient is restricted to bed and wheel chair, unless aided.

Q. What is 'Parkinsonism-plus' syndrome?

In parkinsonism-plus syndrome, classical parkinsonian features (akinesia-rigidity) are seen in combination with autonomic, cerebellar, oculomotor and cortical dysfunction in various heterogeneous neuro-degenerative disorders like:

1. Progressive supranuclear palsy (Steele-Richardson syndrome): Commonest.
2. Multiple system atrophy, e.g. Shy-Drager syndrome, striatonigral degeneration, olivopontocerebellar atrophy.
3. Wilson's disease.
4. Huntington's disease.
5. Normal pressure hydrocephalus (triad of dementia, ataxia and urinary incontinence).
6. Alzheimer's disease, Pick's disease.

Q. Features of atherosclerotic parkinsonism:

1. Age: Usually above 60 years.
2. Higher function: Loss of memory is very common (due to multiple infarction in brain).
3. Bradykinesia is the prominent feature. Tremor and rigidity are less pronounced.
4. Clinical evidences of atherosclerosis (*see* the section on 'Hemiplegia').
5. Bilateral UMN signs may be seen, e.g.
   i. Jaw jerk: Present.
   ii. Plantar response: Bilaterally extensor.
6. Course of the disease is more rapid in comparison to other types.
7. Little or no response to L-dopa therapy.

Q. What are the differential diagnosis of your case?

a. Causes of tremor: Read the section on 'tremor'.
b. Causes of hypertonia: Read the section on 'Paraplegia'.
c. Causes of 'parkinsonism-plus' syndrome (described above).

Q. What is the basic pathology in parkinsonism?

Melanin is lost from the dopaminergic nerve cells in **substantia nigra**, and there is nerve cell loss with gliosis and formation of Lewy body (intracytoplasmic inclusion body). It is seen that the **nigro-striatal pathway** utilise dopamine as a neurotransmitter and subsequently dopamine loss produces parkinsonism. It is a disease of extrapyramidal systern (basal ganglia) due either to an increase in acetylcholine or decrease in dopamine.

There is degeneration of nigro-striatal pathway. Ultimately dopamine level in corpus striatum gets depleted, which is the major pathological change in parkinsonism.

Q. Investigations you like to perform in a case of parkinsonism:

Diagnosis of parkinsonism is essentially made on clinical grounds though investigations may be required in exceptional situations. There is no specific laboratory test.

a. Blood: Serum copper, ceruloplasmin, VDRL, Kahn test.
b. Urine: Urinary copper estimation (in 24 hours).
c. Liver function tests (for detection of Wilson's disease).
d. CT or MRI scan of brain is done in:
   i. Patients <50 years.
   ii. Unilateral disease.
   iii. Signs of UMN, cerebellar or autonomic involvement.
   iv. Diagnosis in doubt.

- Patients <50 years of age are screened for Wilson's disease.
- Dopamine transporter (DaT) imaging may be used to assess the extent of nigro-striatal cell loss.

Q. Outline of treatment of parkinsonism:

A. Stage I and II (mild): Medication may be required. Only anticholinergic drugs and selegiline are used; amantadine may be tried.

B. Stages II, III and IV (moderate and severe):

a. Levodopa, carbidopa or benserazide, bromocriptine, pergolide, lisuride, pramipexole, ropinirole, cabergoline, different COMT inhibitors (tolcapone, entacapone).
b. Stereotactic surgery (e.g. pallidotomy).
c. Physiotherapy, occupational therapy and speech therapy.

- Tremor and rigidity are best controlled by anticholinergic drugs. Akinesia and postural instability are improved by levodopa. Selegiline (MAO-B inhibitor) reduces the free-radical formation generated from the oxidation of catecholamines. COMT stands for catechol-O-methyl-transferase; COMT inhibitors (tolcapone, entacapone) enhance the benefits of levodopa therapy and are useful in patients with response fluctuation to levodopa.
- Other drugs used: rasagiline (MAO-B inhibitor), rivastigmine (used in significant dementia), antioxidants (vitamin C and E), and apomorphine (in advanced disease).

Q. Name some anticholinergic drugs used in parkinsonism:

1. Trihexyphenidyl, 2. Benztropine, 3. Orphenadrine, 4. Biperiden, 5. Procyclidine.

Q. Indications of surgery in parkinsonism:

Stereotactic surgery is done in globus pallidus or ventrolateral thalamus. *Indications of operation* are (obviously with no response to drugs):

1. Relatively young patient.
2. Good general health with sound mental health.
3. Unilateral tremor or rigidity (akinesia is less responsive to surgery).

- Newer treatment: **Deep brain stimulation (DBS)** by stereotactic insertion of electrodes into the brain, or continuous infusion of levodopa gel into the small intestine via a jejunostomy and monitored by a self-operated pump, or direct transplantation of embryonic mesencephalic dopaminergic cells into the putamen. Stem cell and gene therapy are still on research stage.

Q. Side effects of drugs used in parkinsonism:

i. Levodopa: Nausea, vomiting, dyskinesia, postural hypotension, 'on-off phenomenon', hallucinations.
ii. Anticholinergic drugs: Dry mouth, constipation, blurring of vision, glaucoma, retention of unine, Involuntary movements and confusion (use anticholinergic drugs cautiously in aged).
iii. Amantadine: Mental confusion, ankle oedema, livedo reticularis, seizures, urinary retention.
iv. Selegiline (deprenyl): Postural hypotension, involuntary movements, psychosis.

- Carbidopa (levodopa with DOPA decarboxylase inhibitor in a ratio of 10:1; DOPA decarboxylase Inhibitor prevents destruction of levodopa in the blood stream) is preferred to levodopa. Propranolol is sometimes used to treat tremor.

Q. What is 'on-off phenomenon'?

After 3–6 years of treatment with levodopa, a short period of dyskinesia may develop (e.g. athetosis of the neck). Akinesia and weakness may last for few minutes to hours and may alternate with dyskinesia. These symptoms are due to narrow therapeutic index of levodopa. The patients are benefited by lowering the dose of levodopa or giving levodopa with selegiline.

SECTION 5: GENITOURINARY SYSTEM

The cardinal symptoms of (genito-) urinary system are:

1. Oliguria.
2. Polyuria.
3. Anuria.
4. Swelling of the face, legs or whole body (i.e. anasarca).
5. Haematuria (i.e. bloody urine).
6. Nocturia (all polyuric states, oedema-forming states, prostatism, salt-losing nephropathy, cystitis, vesico-ureteric reflux, autonomic dysfunction, and insomnia even without renal disease produce nocturia). In CCF and other oedema-forming states, there is increase in renal blood flow during recumbency. See also page 178.
7. Dysuria (pain or discomfort during micturition), strangury, burning micturition, increased frequency of micturition (passing urine more often than usual) and urgency (sudden urge or need to pass urine); hesitancy (delay in initiation of micturition) or precipitancy (sudden voiding of urine), post-micturition dribbling (e.g. benign hypertrophy of prostate—BHP), impaired flow of urine, or urethral discharge.
8. Retention of urine (coma due to any cause, myelopathy, BHP, anticholinergic drugs usage).
9. Incontinence of urine (stress, urge, true or overflow incontinence): Vide page 159.
10. Enuresis (bed-wetting at night or during sleep).
11. Increased nocturnal frequency (BHP, diabetes mellitus, nocturia).
12. Fork urine (bifid) in stricture urethra, pneumaturia (bubbly urine) in vesico-enteric fistula (e.g. in Crohn's disease) or in gas-producing organisms in the urinary tract in diabetes mellitus.
13. Passage of milky urine: Chyluria; smoky urine (AGN); foul smell in urine (UTI) or discharge per urethra (gonococcal urethritis).
14. Renal colic: It is the colicky pain caused by urinary tract stone, where pain moves from loin to groin.
15. Pain (urinary): It can be of renal (in loin region), ureteric or bladder origin. Renal pain is due to stretching of renal capsule. Pain radiating from loin to groin, and to testis or labia is due to ureteric stone. Acute glomerulonephritis (AGN) is a painless condition.
16. Swelling of abdomen (ascites, renal lump).

17. Sexual problems like frequency of sex, number of partners, whether hetero-/homo-/bisexual, using condom every time or not, lack of libido, impotence, trouble with ejaculation; dyspareunia, details menstrual problems, vaginal discharge and contraception in female. Any symptom related to sexually transmitted diseases (STD).
18. Any complaint regarding male or female genitalia.
19. Fever (UTI, pyelonephritis, renal tuberculosis).
20. General symptoms: Nausea/vomiting/hiccough (from renal failure), appetite, weight loss/gain (i.e. oedema), sleep, fatigue, bowel, etc.
21. Miscellaneous: Pruritus, breathlessness, paraesthesia, restless legs are symptoms in renal failure.

- **BHP** or bladder neck obstruction is manifested by nocturia, increased frequency, reduced size and force of urinary stream, straining to urinate, dribbling at the end, or retention of urine.
- *Dysuria* is difficulty in passing urine which may be associated with pain or discomfort (commonly due to severe bacterial infection, or inflammation of urethra or bladder neck). *Strangury* is severe form of dysuria where there is painful passing of urine drop by drop with severe suprapubic pain.
- *Increased frequency of micturition* (without increase in urine volume) in due to cystitis, BHP, calculus/ foreign body/tumour in bladder, or reduced bladder capacity.

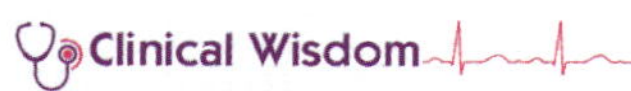

Clinical Wisdom

Nephron is the functional unit of kidneys where each kidney contains approximately one million nephrons.

Scheme of Examination (Proforma)

This system may be written separately though few clinicians prefer the combined system of GI tract plus genitourinary system. While writing this system, proforma of GI system should be followed with special reference to:

A. General survey:

1. **Pallor** with yellow complexion (e.g. CRF).
2. Face: Puffiness of the face (especially periorbital) or moon face, present or not.
3. **Oedema:** Pitting or non-pitting, localised or generalised, parietal oedema present or not.
4. Nutrition: Cannot be assessed properly due to presence of anasarca (if present).
5. **Pulse:** Condition of the arterial wall may be thickened rarely in nephrotic syndrome (due to accelerated atherosclerosis). Sometimes, an arteriovenous fistula (Brescia-Cimino fistula: vascular access, artificially made for haemodialysis) with a continuous thrill may be present in the anterior aspect of lower part of forearm.
6. **BP:** Measurement should be done in all patients as hypertension is common in AGN and CRF.
7. Skin: Whether scabies with pyoderma present (acute nephritis) or not.

B. GI system: In details (**tonsils** should be examined in a patient with acute nephritis; **prostate** should be examined per rectally in suspected obstructive uropathy).

C. Genitourinary system:

I. ***Inspection:***

Genitalia: Penile swelling, vulval oedema or vaginitis, scrotal swelling, contact ulcer, etc.

Observe the **skin** for renal biopsy mark (benzene seal or leucoplast strap in the loin), nephrectomy scar (in the loin), renal transplant scar (in either of iliac fossa), and small scar or catheter *in situ* in the centre of lower abdomen for peritoneal dialysis. Watch for any visible mass (including mass of transplanted kidney) and abdominal distension (ascites).

- **Testes:** Small—hypogonadism, absent—cryptorchidism, tenderness—orchitis, tumour—teratoma, seminoma; also look for hydrocele and inguinal hernia.
- **Penis:** Adult size is approximately 8–12 cm in length. In hypogonadism, the size is <2.5 cm.

II. ***Palpation:***

1. Examination of genitalia for **phimosis** (tight foreskin over glans penis), penile meatus, glans penis, smegma (secretion under the foreskin), scrotal oedema, hydrocele, contact ulcer in genitalia, palpation of vas deferens and **testes**, etc.
2. Parietal oedema.
3. Fluid thrill.
4. Detailed examination of kidneys (palpation with special reference to bimanual palpation and ballottement to find out a **renal mass.**
5. **Renal angle:** Tender or not; fullness of renal angle in perinephric abscess.

III. ***Percussion:***

1. Shifting dullness in abdomen.
2. Upper border of liver dullness (as hydrothorax may be present).
3. **Band of colonic resonance over the left renal mass.**
4. **Percussion of the urinary bladder, if distended.**

IV. ***Auscultation:***

1. Peristalsis.
2. **Renal artery bruit** (heard on either side of the midline in the mid-abdomen in renal artery stenosis) **(Fig. 1.55)**.
3. Venous hum.

V. ***In detail examination*** of genitalia, hernial orifices, per rectal or per vaginal examination (if indicated) with consent of the patient.

D. CVS:

1. Neck veins may not be properly visualised due to anasarca, or neck veins remain engorged due to fluid overload or cardiac tamponade.
2. Apex: Site (for LVH arising out of renal hypertension), murmur (haemic), gallop, etc.

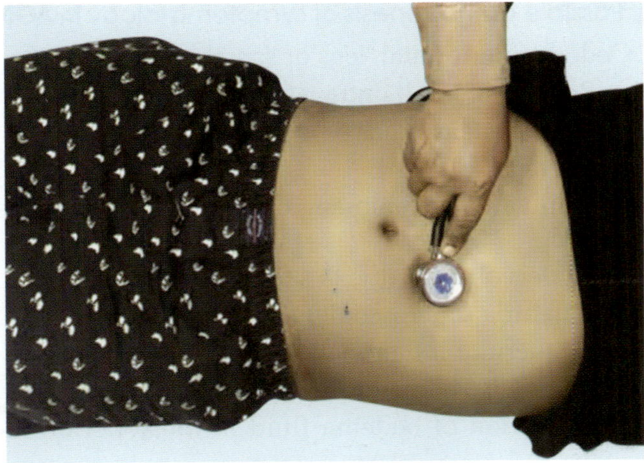

Fig. 1.55: Auscultating **renal artery bruit**

3. **Pericardial rub** (uraemia).
4. Pericardial effusion (percussion of the heart may be necessary).

- CCF due to renal diseases are common as a result of fluid overload and hypertension.

E. Respiratory system:
1. Hyperpnoea due to metabolic acidosis in renal failure.
2. Parietal oedema in the chest wall (i.e. intercostal fullness).
3. Type of respiration: May be thoraco-abdominal due to the presence of ascites.
4. Features of **hydrothorax**.
5. Features of lower respiratory tract infections.

F. Nervous system: Nothing particular. The patient may be drowsy in uraemia or may show flapping tremor or myoclonus rarely. Sometimes, the patient may be restless due to hypertensive encephalopathy. Features of peripheral neuropathy may be present in chronic renal failure.

Fundoscopy may reveal retinopathy, central retinal artery or retinal vein thrombosis.

G. Lymphoreticular system: Examine for anaemia (pallor), sternal tenderness, bleeding spots, lymphadenopathy, etc.

H. 'Urine examination' (optional): To complete the clinical examination, urine should be examined in detalis, i.e. macroscopic, chemical and microscopic examination; especially for the presence of albumin (e.g. nephrotic syndrome) and sugar (e.g. diabetic nephropathy).

- Examination of **penis:** Purulent discharge (may indicate urethritis), balano-posthitis (may suggest underlying diabetes mellitus), meatal ulcer (may be responsible for dysuria and haematuria), pinhole meatus (may produce obstructive uropathy), hypospadias and phimosis (infection underneath tight foreskin may be responsible for ascending UTI). Pruritus vulvae may suggest diabetes.
- Always look for **biopsy mark** in the loin (for kidney) in a patient with nephrotic syndrome.

- In history taking, past history (diabetes, hypertension, anaemia, recurrent infection), family history (polycystic renal disease, Alport's syndrome), and drug history (aminoglycosides, NSAIDs, ACE inhibitors) are especially asked for.
- In a patient with **renal transplant** there will be history of CRF, may have H/o haemodialysis, or presence of an arteriovenous fistula in forearm with a laparotomy scar in abdomen along with transplanted kidney in either right or left iliac fossa. Commonly *renal transplant is performed* due to diabetes with renal failure, hypertensive renal diease, SLE nephropathy or glomerulonephritis.
- A patient of **haemodialysis** will have artificial artiriovenous fistula in forearm or haemodialysis catheters in the subclavian region along with features of uraemia.
- An **artificial arteriovenous fistula** (Fig. 1.56) for haemodialysis will have features like: a) prominent dilated and tortuous veins in the forearm, b) hypertrophy of forearm and arm, c) continuous thrill and continuous bruit over the fistula, d) collapsing pulse indicating hyperdynamic circulation, e) incision mark for operation and puncture mark for dialysis, and f) Branham's sign: Slowing of the pulse rate on occluding the feeding artery of the fistula.

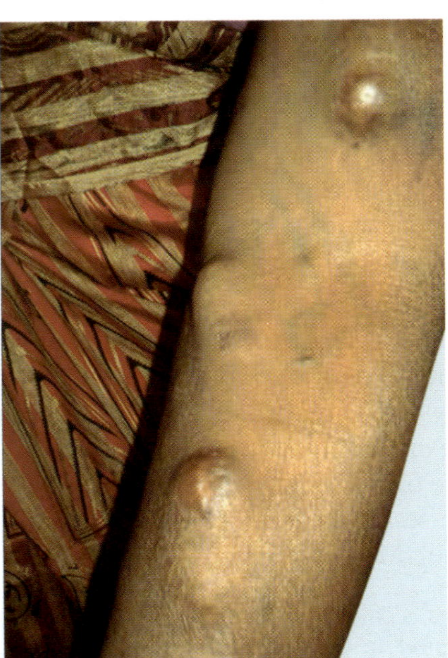

Fig. 1.56: **Artificial arteriovenous shunt** made for haemodialysis resulting in dilated and tortuous veins in the left forearm

ACUTE GLOMERULONEPHRITIS — CASE 20

Q. What is your diagnosis?

It is a case of acute glomerulonephritis, probably post-streptococcal in aetiology.

Q. Why do you say so?

This is a case of acute glomerulonephritis (AGN) because:

1. This boy aged 12 years presented with swelling of his face, scanty micturition with haematuria (or smoky urine but there was absence of frank blood) for last four days. The disease was acute in onset and progressive in nature. He was absolutely normal prior to four days. His mother first noticed the puffiness of

her son's face (mainly periorbital) in the morning after getting up from the bed. He complained of oliguria and haematuria from the same day. There was no H/o respiratory distress, convulsions or anuria. He did not complain of any burning micturition or loin pain (due to stretching of renal capsule). There was presence of low grade fever at the initial period with anorexia, headache and malaise but H/o vomiting was absent.

2. Though he did not suffer from any sore throat (e.g. tonsillitis, pharyngitis) 1–3 weeks back, he gave H/o generalised itching all over the body for last 3 weeks which was probably due to scabies infection. There was neither any H/o viral hepatitis B or C, chickenpox, mumps, measles infection in the recent past nor there was any past history suggesting collagen vascular disease, drug hypersensitivity, type I diabetes or hypertension.
3. On examination, the **face** is pale and puffy **(nephritic facies)**. The swelling is seen more in the eyelids and around the eyes (periorbital) causing narrowing of the palpebral fissure. There is presence of mild pitting, pedal oedema at present. Pyoderma (infected scabies) is seen in the classical distribution like webs of fingers, elbow, below the nipple, umbilicus and groin regions. Pulse shows tachycardia and the BP is 150/90 mm of Hg (definitely hypertensive at the age of 12 years). Jugular veins are engorged (due to hypervolaemia).
4. Neither scrotal oedema nor ascites is detected. Liver, spleen and kidneys are not palpable, and the renal angles are non-tender.
5. Other systems are essentially within normal limit.
6. Urine examination done at the bedside revealed presence of albumin (moderate) but there is absence of sugar (test to detect blood in urine sample is usually not done): May be performed for corroboration.

❍ Sometimes, a patient of AGN may present with anasarca. The 'latent period' in case of pharyngeal infection is usually 1–3 weeks and in cutaneous infection (pyoderma from scabies, furunculosis or impetigo), it is averaging about 2–6 weeks.

Q. What is your case?

Say the summary as mentioned above.

Q. What is acute glomerulonephritis (AGN) or acute nephritic syndrome?

It consists of sudden onset symptom complex like:

1. Periorbital puffiness.
2. Oliguria.
3. Haematuria.
4. Oedema and hypertension.
5. Proteinuria (non-nephrotic range).
6. RBC and RBC cast in urine.
7. Tendency to early renal failure (acute) or acute kidney injury (AKI).

Q. Possible pathogenesis of symptomatology in AGN:

1. Oedema (periorbital, legs or sacral):
   - Retention of salt and water, and
   - Hypoproteinaemia.
2. Hypertension:
   - Stimulation of renin-angiotensin-aldosterone axis, and
   - Hypervolaemia due to salt and water retention.
3. Haematuria (microscopic):
   - Glomerular inflammation.
4. Periorbital swelling or puffiness:
   - Collection of oedema fluid in loose periorbital tissue.
5. Oliguria:
   - Reduction in glomerular filtration rate (GFR).
6. Uraemia or renal failure:
   - Retention of urea, creatinine and other nitrogenous waste products.

Q. Relevant 'past history' in acute nephritis:

1. Sore throat (streptococcal) } Poststreptococcal glomerulonephritis (PSGN)
2. Scabies (complicated by pyoderma) } Poststreptococcal glomerulonephritis (PSGN)
3. Infections like: Hepatitis B or C, mumps, measles, chickenpox, infectious mononucleosis, malaria, pneumococcal pneumonia, infective endocarditis, syphilis (secondary).
4. Collagen vascular diseases (SLE, vasculitis, Henoch-Schönlein purpura, etc.).
5. Drug hypersensitivity, GB syndrome.
6. 'Shunt nephritis' (infection of ventriculo-peritoneal shunt done in hydrocephalus).
7. H/o diabetes and hypertension.
8. H/o prolonged steroid therapy (D/D of moon face) or urticaria (angioneurotic oedema as a D/D of moon face).

❍ Actually 1 to 6 are the different causes of AGN: poststreptococcal aetiology is the commonest.

Q. Physical findings in other systems in acute nephritis:

a. CVS:
   i. JVP may be raised; systemic hypertension.
   ii. Apex may shift down and out (due to LV dilatation), and forceful in nature.
   iii. Loud A_2 (due to hypertension).
   iv. There may be presence of mitral systolic murmur (functional murmur due to LV dilatation).
   v. Gallop rhythm may be present (LVF).
   vi. Rarely, pericardial rub in acute renal failure.
b. Respiratory system:
   i. Bilateral basal crepitations (due to LVF).
   ii. Usually, there is absence of hydrothorax (to differentiate it from nephrotic syndrome).

c. Nervous system:
   i. Features of hypertensive encephalopathy.
   ii. Fundoscopy: Usually normal (not done).
d. GI tract: Tonsils may be enlarged with tender cervical adenopathy due to acute streptococcal tonsillitis. Ascites may be evident.
e. Skin (in general survey): Scabies with pyoderma.

- Never forget to examine the patient for phimosis.

Q. Common features in adults with AGN:

There are some differences in presentation of adult AGN, which are:

1. There may not be any H/o preceding infection (i.e. sore throat or skin infection).
2. Oedema is not marked.
3. Hypertension may or may not be present.
4. Presence of oliguria, haematuria and proteinuria (as occurs in a child).

Q. Pathogenesis and types of streptococci involved in AGN:

Poststreptococcal AGN is produced due to infection by Lancefield group A beta-haemolytic *streptococci* (nephritogenic strains). *Remember, streptoccocal pharyngitis may produce AGN or acute rheumatic fever while streptococcal skin infection produces AGN only.*

M types of streptococci (nephritogenic strains), e.g. types 2, 49, 55, 57 and 60 are seen following skin infections, and types 1, 3, 4, 12, 25 and 49 after pharyngitis (throat infection).

Actually, AGN or acute nephritic syndrome is an immune complex glomerulonephritis where there is production of antibodies against glomerular antigen and thereby leading to deposition of immune complexes in the walls of glomerular capillaries, and ultimately developing into inflammation of the glomeruli.

Q. Causes of acute glomerulonephritis:

i. Infectious diseases:
   A. Poststreptococcal glomerulonephritis (PSGN).
   B. Non-poststreptococcal glomerulonephritis:
      a. Bacterial: Staphylococcal and pneumococcal infection, infective endocarditis, meningococcaemia, typhoid.
      b. Viral: Hepatitis B and C, mumps, measles, varicella, infectious mononucleosis, coxsackievirus.
      c. Parasitic: Malaria, toxoplasmosis.
ii. Systemic disorders: Vasculitis, SLE, Henoch-Schönlein purpura, cryoglobulinaemia, Goodpasture's syndrome.
iii. Primary glomerular disease: Membranoproliferative glomerulonephritis, mesangial proliferative glomerulonephritis, IgA nephropathy (Berger's disease).
iv. Miscellaneous: GB syndrome, serum sickness, infective endocarditis, shunt nephritis, DPT vaccination.

Q. Causes of red urine in clinical practice:

1. Hematuria (presence of intact RBC under microscope).
2. Haemoglobinuria (in haemolytic disorders; urine gives chemical tests for haemoglobin but there is no RBC present in the centrifuged deposit of fresh sample of urine) and myoglobinuria (in rhabdomyolysis; very dark urine, no RBC on M/E)*.
3. Ingestion of beet root (beeturia), senna and dyes used to colour sweets.
4. Phenolphthalein (used in purgatives) in alkaline medium (after use of systemic alkaliser) of urine.
5. Acute intermittent porphyria (presence of porphobilinogen may be detected by addition of Ehrlich's aldehyde reagent. Freshly voided urine appears normal but may take dark red or Burgundy-wine colour on standing for few hours).
6. Drugs: Phenazopyridine (pyridium), phenindione, clofazimine, rifampicin (it actually changes the unine to dark orange colour).
7. Alkaptonuria (becomes dark-brown or black due to presence of homogentisic acid, if kept for long time).

- If blood from these patients* are kept in a test-tube for few minutes, the supernatent serum will be reddish in myoglobinuria while it will be clear in patients with haemoglobinuria.

Q. (Medical) causes of haematuria:

1. Acute glomerulonephritis.
2. Malignant hypertension.
3. SBE (generally microscopic haematuria).
4. Snake bite.
5. Henöch-Schonlein purpura or other coagulation disorders.
6. Weil's disease.
7. Anticoagulant therapy.
8. Renal tuberculosis.
9. Papillary necrosis (diabetes, sickle cell disease, analgesic-induced).
10. SLE (microscopic haematuria).
11. Renal ischaemia (renovascular disease).
12. Tumours of kidney, ureter, bladder or prostate.
13. Goodpasture's syndrome.
14. Disseminated intravascular coagulation (DIC).

- *Painless haematuria:* AGN, SBE, IgA nephropathy, hypernephroma, papilloma of urinary bladder, adult polycystic kidney disease, coagulation disorder, renal tuberculosis, hypertension.
- *Painful haematuria:* Urinary tract infection, renal calculus, papillary necrosis and trauma.

Q. Definition of polyuria, oliguria and anuria:

1. **Polyuria:** Urine output persistently above 3 litres per day. The normal urine output for a healthy adult is approximately 1.5 litres (400 mL–3 litres) per day. The common causes are:
   a. Chronic renal failure.
   b. Diabetes mellitus.
   c. Diabetes insipidus.
   d. Psychogenic polydipsia (compulsive water drinking).
   e. Use of diuretics in patients with oedema.
   f. Diuretic phase of ARF.
   g. Hypercalcaemic nephropathy.
   h. Hypokalaemic nephropathy.
   i. 'Post-obstructive uropathy'.
   j. Drugs: Alcohol, caffeine.
   k. High-altitude diuresis (i.e. >10000 feet)
   l. Transient polyuria (after epileptic seizure, paroxysmal atrial tachycardia).
2. **Oliguria:** Urine volume <400 mL per day. Common causes are acute gastroenteritis, high fever, acute glomerulonephritis, congestive heart failure (decompensated), renal failure (acute and chronic), hypovolaemia and shock, *'third space' loss* in acute peritonitis, burn and acute pancreatitis.
3. **Anuria:** Ne urine formation for 12 hours (some nephrologists define anuria as <50 mL urine output per day). Complete anuria, i.e. no urine formation by catheterisation occurs in bilateral ureteric obstruction, rapidly progressive glomerulonephritis, diffuse cortical necrosis and bilateral renal artery stenosis.

- Passing of more than one-third of the total daily output by night is **nocturia**, and diabetes mellitus and benign hypertrophy of prostate (BHP) are two prime causes in clinical practice. Like tachypnoea in respiratory disorders, nocturia may be an early manifestation of renal disorder, cardiac failure or hepatic failure. Nocturia is usually assessed as pathological.

Q. Why this is not a case of nephrotic syndrome?

As there is:

1. History of scabies with secondary infection.
2. Acute onset of oliguria.
3. Absence of anasarca.
4. Presence of haematuria.
5. Presence of hypertension.
6. A classical history.
7. Microscopical examination of urine (if allowed to do) shows presence of mild to moderate proteinuria, RBC and RBC cast.

All the above mentioned points are against nephrotic syndrome.

Q. Differential diagnosis of your case:

1. Angioneurotic oedema: Itchy swelling of eyelids, lips and tongue; absence of pyrexia, hypertension, oliguria and haematuria. H/o atopy present.
2. Acute pyelonephritis: Fever with chill and rigor, H/o loin pain with tender renal angles. Oedema is absent and there is no hypertension. Increased frequency of micturition is often present.
3. Other causes of haematuria are to be differentiated.
4. Nephrotic syndrome: Already mentioned above.
5. Acute exacerbation of chronic nephritis: H/o previous attacks of nephritis, severe hypertension and renal functional impairment are present.

Q. Investigations you like to do:

1. Urine examination:
   i. Smoky urine.
   ii. 300–600 mL in 24 hours.
   iii. High specific gravity (due to increased tubular reabsorption).
   iv. **Mild to moderate proteinuria.**
   v. Presence of RBC, RBC cast, WBC, granular cast (present lately), epithelial cell and cast **(RBC cast is diagnostic of acute nephritis)**.
   vi. Urine is sterile on culture.
2. Blood examination:
   i. Anaemia (haemodilution).
   ii. Leucocytosis.
   iii. Raised ESR.
   iv. Raised ASO titre in poststreptococcal AGN (more common with throat infection).
   v. Hypocomplementaemia C_3 and C_4.
   vi. Others (in search of aetiology): ANF, anti-ds DNA, p-ANCA, c-ANCA; HB_SAg, anti-HCV.
3. Blood biochemistry:
   i. Urea and creatinine levels may be elevated (if progresses to acute renal failure).
   ii. Normal cholesterol level (differentiates nephrotic syndrome).
4. Chest X-ray:
   i. Cardiac enlargement, or
   ii. Features of pulmonary congestion (indicates hypervolaemia).
5. Renal function test: Diminished GFR.
6. Cultures of throat swab or swab from infected skin may grow group A beta-haemolytic *streptococci*.
7. Ultrasonography of kidneys shows normal or large kidneys in 'acute' glomerulonephritis.

- **Characteristic cast in AGN is RBC cast, in nephrotic syndrome it is fatty cast, granular cast in CRF, and WBC cast in chronic pyelonephritis. Presence of hyaline cast is a normal finding.**
- **'Azotaemia'** is increase in the concentration of urea and creatinine in blood resulting from a fall in the glomerular filtration rate (GFR).
- Renal biopsy is usually not done in acute glomerulonephritis.

Q. Complications of acute nephritis:

1. Acute renal failure (ARF) or acute kidney injury (AKI).

2. Hypertensive encephalopathy.
3. Acute left ventricular failure (LVF).
4. Infections: Urinary tract, respiratory tract, etc.
5. Fluid and electrolyte imbalance, nephrotic syndrome, chronic glomerulonephritis (CGN).
6. Fluid overload.
7. Rapidly progressive glomerulonephritis (RPGN).

Q. How to recognise the major complications of AGN?

A. Acute renal failure (ARF) or acute kidney injury (AKI):

i. Severe oliguria to anuria.
ii. Drowsiness, confusion, delirium and even coma may supervene.
iii. Hypertension.
iv. Acidotic breathing (deep sighing, rapid breathing at a regular rate and with a hissing sound is called Kussmaul's breathing).
v. Blood urea, creatinine and potassium levels are invariably high with acidosis.

B. Hypertensive encephalopathy:

i. Features of increased intracranial tension, i.e. headache, vomiting, convulsions or coma.
ii. Hypertension.
iii. Confusion, delirium.
iv. Though rare, focal neurological signs like temporary blindness, aphasia, hemiparesis or extensor plantar response may be present.
v. Papilloedema with retinal exudates and haemorrhages may be evident.

C. Acute left ventricular failure:

i. Acute respiratory distress, orthopnoea; H/o PND.
ii. Cough with copious, pinkish, frothy sputum.
iii. Central cyanosis.
iv. Hypertension.
v. Gallop rhythm, crepitations at lung bases and pulsus alternans.

- *These 3 are the major complications of AGN.* Prognosis of (A), (B) and (C) are very bad. All the complications should be treated promptly as soon as they are recognised.

Q. What is RPGN?

It is known as rapidly progressive glomerulonephritis (RPGN). This term is often applied to a group of acute nephritis patients who develop persistent renal failure in a period of weeks to months and show little tendency for spontaneous recovery. Usually the pathology is extensive extracapillary (crescentic) glomerulonephritis. Clinically there are presence of nausea, vomiting, weakness, persistent hypertension, haematuria, proteinuria and azotaemia. Common causes are systemic vasculitis, SLE, poststreptococcal AGN, Goodpasture's syndrome. The prognosis is poor. Steroids, cytotoxic agents or intensive plasma exchange may be useful. Fifty percent of patients may require dialysis within 6 months.

Q. Common causes of acute renal failure (ARF) or AKI in your hospital:

1. Hypovolaemia due to acute gastroenteritis, severe haemorrhage, pancreatitis, peritonitis or extensive burns.
2. Acute glomerulonephritis.
3. Septicaemia, endotoxic shock.
4. Malignant hypertension.
5. Mismatched blood transfusion.
6. Snake bite (Viperidae group).
7. Septic abortion, eclampsia.
8. Acute myocardial infarction.
9. Hepato-renal syndrome.
10. Acute interstitial nephropathy.

Q. Prognosis of acute nephritis:

1. Complete recovery: 85% of children and 50% of adults (within 2 weeks).
2 Complications: 5% cases produce complications mentioned above; few suffer from RPGN.
3. Apparent recovery: 10% cases live with persistent proteinuria and haematuria for long periods.

- As a whole, the prognosis is good and the prognosis in children is better than adults.

Q. How do you like to manage a case of AGN?

1. Strict bed rest: Continued until the signs of glomerular inflammation and circulatory congestion subside (i.e. disappearance of oedema, oliguria, haematuria, hypertension, high blood urea, RBC cast in urine).
2. Diet: Mild protein restriction is done in azotaemic patients. When oliguria is moderate, 0.5 mg/kg/day of protein should be given. Mainly carbohydrate diet is preferred.
3. Salt and water balance: Salt-free foods are given. The fluid intake is restricted to previous days urine output plus 500 mL of extra fluid. Salt and fluid restriction are most important.
4. Diuretics: Tablet furosemide (40 mg/tab) 1 tab daily is given to relieve oedema and hypertension.
5. Antihypertensives: Nifedipine, amlodipine, hydralazine and diazoxide may be of help.
6. Antibiotics: 7–10 days course of crystalline penicillin (5 lakh, IM, BD) or erythromycin (250 mg QDS, orally) is given, if streptococcal infection is documented.
7. Treatment of complications (e.g. AKI, LVF, and hypertensive encephalopathy).
8. Dialysis may be required in severely azotaemic or fluid overloaded patients.
9. Steroid, cytotoxic drugs, long-term chemoprophylaxis like rheumatic fever are not needed.
10. Tonsillectomy may be done afterwards.

Conclusion

1. Always measure the BP of the patient (commonly hypertensive).
2. Examine for phimosis, scabies infection and swelling of tonsils.
3. Percuss the urinary bladder for retention of urine (to make D/D with oligo-anuria).
4. Search for gallop rhythm and pericardial rub.
5. Note the colour of the urine carefully (red, smoky or coca-cola urine): Send the patient to toilet with a test tube to collect urine.

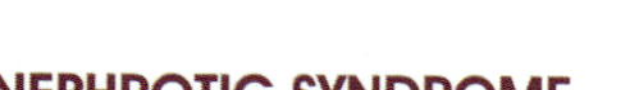

Acute glomerulonephritis in also known as acute nephritis, Type I nephritis, acute glomerulonephritis syndrome or acute nephritic syndrome.

NEPHROTIC SYNDROME — CASE 21

Q. What is your diagnosis?

The diagnosis may be delivered in one of the two ways:

1. This is a patient of nephrotic syndrome probably due to minimal lesion nephropathy, or
2. This is a patient of anasarca probably due to nephrotic syndrome.

Q. Why do you say so?

This is because of:

1. This male child aged 14 years presented with gradual swelling of the whole body for last one month. He was absolutely normal one month back. The disease was insidious in onset and gradually progressive. His father first noticed the puffiness of his son's face (mainly periorbital) in one morning when the swelling gradually involved the whole body (descending oedema) in course of time. The swelling was a bit posture-dependent. Lately, swelling involved the abdomen and the scrotum; it was painless and pitting in nature according to the patient. The boy also complained of increasing weakness. The output and colour of urine were within normal limit, and there was no H/o haematuria, burning micturition, renal colic. He did not give any H/o respiratory distress.
2. There was no past H/o sore throat, skin infection, diabetes mellitus, facial rash (i.e. SLE), drug intake or jaundice; no family H/o diabetes or hypertension was present, and no other family member was suffering from the same type of illness.
3. On examination, the **face** is puffy with baggy lower eyelids and it seems a **'moon face'** (also there is waxy pallor in the face) **(Fig. 1.57)**. There is presence of generalised, massive, posture-dependent, descending pitting oedema. BP is within normal limit (110/80 mm of Hg). Scrotal oedema with contact ulcers and parietal oedema are present **(Fig. 1.58)**. Huge swelling of penis is seen. There is mild anaemia.

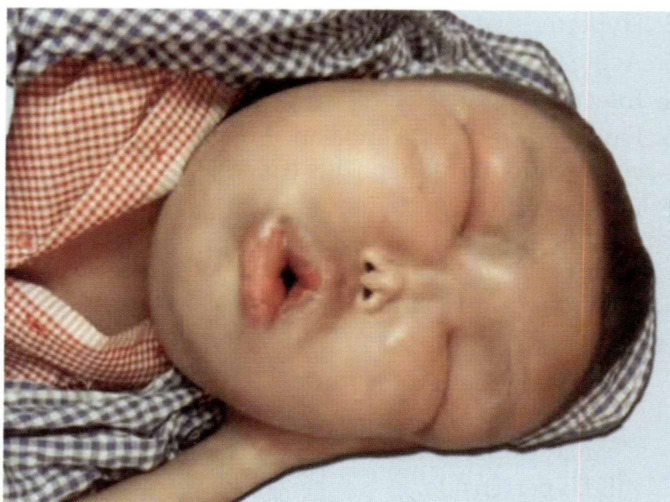

Fig. 1.57: Nephrotic syndrome. Note the extremely puffy and rounded face

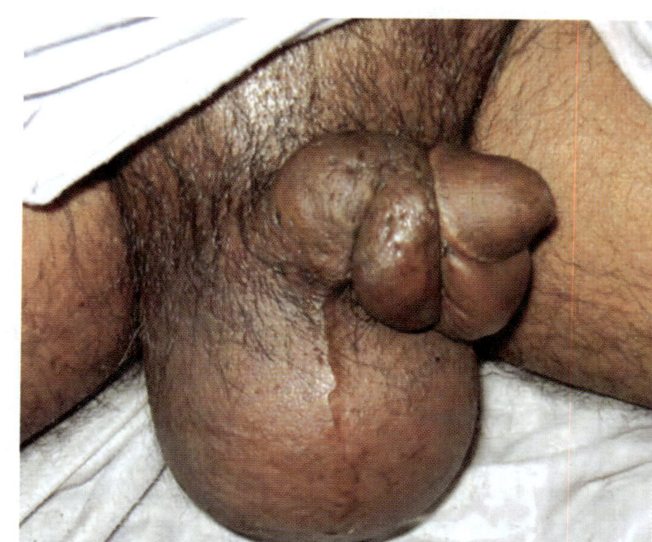

Fig. 1.58: Oedema of the genitalia (scrotum and penis) in nephrotic syndrome

4. Fluid thrill and shifting dullness are present, i.e. there is presence of ascites. Liver, spleen, gallbladder and kidneys are not palpable by dipping method. Renal angles are non-tender.
5. On examination of the other systems there is no pericardial rub, hydrothorax or pericardial effusion present
6. Urine examination done at the bedside revealed presence of albumin (massive) but there is absence of sugar in the sample: May be performed for corroboration.

- Renal oedema: periorbital + genital + generalised oedema.

Q. Causes of anasarca and moon face:

Read the sections on 'Oedema' and 'Moon face', respectively.

Q. What is nephrotic syndrome?

It is a clinical syndrome (or symptom complex) characterised by undermentioned four criteria:

a. Massive proteinuria, i.e. >3.5 g/day (albuminuria).
b. Hypoalbuminaemia (hypoproteinaemia, i.e. serum albumin <3 g/dL).
c. Generalised oedema or anasarca, and
d. Hyperlipidaemia (e.g. hypercholesterolaemia, i.e. serum cholesterol >300 mg/dL).

- Proteinuria >3.5 g/1.73 m² per day is considered to be in the nephrotic range. Normal body surface for a reference man is 1.73 m². *Proteinuria is the hallmark of nephrotic syndrome.*
- Nowadays, lipiduria and hypercoagulability are new additions in the clinical complex of nephrotic syndrome (though not essential for diagnosis).

Q. Importance of 'past history' in nephrotic syndrome:

A. Relating to aetiology:

1. Jaundice (hepatitis B or C infection).
2. Sore throat (poststreptococcal).
3. Diabetes mellitus.
4. Diseases like leprosy, syphilis, malaria.
5. Drug intake: Anti-snakevenom, penicillamine, troxidone, probenecid, organic gold.
6. Swelling in the neck or axilla (lymphoma).
7. Skin rash, arthralgia, arthritis, alopecia (collagen vascular disease, e.g. SLE).

B. Relating to cause of anasarca:

1. Jaundice, alcoholism, H/o haematemesis or melaena (indicates cirrhosis of liver).
2. H/o respiratory distress or palpitations (cardiac disorder).
3. H/o chronic diarrhoea (malabsorption and malnutrition).
4. H/o tuberculosis (tuberculous pericardial effusion or constrictive pericarditis).
5. Hoarseness of voice and constipation (hypothyroid).
6. H/o long-standing corticosteroid therapy (D/D with moon face and swelling of body).

Q. How nephrotic syndrome is classified?

1. Primary glomerular diseases:
   a. Minimal lesion or minimal change disease.
   b. Membranous glomerulonephritis.
   c. Focal and segmental glomerulosclerosis.
   d. Membranoproliferative glomerulonephritis (or mesangiocapillary glomerulonephritis).
   e. Mesangial proliferative glomerulonephritis.
2. Secondary to other diseases:
   a. Infections: Poststreptococcal, hepatitis B or C, malaria, lepromatous leprosy, secondary syphilis, infectious mononucleosis, infective endocarditis, HIV infection and AIDS.
   b. Drugs: Anti-snakevenom, penicillamine, troxidone, probenecid, bismuth, gold, mercury, captopril, α-interferon, street heroin, contrast media.
   c. Multisystem disease: SLE, Henoch-Schönlein purpura, vasculitis due to any cause, rheumatoid arthritis, Goodpasture's syndrome.
   d. Neoplasm: Lymphoma, leukaemia, carcinoma, melanoma.
   e. Heredo-familial: Diabetes mellitus, congenital nephrotic syndrome, Alport's syndrome, sickle cell disease, nail-patella syndrome.
   f. Miscellaneous: Pre-eclamptic toxaemia, amyloidosis, snake bite, bee-stings.

Q. What is Kimmelstiel-Wilson (K-W) syndrome?

1. It is a variety of nephrotic syndrome commonly arising from type I diabetes mellitus (30–40% in type I and 3–10% in type II diabetes mellitus).
2. Histological lesion is nodular glomerulosclerosis.
3. Usually develops in a long-standing diabetes mellitus (>10 years approximately).
4. Commonly starts with proteinuria.
5. The requirement of insulin becomes less with the development of K-W syndrome (as with development of nephropathy, insulin antibodies come out with urine).
6. Lately hypertension may be present.
7. End-stage renal disease can be expected to occur within 5–7 years.

- K-W lesion: Nodular glomerulosclerosis (K-W nodules, reasonably specific for diabetes mellitus).
- K-W disease: Any manifestation of glomerulonephropathy in diabetes mellitus.
- K-W syndrome: Nephrotic syndrome from diabetes mellitus.

Q. Common causes (histopathological) of nephrotic syndrome in different age group:

A. Children:

1. Minimal lesion: 70%
2. Mesangial proliferative: 15%
3. Focal glomerulosclerosis: 10%
4. Secondary: 5%
5. Membranous, membranoproliferative: Rare.

B. Adults:

1. Membranous: 35%
2. Secondary: 30%
3. Minimal lesion: 15%
4. Focal glomerulosclerosis: 10%
5. Mesangial proliferative: 5%
6. Membranoproliferative: <5%.

Clinical Wisdom

In children, primary disease is 95% and secondary is 5%. In adults, primary disease is 70% while secondary (commonest is diabetic nephropathy) is 30%.

Q. Possible pathogenesis of different features in nephrotic syndrome:

- Proteinuria: Either due to change in pore size or ↓ in anion barrier in lining of foot process of the epithelium.
- Hypoalbuminaemia: Proteinuria plus renal catabolism of filtered albumin.
- Oedema and anasarca: Hypoalbuminaemia →↓ in oncotic pressure →↑ in extracellular fluid volume. Moreover, there is ↓ in intracellular fluid →↑ renin-angiotensin-aldosterone axis →↑ Na^+ and water retention in extracellular compartment → oedema and anasarca.
- Hyperlipidaemia and lipiduria: Hypoalbuminaemia →↓ oncotic pressure → stimulate liver for lipoprotein synthesis →↑ cholesterol, ↑ LDL, ↑ TG and ↑ VLDL (no change in HDL or ↓ HDL) → hyperlipidaemia may be responsible for accelerated atherosclerosis and progression of renal disease.
- Hypercoagulability: ↓ antithrombin III, protein C and S, ↓ fibrinolysis, hyperfibrinogenaemia and ↑ platelet aggregation →↑ coagulability of blood with thromboembolic manifestations.

Q. Differential diagnosis of nephrotic syndrome:

A. Causes of anasarca:

1. CCF: Read the section on 'Oedema'.
2. Cirrhosis of liver:
   i. H/o haematemesis and melaena may be present.
   ii. Usually the face is not puffy.
   iii. Ascites appears first; pedal oedema appears next.
   iv. Splenomegaly and venous prominence in the abdomen with venous flow away from the umbilicus.
   v. Signs of hepato-cellular failure may be present.
3. Anaemia with hypoproteinaemia:
   i. Pallor.
   ii. Signs of malnutrition like glossitis, angular stomatitis, cheilosis, koilonychia may be present.
   iii. Oedema appears first in ankles (or face); ascites appears late.
   iv. Systolic murmur may be present over the pulmonary area.
4. Constrictive pericarditis: Read the section on 'Examination of neck veins'.
5. Pericardial effusion: Read the section on 'Pericardial rub'.
6. Myxoedema:
   i. Absence of urinary problem.
   ii. Hoarseness, constipation, cold sensitivity, lethargy, menorrhagia.
   iii. Bradycardia, hypertension.
   iv. Oedema is non-pitting in nature.
   v. Delayed relaxation of ankle jerk.

B. Causes of moon face: Read the sections on 'Moon face' and 'Acute glomerulonephritis'.

Q. Common complications of nephrotic syndrome:

1. Protein catabolism: May lead to wasting, striae and osteoporosis.
2. Impaired resistance to infections like cellulitis, respiratory tract infections, peritonitis.
3. Thromboembolic manifestations (due to loss of antithrombin III in urine, hyperfibrinogenaemia, impaired fibrinolysis, reduced activity of protein C or protein S, hyperlipidaemia, and enhanced platelet aggregation): Arterial thrombosis (especially pulmonary artery thrombosis), venous thrombosis (especially renal vein thrombosis).
4. Hypovolaemia may produce syncope, postural hypotension, renal failure.
5. Renal failure (chronic).
6. Accelerated atherosclerosis (may lead to 'strokes in young' and early coronary artery disease).
7. Fluid retention, hydrothorax, pericardial effusion.
8. Consequences of loss of specific binding proteins (*see later*).

Q. Renal vein thrombosis in nephrotic syndrome:

Previously it was thought to be a cause of nephrotic syndrome but nowadays it is regarded as a consequence. The condition is treated by long-term oral anticoagulation. It is commonly found in:

1. Membranous nephropathy
2. Membranoproliferative glomerulonephritis, and
3. Amyloidosis.

It is diagnosed by:

a. Unilateral or bilateral loin pain.
b. Haematuria.
c. Left-sided varicocele.
d. Widely fluctuating urine volume.
e. Asymmetry of renal size in ultrasonography.
f. Best documented by renal venous angiography.

Q. Nephrotic syndrome with hypertension:

Usually hypertension is not a feature of nephrotic syndrome. If present, one should think of:

1. K-W syndrome (i.e. diabetic nephropathy), SLE or polyarteritis nodosa as aetiology.
2. The patient is on long-term corticosteroid therapy.
3. 'Nephritic-nephrotic syndrome'—it is nephrotic syndrome with atypical features of hypertension, microscopic or gross haematuria, early renal failure and low complement C_3. The common aetiologies are SLE, IgA nephropathy and Henoch-Schönlein purpura.
4. The patient has developed early CRF.

Clinical Wisdom

Hypertension in renal diseases: AGN and CGN, chronic pyelonephritis, obstructive uropathy, renovascular hypertension, vasculitis, lupus nephritis and renal stone disease. Focal glomerulosclerosis is commonly associated with hypertension while patients with interstitial nephritis usually have normal BP.

Q. Physical signs in different systems in nephrotic syndrome (Table 1.24):

1. **GI tract and renal system:** Skin of the abdomen is shiny, ascites, neither hepatosplenomegaly nor any renal lump felt, non-tender renal angle, scrotal (or vulval) oedema or presence of hydrocele (Fig. 1.58), urinary bladder is generally empty. Phimosis should be looked for.
2. **Respiratory system:** Respiration is thoraco-abdominal in type (due to presence of ascites), parietal oedema in the chest wall, bilateral hydrothorax, crepitations at lung bases may be audible. Sometimes, evidences of pneumonia are present.
3. **CVS:** The patient may be orthopnoeic. BP is usually normal. Neck veins may not be properly visualised due to oedema (usually JVP is normal); presence of pericardial rub (in renal failure), rarely pericardial effusion; condition of the arterial wall (in peripheral pulse) may reveal thickening of arteries due to accelerated atherosclerosis (press the oedema fluid for few seconds for better palpation of pulse).
4. **Nervous system:** Nothing particular (patient may be lethargic or drowsy in renal failure).
5. **Reticulo-endothelial system:** Examine the patient for lymphadenopathy (as lymphoma, SLE and infectious mononucleosis may be the aetiology). Absence of sternal tenderness.

- Xanthelasma around the eyes may be occasionally seen because of hypercholesterolaemia. Bilateral hydrothorax and pericardial effusion should be carefully looked for, as they are commonly missed.

Table 1.24: Differentiation of AGN from nephrotic syndrome at the bedside

Features	AGN	Nephrotic syndrome
1. Age	5–15 years	1–5 years, adults too
2. H/o pharyngitis or skin infection	+	–
3. Haematuria	+	–
4. Hypertension	+	– (rarely present)
5. Anasarca	–	+
6. Oliguria	+	–
7. Hydrothorax and scrotal oedema	–	+

Q. In nephrotic syndrome, consequences of plasma proteins lost in urine:

Specific binding plasma proteins are lost in urine of nephrotic syndrome and they are:

1. Albumin (oedema, anasarca and increased susceptibility to infections).
2. Antithrombin III (causes increased coagulability and thromboembolic complications).
3. Thyroxine-binding globulin (produces abnormal thyroid function tests).
4. Cholecalciferol-binding protein (osteomalacia may be precipitated).
5. Transferrin (produces iron-resistant microcytic-hypochromic anaemia).
6. Metal binding proteins (may produce Zn- and Cu-deficiency states).
7. Globulin (severe IgG deficiency may lead to bacterial peritonitis).
8. Drug-binding proteins (may result in altered drug pharmacokinetics).

Q. How do you classify proteinuria?

Normal adults may excrete up to 150 mg protein in 24 hours of which 15 mg is albumin and 25 mg is 'Tamm-Horsfall mucoprotein' produced by the renal tubules. Proteinuria (pathological) is classified into:

a. Mild: 150–500 mg/day (+)
b. Moderate: 500 mg–2 g/day (++)
c. Massive: >2 g/day (+++); if it crosses 3.5 g/day, it is designated as 'nephrotic range'.

- Proteinuria may be divided into selective (responsive to corticosteroid) and non-selective types.
- **Microalbuminuria:** It is defined as daily excretion of albumin of 20–200 microgram/min (i.e. 30–300 mg/day) and is commonly found in diabetes mellitus with early renal involvement.
- Proteinuria often makes the urine frothy or foamy (i.e. full of tiny air bubbles).

Q. Characteristics of minimal change disease:

1. It is also known as lipoid nephrosis, nil lesion or foot process disease. No alterations are demonstrable by light microscopy (so, nil lesion) but electron microscopy shows diffuse epithelial foot process effacement.
2. It is the commonest cause of nephrotic syndrome in children (70%); male > female.
3. Highly selective proteinuria.
4. Progression to ARF is rare and the prognosis is good as 10 years survival rate exceeds 90%.
5. Generally steroid or cytotoxic drug-responsive.

Q. Characteristics of membranous nephropathy:

1. It is the commonest form of nephrotic syndrome in adults (35%).
2. Commonly due to SLE, carcinoma of lung or penicillamine therapy.
3. Light microscopy shows thickening of glomerular basement membrane (GBM): So 'membranous'.
4. Non-selective proteinuria. Haematuria may be evident.
5. Renal vein thrombosis is common, as common is the progression to chronic renal failure.
6. Prognosis is bad. Treated by steroid but the response is inconsistent.

Q. Neuromuscular complications of chronic renal failure (azotaemia):

1. Fatigue, 2. Headache, 3. Lethargy, 4. Difficulty in concentration, 5. Drowsiness, 6. Muscular irritability, 7. Flapping tremor (asterixis), 8. Hallucinations, 9. Convulsions, 10. Peripheral neuropathy, 11. Myoclonus, 12. Muscle cramps, 13. Restless leg syndrome, 14. Coma.

Q. How do you like to investigate your case?

a. Urine examination: Urine volume is normal or low, **massive proteinuria** (24-hours urinary protein estimation is essential for diagnosis which reveals 'nephrotic range' proteinuria, i.e. >3.5 g/24 hours), normal specific gravity, shows hyaline and **fatty cast**.

b. Blood examination:

   i. Mild normocytic normochromic anaemia.

   ii. Albumin level <3 g/dL (normal level of albumin is 3.5–5.5 g/dL and that of globulin is 2–3.5 g/dL). Often the α_2 and β globulin are elevated inspite of low total globulin level.

   iii. Urea and creatinine levels are usually normal but may be elevated in renal failure.

   iv. Serum cholesterol is high and is usually >300 mg/dL (normal desirable value <200 mg/dL).

   v. Investigations for primary disease: Blood sugar, ANF, ANCA, anti-GBM antibody, HB_SAg, anti-HCV, complement C_3; selective protein clearance.

c. Chest X-ray: May show evidence of hydrothorax or pneumonitis.

d. Ultrasonography of kidneys reveal normal, small or enlarged kidney size. Kidneys in chronic glomerulonephritis are small, while diabetic and amyloid kidneys are large in size.

e. Renal biopsy: For histological diagnosis, and also in assessing the treatment and prognosis.

Q. How to diagnose that CRF has developed from nephrotic syndrome?

1. Beginning of polyuria.
2. Diminution of anasarca.
3. Appearance of hypertension.
4. Development of anaernia.
5. Specific gravity of urine: Low and fixed (1010).
6. Blood urea and creatinine levels increase.

Q. What is pulmonary-renal syndromes?

Symptom complexes like catastrophic haemoptysis and glomerulonephritis associated with varying degree of renal faiure constitute this syndrome. The causes are Goodpasture's syndrome, Wegener's granulomatosis, Churg-Strauss syndrome, microscopic polyangiitis or cryoglobulinaemia. Haemoptysis may be life-threatening; dialysis is mandatory in renal failure. Plasmapheresis and methylprednisolone are often tried.

Q. Conditions associated with hypercholesterolaemia:

1. Pregnancy.
2. Diabetes mellitus (uncontrolled).
3. Myxoedema.
4. Nephrotic syndrome.
5. Obstructive jaundice.
6. Familial hypercholesterolaemia.
7. Prolonged intake of glucocorticoids, β-blockers, thiazides and oral contraceptive pills.

Q. Overall outcome of nephrotic syndrome:

The course may vary from complete recovery to death.

1. 30% recover completely.
2. 40% may die within a year or two after relapses and remissions (due to renal failure commonly).
3. 30% pass on to chronic renal failure.

- The long-term prognosis for minimal lesion nephropathy is excellent.

Q. Common causes of chronic renal failure (CRF) in your hospital:

1. Chronic glomerulonephritis, nephrotic syndrome.
2. Malignant hypertension.
3. Diabetes mellitus.
4. Chronic pyelonephritis.
5. Polycystic kidney disease.
6. Collagen vascular diseases.
7. Obstructive uropathy.
8. Interstitial nephritis.
9. Analgesic nephropathy.
10. Renal tuberculosis.
11. Gout, multiple myeloma.
12. Renal artery stenosis.
13. Amyloidosis.

Clinical Wisdom

In a long case of chronic kidney disease (CKD), write diagnosis like: It is a patient of CRF developing from diabetes mellitus who is in stage 5, and is having continuous haemodialysis.

Q. How do you like to manage your patient (minimal lesion)?

1. To maintain an intake-output chart; intake = previous days urine output+ 500 mL.
2. High protein intake is not advised. Increased intake of protein may cause hyperfiltration in the living nephrons which may end in glomerulosclerosis and renal failure. Nowadays, modest protein restriction (e.g. 0.6 mg/kg of body weight/day) is advocated, particularly in an azotaemic patient. Dietary proteins should be of high biological value and can be supplemented by amino acids.
3. No added salt in diet, i.e. 100 mEq of sodium/day is allowed and often it may be as low as 30–50 mEq/day.

4. Diureties: Bendroflumethiazide 5–10 mg/day (in mild oedema), furosemide 80–120 mg/day or bumetanide (2–3 mg/day) or spironolactone (100–200 mg/day) in moderate oedema may be used singly or in combination (in severe oedema). The targeted weight loss should be <1 kg/day as aggressive diuretic therapy may lead to ARF or AKI as a result of contraction in intravascular volume.
5. IV salt-free abumin is given to increase the plasma oncotic pressure (a transient effect): 20 g in 100 mL is used in 1 hour. It is costly and in hospitals, 'plasma' or blood transfusion is used for this purpose.
6. Corticosteroids and cytotoxic drugs: Prednisolone 60 mg/m^2 in children and 1–1.5 mg/kg of body weight in adults is used daily for 4 weeks or until proteinuria disappears. After the urine is totally protein-free, the dose of prednisolone is gradually tapered to zero over next 4 weeks. But for those who show no response to initial 4 weeks' therapy, alternate-day prednisolone (35–40 mg/m^2 in children, 1 mg/kg in adults) for 4 additional weeks is advocated. Majority responds by the initial 4 weeks' treatment. Absence of response within 8 weeks is usually indicative of error in diagnosis and should be reviewed by a renal biopsy. Those who show relapse (within first year mainly), may be continued with low dose prednisolone, i.e. 5–10 mg daily or on alternate days for 3–6 months. Those who have frequent relapses or show side-effects with prednisolone, may be given a brief course of cyclophosphamide (1.5–2 mg/kg daily) or chlorambucil (0.1–0.2 mg/kg daily) daily for 2–3 months to induce subsequent remissions.
7. 'Statins' are used for the treatment of hyper-cholesterolaemia (e.g. atorvastatin 10 mg daily at bed time).
8. ACE inhibitors or angiotensin II receptor antagonists may be used for their anti-proteinuric properties.
9. General measures: Multivitamins, antibiotics for secondary infections (as a result of hypo-gammaglobulinaemia), paracentesis for hydrothorax or ascitic fluid, metoclopramide for nausea and vomiting, packed red cells transfusion for aneamia, long-term oral anticoagulation in renal vein thrombosis, vitamin D supplementation in biochemical evidence of deficiency.
10. Emotional and psychological support to the child and his parents.

[11. In other histological varieties: Steroids, cytotoxic drugs (cyclosporin, cyclophosphamide, etc.), anticoagulants and antiplatelet drugs are tried. Plasmapheresis is beneficial in Goodpasture's syndrome and immune complex nephritis. Dialysis is advised if the patient goes into renal failure.]

Q. Decoding of few terminologies in minimal lesion nephropathy:

1. Steroid resistant: Poor response with full dose of corticosteroid for 8 weeks.
2. Steroid dependent: When symptoms appear after withdrawal of steroid.
3. Steroid toxic: When side-effects of corticosteroid appear (like moon face, hypertension, peptic ulcer, stunted growth, behavioural changes, etc). These are the commonly encountered complications while treating rephrotic syndrome.
4. Steroid responsive: Urine is free of protein within 3–4 weeks.

 *Conclusion*

1. Always measure the BP of the patient (usually normotensive).
2. Take the H/o diabetes and hypertension routinely (past and family history).
3. Never forget to see the scrotal or vulval oedema, hydrocele, contact genital ulcers and phimosis. Examination of sacral oedema is mandatory.
4. Always percuss the urinary bladder for retention of urine (to make D/D with oligo-anuria).
5. Palpate the abdomen by 'dipping method' in the presence of ascites.
6. Examine for presence of hydrothorax (often bilateral).
7. Accurate drug history should be taken in all renal patients.

SECTION 6: LOCOMOTOR SYSTEM

The locomotor system or **rheumatology** (or musculo-skeletal system) comprises muscles, bones, joints and soft tissue structures (e.g. ligaments and tendons).

The cardinal points in the history:

1. **Chief complaints:** Onset, duration; pain and swelling of joint (arthritis) or only pain (arthralgia); axial or appendicular skeleton involved; big joints or small joints; mono-, pauci- or polyarticular involvement; fleeting, additive or intermittent arthritis; morning stiffness, limitation of joint movements, muscle weakness, any deformity, any pain during walk up and down the stairs, any associated H/o fatigue, loss of appetite, weight loss, conjunctivitis, iritis, skin rash, skin nodule, skin or oral or penile ulcer, lymphadenopathy, alopecia, dry mouth, previous miscarriage.
2. **Past H/o** trauma, tuberculosis, bacillary dysentery, bleeding diathesis, enteric fever, sore throat, sexual exposure (STD-induced arthritis or reactive arthritis), fever (non-organ specific like in RA and SLE, or organ-specific like pleurisy, nephritis), urethritis, bronchial asthma, diabetes, hypertension.
3. **Family H/o** tuberculosis, ankylosing spondylitis, haemophilia or gout; occupational history.

Scheme of Examination (Proforma)

Examination of each joint can be simply summarised as 'look, feel and move'.

A. Inspection:
  a. Mono-, pauci- or polyarticular: Joint/joints involved, 'attitude' of the limb.
  b. Swelling.
  c. Deformity (fixed or reducible; varus, valgus, ulnar, radial, flexion).
  d. Signs of inflammation over the involved joint (e.g. erythema).
  e. Wasting of muscles.
  f. Skin changes (e.g. psoriatic patch or facial butterfly rash in SLE).

B. Palpation:
  a. Temperature of the local part (↑ warmth in inflammation, e.g. synovitis).
  b. Tenderness (in joint line or periarticular); squeeze test (squeeze the hand and foot, and ask for tenderness **(Fig. 1.59A and B)**.
  c. Corroboration of the findings of inspection.
  d. Any swelling: Fluctuant or non-fluctuant; boggy feeling of thickened synovium.
  e. Tendons, ligaments, bursae, synovium and muscles around the joint.
  f. Muscle power, e.g. grip strength.

C. Movements (passive as well as active joint movements are tested for pain and range of motion):
  a. Restricted movement (i.e. range of movement—active and passive), instability or excessive mobility.
  b. Any pain on movement.
  c. Crepitus or grating sensation felt during joint movement (e.g. osteoarthiritis of knee joint).
  d. Any associated muscular spasm.

D. Measurements:
  a. Length and circumference of the limb.
  b. Measurement in relation to various body points.
  c. Thoracic ankylosis by chest expansion measurement and lumbar ankylosis by Schober's test.
  d. To measure the range of joint movement with the help of goniometer.

E. Examination of the **spine** for tenderness, mobility, kyphoscoliosis, lordosis, gibbus. Spine movement (e.g. in SpA): Cervical—occiput to wall distance (normally occiput touches the wall), thoracic—expansion of chest, lumbar—Schober's test

F. Gait.

G. Systemic examination (with functional assessment of joint): To search for evidences of pleurisy, pericarditis, vasculitis, iritis, hepatosplenomegaly, aortic incompetence or lymphadenopathy.

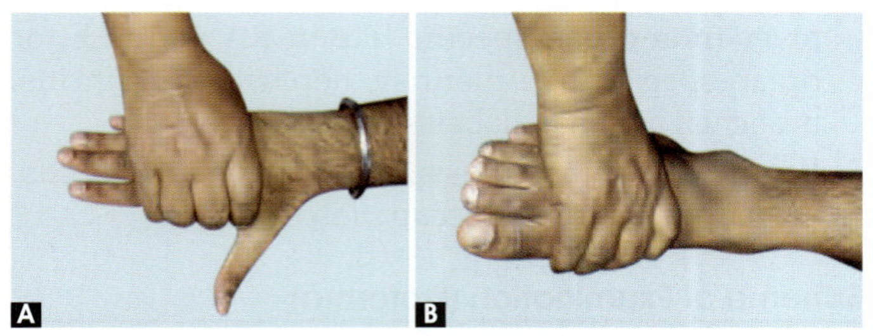

Fig. 1.59A and B: MCP **Squeeze test** (A) and MTP Squeeze test (B)

- **Schober's test (Fig. 1.60A and B)**: It is performed to make out flexion movement of lumbar spine. The patient stands erect. Give two skin marks at the back in the midline, one 10 cm above and the other 5 cm below the lumbosacral junction (lumbosacral junction is marked by a horizontal line joining the 'Dimple of venus' on the sacral promontory). On full forward flexion, these marks distract >5 cm (i.e. >20 cm from upper to lower line) but no distraction of skin marks is seen in ankylosing spondylitis.
  In modified Schober's test, only the upper marking is taken (as the lower part, lumbosacral junction remains fixed). So, on full forward flexion, distance between two lines will be >15 cm; if <15 cm, it indicates restricted movement of lumbar spine.
- Read gout, different arthritis like rheumatic, rheumatoid, septic and osteoarthritis from standard textbooks. Vide the sections on 'Aortic stenosis', 'Examination of the hands' and 'Charcot joint' too.

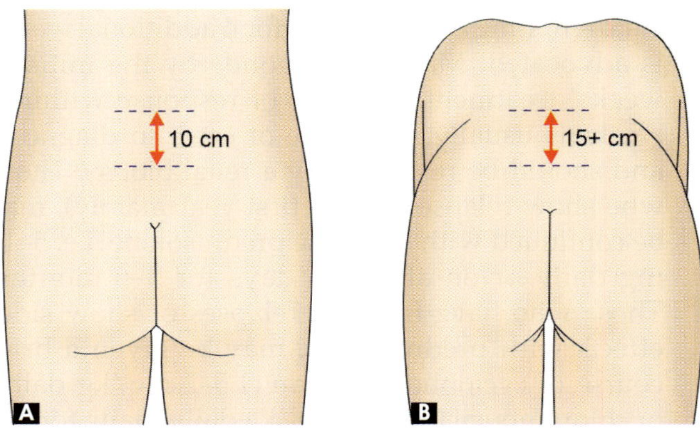

Fig. 1.60A and B: **Modified Schober's test** [A] and [B]

POLYARTHRITIS — CASE 22

Q. Clinical pressentation:

A middle-aged female presents with H/o long-duration of joint pain, disability and deformity. She has bilaterally symmetrical involvement of small as well as large joints with active synovitis in few joints, along with deformities of hands and feet. It is an additive arthritis of peripheral joints while the axial joints are not affected. So, *it is a chronic symmetrical inflammatory polyarthritis with deformity.*

The most probable provisional diagnosis is rheumatoid arthritis.

Q. How to approach in a patient of musculoskeletal (MSK) disorder?

Pain is the commonest manifestation and a near universal feature of MSK disorders. Since a wide variety of conditions give rise to MSK complaints (i.e. arthralgia, myalgia, or bone pain), a systemic approach is necessary to make a provisional diagnosis. A careful history, meticulous clinical examination and judicious use of laboratory investigations help to arrive at a definitive diagnosis. The approach should be **(Flowchart 1.2)**:

Flowchart 1.2: Stratification of MSK diseases

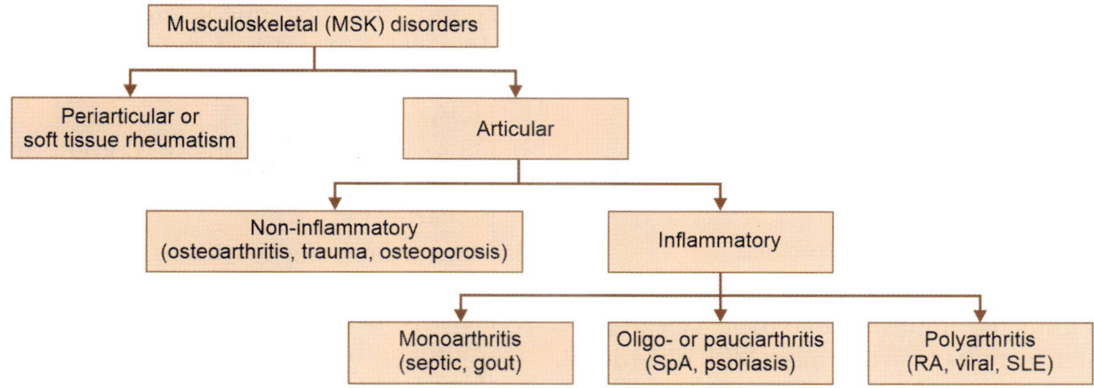

- **Decoding of few terminology:** RA: Rheumatoid arthritis, SpA: Spondyloarthropathy, ReA: Reactive arthritis, SLE: Systemic lupus erythematosus, OA: Osteoarthritis, CRP: C-reactive protein, ANA: Antinuclear antibodies, RF: Rheumatoid factor, MCP: Metacarpophalangeal, MTP: Metatarsophalangeal, PIP: Proximal interphalangeal, DIP: Distal interphalangeal, DMARDs: Disease-modifying anti-rheumatic drugs, NSAIDS: Non-steroidal anti-inflammatory drugs, TNF-α: Tumour necrosis factor-alpha.

Q. Characteristics of inflammatory joint disorders:

Inflammatory joint disorders (RA, SpA, ReA) will have:

1. Significant early morning stiffness >30 minutes.
2. Pain aggravation on resting the joints.
3. Symptomatic improvement on gentle use of joints.
4. Spontaneous flares (up-and-down course) are common.
5. Constitutional symptoms: Fatigue, loss of appetite, weight loss, low-grade fever, night sweats.
6. Increased acute phase reactants, e.g. high ESR and CRP.

- In non-inflammatory disorders, from No. 1 to 6, respectively they are <30 minutes, pain on moving the joints, no improvement, uncommon, absent, and normal acute phase reactants.

Q. What is soft tissue rheumatism (STR)?

'Soft tissue rheumatism' is a term restricted to inflammatory or painful conditions which are, in general, non-articular in origin, and refers to aches or pains arising from structures surrounding the joint such as muscles, tendons, ligaments and bursae. This group accounts for the major chunk of musculoskeletal disorders in any general outpatient clinic.

The anatomical basis of pain in MSK system could be due to:

Joint:

- Synovium: Synovitis
- Joint capsule: Capsulitis

Periarticular soft tissue:

- Bursa: Bursitis
- Tendon: Tendonitis
- Tendon sheath: Tenosynovitis
- Insertion of tendon, ligament: Enthesitis

Bone:

- Osteoporosis, osteomalacia, multiple myeloma, osteonecrosis.

Q. Differentiation of articular from non-articular/periarticular disorders?

A careful clinical examination should be performed to differentiate soft tissue rheumatism (i.e. periarticular disorders) from articular disorders. Bedside examination should follow:

1. Inspection: 'local' swelling around a joint (periarticular) favours STR rather than articular disorders whereas the joint (articular) swelling looks globular or fusiform surrounding a joint.
2. Palpation: In STR, tenderness is localised and usually away from joint-line margin. Articular disorders are conspicuous by the presence of joint-line tenderness, crepitus over the joint and/or joint effusion.
3. Movements: Active (the patient moves the joint) and passive (the physician moves the joint while the patient relaxes the limb) movements are equally impaired in articular disorders. In STR, pain is aggravated on active than on passive movement, and limitation of motion is always greater in active movement rather than passive one.
4. Dramatic relief of pain with local injection of corticosteroid in STR or periarticular diseases.

Q. Common types of soft tissue rheumatism:

The common examples are:

- Shoulder: Frozen shoulder, rotator cuff syndrome, bicipital tendonitis
- Elbow (epicondylitis): Tennis elbow, golfer's elbow
- Bursitis: Pre- and infrapatellar bursitis, olecranon bursitis, trochanteric bursitis
- Tenosynovitis: de Quervain's tenosynovitis
- Entrapment syndromes: Carpal tunnel syndrome (median nerve), tarsal tunnel syndrome (posterior tibial nerve), meralgia paraesthetica (lateral femoral cutaneous nerve)

Q. Disease differentiation by nature of pain:

- Pain on use: Worse on usage and relieved by rest (e.g. mechanical strain, osteoarthritis)
- Rest pain: Worse after rest and improved by movement (e.g. inflammatory arthritis like RA)
- Nocturnal pain: Commonly at night and poorly related to movement (e.g. of 'bone' origin)

Q. Pattern recognition in MSK disorders:

Pattern recognition in MSK disorders or rheumatological diseases is of immense importance to have a clean-cut diagnosis. Often features of two or more MSK disorders are present in a single patient to build up a diagnosis of 'overlap syndrome'. If the pattern of involvement is not recognized clinically, it is very difficult to clinch a diagnosis of rheumatological disease only by ordering of RF, ANA, autoantibodies or other immunological markers. Ask the patient about:

1. Mode of onset: Acute or insidious.
2. Duration of joint pain: Acute (<6 weeks) or chronic (>6 weeks).
3. Number of joints affected: Monoarthritis, oligo- or pauciarthritis, polyarthritis.
4. Pattern of involvement: Axial (spine, sacroiliac, anterior chest wall, and shoulder and hip joint) or appendicular (peripheral joints), or overlap. Shoulder and hip joint are known as root joints.
5. Distribution of joint involvement: Symmetrical or asymmetrical, small or large joint, lower limbs or upper limbs, involvement of any specific joint (e.g. first metatarsophalangeal joint in gout, haemarthrosis of knee joint in haemophilia, DIP joints of hands in osteoarthritis).
6. Order or sequence of affection: Intermittent (gout or relapsing polychondritis) or progressive (classical RA), migratory (rheumatic arthritis, SLE, serum sickness) or additive (RA, ReA).
7. Pain worse by activity and eased by rest (mechanical strain, osteoarthritis) or worse after rest (inflammatory arthritis). Whether deformities present or not.
8. Extra-articular manifestations: Constitutional symptoms (e.g. fever, weight loss), anaemia, skin rash, subcutaneous nodule, oral ulcer, conjunctivitis or episcleritis, penile ulcer, nail changes (e.g. psoriasis), pleural effusion (e.g. SLE) or Raynaud's phenomenon (e.g. scleroderma).

Clinical Wisdom

Diagnostic format in rheumatology: Includes No. 1–8 above (i.e. acute or chronic, inflammatory or non-inflammatory, mono-/oligo-/polyarthritis, symmetrical or asymmetrical, axial or appendicular, and with or without extra-articular manifestations) *plus* disease activity (i.e. DAS 28 score).

Q. Possible causes of polyarthritis, oligoarthritis and monoarthritis:

a. Polyarthritis: RA, viral arthritis (Parvovirus B19, hepatitis B and C, HIV, chikungunya), SLE, psoriasis, juvenile idiopathic arthritis (JIA), ReA, ankylosing spondylitis, systemic sclerosis, adult-onset Still's disease, generalized osteoarthritis, rheumatic arthritis, chronic gout, sarcoidosis (chronic) and HOA.
b. Oligo- or pauciarthritis: JIA, gout, SpA, psoriatic arthropathy, OA, oligoarticular presentation of polyarthritis.
c. Monoarthritis: Septic arthritis (*S. aureus*, *N. gonorrhoeae*), crystal arthropathy (gout and pseudogout) (Fig. 1.61A and B), tuberculous arthritis, osteoarthritis (OA), SpA, traumatic, haemarthrosis (e.g. trauma, haemophilia) (Fig. 1.62), monoarticular flare of polyarticular disease, palindromic RA, Charcot joint.

- **Few terminology: Arthralgia:** Joint pain without obvious inflammation (i.e. only pain, no swelling)—**arthritis** pain and swelling in the joints, i.e. demonstrable features of inflammation; monoarthritis—affection of single joint, oligo- or pauciarthritis—affection of 2–4 joints, **polyarthritis**—involvement of 5 or more joints, synovitis—clinically apparent inflammation of synovium, enthesopathy/enthesitis—inflammation of an enthesis (i.e. the site of ligament, tendon, or articular capsule insertion into periosteum and bone),

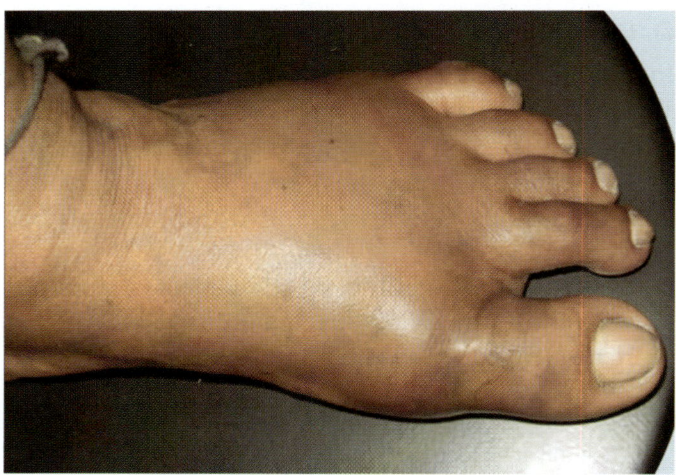

Fig. 1.61A: Swelling of left first metatarsophalangeal joint in **acute gout**—red, hot, swollen, painful joint with shiny overlying skin

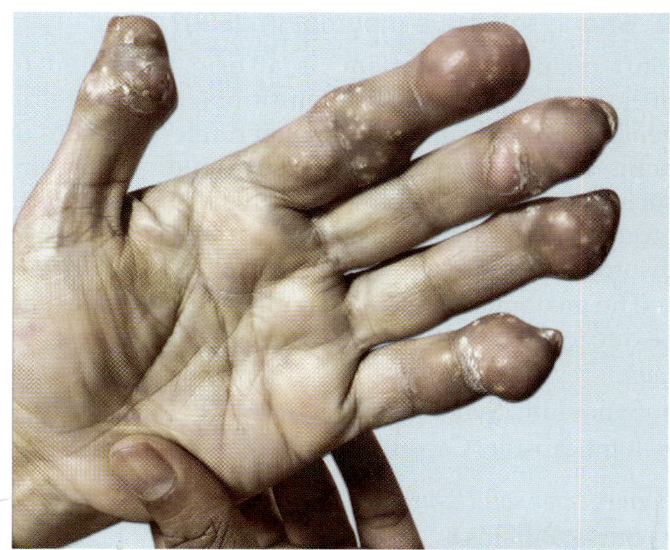

Fig. 1.61B: **Chronic** tophaceous **gout** in hand

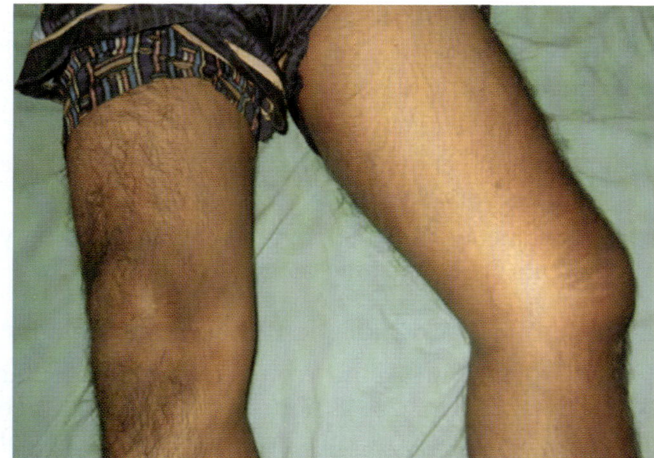

Fig. 1.62: Muscle haematoma (left thigh) and monoarthritis of left knee joint in **haemophilia**

periarthritis—involvement of joint capsule and other structures like ligament, tendon, bursa; **GALS screen** (**G**lobal **A**ssessment of **L**ocomotor **S**ystem): It is a quick reliable screen of gait, arms, legs and spine of the locomotor system.

Q. Small and large joint involvement in MSK diseases:

a. Small joint arthropathy: RA, SLE, ReA, gout, nodular osteoarthritis, psoriasis, enteropathic arthritis (i.e. associated with inflammatory bowel disease or IBD, i.e. ulcerative colitis and Crohn's disease), sarcoidosis.
b. Large joint arthropathy: RA, ReA, ankylosing spondylitis, rheumatic arthritis, generalised osteoarthritis, psoriatic and enteropathic arthritis.
c. Both large and small joints arthropathy: RA, SpA, osteoarthritis.

Q. Symmetrical versus asymmetrical involvement:

Symmetrical involvement refers to affection of same joints on both the sides though it may not be mirror-image symmetry. For example, involvement of left-sided 2nd and 3rd, and right-sided 2nd and 4th MCP joints of hands in RA is deemed symmetrical involvement of MCP joints.

a. Symmetrical: RA, SLE, PSS, nodular osteoarthritis of hands, JIA and haemochromatosis.
b. Asymmetrical: Gout, SpA, metabolic arthropathy (acromegaly).

- Psoriasis may be symmetric or asymmetric at presentation.

Q. Arthritis in relation to age and sex of the patient:

A. Age:
   a. Children: JIA (juvenile idiopathic arthritis), haemophilia, trauma.
   b. Adolescents: RA, SPA, JIA, trauma, poststreptococcal reactive arthritis.
   c. Young: Trauma, gonococcal.
   d. Adults: SpA, ReA, SLE, psoriasis, gout.
   e. Middle age: RA, gout, osteoarthritis, scleroderma.
   f. Old age: Osteoarthritis, polymyalgia rheumatica.

B. Sex: Majority of arthritides are dominant in females except gout, ankylosing spondylitis, ReA (Reiter's syndrome) and polyarteritis nodosa which are common in males.

Q. Possible causes of fleeting or migratory arthritis:

Here, arthritis shifts from one joint to another after remission of the existing joint's inflammation.

1. Rheumatic arthritis (commonest).
2. SLE.
3. Drug reaction/serum sickness.
4. Arthritis following gonococcal or meningococcal bacteraemia; brucellosis.
5. Viral arthritis (Lyme arthritis, chikungunya).
6. Arthritis associated with inflammatory bowel disease or Whipple's disease.
7. 'Seroconversion' phase in AIDS.
8. Septicaemia.
9. Following intestinal by-pass surgery.
10. Sarcoidosis.

Q. Define rheumatoid arthritis and criteria for its diagnosis:

Rheumatoid arthritis is an autoimmune disorder of unknown aetiology characterized by chronic symmetrical polyarthritis, joint erosions and destruction. It is the commonest inflammatory joint disease seen in clinical practice, and in its world-wide distribution it affects 0.5–1% of the population. The course is extremely variable and sometimes associated with extra-articular features. RA is notorious for development of joint deformities, especially the small joints of hands and feet. The age of onset is commonly in between 30–50 years, and in gender predilection F: M = 3:1 before menopause while F:M = 1:1 post-menopause. RA was previously diagnosed by **ACR criteria** (American College of Rheumatology, 1987 revision).

- Read new criteria (2010) made by ACR and EULAR (European League Against Rheumatism) for diagnosis of RA, from any standard textbook. These criteria are based on four parameters like number of joint involvement, serology (RF and ACPA), acute phase reactants (CRP and ESR) and duration of symptoms (<6 weeks or >6 weeks).
- Other common **autoimmune disorders** are Hashimoto's thyroiditis, Graves' disease, Addison's disease, SLE, myasthenia gravis, pernicious anaemia, type 1 diabetes, vitiligo, pemphigus vulgaris and scleroderma.

Q. How a patient of rheumatoid arthritis presents?

A patient of RA (prototype of inflammatory polyarthritis) usually presents with:

1. Aches and pains in the joints.
2. Insidious onset of polyarthritis.
3. Prolonged early morning stiffness.
4. Bilaterally symmetrical involvement.
5. Small joints of hands (and feet) are always involved in addition to large joint involvement. In small joints

of hand (and feet), MCP (MTP) and PIP joints are commonly involved; DIP joints are spared in RA. Large joints commonly involved are wrists, elbows, shoulders, knees and ankles.

6. Signs of inflammation may be seen in joints in the early part of the disease, e.g. swelling (synovitis), erythema, warmth, and pain and tenderness.
7. As the disease progresses, deformity of hand and foot joints may develop in the absence of treatment.
8. The patient may suffer from different **extra-articular manifestations** along with joint involvement. There may be systemic (fever, loss of appetite, weight loss, fatigue), musculoskeletal (tenosynovitis, bursitis, wasting of muscles), dermatological (nodules, pyoderma gangrenosum, leg ulcer, vasculitis) (Fig. 1.63), pulmonary (pleural effusion, bronchiolitis, fibrosing alveolitis, pulmonary nodules, Caplan's syndrome, tuberculosis from DMARD therapy), cardiac (pericarditis, myocarditis, endocarditis, aortic regurgitation, conduction defects), ophthalmic (episcleritis, scleritis, keratoconjunctivitis sicca, scleromalacia), neurological (mononeuritis multiplex, cervical cord compression, entrapment neuropathy, peripheral neuropathy), lymphoreticular (anaemia, eosinophilia, thrombocytosis, Felty's syndrome, splenomegaly), and miscellaneous (Raynaud's phenomenon, amyloidosis, dry mouth, lymphadenopathy) involvement.

Q. A 'must' to remember in diagnosing rheumatoid arthritis:

A clinician should always remember that RA is:

- Entirely a clinical diagnosis.
- Typically bilaterally symmetrical.

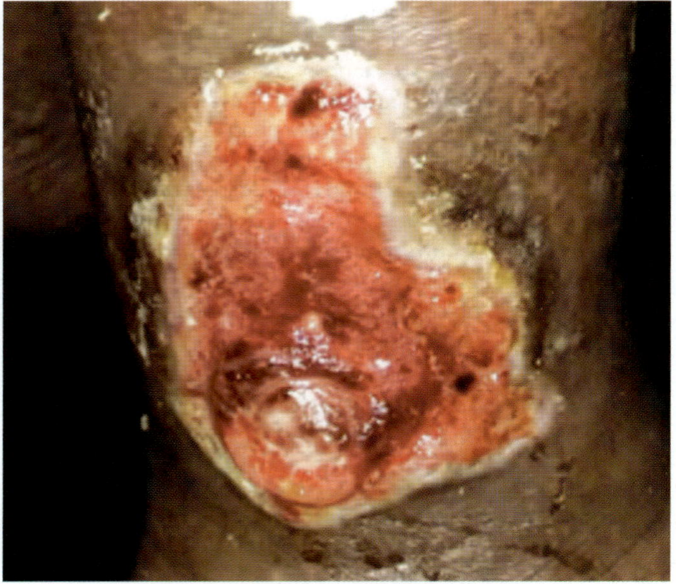

Fig. 1.63: **Pyoderma gangrenosum**—chronic painful necrotic ulcer with under-mined purplish border, commonly in legs; usually associated with ulcerative colitis, rheumatoid arthritis, multiple myeloma and immunodeficiency (HIV disease)

- Classically presents as polyarthritis (may present as oligoarthritis rarely).
- Do not diagnose if hands are not involved.
- DIP joint involvement is extremely rare.
- Lumbar spine is not involved in RA; cervical spine affection is very rare.
- Mucocutaneous rash, high pyrexia and active urinary sediments are against the diagnosis.

Q. 'Palindromic' and 'malignant' rheumatoid arthritis:

- Palindromic RA: Acute recurrent monoarticular attacks lasting for 24–48 hours with symptom-free interval for days to months between attacks; 50% of them progress to other types of RA.
- Malignant RA: Severe and progressive disease associated with systemic features, severe extra-articular manifestations and vasculitis.

Q. What is 'early' rheumatoid arthritis and what is its importance?

It is the early disease having duration of persistent synovitis of around 3 months to 2 years. Different studies show that 10–26% patients of RA have radiographic bone erosion at 3 months, while 60% have it at 1 year, and 75% within 2 years. Unfortunately, bony erosions and deformities are largely irreversible. Hence, early disease represents a potential 'window of opportunity' for therapeutic interventions with DMARD, which has shown beneficial short and long-term effects. So, present day goal is to diagnose RA as early as possible, i.e. 'catch them young'. Early RA is diagnosed by RF, antibodies to cyclic citrullinated peptide (anti-CCP), high resolution ultrasonography (USG) with colour and power Doppler, and MRI scan of joints along with suggestive clinical features.

Q. Describe different hand deformities in rheumatoid arthritis:

Read the section on 'Examination of the hands'.

Q. What is 'seronegative spondyloarthropathy' (SpA)?

These are group of inflammatory joint diseases which are characterised by inflammatory low back pain in addition to peripheral arthritis. They suffer from asymmetrical oligoarthritis (lower limb affected more than upper limb), sacroiliitis and inflammatory spondylitis. There may have a positive family history and an **association with HLA-B27** allele. The rheumatoid factor is always negative (seronegative). SpA encompasses 5 disorders like:

1. Ankylosing spondylitis (prototype of SpA).
2. Reactive arthritis (including Reiter's syndrome).
3. Psoriatic arthropathy.
4. Arthritis associated with inflammatory bowel disease (enteropathic arthritis), and
5. Undifferentiated SpA.

- The sixth group (according to some rheumatologists) is juvenile-onset SpA. Non-radiographic axial spondyloarthritis is a new entity.

Q. Differentiate arthritis according to serology:

a. Seropositive (RF positive): Sjögren's syndrome, RA (70%), Felty's syndrome, SLE, polymyositis-dermatomyositis, systemic sclerosis, MCTD, sarcoidosis, vasculitis (polyarteritis nodosa). The higher the titre of RF, the more severe is the disease.
b. Seronegative (RF negative): SpA (the whole group), gout, osteoarthritis, juvenile idiopathic arthritis (JIA; majority are RF negative), RA (30%), rheumatic arthritis, Still's disease.

- RF: Rheumatoid factors are antibodies (IgM immunoglobulin commonly) against the Fc portion of IgG.
- RF is also positive in certain non-rheumatic diseases like fibrosing alveolitis, leprosy, tuberculosis, infectious mononucleosis, syphilis, kala-azar, chronic hepatitis, infective endocarditis, cryoglobulinaemia, malignancy, and in normal population (5–20% women aged above 65 years).

Q. Polyarthritis affecting hands—pattern of involvement:

1. Rheumatoid arthritis: MCP, PIP but spares DIP.
2. Osteoarthritis: DIP but spares MCP; affects 1st carpometacarpal joint (base of the thumb).
3. Psoriatic arthropathy: Commonly DIP.
4. Chronic gout: MCP, interphalangial joints.
5. SLE: MCP joints commonly (Jaccoud's arthritis).

- **DIP joints in hands** are affected in osteoarthritis (Heberden's node), psoriasis, scleroderma, sarcoidosis, gout and adult-onset Still's disease.
- **PIP joints in hands** are affected in RA, SLE, scleroderma and osteoarthritis (Bouchard's node).
- **MCP joints** are commonly involved in RA, SLE, scleroderma and haemochromatosis.

Clinical Wisdom

Osteoarthritis (OA): It is the commonest form of arthritis in clinical practice which is regarded as a degenerative process due to old age. OA is a non-inflammatory, painful, slowly progressive disease which usually affects the cartilage. It commonly affects hands (see above), knee, hip and spine (cervical and lumbar spondylosis).

Q. Rheumatic disorders with subcutaneous nodule formation:

Rheumatoid arthritis (commonest), rheumatic fever, erythema nodosum, gout (tophi), SLE, sarcoidosis (granuloma) and xanthoma (from hyperlipidaemia).

Q. Rheumatic diseases with oral and genital ulcerations:

Behcet's syndrome, Reiter's syndrome (reactive arthritis), Crohn's disease, SLE (oral ulcer only).

Q. Rheumatic disorders with skin rash:

SLE, psoriasis, dermatomyositis, Still's disease, sarcoidosis, Henoch-Schönlein purpura, viral infection (rubella or chikungunya), rheumatic fever, leprosy and reactive arthritis.

Q. Skin changes in rheumatological disorders:

Hard skin (scleroderma), palpable purpura (vasculitis), heliotrope rash (dermatomyositis), livedo reticularis (APS), pyoderma gangrenosum (RA), keratoderma blennorrhagica (reactive arthritis), nodules (RA), digital gangrene (Raynaud's phenomenon, vasculitis), salt-pepper appearance (scleroderma), Gottron's papules (dermatomyositis), etc.

Q. Arthritis associated with cardiac murmurs:

Rheumatic fever, ankylosing spondylitis, RA, SBE, SLE with Libman-Sacks endocarditis, cardiac myxoma.

Q. Arthritis in haematological disorders:

Haemophilia, sickle cell disease, multiple myeloma, leukaemias.

Q. Arthritis with diarrhoea:

Inflammatory bowel disease (enteropathic arthritis), enterogenic (bacterial) reactive arthritis, coeliac disease, Whipple's disease.

Q. Arthritis with lymphadenopathy:

Still's disease, SLE, sarcoidosis and brucellosis.

Q. Rheumatic disorders with nail changes:

Pitting and onycholysis (psoriasis), splinter haemorrhages (vasculitis) and clubbing (interstitial lung disease developing from RA).

Q. Specific eye changes in rheumatic diseases:

Conjunctivitis in Reiter's syndrome, episcleritis and scleritis in RA, uveitis in ankylosing spondylitis (Fig. 1.64), iridocyclitis in JIA and scleromalacia perforans in RA.

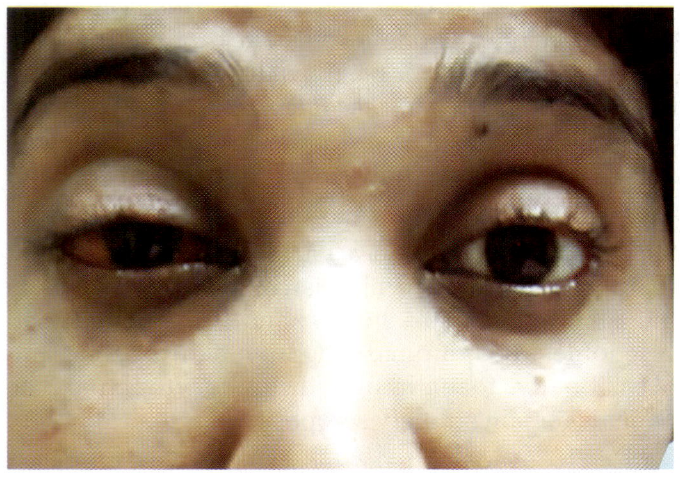

Fig. 1.64: **Uveitis** in ankylosing spondylitis

Q. Rheumatic diseases with involvement of eye:

Spondyloarthropathy, rheumatoid arthritis, Sjögren's syndrome (xerophthalmia), vasculitis, Wegener's granulomatosis, sarcoidosis, Behçet's syndrome, giant cell arteritis, Takayasu's arteritis.

- **A must to examine in rheumatic diseases:** Skin, eyes, nails, oral cavity and mucous membrane.

Q. Overnight joint swelling is seen in:

Haemophilia, trauma and gonococcal arthritis.

Q. 'Stooped posture' (increased thoracic kyphosis) in clinical medicine:

1. Ankylosing spondylitis.
2. Parkinsonism.
3. Osteoporosis of spine with collapse (widow's stoop).

Q. 'Bone deformities' encountered in clinical practice:

1. Developmental and inherited disorders.
2. Malunion of fracture.
3. Rickets.
4. Rheumatoid arthritis, psoriasis.
5. Osteoporosis.
6. Osteogenesis imperfecta.

- Sausage digits (dactylitis)—SpA (especially, ReA), gout (polyarticular) and sarcoidosis.

Q. What are Reiter's syndrome, Felty's syndrome, Still's disease and Caplan's syndrome?

Reiter's syndrome: In the year 1916, Hans Reiter, the physician leader of the Nazi party in Germany during World War II, first described this syndrome. At present, the older term Reiter's syndrome is being used less frequently, and has been replaced by 'reactive arthritis'. The *classical triad of urethritis, conjunctivitis and arthritis* following a gastrointestinal (mainly *Salmonella, Shigella, Campylobacter, Yersinia*-induced) or genitourinary infection (non-gonococcal urethritis or sexually acquired infection with *Chlamydia*), previously referred to as Reiter's syndrome, is now considered part of the spectrum of reactive arthritis. The extra-articular manifestations are circinate balanitis (painless superficial ulceration of glans penis), keratoderma blennorrhagica (painless, red, raised pustules and plaques in sole of feet and palmar surface of hands), nail dystrophy (onycholysis and hyperkeratosis) and buccal erosions.

Felty's syndrome: It is a variety of long-standing rheumatoid arthritis which is common in females in the age group of 50–70 years, and is associated with splenomegaly, lymphadenopathy, neutropenia, and occasionally anaemia and thrombocytopenia. The patients remain strongly seropositive.

Still's disease: This is the seronegative variant of RA in children, which also occurs rarely in young adults. The presenting features are high rise of swinging pyrexia associated with evanescent maculopapular rash, arthralgia and arthritis, myalgia and generalised lymphadenopathy. Hepatosplenomegaly and pleurisy/pericarditis are also evident. Anaemia, neutrophilia, thrombocytosis with high ESR and CRP are common. Serum ferritin may be enormously elevated in adult-onset Still's disease.

Caplan's syndrome: This is the coexistence of seropositive rheumatoid arthritis and pneumoconiosis of the lung (shows rounded fibrotic nodules 0.5–5.0 cm in diameter in lung). It is seen in coal miners suffering from RA, along with cough, breathlessness and haemoptysis.

Q. Common laboratory findings in rheumatoid arthritis:

No tests are specific for RA; however, following tests are commonly performed:

1. Anaemia (normocytic normochromic), eosinophilia, thrombocytosis.
2. Raised ESR and CRP. Plasma viscosity is also increased.
3. RF is positive in approximately 70% patients (ANA is positive at low titre in 30%).
4. Positive antibodies to cyclic citrullinated peptide (anti-CCP) or anti-citrullinated peptide antibody (ACPA) having high specificity (90–98%); commonly done in seronegative patients to confirm the diagnosis.
5. Acute phase response: High ferritin, reversed albumin globulin ratio, moderate elevation of alkaline phosphatase. Raised ESR and CRP are also acute phase responses.
6. Radiology: Early RA may show only soft tissue swelling in X-ray. Stages of radiological (X-ray) progression in RA are periarticular osteopenia, marginal erosions, loss of articular cartilage, and subluxation or ankylosis. High resolution USG with colour and power Doppler picks up synovitis, effusion and erosion earlier than conventional X-ray. The MRI scan exhibit bone marrow oedema, synovitis and tendonitis. USG and MRI are rarely performed.
7. Joint fluid study (in effusion): This is rarely performed. Due to presence of white cells, the aspirate often looks cloudy.

Q. Common investigations performed in rheumatological disorders:

1. Full blood count (including platelet count).
2. ESR and CRP.
3. Unine for R/E (protein, RBC, cast) and special test (Bence Jones protein).
4. Rheumatoid factor (a titre >1: 40 or unit value >20 U is considered positive, although this may vary with methods used). It is Rose-Waaler test.
5. Anti-CCP or ACPA.

6. Antinuclear antibody (ANA) or antinuclear factor (ANF): A titre >1: 80 is usually considered positive using HEp-2 cell lines (i.e. human epithelial type-2; HEp-2000 substrate may be used).
7. Anti-ds DNA (for SLE).
8. Anti-extractable nuclear antigen (ENA) antibodies: Anti-histone, anti-Sm, anti-Ro, anti-La, anti-U_1 RNP, anti-Jo, anti-topoisomerase 1, anti-centromere antibody.
9. Anti-neutrophil cytoplasmic antibody (ANCA). Commonly c-ANCA (antibodies directed against PR-3) and p-ANCA (antibodies directed against MPO) are estimated.
10. Antiphospholipid antibody.
11. Complement, immune complexes.
12. Others: Ca, PO_4, alkaline phosphatase, PTH, 25-OH vitamin D, creatinine kinase (CK).
13. ASO titre, serum uric acid, serum ferritin (↑ in adult-onset Still's disease) and protein electrophoresis.
14. HLA-B27 assay.
15. Radiology (X-ray, USG, CT, MRI, bone scintigraphy, DEXA scan for BMD, PET scan).
16. Synovial fluid analysis.
17. Arthroscopy.
18. EMG and NCV.
19. Viral titres against parvovirus, chikungunya or coxsackievirus.
20. Biopsy: Synovium, temporal artery, sural nerve (for vasculitis), bone (iliac crest for renal osteodystrophy or osteomalacia), lip minor salivary gland (for Sjögren's syndrome) and muscle (deltoid or quadriceps).

Q. How the disease activity is monitored in rheumatoid arthritis?

This is assessed by:

1. Duration of early morning stiffness (measured by minutes).
2. Visual analogue scale for general health (e.g. pain) as subjectively estimated by the patient.
3. Global assessment by observer as well as patient.
4. Joint count (number of swollen and tender joints).
5. Acute phase response: ESR and CRP.
6. NSAID pill count (i.e. number of analgesics consumed by the patient).
7. DAS (disease activity score): A complex formula encompassing four criteria, i.e. 28 tender joint count, 28 swollen joint count, ESR, and general health assessment by the patient on a visual analogue scale (VAS) from 0 to 100 (i.e. **DAS 28 score)**. It is measured by a DAS calculator.

   The 28 joints are 20 in hand joints (MCPs and PIPs), 2 each for shoulder, elbow, wrist and knee joints. DAS score: >5.1: high disease activity, 3.2–5.1: moderate disease activity, 2.6–3.2: low disease activity and <2.6: disease remission.

Q. Common imaging modalities done in musculoskeletal disorders:

1. X-ray: To demonstrate fracture, bony erosion, osteophytes, ankylosis, etc.
2. Ultrasonography: To visualize soft tissue/periarticular structures/tendon, Baker's cyst, rotator cuff tear, thickened Achilles tendon. USG also guides local injections.
3. Radionuclide scintigraphy: ^{99m}Tc-bisphosphonate (used to see bone turnover, i.e. metastases, bone tumour, Paget's disease); ^{67}-gallium and ^{111}-indium scans are occasionally used to localize infections.
4. CT scan: For sacroiliitis, prolapsed intervertebral disc, trauma to the spine, etc.
5. MRI scan: To visualize vessel, nerve, fascia, muscle, cartilage, ligament, synovial effusion, bone marrow oedema (e.g. early RA or early sacroiliitis). Commonly used in spinal cord compression, prolapsed intervertebral disc, early avascular necrosis, etc.
6. PET scan: Useful in diagnosis of Takayasu's arteritis.
7. Bone mineral density (BMD) measurement: Dual energy X-ray absorptiometry (DEXA) is the current method of choice to diagnose osteopenia and osteoporosis (T-score and Z-score). T-score in BMD may be above –1.0 (normal), lie between –1.0 and –2.5 (osteopenia), or falls to –2.5 or below (osteoporosis).

Q. Outline of management of rheumatoid arthritis:

The treatment paradigms of RA have shifted much from the past. In the past, traditional pyramidal approach (empirical) was go slow, go low but the present era is for early and universal use of DMARDs (evidence-based) though the future is waiting (hopefully, we have reached) for combination therapy with DMARDS and biological agents (mechanism-based). Treatment needs coordination of a team of medical specialists (rheumatologist, orthopedic surgeon, physiatrist, physiotherapist, social worker, trained nurse, occupational therapist) who deliver an integrated programme of multidisciplinary care and rehabilitation. The **goal** is achieved by drugs, rest, physiotherapy, surgery, aids and appliances, and occupational and social services.

Aim of treatment: Relief of symptoms, restoration of function and control of systemic involvement. Different **modalities of management** are:

I. Pharmacological:
   a. NSAIDs (for relief of pain): Used as and when necessary.
   b. Corticosteroids (for 'bridge therapy' before the onset of action of DMARDs, in rheumatoid flare, for extra-articular manifestations, and pregnancy).
   c. DMARDS: Commonly used drugs are sulphasalazine, hydroxychloroquine, methotrexate (Fig. 1.65) and leflunomide. Less frequently

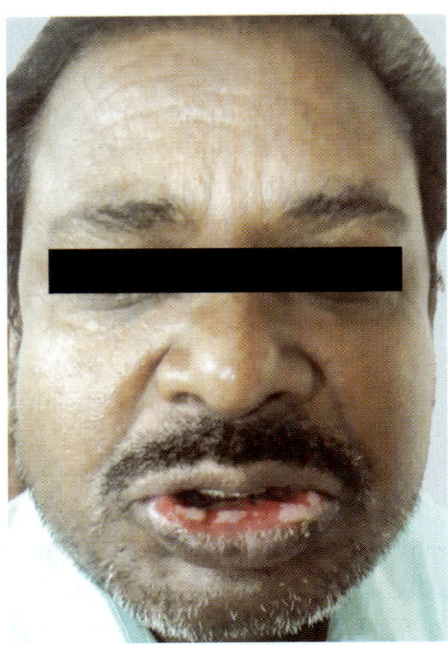

Fig. 1.65: **Stomatitis** following methotrexate overdose in treatment of rheumatoid arthritis

used drugs are iguratimod, azathioprine, gold (oral and parenteral), cyclosporine A, chloroquine, cyclophosphamide, D-penicillamine, minocycline, chlorambucil and levamizole; except azathioprine and cyclosporine A, others are not in use now.

d. Biological response modifiers (biologics): These are genetically engineered treatment which basically acts by blocking TNF-α. Biologics are very costly and often out of reach of common people. The commonly used agents are etanercept (in psoriasis), infliximab (in SpA) and adalimumab (in SpA and RA). Rituximab (causes lysis of CD-20 B cells), tocilizumab (intuleukin-6 angatonist) and abatacept are promising in RA. The effect of Janus kinase (JAK) inhibitors like tofacitinib (oral) is very encouraging.

II. Surgical: Decompression (in carpal tunnel syndrome), synovectomy, osteotomy, arthrodesis, arthroplasty, replacement of joints, joint fixation (atlanto-axial subluxation), etc.

SECTION 7: LYMPHORETICULAR SYSTEM

The cardinal symptoms of lymphoreticular system are:

1. Painless or painful enlargement of lymph nodes.
2. Pallor (resulting in weakness, palpitations, postural dizziness, ankle oedema, lassitude, anorexia, lightheadedness, breathlessness, etc.).
3. Dragging pain or heaviness in the left hypochondrium (e.g. massive splenomegaly).
4. Haemorrhagic spots (e.g. petechiae, purpura, etc.) in the mucous membrane or skin
5. Epistaxis, gum bleeding, menorrhagia, haemarthrosis, H/o prolonged bleeding.
6. Bone pain (multiple myeloma, acute leukaemia) and joint pain (Henoch-Schönlein purpura).
7. Jaundice (e.g. haemolysis).
8. Recurrent respiratory tract infections (due to impaired immunity).
9. Loss of body weight.
10. Mass in the abdomen (abdominal lymphoma).
11. Sore throat (agranulocytosis), non-healing wounds (leucopenia).
12. Fever (leukaemia, lymphoma, neutropenia, infection with immunosuppression).
13. Skin rash, urticaria (e.g. polycythemia vera).
14. Paraesthesia (e.g. vitamin B_{12} deficiency), palpitations or anginal pain (from anaemia).

Scheme of Examination (Proforma)

This system is also known as **haemopoietic system** or **reticulo-endothelial system**.

1. Anaemia (it is better to examine the patient for jaundice too).
2. Haemorrhagic manifestations (haemorrhages into skin, conjunctival or buccal mucosa; epistaxis, gum bleeding, haemarthrosis, menorrhagia).
3. Oral cavity (ulcers; gum for bleeding or hypertrophy, tongue, tonsils, involvement of Waldeyer's ring) and skin (e.g. skin infiltration in lymphoma and leukaemia, telangiectasis).
4. Lymph nodes examination (in details) including mediastinal percussion (for mediastinal lymphadenopathy).
5. Examination of liver and spleen (in details).
6. *Sternal tenderness.*
7. Ophthalmoscopy or fundoscopy (for retinal haemorrhage, papilloedema, Roth spots, etc.).

Clinical Wisdom

While examining haemopoietic system, **examine the other systems** for:

I. CVS: Haemic murmur and ejection systolic murmur for progressive anaemia, venous hum from severe anaemia, venous/arterial thrombosis from polycythemia vera.
II. Nervous system: LMN type VIIth nerve palsy (leukaemic or lymphomatous deposits), spinal cord compression from multiple myeloma, subacute combined degeneration from vitamin B_{12} deficiency.
III. Respiratory system: Pleural effusion (e.g. lymphoma), pneumonia (due to immunocompromisation).
IV. GI tract and hepatobiliary system: Other than hepatosplenomegaly, search for any abdominal mass or lymphadenopathy, or ascites.
V. Genitourinary system: With special reference to examination of testes (ALL or NHL); renal mass.
VI. Locomotor system: Bone pain, joint swelling (haemophilia, gout), spine examination.
VII. Skin and appendages: Pruritus (lymphoma), pigmentation (lymphoma, busulfan therapy in CML), leg ulcers (sickle cell anaemia, paraproteinaemia), splinter haemorrhage (acute leukaemia), koilonychia (iron deficiency anaemia), alopecia (cytotoxic therapy).
VIII. Eye: Pallor, Jaundice, subconjunctival haemorrhage (from bleeding diathesis), conjunctival congestion (polycythemia), chloroma (AML).

Q. What is your diagnosis?

The diagnosis may be stated in one of the four ways. This is a case of:

1. Congenital haemolytic anaemia probably due to thalassaemia major, or
2. Moderate anaemia with hepatosplenomegaly probably from thalassaemia major, or
3. Huge splenomegaly probably due to thalassaemia major, or
4. Hepatosplenomegaly for discussion (if aetiological diagnosis cannot be reached).

Q. Why do you say so?

This is a case of thalassaemia major because of the following:

a. Young patient (18 years male patient) with positive family history, and there are presence of,
b. Anaemia (moderate to severe).
c. Jaundice (mild).
d. Stunted growth.
e. Mongoloid facies.
f. Mild (to moderate) hepatomegaly with huge splenomegaly, and
g. Past H/o repeated blood transfusions.

- **Features of chronic haemolytic anaemia are: anaemia, jaundice and splenomegaly.**

Q. Chief complaints of your patient:

1. Repeated cough and cold, palpitations, ill-health and weakness since childhood.
2. Yellowish discolouration of the eyes (from time to time) for last 5 years.
3. Dragging pain in the left hypochondrium with a mass present there for last 4 years.
4. Respiratory distress with respiratory tract infections since childhood and more for last 2 weeks.

Q. What is the H/o present illness?

1. Insidious in onset and gradually progressive illness.
2. Blood transfusion alleviates his sufferings.
3. Respiratory distress is exertional and often associated with purulent expectoration. There is neither any H/o PND nor any H/o seasonal variations.
4. Palpitations are exertional. There is no H/o fainting (black-out).
5. Dragging pain in the left hypochondrium is associated with a palpable mass in that region.
6. Mild jaundice which increases from time to time. Anorexia is profound.
7. There is no H/o gum bleeding, epistaxis, haematemesis, melaena or haemoptysis. The patient does not give any H/o leg ulcers or bipedal swelling. Occasionally he suffers from fever without any chill and rigor.
8. He has left school at 12 years of age. Till now he has been admitted several times in different city hospitals and each time he has been treated with blood transfusions by different doctors.

- Irregular fever in thalassaemia is due to increased metabolic activity or intercurrent infections.

Q. What 'past history' you have enquired for?

1. Whether the patient was admitted previously in any hospital for the same ailments?
2. Whether he has received blood transfusions during his past admissions in hospital?
3. Past H/o fever (chronic malaria and chronic kala-azar to analyse splenomegaly).
4. Any H/o pain abdomen (pigment stone-induced or haemolytic crises)?
5. Had he ever resided in Bihar or UP of India (endemic zone for chronic kala-azar)?
6. As a routine: H/o diabetes, hypertension, rheumatic fever (joint pain, dyspnoea, palpitations), past history of jaundice, malaria or kala-azar (due to hepatosplenomegaly), tuberculosis should be enquired for.

- In thalassaemia, one should enquire the presence of similar disorder in brothers, sisters, parents and other family members. Is there any H/o death in the family due to jaundice?

Q. What is a hereditary or familial disease?

This is caused by:

a. Mutant genes.
b. Follows the Mendelian law of inheritance and is transmitted from one generation to other.
c. May not be present at brith.

Examples are: Diabetes mellitus, hypertension, bronchial asthma, schizophrenia.

Q. What is a congenital disease?

This is:

a. Not produced by mutant genes.
b. Not follows Mendelian law of inheritance.
c. Present since birth.

Examples are: Congenital heart disease, cleft lip, imperforate anus.

Q. Points noted in the 'treatment history' of thalassaemia:

1. H/o blood transfusion.
2. Any specific drug used for the present disease (e.g. desferrioxamine).
3. Any surgery done in the past (pigment stone removal or splenectomy).

Q. 'General survey' in thalassaemia major (or any haemolytic anaemia):

In the **'general survey'**, the important points in favour of thalassaemia are:

1. Apparent age (often looks younger than actual age).
2. Build (there may be stunted growth).
3. Facies (mongoloid facies).
4. Anaemia (moderate to severe).
5. Jaundice (mild).
6. Pulse (may get water-hammer pulse due to severe anaemia).
7. Neck veins (may be engorged and pulsatile due to CCF).
8. Legs: Chronic leg ulcer over malleoli (common in sickle cell anaemia).
9. Secondary sexual characters (there may be delayed development).
10. Splenectomy scar (if there is absence of splenomegaly), and
11. Cholecystectomy scar (pigmented gallstones due to increased haemolysis).

Q. What is thalassaemia?

This is an inherited (genetic basis is heterogeneous) impairment of haemoglobin synthesis, in which there is partial or complete failure in the synthesis of a specific type of globin chain. It is a quantitative defect in the production of haemoglobin (qualitative defect is seen in sickle cell anaemia).

Thalassaemia is of two types:

- α (reduction or absence of α-chain synthesis), and
- β (reduction or absence of β-chain synthesis): **Commonest amongst thalassaemic patients.**

a. **α-thalassaemia:** 4 types (seen in South East Asia, Southern China, Middle East),
   i. Silent carrier.
   ii. α-thalassaemia trait.
   iii. HbH disease.
   iv. Hydrops fetalis (Hb Barts).

b. **β-thalassaemia:** 3 types (seen in mediterranean area),
   i. Heterozygous (thalassaemia minor or trait): One of the parents has thalassaemia minor.
   ii. Homozygous (thalassaemia major) or double heterozygous: Both parents have thalassaemia minor.
   iii. Intermedia (homozygous who survive into adulthood are likely to have this milder from of disease: Haemolysis occurs but the patient is not transfusion-dependent).

- 'Intermedia' is more severe than 'minor' but milder than transfusion-dependent 'major'. Usually the patients suffer from moderate anaemia.
- HbE disorders and HbD-Punjab are common in India.

Q. Normal haemoglobin pattern in human being:

a. Adult haemoglobin:

1. HbA (97%)	$\alpha_2\beta_2$
2. HbA_2 (1.5–3.5%)	$\alpha_2\delta_2$
3. HbF (<2%)	$\alpha_2\gamma_2$

b. Abnormal haemoglobin (in intrauterine life and neonates):

1. HbF	$\alpha_2\gamma_2$
2. Hb Barts	γ_4
3. HbH	β_4
4. Hb portland	$\Sigma_2\gamma_2$

At term, HbF accounts for 70–90% of total Hb in the fetus. HbF then fails rapidly and it becomes 25% at 1 month, and 5% at 6 month. The adult level (<2%) may not be reached in some children until puberty.

In an adult, the major haemoglobins seen are HbA and HbA_2 while in foetus, it is HbF and Hb Barts.

Q. Why HbF is increased in thalassemia major?

Thalassaemia is an inherited abnormality (autosomal recessive) in haemoglobin production, where there is partial or toal failure to synthesise a specific type of globin chain. In β-thalassaemia major, there is reduction or absence of β-chain production (defect within globin part) and thus, relative excess of α-chain synthesis occurs. Free α-chains have decreased solubility and will form inclusions within the RBC precursors in bone marrow. As a result of this, there is abnormality in membrane permeability as well as destruction of RBC by the macrophages. So thalassaemia major is characterised by both intramedullary erythroid destruction (ineffective erythropoiesis) and also a marked shortening of the life span of circulating RBC (peripheral haemolysis). Double injury to RBC results in expansion of red marrow (produces typical facial changes) and extramedullary haematopoiesis in the liver and spleen (i.e. in organs outside of the bone marrow). There is also compensatory increase in synthesis of γ-chain which combines with excess of free α-chains and form a stable tetramer of HbF ($\alpha_2\gamma_2$).

Patients with thalassaemia major who have relatively high rate of α-chain synthesis (i.e. more HbF), have less severe clinical course. Patients suffering from thalassaemia major have HBF ranging from 10 to 80%. Thalassaemia major patients (where both parents have thalssaemia minor or trait) may prove fatal, if left untreated.

Q. How do you classify haemolytic anaemia?

A. Acquired:

I. Environmental factors:
   a. Antibody: Immune haemolytic anaemia (lymphoma, SLE, drugs).
   b. Mechanical trauma: Microangiopathic haemolytic anaemia (prosthetic valves, haemolytic-uraemic syndrome, thrombotic thrombocytopenic purpura, eclampsia).
   c. Direct toxic effect: Malaria, claustridial infection.
   d. Splenomegaly.

II. Membrane abnormalities:
   a. Spur cell anaemia (associated with portal cirrhosis).
   b. Paroxysmal nocturnal haemoglobinuria (PNH).

B. Hereditary:

I. Membrane abnormalities:
   a. Hereditary spherocytosis.
   b. Hereditary elliptocytosis.

II. Haemoglobinopathies:
   a. Thalassaemia (quantitative defect).
   b. Sickle cell disease (qualitative defect).

III. Enzymopathies (metabolic defects):
   a. G_6PD deficiency
   b. Pyruvate kinase deficiency.

- Extracorpuscular defects: All 'acquired' causes except PNH. Intracorpuscular defects: All 'hereditary' causes plus PNH.
- Haemolysis: a) Intravascular: All acquired causes above plus transfusion reactions, DIC, snake bite, b) Extravascular: All hereditary casuses plus drug-induced (e.g. methyl dopa).

Q. Describe thalassaemic or mongoloid facies (Fig. 1.66A):

In thalassaemia, there is $\uparrow O_2$ affinity of HbF → resulting in tissue hypoxia → which in turn, stimulates erythropoiesis → expansion of marrow space → gives rise to characteristic facial appearance.

1. Frontal bossing (prominent forehead due to marrow hyperplasia).
2. Depressed bridge of the nose.
3. Hypertelorism (widely set eyes due to hyperplasia of lesser wing of sphenoid).
4. Apparent mongoloid slant of the eyes (mimics the eyes of Hindu Goddess 'Durga').
5. Malar prominence (due to maxillary marrow hyperplasia)—'Chipmunk' facies.
6. Dental malocclusion with prominent upper incisors (due to expansion of marrow of upper jaw).
7. Associated with mild icteric tinge of the conjunctiva, and pallor.

- Chipmunk is small, stripped squirrel.

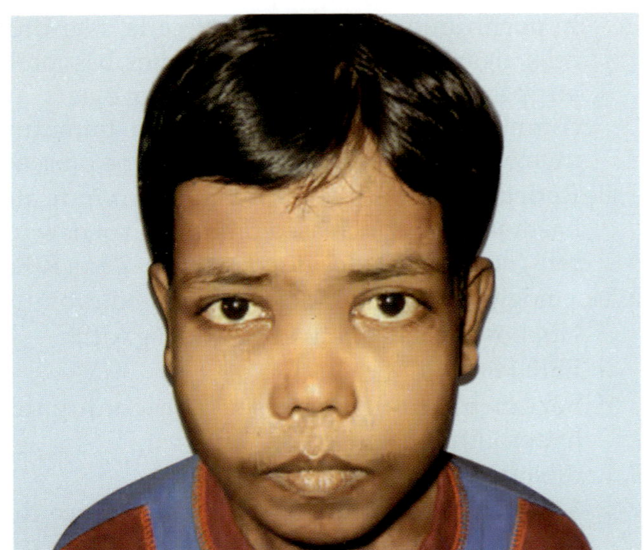

Fig. 1.66A: Thalassaemia with frontal bossing, depressed bridge of the nose, malar prominence and mild icterus

Q. Why there is anaemia in thalassaemia major?

1. Impaired haemoglobin production.
2. Ineffective erythropoiesis.
3. Haemolysis.
4. Haemodilution.
5. RBC destruction from hypersplenism.

Q. Why there is jaundice in thalassemia major?

1. Haemolysis (classically it is haemolytic jaundice).
2. Viral hepatitis (type C or B infection due to repeated blood transfusions).
3. Rarely, due to iron deposition in liver.

Q. Why there is cardiomegaly or heart failure seen in thalassemia major?

1. Persistent hypoxia (as progressive anaemia is always present).
2. Volume overload due to repeated blood transfusions.
3. Rarely, there is cardiomyopathy by haemosiderosis/ haemochromatosis.

Q. Description of splenomegaly in your patient:

1. Enlarged 18 cm below the left costal margin along its long axis (or along the splenic axis) and has crossed the umbilicus. It has enlarged towards the right iliac fossa.
2. Non-tender (rarely it may be tender due to splenic infarction, especially in a very big spleen).
3. A notch is present in the superior border.
4. Firm in consistency.
5. It is freely moving with respiration.
6. Surface is smooth.
7. Margin is sharp.
8. Fingers cannot be insinuated between the spleen and the left costal arch.
9. It is neither bimanually palpable nor ballottable.
10. There is no (colonic) resonance over the mass (differentiates left renal mass).
11. No palpable splenic rub (present in case of splenic infarction).

- Never forget to auscultate over a hugely enlarged spleen for audible splenic rub.

Q. Describe the hepatomegaly in your patient:

1. Enlarged 5 cm below the right costal margin at right MCL
2. Moving with respiration.
3. Firm in feel.
4. Non-tender.
5. Smooth surface.
6. Margin is sharp and regular
7. Left lobe is not palpable.
8. Upper border of liver dullness is at right 5th ICS at right MCL
9. No pulsation, no rub, no bruit.

- Splenohepatomegaly in thalassaemia is mainly due to extramedullary haematopoiesis and rarely transfusional haemosiderosis. Extensive erythropoiesis results in extramedullary haematopoiesis (i.e. ectopic haematopoietic activity) in liver, spleen, skull, pelvis and paraspinal region (as a mass).

Q. Features in other systems in thalassaemia major:

A. CVS: Effect of anaemia on CVS with special reference to haemic murmur. Read the section on 'Anaemia'. There may be features of high output heart failure. Look for neck veins carefully.

B. Respiratory system:
   1. Occasional rhonchi, and
   2. Crepitations due to respiratory tract infections.

C. Nervous system: Rarely, there may be spastic paraplegia due to 'extramedullary haematopoiesis' in the paravertebral region in thorax.

D. Reticulo-endothelial system:
   a. Anaemia.
   b. Tonsils may be enlarged.
   c. No lymphadenopathy.
   d. No bleeding manifestations into skin.
   e. Hepatosplenomegaly.
   f. Rarely, sternal tenderness may be present (due to severe anaemia).

- Ascites is not a feature of thalassaemia. In a **long case of thalassaemia**, first examine the GI system, next the CVS, respiratory system and so on. One may examine the reticulo-endothelial system after the examination of GI system.

Q. How thalassaemia minor (trait) presents?

They are rarely associated with significant clinical manifestations, i.e. the patients can lead normal life with normal life expectancy. Usually they spend their life without diagnosis. Twenty percent patients have splenomegaly and few may have pallor or mild icterus. The diagnosis is generally made when they are evaluated for persisting mild anaemia or during pre-marital check up. Reticulocyte count is normal. HbA_2 is usually raised up to 5% and 50% patients have HbF elevated.

Q. Differential diagnosis you will consider:

Basically one has to consider the **causes of huge splenomegaly**. For the discussion, read the section on 'Hepatosplenomegaly'. Actually, the task is to differentiate thalassaemia from chronic kala-azar, chronic malaria, CML, cirrhosis of liver (with hyper-splenism) and tropical splenomegaly syndrome.

Q. 'Crises' described in haemolytic anaemias:

The 'crises' are very common in sickle cell anaemia. There are 4 types:

1. Haemolytic crisis (sudden hepatosplenomegaly with rapidly developing anaemia): Relatively rare.
2. Aplastic crisis or aregenerative crisis (temporary marrow suppression): Occurs in the presence of infection (particularly with human parvovirus B_{19}) and/or folic acid deficiency, and may be seen even in thalassaemia major.
3. Vaso-occlusive or thrombotic crisis **(commonest)**: Acute and severe bone pain results from plugging of small vessels in bone (bone necrosis). Various part of the body like hands and feet in children (resulting in dactylitis), or humerus, femur, ribs, vertebrae and pelvis in adults may be affected; acute abdomen, neurological disorders and retinopathy are not uncommon. Sweating, pyrexia and tachycardia are common.
4. Sequestration or infarction crisis: Thrombosis of the venous outflow results in crisis in an organ. Splenic infarction in sickle cell anaemia (autosplenectomy) is a classical example.

- In haemolytic crisis, reticulocyte count increases but in other crises reticulocyte count does not increase from the basal level. By about 8 years of age, in sickle cell disese, spleen is no longer palpable due to repeated episodes of splenic infarcts leading to 'autosplenectomy'.
- Sickling in sickle cell anaemia is precipitated by infection (fever), dehydration, cold (e.g. in high altitude), acidosis, sluggish blood flow or hypoxia.

Q. Pain abdomen in thalassaemia major:

1. Dragging pain due to huge splenomegaly.
2. Vaso-occlusive crisis (rare).
3. Biliary colic (due to production of pigment stones from haemolysis).
4. Rarely due to splenic infarction.

Q. How to establish the diagnosis of thalassaemia major?

1. Peripheral blood smear (first test to be done):
   i. Anisocytosis (variation in size of RBC), poikilocytosis (variation in shape of RBC), **microcytic hypochromic aneemia, target cells**, tear-drop cells, cigar-shaped cells, Heinz bodies, basophilic stippling, polychromasia, normoblasts are commonly seen. Small number of immature myelocytes or metamyelocytes may be present.
   ii. **Reticulocytosis** (by supravital stain) indicates haemolysis and increased production of new red cells; normal reticulocyte count is 0.2–2% of RBC).
2. Haemoglobin concentration, ESR and bilirubin:
   i. Hb: Low (usually between 2 and 6 g/dL).
   ii. ESR: High
   iii. Serum bilirubin is raised (un-conjugated hyperbilirubinaemia).
3. Radiology:
   i. **X-ray of skull: 'Hair on end'** appearance due to the separation of two tables of skull (i.e. widened diploic space with cortical thinning) with perpendicular trabeculae in-between.

ii. **X-ray of small bones of hands: 'Mosaic-patterns'** due to widening of medullary space with thinning of cortex and criss-cross trabeculae in between **(Fig. 1.66B)**.
iii. Chest X-ray (PA view): Cardiomegaly, pneumonitis or paravertebral shadow as a result of extra-medullary haematopoiesis.

4. **Haemoglobin electrophoresis:** Diagnostic and confirmatory. Shows presence of **HbF (>2% of total Hb)** and variable amount of HbA_2 and HbA (HbA_2 is increased more in thalassaemia minor than in major, and is usually >3.5%).
5. Alkali denaturation test: HbF is resistant to alkali denaturation (i.e. the test is positive).
6. Osmotic fragility test: It is decreased, i.e. there is increased resistance of red cells to osmotic lysis (osmotic fragility is increased in hereditary spherocytosis).
7. Ferrokinetics: **Serum iron concentration is increased**, and TIBC usually remains normal or reduced.
8. Red cell survival study: Shortened red cell survival measured by different techniques.
9. Bone marrow: Hyperplastic bone marrow with hyperplasia of erythropoietic and leucopoietic tissue. Myeloid and erythroid ratio (M : E) becomes 1 or less (normal M : E = 3 : 1 or 4 : 1). Granulopoiesis and thrombopoiesis are preserved.

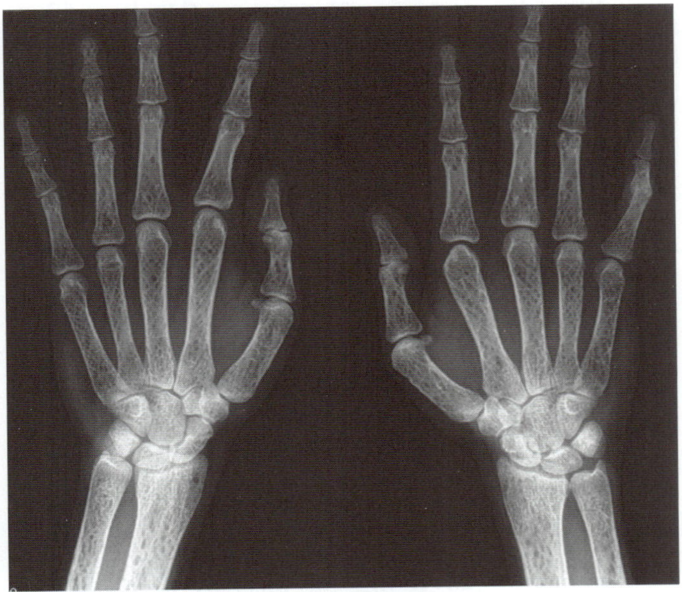

Fig. 1.66B: The **'mosaic-patterns'** in X-ray hand

10. Both the parents have thalassaemia minor (↑ HbA_2 in both the parents).

Clinical Wisdom

The other names of thalassaemia major are Cooley's anaemia, target cell anaemia, mediterranean anaemia (Greek *'thalassa'* means 'the sea') and splenic anaemia.

Q. Laboratory features of 'haemolysis':

1. Fragmented red cells in peripheral blood. Peripheral smear may show spherocytes, target cells.
2. **High serum bilirubin, usually <6 mg/dL (unconjugated > conjugated).**
3. **High urinary urobilinogen.**
4. Low plasma haptoglobin and haemopexin.
5. Haemoglobinaemia and haemoglobinuria.
6. Increased methaemalbumin in blood (detected by Schumm test).
7. High urinary haemosiderin.
8. **Reticulocytosis.**
9. Reduced RBC survival.
10. Hyperplastic bone marrow (i.e. erythroid hyperplasia).
11. Increased plasma LDH.

- 5, 6 and 7 are classically seen in intravascular haemolysis.

Q. Features of iron overload in thalassaemia major:

In thalassaemia, iron overload is due to:
a. Haemolysis.
b. Repeated blood transfusions, and
c. Increased absorption of iron from gut.

Features of **iron deposition (haemosiderosis)** in different systems are **(Table 1.25)**:

1. CVS: Pericarditis, cardiomyopathy, ventricular ectopics, heart blocks, pump failure.
2. Hepatic: Hepatomegaly (prothrombin time and liver enzymes may ↑), rarely cirrhosis of liver.
3. Endocrine:
   i. Pancreas: Diabetes mellitus.
   ii. Adrenal gland: May have adrenal crisis.
   iii. Due to ↓ gonadotropin release: Delayed development of secondary sexual characters (due to impaired hypothalamo-pituitary-gonadal function), i.e. features of hypogonadism.
4. Skin: Hyperpigmentation.

Table 1.25: Differences between haemosiderosis and haemochromatosis

Features	Haemosiderosis	Haemochromatosis
1. Inheritance	1. Always acquired	1. Genetic or acquired
2. Tissues affected	2. Reticulo-endothelial cells	2. Parenchymal cells
3. Damage	3. Less tissue damage	3. Obvious tissue damage
4. After desferrioxamine application	4. Urinary excretion of iron does not exceed 4 mg/24 hours	4. Urinary excretion of iron exceeds 4 mg/24 hours

5. Joints: Chondrocalcinosis (pseudogout), arthritis, osteopenia.

❍ Liver biopsy in thalassaemia major shows both reticulo-endothelial and parenchymal iron.

Q. Causes of iron overload in internal medicine:

1. β-thalassaemia major.
2. Haemochromatosis.
3. Sideroblastic anaemia.
4. Alcoholic liver disease.
5. Repeated blood transfusions.
6. Iron-dextran infusions.
7. Chronic haemodialysis.

Q. Complications of thalassaemia major:

1. Stunted growth with facial disfigurement.
2. Pigment gallstones (due to haemolysis).
3. Iron overload complications (described above): Haemosiderosis.
4. Leg ulcers.
5. Hypersplenism.
6. Repeated respiratory tract infections.
7. Compressive myelopathy (due to extramedullary haematopoiesis).

❍ Thalassaemic patients experience serious iron-induced toxicity and death, while the main cause of death is due to congestive cardiac failure. Death commonly results from ischaemic or restrictive cardiomyopathy, and infections.

Q. Causes of microcytic hypochromic anaemia:

1. Iron deficiency anaemia (commonest).
2. Thalassaemia.
3. Sideroblastic anaemia (often responses to pyridoxine).
4. Sometimes seen in lead poisoning.
5. Anaemia of chronic diseases (e.g. rheumatoid arthritis).

❍ Sideroblast: These are nucleated RBC having excess of iron-containing granules in the cytoplasm.

Q. MCV, MCH, MCHC in thalassaemia:

1. Normally MCV is 87 ± 7 cubic μ (low in thalassaemia).
2. Normally MCH is 29.5 ± 2.5 picogram (low in thalassaemia).
3. Normally MCHC is 35 ± 3 g/dL (low in thalassaemia).

Q. Severe anaemia without splenomegaly—possibilities in clinical medicine:

1. Anaemia due to acute or chronic blood loss.
2. Aplastic anaemia.
3. Sickle cell anaemia (autosplenectomy).
4. Anaemia due to hookworm infestation.
5. Chronic renal failure.
6. Rheumatoid arthritis.

Q. What is the outline of treatment in thalassaemia major?

1. **No oral or parenteral iron therapy.**
2. **Repeated transfusions** to keep the haemoglobin in the range of 9–10.5 g/dL with desferrioxamine therapy.
3. Folic acid: 5 mg daily, orally for life-long.
4. Antibiotics for infections.
5. Splenectomy in some cases.

❍ **Thalassaemia minor** is, many a time, confused with iron deficiency anaemia. It needs no treatment other than folic acid supplementation (5 mg/day). The patient should be reassured with explanation of genetic counselling. α-thalassaemia requires only genetic counselling.

Q. Recent trends in the management of thalassaemia major:

To maintain the most beneficial Hb level, it requires an individualised programme of transfusion with iron chelation and careful attention to the development of skeletal, endocrine and cardiac abnormalities.

1. Transfusion therapy: The key intervention in the management of thalassaemia major is chronic blood transfusion therapy to a target Hb concentration of 9–10.5 g/dL. Regular transfusions result in improvement of hepatosplenomegaly, cardiac dilatation and sketetal abnormalities. Previous mode of treatment of hypertransfusion (Hb kept >10 g/dL) and supertransfusion (Hb kept 12 g/dL) is not popular nowadays. Transfusion therapy should always be accompained by iron chelation therapy (*see* below).
2. Iron chelation is achieved by desferrioxamine which delivers drug by a small portable pump. The dose is 20–40 mg/kg/day and is given by subcutaneous continuous infusion. 1 g of desterrioxamine chelates 85 mg of iron. Nowadays, it is started at 5 years of age when the child can use the 'infusion pump' of his own. Infusion lasts 10–12 hours (overnight) and is given for 5–7 nights per week with a goal to keep serum ferritin <1000 ng/mL. Common side effects are pruritus, local swelling, sore arm, etc. Excessive doses may give rise to cataract, optic neuritis, nerve deafness and retinal damage. Oral iron chelation therapy with deferiprone (25 mg/kg, tds) and deferasirox (20–40 mg/kg/day) are used in many countries.
3. Splenectomy (*see* below) which is preceded 4–6 weeks by pneumococcal, *H. influenzae* and meningococcal vaccine.Thrombotic events may increase after splenectomy.
4. Vitamin E: Can be used as an antioxidant drug; excretion of iron is enhanced by vitamin C (low dose, i.e. usually 3 mg/kg daily is used to avoid cardiotoxicity).
5. Vitamin D and calcium may be used regularly to control osteoporosis.

6. Local irradiation of face to minimise facial disfigurement.
7. Neocyte transfusion, i.e. transfusion of young low-density RBC (average life span 90 days); the neocytes reduce the rate of iron accumulation. Gerocytes (old RBC) may be removed by pheresis to reduce iron load.
8. Genetic manipulation is done by azacitidine or butyrate which increases the production of HbF (increased HbF in thalassaemia is associated with less severe clinical course). Hydroxyurea (1–2 g/day) may prevent ineffective erythropoiesis. Sotatercept is a promising new drug to improve anaemia.
9. Allogenic bone marrow transplantation is done from HLA compatible sibling **(definitive therapy)**. Globin gene therapy, achieved through manipulation of autologous stem cells, is an attractive alternative.
10. Life-long folic acid supplement (5 mg daily, orally) and antibiotics, as and when necessary. Chronic leg ulcers may be managed with elevation of the affected leg and daily dressings with zinc sulphate.
11. Gene therapy is promising.
12. Prevention (prenatal) is possible by identifying a fetus with β-thalassaemia by DNA analysis (PCR amplification) of chorionic villus in early pregnancy (8–10 week) and also by amniocentesis (14–18 week). Fetal cord blood in the womb can also be tested in 18–20 weeks of pregnancy. This is appropriate if both the parents are known to be carriers, i.e. β-thalassaemia minor, and always terminate the pregnancy in these cases. Genetic counselling is a must.

    Premarital blood should be tested to identify thalassaemia minor.

- If both the parents are thalassaemia minor:
  - 25% chance to have thalassaemia major
  - 50% chance to have thalassaemia minor
  - 25% chance to have a normal child

Q. Indications for splenectomy in thalassaemis major:

1. Mechanical problems due to massive splenomegaly (dragging pain in abdomen, or early satiety).
2. To decrease the requirement of excessive blood transfusions (normal requirement is 1–3 units of packed RBCs/4–6 weeks to maintain the Hb level in the range of 10 g/dL).
3. Features of hypersplenism.

- Splenectomy should be done in a child who is >5 years of age.
- **If spleen is not palpable in thalassaemia, always look for the splenectomy scar.**

Q. Peripheral blood film after splenectomy (or asplenia):

1. Marked anisocytosis, poikilocytosis.
2. Howell-Jolly bodies.
3. Target cells.
4. Thrombocytosis.
5. Pappenheimer bodies (sideroblastic granules).
6. Heinz bodies.
7. Nucleated RBCs.
8. Basophilic stippling.

- Remnants of nuclear material in RBC (No. 2).
- Formed from denatured aggregated Hb (No. 6).

Q. Indications (medical) of repeated blood transfusions in a city hospital:

1. Thalassaemia.
2. Aplastic or hypoplastic anaemia.
3. Haemophilia.
4. ITP (immune thrombocytopenic purpura).
5. Recurrent haematemesis or melaena.
6. Chronic renal failure.

Q. Drawbacks of repeated blood transfusions:

1. Risk of iron overload and heart failure.
2. Chance of isoimmunisation.
3. Entry of infections through blood like malaria, hepatitis C and B; HIV, toxoplasmosis, brucellosis, cytomegalovirus infection, syphilis; citrate toxicity.

- Acute (<72 hours) complications after blood transfusion are anaphylaxis, transfusion reactions (chills, urticaria, breathlessness, etc.), febrile reactions, fluid overload resulting in LVF, mismatch (haemolysis), hypothermia. Delayed (>72 hours) complications are thrombophlebitis and entry of different infections.

Q. Causes of target cell in peripheral blood film:

1. Thalassaemia.
2. Iron deficiency anaemia.
3. Cholestatic jaundice.
4. After splenectomy or hyposplenism.

Q. Common causes of refractory anaemia in clinical practice:

It is the non-response to appropriate treatment of anaemia given for optimal period. They are:

1. Aplastic anaemia.
2. Sideroblastic anaemia.
3. Erythroleukaemia (M_6 variety of AML).
4. Aleukaemic leukaemia.
5. Myelodysplastic syndrome.
6. Chronic renal failure.

Conclusion

H/o repeated blood transfusions and previous hospital admissions of the patient should always be enquired. Menstrual history should be taken with care as in many patients menarche may not be attained.

Typical facies, pallor, jaundice and a big palpable spleen are essential bedside clue to diagnosis. Never forget to examine for cardiomegaly, CCF and systolic murmur over the precordium.

CHRONIC MYELOID LEUKAEMIA — CASE 24

Q. What is your diagnosis?

The diagnosis may be delivered in one of the three ways:
1. This is a patient of huge splenomegaly and moderate hepatomegaly probably due to chronic myeloid leukaemia (CML), or
2. This is a patient of anaemia with hepatosplenomegaly probably due to chronic myeloid leukaemia, or
3. Huge splenomegaly probably due to chronic myeloid leukaemia.

Q. Why do you say so?

This is a case of CML because of the following:
1. This is an adult patient (majority are in the age group of 30–80 years with peak age at 55 years) who complains of gradual onset of dragging pain along with heaviness in the abdomen, mainly the left upper quadrant with a palpable, non-tender swelling present there (ie, feeling of a lump). This is associated with loss of appetite and early satiety, vague ill-health, abdominal fullness, tiredness, marked weight loss, and occasional rise of temperature with night sweats but without chill and rigor for last 6 months. The onset of the disease is insidious and the progress is slow.
2. There is neither any past H/o haematemesis, melaena, jaundice, blood transfusion, oedema feet nor it is associated with positive family history with similar type of illness.
3. On examination there is mild anaemia, absence of jaundice, moderate hepatomegaly with huge splenomegaly as well as there is presence of sternal tenderness. Lymphadenopathy, signs of hepatocellular failure or bleeding manifestations into skin are absent.

Clinical Wisdom

At the onset, one should know that there are four main types of leukaemia like acute myeloid leukaemia (AML), acute lymphoblastic leukaemia (ALL), chronic myeloid leukaemia (CML) and chronic lymphocytic leukaemia (CLL).

Q. Chief complaints of your patient:

1. Gradually progressive swelling with dragging pain in the left upper abdomen, especially in upright posture for last 6 months.
2. Loss of appetite, tiredness, weakness, fever and loss of weight for the same duration.

Q. Presence of sternal tenderness—conditions associated:

Clinical method (Fig. 1.67): Press the upper part of the body of sternum with the **ball of the right thumb** for

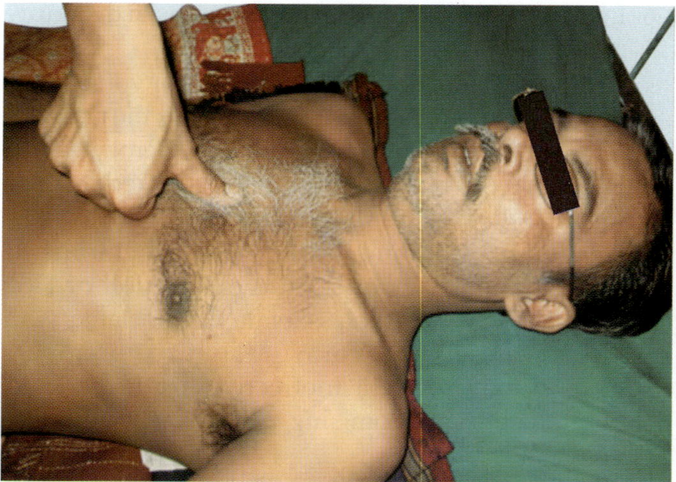

Fig. 1.67: Detection of sternal tenderness—pressing the upper part of body of sternum with the ball of the right thumb

2–3 seconds. In the presence of sternal tenderness, the patient winces with pain (also see the facial grimace) or complains of pain. Sternal tenderness is found in:
1. Acute leukaemias (AML and ALL) (**Table 1.26**).
2. Chronic myeloid leukaemia.
3. Severe anaemia due to any cause (except aplastic anaemia).
4. Multiple myeloma or secondary metastases in bones.
5. Rarely, in osteomalacia and osteoporosis.
6. After sternal puncture.

Clinical Wisdom

When sternal tenderness is present, examine the patient for tenderness in other bones like pelvic bones, ribs, vertebrae, long bones (press the upper part of shin bone) and frontal bone (press the forehead). Look for the evidence of sternal puncture or posterior iliac crest puncture (benzene stain or cotton seal over the puncture site) in these cases. **Sternal tenderness is due to proliferation as well as hypercellularity of bone marrow. 1 and 2 are most common causes.** Bone tenderness may also be examined by taping over the spine or gently pressing both clavicles with the heel of the hands. Remember, diffuse bone pain is common in osteomalacia and multiple myeloma.

Q. Causes of swelling in the left upper abdomen:

1. Splenomegaly.
2. Kidney lump (left).
3. Tumour of splenic flexure.
4. Growth from stomach.
5. Tumour of left adernal gland.
6. Rarely, tumour of the tail of pancreas.
7. Enlarged left lobe of liver.
8. Omental mass.

Q. 'Past history' you have enquired for:

1. Haematemesis or melaena.
2. Jaundice.
3. Fever (ref: malaria or kala-azar).
4. Repeated blood transfusions.

5. Bone pain.
6. Ankle oedema.
7. Bleeding manifestations, e.g. purpura.
8. Haematuria (ref: kidney lump).
9. Diabetes mellitus.
10. Systemic hypertension.

Q. Causes of huge splenomegaly:

Read the section on 'Hepatosplenomegaly'.

Q. What is the classical description of the spleen of CML:

Splenomegaly in CML is present in 90% cases and approximately in 10%, the enlargement is massive and the spleen goes towards the right inguinal ligament. Splenic rub may be present.

For typical description: Read the section on 'Thalassaemia' as the description of splenic enlargement is the same in both the conditions. The spleen of CML is very hard and is known as *'cast iron spleen'*. Hepatomegaly occurs in 50% cases. Hepatosplenomegaly in CML is due to myeloid metaplasia.

Q. Phases of CML (in natural history of the disease):

1. Chronic or stable phase: Easily controlled by treatment. Usually lasts for 3–5 years.
2. Accelerated phase: Control of the disease is difficult (progressive anaemia, organomegaly, fever, thrombocytosis or thrombocytopenia develop).
3. Blastic (blast crisis) phase: It is a dreadful condition where the patient transforms into acute leukaemia (AML in 75% and ALL in 25%). **The blast cell of AML contains Auer rods which are not seen in blast crisis of CML.** This is the cause of death in majority of patients.

- *CML is a monoclonal stem cell disorder* or myeloproliferative disorder characterised by an overproduction of myeloid cells with fairly normal maturation, possessing a reciprocal translocation between chromosome 9 and 22.

Q. Why it is not a case of chronic malaria, chronic kela-azar or thalassaemia?

Read the sections on 'Hepatosplenomegaly' and 'Thalassaemia'.

Q. Why it is not a case of chronic lymphocytic leukaemia (CLL)?

The salient features of CLL are:

1. Peak age for the disease is 65 years.
2. Onset is very insidious.
3. Anaemia develops slowly and lately.
4. Absence of sternal tenderness.
5. Presenting complaint is painless, discrete, firm and moderate enlargement of lymph nodes all over the body (important bedside finding).
6. Moderate splenomegaly.

These features are absent here and this is why it is not a case of CLL.

Q. How will you recognise the 'blast crisis'?

It means that the disease has been transformed to acute leukaemia. The features of blast crisis are:

1. The stable patient will deteriorate (there is refractoriness to treatment).
2. Anaemia progresses rapidly; bone pain and sternal tenderness increase.
3. Severe bleeding starts, e.g. petechiae, purpura, bruise, epistaxis, gastrointestinal bleeding, bleeding from urogenital tract; fever appears.
4. Generalised lymphadenopathy may be present (due to transformation into ALL).
5. Abrupt increase in splenic size and tenderness.
6. Peripheral blood film shows >10% blast cells.

Q. Manifestations at the late stage of CML:

1. Bleeding into the skin or from mucous membrane of internal organs.
2. Acute pain in the left hypochondrium: Due to splenic infarction with audible splenic rub.
3. Persistent rise of temperature.
4. Leukaemic infiltrations in cranial nerves with their paralysis, pleural effusion, ascites or peripheral neuropathy.
5. Respiratory tract infections.

Q. Differential diagnosis you will consider in this case:

Consider causes of massive splenomegaly.

Q. How your diagnosis will be established?

1. Blood examination (first and foremost investigation):
   a. Hb and RBC: RBC count is low with anisocytosis, poikilocytosis, few normoblasts, normocytic normochromic anaemia, low Hb (mean Hb level is 10.5 g/dL).
   b. WBC:
      i. Average total count (TC) is 1.5–2.5 lac/mm^3 (1–5 lac/mm^3).
      ii. Differential count (DC) includes myelocytes 20–30%, metamyelocytes 25%, promyelocytes 2–3%, polymorphs 40%, eosinophils 4%, basophils 2%, lymphocytes 5%, monocytes 1%, myeloblasts 1–2% (usually <10%).
   c. Platelets: Initially normal or increased, but diminished gradually.
   d. ESR Increased.

Clinical Wisdom

In the accelerated phase, more primitive cells appear and in the blastic phase, there is dramatic increase in blast cells (>10%) in the peripheral blood film.

2. Bone marrow examination: It is not mandatory (though gives definitive diagnosis) because **peripheral blood**

picture is the most useful diagnostic aid. It shows increased myelocyte series with increased myeloid and erythroid ratio (as high as 20:1) in a hypercellular marrow. Often prominent megakaryocytes are seen (in acute leukaemias, bone marrow is hypercellular and there is >30% of leukaemic blast cells). Cytogenetics show t(9;22) translocation.

3. Philadelphia (ph) chromosome is seen in myeloid and erythroid series of blood and bone marrow.
4. Other findings:
   a. High serum uric acid and LDH level (due to increased cell breakdown).
   b. High serum vitamin B_{12} level (due to ↑ in transcobalamin III present in neutrophil granules).
   c. Low leucocyte alkaline phosphatase (LAP score).
5. Special investigation: Fluorescence-*in situ* hybridisation (FISH) or reverse transcriptase polymerase chain reaction (RT-PCR) helps demonstrating cytogenetic/molecular abnormality.

- A **hypermetabolic state** is found in CML, lymphoma, tuberculosis, thalassaemia, malignancy and myelofibrosis.
- **LAP score is diminished** in CML and paroxysmal nocturnal haemoglobinuria (PNH). It is **increased** in infection (leukaemoid reaction), pregnancy, after steroid administration, stress, Hodgkin's disease, polycythemia vera, essential thrombocythemia and myelosclerosis.
- The mean haemoglobin level is 10.5 g/dL (i.e. mild anaemia). Anaemia in CML is never severe in degree. **Basophilia often points towards the diagnosis** and tends to increase as disease progresses.
- RNA analysis in CML demonstrates the presence of the chimeric **BCR-ABL oncogene**. ABL stands for abelson (named after the abelson murine leukaemia virus), and BCR for breakpoint cluster region (BCR gene on chromosome 22).

Q. Hypercatabolic (hypermetabolic) symptoms of CML:

1. Weight loss (wasting).
2. Fever.
3. Sweating (night).
4. Malaise and anorexia.
5. Gout.
6. Heat intolerance.

Q. What is philadelphia (Ph) chromosome?

1. Diagnostic of CML; detected by cytogenetics analysis.
2. Shortening of long arms of chromosome G 22 (due to balanced reciprocal translocation of genetic material with chromosome 9).
3. Found in 95% cases of CML. Thus, 5% patients are Ph-chromosome –ve.
4. Ph-chromosome +ve cases have a better prognosis than Ph-chromosome –ve cases.
5. Found in myeloid and erythroid series of blood and bone marrow (never seen in lymphocytes).
6. Present in all the phases throughout the course of the disease and even after therapy; however, Ph +ve cells decrease with α-interferon and imatinib therapy.
7. Helps in differentiation between AML and blast crisis of CML.

- By polymerase chain reaction (PCR), Ph-chromosome is present in almost all patients of CML.

Q. Confirmation of diagnosis of CML:

1. Peripheral blood film with bone marrow examination.
2. Ph-chromosome: Pin-points the diagnosis.
3. RNA analysis for presence of BCR-ABL oncogene.
4. Low LAP score.

Q. Aleukaemic and subleukaemic leukaemia:

In acute leukaemia, an increase in total WBC count is expected but in:

a. Aleukaemic leukaemia: The total WBC count remains normal or subnormal, and there is absence of abnormal cells in the peripheral blood.

Table 1.26: Bedside differentiation between acute leukaemias

Features	AML	ALL
1. Symptoms	Fever, tiredness, haemorrhagic manifestations, ulcers in the mouth, recurrent infection	Same as AML. Bone and joint pain are more common. Bleeding as presentation is less common
2. Age	Relatively uncommon in children (common in adults), median age at presentation is 60 years	Mainly a disease of childhood (peak incidence: 3–7 years)
3. Lymphadenopathy and enlarged tonsils	Rare	Common
4. Gum hypertrophy	Seen (especially in M_5 variety)	Not seen
5. Splenomegaly	Less common (50%)	More common (70%)
6. Chloroma	Common	Usually not seen
7. Anaemia	++	+++
8. Leukaemic meningitis	Less common	More common

- Sternal tenderness is present in both the types of acute leukaemia.
- **Chloroma:** Localised greenish tumour masses in orbit, skin and other tissues.

b. Subleukaemic leukaemia: The total WBC count is within or below normal limit but few immature cells are seen in the peripheral blood.

Both a) and b) present as acute leukaemia. The confused **diagnosis is confirmed by bone marrow examination**.

Q. What is juvenile CML?

This rare form of CML is characterised by:

1. Affection below 4 years of age.
2. Absence of Ph-chromosome.
3. Increased level of HbF.
4. Normal cytogenetic karyotype.
5. Paucity of blastic transformation.
6. Prominent monocytosis and thrombocytopenia.

Q. What is myelodysplastic syndrome (MDS)?

These are a group of acquired clonal abnormalities of haematopoietic stem cells with varying degrees of cytopenia which represent steps in the pathway of development of leukaemia. Often it is called 'preleukaemia' or oligoblastic leukaemia as these patients are at increased risk of developing acute leukaemia. People over 50 years of age are usually affected (median age 69 years). Blast cells in marrow are increased but never cross 30% (>30% blast cells in marrow indicates acute leukaemia). Bone marrow examination shows hypercellularity with evidence of dysplasia. Though the exact cause is unknown, exposure to benzene or chemotherapeutic agents, or radiation may lead to MDS. Chromosomal abnormality is seen in up to 80% of cases. There is high morbidity and mortality due to bone marrow failure (symptoms of anaemia, bleeding or recurrent infections) or transformation into acute leukaemia. Supportive care (RBC and platelet transfusion), chemotherapy, lenalidomide (a thalidomide analogue) and bone marrow transplantation are proposed line of treatment. Other drugs tried are azacitidine, decitabine and luspatercept.

The *six distinct clinical syndromes* under MDS (WHO classification) are refractory anaemia, refractory anaemia with excess blasts (RAEB), refractory anaemia with ring sideroblasts (RARS), refractory cytopenia with multilineage dysplasia (RCMD), myelodysplastic syndrome with isolated del(5q-) (5q-syndrome), and myelodysplastic syndrome unclassified (MDS-U).

Q. Prognosis of CML:

1. Median survival of treated CML is 3 years (in imatinib era, it is approximately 5 years).
2. Median survival is about 1 year after blast crisis and <1 year in Ph-ve variety.
3. Few patients survive over 10 years.

Q. Complications of CML:

1. Blast crisis.
2. Haemorrhages into skin or mucous membrane of internal organs.
3. Recurrent infections (commonly in respiratory tract).
4. Hyperuricaemia (C/o joint pain due to gout).
5. Leukaemic infiltrations in cranial nerves, pleura (effusion), bones (paraplegia).
6. Rupture of the spleen.
7. Infarction of the spleen.
8. Priapism (persistent painful erection of penis).

- **'Leucostasis'** in CML may produce priapism, blurred vision or respiratory distress.
- **'Priapism'** may also be due to sickle cell anaemia, rabies, paraplegia (in flexion), spinal cord injury and local causes (thrombosis or haemorrhage).

Q. Physical findings in different systems in CML:

a. General survey: Mild anaemia, emaciation; pedal oedema due to anaemia or pressure over IVC by big spleen, haemorrhagic spots into skin may be present; very rarely jaundice may appear due to hepatic involvement, or type B or C hepatitis from blood transfusion.

b. GI tract: Huge splenomegaly, mild-to-moderate hepatomegaly. Usually there is absence of ascites. **The hallmark physical finding in CML is huge or massive splenomegaly.**

c. Lymphoreticular system: Presence of sternal tenderness; rarely lymphadenopathy in blastic transformation into ALL. Bone pain due to infiltration of marrow by leukaemic cells may be present.

d. Respiratory system: Basal crepitations due to pulmonary congestion; pleural effusion or rarely pneumnic consolidation.

e. CVS: Rarely, pericardial effusion.

f. Nervous system: Cranial nerve involvement (e.g. Bell's palsy), paraplegia; rarely meningeal signs may be seen. Retinal haemorrhage due to leucostasis may be evident on fundoscopy.

g. Genitourinary system: Sometimes, there is presence of priapism.

Q. How do you like to manage this case?

a. Imatinib mesylate: It is recommended as first-line treatment in chronic or stable CML. Treatment of CML has been totally transformed after advent of imatinib. It is a tyrosine kinase inhibitor that blocks the enzymatic action of the BCR-ABL fusion protein, and thereby reduces proliferation of WBC. Majority of patients after 18 months of therapy show complete 'cytogenetic' response (proved by disappearance of Ph-chromosome), and a proportion of patients will lose molecularly detectable BCR/ABL transcripts from blood (complete 'molecular' remission). The complete 'haematologic' response with imatinib is far superior than interferon (IFN)-α and cytarabine. *This drug is also indicated in accelerated or blastic phase.* The recommended daily dose is 400 mg/day (taken after a meal with a large glass of water). The side effects encountered are nausea, headache, skin rash, diarrhoea, muscle cramps, fluid retention, periorbital swelling and myelosuppression. Second-generation tyrosine kinase inhibitors like dasatinib or nilotinib are used in imatinib-resistant cases; asciminib, bosutinib and ponatinib are promising drugs.

b. Interferon-α: It was the treatment of choice before introduction of imatinib. It is used in doses of 1.5 million unit, subcutaneously on alternate days. It can induce control and maintain the control in chronic phase. There may be elimination of Ph-chromosome in 20% cases. Common side effects are flu-like syndrome, myelosuppression and neurotoxicity (fatigue, depression, myalgia, severe weight loss). IFN-α still has a role in the treatment.

c. Chemotherapy: Hydroxyurea (1–4 g/day) and busulfan (2–4 mg/day) are usually reserved for patients for rapid lowering of WBC, reduction of symptoms and reversal of symptomatic splenomegaly. As cytogenetic remissions with hydroxyurea is uncommon and busulfan produces serious side effects, *these drugs are not recommended nowadays to treat CML*. However, hydroxyurea is still being used in many countries.

d. Splenectomy (or irradiation of the spleen): Done to alleviate symptoms of discomfort and pain as a result of repeated splenic infarction, and to correct prolonged thrombocytopenia.

e. Blood transfusion: Low platelet count is raised by repeated fresh blood transfusions.

f. Allogenic haematopoietic stem cell transplantation (HSCT) can cure 70% patients, and is used in imatinib-failure patients or in progressive disease on therapy.

g. Good nutrition, antibiotics for infections and maintenance of proper oral hygiene.

h. Others: Oral hydroxycarbamide (used in palliative situations), arsenic trioxide, leukapheresis for symptomatic leucostasis (pulmonary failure or CVA).

i. Accelerated or blastic phase:
   1. Accelerated phase: Imatinib, hydroxycarbamide, low-dose cytarabine.
   2. Blast crisis: Blastic transformation to ALL responses better than AML. Most patients have a short-lived response to imatinib. However, ultimatily HSCT may be necessary. Blast crisis has a poor response with all modalities of treatment.

Q. Complications of busulfan:

1. Increased skin pigmentation.
2. Sterility.
3. Dryness of skin and mucous membrane.
4. Pancytopenia (myelosuppression, as it acts on early progenitor cells).
5. Interstitial pulmonary fibrosis (busulfan lung) and retroperitoneal fibrosis. Endocardial and marrow fibrosis have been reported.
6. A wasting syndrome similar to that seen in adrenal insufficiency.

- Complications of hydroxyurea are diarrhoea, mucositis or rash.

Q. Features of aplastic anaemia:

It is characterised by hypocellular bone marrow with pancytopenia:

a. Precipitating factor or the aetiological factor is very often present (drugs, chemicals, radiation).
b. **Severe anaemia** and its manifestations: Fatigue, lassitude, vertigo, black-out, tingling and numbness of extremities, palpitations, dyspnoea, chest pain, anorexia.
c. **Leucopenia** and its manifestations: Sore throat, fever with chill and rigor due to infection, fatigue, features of depressed immunity.
d. **Thrombocytopenia** and its manifestations: Bleeding manifestations into skin as petechiae, purpura, bruise; epistaxis; gum bleeding.
e. There is **absence of splenomegaly**, lymphadenopathy, jaundice or sternal tenderness in aplasic anaemia.

- Diminusion of the count of RBC series, WBC series and platelets are known as tricytopenia (i.e. pancytopenia); if any two of the series are affected, it is called bicytopenia.

Q. Drugs producing agranulocytosis:

1. Chloramphenicol, 2. Sulphonamides, 3. Chlorpropamide, 4. Chlorpromazine, 5. Propylthiouracil, 6. Cytotoxic drugs, 7. Oxyphenbutazone, 8. Phenytoin, 9. Carbimazole.

Conclusion

1. An adult person with swelling in left hypochondrium but without any suggestive facies.
2. Huge splenomegaly (usually feels hard).
3. Fever (neither double quotidian like kala-azar nor associated with chill and rigor like malaria).
4. Presence of sternal tenderness.
5. Absence of hepato-cellular failure, no jaundice, no lymphadenopathy.
6. Mild anaemia.

LYMPHOMA — CASE 25

Q. What is your diagnosis?

The diagnosis may be told in one of the two ways:

1. It is a case of lymphoma, probably Hodgkin's disease, or
2. It is a patient of generalised lymphadenopathy (for discussion).

Q. Why do you say so?

This is a patient of lymphoma because of the following:

1. There are presence of persistent fever, malaise, fatigability, night sweats, loss of body weight and pruritus for last 6 months.

2. Gradual painless swelling of lymph nodes (lumps) on both sides of the neck, right axilla and both inguinal regions for last 4 months.
3. On examination there are presence of:
   a. Anaemia (moderate).
   b. Lymph node enlargement: Cervical, axillary and inguinal nodes are enlarged. The lymph nodes are discrete (not matted), non-tender, rubbery in feel, neither fixed to deeper structures nor to the overlying skin, and without any sinus formation. Local temperature over the lymph nodes are not raised.
   c. Spleen: Moderately enlarged and non-tender.
   d. Liver: Moderately enlarged and non-tender.
   e. Absence of features of superior mediastinal syndrome, bone pain, paraplegia, intestinal obstruction, lump in the abdomen, ascites, pleural effusion at present.
   f. Absence of sternal tenderness.

Q. Can you specify the type of lymphoma?

No. Final diagnosis can be given after biopsy of the lymph nodes but the clinical features in this patient suggest that probably it is a case of Hodgkin's disease (see the differentiation between two types in page 213).

Q. What is lymphoma?

These are heterogenous group of malignant diseases of lymphoreticular origin (previously, known as reticulosis). The major types are Hodgkin's disease (HD) and non-Hodgkin's lymphoma (NHL).

Q. B-symptoms of lymphoma:

Presence of at least one of:
1. Recurrent unexplained fever above 38°C,
2. Drenching night sweats, and
3. Unexplained loss of more than 10% of body weight within the previous 6 months.

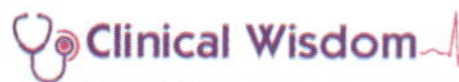

'A' indicates absence, and 'B' indicates presence of these symptoms. B-symptoms indicate bad prognosis too.

Q. Describe the different patterns of fever in lymphoma:

1. Usually it is a low grade fever unaccompanied by chill and rigor. The fever may be remittent in type like tuberculosis or continued in type resembling enteric fever.
2. Occasionally it is a swinging fever (with ups and downs).
3. Classical 'Pel-Ebstein' fever (10% cases of Hodgkin's disease) is not seen nowadays. It is a cyclical fever where several days or weeks of fever alternates with afebrile period.

- Pel-Ebstein fever is also noted in brucellosis and hypernephroma.

Q. How to examine the lymphoreticular system?

This system should be **examined first** in lymphoma. Follow the 'Scheme of examination' in 'Lymphoreticular system'. Ophthalmoscopic examination, though essential, is not in the curriculum of undergraduate students; only mention the heading and write 'not done'.

Q. Method of lymph nodes examination

Lymph nodes support the immune system (**Fig. 1.68**). Normal adults have more than 500 lymph nodes connected through a network of lymph vessels, of which >100 are in neck region. In health, usually the lymph nodes are not palpable (inguinal and cervical nodes are sometimes palpable like the size of a small bean) unless it is enlarged. Nodes are palpated symmetrically on **both sides** of the body **from above downwards**.

A. Lymph nodes in the neck:

Method: These lymph nodes are **always palpated from 'behind'** when the patient is sitting or standing with the head bending forward (to relax the muscles in the anterior part of neck).

a. The upper circular group is palpated symmetrically by both hands (using right hand for right side and left hand for left side) in the following order from front to back (**Fig. 1.69**):
   i. Submental (in the midline, just behind tip or mental protuberance of the mandible).
   ii. Submandibular (midway between tip and angle of the mandible).
   iii. Tonsillar (under the angle of the mandible).
   iv. Preauricular (immediately in front of the tragus).

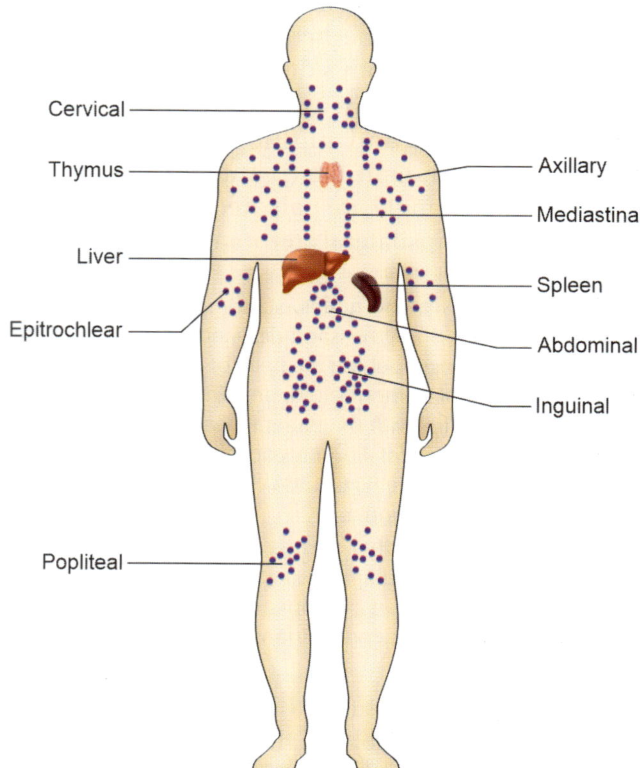

Fig. 1.68: Lymph nodes and immune system in human body

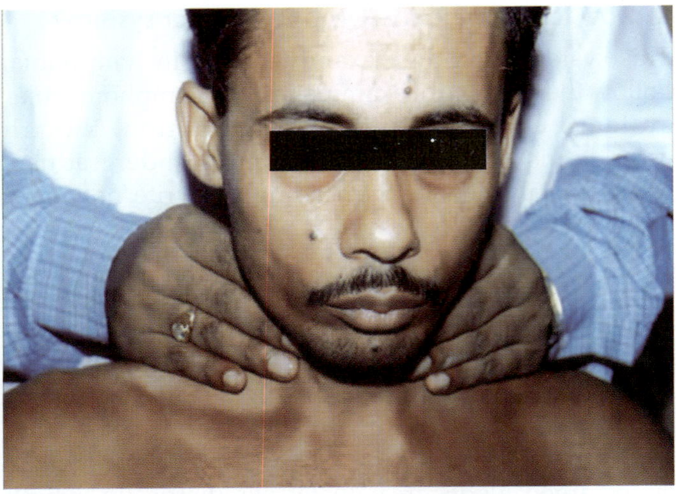

Fig. 1.69: Palpation of **cervical glands** from behind using both hands

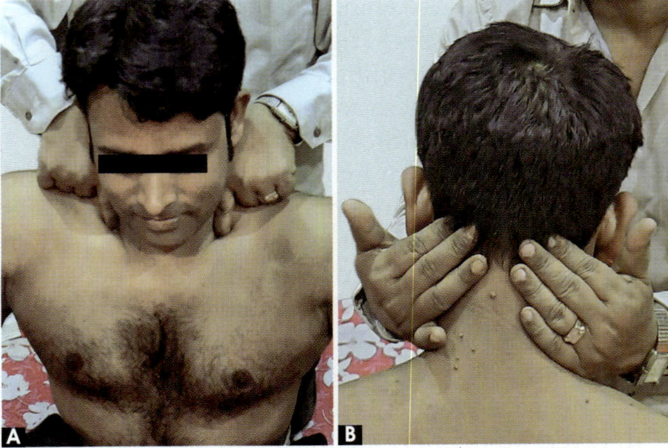

Fig. 1.70A and B: A) Palpation of **scalene nodes** in neck; B) Palpation of lymph nodes in **posterior triangle** of neck

v. Postauricular (behind the ear, over mastoid process), and
vi. Occipital gland—back of the head, above the hairline on both sides.

- From (i) to (vi) constitute Waldeyer's outer ring.

Clinical Wisdom

If one side of the neck is palpated at a time, the neck should be flexed to that side.

b. Lower horizontal or supraclavicular group of lymph nodes: These are arbitrarily divided into medial, intermediate and lateral groups. Special attention should be paid in palpating left-sided medial group of nodes **(Virchow's)** and **scalene nodes** (present above and behind the head of clavicles, deep to sternomastoids on both sides of the neck).
c. The vertical chain in the middle of the neck (jugulodigastric and jugulo-omohyoid lymph nodes): The glands in the (i) anterior triangle, and (ii) posterior triangle are palpated (the triangles are divided by the ipsilateral sternomastoid muscle).

- For palpation of **scalene nodes**, standing behind the sitting patient ask him to shrug his shoulder, and then dip down the palpating index finger behind the head of clavicle through the clavicular origin of sternomastoid, pressing gently downwards towards the first rib, with the patient's neck slightly flexed to that side. Scalene nodes lie in a pad of fat on the surface of scalenus anterior muscle (Fig. 1.70A). These nodes are enlarged in bronchogenic carcinoma.
- Few clinicians opine that glands in the posterior triangle (Fig. 1.70B), postauricular and occipital group of nodes are better palpated from front. Occipital nodes are present in the apices of the posterior cervical triangle.

B. Axillary lymph nodes (Fig. 1.71)*:* There are 5 groups. The patient sits on a stool and the examiner sits in front of the patient (only the subscapular group is palpated from behind).

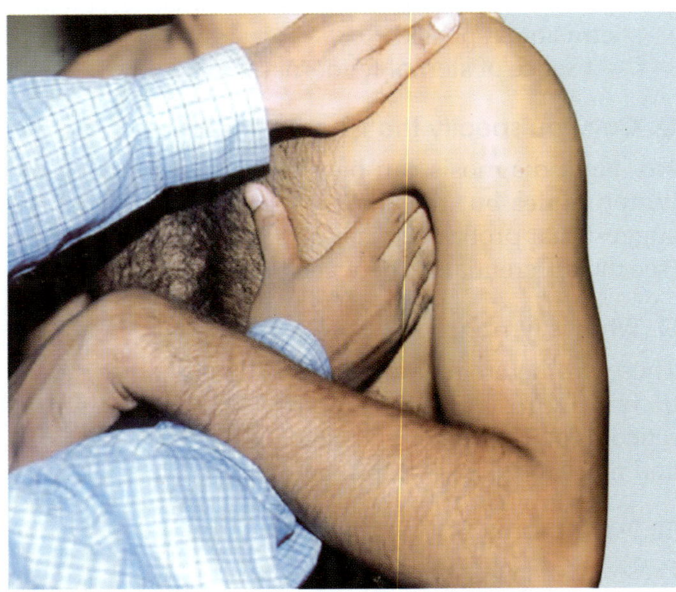

Fig. 1.71: Palpation of **axillary lymph nodes** of left side

a. *Central group:* The left side is palpated by right hand and *vice versa* for the right side. The patient's arm is abducted, and the hand of the examiner is placed in the axilla in such a way that the palm is directed towards the chest. Now the arm of the patient is adducted and allowed to rest 'comfortably' (complete relaxation of muscles is necessary) on the examiner's forearm. The other hand of the examiner is placed on the patient's same shoulder. The central group is palpated by sliding the fingers upwards to reach the highest limit of axilla.
b. *Apical group:* The same method as described above is applied here but the fingers are pushed as high as possible.
c. *Pectoral (anterior) group:* These glands are situated under the anterior axillary fold. For the left axilla, the fingers of right hand are insinuated under the pectoralis major and vice versa for the right axilla. The nodes are palpated with the help of the thumb and fingers.
d. *Brachial (lateral) group:* Here the left hand is used for the left side and the right hand for the right side. This

Clinical Wisdom

Relaxation of muscles is a must during palpation of all the groups of axillary nodes. After examination of one axilla, start examining the other side.

group of nodes are palpated against the upper part of the humerus when the examiner's palm directs laterally.

e. *Subscapular (posterior) group:* This group lies on the posterior axillary fold. It is *palpated from behind* when the hand insinuates within the latissimus dorsi, keeping the patient's arm horizontally forward (during palpation examiner's palm looks backwards).

C. Epitrochlear lymph nodes (Fig. 1.72)*:* Make the elbow slightly flexed and forearm supinated. The epitrochlear group of nodes are palpated under the thumb if the patient's left elbow is grasped by the examiner's left hand and *vice versa* for the right. It is better to fix the patient's forearm at the wrist by the examiner's opposite hand. The glands are palpated in the antero-medial region of the lower part of arm (in-between the groove of biceps and brachialis muscle) adjacent to the elbow. Both the sides should be examined. Palpable epitrochlear nodes almost always indicate some pathology.

D. Mediastinal group of lymph nodes: It is not possible to examine physically this group of nodes. Their presence can be detected indirectly by percussion of the sternum (read the section on 'Percussion of the sternum or base of the heart'). d'Espine's sign indirectly indicates mediastinal lymphadenopathy. This group comprises paratracheal, subcarinal, tracheobronchial and hilar lymph nodes. Chest X-ray and CT scan of thorax can detect these nodes in a better way.

E. Abdominal lymph nodes (pre- and para-aortic, coeliac, retroperitoneal, mesenteric)*:* This group, if enlarged will present as lump in the abdomen, or felt as nodular discrete or matted mass (read the section on 'Abdominal lump'). USG and CT scan of abdomen help in detecting these nodes satisfactorily.

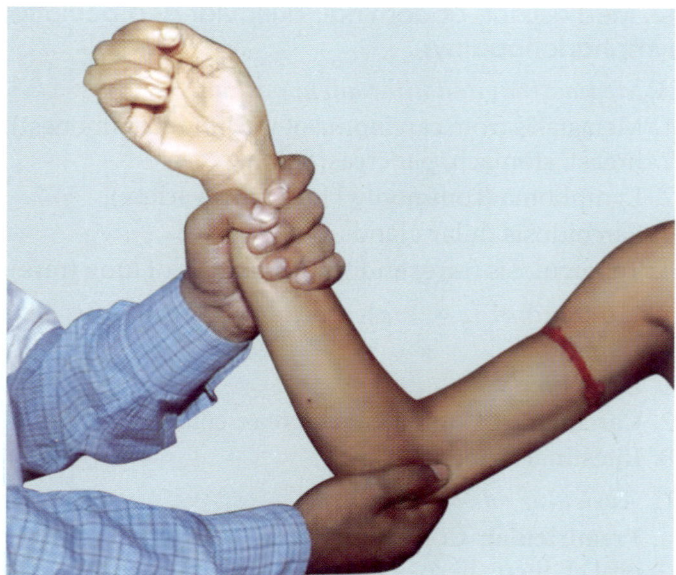

Fig. 1.72: Palpation of **epitrochlear lymph nodes** of right side

F. Inguinal lymph nodes: This group is commonly enlarged and especially palpable in bare-footed persons due to repeated trauma and infections of the lower limbs. Horizontal chain lies below inguinal ligament and vertical chain lies along upper part of saphenous vein. Both the sides are palpated one after another in supine position *after extending the thighs*.

G. Popliteal group of lymph nodes: The patient lies in supine position with semiflexed legs. The popliteal fossa is felt with the fingertips of either hand, when the fingers of both hands being curled into the popliteal fossa and both thumbs rest on tibial tuberosity (just like palpation of popliteal artery).

- Local examination is incomplete without the examination of the lymph nodes draining the affected area.

Q. What are lymph node 'levels' and 'stations'?

These are radiologically useful boundaries required for oncologic staging and planning. In neck, cervical nodes have been divided into at least six anatomic levels for the purpose of head and neck cancer staging (e.g. submental, submandibular, poisterior triangle, etc). Thoracic lymph nodes are divided into fourteen stations for lung cancer staging (e.g. superior mediastinal, aortic, etc.).

Q. Ideal description of a lymph node enlargement:

In lymphadenopathy, points to be noted at the bedside are:

1. Position or anatomical region affected (situation and extent).
2. Number and size.
3. Discrete or matted (margin).
4. Tenderness (i.e. infection within oral cavity, e.g. tonsillitis, dental sepsis).
5. Consistency (texture): Soft (cold abscess) (Fig. 1.73), rubbery and elastic (Hodgkin's disease), firm and shotty (syphilis), firm and matted (tuberculosis), and hard (malignancy). The normal lymph nodes are firm in feel.
6. Surface.
7. Mobility: Fixity to skin and surrounding structures (muscles, vessels, nerves or with any viscus) should be examined, i.e. fixed or mobile.
8. Rise of local temperature (i.e. indicates inflammation).
9. Skin changes [sinus, peau d'orange (orange skin appearance) or any sign of inflammation].
10. Lymphangitis (red, linear, tender lymph vessels radiating proximally): Present or not.
11. Draining area (e.g. in epitrochlear lymphadenopathy, examine the hand): It is a must.

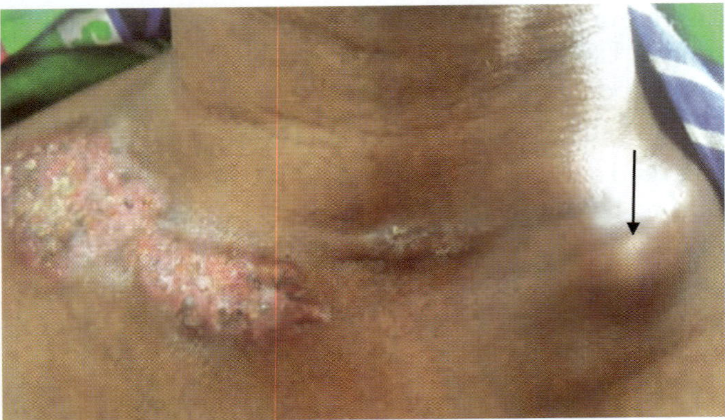

Fig. 1.73: Formation of **cold abscess** over lower part of neck (left). Scars of healed tuberculous lymphadenitis are also noted (right)

- **Matted** (means periadenitis) nodes are *most commonly found in tuberculosis*, and rarely in chronic lymphadenitis and NHL. 'Matted' means nodes are adhered together to form a mass.

Q. Common causes of cervical lymphadenopathy:

1. Infection (tonsillitis or impacted wisdom tooth), malignancy or ulcer in the oral cavity.
2. Infection in the ear, eye and nose.
3. Scalp infection by louse, dandruff.

- These (mentioned above) are common causes of cervical adenopathy which are very often missed.

4. Lymphoma.
5. Lymphatic leukaemia (acute and chronic).
6. Tuberculosis (pulmonary or miliary).
7. Metastasis in lymph nodes (from head, neck, breast, thyroid, stomach and lung malignancy).
8. Infectious mononucleosis, cytomeglovirus (CMV) infection, toxoplasmosis, HIV infection .
9. Sarcoidosis.
10. Rubella infection (postauricular and occipital nodes mainly).

- **Bull-neck:** This is classically seen in malignant diphtheria where the space between the mandible and the clavicles bulges with enlarged lymph nodes and oedema.
- Common viral infection producing lymphadenopathy: Rubella, CMV, Epstein-Barr virus, HIV.

Q. Causes of axillary and epitrochlear lymphadenopathy:

A. Axillary adenopathy:

1. Breast carcinoma (Fig. 1.74).
2. Infections of the upper extremity.
3. Lymphoma, melanoma.
4. ALL or CLL.
5. Tuberculosis.
6. Brucellosis.
7. Cat-scratch disease.

B. Epitrochlear adenopathy:

1. Hand infections.

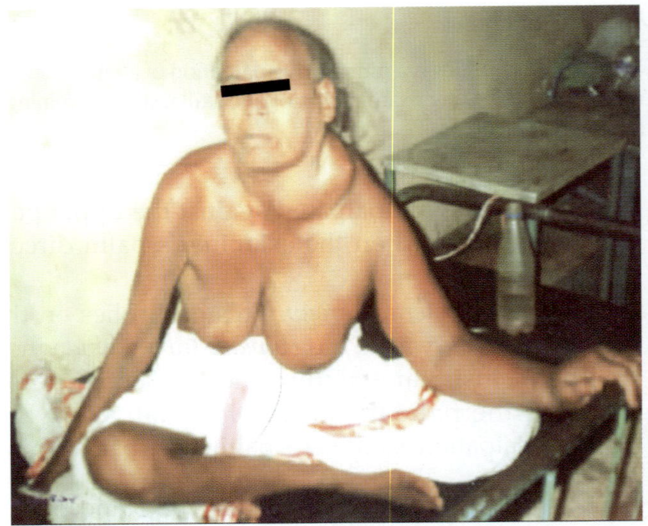

Fig. 1.74: **Carcinoma of left breast** with metastatic cervical lymphadenopathy and **lymphoedema** of left upper extremity

2. Lymphoma (especially NHL).
3. ALL or CLL.
4. Sarcoidosis.
5. Cat-scratch disease.
6. Tularaemia, infectious mononucleosis.
7. Secondary syphilis, HIV infection.

Q. Causes of inguinal lymphadenopathy:

1. Infection, injury or cellulitis of lower limb (commonly the vertical chain).
2. Filariasis.
3. Syphilis (primary), tuberculosis, plague.
4. Metastasis from genital malignancy, carcinoma of the uterus and rectum.
5. Chancroid, lymphogranuloma venereum (bilateral inguinal 'bubo'), genital herpes.
6. Acute lymphoblastic or chronic lymphocytic leukaemia, i.e. ALL or CLL.
7. Lymphoma.

Q. Mediastinal, abdominal, auricular and occipital lymphadenopathy:

A. Mediastinal and hilar adenopathy:

1. Metastasis from carcinoma of the lung (commonest), breast, stomach, pancreas, colon.
2. Lymphoma (commonly Hodgkin's variety).
3. Sarcoidosis (hilar glands ↑).
4. Tuberculosis (rare) and fungal disease of lung (rare).

B. Abdominal (e.g. mesenteric) and retroperitoneal adenopathy:

1. Lymphoma.
2. Carcinoma of stomach, pancreas, colon.
3. Intestinal tuberculosis.

C. Auricular adenopathy:

a. **Preauricular:** Conjunctivitis, rodent ulcer, primary oral chancre, herpes zoster ophthalmicus.
b. **Postauricular:** Leprosy, rubella, sarcoidosis.

D. Occipital (or posterior triangle) adenopathy: Scalp infection, rubella, pediculosis capitis, measles, infectious mononucleosis, secondary syphilis.

Q. What is Virchow's node (or sentinel node/Ewald's node/signal node)?

These are medial group of left-sided supraclavicular lymph nodes which lie in between two heads of sternomastoid muscle. They receive lymphatics from:

1. Upper limb (left).
2. Breast (left).
3. Lung (left).
4. Stomach (Troisier's sign), and
5. Testes.

Clinical method for palpation (Fig. 1.75): Stand behind the sitting patient. Put your right hand over the right side of patient's face and ask him to turn the face to right against your resistance. Two heads of left sternomastoid become prominent and now put your left index finger in between the two heads.

Clinical Wisdom

Bronchogenic carcinoma commonly produces scalene node enlargement. Supraclavicular nodes (e.g. Virchow's node) are important in relation to malignancy of lung, breast, GI tract and genitals.

- **Breast** should always be examined in a case of cervical and axillary lymphadenopathy for symmetry, ulcers, redness, peau d'orange appearance, dimpling of skin and nipple discharge. Palpate all the quadrants with flat of the hand, and lastly examine the axillary and cervical lymph nodes.
- **Virchow's triad (law):** Hypercoagulability + haemodynamic changes (stasis, turbulance) + endothelial injury or dysfunction. It is the basis of formation of deep vein thrombosis (DVT).

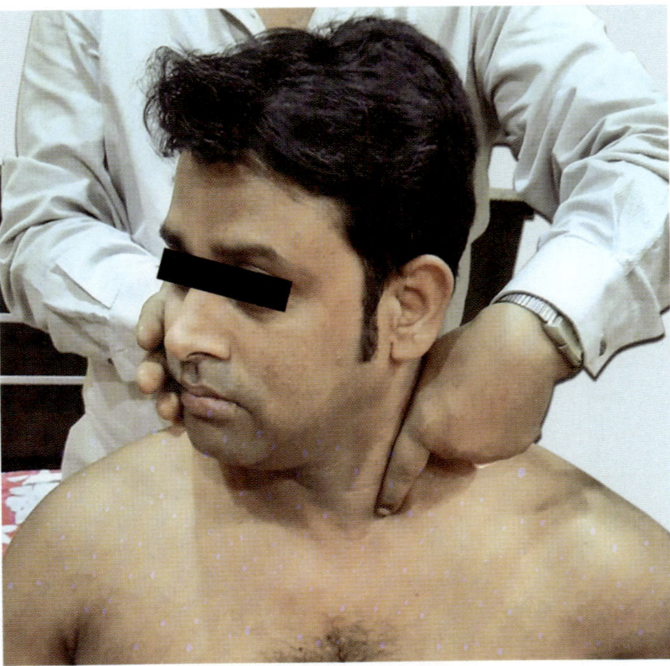

Fig. 1.75: Palpation of **Virchow's gland** in neck

- Delphian node: A midline pre-laryngeal lymph node seen in thyroid disorder, lymphoma or laryngeal malignancy.
- Rudolf Ludwig Carl Virchow (1821–1902) was a German pathologist, and anatomist of Wurzburg and Berlin. He was known as 'Father of modern pathology'.

Q. When the enlarged nodes are of pathological significance?

It is said that lymph nodes are pathologically significant when they are:

1. (Usually) greater than 1 cm in diameter.
2. Firm or hard in consistency.
3. Round in shape.
4. Matted (nodes become adherent).
5. Tender on palpation.
6. Fixed to underlying tissue or skin.

However, in assessing the significance of enlarged lymph nodes, following factors should always be considered like a) age of the patient, b) the physical characteristics of the nodes, c) anatomical sites involved, and d) the clinical setting.

- Inguinal lymph nodes ≥2 cm in size may be considered as 'significant'.
- Small, soft, discrete, non-tender lymphadenopathy is usually 'benign' while hard, fixed, non-tender (may be tender) lymphadenopathy is 'malignant' in nature. After age 50, incidence of benign disorder decreases and that of malignant disorder increases.

Q. Lymph nodes fixed to surrounding structures:

1. Metastases in the lymph nodes (i.e. malignancy)—hard, 'craggy' lymph nodes.
2. Tuberculosis.

Q. Painful and tender lymph nodes:

1. Pyogenic infections, diphtheria, infectious mononucleosis, fungal infections.
2. Metastases in the lymph nodes (may or may not be tender).

Q. Lymphadenopathy with sinus formation:

1. Tuberculous lymphadenitis (Fig. 1.73).
2. Malignancy.
3. Actinomycosis.

Q. What is Waldeyer's ring?

There are two rings—outer (described in page 208) and inner. The **inner one** is the ring of lymphoid tissue within the oral cavity (in posterior part of oropharynx and nasopharynx) and is composed of: 1. Adenoids, 2. Faucal tonsils and 3. Lingual tonsils. This ring is commonly involved in NHL.

Q. What is generalised lymphadenopathy?

Lymphadenopathy is defined as inflammatory or non-inflammatory enlargement of lymph nodes. **'Generalised lymphadenopathy'** is characterised by the involvement of three or more non-contiguous lymph node areas—for example, when the right axilla and both sides of the neck (contiguous affection) are involved, it is not designated as generalised lymphadenopathy. The present case on discussion has involvement of neck, axillary and inguinal lymph nodes, and thus it is a case of generalised lymphadenopathy.

When a single anatomical area is involved, it is known as 'localised (regional) lymphadenopathy'.

❍ Each side of the neck is considered as single lymph node area.

Q. Description of lymph node enlargement in lymphoma (Table 1.27):

A. **Hodgkin's disease (HD):** Cervical nodes are initially affected. Other nodes are involved in course of time and rarely, abdominal and inguinal nodes are involved.

Description: Enlarged, non-tender with *India-rubbery feel*, smooth surface, not fixed to skin or deeper structures, discrete, no sinus or no rise of temperature in the overlying skin, and there is no softening or any suppuration.

B. Non-Hodgkin's lymphoma (NHL): Enlargement of lymph nodes may affect any area initially. There is more chance of involvement of epitrochlear nodes and inner Waldeyer's ring.

Description: Enlarged, non-tender (rarely tender) with *firm or variegated feel*, smooth or nodular surface, may fix to deeper structures, discrete, without any sinus in the overlying skin, sometimes with elevated local skin temperature, and there is neither softening nor any suppuration.

❍ Thomas Hodgkin (1798–1866) was the curator of the museum of Guy's Hospital, London, UK.

Q. Pathological classification of lymphoma:

A. **Hodgkin's disease** (WHO pathological classification, which is a minor modification of previous *Rye classification)*:
- Nodular lymphocyte-predominant HD (5%; slowly growing, localised, rarely fatal).
- Classical HD (95%):
  - Nodular sclerosis HD (70%).
  - Mixed cellularity HD (20%).
  - Lymphocyte-rich HD (5%).
  - Lymphocyte-depleted HD (rare).

Table 1.27: Clinical differentiation between HD and NHL

Features	Hodgkin's disease (HD)	Non-Hodgkin's lymphoma (NHL)
1. Frequency	Less common (30%)	More common (70%)
2. Age	Bimodal peaks seen: larger peak between 15–35 years and smaller peak over 50 years	Any age; more frequent with increasing age
3. B-symptoms	Early and prominent	Late and non-prominent (only in 20% cases)
4. Anaemia	Late	Early
5. Dissemination	Unifocal in origin; well localised at diagnosis	Multicentric in origin; widespread at diagnosis
6. Lymph node involvement		
a. Presentation	90% nodal and 10% extranodal	60% nodal and 40% extranodal
b. Size	Smaller	Larger
c. Rate of growth	Slow	Fast
d. Consistency	Rubbery elastic	Variegated or firm
e. Matting	Rare	May be seen
f. Local temperature	Normal	May be raised
g. Tenderness	Absent	May be present
h. ↑ Epitrochlear nodes	Less common	Common
i. ↑ Waldeyer's ring (inner)	Less common	Common
j. ↑ Mediastinal lymph node	More comman	Less common
k. ↑ Abdominal lymph nodes	Early involvement of para-aortic nodes	Early involvement of mesenteric nodes
7. Pruritus	Common	Less common
8. Splenomegaly	More common	Common
9. GI tract involvement	Uncommon	Common
10. CNS involvement	Uncommon	Common
11. Bone marrow involvement	Late	Early
12. Alcohol test	Common	Uncommon

❍ **Alcohol test:** After intake of alcohol, there may be pain in the area of nodal involvement.
❍ In HD, the disease spreads by contiguity and in NHL, it is non-contiguous (haematogenous) spread.

- The prognosis of a), b), c) and d) are respectively a) very good, b) good, c) fair, and d) poor.
- Nodular sclerosis variety is most commonly encountered, followed by mixed cellularity, lymphocyte-rich and lymphocyte-depleted type. Mixed cellularity is most common type of HD in India.

B. **Non-Hodgkin's lymphoma** (*Rappaport's classification*):

a. Nodular:

i. Lymphocytic: Poorly differentiated.

ii. Mixed: Lymphocytic and 'histiocytic'.

iii. 'Histiocytic'.

b. Diffuse:

i. Lymphocytic: Well differentiated and poorly differentiated.

ii. Mixed: Lymphocytic and 'histiocytic'.

iii. 'Histiocytic'.

iv. Lymphoblastic.

v. Undifferentiated: Burkitt's and non-Burkitt's lymphoma.

Clinical Wisdom

Lukes and Collins made the most modern classification of NHL according to cytologic types: T cell, B cell, U cell, histiocytic. NHL in 1982 was classified into high-grade, intermediate-grade and low-grade lymphoma (International Working Formulation). Nodular lymphomas are mainly of low-grade (prognostically better) and diffuse lymphomas are mostly of high-grade (prognostically worse).

- REAL (Revised European-American Lymphoma), a new pathologic classification of NHL, was introduced in 1984, and the new entries over International Working Formulation were mucosa-associated lymphoid tumours (MALT), mantle cell lymphoma and anaplastic large cell lymphoma (Ki-1 lymphoma).
- The classification of NHL is most controversial and has been changed 6 times in past 40 years, like:
  1. Rappaport's classification (1966).
  2. Lukes and Collins classification (1972).
  3. Kiel's classification (1981).
  4. International Working Formulation (1982).
  5. REAL classification (1984, and revised in 1990).
  6. WHO classification (2001, and modified in 2008): Most accepted worldwide (based on precursor B, mature B, precursor T and mature T/NK cell).
- NHL is finally subclassified according to its cell of origin, i.e. T or B cell, and the stage of lymphocytic maturity (i.e. precursor or mature) at which they develop. Diffuse large B-cell lymphoma is most common NHL in India.

Q. Describe the splenic enlargement in lymphoma:

The spleen is the largest lymphatic organ in the body. Spleen has no afferent lymphatics and its involvement indicates vascular invasion even in an apparently localised disease. In 30% patients with normal spleen, Hodgkin's disease was found in the spleen removed at surgery. Again, it is said that splenomegaly does not always indicate involvement by Hodgkin's disease (25% patients with splenomegaly have only reactive hyperplasia). As a whole, spleen is enlarged in 45% patients of Hodgkin's disease. It is of moderate enlargement, firm to hard in consistency, non-tender and at times with irregular surface (previously known as 'hard bake spleen').

In NHL, spleen is often enlarged at the onset of the disease and subsequently may show marked enlargement with features of hypersplenism. *Splenomegaly in NHL usually indicates splenic involvement.* The description of palpable spleen is more or less same in both HD and NHL. **Spleen is less commonly involved in NHL than in HD.**

Q. Clinical staging (Ann Arbor classification) of your case:

In stage IIIB (as both sides of diaphragm are involved with systemic symptoms).

Q. 'Ann Arbor staging classification' of lymphoma (especially Hodgkin's disease):

Stage I: Involvement of a single lymph node region (I) or of a single extralymphatic organ or site (IE).

Stage II: Involvement of two or more lymph node regions **on the same side of the diaphragm** (II), or localised affection of an extralymphatic organ or site and of one or more lymph node regions on the same side (above or below) of diaphragm (IIE).

Stage III: Involvement of lymph node regions **on both sides of the diaphragm (III)**, which may also be associated with splenic involvement (IIIS) or by localised involvement of an extralymphatic organ or site (IIIE) or both (IIISE).

Stage IV: Diffuse or disseminated involvement of one or more extralymphatic organs or tissues, with or without associated lymph node involvement (e.g. involvement of *extralymphatic organ or site* like lung, liver, pleura, bone, bone marrow, skin and subcutaneous tissue).

Clinical Wisdom

All the four stages are associated with A or B-symptoms. The *lymphatic structures* are lymph nodes, spleen, Waldeyer's ring, thymus, Peyer's patches and appendix. Recently few modifications (e.g. both-sided hilar node involvement is categorised as stage II) of this classification has been done **(Cotswolds modification)**, 'A' (no symptoms) and 'B' (presence of fever, drenching night sweats and weight loss) are added accordingly.

- New designations applicable to clinical staging are: A: asymptomatic, B: with symptoms, X: bulky nodal disease, E: involvement of single extranodal site, and S: splenic involvement.

Q. Importance of staging in lymphoma:

Staging is important to establish the extent of the disease and to plan for therapeutic approach. There are two types of staging (i.e. extent of the disease): Clinical stage (CS) and pathologic stage (PS). The **clinical stage** (Ann Arbor staging classification) is based on physical examination and different noninvasive tests (chest X-ray, USG of abdomen, CT scan). The **pathologic stage** is determined by the information obtained from invasive tests which include the collection of biopsy specimens from different sites (usually during a staging laparotomy). As NHL frequently disseminate haematogenously and becomes widespread at the time of diagnosis, Ann Arbor staging system has little impact on this variety of lymphoma. *One should never forget that the treatment and prognosis in HD depend largely on stage of the disease, whereas in NHL the therapy is usually based on its histological type.*

Staging evaluation for NHL is usually done by:

- Physical examination .
- Presence of B-symptoms.
- Laboratory tests (CBC, LFT, uric acid, LDH, β_2-microglobulin).
- Chest X-ray.
- CT scan (abdomen, pelvis, chest).
- Bone marrow biopsy.
- Lumbar puncture.

Q. Confirmation: HD or NHL?

It is done by biopsy of the lymph nodes. Presence of Reed-Sternberg (R-S) cells confirms the diagnosis of Hodgkin's disease (absence of R-S cells does not exclude Hodgkin's disease).

Q. How to diagnose Reed-Sternberg (R-S) cell or Dorothy Reed cell ?

A. Features of R-S cell (a giant cell which looks like owl's eye):
   1. Large giant cell with abundance of acidophilic cytoplasm.
   2. Mirror image nuclei with vesicular pattern.
   3. Chromatin is loosely wooven.
   4. Multiple nucleoli with perinuclear halo.
   5. On immunophenotyping, they are usually CD 15+ and CD 30+.

B. R-S cells or cells simulating R-S cells are found in: 1. Hodgkin's disease (hallmark of diagnosis; not found in NHL), 2. Infectious mononucleosis, 3. Breast carcinoma, 4. Burkitt's lymphoma, 5. Mycosis fungoides (Fig. 1.76), 6. Malignant melanoma.

Q. Infecting agents associated with lymphoid malignancy:

Epstein-Barr virus (Burkitt's lymphoma), HIV (diffuse large B-cell lymphoma), HTLV-1 (adult T-cell lymphoma), Hepatitis C (lymphoplasmacytic lymphoma), *H. pylori* (gastric MALT lymphoma) and human herpesvirus-8 (primary effusion lymphoma).

Q. Importance of examination of other systems in lymphoma:

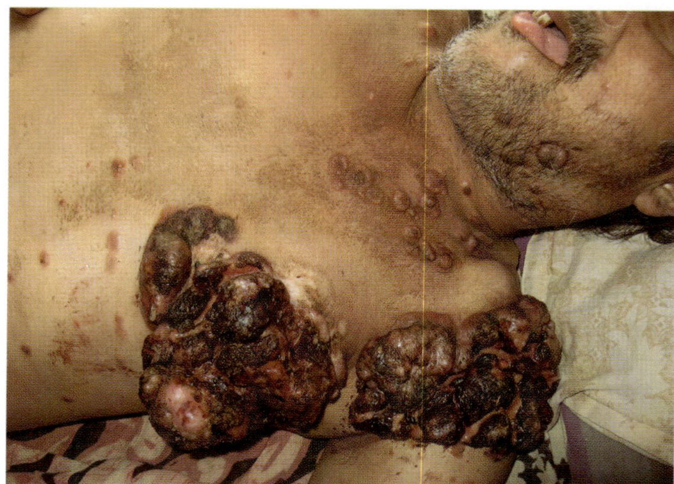

Fig. 1.76: **Mycosis fungoides** (cutaneous T-cell lymphoma)–multiple tumour-like lesions in ulcerated base

1. General survey: Anaemia, lymphadenopathy, pyrexia, puffy face (e.g. SVC syndrome).
2. Respiratory system: Pleural effusion (often bilateral), collapse of the lung due to mediastinal lymphadenopathy. Always perform the 'mediastinal percussion' and look for the features of superior mediastinal syndrome.
3. CVS: Pericardial effusion.
4. Nervous system: Cranial nerves involvement, paraplegia, proptosis, LMN type facial palsy.
5. GI tract: Other than hepatosplenomegaly there may be lump abdomen (lymph node lump), jaundice, ascites or signs of intestinal obstruction.
6. Genitourinary system: Haematuria, renal lump, hydronephrosis; occlusion of renal vein may produce nephrotic syndrome; renal failure from ureteric obstruction; testicular mass.
7. Skin: Skin lesions of lymphoma (lymphoma cutis), signs of generalised pruritus, herpes zoster, erythroderma, etc.
8. Bones: Diffuse bone pain, swelling of bones.

Q. Drugs producing lymphadenopathy (pseudo-lymphoma):

1. Phenytoin, 2. Cyclosporin A (used in organ transplantation), 3. Carbamazepine, 4. Cephaloridine, 5. PAS (used in multi-drug resistant tuberculosis), 6. Primidone, 7. Hydralazine, 8. Allopurinol.

Q. Anaemia in lymphoma:

1. Ineffective erythropoiesis.
2. Haemodilution.
3. Hypersplenism.
4. Haemolysis (rare).

Q. How paraplegia is produced in lymphoma?

Involvement of thoracic vertebrae is common in lymphoma. It may be produced by:

1. Involvement of body of the vertebra with collapse.

2. Invasion of the epidural space from retroperitoneal lymph nodes with cord compression.
3. Jeopardized vascular supply of the spinal cord.

Q. Jaundice in lymphoma:

1. Hepatic involvement.
2. Extrahepatic biliary obstruction (lymph nodes pressing porta hepatis).
3. Hepatitis due to repeated blood transfusion (type B or C).
4. Haemolysis (autoimmune and rare).

Q. Symptoms relating to GI tract:

These symptoms are common in NHL variety. Symptoms may be:
1. Anorexia.
2. Nausea, vomiting.
3. Haematemesis and melaena.
4. Diarrhoea (malabsorption syndrome).
5. Swelling of the abdomen (lump abdomen formed due to adenopathy, or presence of ascites).

Q. Is it possible to have lymphoma without palpable lymphadenopathy?

Yes, it is possible in abdominal lymphoma.

Q. Possible associations of 'night sweats' in clinical medicine:

1. Tuberculosis.
2. Lymphoma.
3. Chronic myeloid leukaemia.
4. Giant cell arteritis.
5. Brucellosis, rheumatoid arthritis.
6. AIDS.
7. Amoebic liver abscess.
8. Nocturnal (sleeping) hypoglycaemia.

- **Excessive sweating** is characteristic of familial or idiopathic, hypoglycaemia (drenching sweat), acute myocardial infarction (drenching sweat), anxiety neurosis (cold and moist hands), thyrotoxicosis (warm and moist hands), acromegaly, pheochromocytoma (paroxysmal sweating), menopausal syndrome, arecoline sensitivity (present in betel nut) and gustatory hyperhidrosis (autonomic neuropathy).

Q. History with special findings in lymphadenopathy pointing towards a disease:

- Fever: Lymphoma, tuberculosis, different bacterial and viral infections, sarcoidosis, ALL, SLE, infectious mononucleosis, AIDS.
- Petechial haemorrhage in palate in a young boy with cervical adenopathy: Infectious mononucleosis.
- Hard lump in breast associated with ipsilateral axillary adenopathy: Breast carcinoma.
- Swelling of feet/legs, non-pitting or solid oedema along with inguinal adenopathy: Filariasis.
- Fever, weight loss, loss of appetite ± night sweats associated with adenopathy: Tuberculosis, lymphoma, malignancy, AIDS, ALL.
- Prolonged medication-induced lymphadenopathy: Commonly phenytoin-induced (search for gum hypertrophy and acne, induced by chronic phenytoin therapy in a patient of epilepsy).
- Lymphadenopathy with skin lesion: SLE (butterfly-rash in face), sarcoidosis (lupus pernio in face), secondary syphilis, amyloidosis.
- With splenomegaly: Lymphoma, leukaemias (ALL and CLL), disseminated tuberculosis, SLE, HIV infection.
- With arthritis: SLE, Still's disease, sarcoidosis, brucellosis, amyloidosis.

Q. Causes of generalised lymphadenopathy:

Lymphadenopathy (or adenopathy) may be an incidental finding. Majority of generalised lymphadenopathy are non-malignant in nature. The causes are:
1. Lymphoma (HD and NHL).
2. Acute lymphoblastic leukaemia.
3. Chronic lymphocytic leukaemia.
4. Disseminated or miliary tuberculosis.
5. Secondary metastasis to lymph nodes.
6. Secondary syphilis.
7. Infectious mononucleosis.
8. Collagen vascular disease, e.g. SLE.
9. Sarcoidosis.
10. Filariasis.
11. Chronic lymphadenitis.
12. HIV infection (AIDS).
13. Amyloidosis.
14. Drug-induced.

- Brucellosis, cytomegalovirus (CMV), toxoplasmosis, Kawasaki's disease, blast crisis in CML and Still's disease may give rise to generalised lymphadenopathy.
- Dermatopathic lymphadenopathy: Generalised lymphadenopathy from psoriasis or eczema evolving as a reactive process.
- Aetiology unknown (lymphadenoapthy): Kawasaki disease, Kikuchi disease, Kimura's disease, Rosai-Dorfman disease, sarcoidosis, Castleman disease and Familial Mediterranean fever.

Q. Differential diagnosis of generalised lymphadenopathy:

A. Lymphoma
1. Any age.
2. Usually cervical group is involved first.
3. SVC obstruction.
4. Fever, night sweats, loss of weight.
5. Hepatosplenomegaly.
6. Pleural effusion (often bilateral) or ascites.
7. Discrete, rubbery or firm, non-tender lymphadenopathy. Epitrochlear nodes are commonly involved in NHL.

B. Acute lymphoblastic leukaemia (ALL)
1. Children or young adults.
2. Fever may be very high; intermittent infections.

3. Descrete, non-tender adenopathy.
4. Moderate splenomegaly with hepatomegaly; severe anaemia.
5. Very short course of disease.
6. Haemorrhagic manifestations (purpura, gum bleeding, epistaxis), mouth ulcers, sore throat.
7. Presence of sternal tenderness.
8. Involvement of eye, CNS and testes are not uncommon.

C. Chronic lymphocytic leukaemia (CLL)

1. Over the age of 45 years (peak 65 years) and M>F; insidious onset.
2. Firm, discrete, non-tender, generalised lymphadenopathy.
3. Moderate splenomegaly with hepatomegaly. *Most common form of chronic leukaemia.*
4. Gradual onset of weakness, slowly developing pallor and presence of irregular fever.
5. Haemorrhagic manifestations into the skin in late stages.
6. Increased frequency of infections (*S. pneumoniae, staphylococcus and H. influenzae*).
7. Absence of sternal tenderness.

- CLL: A neoplastic disorder of lymphocytes, usually affecting the B-lymphocytes (95%), and rarely T-lymphocytes (5%).

D. Disseminated or miliary tuberculosis

1. Children or young adults.
2. High rise of temperature with night sweats, loss of weight, progressive anaemia and cough.
3. Glands are palpable, matted (means perladenitis), usually painless but may be painful, firm, without any rise of local temperature; rarely there may be a sinus present in the skin with formation of cold abscess underneath (Fig. 1.73). Early disease may be with discrete nodes. Hard and craggy nodes (with calcification) are found in healed tuberculosis. Nodes in the posterior triangle of neck are commonly affected.
4. Paucity of signs in the chest (miliary). Often few crepitations are heard late in the disease
5. Mild hepatomegaly with mild, tender splenomegaly.
6. Choroidal tubercles may be seen (25%) in the retina by ophthalmoscopy (miliary tuberculosis).
7. Mantoux test may be negative, miliary mottlings may be seen in chest X-ray, while caseating granuloma in lymph node biopsy may prove the diagnosis.

- Choroidal tubercles are yellowish and slightly shiny lesions with a diameter of <1/4th of optic disc.

E. Secondary metastasis to lymph nodes

1. Middle or old age commonly.
2. Lymph nodes are stony hard or craggy, fixed, non-tender; generally localised, rarely generalised.
3. H/o haemoptysis, melaena, sore throat, breast lump, etc.
4. Anaemia with emaciation (cachexia).
5. Presence of primary source like carcinoma of head, neck, thyroid, lung, breast or stomach.

- Though initially non-tender, pain and tenderness of variable intensity may appear lately (metastatic lymph nodes).

F. Secondary syphilis

1. Usually in young adults.
2. Past H/o exposure and primary syphilis (e.g. genital ulcers).
3. Moderately enlarged, discrete, *firm and shotty*, painless and non-tender adenopathy. Though the distribution is generalised, there is predilection for affection of occipital and epitrochlear nodes.
4. Skin rash, condylomata lata and snail track ulcers (mucous patches) in mouth may be seen

Clinical Wisdom

Secondary syphilis is not seen nowadays because of the early use of antibiotics in the treatment of 'chancre' (primary syphilis). There may be hepatosplenomegaly.

G. Infectious mononucleosis

1. Children or young adults.
2. Adenitis is mostly cervical (posterior cervical group), may be generalised. Glands are palpable, a bit tender with moderate enlargement.
3. Fever of short duration, malaise, headache, sore throat may be present.
4. Acute onset with a maculopapular rash (like drug rash), especially with amoxycillin.
5. Petechial haemorrhages may be seen at the junction of the hard and soft palate.
6. Spleen is often palpable.
7. Atypical lymphocytes in peripheral blood. Positive Paul-Bunnell test and monospot test.

H. Systemic lupus erythematosus (SLE)

1. Young or middle-aged female patients.
2. Present with arthralgia, arthritis, PUO, myalgia, butterfly rash in face, palatal ulcer or oliguria
3. Moderate splenomegaly with hepatomegaly.
4. Non-tender, discrete adenopathy.
5. Pleurisy, pleural effusion, pericarditis or renal failure may develop.

I. Sarcoidosis

1. Usually in children or young adults.
2. Generalised adenopathy with frequent involvement of pre- and postauricular, submandibular, epitrochlear and paratracheal nodes.
3. Mild splenomegaly.
4. Classical skin lesions around nose/eye/cheeks (lupus pernio), uveitis or parotid swelling may be seen. Patient may have cough, dyspnoea, fatigue or presence of erythema nodosum.
5. **Lofgren's syndrome** (erythema nodosum, arthritis and hilar adenopathy), and **Heerfordt syndrome**

(anterior uveitis, parotid swelling, facial palsy) are characteristic.

6. Bilateral hilar adenopathy in chest X-ray, positive Kveim test, elevated serum angiotensin-converting enzyme (SACE) and negative Mantoux test are characteristic features.

J. Filariasis (Fig. 1.77)

1. Any age.
2. Fever with chill and rigor intially with every full moon and new moon. There may be pain felt in the scrotum, breast, vulva, or erythematous and painful cord like swelling in the limbs. Spermatic cord may be thick and tender. Non-pitting oedema of legs with peau d'orange appearance of the skin may be seen.
3. In the chronic stage elephantiasis (lymphoedema as well as increased thickness of skin) of scrotum, vulva or legs with pleural effusion (chylous), ascites (chylous) and chyluria may develop.
4. Discrete, non-tender palpable lymph nodes in the inguinal region may be generalised.

- Peau d'orange appearance and lymphoedema are often associated with filariasis and malignancy.

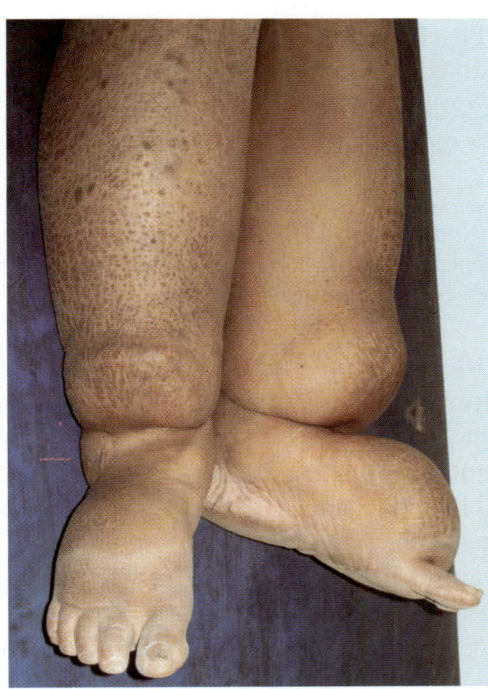

Fig. 1.77: Elephantiasis of legs from **filariasis**

K. Chronic lymphadenitis

1. Any age. Common in cervical and inguinal lymph nodes.
2. Primary focus is in the oral cavity, scalp, genitalia or in the neighbourhood of the affected glands.
3. Moderately enlarged, firm, mildly tender (rarely matted).
4. There may be rise of body temperature.

L. HIV infection (AIDS) (Fig. 1.78)

1. Any age, young adults commonly

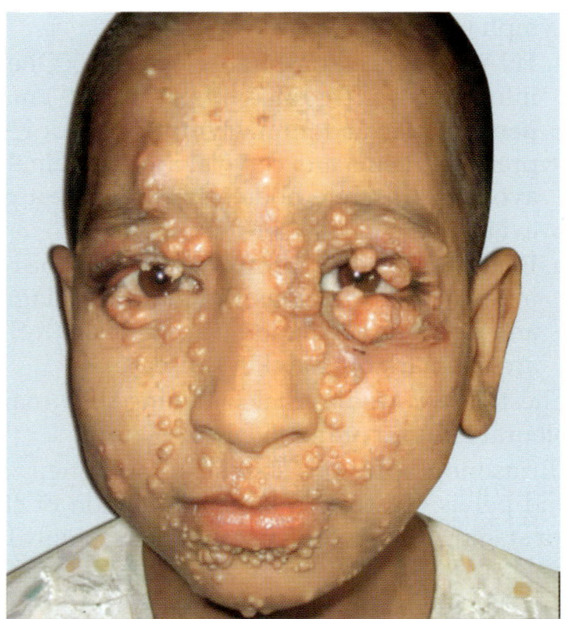

Fig. 1.78: **Molluscum contagiosum:** Multiple, glistening pale, poxvirus-induced, umbilicated, dome-shaped, pinhead to 1 cm papules. The child is **HIV positive**

2. H/o homosexuality, promiscuous sex or receiving blood transfusion.
3. Patient may present with infectious mononucleosis-like illness with pyrexia, rash and lymphadenopathy.
4. A subgroup of patients with asymptomatic infection may present with *persistent generalised lymphadenopathy (PGL)* or AIDS-related complex (ARC). Patient with ARC may have chronic diarrhoea, night sweats, fever, weight loss and oral candidosis. PGL is defined as the presence of enlarged lymph nodes (>1 cm) in 2 or more extrainguinal non-contiguous sites for more than 3 months. The lymph nodes are symmetrical, firm, mobile and non-tender. Lymphadenopathy in AIDS may be due to diseases like tuberculosis or lymphoma.
5. Rapid downhill course.
6. Biopsy of the lymph nodes show reactive hyperplasia.
7. ELISA test for HIV antibody (screening test) and Western Blot test to identify antibodies to specific viral protein (confirmatory test) are positive.

M. Amyloidosis: Read the section on 'Hepatosplenomegaly'.

N. Drug-induced: *See* page 214, also known as pseudo-lymphoma.

Q. How do you like to investigate a case of lymphoma?

1. Blood examination:
   a. Anaemia (normocytic normochromic).
   b. Leukaemoid reaction may be seen (common in Hodgkin's disease).
   c. Mild eosinophilia (10–15% cases) in Hodgkin's disease.
   d. Lymphocytopenia (bears a bad prognosis).
   e. High ESR (Indicates disease activity).

2. Lymph node biopsy:
   a. FNAC (fine needle aspiration cytology): Often not informative. CT-guided biopsy (FNAC) may be performed in abdominal lymphoma. For FNAC, preferred items are: cervical area (inguinal area avoided), discrete node with the largest gland available.
   b. **Excision (open) biopsy:** 'Most important' investigation. **It gives the accurate diagnosis** and helps in evaluation of prognosis (R-S cells are hallmark of Hodgkin's disease).
3. Chest X-ray: Mediastinal widening (HD mainly), pleural effusion or involvement of lung.
4. Ultrasonography or CT scan of abdomen, chest and pelvis: CT scan is the investigation of choice for staging although PET scan is increasingly being used.
5. Pleural aspiration, paracentesis abdominis or lumbar puncture (in paraplegia).
6. Biopsy of pleura, liver or skin lesions.
7. Endoscopy of upper GI tract (for haematemesis and melaena) or barium meal X-ray of stomach and duodenum with follow through.
8. Bone marrow examination (aspiration or trephine biopsy): Helps in the diagnosis and staging of the disease (bone marrow involvement indicates stage IV disease).
9. Bipedal lymphangiography will demonstrate pre- and para-aortic, or retroperitoneal lymph nodes involvement.
10. Liver function tests (may be abnormal with or without hepatic involvement).
11. Biochemical:
    a. Serum calcium or alkaline phosphatase may be elevated due to involvement of bones.
    b. Serum copper, LDH and uric acid are often increased in NHL variety.
    c. Blood surgar, urea and creatinine as a routine investigation.
12. Intravenous pyelography (IVP) for renal involvement.
13. Skeletal survey by X-ray or Gallium scan (usually osteosclerotic lesion is seen in HD: 'Ivory vertebra', and osteolytic lesion in NHL variety).
14. Laparotomy (mainly for staging purpose): Rarely required.

- As high-grade NHL may be associated with AIDS, do the HIV testing. For modern classification, send the lymph node biopsy material for immunophenotyping of surface antigens and cytogenetic/molecular analysis. Immunophenotyping may be done on blood, bone marrow or nodal material.
- In leukaemia, peripheral blood smear and bone marrow examination are more important than lymph node biopsy.

Q. How do you treat a case of lymphoma?

A. Hodgkin's disease:

Therapeutic guidelines are:

a. Indication of **radiotherapy**:
   i. Stage I and II A with 3 or less areas of involvement.
   ii. To lesions causing serious pressure symptoms, e.g. SVC syndrome.
b. Indication of **chemotherapy**:
   i. All patients with B-symptoms.
   ii. Stage II with > 3 areas of involvement, stage III and stage IV diseases.

Radiotherapy is used in a dose of 3600 to 4400 cGy (daily dose of 200 cGy over 4 weeks).

Different modes like involved-field radiotherapy (IF), inverted Y-field radiotherapy, mantle-field radiotherapy, extended-field radiotherapy (EF) and total axial lymph node irradiation (TANI) are used.

Regimens of chemotherapy are:

1. MOPP (mustine hydrochloride, vincristine, prednisolone and procarbazine): Previously used.
2. MVPP (only vinblastine replaces the vincristine of MOPP regimen): Previously used.
3. ABVD (adriamycin, bleomycin, vinblastine and decarbazine): Preferred regimen.
4. SCAB (streptozotocin, CCNU, adriamycin and bleomycin): Active regimen.
5. ChlVPP (chlorambucil, vinblastine, prednisolone and procarbazine): Preferred regimen.
6. BEACOPP (BACOP + etoposide + procarbazine): Newer regimen for ABVD-failure cases.

- Combined modality (chemotherapy followed by radiotherapy) is applied in *bulk disease*. Autologous bone marrow transplantation is tried after failure of chemotherapy. Treatment response is monitored by CT or PET scan.

B. Non-Hodgkin's lymphoma:

Radiotherapy is usually given by involved-field treatment (IF) or total body irradiation (stage I).

Chemotherapy is used in stages II, III, IV in high-grade NHL and in stages IIB, III, IV in low-grade NHL. Regimens of chemotherapy are:

1. Chlorambucil: As single drug oral therapy (in low-grade NHL).
2. CVP (cyclophosphamide, vincristine and prednisolone).
3. CHOP (cyclophosphamide, hydroxyadriamycin, vincristine and prednisolone).
4. BACOP (bleomycin, adriamycin, cyclophosphamide, vincristine and prednisolone).

- R-CHOP therapy is rituximab combined with CHOP regimen. Addition of rituximab increases the complete response rates and improves overall survival. R-CVP (rituximab + CVP) therapy and R-Bendamustine (gaining popularity) regimens are also used. There is dramatic improvement in survival after addition of rituximab.
- Other drugs tried are bortezomib, temsirolimus, ibrutinib, idelalisib, etc.

Clinical Wisdom

These drugs are given on a 28-day cycle (one pulse) for a total of **6–8 'pulses'** 'in both HD and NHL'. Autologous bone marrow transplantation is a new modality of treatment in NHL. Blood is transfused in severely anaemic patients along with supportive care.

Conclusion

1. Palpate all the anatomical areas for lymph node enlargement.
2. In a patient with lymphadenopathy, one should be careful about examination of inner Waldeyer's ring, *breast*, *testes*, non-pitting oedema in legs, sternal tenderness, hepatosplenomegaly, ascites, pleural effusion and tenderness in spine (i.e. paraplegia in a case of lymphoma).
3. Other systems should be examined carefully, especially the abdomen.
4. In a patient with inguinal lymphadenopathy, examine the legs and sole of the foot for the presence of any ulcer, infection, etc.

- **A case of lymphoma may be given as superior mediastinal syndrome in the examination.**

SECTION 8: MISCELLANEOUS

CHRONIC KALA-AZAR — CASE 26

Q. What is your diagnosis?

The diagnosis may be delivered in one of the two ways:

1. It is a case of huge (sometimes, moderate) splenomegaly with mild (to moderate) hepatomegaly and fever, probably due to chronic kala-azar, or
2. It is a patient of hepatosplenomegaly with pyrexia for discussion (if not properly diagnosed).

Q. Why do you say so?

This is a case of chronic kala-azar because:

1. The patient comes from an endemic zone (kala-azar is endemic in Bihar, Gangetic belt of West Bengal, along the coast of Brahmaputra in Assam, coastal Odisha and in eastern part of UP in India).
2. Intermittent rise of temperature for last 6 months which occasionally peaks twice in 24 hours.
3. Weakness, malaise, easy fatigability with substantial loss of body weight (6 kg over last 6 months) for the same duration in spite of good appetite and persistent fever **(Table 1.28)**.
4. Massive non-tender, 'soft' to firm (often with doughy feel) splenomegaly.
5. Moderate enlargement of liver which is firm and non-tender.
6. The ratio of liver and spleen is 2 : 5 or 1 : 2½.
7. Presence of moderate anaemia, alopecia and diffuse blackish pigmentation (forehead, perioral and temple region mainly).
8. Received 10 injections of sodium antimony gluconate so far in another city hospital (according to the patient).
9. There is no H/o chill and rigor, cough, haemoptysis, haematemesis or melaena.

Q. Pattern of fever in kala-azar:

1. May be of any type but usually intermittent in nature.
2. To start with, it is of quotidian variety but without definite chill and rigor (mild chill may be present). Fever is usually nocturnal and without signs of toxaemia.
3. Later on, the fever may be of double quotidian (camel hump fever; 20% cases) in nature (i.e. double rise in 24 hours). This type of fever is very specific for kala-azar.
4. The fever is not very high and ranging between 101° and 102°F.
5. Chronic cases may be apyrexial. Though the fever is associated with tachycardia, pallor and weight loss, the patient remains ambulatory (in spite of fever).

Table 1.28: Relationship of appetite with weight loss

Weight loss + appetite ↑	Weight loss + appetite ↓
1. Diabetes mellitus (uncontrolled)	1. Malignancy (advanced)
2. Thyrotoxicosis	2. Infections (tuberculosis, HIV)
3. Chronic kala-azar	3. Depression (endogenous)
4. Malabsorption syndrome	4. Anorexia nervosa
5. Worm infestation in children	5. Addison's disease
6. Pheochromocytoma	6. Chronic renal failure

- ↑ appetite is also characteristic of hypothalamic disorder and bulimia nervosa.

Q. Chief complaints of your patient:

1. Fever, weakness and loss of weight for 6 months, and
2. Heaviness in the left upper abdomen for 2 months.

Q. Other features of chronic kala-azar:

1. GI tract: Diarrhoea or dysentery, rarely jaundice in late stage, gingivitis.
2. Respiratory system: Dry cough, chest pain or bronchopneumonia due to superadded infection. Haemoptysis, if complicated by pulmonary tuberculosis.
3. CVS: Palpitations.
4. Haemorrhagic manifestations: Bleeding gum or epistaxis (due to pancytopenia).
5. Skin: Cancrum oris and diffuse blackish pigmentation of the whole body.
6. Reticulo-endothelial system: May present with lymph node swelling (very rare in India), pallor.

Q. Physical findings in different systems:

1. General appearance: Dry rough pigmented skin, emaciation, moderate anaemia, scanty hair in scalp, protuberant abdomen, thin legs with occasional oedema feet.
2. GI tract: Hepatosplenomegaly, jaundice (in late stage).
3. Respiratory system: Occasionally crepitations are heard in the presence of secondary pulmonary infection.
4. CVS: Tachycardia, low BP, murmur in the pulmonary area due to severe anaemia.
5. Haemorrhagic manifestations: Gum bleeding and epistaxis may be there.
6. Skin: Increased black pigmentation (so the name kala-azar, which is Hindi version of 'black-sickness'), dry, thick, rough, scaly skin, or rarely cancrum oris (ulcerative lesion around mouth).
7. Reticulo-endothelial system: Rarely, there are presence of sternal tenderness (due to severe anaemia) and palpable lymph nodes (very rare in India, found in African form).

Q. What is cancrum oris (noma)?

This is a form of sloughing ulcerative gingivitis (orofacial gangrene) which spread to buccal mucosa, cheek, mandible or maxilla resulting in widespread destruction of bone and soft tissue. It is thought to be due to invasion of tissues by *Bacteroids*, *Borrelia vincentii*, *Fusobacterium* and other normal commensals of the mouth. **The causes are:** 1. Kala-azar (due to neutropenia), 2. Acute leukaemia, 3. Measles, 4. Enteric fever, 5. Immunosuppression, 6. Children with malnutrition, 7. Poor oral hygiene.

Q. Points in the past history you have enquired for:

1. Jaundice (as cirrhosis of liver and thalassaemia may be present with hepatosplenomegaly).
2. Repeated blood transfusions (indicate thalassaemia).
3. Haematemesis or melaena (indicate cirrhosis of liver).
4. Tuberculosis (ask for cough and haemoptysis, as kala-azar may be complicated by tuberculosis).
5. Swelling anywhere in neck, axilla or groin (indicates lymphoma).
6. IV drug abuse (may give rise to prolonged fever).
7. Bleeding manifestations (for leukaemias).
8. Diabetes mellitus and hypertension as a routine enquiry.

Q. Importance of treatment history:

Whether the patient has received any injection for 21–28 days (sodium antimony gluconate) or directly ask the patient if he knows the name of the drugs used so far. Usually a patient of chronic kala-azar is treated by too many doctors with too many drugs.

Q. Describe the splenic enlargement in kala-azar:

It is just like thalassaemic spleen (read the section on 'Thalassaemia'). The difference is that the spleen of chronic kala-azar is 'soft' to firm in consistency and not very firm like thalassaemia. At the end of 1 month of illness, splenic enlargement is about 2–3 cm below the left costal margin and then the spleen enlarges at the rate of 1 cm per month. Spleen may be tender in splenic infarction. [In case of acute malaria, spleen is usually palpable after second paroxysm of fever (i.e. after 3rd day of illness) and the spleen of enteric fever is palpable after 7 days of illiness]. The spleen of chronic kala-azar is not so firm like chronic malarial spleen. The spleen of acute kala-azar (and acute malaria) is always soft in consistency.

Clinical Wisdom

In Kala-azar, splenic size often determines the duration of the disease.

Q. Anaemia in kala-azar:

1. Hypoproteinaemia (malnutrition), bleeding, haemo-dilution.
2. Bone marrow depression (due to proliferation of parasitised reticulo-endothelial cells).
3. Haemolysis (autoimmune and rare).
4. Hypersplenism (sequestration and splenic pooling).

- **Anaemia in malaria** is due to haemolysis, impaired erythropoiesis, splenomegaly with hypersplensim, and folate deficiency (↑ demand).

Q. Causes of jaundice in kala-azar (though rare):

1. Blood transfusion causing jaundice by hepatitis B or C virus.
2. Portal hypertension with cirrhotic change in liver.

Q. Why there is bleeding in kala-azar?

1. Before treatment: due to thrombocytopenia.
2. During treatment: with sodium stibogluconate.

Q. How kala-azar is produced?

1. Kala-azar is also known as visceral leishmaniasis and is caused by Leishmania donovani.
2. Incubation period averages 1–2 months, but may be several years.
3. Transmitted by:
   i. Bite of female sand fly (*Phlebotomus argentipes*, the Indian vector).
   ii. Blood transfusion (very rare).
   iii. Rarely, inoculation of cultures of *Leishmania donovani*; or transplacental (congenital).

- The term 'leishmaniasis' encompasses multiple clinical syndromes, i.e. visceral, cutaneous and mucosal leishmaniasis. Human is the only reservoir in subcontinent of India.

Q. What are the differential diagnosis?

Discuss the differential diagnosis of moderate or huge splenomegaly as your case is. Read the section on 'Hepatosplenomegaly'.

Q. How will you diagnose (chronic) kala-azar?

A. Indirect evidences:

1. Blood examination: Low Hb with normocytic normochromic anaemia. Leucopenia (neutropenia and eosinopenia) with relative lymphocytosis and monocytosis. Agranulocytosis and thrombocytopenia may occur. *Pancytopenia is seen*. It repeated, there is *progressive leucopenia*.
2. **Aldehyde test (Napier's):** Positive after 3 months of illness. About 1–2 mL of serum is taken and one to two drops of 40% formalin is added to it. A positive result is indicated by 'jellification of milk white opacity' within 20 minutes. This test is falsely positive in multiple myeloma and cirrhosis of liver. Positivity depends upon increase in serum gamma globulin.
3. Antimony test (Chopra's): Positive after 6 weeks of illness (due to high IgG).
4. Complement fixation test (CFT) with WKK (Witebsky, Klingenstein and Kuhn) antigen becomes positive within 3 weeks. Nowadays, Kedrowsky's antigen is preferred to WKK antigen.
5. Immunofluorescence test (indirect).
6. Haemagglutination test (indirect).
7. Counterimmunoelectrophoresis.
8. ELISA (enzyme-linked immunosorbent assay) test.
9. Others: Direct agglutination test (DAT) with freeze-dried antigen is a simple, cheap and quick test which can be used in the field conditions. Dot-enzyme immunoassay (EIA) and reverse Western blotting also detect antigen. DNA detection by PCR may be done. Another field-tested technique is *immunochromatographic dipstick testing* of fingerstick blood for antibody to recombinant Leishmanial antigens or synthetic peptides (also called rapid dipstick rK-39 test). Detection of leishmanial antigen (done by latex agglutination test) in urine is found within a week.
10. **Serum electrophoresis:** *Hypoalbuminaemia with marked hyperglobulinemia (IgG).*

B. Direct evidences (definitive diagnosis): **LD bodies (Leishman-Donovan bodies)** may be demonstrated by:

1. Preparation of buffy coat in blood: The yield is better (83%) if a thick blood film is made or a straight leucocyte edge is produced in the slide, or by using centrifuged citrated blood. The smear is stained by Giemsa's or Romanowsky's stain, and examined under oil-emersion lens to see the amastigote form of the parasite containing nucleus and kinetoplast.
2. **Splenic puncture or aspiration:** Yield is maximum (>98%), and *gold standard in diagnosis*.
3. Bone marrow aspiration or biopsy: Either taken from sternum or illac crest (carefully observe for evidence of marrow puncture in your patient). Yield is 80–98%.
4. Hepatic aspiration (yield is 75–85%).
5. Lymph node biopsy (if palpable) or FNAC: Yield is 64%.
6. Culture in NNN (Novy-MacNeal-Nicolle) medium in a cool incubator at 22°C.
7. Skin biopsy in cases of post kala-azar dermal leishmaniasis (PKDL).

Clinical Wisdom

Multiplication of leishmania takes place in macrophages in the liver, spleen and bone marrow. *Culture shows promastigote (flagellar) form and stained films show amastigote (non-flagellar) form*. The fully developed promastigote form looks like long slender spindle-shaped bodies while the amastigote form is round or oval; amastigote form is found in human, while promastigote form is found in sandfly. Leishmanin skin test is not much informative (negative in acute kala-azar reflecting a poor cell-mediated immunity).

HIV patients may be infected with Leishmania donovani if ever been in leishmaniasis-endemic areas. The sensitivity of serologic tests for kala-azar is lower in HIV-infected patients than in non-HIV-infected patients.

Q. What is acute kala-azar and how it is diagnosed?

Early kala-azar of 2–6 weeks duration is **'acute kala-azar'**, which is diagnosed by:

1. Blood examination: Progressive leucopenia with relative lymphocytosis and monocytosis.
2. Complement fixation test (CFT).
3. Direct agglutination test (detects IgM antibody and is a sensitive indicator of acute disease).
4. Counterimmunoelectrophoresis.
5. Demonstration of LD bodies from:
   a. Buffy coat preparation, and
   b. Bone marrow aspiration or biopsy, from sternum or iliac crest.

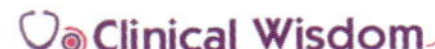

Clinical Wisdom

Aldehyde test is negative in acute kala-azar.

Q. Why splenic puncture is not advocated in acute kala-azar?

In acute kala-azar, spleen is not sufficiently enlarged to be punctured.

Q. Complications of kala-azar:

1. Pulmonary tuberculosis or intercurrent infection (pneumococcal pneumonia) in lung.
2. Pancytopenia with its consequences.
3. PKDL (post kala-azar dermal leishmaniasis): Skin lesions (macules, papules, nodules, patches) are most prominent in nose, cheek and ear lobule (with thick skin) that develops during or after therapy. *D/D of PKDL* are syphilis, leprosy and yaws. PKDL may improve by treatment with miltefosine.

4. Malabsorption syndrome, bacillary dysentery.
5. Portal hypertension (10%).
6. Splenic rupture (rarely).
7. Cancrum oris.
8. Severe epistaxis, malnutrition, uveitis, measles, amyloidosis.

- Death is usually due to bacterial infection or uncontrolled bleeding.

Q. How do you like to treat kala-azar?

1. Sodium antimony gluconate or sodium stibogluconate (pentavalent antimonial): It is the drug of choice; 1 mL of injection contains 100 mg of the drug. The dose is 20 mg/kg by rapid IV infusion (preferred) or deep IM route (painful) as single daily dose, for minimally 28 days (maximum daily dose 850 mg). The dose may be repeated after 2–4 weeks for 40–60 days in patients with relapse or incomplete responses.
2. Meglumine antimoniate (pentavalent antimonial): 50 mg/kg daily for 15 days (alternative drug).
3. For resistant cases:
   i. Amphotericin B (deoxycholate): 0.5–1 mg/kg, IV by slow infusion daily or on alternate days (for 15 days). The drug is nephrotoxic and more protein bound.
   ii. Pentamidine isethionate: 2 mg/kg, IM or IV, three times a week for 7 days.
4. Recent advances:
   i. AmBisome, the lipid formulation of amphotericin B or liposomal amphotericin B may be used, IV in resistant kala-azar in a dose of 3 mg/kg/day over a short period of time (given on days 1 to 5, 14 and 21; may be repeated). This expensive drug takes the advantage of 'target-specific drug delivery system' (less toxic, more effective, less protein bound and retained in macrophage-rich organs).
   ii. Miltefosine: It is a cytotoxic drug which is used in a daily dose of 2.5 mg/kg/day, **orally** in two divided doses for 28 days (i.e. 50 mg capsule twice daily). The drug gives excellent results in areas resistant to antimonials, especially in India (particularly in Bihar and North-East parts).
   iii. Aminosidine (aminoglycoside paromomycin): 11 mg/kg, IM for 21 days; cheaper drug.
   iv. Sitamaquine (an 8-aminoquinoline): Being field-tested in various regions and has a narrow therapeutic window.
   v. Addition of allopurinol: 20–30 mg/kg, daily in three divided doses with sodium antimony gluconate.
   vi. Recombinant human interferon-γ (in seriously ill patients or treatment failures) in a dose of 100 µg/m^2 body surface/day given by SC route for 28 days along with standard dose of sodium antimony gluconate.
   vii. Fluconazole or ketoconazole may be used orally, in a dose of 3 mg/kg daily.
   viii. Adjunctive splenectomy is done in some drug-resistant kala-azar.
5. Treatment of anaemia, secondary infections in lung, pulmonary tuberculosis, intercurrent bacterial infections, bleeding manifestations and malnutrition are done accordingly.

- Urea stibamine [discovered by an Indian, **Dr (Sir) Upendra Nath Brahmachari**], the first drug for kala-azar, is not used now. Remember, incomplete therapy of initial illness results in relapse with drug-resistant organisms, which is a burning problem in India.
- **First-line drugs** are pentavalent antimonials and lipid formulation of amphotericin B.
- *Relapse* (reappearance after cure): Treated by sodium stibogluconate for 40–60 days (i.e. same dose with doubling the duration). *Resistant* kala-azar (no response to therapy): treated by pentamidine isethionate, liposomal amphotericin B, miltefosine, interferon-γ and ketoconazole.

Q. Side effects of different drugs used in kala-azar:

a. Antimony preparations: Nausea, vomiting, diarrhoea, arthralgia, myalgia, fever, metallic taste, hepatitis, pancreatitis, arrhythmias, Q-Tc prolongation (monitoring should include ECG) or even death; cyanosis, rapid and irregular pulse, dyspnoea and shock are known as 'Nitritoid crisis'; anaphylaxis after 6th or 7th injections.
b. Amphotericin B: Fever with chills, hypokalaemia, arrhythmias, renal toxicity, myocarditis.
c. Pentamidine isethionate: Hypoglycaemia, hypotension, tachycardia, irreversible induction of diabetes mellitus and even sudden death.
d. Miltefosine: GI symptoms like vomiting and diarrhoea, reversible hepatotoxicity and nephrotoxicity. It should be used with caution in females as it is abortifacient and teratogenic in animals.
e. Sitamaquine: Methaemoglobinaemia, nephropathy.

Q. Assessment of progress (monitoring) in kala-azar:

It is assessed by, 1. Body weight, 2. Splenic size, 3. Hb estimation, and 4. Serum albumin level.

DIABETES MELLITUS — CASE 27

Q. What is your diagnosis?

This is a case of type 2 diabetes mellitus (DM) with hypertension and obesity along with evidences of renal involvement (K-W syndrome) and peripheral neuropathy.

Q. What are the chief complaints?

1. Increased volume with frequency of urine, increased thirst and appetite for last 15 years.
2. Dimness of vision for last 4 years.
3. Tingling and numbness of the extremities for last 2 years.
4. Gradual swelling of the whole body for last 6 months, and more for last 2 weeks.

Q. What is the H/o present illness?

This 55-years non-smoker and non-alcoholic but hypertensive and diabetic obese male businessman was normal till 15 years back, and has been admitted in the hospital for swelling of the whole body. The onset of the disease was insidious and it was gradually progressive. He was admitted in this hospital 10 days back and has improved slightly with treatment.

All the symptoms regarding increased appetite, thirst and urination started 15 years back. The patient used to drink 3–4 litres of water daily. He had to wake up 3–4 times every night for urination and total urinary output per day was approximately 3.5 litres. There is no burning sensation during micturition at present. Though he had a good appetite, he had lost substantial body weight for the last few years. He also complained of increased fatigability and exhaustion even while at rest.

For last 6 months (more for last two weeks), he has observed gradual swelling of the whole body which started from the face. The swelling was a bit posture-dependent and pitting in nature. He also complained of swelling in the abdomen. There was no H/o rise of temperature (tuberculosis, UTI) for last couple of months. For the last two weeks, the total daily urine output was approximately 1.5 litres. The patient was admitted in the hospital for these ailments.

For last 4 years, he had dimness of vision and after using spectacles it was not corrected much. He complained of tingling sensation of the extremities (hands and feet) with weakness of the limbs for last two years. For last one year, he was suffering from retrosternal chest pain (IHD). For last 15 years, he was on oral hypoglycaemic agents (not too regularly) prescribed by different physicians. Once he received inj. insulin for treatment of perianal abscess.

There was no H/o fever, palpitations (thyrotoxicosis), tremor (thyrotoxicosis), haemoptysis (pulmonary tuberculosis), cough (respiratory tract infections), leg pain during walking (large vessel involvement), skin lesions (diabetic dermopathy), dizziness or giddiness (postural hypotension), pain abdomen (pancreatitis), impotence or nocturnal diarrhoea (autonomic neuropathy), itching or any foot ulcer. He has suffered from repeated attacks of burning micturition during last fifteen years (UTI). He did not give any H/o unconsciousness (hypoglycaemia, CVA, etc.) though a hypertensive for last 8 years.

- Add past, personal and family history as described below.
- Exclude the causes of substantial weight loss (e.g. thyrotoxicosis or tuberculosis).

Q. Importance of past, personal, family and treatment history:

A. Past history:

1. No H/o tuberculosis (as a complication of DM).
2. No H/o recurrent pain abdomen (occurs in chronic pancreatitis).
3. IHD present. No other significant serious illness in the past (e.g. recurrent pneumonia, TIA, etc.)
4. All the symptoms started when he was on 40 years (type 2 DM).
5. H/o frequent boils and abscess at various parts of body; delayed wound healing.
6. H/o frequent change of refractory error in eye.
7. Hypertensive for last 8 years.

B. Personal history:

1. Married with three children (two daughters and one son): All are well at present.
2. No addiction (non-smoker, non-alcoholic).
3. Sedentary habit, obese: Businessman by profession.

C. Family history:

1. Father was diabetic and died of IHD, 10 years back. Mother is not suffering from DM.
2. Brothers (two) and sisters (one) are healthy and not suffering from DM.
3. No H/o hypertension in the family.

D. Treatment history:

1. Received glipizide, pioglitazone, sitagliplin and metformin in varying combinations for last 15 years, the intake of drugs was not too regular. He was once prescribed inj. insulin.
2. Treated by norfloxacin from time to time during the attacks of UTI.
3. Received telmisartan and amlodipine for treatment of hypertension.
4. Received multivitamins, gabapentin and methyl_ cobalamin for tingling sensation of the extremities.
5. He had never received corticosteroid and thiazides (may cause secondary diabetes).

Q. Special points in the physical examination of your patient:

A. General survey:

a. Decubitus: Of choice.
b. Facies: Moon face (puffy with baggy lower eyelids).
c. Nutrition: Oedema hampers assessment of nutrition (Ref: BMI, waist-hip ratio).
d. Thyroid gland: Not enlarged.
e. Neck veins: Could not be properly visualised due to the presence of oedema.
f. Oedema: Pitting, generalised, parietal oedema present.
g. Skin: Within normal limit except some papular skin lesions over shins.
h. Pulse: Condition of the arterial wall is thickened. All the peripheral pulses are palpable (press the oedema fluid for few seconds for better palpation of pulse and describe all the points inpulse).
i. BP:
   i. 180/100 mm of Hg: In lying position.
   ii. 170/95 mm of Hg: In standing position.

j. Respiration: 20/min, thoraco-abdominal in type; other points—within normal limit.
k. Temperature: Normal at present.
l. Scrotum: Absence of scrotal oedema and hydrocele at present; penis—within normal limit.
m. Feet: Absence of trophic ulcer; presence of oedema.
n. Dehydration: Absent (to exclude ketoacidosis).
o. Height and weight: Essential to calculate body mass index (BMI).

- Mention all the points in general survey.
- In general examination of DM, carefully look for pallor (renal failure), xanthelasma or xanthoma (hyperlipidaemia), intertrigo/ nail or oral candidosis (fungal infection), foot ulcers or limb amputation, and sternotomy scar (previous coronary artery by-pass surgery).

B. Genitourinary system:

a. No renal lump felt.
b. Renal angle: Non-tender.
c. Urinary bladder: Empty (by percussion).
d. Scrotal oedema: Absent.
e. Prepuce, glans penis, anus: Within normal limit.
f. Genital discharge per urethra: Absent.
[g. Examine vulva, vagina, and per vaginal examination in females, if necessary].

C. Nervous system:

a. The patient is conscious, alert, oriented and co-operative.
b. Higher functions with speech: Normal.
c. Cranium and spine: Within normal limit.
d. Neck rigidity: Absent; SLR test—within normal limit.
e. Cranial nerves: Normal (sometimes, there is IIIrd, IVth or VIth nerve palsy in diabetes). Ophthalmoscopy: Not done.
f. Motor functions:
   1. Nutrition: Could not be assessed properly due to the presence of oedema. No foot drop.
   2. Tone: A bit diminished in all four limbs.
   3. Power: Grade IV in all four limbs.
   4. Coordination: Within normal limit.
   5. Involuntary movements: None.
g. Sensory functions:
   1. Superficial: Pain, touch and temperature sensations are lost over the distal parts of all limbs. Impaired sensation in the proximal part of all limbs and the involvement is rather patchy in nature.
   2. Deep:
      i. Vibration sense: Lost bilaterally (mostly over the medial malleoli).
      ii. Joint sense: Impaired distally (bilaterally).
      iii. Position sense: Impaired distally (bilaterally).
      iv. Muscle sense: Calf muscles are tender on palpation and squeezing.
   3. Cortical: Impaired (in a patient of peripheral neuropathy, cortical sensations can not be tested properly).
h. Reflexes:
   1. Superficial reflex:
      i. Abdominal: No response bilaterally (due to peripheral neuropathy/ascites).
      ii. Cremasteric: No response bilaterally.
      iii. **Plantar response: No response bilaterally.**
   2. Deep reflex:

	Right	*Left*
i. Biceps jerk	Normal	Normal
ii. Triceps jerk	Normal	Diminished
iii. Supinator jerk	Normal	Normal
iv. Knee jerk	Diminished	Lost
v. Ankle jerk	Lost	Lost
vi. Clonus	Absent	Absent

   3. Visceral reflex (swallowing, bladder and bowel): Within normal limit.
   4. Other reflexes (glabellar tap, grasp reflex, palmo-mental reflex): Within normal limit.
i. Trophic changes: Absent (no bed sore, no trophic ulcer in sole of feet). Charcot joint absent.
j. Cerebellar functions: Normal.
k. Autonomic functions:
   i. Tachycardia: Absent.
   ii. Postural hypotension: Absent.
   iii. Sweating: Normally present all over the body.
l. Stance and gait: Could not be tested.

Romberg's sign: Could not be tested properly (due to anasarca and weakness).

D. GI system:

a. Teeth, gum, tongue, oral cavity and breath (odour) within normal limit.
b. Venous prominence over abdomen: Absent.
c. Parietal oedema in abdomen: Present.
d. No hepatosplenomegaly.
e. Ascites: Present (moderate).

E. CVS:

a. Resting tachycardia and orthostatic hypotension: Absent. Systemic hypertension: Present.
b. Procordium: No deformity; thrill: Absent.
c. Apex: Left 5th ICS, on the left MCL with normal character (i.e. mild cardiomegaly).
d. Heart sounds: Normal.
e. Murmur: Absent.
f. Pericardial rub/opening snap/split/click: Absent.

F. Respiratory system:

a. Respiration: 20/min, thoraco-abdominal (due to ascites), regular; absence of air hunger.
b. Trachea: Central in position.
c. Parietal oedema in the chest wall: Present.
d. Percussion: Normal resonant note on both sides.
e. Breath sound: Vesicular in type (try to exclude pneumonia and tuberculosis).
f. Added sounds: Nil (i.e. no crepitations → usually excludes LVF or infection).
g. Vocal resonance: Normal on both sides.

G. Musculoskeletal system: Cheiroarthropathy, frozen shoulder, Charcot joint, OA of knee are absent.

H. Lymphoreticular system:

a. Anaemia: Absent.
b. Lymphadenopathy: Absent.
c. Sternal tenderness: Absent.
d. Haemorrhagic spots: Absent.

I. Examination of the skin: Abscess, balano-posthitis, candidosis, xanthoma, xanthelasma, acanthosis nigricans or trophic ulcers are absent; diabetic dermopathy is present over shins bilaterally.

J. Examination of the eyes:

a. Visual acuity, ocular movements and pupillary reactions: Within normal limit
b. No stye.
c. Pseudo Argyll Robertson pupil: Absent.
d. Cataract (early) in both eyes.
e. Glaucoma: Absent.
f. Ophthalmoscopy: Not done (Ref: diabetic and hypertensive retinopathy).

K. Urine examination done at the bedside:

a. Sugar: Present, b. Protein: Present.

Clinical Wisdom

Ophthalmoscopy (fundoscopy): Not for UGs, essential for PGs.

Q. What is diabetes mellitus (DM)?

It is a clinical syndrome characterised by high blood sugar level (hyperglycaemia) and glycosuria due to relative or absolute deficiency of insulin secretion and/or action, or insulin resistance that leads to disturbances in carbohydrate, protein, fat metabolism, and water and electrolyte homeostasis.

The WHO diagnostic criteria for diabetes mellitus:

- Symptoms of diabetes plus 'random' blood glucose concentration ≥200 mg/dL, or
- 'Fasting' plasma glucose ≥126 mg/dL, or
- '2h-postload' plasma glucose ≥200 mg/dL during an oral GTT, or
- HbA_{1C} ≥6.5%

The diagnostic criteria for pre-diabetes and diabetes are:

In these criteria, the categories of FPG are:

- FPG <100 mg/dL = Normal fasting glucose
- FPG ≥100 mg/dL and <126 mg/dL = Impaired fasting glucose (IFG)
- FPG ≥126 mg/dL = Provisional diagnosis of diabetes (on more than one occasion)

The corresponding categories when the oral GTT is used, are as follows:

- 2 hPG <140 mg/dL = Normal glucose tolerance
- 2 hPG ≥140 mg/dL and <200 mg/dL = Impaired glucose tolerance (IGT)
- 2 hPG ≥200 mg/dL = Provisional diagnosis of diabetes (must be confirmed on a subsequent day)

- FPG = Fasting plasma glucose; 2 hPG = 2-h postload glucose.
- The prognostic significance and outcome (i.e. accuracy) are same whether it is the FPG ≥126 mg/dL or 2 hPG ≥200 mg/dL (i.e. in diabetes). This is why, in clinical practice, the FPG test is now mostly preferred because of ease of administration, convenience, acceptibility to patients and its lower cost.
- 2-h postload glucose is done by taking 75 g of anhydrous glucose dissolved in 300 mL water.
- Results are for venous plasma, while the whole blood values are lower.
- 'Fasting' is defined as no calorie intake (i.e. overnight) for at least 8 hours. 'Random' is defined as any time of the day without regard to time since the last meal. HbA_{1C} is currently the gold standard of glucose monitoring.

Q. Classification of diabetes mellitus:

Read the modern aetiological classification from 'Bedside Clinics in Medicine, Part II'. In the recent classification, IDDM has been replaced by the term type 1 and NIDDM by type 2 diabetes mellitus.

Q. Who is a potential diabetic?

These patients usually have no symptoms, and show no abnormality on examination or by GTT but are susceptible to develop diabetes in any time of their life.

1. When one parent is diabetic and the other have a family history of diabetes.
2. Diabetes present in both the parents.
3. Mother of a 'Herculean baby' (>9 lbs).
4. Non-diabetic member of a monozygotic twin, where the other is diabetic.

- Patients with IGT (140–199 mg/dL), and/or IFG (100–125 mg/dL), and/or HbA_{1C} of 5.7–6.4% are now regarded as **'pre-diabetes'**.
- **Latent diabetics** are persons who show impaired GTT under stressful conditions like pregnancy, infections, physical and mental stress or when overweight.

Q. Characteristics of Type 1 DM:

1. Age of onset is usually below 30 years.
2. Usually wasting is prominent (or lean patients).
3. Abrupt onset with rapid progress.
4. Pancreatic islet cells (of Langerhans) are almost destroyed. Plasma insulin is low to absent.
5. Polyphagia, polyuria and polydipsia are classically present.
6. Always responsive to insulin.
7. Unresponsive to oral hypoglycaemic agents.
8. Diabetic ketoacidosis occurs very often.
9. Family H/o diabetes mellitus is usually absent.
10. Presence of other autoimmune diseases with autoantibodies.
11. HLA-DR3 or DR4 in >90%.
12. Disappearance of C-peptide.
13. High mortality, if untreated.

Q. Characteristics of type 2 DM:

1. Usually starts after the age of 30 years.
2. Obese persons (or overweight).
3. Insidious onset with gradual progress.
4. Pancreatic islet cells are not totally destroyed. Plasma insulin is normal to high.
5. Polyphagia, polyuria and polydipsia: Not so classically seen as in type 1 DM.
6. Responsive to oral hypoglycaemic agents.
7. Insulin therapy: Responsive to resistant.
8. Hyperosmolar hyperglycaemic non-ketotic coma occurs very often.
9. Family H/o diabetes mellitus is usually present.
10. Absence of other autoimmune diseases and auto-antibodies.
11. No HLA links; 50% concordance in idential twins.
12. C-peptide persists.
13. Low mortality, if untreated.

Q. Causes of polyuria:

Read the section on 'Acute glomerulonephritis'.

Q. Causes of polyphagia (increased appetite) (*see* **Table 1.28**):

1. Diabetes mellitus, 2. Thyrotoxicosis, 3. Obesity, 4. Hungry individuals, 5. Binge eating (bulimia), 6. Sometimes, in malabsorption syndrome.

Q. Causes of polydipsia (increased thirst):

1. Polyuria (all causes), 2. Psychogenic polydipsia (compulsive water drinking), 3. Anxiety, tension, phobia, 4. Orators, 5. Anticholinergic or antidepressant medication, 6. After heavy protein meal.

- Pathophysiology of P_3 symptoms (or 'osmotic symptoms'): In diabetes, there is hyperglycaemia → glycosuria → osmotic diuresis → **polyuria** → **polydipsia**. Continuous glycosuria leads to neoglucogenesis from protein which results in wasting of muscles (resulting in loss of weight). Non-utilisation of sugar (in the presence of hyperglycaemia) for energy expenditure is responsible for **polyphagia** or excessive hunger. The classic triad of DM is often polyuria, polydipsia and weight loss (due to fluid depletion, and accelerated breakdown of muscle and fat, secondary to lack of insulin).

Q. Drugs provoking hyperglycaemia:

Corticosteroids, thiazides, diazoxide, dopexamine, protease inhibitor, clozapine, non-selective beta blockers, cyclosporin, pentamidine, nicotinic acid, α-interferon.

Q. How to suspect DM clinically in an outdoor or OPD patient?

1. Classical triad of symptoms (polyphagia, polyuria and polydipsia—the P_3 *symptoms*).
2. Recurrent abscess, boils, carbuncles or fungal infections; recurrent urinary tract infections.
3. Recurrent stye or chalazion.
4. Unexplained emaciation; undue tiredness or fatigue.
5. Delayed wound healing.
6. Frequent change of glasses due to error of refraction.
7. Cataract appearing at an early age.
8. Sudden, isolated IIIrd cranial nerve palsy.
9. Resistant pulmonary tuberculosis.
10. Non-resolving pneumonia.
11. Silent myocardial infarction.
12. Generalised pruritus, balanitis or pruritus vulvae.

Q. Effects of diabetes on pregnancy:

1. Hydramnios.
2. Toxaemia of pregnancy.
3. Maternal infections.
4. Difficult labour.
5. Recurrent abortions.
6. Postpartum haemorrhage.
7. Puerperal sepsis.

Q. Effects of diabetes on the fetus:

1. Prematurity.
2. Stillbirth.
3. Macrosomia (large baby).
4. Postpartum hypoglycaemia.
5. Respiratory distress syndrome.
6. Hyperbilirubinaemia.
7. Congenital heart diseases.
8. Open neural tube defects.

Q. Differential diagnosis (D/D) of your case:

If the history and presentation are so classical, no D/D are required. Otherwise, differentiate among the causes of polyuria, nephrotic syndrome or peripheral neuropathy.

Q. Complications of DM:

The life-history of diabetes mellitus is full of complications. The patient presents to different specialists or subspecialists with different organs/systems involvement. The **common cause of death** in treated patients are cardiovascular ailments (70%), followed by renal failure (10%) and infections (6%).

A. Acute (early)

1. **Hypoglycaemia.**
2. **Diabetic ketoacidosis (DKA).**
3. Hyperosmolar hyperglycaemic non-ketotic coma.
4. Lactic acidosis (rare).
5. Infections (boils, abscess, cellulitis, carbuncle, tuberculosis).
6. Acute circulatory failure.

B. Late

1. **Circulatory abnormalities (macro- and micro-angiopathy).**
2. **Retinopathy (microangiopathy).**
3. **Neuropathy (peripheral and autonomic).**
4. **Nephropathy (microangiopathy).**

5. Gastrointestinal disorders.
6. Recurrent infections.
7. Diabetic foot (ulcer, gangrene).
8. Dermatological complications.
9. Miscellaneous: Malignant otitis externa, emphysematous cholecystitis, rhinocerebral mucormycosis, hypertriglyceridaemia, platelet aggregate abnormality, etc.

Q. Common infections encountered in DM:

In uncontrolled DM, various bacterial, fungal or viral infections occur. Commonly they are cellulitis, boils (*Staphylococcus, Streptococcus*, gram-negative bacilli), carbuncle, stye, pulmonary tuberculosis, otitis externa or media, brain abscess, osteomyelitis, diabetic foot, cholecystitis, meningitis, rhinocerebral mucormycosis. They are treated with proper antibiotics along with tight control of blood sugar with insulin.

Q. Ocular complications of DM:

A. Non-retinopathic (diagnosed by bedside examination)

1. Recurrent stye and chalazion.
2. Signs of dyslipidaemia (corneal arcus and xanthelasma) may be present.
3. Anterior uveitis (hypopyon).
4. Rubeosis iridis (moth-eaten appearance of iris).
5. Pseudo Argyll Robertson pupil.
6. Frequent change of glasses due to error of refraction.
7. Snow flake cataract (specific of DM): Rare.
8. Senile cataract: Accelerated senile cataract.
9. Glaucoma.
10. IIIrd, IVth and VIth cranial nerve palsy.

B. Retinopathy (diagnosed by fundoscopy)

1. Simple, background or non-proliferative:
   a. Increased capillary permeability.
   b. Capillary closure and dilatation.
   c. Microaneurysms (earliest change observed by ophthalmoscopy and is known as 'dots').
   d. Arteriovenous shunts.
   e. Venous dilatation.
   f. Haemorrhages (occur in deeper layer of retina and is known as 'blots').
   g. Hard exudate (due to leakage of protein and lipids from damaged capillaries, and is very characteristic of DM).
   h. Cotton-wool spots (superficial exudates formed due to 'microinfarction' and is usually seen in diabetes with hypertension).

- c) and f) are collectively known as 'dots and blots' in diabetic retinopathy.

2. Proliferative:
   a. Neovascularisation (new vessel formation in response to retinal hypoxaemia).
   b. Pre-retinal haemorrhage (sub-hyaloid).
   c. Retinitis proliferans
   d. Vitreal haemorrhage.
   e. Retinal detachment.

- Other causes of **microaneurysms** are systemic hypertension, SLE, hyperviscosity syndrome and Coats disease (rare). *Microaneurysms are the hallmark of diabetic retinopathy.* **Neovascularisation** is also seen in sickle cell retinopathy, central retinal vein occlusion and Eales' disease.
- Medical causes of **cataract** are diabetes, hypoparathyroidism, galactosaemia, myotonic dystrophy, Down syndrome, Marfan's syndrome, Cushing's syndrome and corticosteroid-induced.
- **DM is a leading cause of blindness in adults.** Vascular endothelial growth factor (VEGF) is increased in proliferative retinopathy.

Q. What is maculopathy?

When the macula is involved, there is sudden loss of visual acuity. Macula may be involved by: 1) Oedema, 2) Haemorrhage, or 3) Exudate (hard).

Clinical Wisdom

Microaneurysm, venous abnormality, haemorrhage or exudate do not interfere with vision unless they are associated with maculopathy. **Sudden loss of vision** in DM may also be due to vitreal haemorrhage, haemorrhage in iris or retinal detachment, retinal vein or artery occlusion.

Q. Neurological complications of DM:

A. Peripheral neuropathy:

1. Distal, symmetrical, sensory polyneuropathy (commonest).
2. Distal, symmetrical, mixed sensory-motor polyneuropathy.
3. Asymmetrical, proximal motor neuropathy (diabetic amyotrophy): Commonly affects quadriceps, adductor magnus muscles.
4. Asymmetric mononeuritis multiplex (painful).
5. Acute mononeuropathy (paralysis of IIIrd, IVth or VIth cranial nerves, or sudden foot drop and wrist drop).
6. Radiculopathy (usually involves spinal nerves, over the chest wall or abdomen).

B. Autonomic neuropathy (involves multiple systems):

1. Hypoglycaemic unawareness (dangerous, due to lack of warning symptoms).
2. Tachycardia (resting), absence of sinus arrhythmia, sudden cardio-respiratory arrest (death).
3. Postural or orthostatic hypotension (sustained drop in systolic pressure by ≥20 mm of Hg or diastolic pressure by ≥10 mm of Hg in standing condition than in lying down position—BP should be measured within 3 minutes of standing). Postural drop may cause syncope (fainting) in erect posture.
4. Sleep apnoea.
5. Gustatory sweating (circumoral sweating during eating), or disturbance of sweating.

6. Gastroparesis diabeticorum (abdominal fullness, vomiting), biliary dyskinesia.
7. Nocturnal and post-prandial diarrhoea.
8. Anhidrosis (loss of sweating) in lower extremity and hyperhidrosis in upper extremity.
9. Impotence (erectile dysfunction), loss of libido and absence of testicular sensation, dyspareunia.
10. Retrograde ejaculation, hesitancy or precipitancy in urination.
11. Charcot joint; cold feet (due to loss of vasomotor response).
12. Pupillary areflexia; pseudo Argyll Robertson pupil.

- **Postural (orthostatic) hypotension** in the community is commonly due to fluid depletion (dehydration, haemorrhage), autonomic neuropathy (diabetes), drugs (vasodilators, diuretics), metabolic (adrenal insufficiency) and idiopathic orthostatic hypotension.
- Causes of **impotence** (erectile dysfunction) in clinical practice are psychological, diabetes mellitus (autonomic neuropathy), atherosclerosis of penile artery (vascular), pituitary and testicular failure (endocrinopathy), β-blockers and antidepressants (drug-induced), and miscellaneous (CRF, hyperprolactinaemia, motor neurone disease, prostatectomy or substance abuse).
- **Loss of libido** is commonly due to psychogenic, autonomic neuropathy (e.g. diabetes), cirrhosis of liver, any chronic debilitating illness or haemochromatosis.

Q. Other causes of autonomic neuropathy:

Other than **diabetes mellitus (commonest cause)**, they are:

1. GB syndrome.
2. Porphyria.
3. Amyloidosis.
4. Uraemia.
5. Peroneal muscular atrophy.
6. Shy-Drager syndrome (orthostatic hypotension with central nervous system disorder).
7. Riley-Day syndrome (familial dysautonomia).
8. AIDS.

Clinical Wisdom

DM never affects brain. Deep-seated, lancinating pain in the lower limbs as a result of peripheral neuropathy is known as diabetic pseudotabes.

Q. Causes of coma in a diabetic:

1. Hypoglycaemia (commonest cause).
2. Diabetic ketoacidosis (DKA).
3. Hyperosmolar hyperglycaemic non-ketotic coma.
4. Lactic acidosis (rare).
5. Other causes of coma (may or may not be associated with diabetes) like:
   a. CVA.
   b. Renal failure.
   c. Hepatic coma.
   d. Drug-induced coma.
   e. Septicaemia.

- Except No.2, all are causes of non-ketotic coma in a diabetic.

Q. Renal lesions in diabetes (diabetic nephropathy):

Diabetic nephropathy is a leading cause of chronic kidney disease (CKD) terminating in renal failure.

The renal lesions in DM are:

1. Diffuse glomerulosclerosis (commonest lesion).
2. Nodular glomerulosclerosis (K-W lesion).
3. Arterionephrosclerosis.
4. Chronic interstitial nephritis.
5. Pyelonephritis, perinephric abscess.
6. Papillary necrosis.
7. Various tubular lesions like fibrin cap, capsular drop and glycogen in renal tubules.

- The 'sequence of events' (time course) in diabetic nephropathy are: Glomerular hyperperfusion and renal hypertrophy result in increase in GFR within 1 year → structural change in glomerulus and mesangium occurs within 5 years with returning of GFR to normal → at 5–10 years some patients develop 'microalbuminuria' (incipient proteinuria) → clinical nephropathy with 'overt proteinuria' develops at 18–20 years → 'end-stage renal disease (ESRD)' is reached at 22–25 years.
- In DM, recurrent UTI is very common. ACE inhibitor therapy may delay the onset of nephropathy.
- **Diabetic nephropathy** (microvascular complication) includes all the lesions occurring in the kidneys of patients suffering from DM; No. 1 and 2 (question above) may lead to K-W syndrome.

Q. Clinical features due to renal involvement :

1. Oedema.
2. Hypertension.
3. K-W syndrome (nephrotic syndrome).
4. Chronic renal failure.
5. UTI (usually recurrent).
6. Acute renal failure (due to acute papillary necrosis—rare).

Q. Insulin requirement in renal involvement in a patient of DM on insulin:

Insulin requirement in DM is usually reduced with advancing renal insufficiency and is due to :

1. Excretion of insulin binding antibodies (with albumin) in the urine.
2. Reduced rate of degradation of insulin.
3. Uraemia tends to impair neoglucogenesis.

- **Daily insulin production** in a normal healthy non-obese adult is 25 units.

Q. Gastrointestinal manifestations in DM:

1. Fungal infection within the oral cavity (e.g. candidosis).
2. Gastroparesis diabeticorum (gastric atony and stasis).
3. Motility disturbance of gallbladder, oesophagus, stomach and colon.
4. Chronic gastritis.
5. Diabetic enteropathy (especially nocturnal diarrhoea).

6. Chronic pancreatitis (steatorrhoea).
7. Fatty liver and increased incidence of pyogenic liver abscess.
8. Acalculous cholecystitis.
9. Periodontitis.
10. Rectal and ischiorectal abscess in poor control of blood sugar.

Q. Why there is diarrhoea and steatorrhoea in DM?

1. Exocrine pancreatic insufficiency.
2. Coexistant coeliac disease.
3. Abnormal bacterial proliferation in intestine, or
4. Autonomic neuropathy (diabetic diarrhoea).

Q. Dermatological manifestations in diabetes:

1. Recurrent boils, abscess, furuncles and carbuncles.
2. Balano-posthitis (inflammation of glans penis and prepuce, respectively).
3. Vulval (pruritus vulvae) and vaginal moniliasis.
4. Delayed wound healing.
5. Candidosis of skin.
6. Blisters (usually on feet or hands), bullae (bullosis diabeticorum), granuloma annulare, vitiligo.
7. *Diabetic dermopathy* (Fig. 1.79): Small rounded brown plaques with a raised border, which are hyperpigmented and scaly, located over anterior tibial surface ('shin spots' or spotted leg syndrome).
8. Xanthomas (eruptive) secondary to hyperlipoproteinaemia.
9. Necrobiosis lipoidica diabeticorum (NLD) (Fig. 1.80): Yellowish plaque-like lesion with a brownish border and atrophic centre over the pretibial region, predominantly in young women.
10. Lipoatrophy and lipohypertrophy (due to insulin injection), or drug rash.
11. Diabetic foot (due to ischaemia and/or neuropathy): Ulcer or gangrene.
12. Dupuytren's contracture.
13. Scleroderma-like skin lesion (tight waxy skin over shoulders and upper back): Scleroderma diabeticorum.
14. Prayer sign (Fig. 1.81): 'Cheiroarthropathy' (stiff hand syndrome or limited joint mobility), i.e. mild, fixed curvature of the fingers making it impossible to place the hand and fingers flat on a surface (vide page 230).
15. Acanthosis nigricans in type 2 DM (in case of insulin resistance).
16. Ulcers (neuropathic or due to arterial disease), especially in legs or sole of feet.
17. Vitiligo, especially in type 1 DM.

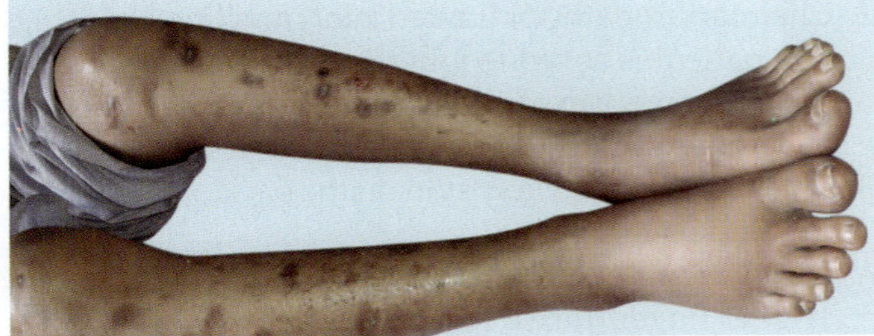

Fig. 1.79: Red-brown flat-topped papules or plaque-like hyperpigmented lesions over both shins in type 2 diabetes mellitus—the **diabetic dermopathy**

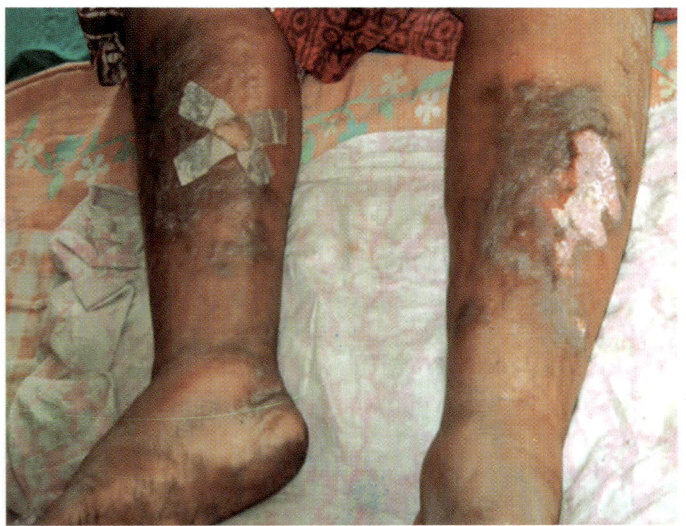

Fig. 1.80: **Necrobiosis lipoidica diabeticorum (NLD)**—yellowish plaque-like lesion which has ulcerated with atrophic centre along with surrounding spreading erythema, classically seen over the shins in diabetes mellitus

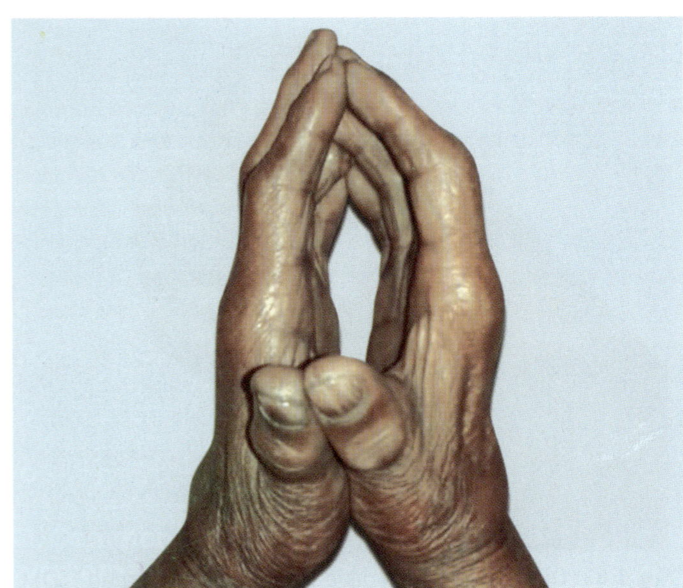

Fig. 1.81: **Prayer sign (Cheiroarthropathy)** in diabetes mellitus with mild, fixed curvature of fingers

- Lipoatrophy or lipohypertrophy (i.e. lipodystrophy): Localised atrophy or hypertrophy of subcutaneous fat, respectively.

Q. Importance of 'examination of foot' in DM:

1. Ulceration (i.e. neuropathic ulcer) and callosity in skin of sole, cracks and fissures, change in colour of skin (may have cyanotic hue), anhidrosis, clawed-up toes (a feature of neuropathy), loss of plantar arch, digital

gangrene, fungal infection in nails and in between toes.

2. Temperature of the skin (in ischaemia, feet become cold).
3. Pulsation in arteria dorsalis pedis and posterior tibial artery (↓ pulsation in angiopathy).
4. Loss of light touch (use monofilaments), proprioception (position of great toe) with distal anaesthesia (in stocking distribution): Peripheral neuropathy.
5. Painful calf muscles: Peripheral neuropathy.
6. Ankle jerk: Lost in peripheral neuropathy. Plantar response: Flexor or no response.
7. Vibration sense: Lost early in DM with neuropathy.
8. Oedema: Present in nephropathy.
9. Foot deformity in Charcot's arthropathy.

- **Diabetic foot** ulcer is due to ischaemia (microangiopathy ± associated atherosclerosis)/neuropathy/both ischaemia and neuropathy ± secondary infection **(Fig. 1.82)**.

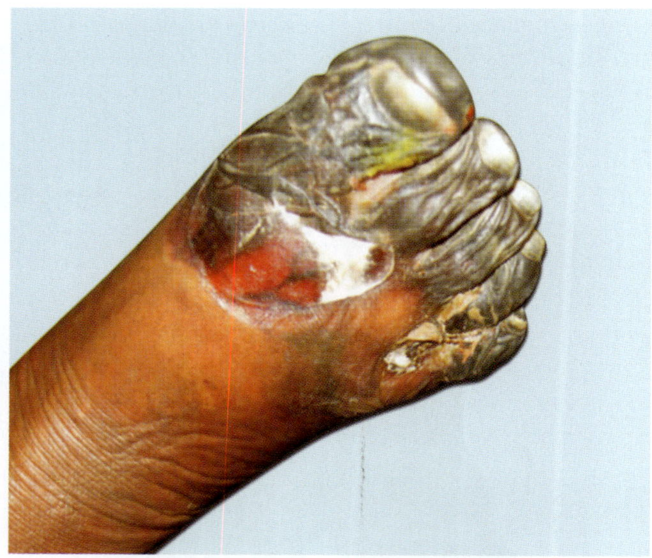

Fig. 1.82: Diabetic foot in a patient of irregularly treated T_2DM

Q. Causes of 'leg ulceration' and their basic investigations:

When the leg ulcers are present on the lower leg, usually it is due to vascular diseases. The site of ulcer on the lower leg often gives an indication of the underlying aetiology. The common causes are:

a. *Venous disease:* Varicose veins, deep venous thrombosis, deep venous obstruction (e.g. from pelvic growth), incompetent valves.
b. *Arterial diseases:* Atherosclerosis, Buerger's disease, vasculitis.
c. *Small vessel disease:* Diabetes mellitus, vasculitis.
d. *Neuropathy:* Diabetes mellitus, leprosy, polyneuropathy due to any cause, syphilis (rare).
e. *Haemorheological:* Sickle cell disease, hereditary spherocytosis, chronic haemolytic anaemia (e.g. thalassaemia), cryoglobulinaemia, thrombocytosis, immune complex disease.
f. *Tumour:* Squamous cell carcinoma, Kaposi's sarcoma, melanoma, basal cell carcinoma.
g. *Trauma:* Trophic ulcer, injury, contact dermatitis, self-inflicted, chronic atopic eczema.
h. *Infections:* Tuberculosis, leprosy, syphilis, mycotic, yaws, tropical ulcer.
i. *Miscellaneous:* Pyoderma gangrenosum, osteomyelitis, lymphoedema.

Basic clinical examination: Temperature of the local skin, site of ulcer (venous—lower leg, medial aspect of leg around ankle with pigmentation; arterial—shin, foot and looks punched-out; vasculitis—shin, upper leg, punched-out and painful; neuropathy—heel, ball of the great toe; painless), peripheral arterial pulses, ankle jerk, vibration sensation, oedema, local cyanotic hue, blood pressure, thickened peripheral nerves.

Clinical Wisdom

In arterial diseases, there is positive H/o intermittent claudication; and the pain in lower extremities are relieved by dependency and increased by elevation of limbs (reverse occurs in pain due to venous obstruction in lower limbs).

Basic investigations:

1. Blood: For anaemia, blood dyscrasias; VDRL; sugar, lipid profile, ANF, ANCA.
2. Urine: For sugar.
3. Bacterial swab: For detection of pathogens.
4. Doppler ultrasound of lower extremities (both venous and arterial system).
5. Ankle-brachial pressure index, or ABPI (in health, the value is ≥ 1.0 in supine position): ABPI in intermittent claudication is <0.9; ABPI of <0.4 is found in critical limb ischaemia. A normal ABPI generally excludes occlusive arterial disease. Detection of ABPI needs a hand-held Doppler and a sphygmomanometer.
6. Venography.
7. Nerve conduction study.

- Treatment—stoppage of smoking, control of DM/hypertension/dyslipidaemia, local care, antibiotics in infection, advice of chiropodist, and surgery (balloon dialatation) or amputation in selected cases.

Q. Importance of 'hand examination' in DM:

1. Pulp infection, blisters, digital gangrene, fungal infection in nails and in between fingers (intertrigo).
2. Cheiroarthropathy or limited joint mobility **(Fig. 1.81)**: The patient is asked to join the hands as if in prayer, and the hands can not be apposed (prayer sign). There is painless stiffness in fingers.
3. Thickened, tight, waxy skin on the back of the fingers (sclerodactyly-like).
4. Dupuytren's contracture.
5. Trigger finger (flexor tenosynovitis).
6. Carpal tunnel syndrome is common in diabetics.
7. Small muscle wasting (due to emaciation or peripheral neuropathy).

- **Rheumatological complications in DM:** Cheiroarthropathy, flexor tendinopathy, adhesive capsulitis, (e.g. in shoulders), osteoarthropathy (e.g. in knees), carpal tunnel syndrome, reflex sympathetic dystrophy, Dupuytren's contracture, Charcot arthropathy and diffuse idiopathic skeletal hyperostosis (DISH).

Q. Circulatory and CVS complications in DM:

DM is designated as 'coronary heart disease risk equivalent' by American Heart Association.

1. **Microangiopathy** (responsible for **'triopathy'**, i.e. retinopathy, nephropathy and neuropathy).
2. Intermittent claudication due to accelerated atherosclerosis (**macroangiopathy**; macrovascular disease includes coronary artery disease, peripheral vascular disease, cerebrovascular disease, diabetic foot and hypertension).
3. Gangrene (peripheral vascular disease).
4. Impotence (on a vascular basis).
5. Resting tachycardia and postural hypotension (autonomic neuropathy); cardiac failure.
6. Angina pectoris.
7. Silent myocardial infarction (involves multiple vessels in diabetics).
8. CVA is common in diabetics (increased by threefold).
9. Cardiomyopathy.
10. Hypertension (macroangiopathy, or following renal involvement). In DM, BP should idealy remain <140/80 mm of Hg.

Q. Causes of painless (silent) myocardial infarction:

It is known that 15–20% of myocardial infarcts are painless. The common causes are:

1. Diabetes mellitus with autonomic neuropathy.
2. Patient under general anaesthesia.
3. Elderly patients with cerebrovascular disease or dementia.
4. Few patients may not have pain (more in women).
5. Inability to recognise the symptom by the patient.

Q. Symptoms of hypoglycaemia:

Prolonged hypoglycaemia may produce permanent brain damage. The symptoms (usually blood glucose becomes less than 55 mg/dL; the lower limit of FPG is 70 mg/dL in health) are due to excessive secretion of catecholamines and dysfunction of CNS. Thus, they are divided into two groups like 'autonomic' and 'neuroglycopenic' symptoms as:

1. Weakness, 2. Hunger, 3. Sweating (drenching), 4. Tremor (trembling), 5. Palpitations (pounding heart), 6. Dizziness, yawning, 7. Headache, 8. Clouding of vision, 9. Abnormal behaviour (aggression), 10. Confusion, inability to concentrate and incoordination, 11. Diplopia, 12. Convulsions, 13. Coma.

Autonomic: 2, 3, 4, 5; neuroglycopenic: 6, 8, 9, 10, 11, 12, 13; non-specific: 1 and 7.

Clinical Wisdom

Common signs in hypoglycaemia are sweating and pallor; tachycardia and high systolic BP are typical. Transient focal neurodeficit may be seen occasionally.

- Remember, autonomic symptoms predominate in rapid onset hypoglycaemia whereas neuroglycopenic symptoms are the chief complaints in gradual onset hypoglycaemia.
- Diurnal hypoglycaemia: Nervousness, sweating, hunger and tremor mainly.
  Nocturnal hypoglycaemia: Night sweats, bad dreams, early morning headache and confusion.
- **Hypoglycaemia is traditionally classified** into a) Fasting hypoglycaemia (occurs in the presence of diseases like hyperinsulinism, liver disease, renal disease, endocrine causes and drug-induced), and b) Reactive (post-prandial) hypoglycaemia (occurs in response to meals like dumping syndrome, galactosaemia).

Q. Important points to diagnose hypoglycaemic coma (or D/D with diabetic ketoacidosis):

Hypoglycaemic coma is always confused with diabetic coma (ketoacidosis). The characteristic features of 'hypoglycaemic coma' are:

1. History of overdose of insulin or oral hypoglycaemic agents, vigorous exercise or missing a meal.
2. Classical symptoms of hypoglycaemia may be present (already described): Drenching sweat is very important.
3. Sudden onset of unconsciousness.
4. a. Dehydration: Absent (rather pallor plus cold sweat are present).
   b. Pulse: Normal volume or full pulse; tachycardia.
   c. BP: Normal or high.
   d. Air hunger: Absent; rather shallow or normal respiration.
   e. Smell of acetone: Absent.
   f. Convulsions: May be present.
   g. **Jerks: May be brisk.**
   h. **Plantar response: Often bilaterally extensor.**
5. Urine: Absence of sugar and ketone bodies.
6. Blood: Blood sugar is low; HCO_3^- level is normal.
7. Lump of sugar (given orally) or infusion of glucose (given in an unconscious patient) helps in regaining consciousness.

- In **diabetic ketoacidosis:** The patient will have polyuria, polydipsia, anorexia, vomiting and abdominal pain. *Dehydration+*; pulse is usually weak, BP is low with dry skin and tongue, air hunger is present with smell of acetone in the breath (Kussmaul's breathing); deep reflexes are dull with flexor plantar response. Sugar and ketone bodies are present in urine; high blood sugar with low HCO_3^- level. The patient needs immediate treatment.

Q. Bedside clinical tests for autonomic neuropathy:

There are battery of tests to diagnose autonomic neuropathy but the commonly practised cardiovascular reflexes are described below. In autonomic neuropathy, there will be:

1. Response of Valsalva manoeuvre on R-R interval in ECG (absence of ↑ in R-R interval).
2. Change of heart beat and BP, in response to change of posture (absence of slight ↑ in pulse and BP on standing).
3. Blood pressure response to sustained handgrip (absence of normal ↑ in BP during handgripping).
4. Heart rate response to deep breathing (absence of ↓heart rate on deep inspiration).
5. Presence of orthostatic hypotension (*see* page 227).
6. Presence of resting tachycardia (i.e. tachycardia at rest).
7. Pupils are mid-dilated with sluggish reaction.

- Simply one can **examine at the bedside** for light reflex, accommodation reflex, pupillary resistance to mydriatics, or disturbance of sweating.

Q. What are the causes of sudden death in diabetes?

Probably it is due to autonomic neuropathy and the different hypothesis put forward are:

a. Patients do not respond normally to hypoxia and sustain cardio-respiratory arrest.
b. Apnoea.
c. Cardiac arrhythmias.

Q. Investigations you like to perform in a case of DM:

1. Blood:
   a. Sugar (fasting and post-prandial; for diagnosis and monitoring) and glycosylated Hb (HbA_1 or HbA_{1C}: Comprising 4–6% of total Hb and reflects blood glucose concentration for preceding 6–8 weeks).
   b. TC, DC and ESR; panel of blood tests like triglycerides, LDL, VLDL, HDL and total cholesterol (lipid profile); urea and creatinine; uric acid.
2. Urine (R/E): With special reference to specific gravity, RBC, pus cells, protein, sugar, ketone bodies, casts. Culture and sensitivity tests are done, and 24-hours protein excretion is measured, if indicated (i.e. in nephrotic syndrome developing as a complication); estimated glomerular filtration rate (eGFR).
3. ECG: To diagnose IHD or to observe the changes due to hypertension (associated).
4. Chest X-ray: Pulmonary tuberculosis and fungal infection of lung are very common in diabetics. Cardiomegaly from hypertension should be looked for. Straight X-ray of abdomen is done to exclude pancreatic calcification (fibro-calculous pancreatic disease—commonly seen in T_1DM).
5. Ophthalmoscopic examination (fundoscopy): For diabetic retinopathy.
6. Barium meal examination of GI tract and endoscopy are done to study motility of the GI tract.
7. Nerve conduction study (in peripheral neuropathy).
8. Doppler studies of peripheral vessels, if indicated.
9. Last but not the least, regular recording of blood pressure.

- Glycosylated haemoglobin is a parameter for assessing long-term glycaemic control, and for tight control of DM it should be kept below 6.5%. ESR may be high in the presence of infection, commonly tuberculosis. Glycated (glycosylated) fructosamine, which measures the amount of total glycated serum protein (mainly albumin), gives an indication of glycaemic control for over the last 2–3 weeks.
- **In all patients of pulmonary tuberculosis check blood sugar and in diabetics, always do a chest X-ray.**

Q. How to classify oral hypoglycaemic agents (OHA)?

A. Sulphonylureas:
   a. 1st generation: Chlorpropamide, tolbutamide, tolazamide, acetohexamide.
   b. 2nd generation: Glimepiride, glipizide, gliclazide, glyburide (glibenclamide).

B. Non-sulphonylurea agents:
   a. Biguanides: Phenformin (not used), metformin, buformin (not used).
   b. Meglitinides (prandial glucose regulators): Repaglinide, nateglinide.
   c. Alpha-glucosidase inhibitors: Acarbose, voglibose, miglitol.
   d. Thiazolidinediones [also known as 'glitazones' or PPARγ agonist (peroxisome proliferator-activated receptor-gamma)]: Troglitazone, ciglitazone, pioglitazone, rosiglitazone. Majority are withdrawn and pioglitazone is the only remaining agent in this class available in India.
   e. Dipeptidyl peptidase-4 (DPP-4) inhibitors: Sitagliptin, vildagliptin, linagliptin, saxagliptin, teneligliptin.
   f. SGLT-2 (sodium-glucose co-transporter-2) inhibitors (so called, 'gliflozins'): Canagliflozin, depagliflozin, empagliflozin, ertugliflozin.

- The OHAs are divided into three categories:
  1. Insulin sensitizers: Metformin, pioglitazone, rosiglitazone.
  2. Insulin secretagogues: Glimepiride, glipizide, gliclazide, tolbutamide, chlorpropamide, glyburide, meglitinide analogues, GLP-1 agonists and DPP-4 inhibitors.
  3. Inhibitors of glucose absorption: Alpha-glucosidase inhibitors, guar gum.
- Parenteral hypoglycaemic agents are:
  • Insulins.
  • Glucagon-like peptide (GLP-1) agonists: 'Incretin mimetics' like exenatide, liraglutide, lixisenatide, dulaglutide, semaglutide.
  • Amylin agonist: Pramlintide.
- Other oral drugs tried in treating DM are: Bromocriptine (dopamine agonist), colesevelam (bile acid sequestrant) and hydroxychloroquine.
- Read the section on 'Insulin syringe' from 'Bedside Clinics in Medicine, Part II' for insulin preperations.

Q. What is glycaemic Index?

It is the rapidity with which a carbohydrate increases the blood sugar level. Patients with DM are advised to avoid foods with high glycaemic index like glucose, potato or white bread; legumes, whole grain cereals and brown bread are of low glycaemic index.

Q. How will you correct the fluid loss in ketoacidosis?

In an established case, the patient usually suffers from a fluid deficit of 7–8 litres. Fluid of choice is normal saline until the blood sugar falls below 250 mg/dL when it may be changed to 5% glucose. It is advisable to correct the fluid loss in this way

Normal saline volume	*Time*
1 litre	in 30 min
1 litre	in next 1 hour
1 litre	in next 2 hours
1 litre	in next 4 hours
4 litres	in next 16 hours

Q. Dawn phenomenon:

When DM patients (type 1 DM mainly) are closely monitored during insulin therapy, it is seen that hyperglycaemia develops in between 3–7 AM. This increase in the insulin requirement in known as Dawn phenomenon and is due to increase in the counterregulatory hormones like cortisol, growth hormone, glucagon and catecholamines. During sleep, there is a surge in the secretion of these hormones. Treatment is aimed to **increase** the overnight insulin dosage.

Q. Somogyi phenomenon:

This is a manifestation of early morning rebound hyperglycaemia following, possibly unrecognised, hypoglycaemia. Often it is seen that the previous night time dose of insulin was in excess. Treatment is aimed to **decrease** the overnight insulin dosage. This is commonly seen in children.

- Early morning (3 AM) blood sampling is necessary to differentiate both the conditions. In Dawn phenomenon, both the 3 AM and morning fasting blood show hyperglycaemia. In Somogyi phenomenon, 3 AM blood sample shows hypoglycaemia and morning fasting blood documents hyperglycaemia.
- The cumulative risk of nephropathy in type 2 DM varies with ethnic origin (may be 50%).

- Though microvascular diseases are the main cause of death in type 1, many patients of type 2 succumb to macrovascular disease prior to development of significant microvascular disease. Advanced age, development of atherosclerosis as a result of co-morbid conditions like physical inactivity, smoking, hypertension and hyperlipoproteinaemia are important causes of death in type 2 diabetes **(Table 1.29)**.
- Majority of diabetics, approximately 90–95% in India, suffer from T_2DM.

Clinical Wisdom

In T_1DM, microalbuminuria is an early predictor of nephropathy while in T_2DM, it usually predicts future development of malignant angiopathy and cardiovascular complications.

Q. Define metabolic syndrome or 'syndrome X':

The **NCEP ATP III criteria** goes like this:

Presence of three or more among five of the following:

- High blood pressure ≥130/85 mm of Hg.
- Hypertriglyceridaemia >150 mg/dL.
- Low HDL cholesterol <40 mg/dL in men and <50 mg/dL in women.
- Abdominal obesity, i.e. waist circumferance >102 cm in men and >88 cm in women.
- High fasting blood glucose ≥110 mg/dL.

- NCEP = National Cholesterol Education Programme; ATP = Adult Treatment Panel

The **International Diabetes Federation (IDF)** criteria (needs central obesity + any other 2 features) are:

- High blood pressure ≥130/85 mm of Hg.
- Hypertriglyceridemia >150 mg/dL.
- Low HDL cholesterol <40 mg/dL in men and <50 mg/dl in women.
- Waist circumferance (ethnic specific values), e.g. >94 cm in men and >80 cm in women.
- High fasting glucose ≥100 mg/dL.

Clinical Wisdom

WHO criteria of metabolic syndrome essentially require insulin resistance to fulfil the criteria. '**Insulin resistance**' is clinically suspected by the presence of acanthosis nigricans, skin tags (acrochordons), central obesity, lipodystrophy and features of polycystic ovarian disease.

Table 1.29: Chronic complications in type 1 versus type 2 DM (with approximate incidence)

Complications	Type 1 DM	Type 2 DM
1. Retinopathy	90% (after 20 years)	15–20% (after 15 years)
2. Nephropathy	30–40%	3–16%
3. Neuropathy	60% (after 30 years)	60% (after 30 years)
4. Ischaemic heart disease	Increases after 30 years	2–3 times of normal
5. Peripheral vascular disease	30%	45% (after 20 years)
6. Hypertension	50% (after 30 years)	50%

Q. Outline of management of the patient described at outset (T_2DM):

1. Diabetic diet. Lifestyle modification. Liaison with a diabetologist.
2. Insulin (insulin requirement is low in renal involvement): Used to improve the glycaemic control.
3. Oral hypoglycaemic agents (reduction or modification of dosage may be necessary in azotaemia).
4. Treatment of hypertension, obesity, dyslipidaemia and coronary heart disease.
5. Treatment of oedema.
6. Management of nephrotic syndrome. Even dialysis may be needed, if azotaemia develops.
7. Control of muscle pain (due to neuropathy) by: Phenytoin, carbamazepine, pregabalin, codeine or tricyclic antidepressants.
8. Control of UTI and skin lesions, if develops.
9. Care of the feet to prevent 'diabetic foot' (consult chiropodist).

Clinical Wisdom

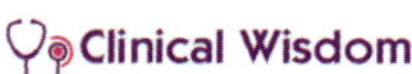

Diabetics should keep away from (i.e. **avoid list**) sugar, sweets, candies, honey, cakes, muffins, pastries, cream, dried fruits, nuts, sweet pickles, bear or wines, carbonated drinks or sweet drinks, bananas, grapes, mangoes, etc.

Conclusion

1. Explore 'all the systems' with examination from 'head to toes' in a patient of DM.
2. Palpate all the peripheral pulses (especially pedal pulses). Measure BP both in lying down and upright position.
3. Search for trophic ulcer in foot.
4. Give attention to retinopathy, nephropathy and neuropathy.
5. Do not forget to test the urine sample for sugar and protein, if possible.

Chapter 2

Short Cases

"The whole art of medicine is in observation."

—**Sir William Osler** (1849–1919), a multifaceted physician functioning as a clinician, pathologist, internist, educator, historian and an author—**'Father of modern medicine'**

CYANOTIC CONGENITAL HEART DISEASES — CASE 28

Q. Clinical presentation:

A young male with history of anoxic spells, breathlessness and syncope is presented. On examination, it reveals central cyanosis, polycythemia, clubbing, tachypnoea and an ejection systolic murmur in the pulmonary area. The most probable provisional diagnosis is Fallot's tetralogy.

Q. How do you classify congenital heart diseases?

A. Cyanotic:

With increased pulmonary blood flow

- Transposition of great vessels (aorta arises from RV while pulmonary artery arises from LV).
- Truncus arteriosus (single common trunk arising from RV and LV).
- Total anomalous pulmonary venous connection (TAPVC) [4 pulmonary veins drain into RA].
- Double-outlet right ventricle (DORV) [aorta connects to RV instead of to LV].
- Hypoplastic left heart.

Normal or decreased pulmonary blood flow

- Tetralogy of Fallot (TOF).
- Tricuspid atresia (absence of orifice between RA and RV).
- Ebstein's anomaly (there is atrialisation of RV with murmur of tricuspid incompetence).
- Pulmonary atresia (here, pulmonary valve does not form properly).
- Single ventricle.

B. Acyanotic:

With shunt (left-to-right)

- Atrial septal defect (ASD), ventricular septal defect (VSD), patent ductus arteriosus (PDA).
- Partial anomalous pulmonary venous connection.
- Ruptured sinus of Valsalva.
- Coronary arteriovenous fistula.
- Aortopulmonary window.

Without shunt

- Coarctation of aorta.
- Congenital aortic stenosis.
- Congenital pulmonary stenosis.
- Left heart malformation (congenital mitral stenosis, congenital mitral regurgitation).
- Idiopathic dilatation of the pulmonary trunk.

> - Common cyanotic congenital heart diseases include 5 'T': Tetralogy of Fallot, Tricuspid atresia, Transposition of great vessels, TAPVC and Truncus arteriosus.
> - Commonest congenital cardiac anomaly is bicuspid aortic valve (affecting 1–2% of the population) which goes unnoticed until later in life when the valve is stenosed due to fibrosis or calcium deposition, or results in significant aortic regurgitation. **VSD is the commonest congenital heart disease.**
> - Colour Doppler echocardiogram confirms the congenital heart diseases.

Q. Components of tetralogy of Fallot (TOF):

It is the commonest cyanotic congenital heart disease in children above the age of 1 year, i.e. who do survive infancy. A baby who is cyanotic at birth is unlikely to have TOF. It has 4 distinct abnormalities:

1. Ventricular septal defect (large, non-restrictive, infracristal)—VSD.
2. Right ventricular outflow tract obstruction—infundibular pulmonary stenosis (PS).
3. Overriding of aorta (aorta arises 2/3rd from left ventricle and 1/3rd from right ventricle), and
4. Right ventricular hypertrophy—RVH.

Q. Give a brief account of tetralogy of Fallot (Fig. 2.1):

Children with TOF may present with H/o dyspnoea, fatigue, deep cyanosis, hypoxic spells (see below), squatting, syncope (due to severe right ventricular outflow tract obstruction, there is increased right-to-left shunt with admixture of venous and arterial blood leading to reduced cerebral oxygenantion), recurrent respiratory tract infections, haemoptysis or impaired growth.

Physical examination reveals prominent a-wave in neck veins, central *cyanosis* (commonest clinical manifestation and depends on the severity of PS; the more severe the PS is, the more is the right-to-left shunt through VSD. Cyanosis is also due to mixing of blood in overridden aorta), *clubbing*, polycythemia (secondary to chronic hypoxaemia), *quiet precordium*, normal sized heart (no cardiomegaly), mild parasternal impulse (due to VSD, there is absence of heave), systolic thrill (rarely felt) and ejection systolic murmur (due to PS) along the left sternal border and in the pulmonary area. *The intensity and duration of the systolic murmur are inversely proportional to the severity of PS.* S_1 is normal, and S_2 is single, loud and represents aortic valve closure (A_2). Continuous murmurs of bronchial collaterals may be heard over the back. As the VSD is large, the systolic pressure difference between two ventricles remains very low, and thus the VSD murmur remains inconspicuous (silent). The right ventricle is effectively decompressed by VSD and this is why CCF does not occur in TOF unless complicated by infective endocarditis or anaemia.

The patient may be complicated by syncope (hypoxic spell), paradoxical embolism with brain abscess, CVA, infective endocarditis, and complications following marked secondary polycythemia, e.g. intravascular thrombosis developing at different sites. *Chest X-ray* (PA view) shows normal-sized heart with a characteristic appearance known as 'Coeur en Sabot' (boot-shaped heart with an upturned apex) with oligaemic lung fields; right-sided aortic arch (25%). ECG and cardiac catheterisation are also done, while echocardiography is diagnostic.

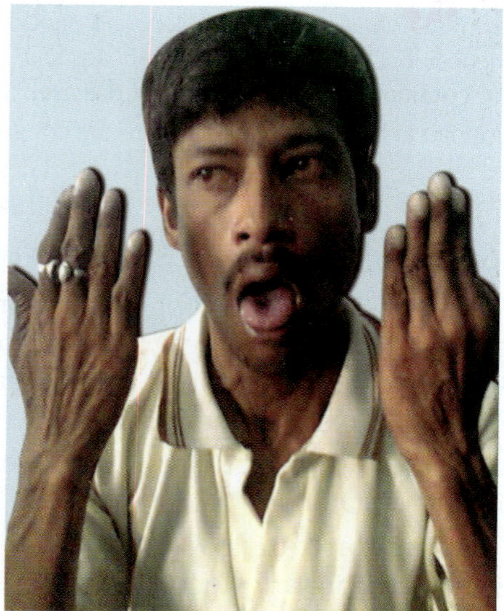

Fig. 2.1: Shadows of respiratory distress in face, **central cyanosis, clubbing** and **polycythemia** (suffused conjunctiva) in **Fallot's tetralogy**

- Mild case: Loud and prolonged murmur, severe case: Reduced murmur.

Clinical Wisdom

E-L Arthur Fallot (1850–1911) was Professor of Hygiene and Legal Medicine in Marseille, France.

Q. Common associations with tetralogy of Fallot:

Other cardiac anomalies associated with TOF are:

1. Patent foramen ovale (present in all).
2. Right-sided aortic arch (25%).
3. Persistent left-sided superior vena cava (10%).
4. Aortic regurgitation.
5. PDA.
6. ASD.
7. Anomalous origin of coronary arteries.
8. Absent left pulmonary artery.

Q. Other terminologies regarding Fallot's type of defects:

- Fallot's trilogy: Pulmonary stenosis (PS) + reversed interatrial shunt (i.e. with ASD) + RVH.
- Fallot's pentalogy: Fallot's tetralogy + ostium secundum ASD.
- Acyanotic (pink) Fallot's: Where right ventricular outflow tract obstruction (PS) is mild, i.e. mild Fallot's.
- Acquired Fallot's: In 5% cases of VSD, jet of blood comes to infundibulum and results in its hypertrophy, and thus the right ventricle is enlarged.

- Fallot sign: In older children, hypoxic spells are uncommon but increasing cyanosis with clubbing and polycythemia are common.

Q. Complications of TOF:

1. Anoxic spells, syncope (due to sudden contraction of pulmonary infundibulum), seizure.
2. Paradoxical embolism (thrombus from systemic veins may enter into arterial system through communication between ventricles, and results in CVA or infective endocarditis).
3. Infective endocarditis (common).
4. Polycythemia (may produce CVA), cerebral thrombosis, cerebral abscess.
5. Growth retardation.
6. Iron deficiency anaemia.
7. Incidence of pulmonary tuberculosis (very rare).

Q. What is hypoxic, anoxic or cyanotic spells?

The child hyperventilates, and suddenly becomes more cyanosed with development of apnoea, syncope, seizures or even sudden death (thus, potentially fatal), especially during waking up, feeding, crying, pyrexia or exercise. Cyanotic spells (*Fallot's spells*) are common between 2 months and 2 years of age. Systemic vasodilatation follows feeding, crying, etc. resulting in an increased right-to-left shunting of blood through VSD with associated decreased pulmonary blood flow. The pulmonary ejection systolic murmur disappears during hypoxic spells.

The child adopts **squatting** posture, i.e. sits with flexed hips and knees (knee-chest position) to reduce the cyanotic spells, and thus peripheral systemic vascular resistance is increased (as femoral artery and abdominal aorta are compressed) which reduces right-to-left shunting with improvement in arterial oxygen saturation and improved cerebral oxygenation; squatting also increases venous return to the heart and thereby increasing pulmonary blood flow. Squatting following physical exertion is almost always pathognomonic of TOF. The hypoxic spells may vary from once in a fortnight/month to multiple attacks in a day.

Q. Management of TOF:

Medical: Iron supplement for anaemia and antibiotic prophylaxis for infective endocarditis are essential. Cyanotic spells are managed by:

1. Squatting or knee-chest position.
2. Humidified 100% oxygen.
3. Morphine (0.1–0.2 mg/kg, IV).
4. Propranolol (0.1 mg/kg, slow IV).
5. Methoxamine (vasopressor) drip.
6. Continuous phenylephrine drip.
7. IV infusion of sodium bicarbonate (1–2 mEq/kg) to combat acidosis.
8. If medical therapy is ineffective, emergency surgical shunts may be considered.

Surgical:

1. Blalock-Taussig shunt (preferred): Left subclavian artery–pulmonary artery anastomosis.
2. Waterston-Cooley shunt: Ascending aorta–right pulmonary artery anastomosis.
3. Potts shunt: Descending aorta–left pulmonary artery anastomosis (not used now).

Q. What is atrial septal defect (ASD)?

It is the most common congenital heart disease in adults, which is 2–3 times more common in females. There are two main types of ASD, *ostium secundum* (75%, commonest type; at the level of fossa ovalis) and *ostium primum* (15%, rare; antero-inferior to foramen ovale). The third type of ASD is sinus venosus type (5–10%, posterior to foramen ovale). ASD is an acyanotic congenital heart disease where there is a defect in the atrial septum with shunting of blood from left atrium to right atrium. ASD should never be confused with patent foramen ovale (PFO); PFO is a normal variant, usually remains asymptomatic and not a true septal defect. In ASD, the right atrium not only receives blood from SVC and IVC but also from the left atrium, and thus enlarged in size.

Most of the children are asymptomatic but may complain of weakness, dyspnoea (effort intolerance), palpitations (due to atrial arrhythmia); the patients are prone to recurrent respiratory tract infections. The pulmonary vascular resistance which is low or normal at childhood goes high up as the patient reaches third or fourth decade, giving rise to pulmonary hypertension. As pulmonary hypertension develops, the initial left-to-right shunt reverses to right-to-left shunt (Eisenmenger's syndrome). The patient may develop right heart failure or atrial fibrillation in the adult life.

- In ASD, atrial fibrillation is common, and infective endocarditis (due to slow flow of blood) is rare.

Q. Associated diseases/anomalies with ASD:

1. Down syndrome (ostium primum).
2. Marfan's syndrome (ostium secundum).
3. Partial anomalous pulmonary venous connection.
4. Persistent left-sided superior vena cava.
5. Pulmonary stenosis.
6. Lutembacher's syndrome (ASD with rheumatic mitral stenosis).
7. Mitral valve prolapse or floppy valve syndrome (mitral regurgitation).
8. Holt-Oram syndrome (upper limb dysplasia, hypoplastic thumb, fingerisation of thumb, absent radius, polythelia or accessory nipple, pectus excavatum).

Q. Basic physical findings in ASD:

1. ASD is an acyanotic congenital heart disease. ASD may have a systolic thrill (10%) in the pulmonary area. If the thrill is very prominent, think of associated PS.
2. Prominent left parasternal lift.
3. Wide and fixed splitting of S_2 (hallmark of diagnosis) with a loud P_2. 'Fixed' means that the splitting does not vary with the phases of respiration because of equal pressure between left and right atrium throughout the respiratory cycle (inspiration and expiration both) as both atria act as a common chamber. It is 'wide' because of delay in RV ejection, which is again due to increased stroke volume.
   Another view: In ASD, there is left to right shunt → increased blood volume in RV → increased pulmonary blood flow → increased capacitance of pulmonary vascular bed in both inspiration and expiration (i.e. pulmonary hangout interval is prolonged and fixed) → wide and fixed splitting of S_2.
4. Mid-systolic pulmonary ejection murmur (grade II or III) due to increased flow across the normal-sized pulmonary valve, which is best audible at left 2nd or 3rd intercostal space. No murmur is produced across the septal defect due to low pressure gradient between two atria.

5. A mid-diastolic flow murmur across the tricuspid valve and right-sided S_3 are audible in lower left parasternal region.
6. If pulmonary hypertension develops, few of the auscultatory findings change (Eisenmenger's syndrome)—see below.

- Pulmonary stenosis (PS) is the nearest D/D of ASD. PS will have systolic thrill in the pulmonary area, soft P_2 and left parasternal heave; VSD is next considered as D/D.

Q. Investigations performed in ASD:

Chest X-ray: It shows a prominent pulmonary artery (a big pulmonary artery segment is seen and can be traced up to diaphragm; end-on view of juicy pulmonary artery is seen as white dots) and pulmonary plethora. ASD also reveals hypoplastic aortic knuckle, mild to moderate cardiomegaly, prominent right atrium and right ventricle. Fluoroscopy demonstrates 'hilar dance' as a result of pulsation of pulmonary artery.

ECG: Usually right axis deviation (ostium secundum, 85%); left axis deviation in ostium primum, and 10% having normal axis. RBBB (right bundle branch block) is seen, which is partial or complete. Complete heart block may be revealed in ostium primum type; large ASD may have prolongation of P-R interval.

Cardiac catheterisation is performed while echocardiography is diagnostic, which demonstrates the defect and the size of the chambers.

Q. Management of ASD:

Medical: Treatment of complications like respiratory tract infections, embolism (pulmonary and systemic) and brain abscess, arrhythmias (e.g. atrial fibrillation), heart failure and infective endocarditis (though rare).

Surgical: Up to 2 years of age, ASD can close spontaneously. However, children in the age group of 3–5 years without complications and having a significant shunt (i.e. pulmonary to systemic flow is >1.5:1) are best candidates for surgery. The defect is repaired by Dacron patch or direct suturing. If shunt is less, continue medial management.

Q. What are the characteristics of ventricular septal defect (VSD)?

Excluding bicuspid aortic valve, VSD is the commonest cardiac malformation occurring once in approximately 500 live births or accounting for 30% of all congenital cardiac defects, either in isolation or with a range of other malformations; VSD may rarely develop from rupture of intraventricular sepum or trauma (acquired). VSD is an acyanotic congenital heart disease where there is a defect in the ventricular septum with shunting of oxygenated blood from high-pressure left ventricle to low-pressure right ventricle. When pulmonary blood flow becomes very large and pulmonary arterial pressure increases, there is reversed shunting of blood from right-to-left (Eisenmenger's complex) with development of central cyanosis. The septal defects may vary in size, shape and number, and can be either in membranous part or in muscular portion of the ventricular septum; perimembranous defects are most common (80%), and may be supracristal (subpulmonic) or infracristal (subaortic or behind the tricuspid valve).

Q. Basic physical findings in VSD:

The apex beat is hyperdynamic. A systolic thrill may be palpable at the left parasternal region. Left parasternal lift or heave may be felt; tachypnoea with indrawing of the lower ribs may be revealed. The S_1 and S_2 are usually masked by the murmur. The murmur is typically rough and pansystolic/holosystolic, best heard in left 3rd and 4th intercostal space close to the sternum but radiating all over the precordium. A mid-diastolic flow murmur across the mitral valve may be audible at the apex in large VSD. The nearest D/D are mitral or tricuspid incompetence.

Complications are recurrent respiratory tract infections, CCF, infective endocarditis, pulmonary hypertension (Eisenmenger's complex) and arrhythmias.

The VSDs are classified as:

Small VSD ('maladie de Roger'): Very often found in routine examination. It is the asymptomatic, small haemodynamically insignificant VSD where thrill and pansystolic murmurs are very prominent. Majority (90%) closes spontaneously by the age of 10 years.

Moderate VSD: The patient comes with fatigue, dyspnoea or pulmonary infections. Cardiac size is enlarged (LVH). Systolic thrill and pansystolic murmur at the lower left sternal edge radiated towards right chest are characteristic finding.

Large VSD: Usually develops CCF at 1 year; at 9–10 years of age, eventually Eisenmenger's complex develops. There is cardiac enlargement. Usually, there is no thrill and murmur is not so rough.

- Signs of closing VSD: Holosystolic murmur gets shorter, softer and gradually disappear.
- *Chest X-ray* reveals enlargement of LA and LV along with pulmonary plethora. *ECG* features biventricular hypertrophy in larger defects. A small VSD shows no abnormality in chest X-ray or in ECG. *Echocardiography* identifies the site, size and haemodynamic consequences of VSD.
- *Management:* Medical treatment is done against infective endocarditis and CCF. Surgical closure of moderate and large VSDs (by Dacron patch or direct suturing) is ideally performed before 2 years of age or before the development of severe pulmonary hypertension. Small VSD is observed for spontaneous closure.

Q. Conditions where VSD is an essential part of the syndrome:

1. Fallot's tetralogy, 2. Double-outlet right ventricle (DORV), 3. Truncus arteriosus, 4. AV canal defects.

Q. Associated syndromes with VSD:

1. Cri du chat syndrome.
2. Fetal alcohol syndrome.
3. Trisomy 13, 18, 21.
4. DORV.

Q. What is patent ductus arteriosus (PDA)?

The ductus arteriosus connects the *left pulmonary artery* just after the bifurcation of the main pulmonary artery with the *descending aorta* just distal to the origin of left subclavian artery. In the fetus, the channel (ductus arteriosus) diverts blood from the pulmonary to systemic circulation. Physiological closure occurs soon after birth (due to high oxygen concentration in lungs and reduced pulmonary vascular resistance) and anatomical closure is completed within 2–3 weeks after birth. In a malformed duct with less elastic tissue, the patient may live with patent ductus arteriosus (PDA). As pressure in aorta is higher than pulmonary artery, blood shunts in PDA from aorta-to-pulmonary artery (left-to-right). Thus, venous return to left heart is increased resulting in left ventricular volume overload and ultimately its failure. Over the time, pulmonary hypertension with reversed shunting (right-to-left), i.e. Eisenmenger's syndrome develops.

PDA is common in females, premature babies, babies born at high altitudes or in continual prenatal hypoxaemia, Down syndrome, and with maternal rubella in first trimester of pregnancy.

Q. Basic physical findings in PDA:

The salient features are:

1. Pulse: High volume, bounding or water-hammer in character; wide pulse pressure.
2. Differential cyanosis, if pulmonary hypertension develops.
3. Apex beat: Hyperdynamic.
4. Thrill: Systolic or systolo-diastolic thrill may be palpable at the left 2nd intercostal space.
5. Heart sounds: S_1 and S_2 are loud, and S_3 may be audible at the apex.
6. Murmurs: The typical continuous 'machinery' murmur ('Train in the tunnel' murmur, Gibson's murmur) with late systolic accentuation is best audible in left infraclavicular area and left 2nd intercostal space. A mid-diastolic apical rumbling murmur may be audible due to increased flow across the mitral valve.

- *Chest X-ray* reveals LVH, LAH, big pulmonary artery, calcification of ductus (in elderly), and rarely huge aneurysmal dilatation of ductus (due to infection in ductus).
- *ECG* shows LVH and LAH; RVH in pulmonary hypertension.
- *Echocardiography* diagnoses PDA while colour Doppler test demonstrates the direction of flow.
- *Management:* Premature infants with PDA are treated medically with indomethacin or ibuprofen (as prostaglandin inhibitor) in the first week of life to stimulate ductal closure. Surgery is done by ligation (<5 years), and ligation as well as excision of the patent duct (>5 years). Coil embolisation of PDA may be done in older children.

Q. Complication of PDA:

Eisenmenger's syndrome, CCF, atrial fibrillation, infective endocarditis, duct calcification or rupture.

Q. Associated anomalies with PDA:

1. Coarctation of aorta.
2. Congenital aortic stenosis.
3. TAPVC and TOF may be associated with.
4. Tricuspid atresia.
5. Pulmonary stenosis.
6. VSD.

Q. PDA is lifesaving in:

1. Aortic atresia.
2. Pulmonary atresia.
3. Severe coarctation of aorta.
4. Incomplete aortic arch syndrome.
5. Hypoplastic left heart syndrome.

Q. Eisenmenger's syndrome:

Pulmonary hypertension with reversal of shunt (right-to-left) from an initial left-to-right shunt is known as Eisenmenger's syndrome and the causes are:

1. VSD (Eisenmenger's complex): Occurs earlier in life.
2. PDA: Develops a little later than VSD.
3. ASD: Develops late in adult life.

Mechanism: Persistently elevated pulmonary flow (left-to-right shunt) → raised pulmonary resistance → pulmonary hypertension → progressive, obliterative and irreversible changes occur in the pulmonary vasculature → persistent pulmonary hypertension → reversed right-to-left shunting of blood.

The **symptoms** are breathlessness, fatigue, dizziness, syncope, angina, cough with haemoptysis or features of CCF. The **developing signs** of Eisenmenger's syndrome are:

1. Central cyanosis (not corrected even by giving 100% oxygen).
2. Polycythemia.
3. Clubbing.
4. Prominent a-wave in neck veins.
5. Pulse: Low volume.
6. Features of RVH (outward apex, left parasternal heave and epigastric pulsation) or RVF.
7. Loud and palpable P_2.
8. Ejection click and ejection systolic murmur due to pulmonary hypertension.
9. Occasionally pansystolic murmur of functional tricuspid incompetence may be audible.
10. Original murmur (VSD, PDA, ASD) decreases in intensity, duration and may disappear.

Conditions provoking systemic vasodilatation like pyrexia, exercise, hot climate may trigger the right-to-left shunt and worsen the systemic desaturation. Pregnancy, vasodilatation and anaesthesia are tolerated very badly by these patients. Haemoptysis is a bad sign in Eisenmenger's syndrome though not very common. The *chest X-ray* is characteristic which reveals enlarged central pulmonary arteries and peripheral 'pruning' of pulmonary vessels (i.e. peripheral ⅓rd of lungs have less arterial markings). The ECG shows features of RVH. Though diuretic and digoxin are prescribed to the patient, heart-lung transplantation remains the only curative treatment.

- Remember, right-to-left shunt gives rise to cyanosis, left-to-right shunt does not.
- Cyanotic congenital heart diseases are usually given as short and spot cases.

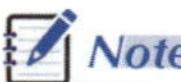

Note

In a **'Short case'**, a student has to examine the patient for general survey and one particular system asked for; the candidate is usually not allowed to take the history and thus, need not write the case history sheet. Commonly, the time alloted is 15 minutes.

FIBROSIS OR COLLAPSE OF THE LUNG — CASE 29

Q. Clinical presentation:

1. Respiratory distress.
2. Dry cough.
3. Pain on the affected chest.
4. Pyrexia (may or may not be present).

Symptomatology basically depends on:

- Rapidity of development.
- Amount of lung parenchyma involved.
- Presence or absence of infection.

Q. Describe the outline of findings in this case:

A. General survey:

1. Dyspnoea, orthopnoea (if a major bronchus is suddenly obstructed).
2. Central cyanosis.
3. Clubbing: Fibrosing alveolitis, or collapse developing from bronchogenic carcinoma.
4. Tachypnoea.
5. Tachycardia.

B. Inspection:

1. Flattened chest with supraclavicular hollowing, infraclavicular flattening and suprascapular wasting.
2. **Crowding of ribs and narrowing of intercostal spaces**, especially in long-standing cases.
3. Restricted movement on affected side.
4. Drooping of the shoulder in case of involvement of apex (seen from back).
5. Shifting of apical impulse towards the affected side.
6. Kyphoscoliosis resulting from extensive fibrosis.

C. Palpation:

1. **Shifting of trachea and apex beat towards the affected side.**
2. Movement of the chest: Diminished movement and reduced expansion on the diseased side.
3. Vocal fremitus:
   i. Fibrosis: Diminished.
   ii. Collapse: Diminished or absent (bronchus is obstructed), or increased (bronchus is patent).

D. Percussion: Impaired resonance or dull note.

E. Auscultation:

a. Collapse with obstructed bronchus, or fibrosis: Diminished vesicular (fibrosis) or absent breath sound (collapse), diminished or absent vocal resonance, fine crepitations and occasionally rhonchi are heard in fibrosis; rhonchi and crepitations are absent in collapse with obstructed bronchus.

b. Collapse with patent bronchus: Tubular breath sound, bronchophony with whispering pectoriloquy, and occasionally coarse crepitations are heard.

- In **fibrosis**, the onset is chronic and the chest wall is retracted in comparison to **collapse** of the lung where the onset is acute and the chest wall is flattened. Drooping of the shoulder, flattening of chest or crowding of ribs (on affected side) are commonly found in fibrosis, and may be seen in collapse of prolonged duration. *Features of collapse are more or less same as fibrosis but is of lesser in degree.*
- Past history: Tuberculosis, mumps/measles/whooping cough in childhood, joint pain, symptoms regarding bronchogenic carcinoma should be enquired into.

Q. Types of fibrosis of the lung:

a. *Focal fibrosis:* Coal-worker's pneumoconiosis, asbestosis, silicosis.

b. *Replacement fibrosis:* Tuberculosis, bronchiectasis, post-radiation fibrosis, lung abscess, pulmonary infarction, necrotizing pneumonia.

c. *Interstitial fibrosis:* This is the fibrosis of the alveolar walls, which affects both lungs diffusely (fibrosing alveolitis). It is commonly associated with systemic collagen diseases like rheumatoid arthritis, scleroderma, etc. 'Interstitial lung disease' is recently better known as **'diffuse parenchymal lung disease' (DPLD)**.

- Patient is more symptomatic in a) and c) but physical signs are more pronounced in b).
- Fibrosis of the lung of cardiac origin are mitral stenosis and multiple pulmonary infarcts.

Q. Fibrosis of the lung—upper versus lower lobe:

- Upper lobe: Tuberculosis, silicosis, ankylosing spondylitis, post-radiation.
- Lower lobe: Progressive systemic sclerosis, rheumatoid arthritis, fibrosing alveolitis.

Q. What is 'diffuse fibrosis' of the lung?

1. Acute: Hamman-Rich disease (acute onset, progressive course, unknown aetiology).
2. Chronic: Fibrosing alveolitis.

Diffuse fibrosis of the lung (chronic) is diagnosed clinically but confirmed by lung biopsy. The findings are bilateral and diffuse (not localised).

Q. Classical features of fibrosing alveolitis at the bedside:

1. Progressive disabling dyspnoea, orthopnoea, tachypnoea; persistent dry cough; weight loss and fatigue.
2. Constitutional symptoms like arthralgia (rare).
3. Central cyanosis, polycythemia.
4. Clubbing.
5. Bilateral diminution of chest movement; diminished vesicular breath sound.
6. Leathery crepitations ('velcro crepitations' linked to unzipping of velcro): Chiefly end-inspiratory crepitations, uninfluenced by cough, heard particularly over both the lower zones at back (bi-basal crepitations).
7. Signs of pulmonary hypertension, RVF or chronic cor pulmonale in late stages.

- These patients are usually corticosteroid-responsive.

Q. How do you classify collapse of the lung?

a. *Absorption or active collapse:* The bronchus is either obstructed by mucus plugs or bronchial casts, foreign body, blood, neoplasm (endobronchial), or compressed from outside by enlarged glands, aneurysm, neoplasm (exobronchial), or by neoplasm arising within the bronchial wall (intrabronchial).
   The trachea is shifted to the same side due to more negative intrapleural pressure.
b. *Compression or passive collapse:* The bronchus remains patent, and is developed as a result of pleural effusion, empyema, pneumothorax, hydropneumothorax, pyopneumothorax or very large neoplasm.
   The trachea is pushed to the opposite side as a result of positive intrapleural pressure.

- **Collapse** is the airlessness with shrinkage of lung volume. Previously absorption collapse was known as **'atelectasis of lung'**.
- In clinical practice, unless or otherwise qualified, collapse means absorption collapse (i.e. the model case described above). Whereas, signs of compression collapse literally means signs of pleural effusion/pneumothorax/hydropneumothorax where the underlying lung remains silent.
- Collapse may again be divided by patency of bronchus:
  - Central (mass lesion): Bronchus is obstructed; all signs of collapse are dampened.
  - Peripheral: Bronchus remains patent; bronchial breath sound and bronchophony present.

Q. Common causes of absorption collapse in relation to age:

a. Neonates: Meconium aspiration.
b. Children: Foreign body aspiration.
c. Adults: Bronchial adenoma.
d. Old age: Bronchogenic carcinoma or bronchial obstruction by foreign body (e.g. dentures).

Q. Position of mediastinum in collapse of the lung:

In a wider sense (as discussed earlier), collapse of the lung means absorption collapse.

a. Absorption collapse: Mediastinum is pulled to the affected side.
b. Compression collapse: Mediastinum is pushed to the opposite side.

- Read the section on 'Pleural effusion' for better understanding.

Q. What is 'middle lobe syndrome'?

It is the recurrent or persistent atelectasis of right middle lobe caused by compression of bronchus as a result of enlarged lymph nodes arising out of tuberculosis or malignancy. The diagnosis is confirmed by CT scan or bronchoscopy.

Q. Clinical features of bronchiectasis:

1. *Symptoms:*
   a. Cough with expectoration: Copious, purulent, foetid, often related to change of posture, most prominent in the early hours of the morning while arising from bed or at the time of retiring to bed.
   b. Haemoptysis (40–70%).
   c. Systemic symptoms like febrile episodes, malaise, anorexia, loss of weight.
   d. Breathlessness and wheezing.
   e. Pain in the chest (due to pneumonia or dry pleurisy).
2. *General survey:*
   a. Dyspnoea.
   b. Clubbing.
   c. Anaemia, fever, halitosis.
   d. Central cyanosis in bilateral and extensive disease.
   e. Undernutrition.
3. *Examination of the chest:* There may be no abnormal sign in the chest. The signs depend on the size of affected bronchi, airway patency and viscosity of secretions. One may get the signs of (i) bronchitis, (ii) fibrosis, iii) consolidation, (iv) collapse, (v) cavitation or, rarely vi) pleural effusion.

The physical signs often **change after a large bout of cough**. Breath sound may be vesicular with prolonged expiration to high-pitched bronchial (tubular) in type. Sharp metallic or bubbling 'leathery', coarse crepitations are characteristic. All the **signs are predominantly basal and bilateral**.

- Read details of bronchiectasis from Radiology section of 'Bedside Clinics in Medicine, Part II'.

Q. Clinical features of pulmonary tuberculosis (post-primary):

A. Symptoms:

a. Evening rise of temperature, anorexia, loss of weight, lassitude, night sweats, palpitations.
b. Persistent cough; sometimes there is sputum production (in advanced stage).
c. Haemoptysis.
d. Chest pain (due to pleurisy).
e. Breathlessness.

B. Signs: Initially there may be no abnormal physical sign in the chest. The earliest sign is often *post-tussive crepitations* heard in the apex of the lung. Gradually the physical signs of tuberculous consolidation, cavitation, fibrosis, pleurisy, pleural effusion or spontaneous pneumothorax may develop.

Q. Clinical stigmata of evidence of past or present tuberculous infection:

Always search for these features in a suspected patient of tuberculosis, especially in India.

- Erythema nodosum (present infection).
- Phlyctenular keratoconjunctivitis (present infection).
- Old scar or sinus reflecting the footprints of tuberculous lymphadenopathy (past infection) (*see* **Fig. 1.73**).
- Scrofuloderma or matted lymph nodes (present or past infection).
- Beaded and thickened spermatic cord (past infection).
- Gibbus (present or past infection).
- Choroidal tubercles (present infection).

Q. Effects of asbestos exposure in respiratory system:

Usually, at least 10 years of moderate to severe exposure to asbestos has occurred before the disease becomes overt. It affects persons working in asbestos mines, textile industries, manufacturer of fireproof, boilerman and shipyard workers. The manifestations are:

1. **Asbestosis** (progressive pulmonary fibrosis): Dry cough, chest tightness, dyspnoea on exertion, clubbing and end-inspiratory crepitations at lung bases.
2. Benign pleural plaques, diffuse pleural fibrosis, benign pleural effusion.
3. Bronchogenic carcinoma: Usually adenocarcinoma.
4. Mesothelioma of pleura (and peritoneum): Produces malignant pleural effusion.
5. Laryngeal carcinoma.

- So, proper attention must be paid while enquiring for **occupational history**, both present and past.
- One year's exposure to asbestos in teens may even result in mesothelioma in the fifth decade.

Q. What is 'pack year'?

While taking **smoking history**, ask for type of smoking (bidi, cigarette, pipe, etc.), amount (number of cigarettes consumed per day) and duration of smoking (i.e. pack year); enquire the duration of cessation of smoking in ex-smokers.

Pack year is the duration of smoking in years multiplied by number of packets of cigarettes smoked per day, e.g. one pack of cigarette (containing 20 cigarettes) smoked per day for 30 years make 30 pack years. The importance lies in the fact that risk for development of bronchogenic carcinoma is much increased when the pack years exceed 40. Chances of development of COPD is increased, if crosses 20 pack years.

- **Drugs used to help stop smoking** are bupropion (slow release), nicotine (gum, lozenges, spray, patch), or nortriptyline; other second-line drugs, e.g. varenicline, NicVax (vaccine) and rimonabant (withrawn from market) may be helpful.

Q. Bronchopulmonary segments in the lung:

Bronchopulmonary segment is a part of lung tissue supplied by one segmental bronchus, along with corresponding branches of pulmonary artery and pulmonary vein. There are 3 lobes (upper, middle and lower) in right, and 2 lobes (upper and lower) in left side of lung. Right lung have 10 and left lung have 9 bronchopulmonary segments (medial basal segment is usually missing in left side).

Q. Investigations you like to perform (fibrosis, or collapse, or fibrosing alveolitis):

1. Blood: Raised ESR, polycythemia; rheumatoid factor, antinuclear antibodies or circulating immune complexes may be found in fibrosing alveolitis. Arterial blood gas analysis shows hypoxaemia, especially in cases of acute onset.
2. Chest X-ray (PA view, lateral view is also required to determine the segment or lobe involved):
   i. Homogeneous shadow of the collapsed lung.
   ii. Displacement of mediastinum towards the affected side.
   iii. Retraction of hemithorax on the affected side.
   iv. Bi-basilar reticular pattern or 'Honeycomb lung' in fibrosing alveolitis.
   v. Tenting of hemi-diaphragm in basal collapse or fibrosis in the base.
   vi. In compression collapse: The aetiology of compression is seen in the X-ray plate, e.g. pneumothorax, pleural effusion, etc.
3. High-resolution CT (HRCT) scan: Investigation of choice which shows ground-glass appearance (alveolitis), thickened interalveolar septa, traction bronchiectasis and honeycombing (fibrosing alveolitis), which are marked peripherally in both the lungs. CT scan helps in early and confirmed diagnosis with extent of the disease.
4. Lung function tests (especially in fibrosis): Show restrictive type of defect, i.e. FEV_1/FVC is

approximately 90% (in obstructive defect, i.e. in bronchial asthma, FEV_1/FVC is near about 40–50%).

5. Bronchoscopy: To identify the cause of obstruction or to get a biopsy.
6. Rarely lung biopsy is needed to diagnose fibrosing alveolitis (i.e. the biopsy specimen shows patchy foci of interstitial fibrosis).

SUPERIOR MEDIASTINAL SYNDROME — CASE 30

Q. Synonyms:

1. Superior vena caval (SVC) syndrome.
2. Superior vena caval obstruction.
3. Reversed congestive cardiac failure (i.e. as upper half of the body is swollen).

Q. What is SVC syndrome (Fig. 2.2)?

SVC is formed by the left and right brachiocephalic vein (also known as innominate veins), which receives blood from head, neck, upper extremity and thorax, and delivers it to the right atrium.

In SVC syndrome, there is obstruction of SVC due to compression and/or infiltration by superior mediastinal tumours which result in characteristic features like headache, breathlessness, plethora with oedema of the face, dilatation of collateral veins in upper thorax and conjunctival oedema.

Q. Common causes of SVC syndrome:

Malignant diseases are the principal cause of this syndrome (90–95%) and therefore, the prognosis is very bad. The causes are:

1. Bronchogenic carcinoma (75%).
2. Lymphoma (20%).
3. Retrosternal goitre.
4. Tumours of the thymus.

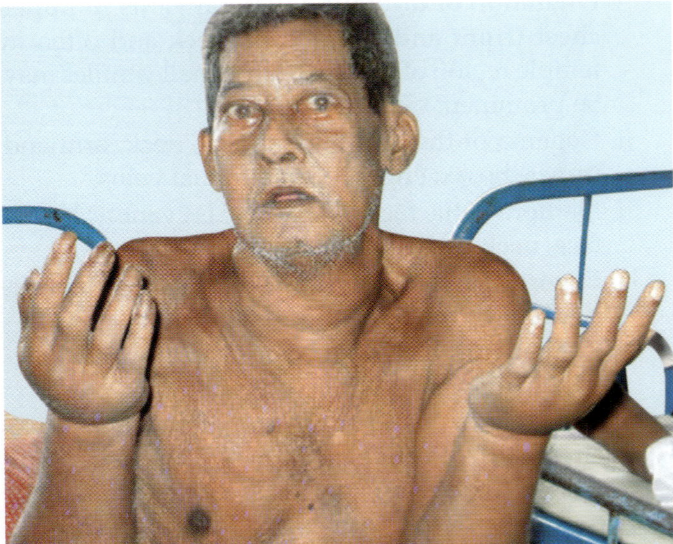

Fig. 2.2: **SVC syndrome**. Note the prominent external jugular veins and veins over the anterior chest wall. The face is puffy, and chest and upper limbs are swollen. The patient had moderate degree of respiratory distress

5. Metastatic tumour, e.g. from carcinoma of breast.
6. Teratoma.
7. Dermoid cyst.
8. Giant aortic aneurysm.
9. Fibrosing mediastinitis (e.g. methysergide-induced)
10. Pericardial cyst.
11. Thrombosis of SVC.
12. Persistent left-sided SVC.
13. Central venous catheter causing thrombosis.
14. Hypercoagulable state.
15. Tuberculous mediastinitis.

Clinical Wisdom

Elderly or middle aged—bronchogenic carcinoma or lymphoma, young or early age—commonly lymphoma; SVC of recent origin—likely malignancy; long-standing SVC syndrome—benign.

Q. Different modes of presentation (symptoms):

The *mediastinal mass usually compresses three tubes, three nerves and three vessels*. In bronchogenic carcinoma and lymphoma, the mediastinal structures are involved by spread to mediastinal lymph nodes and sometimes by direct extension of the tumour itself.

A. Tubes:

a. Oesophagus: May present with dysphagia and as it is a mechanical compression of the oesophagus, patient complains of difficulty in swallowing food mainly with solids (later on solid plus liquid).
b. Trachea: Respiratory distress, stridor and paroxysmal cough.
c. Bronchus: As such, obstruction of the bronchus from a mediastinal mass (due to bronchogenic carcinoma) is not very common. *The manifestations of obstruction depend on the nature of obstruction (complete or partial), absence or presence or secondary infection, and its effect on pulmonary function*. When a large bronchus is **'completely'** obstructed, there is absorption collapse or atelectasis, and the patient may complain of breathlessness and pain chest. If the collapse involves a smaller portion of lung, there may be no respiratory difficulty. In case of **'partial'** obstruction of bronchus, there is development of obstructive emphysema (the airflow resistance is increased in expiration than during inspiration and causes overdistension of the lung, lobe or segment) and thus, respiratory embarrassment may be present. Secondary infection of the lung is very common in this situation and the patient may have pneumonia.

B. Nerves:

a. Recurrent laryngeal nerve: The left-sided nerve is commonly involved due to its lower station than the right. The right-sided recurrent laryngeal nerve remains high up and is usually not compressed by the mediastinal mass. The patient presents with:

i. Hoarseness of voice.
ii. Bovine cough (explosive nature of cough is lost), and
iii. Stridor (common in bilateral palsy).

b. Phrenic nerve: There may be breathlessness (mainly in supine position) and sometimes, respiratory failure is present due to diaphragmatic paralysis.

c. Cervical sympathetic trunk (Horner's syndrome): Patient complains of partial drooping of the upper eyelid and loss of sweating on the affected side of face. Usually this happens to occur from Pancoast's tumour (apical bronchogenic carcinoma).

C. Vessels:

a. Superior vena cava: The patient usually complains of:
i. **Swollen and puffy face.**
ii. Headache (mostly at vertex, which is aggravated by cough).
iii. Visual disturbances.
iv. Alteration in the state of consciousness, syncope, black-out, and
v. Rarely convulsions.

b. Azygos vein: Symptoms of pleural effusion (on the side of compression, i.e. right-sided).

c. Lymphatics: Thoracic duct or small lymph channels may be obstructed. There are presence of:
i. Parietal oedema (non-pitting) of upper thorax, and
ii. Symptoms of pleural effusion (chylothorax).

Q. Physical findings in a case of SVC syndrome (signs):

The relevant signs are:

A. Tubes:

a. Oesophagus: Dysphagia may be demonstrated if the patient is allowed to eat some biscuits.

b. Trachea: There may be intercostal suction, central cyanosis and presence of stridor.

c. Bronchus:
i. Signs of absorption collapse (in obstructed bronchus) is found, i.e. there is diminished movement on the affected chest, shifting of the mediastinum to the affected side, impaired note on percussion, absent breath sound with diminished or absent vocal resonance, and usually without any adventitious sound.
ii. Rarely, the cause of SVC syndrome (e.g. bronchogenic carcinoma or lymphoma) may produce pleural effusion and thus, there may be compression collapse. The signs are diminished movement on the affected chest, shifting of the mediastinum to the opposite side, stony dullness on percussion, diminished vesicular or tubular breath sound, diminished vocal resonance or bronchophony, aegophony, whispering pectoriloquy with few coarse crepitations (in malignant pleural effusion, usually the mediastinum remains in the middle or on the same side, and rarely on the opposite side—for better understanding read the section on 'Pleural effusion').
iii. Rarely, a large mediastinal lymph node (at bifurcation of trachea) in lymphoma or the mass in bronchogenic carcinoma may transmit the tracheal sound and as a result of this, there is production of tubular (bronchial) breath sound, whispering pectoriloquy and rarely aegophony (heard in the interscapular region). This is known as **d'Espine's sign (posterior)**.

- Dull note on percussion over 2nd intercostal space anteriorly (right or left) with presence of tubular (bronchial) breath sound, is **anterior d'Espine's sign**.

B. Nerves:

a. Recurrent laryngeal nerve:
i. Ask the patient his name or address, and observe the hoarseness of voice.
ii. Ask the patient to cough for demonstration of bovine cough.
iii. Indirect layngoscopy shows the position of the affected vocal cord (commonly left-sided) in paramedian position (i.e. cadaveric position) during phonation.

b. Phrenic nerve: Read the section on 'Hydropneumothorax' for features of phrenic nerve palsy.

c. Cervical sympathetic trunk: **Horner's syndrome** is characterised by:
i. Pseudoptosis.
ii. Constriction of pupil (miosis).
iii. Anhidrosis (lack of sweating) of ipsilateral face, neck, arm and upper chest.
iv. Enophthalmos, and
v. Loss of ciliospinal reflex.

C. Vessels:

a. Superior vena cava:
i. **Dilatation of tortuous collateral veins in upper chest (front and back), arm, neck** and often in temple region of the face; even small venules may be prominent over chest wall.
ii. Oedema of the face (moon face), neck, arm and upper thorax; engorged sublingual veins.
iii. Plethora of the face (often there is cyanotic hue of face, neck, arm and hands).
iv. **Engorged and non-pulsatile internal jugular vein (with negative hepato-jugular reflux).**
v. Conjunctival oedema (chemosis) and subconjunctival haemorrhage.
vi. The flow of blood in the collateral veins over chest is from 'above downwards' (read the section on 'Prominent veins with venous hum' for demonstration of venous flow).
vii. There may be disturbed sensorium.

b. Azygos vein: Rarely, there may be signs of pleural effusion (on the side of compression of the azygos vein, i.e. right-sided).

c. Lymphatics:
   i. Non-pitting parietal oedema of upper thorax (front and back).
   ii. Signs of chylothorax.

- Two other features of SVC syndrome are bilateral papilloedema and exophthalmos. Remember, all the features in this syndrome increase after sitting and leaning forward (ref: breathlessness in pericardial effusion often diminishes after adopting Mahammedan's prayer position).
- Pre-azygos or supra-azygos SVC obstruction: If obstruction occurs above the joining of azygos vein, there is venous prominence and oedema of face, neck and upper extremity; post-azygos or infra-azygos SVC obstruction: Features of pre-azygos obstruction along with dilatation of superficial veins over the chest, abdomen, back and groin (more severe variety).
- One must look for cervical lymphadenopathy, clubbing, radiation mark in the chest and pulsus paradoxus.

Q. Important physical findings is SVC syndrome:

a. General survey: Decubitus, facies, pallor, neck veins, thyroid (ref: retrostemal goitre), lymph nodes, respiration, clubbing and nicotine stain in fingers, radiation mark in the chest.
b. Systemic examination: Chest (mediastinal percussion), hepatosplenomegaly (for lymphoma), nervous system (e.g. Horner's syndrome, fundoscopy).

Q. Differential diagnosis you will consider:

Mention the causes of 'Moon face'. Other D/D of SVC syndrome are constrictive pericarditis, CCF and chronic cor pulmonale.

Q. How do you like to investigate the patient?

1. Blood examination: Hb, TC, DC, ESR, sugar (F).
2. Chest X-ray: PA and lateral view (single investigation which gives a clue to SVC obstruction).
   i. **Mediastinal widening.**
   ii. Atelectasis.
   iii. Dense irregular hilar opacity which is extending peripherally (bronchogenic carcinoma).
   iv. Pulmonary parenchymal opacity (bronchogenic carcinoma).
   v. Pleural effusion, elevation of the hemidiaphragm (phrenic nerve palsy), rib erosion.
   vi. Rarely, pericardial effusion.
3. Indirect laryngoscopy to see the paramedian position of left-sided vocal cord on phonation in a patient with hoarseness of voice.
4. Cytological examination of sputum, bronchial brushings or washings for malignant cells.
5. FNAC or excision biopsy of scalene node, Virchow's gland or any palpable lymph node.
6. Pleural fluid aspiration and pleural biopsy.
7. Scanning of lung or thyroid (by using I^{131} or technetium 99 m for retrosternal goitre), or **CT scan of the thorax with FNAC**, if possible.
8. Barium swallow examination shows oesophageal displacement or compression.
9. Echocardiography in selected cases.
10. Bronchoscopy, oesophagoscopy and mediastinoscopy are usually contraindicated in the acute stage due to risk of bleeding. If the obstruction is relieved by treatment (radiotherapy or corticosteroid), one skilled clinician may go through the investigations for tissue diagnosis.

Clinical Wisdom

Rarely, there is presence of pericardial effusion in SVC syndrome. On an anatomical basis, right-sided tumours produce this syndrome much more frequently.

Q. How you are going to manage a patient of SVC syndrome?

The SVC syndrome is a serious medical problem and should be managed promptly. Unless the clinical examination and non-invasive diagnostic procedures suggest a benign cause of obstruction, or unless there is availability of tissues elsewhere in the body for biopsy (e.g. lymph node biopsy), the patient should receive irradiation or chemotherapy (cyclophosphamide) before attempts are made to come to a tissue diagnosis. Elevation of head and oxygen therapy may give temporary symptomatic relief; ventilatory support may be necessary. Corticosteroids and diuretics are often used initially to reduce oedema at the site of obstruction. Tracheal obstruction needs emergency radiotherapy. Endovascular placement of stent may be done. Anticoagulation may be given, if needed. When a tissue diagnosis is made afterwards, the patient is managed accordingly.

Q. What is inferior vena caval (IVC) syndrome (Fig. 2.3)?

It is the IVC obstruction as a result of:

a. Extraluminal compression: Ascites, tumours in the abdomen and pelvis, tuberculous plastic peritonitis, pregnancy.

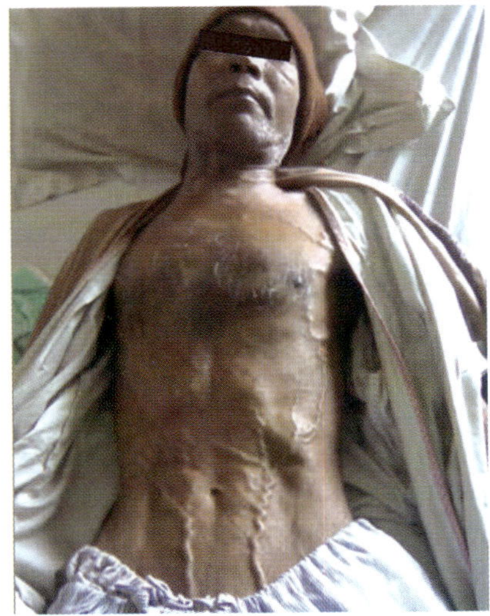

Fig. 2.3: **IVC obstruction.** Prominent collateral veins are seen over the anterior abdominal walls and flanks. There is absence of ascites

b. Intraluminal compression: Malignancy of kidney or adrenals, thrombosis extending from pelvic veins, membranous obstruction of IVC, OC pills, myeloproliferative diseases, hypercoagulable states.

Clinical features:

1. Pitting oedema of legs with dilated varicose veins, local cyanotic hue.
2. Collateral veins are seen over the abdomen, flanks and back.
3. Swollen and oedematous buttocks and groin.
4. Sometimes, there is presence of ascites (ascites follows pedal oedema).
5. Direction of blood flow is from 'below upwards'.
6. Stasis ulcer on the legs with pigmentation in chronic cases.

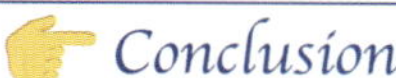

In a patient of SVC syndrome, obstruction of bronchus is lately seen in comparison to compression of vein and nerve (early and common). In the SVC syndrome, both **direct** (dull note on sternal percussion and d'Espine's sign) and **indirect** (vein and nerve compression) effects are observed though the indirect effects are more commonly encountered. Engorged and non-pulsatile neck vein is a very important bedside clinical clue. Always percuss the sternum in a suspected case of SVC syndrome.

The typical patient presents with dyspnoea (more on exertion), stridor, puffy and plethoric face with periorbital oedema, and tortuous veins over chest wall.

ASCITES — CASE 31

Q. What is ascites?

Ascites refers to collection of 'free' fluid within the peritoneal cavity (Fig. 2.4). Normally, there is virtually no fluid present in the peritoneal cavity. The Greek word 'askitos' means bag or sac.

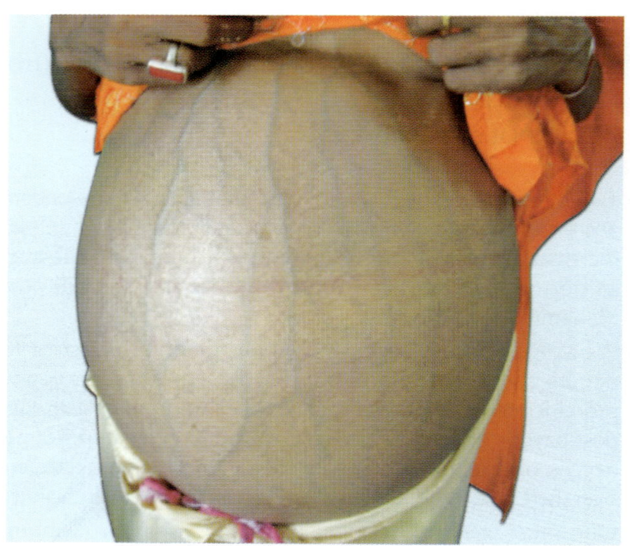

Fig. 2.4: Football-like **distension of abdomen by ascites** in cirrhosis of liver. Venous prominence of portal hypertension is also evident; distance between xiphisternum to umbilicus is more than distance between umbilicus to symphysis pubis

Q. Causes of ascites:

A. Ascites with anasarca

1. Congestive cardiac failure (CCF).
2. Nephrotic syndrome.
3. Hypoproteinaemia with severe anaemia (nutritional).
4. Pericardial effusion.
5. Constrictive pericarditis.
6. Myxoedema.
7. Filariasis.
8. Protein-losing enteropathy (due to hypoproteinaemia).
9. Epidemic dropsy (due to consumption of edible oils adulterated with argemone oil).

B. Ascites without anasarca (only ascites)

1. Cirrhosis of liver (may lead to anasarca).
2. Peritonitis:
   i. Acute pyogenic peritonitis.
   ii. Tuberculous peritonitis.
   iii. Malignant peritonitis.
   iv. Spontaneous bacterial peritonitis (SBP).
3. Lymphoma or leukaemias.
4. Pancreatic ascites (e.g. from acute pancreatitis).
5. Hepatic vein thrombosis (i.e. Budd-Chiari syndrome).
6. Meigs' syndrome.
7. Portal vein thrombosis.
8. Rupture of hollow viscus within abdomen.
9. Chylous ascites.
10. Haemoperitoneum following trauma.
11. Rare: Vasculitis, peritoneal dialysis, IVC obstruction, HIV peritonitis, familial Mediterranean fever.

- Common causes of ascites are 1, 2, 3 of (A) and 1, 2 of (B).
- In hypoproteinaemia with severe anaemia, oedema is out of proportion to ascites.
- *Ascites in cirrhosis of liver is mainly due to hepato-cellular failure (i.e. hypoalbuminaemia) and partly due to portal hypertension.*

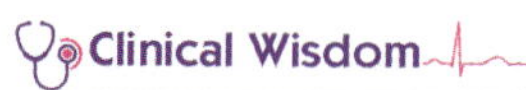

Common causes of ascites in community: Cirrhosis, tuberculous and malignant peritonitis, and CCF.

Q. Points to be asked in history for a patient with ascites:

1. Onset (sudden or gradual) and progress (slowly growing, stationary or progressive).
2. Past history of jaundice, haematemesis or melaena, alcoholism, fever (see below).
3. Pain and tenderness (tuberculous peritonitis, acute pancreatitis).
4. Loss of appetite (tuberculous or malignant ascites).
5. Loss of weight (tuberculosis, malignancy, cirrhosis).

6. Cough with or without haemoptysis.
7. Swelling of legs or face.
8. Respiratory distress (huge ascites, CCF, pericardial diseases).
9. Prolonged diarrhoea (protein-losing enteropathy), alteration of bowel habit (large gut malignancy), or alternate diarrhoea and constipation (intestinal tuberculosis).
10. Any sort of oliguria, paraesthesia in lateral thigh, or heartbum present or not.

Q. Important past history in a patient with ascites:

1. Alcoholism.
2. Jaundice.
3. Haematemesis or melaena.
4. Alteration in bowel habit.
5. Tuberculosis.
6. Haematochezia.
7. Pain abdomen (acute pancreatitis).
8. Loss of weight (malignancy).
9. Past H/o rheumatic fever or respiratory distress.
10. Fever (tuberculous or pyogenic peritonitis).

Q. Why do you say ascites in this case?

1. There is generalised swelling of abdomen; particularly the flanks are full; umbilicus is everted (or flushed with the abdominal wall) with a transverse slit. Maximum girth of abdomen is at the level of umbilicus.
2. Fluid thrill is present.
3. Shifting dullness confirms the diagnosis of ascites.

Q. What are the clinical features of ascites?

Symptoms

1. Progressive swelling and fullness of abdomen with gain in weight.
2. Aching pain all over the abdomen due to stretching; bloated feeling in abdomen.
3. Dyspnoea and even orthopnoea (in massive and rapid collection of fluid).
4. Swelling of lower limbs (due to CCF, cirrhosis of liver or functional IVC obstruction).
5. Paraesthesia in the distribution of lateral femoral cutaneous nerve (meralgia paraesthetica).
6. Oliguria.
7. Dyspepsia, heartburn (due to GERD).

Signs

a. General survey:

1. The patient may be in propped-up position due to dyspnoea.
2. Neck veins may be engorged (due to hypervolaemia).
3. Bipedal pitting oedema.
4. Obvious swelling of abdomen.

b. GI tract (abdomen):

1. Generalised swelling of abdomen with more fullness of flanks. The skin looks stretched and shiny (Fig. 2.4).
2. **Divarication of recti** [if the patient tries to get up from supine position against resistance (rising test), the linea alba bulges between the two recti as a result of protrusion of abdominal contents] may be present; there may be presence of abdominal (umbilical) herniation or abdominal striae (striae albicantes) (Fig. 2.5). Subcostal angle is wide, and lower ribs are pushed upward and outward. There is prominence of hypogastrium in erect posture.
3. There may be prominent veins around umbilicus or in epigastrium where the blood flow is away from the umbilicus (i.e. portal hypertension—in case of cirrhosis of liver): More common. Prominent veins in flanks of abdomen may also be seen where the blood flow is from below upwards (functional IVC obstruction caused by ascites itself—less common). *Abdominal veins are examined in sitting position while the patient is asked to cough.*
4. Cystic feel of the abdomen on palpation.
5. Umbilicus: Flushed or everted with transverse slit (laughing umbilicus); may have umbilical hermia.
6. Fluid thrill: Present.
7. Shifting duliness: Present.
8. Measurements:
   a. Maximum girth of abdomen is at the level of umbilicus.
   b. Spino-umbilical distance (line joining anterior superior iliac spine and umbilicus) is more or less equal on both sides.
   c. The distance between xiphisternum and umbilicus is more than the distance between umbilicus and symphysis pubis (Fig. 2.4).
9. Auscultation: Venous hum over the distended veins around umbilicus may be audible in cirrhosis with portal hypertension.

c. Respiratory system:

1. Basal collapse of lung: Diminished movement, impaired note on percussion, diminished vesicular

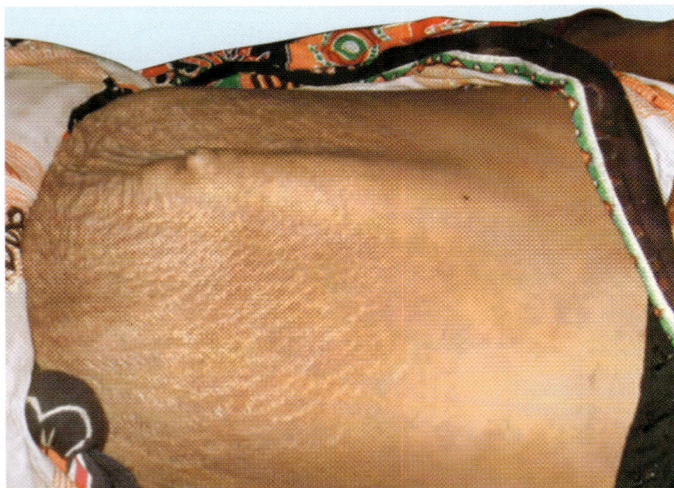

Fig. 2.5: Divarication of recti (bulging of linea alba in-between two recti) and Malgaigne's bulgings (abdominal wall bulging above the iliac crests due to poor tone of external oblique muscles) seen **on attempted 'rising test'**

breath sound and crepitations may be heard in the lower part of chest on both sides.

2. Hydrothorax (commonly right-sided; 10% cases) due to leakage of ascitic fluid through defects (pores) in the right dome of diaphragm for lymphatic channels; may be bilateral.

d. CVS:

1. Apex beat: Deviated upward and outward.
2. There may be diffuse pulsation over the precordium.
3. Soft systolic murmur in pulmonary area may be present (due to associated severe anaemia).

e. Nervous system: Nothing particular. There may be features of hepatic encephalopathy (e.g. flapping tremor).

f. Genitourinary system: Scrotal oedema or hydrocele may be evident as secondary effects of ascites (very rare) or as a clue to aetiological (e.g. nephrotic syndrome) diagnosis of ascites.

Clinical Wisdom

With the above mentioned signs (for ascites *per se*), there are presence of other features due to specific aetiology of ascites. Thus, one should always be careful in searching the other stigmata of cirrhosis of liver, CCF, etc. in a case of ascites. P/R and P/V examinations should be done.

- A **long-standing ascites** is recognised by striae albicantes, divarication of recti (may be associated with visible peristalsis underneath), umbilical hernia and puncture marks.
- Palpate liver, spleen or any other abdominal viscera by dipping method, in the presence of ascites.

Q. Examination for fluid thrill (Fig. 2.6):

If one of the flanks of abdomen is tapped in the presence of fluid in abdomen, three waves are transmitted, i.e. one through anterior abdominal wall, second through posterior abdominal wall, and third through the fluid inside abdomen. Presence of fluid thrill means *appreciation of transmitted impulse through the fluid* after tapping. The procedure goes like this:

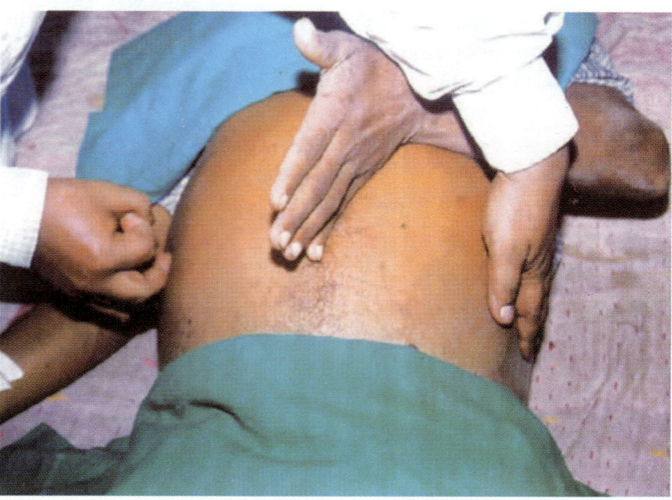

Fig. 2.6: Elicitation of **fluid thrill**

1. The patient lies supine with thighs flexed. The bladder should be evacuated. Either the patient or a third person (in the case of a child patient) will *put his ulnar border of right hand vertically, with fingers directing caudally, over the abdomen in the midline* (sagittal plane) firmly to prevent transmission of impulse or vibration through the anterior abdominal parietis. The impulse passing through the posterior abdominal wall is dampened by the bed.
2. Place the left palm over the left flank and sharply tap or flick the right flank with the fingers of right hand; a fluid wave or unmistakable 'shock wave' is felt by the left palm as a definite impulse. The same manoeuvre is now done by tapping the left flank while the impulse is felt over the right flank.

Q. Where do you get fluid thrill?

Fluid thrill is present in the presence of fluid in the peritoneal cavity **whether it is encysted or free.** Thus, fluid thrill may be found in.

1. Ascites (tense).
2. Ovarian cyst.
3. Pregnancy with hydramnios.
4. Rarely in large hydronephrosis.
5. Any large intra-abdominal cyst.
6. Obesity (false positive).

Q. Essential criteria for positive fluid thrill (Table 2.1):

1. Fluid should remain **under tension** (most important).
2. Large amount of fluid (it is often said that at least 2 litres fluid is necessary to elicit fluid thrill).

Clinical Wisdom

Fluid thrill may not be present if there is small collection or the fluid is not under tension.

Q. Is fluid thrill a definite sign for ascites?

No.

Q. Surest bedside sign for presence of free fluid in the peritoneal cavity (ascites):

'Shifting dullness' (in addition, paracentesis abdominis also confirms the diagnosis).

Q. How do you elicit shifting dullness?

Principle: The presence of ascites can be confirmed by altering the posture of the patient and demonstrating

Table 2.1: Minimal fluid for clinical detection

Clinical entity	Amount of fluid
A. Ascites:	
• Puddle sign	≥120 mL
• Fluid thrill	≥2 litres (tense ascites)
• Shifting dullness	≥1 litre
• Fullness of flanks	≥500 mL
B. Pleural effusion:	
• Clinical detection	≥500 mL
• Mediastinal shifting	≥1.5 litre

a change in the position of air-fluid interface (i.e. the distinct transition zone between tympany and dullness). Shifting dullness has both good sensitivity and specificity.

This method may also be called as 'shifting tympanicity'.

1. The patient lies supine with thighs flexed. The patient is asked to evacuate his/her bladder (full bladder will unnecessarily hamper the midline percussion). Try to exclude pregnancy.
2. Now palpate the abdomen (by dipping method) for any visceromegaly (liver, spleen, kidney lump, etc.). If any viscus is enlarged, try to avoid percussion over them.
3. Starting from the epigastrium, percuss (usually light to medium percussion) in the midline from above downwards. Note the maximum point of tympanicity. Usually it is somewhere around the umbilicus.
4. Now percuss laterally to one side (suppose, the right side) from the maximum point of tympanicity noted in the midline, keeping the pleximeter finger parallel to long axis of abdomen or arbitrary border of the fluid level. When you get a dull note, mark it with a skin pencil but keep on percussing towards the flanks to diagnose that the dullness is continuous and not a localised one due to colonic growth, faecolith, etc. and again return to the first noted point of dullness.
5. Now turn the patient to left lateral position (i.e. turn to the opposite side), keeping the fingers in the point of dullness noted in the right flank. Turning is done in such a way that your fingers in the right flank become the highest point of the patient's body. Now wait for few seconds (at least 10 seconds, usually 30 seconds) for the intestine to float up.
6. Percuss the dull point noted in the right flank, which will now reveal tympanitic resonance. Go on percussing up to the end point of the right flank which also shows tympanitic resonance; next go up to the midline and now the midline which was tympanitic initially will be dull on percussion. So, the dullness in the right flank changes to tympanitic note and the midline becomes dull from the original tympanicity—This is shifting dullness.
7. The same procedure is repeated in the left flank starting from the midline.

Q. Minimal fluid required for demonstration of shifting dullness (Table 2.1):

It is said that at least ½ to 1 litre of fluid is required to demonstrate shifting dullness.

Q. Absent shifting dullness in the presence of fluid in the abdomen:

The possibilities are:

1. Fluid is encysted, i.e. ovarian cyst or 'loculated ascites' in tuberculous peritonitis.
2. 'Small collection' of free fluid.
3. Rarely in massive tense ascites.
4. Short mesentery.
5. Adherent bowel.

Q. Massive splenomegaly or hepatomegaly with ascites: how to elicit fluid thrill?

It is often very difficult to form an opinion regarding fluid thrill in the presence of visceromegaly. One should not place the palm over the enlarged organ (may dampen the 'shock wave' of positive fluid thrill), rather one should tap from that side while the palpating hand is kept on the other side (patient's hand should remain vertically in the midline). In gross hepatosplenomegaly, fluid thrill may remain inconclusive.

Q. Shifting dullness present but there is no free fluid in the abdomen:

False positively in paralytic ileus (rare).

Q. What is meant by 'free fluid' in ascites:

The fluid shifts or changes its position with the intestinal air with change of posture which never occurs in encysted fluid and thus, shifting dullness is never found in encysted fluid (e.g. ovarian cyst) in the abdomen.

Q. In performing shifting dullness why do we percuss the midline first ?

While the patient lies supine, the intestine floats in the midline (in health as well as in ascites), which gives tympanitic note on percussion. To follow the cardinal rules of percussion, we percuss the midline first (tympanitic) and then the flanks (dull)—i.e. we percuss from 'more resonant to less resonant' area.

Q. Result of percussion over an ovarian cyst:

Fluid thrill may be present but shifting dullness is always absent. *In a large ovarian cyst, the midline will be totally dull on percussion.* But in a moderate ovarian cyst, upper part of the midline may be tympanitic though the shifting dullness is always absent. In an ovarian cyst, flanks are tympanitic on percussion.

- If the midline is totally dull on percussion (e.g. large ovarian cyst), it is not necessary to perform the next steps of shifting dullness, i.e. if the midline is dull on percussion, shifting dullness will be absent.
- Absence of fluid thrill and/or shifting dullness does not exclude the presence of ascites.

Q. Clinical detection of 'minimal' or 'small amount' of free fluid:

a. ***Puddle sign*** (Fig. 2.7): First percuss the abdomen in supine position where you will get a tympanitic note in the midline. Now place the patient on the hands and knees (knee-elbow position) for 5 minutes and percuss (with difficulty) over the most dependent part of abdomen (near umbilicus) which now reveals a dull note due to shifting of fluid. Generally

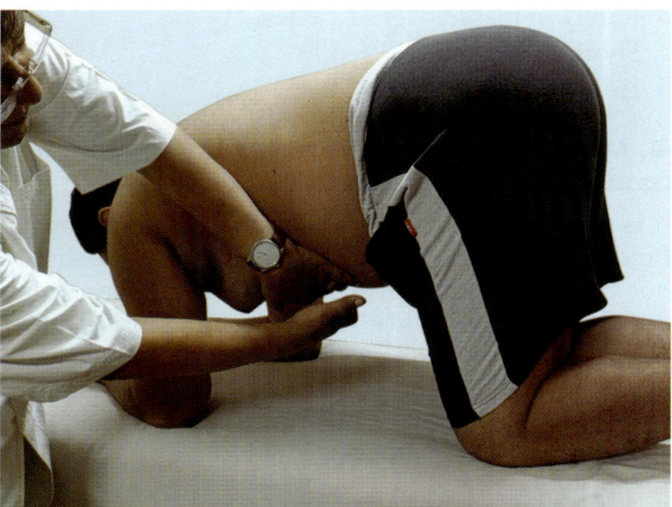

Fig. 2.7: Elicitation of **puddle sign** in minimal ascites

300–400 mL of fluid may be clinically elicited by puddle sign and even as little as 120 mL of fluid can be detected by this method. This sign is actually elicited by ausculto-percussion (placing the stethoscope over the dependent part and flicking the abdominal wall repeatedly to elicit changes in character of percussion note) which is a very complicated method. 'Puddle' literally means 'a small pool of muddy water'.

b. *Per rectal examination:* Boggy and fluctuant swelling in the dependent part due to presence of free fluid.
c. *Same-sided shifting dullness:* Very difficult to demonstrate. During the examination by conventional method of shifting dullness, turn the patient to the side of flank percussion and not to the opposite side. Now percuss the flank with difficulty which gives a dull note (here, flanks are originally resonant in supine position due to 'small' collection of free fluid).

Q. Massive hepatosplenomegaly with ascites: how to elicit shifting dullness?

First percuss the midline in supine position, which will elicit a tympanitic note. Now ask the patient to sit and again percuss the midline from above downwards. In the presence of free fluid in the abdomen, the lower part of midline will be dull on percussion in sitting position which was tympanitic initially (bladder must be evacuated) Actually, in the presence of gross visceromegaly, clinical detection of ascites becomes very difficult.

Q. What is 'horse-shoe shaped' dullness in ascites?

In moderate ascites, the distribution of fluid in supine position of the patient is confined to the flanks, dependent parts and the hypogastrium. Thus, in supine position the epigastrium and umbilical areas are tympanitic on percussion (due to floating of intestine) but a horse-shoe shaped dullness with concave upper broder is elicited due to dull flanks and dull hypogastrium.

Percuss the abdomen in various directions from the central area of tympanicity (i.e. the umbilical region) to outwards, and demonstrate the horse-shoe shaped dullness.

Q. Unilateral shifting dullness:

This is found in splenic rupture and is known as Ballance's sign. The blood present in the left flank becomes clotted (near the spleen) and does not shift to right side in right lateral position but the blood present in the right side (haemoperitoneum) is shifted to the left side.

Q. Abdominal measurements in ascites (Table 2.2):

1. Abdominal girth at the level of umbilicus (maximum girth is at this level in ascites; in ovarian cyst, it is below umbilicus): Periodic measurement is helpful to assess prognosis in ascites.
2. Spino-umbilical distance: Measurement is taken from umbilicus to anterior superior iliac spine on either side. Normally they are equidistant (also in ascites). Unequal distance is characteristic of tumour originating from pelvic organ (e.g. ovarian cyst).
3. Distance between xiphisternum to umbilicus, and umbilicus to symphysis pubis: In health, umbilicus lies in midposition of xiphisternum and symphysis pubis. Umbilicus is displaced down in ascites and upper abdominal mass, and displaced up in ovarian cyst or pelvic tumours.

Q. Why do you say it is ascites (clinical signs)?

1. Generalised swelling of abdomen with fullness of flanks.
2. Fluid thrill.
3. Shifting dullness (surest sign).
4. Puddle sign (in small amount of fluid).
5. Horse-shoe shaped dullness.

Q. D/D of bulging or distension of abdomen:

Commonly this is due to '8 F' (acronyms):

1. Fat: Obesity (inverted umbilicus with absent fluid thrill and shifting dullness).
2. Faeces: Megacolon or low gut obstruction (symmetrical enlargement of abdomen with visible peristalsis).
3. Foetus: Pregnancy (foetal parts are palpable, central dullness).
4. Flatus: Gaseous distension (flanks are not bulged, tympanitic note all over the abdomen).
5. Fluid: Ovarian cyst, ascites, distended urinary bladder.
6. Full (urinary) bladder (flanks are tympanitic, palpation causes pain or discomfort and desire for micturition; usually rounded cystic swelling in hypogastrium which is dull on percussion; shifting dullness is absent).
7. Fibroid ulterus or any fatal tumour (e.g. polycystic kidney or massive splenomegaly).

Table 2.2: Bedside differentiation between ascites and ovarian cyst

Features	Ascites	Ovarian cyst (Fig. 2.8)
1. Uniformity of swelling	1. Symmetrical	1. Asymmetrical
2. Any border seen	2. Never	2. Definite upper border is visible
3. Measurements i. Maximum girth ii. Spino-umbilical distance	3. i. Around umbilius ii. Equal on both sides	3. i. Usually below the umbilicus ii. Not equal
4. Distance between: a. Xiphisternum to umbilicus, and b. Umbilicus to symphysis pubis	4. a > b (Fig. 2.4)	4. b > a
5. Flanks	5. Full	5. Not full
6. Umbilicus	6. Everted and the slit is transverse	6. Everted and the slit is vertical
7. To 'get above' the swelling	7. Not possible	7. Usually possible
8. Percussion over flanks	8. Dull	8. Tympanitic
9. **Shifting dullness**	9. **Present**	9. **Absent**
10. Per vaginal examination	10. Nothing characteristic	10. Ovarian cyst is diagnosed

- Rarely, it is seen that midline percussion evokes dull note in a case of very tense ascites where the intestine is compressed (may have short mesentery too) and cannot come in front. Remember, the maximum bulge in ascites is transverse in contrast to ovarian cyst where the prominence is antero-posterior.
- 'Laughing umbilicus': When the slit of umbilicus becomes transversely stretched.
- Ascites may be classified into **mild, moderate, or tense** according to the amount of fluid collected. In tense ascites, peritoneal cavity is totally filled with free fluid, which may give rise to cardio-respiratory embarrassment.

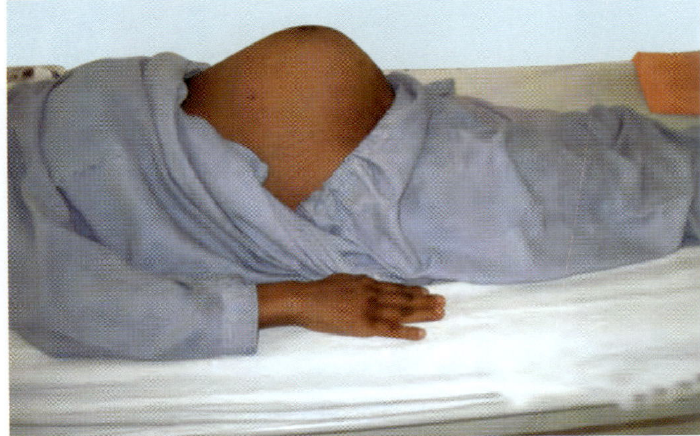

Fig. 2.8: Ovarian cyst. The abdominal swelling is not symmetrical and diffuse like ascites

8. Functional: Irritable bowel syndrome (often associated with bloating).

Distension of abdomen is of two types:
a. Generalised (mentioned above), and
b. Localised (visceromegaly, neoplasm).

Q. Percussion note in distension of abdomen (Fig. 2.9):

1. Ascites: Midline tympanitic, flanks dull.
2. Ovarian cyst, distended bladder and gravid uterus: Midline dull, flanks tympanitic.
3. Gaseous distension (e.g. intestinal obstruction): Midline as well as flanks are tympanitic.
4. Obesity: Midline as well as flanks are dull.

Q. Ascites appearing before oedema feet, or ascites > oedema feet (ascites praecox):

1. Cirrhosis of liver.
2. Constrictive pericarditis or restrictive cardiomyopathy.
3. Tuberculous or malignant peritonitis.
4. Hepatic vein thrombosis.

- In other conditions (CCF, nephrotic syndrome, etc.), oedema precedes ascites.

Q. Describe the normal position of umbilicus:

1. Umbilicus lies more or less in the midway between xiphisternum and symphysis pubis.
2. Normally it is inverted and slightly retracted.
3. Normal umbilicus is a puckered depressed scar and the slit is circular, i.e. neither horizontal nor vertical (the slit is transverse in ascites, and vertical in the presence of ovarian cyst).

Q. Causes of inverted and everted umbilicus:

a. **Everted:** Seen in any condition giving rise to increased intra-abdominal tension like ascites, ovarian cyst, pregnancy, umbilical hernia, hydramnios, severe gaseous distension, etc.
b. **Inverted:** Normally in health and in obesity (in obesity, umbilicus is buried in fat).

Q. Observations on skin over abdomen (inspection):

1. Moles, seborrhoeic warts, angiomas (considered normal changes).

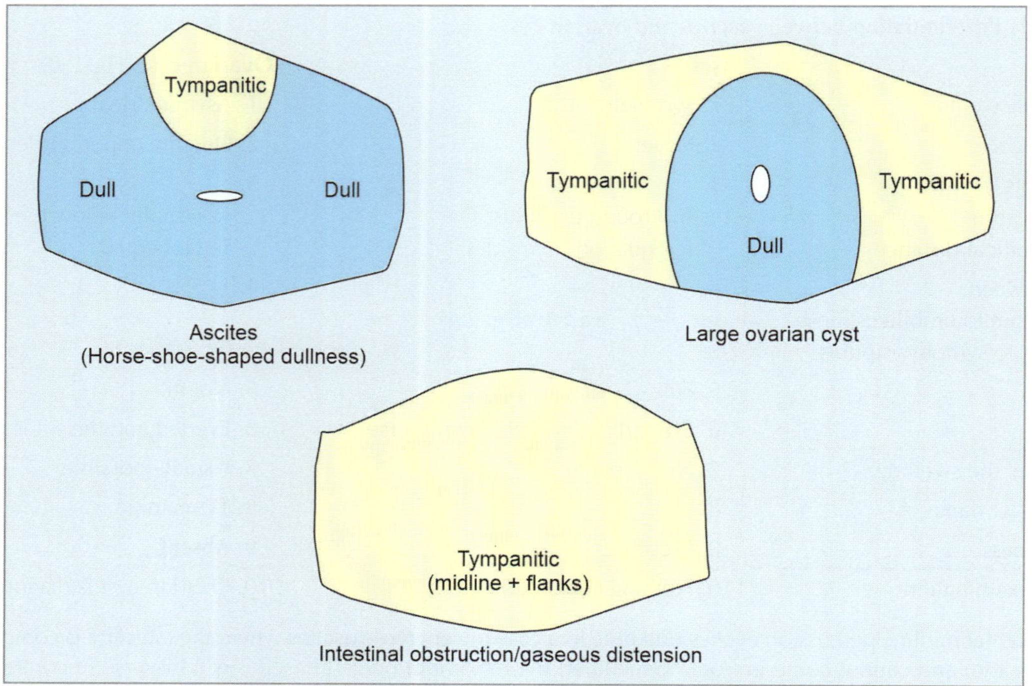

Fig. 2.9: Diagrammatic representation of diffuse **enlargement of abdomen**

2. Scars (especially of previous surgeries—large scars, and in minimal access surgery—sites of port and a small scar of laparoscopic cholecystectomy), haemorrhagic spots, stoma (ileostomy), hypo- or hyperpigmentation (e.g. linea nigra—midline pigmentation below umbilicus seen in pregnancy), bruising periumbilically (Cullen's sign) and in flanks (Grey Turner's sign) in acute pancreatitis, vesicles of herpes zoster (may produce abdominal pain), marking for paracentesis abdominis (benzene stain or cotton seal), parietal oedema, cold abscess, sinuses (e.g. tuberculosis, Crohn's disease), erythema ab igne (by constant heat application) or increased shininess (tense ascites).
3. **Striae:** *White* striae or striae albicantes (obese persons who lost weight rapidly, following pregnancy or relieving ascites) **(Fig. 2.10)**; *purple* striae (usually represent the rupture of subepidermal connective tissue, Cushing's syndrome or prolonged steroid therapy) **(Fig. 2.11)**; broad silvery lines (striae gravidarum) are stretch marks following repeated pregnancies.

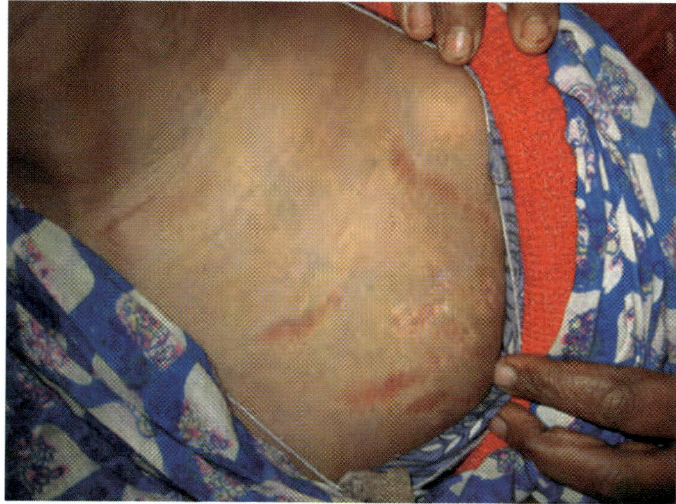

Fig. 2.11: Purple striae developed after long-continued cortico-steroid therapy

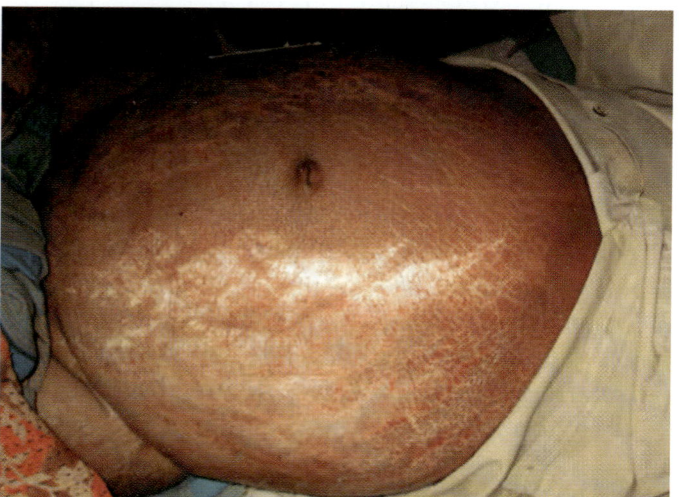

Fig. 2.10: White striae noted after repeated paracentesis abdominis in ascites

Q. Signs of 'peritonitis':

The bedside findings of **peritonitis** are:

a. Inspection: Distension, absence of abdominal movements, absent visible peristalsis.
b. Palpation: Tenderness, rebound tenderness, 'board-like' rigidity.
c. Percussion: Loss of liver dullness (e.g. in perforation of hollow viscus); very tender abdomen (avoid percussion).
d. Auscultation: Absence of bowel sounds.

Table 2.3: Basic differentiation between transudate and exudate

Features	Transudate	Exudate
1. Appearance	Clear, thin; does not clot on standing	Turbid, straw-coloured, haemorrhagic, chylous, mucinous or purulent
2. Specific gravity	<1.016	>1.016
3. Proteins	<3 g/dL	>3 g/dL
4. Cells	<250/mm³ (i.e. low). Endothelial cells or mesothelial cells, and occasionally lymphocytes are seen	>250/mm³ (i.e. high). Lymphocytes, neutrophils or malignant cells
5. Process	Passive	Active
6. Clot formation	Nil	Possible
7. SAAG	≥1.1 g/dL	<1.1 g/dL

- In pancreatic ascites, amylase activity in the fluid is >1000 U/L; and low glucose concentration is found in tuberculous and malignant peritonitis.

Q. Causes of transudative and exudative ascites:

a. Transudate

1. Cirrhosis of liver.
2. CCF.
3. Nephrotic syndrome.
4. Hypoproteinaemia with severe anaemia.
5. Protein-losing enteropathy.
6. Constrictive pericarditis.
7. Pericardial effusion.
8. Meigs' syndrome.
9. Myxoedema.
10. IVC obstruction.

b. Exudate

1. Peritonitis:
   i. Pyogenic
   ii. Tuberculous
   iii. Malignant
   iv. Spontaneous bacterial (SBP).
2. Pancreatic ascites.
3. Budd-Chiari syndrome.
4. Lymphoma or leukaemias.
5. Rupture of hollow viscus.
6. Injury or obstruction to the thoracic duct.

- Myxoedema, Meigs' syndrome and chylous ascites may be exudative.

Q. What is chylous ascites?

1. *Chylous:* Turbid, creamy or milky peritoneal fluid due to presence of lymph. It shows Sudan III-staining fat globules and contains a large amount of triglycerides. Ether dissolves the turbidity of chylous ascites.
2. *Chyliform ascites:* Turbid fluid due to large number of leucocytes, degenerated cells or tumour cells. Addition of alkali clears the turbidity.
3. *Pseudochylous ascites:* Turbid fluid due to increased amount of lecithin, globulin and calcium phosphate (in the ascitic fluid) due to persistent ascites.

Q. Causes of chylous ascites:

1. Tuberculosis, 2. Filariasis, 3. Trauma to the abdomen with rupture of lymphatics, 4. Intra-abdominal malignancy, 5. Nephrotic syndrome, 6. Congenital lymphangiectasia or obstruction of the thoracic duct (e.g. lymphoma).

Q. Ascites with lymphadenopathy:

1. Disseminated tuberculosis.
2. Disseminated malignancy.
3. Lymphoma, and
4. ALL and blast crisis of CML.

Q. Causes of purulent and haemorrhagic ascites:

A. Purulent ascites:

1. Pyogenic peritonitis.
2. Pyaemia and septicaemia.
3. Ruptured amoebic liver abscess.
4. Penetrating injury to the abdomen.
5. Rarely, from pelvic inflammatory disease.

B. Haemorrhagic ascites:

1. Abdominal trauma or traumatic tap.
2. Intra-abdominal malignancy.
3. Tuberculous peritonitis.
4. Bleeding diathesis.
5. Acute haemorrhagic pancreatitis.
6. Ruptured ectopic pregnancy.

Q. Rapidly developing ascites:

1. Malignant peritonitis.
2. Tuberculous peritonitis.
3. Budd-Chiari syndrome.
4. Spontaneous bacterial peritonitis.
5. Lymphoma and leukaemias.
6. Chylous ascites.

- No. 1–5 may develop into **'tender ascites'**.

Q. Hepatomegaly with ascites:

1. Cirrhosis of liver with portal hypertension.
2. Malignancy of liver.
3. Congestive cardiac failure (CCF).
4. Constrictive pericarditis.
5. Disseminated tuberculosis.
6. Budd-Chiari syndrome.
7. Lymphoma.

Q. Splenomegaly with ascites:

1. Cirrhosis of liver with portal hypertension.
2. Lymphoma.
3. Systemic lupus erythematosus (SLE).
4. Disseminated tuberculosis.
5. Budd-Chiari syndrome.
6. Acute leukaemia.
7. Constrictive pericarditis.

Q. Possible causes of refractory ascites:

Medical therapy does not give relief in 10–20% cases of ascites and the contributing factors are: 1. Non-compliance (not following the adequate restriction of sodium), 2. Functional renal failure in cirrhosis of liver, 3. Infection, 4. Spontaneous bacterial peritonitis, 5. Conversion to hepatoma, 6. GI bleeding, 7. NSAID (depresses diuretic effect of furosemide and spironolactone), 8. Portal or hepatic vein thrombosis, 9. Superimposed cardiac or renal disease.

Management: Insufficient response to dietary and diuretic regime indicates development of refractory ascites, and is managed by salt-free albumin infusion (25 g in 3 hours), large volume paracentesis abdominis, LeVeen shunt or side to side porto-caval shunt, and liver transplantation.

Q. Ascites formation in cirrhosis:

1. Hypoalbuminaemia (principal cause): Decreases the plasma oncotic pressure.
2. Portal hypertension (only localises the fluid in the peritoneal cavity).
3. Secondary hyperaldosteronism.
4. Increased level of ADH (due to failure to metabolise ADH by the liver).
5. Increased oozing of 'hepatic lymph' from the surface of liver ('weeping liver'): Lymphorrhoea as a result of peritoneal lymphatic obstruction.

Recent theory: Cirrhotic patients are always in a state of peripheral arterial vasodilatation → diminished arterial blood volume → rise in renin, aldosterone, vasopressin and noradrenaline → leads to renal vasoconstriction, and sodium plus water retention. Moreover, the combination of splanchnic arterial vasodilatation and portal hypertension → alters intestinal capillary permeability → promoting formation of ascites. Vasodilators are of intestinal origin (NO, substance P) and are produced in response to endotoxin and cytokines.

- It is important to remember that in the absence of concomitant hypoalbuminaemia (i.e. hepato-cellular failure), portal hypertension alone does not lead to ascites in cirrhosis.

Q. Ascites—clinical clues on aetiology:

- With dyspnoea: Tense ascites, CCF, chronic cor pulmonale.
- With pedal oedema: Cirrhosis, nephrotic syndrome, constrictive pericarditis.
- Only ascites: Peritoneal disease (e.g. tuberculous or malignant peritonitis).
- With jaundice: Chronic liver disease (e.g. cirrhosis of liver).
- With pain (e.g. peritoneal disease) or without pain (e.g. cirrhosis).
- Onset is acute (Budd-Chiari syndrome), subacute (CCF) or insiduous (tuberculous peritonitis).
- With pyrexia: Peritonitis, malignancy.
- With bleeding manifestations: Chronic liver disease.
- With lymphadenopathy: Disseminated tuberculosis, lymphoma.
- With hepatosplenomegaly: Cirrhosis, lymphoma, disseminated tuberculosis.

Q. Important physical findings for aetiological diagnosis in ascites:

1. Virchow's gland: Gastrointestinal malignancy; gland in other anatomical areas in lymphoma.
2. Skin changes of hepato-cellular failure: Usually from cirrhosis of liver.
3. Engorged and pulsatile neck vein: CCF, pericardial effusion, constrictive pericarditis.
4. Prominent abdominal veins: Portal hypertension.
5. Sister Marie Joseph's nodule around umbilicus: Intra-abdominal malignancy.
6. Non-pitting oedema in feet: Myxoedema, filariasis
7. Splenomegaly: Favours the diagnosis of portal hypertension (cirrhosis of liver) mainly; also found in lymphoma, leukaemias, disseminated tuberculosis and Budd-Chiari syndrome.
8. Hepatomegaly: Firm liver indicates cirrhosis and a hard, tender liver indicates malignancy.
9. Tenderness in ascites: Peritonitis (tuberculous, pyogenic, malignant ascites or SBP).
10. Rectal and vaginal examination: For any rectal or pelvic malignancy, haemorrhoids.

Q. Ascitic fluid in cirrhosis and tuberculous peritonitis (Table 2.3):

A. Cirrhosis of liver: It is transudate in nature.

1. Clear, straw-coloured, light green or bile-stained fluid.
2. Specific gravity <1.016.
3. Protein content <3 g/dL.
4. Cells <250 cells/mm^3, mostly endothelial; Gram's stain and culture—negative.
5. Serum-ascites albumin gradient (SAAG) ≥1.1 g/dL.

B. Tuberculous peritonitis: It is exudate in nature.

1. Straw-coloured, haemorrhagic, mucinous or chylous fluid.
2. Specific gravity >1.016.
3. Protein content >3 g/dL.
4. RBC may be present.
5. Cells: 1000/mm^3, >70% lymphocytes.
6. Serum-ascites albumin gradient (SAAG) <1.1 g/dL.
7. Centrifused deposits stained by Ziehl-Neelsen's method may show tubercle bacilli. The tubercle bacilli may be cultured from ascitic fluid or mycobacterial DNA may be detected by PCR technology. The adenosine deaminase level (ADA) in fluid is increased. The diagnosis is confirmed by peritoneal biopsy under laparoscopy.

Q. What is 'serum-ascites albumin gradient' (SAAG)?

In ascites, routine transudate-exudate system is no longer used and it is prudent to calculate SAAG as:

a. It is the difference of albumin between serum and ascitic fluid, from samples taken at the same time. If the 'serum albumin' minus 'ascitic fluid albumin' (gradient) is equal to or greater than 1.1 g/dL, it suggests underlying portal hypertension. Other than cirrhosis of liver SAAG ≥1.1 g/dL is a feature of CCF, Budd-Chiari syndrome, portal vein thrombosis, myxoedema and constrictive pericarditis.

b. If the gradient is less than 1.1 g/dL, it suggests malignant ascites, tuberculous ascites, pyogenic peritonitis, pancreatic ascites or nephrotic syndrome.

- SAAG is based on oncotic-hydrostatic balance and the gradient directly correlates with portal pressure. SAAG ≥1.1 g/dL and ascitic fluid protein <3 g/dL are usually suggestive of portal hypertension.

Q. Indications of abdominal paracentesis:

Paracentesis literally means removal of fluid or gas. Actually this is divided into **diagnostic** (No. 1 below) and **therapeutic** (No. 2, 3, 4, 5 below) indications. As a whole, they are:

1. Diagnostic paracentesis (approximately 20–50 mL fluid is required).
2. Marked abdominal discomfort or cardio-respiratory embarrassment.
3. Refractory to medical therapy.
4. Danger of strangulation of umbilical hernia, if present (Fig. 2.12).
5. Paracentesis may allow better abdominal examination, needle biopsy of liver, scanning or USG.

Q. Dangers of abdominal paracentesis:

1. Acute cardio-respiratory distress or shock appearing as a result of sudden and rapid withdrawal of large amount of fluid (if appears during the paracentesis, immediately stop tapping the fluid).
2. Introduction of infection (peritonitis).

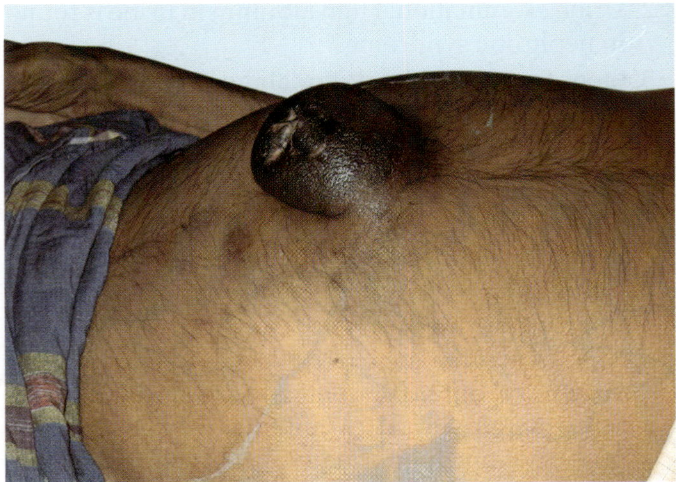

Fig. 2.12: **Ascites with umbilical hernia.** Abdominal paracentesis should be done to avoid strangulation of hernia

3. Precipitation of hepatic coma (the compressed porto-caval shunts open up and nitrogenous materials reach the brain by-passing the liver).
4. Perforation of hollow viscus.
5. Protein depletion (5 litres of ascitic fluid may contain 50–100 g of protein).
6. Constant oozing of fluid (especially in tense ascites or malignant ascites).

Q. Complications of ascites:

1. Collection of fluid in the pleural sac (commonly right-sided).
2. Spontaneous bacterial peritonitis.
3. Hernia (umbilical, inguinal, femoral); divarication of recti in tense and long-standing ascites.
4. Mesenteric venous thrombosis.
5. Functional renal failure.

Q. How USG of abdomen helps in the diagnosis of aetiology of ascites?

USG diagnoses the presence of free fluid in the abdomen and also detects the:

1. Presence of any mass, enlarged pre- or para-aortic lymph nodes (lymphoma/tuberculosis).
2. Splenic enlargement (cirrhosis/lymphoma).
3. Liver: Heterogenous echo-pattern in cirrhosis of liver or diagnose malignancy of liver; oedema or inflammation of pancreas in acute pancreatitis.
4. Increased size of portal vein (≥13 mm) in portal hypertension; presence of collaterals.
5. Any cyst: There may be malignant ascites with malignant ovarian cyst.
6. Enlargement of caudate lobe: Seen in Budd-Chiari syndrome.

Q. Investigations you like to perform in a case of ascites:

1. Routine blood examinations: Hb, TC, DC, ESR; neutrophilia indicates infection.

2. Urine examination: High albumin in urine is found in nephrotic syndrome.
3. Stool for occult blood: For abdominal malignancy and cirrhosis of liver.
4. Serum cholesterol: It is increased in nephrotic syndrome and myxoedema; diminished in cirrhosis.
5. Plasma proteins: Low albumin level is seen in nephrotic syndrome, cirrhosis of liver, hypoproteinaemia with anaemia, and protein-losing enteropathy.
6. X-ray of the abdomen in erect posture: Ground-glass opacity, i.e. diffuse abdominal haziness with loss of psoas margins in ascites (minimally requires 800 mL fluid); not much informative.
7. **Ultrasonography (USG) of the abdomen is the best means to confirm ascites**; CT scan of the abdomen provides similar information. USG can detect as little as 30 mL of ascitic fluid.
8. Examination of ascitic fluid [physical, biochemical, cytological and bacteriological study (detection of AFB, micobacterial C/S, and exfoliative cytology for malignant cells)]: Gram's stain, acid-fast stains and culture should be performed. SAAG should be determined.
9. Biopsy of Virchow's gland or any palpable lymph node: Informative in tuberculosis, lymphoma and malignancy.
10. Tests of portal hypertension: See the section on 'Cirrhosis of liver'.
11. Liver function tests (bilirubin, AST, ALT, alkaline phosphatase, albumin, globulin, etc.).
12. Laparoscopy (peritoneoscopy): May reveal peritoneal deposits of tuberculosis or malignancy.
13. Liver biopsy (cirrhosis/malignancy) or needle biopsy of peritoneum (especially in exudative ascites).
14. Laparotomy.

- *Routine investigations* like chest X-ray (pulmonary tuberculosis, cardiomegaly from CCF), ECG and echocardiography (CCF, pericardial effusion, constrictive pericarditis) should also be performed.

Q. How to manage a case of ascites?

Maximally, 500–700 mL fluid can be mobilised in 24 hours by the following:

1. Rest in bed mobilises ascitic fluid and helps in diuresis as renal perfusion increases in recumbency.
2. Diet: Salt restricted diet is given (also avoid salt-retaining drugs, e.g. steroid, NSAID). In severe cases, sodium in the diet should be less than 10 mEq/day, i.e. 200 mg (in an average case 22 mEq or 440 mg of sodium is allowed daily, i.e. no extra salt, only minimum addition of salt during cooking is allowed).
   Total calories given daily are 2000–2200. One must be cautious while giving high protein diet, if the patient shows features of neuro-psychiatric manifestations (from cirrhosis of liver). 1 g/kg of body weight of protein (only vegetable protein) is allowed unless there is any evidence of hepatic pre-coma.
3. Diuretics: They are introduced in a step-wise manner:
   i. Spironolactone (drug of choice): 100–400 mg/day in divided doses. Start with 25 mg thrice daily and gradually increase the dose (remember, it may produce hyperkalaemia).
   ii. Furosemide: 40–80 mg/day, if good response is not obtained by spironolactone alone. Overzealous treatment with furosemide may lead to hypokalaemia, which may precipitate hepatic coma.
   iii. Combination of i) and ii).
   iv. Other drugs like amiloride, bumetanide (1 mg/day), torsemide (5–10 mg/day) may be tried.
4. Water intake: Restrict the intake to 1–1.5 litres daily.
5. Regular monitoring of serum electrolytes, creatinine, weight, abdominal girth and urinary output.
6. Salt-free albumin infusion may be helpful.
7. Paracentesis abdominis: Done, whenever indicated (nowadays, large volume paracentesis is done in cirrhosis of liver; 3–5 litres fluid is aspirated in one sitting with 6–8 g/L of salt-free albumin infusion). Dextran 8 g/L of ascitic fluid or haemaccel 125 mL/L of ascitic fluid may be infused instead of albumin to maintain the circulation.
8. Antituberculosis treatment is started in tuberculous peritonitis.
9. Treatment of other aetiologies: CCF, pericardial effusion, myxoedema, nephrotic syndrome, malignancy.
10. Peritoneo-venous shunt: Ascitic fluid is drained directly into internal jugular vein and is known as LeVeen shunt.
11. Transjugular intrahepatic portosystemic stent shunting (TIPSS) may relieve resistant ascites in cirrhosis: A stent is placed between portal vein and hepatic vein in liver under radiological control. Porto-systemic shunt surgery may be tried (rarely done nowadays).
12. Liver transplantation: In patients with cirrhosis of liver refractory to medical treatment.

Clinical Wisdom

Guide to progress in ascites: By weighing the patient (should not fall >1 kg/day if ascites and oedema are present, and should not fall >0.5 kg/day in ascites alone) with measuring the girth of abdomen daily (often unreliable due to gaseous distention) and checking the serum electrolytes twice weekly.

Q. How do we divide the abdomen for clinical examination?

Abdomen is conveniently divided by two horizontal and two vertical lines into **nine distinct areas**. The **vertical lines** pass from the femoral artery below to cross the lower costal margins close to the tip of the ninth costal cartilage (or, midinguinal point below to midclavicular point above). The two **horizontal lines** are:

i. Subcostal or transpyloric (upper one), and
ii. Inter-tubercular (lower one).

The *subcostal line* is formed by joining the tips of the tenth costal cartilages on either side, the *transpyloric plane* lies midway between suprasternal notch and symphysis pubis, and the *inter-tubercular line* is formed by joining the tubercles on the iliac crests.

The different areas with contents are (clockwise):

1. Right hypochondrium (right lobe of liver, gall-bladder, hepatic flexure of colon).
2. Epigastrium (left lobe of liver, stomach, transverse colon, lower end of oesophagus).
3. Left hypochondrium (fundus of stomach, spleen, tail of pancreas, splenic flexure of colon).
4. Left lumbar (left kidney and adrenal gland, left ureter, descending colon).
5. Left iliac fossa (part of descending and sigmoid colon, left ovary and fallopian tube).
6. Hypogastrium or suprapubic (urinary bladder, uterus, sigmoid colon, rectum).
7. Right iliac fossa (caecum, appendix, part of ascending colon, right ovary and fallopian tube).
8. Right lumbar (right kidney and adrenal gland, right ureter, ascending colon).
9. Umbilical area in the middle (aorta, IVC, part of stomach, duodenal loop, small intestine, head and body of pancreas, and mesentery).

Q. Normal shape or contour of the abdomen:

Normal shape of the abdomen is neither scaphoid nor distended. Some clinicians describe the normal shape as flat or slightly globular.

The shape of the abdomen may be normal, scaphoid or distended.

Q. Causes of scaphoid (sunken or boat-shaped) abdomen (Fig. 2.13A):

1. Severe dehydration.
2. Emaciation or cachexia.
3. Advanced starvation.
4. Tuberculous peritonitis.
5. Malignant peritonitis.
6. Meningitis.

- For causes of 'distension' of abdomen, read the section on 'Ascites' (page 250).

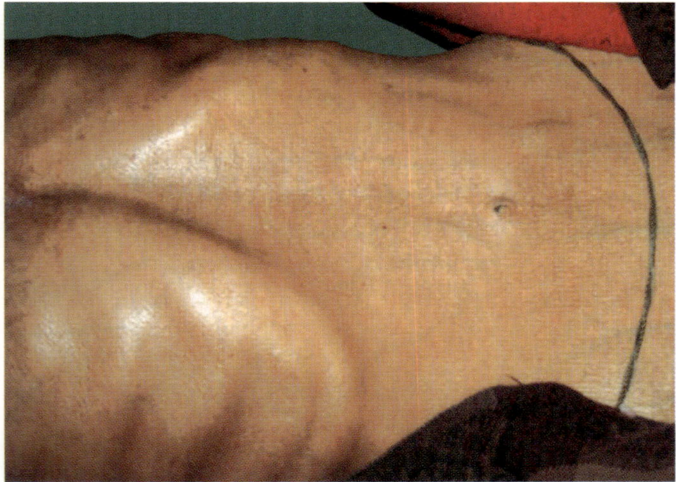

Fig. 2.13A: **Scaphoid abdomen** (sunken or boat-shaped) in advanced starvation; wasting of intercostal muscles (due to loss of subcutaneous fat) is also noted

Q. Points noted during 'superficial palpation' of abdomen:

Prerequisites:

1. The patient should lie supine comfortably with knees bent, and ask him to breathe deeply but regularly. Warm your hands by rubbing (especially in winter) and trim your nails for satisfactory abdominal palpation. Stand on the right side of the patient.
2. Use the flat of the right hand (do not poke with fingers—wrist and forearm should be in same horizontal plane).
3. Prepare the patient with thigh flexed, face turned to the opposite side. Exposure of abdomen is the same as done during palpation of liver.
4. Movements of the right hand should be gentle and come from slight flexion of metacarpophalangeal joints. The hand is held flat and relaxed, and 'moulded' to the abdominal wall.
5. Start unhurried palpation from left iliac fossa (or from an area which is far away from site of pain) and move anti-clockwise to end in suprapubic and umbilical region. Try to examine the tender area (according to the patient) at the last. Always look at the patient's eyes to note whether he or she winces in pain.

Points to note:

1. Surface temperature.
2. Tenderness or hyperaesthesia.
3. Parietal oedema.
4. Consistency or feel (normal elastic feel, or muscle guard or rigidity).
5. Any localised lump.
6. Divarication of recti (detected by rising test).
7. To determine the direction of blood flow in prominent abdominal wall veins.
8. Pulsation (transmitted or expansile).
9. Fluid thrill with girth of the abdomen at the level of the umbilicus.
10. Cough impulse at hernial orifices.

Q. Normal consistency of the abdomen:

Normally the abdomen is elastic in feel (doughy in tuberculous peritonitis); 'board-like' rigidity is found in peptic perforation, tetanus and black widow spider bite.

- *Local guarding:* Tender, inflammed viscus underneath (e.g. acute cholecystitis produces guarding in right hypochondrum) or localised peritonitis.
- *Generalised guarding:* Due to anxiety.
- *Rigidity:* Indicative of peritonitis, pancreatitis, ruptured ectopic gestation.

Q. How to describe the lump or mass present in the abdomen (Fig. 2.13B)?

Preliminary preparations of the patient are the same as done during palpation of liver. Palpation of a lump falls within the purview of 'deep palpation' of the abdomen. Following points are to be described:

1. Site.
2. Size.
3. Shape.
4. Overlying skin (whether red, tense, shiny or pigmented).
5. Consistency (soft, firm, hard or cystic).
6. Margin (sharp or rounded).
7. Surface (smooth or nodular).
8. Mobility.
9. Tenderness.
10. Movement with respiration.
11. Parietal or intra-abdominal.
12. Pulsatile or not.
13. Bimanually palpable or not; ballottable or not.

[14. Lastly palpate the liver, spleen and other viscera areawise, and examine the deep tender spots (McBurney's point, duodenal point, renal angle, gallbladder point). Also examine the hernial sites, detect the presence of free fluid in the abdomen and do the P/R, P/V examinations].

Q. An abdominal mass is palpable: what to do?

So far as lump abdomen is concerned, the abdomen is a temple of surprise. First **aim** is to decide the organ of origin and secondly, the pathological nature of the lump.

1. **Intra-abdominal or parietal?**
   i. Ask the patient to raise the shoulders from the bed with arms over the chest, and then press firmly against the forehead **(rising test)** (*see* Fig. 1.45), or
   ii. Ask the patient to raise both extended legs from the bed (leg lifting test). Now one has to observe whether the swelling becomes less visible or disappears (intra-abdominal), or becomes more prominent or remains same (parietal). Parietal swelling like lipoma, fibroma, neurofibroma or large sebaceous cyst are of surgical interest.

   In case of an intra-abdominal swelling, place the patient on **knee-elbow position**. An intra-abdominal swelling becomes more prominent but not a retroperitoneal one.
2. Next, note the **region** where the swelling is present and think of the anatomical organs which are normally present there. For example, a mass palpable in the right hypochondrium may arise from liver, gallbladder, right kidney or hepatic flexure of colon.
3. Now try to **'get above the swelling'** if the mass is in the upper abdomen and try to 'get below' the swelling if it is present in the lower abdomen. For example, in case of a hepatic, splenic, renal or gastric mass, one cannot 'get above' the swelling. Similarly one cannot 'get below' a lower abdominal mass if it arises from uterus, urinary bladder, or upper recturn.
4. **Size and shape:** Swelling arising from liver, spleen, kidney, uterus or urinary bladder does not produce any problem for diagnosis in majority of cases. But if the swelling arises from stomach, small or large gut, pancreas (retroperitoneal structure) or peritoneum, it may be very difficult to diagnose; a large mass growing from the above mentioned organs (i.e. stomach, etc.) usually distort their normal anatomical configuration. Note the site, shape, size by proper deep palpation.
5. **Margin, surface, tenderness, consistency and pulsation:** Smooth, round, non-tender, regular and tense swelling is usually cystic and benign whereas a hard, irregular, nodular and tender swelling is likely to be malignant in nature. A solid, ill-defined very tender mass suggests an inflammatory lesion. Note the overlying skin (any ulcer, sinus, peau d'orange appearance, redness, pigmentation) and examine for any pulsation (transmitted or expansile, judged by "Two fingers' test") present in the swelling.
6. **Movement with respiration and mobility:** Place the hand over the lower margin of the swelling and ask the patient to take deep breath. If the swelling moves up and down with respiration, it is obviously an intra-abdominal swelling (never parietal). Swelling arising from fixed organs like liver, spleen, kidneys, gallbladder and distal stomach show downward movement with respiration, however,

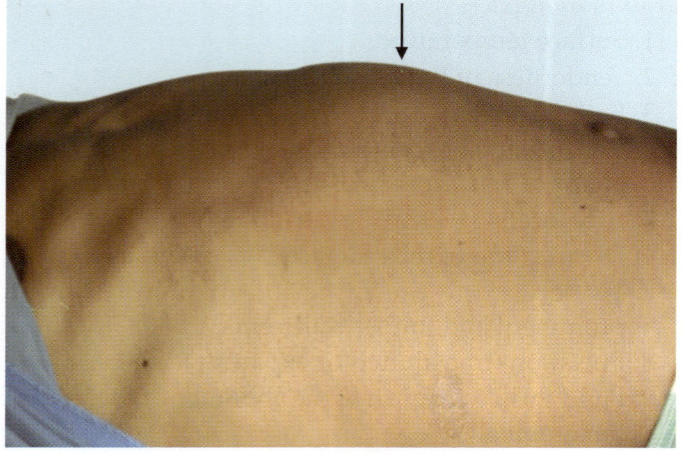

Fig. 2.13B: Lump abdomen in the left hypochondrium

one cannot move the structures with the hand. But the swelling arising from structures having a broad base (mesentery or peritoneum) can be made to move freely by hands but they show no movement with respiration, e.g. tumour of small and large gut, mesenteric cyst, secondary deposits in greater omentum. Look for peristaltic movement, if any.

A totally fixed mass is usually of retroperitoneal origin, like the pancreatic mass. A side to side mobility is present in fibroid uterus which is not a feature of full bladder or swelling arising from ovary. An ovarian tumour with long pedicle is mobile in all directions.

7. **Bimanually palpable or ballottable:** *Renal mass is always bimanually palpable and ballottable.* Even rarely a posteriorly situated gallbladder or a mass in the postero-inferior part of right lobe of liver may be bimanually palpable (but not ballottable).

- For palpation of viscera of pelvic origin, empty the urinary bladder.
- For a pulsatile mass, perform "Two fingers' test": Place two index fingers on two sides of the mass as far apart as the mass allows and observe whether the fingers are raised and separated (expansile pulsation due to aortic aneurysm), or only raised (transmitted pulsation due to a mass where the mass lies over the aorta).

Q. D/D of cystic swellings in the abdomen:

1. Full bladder: Probably the commonest cause (read the section on 'Ascites' and see page 261).
2. Ovarian cyst: See the section on 'Ascites'.
3. Encysted ascites (commonly seen in a patient with abdominal tuberculosis).
4. *Mesenteric cyst:* It is a well defined cystic swelling in the abdomen, usually lying in the umbilical region. It *moves freely at right angles to the line of attachment of the mesentery* than along the line. The line of attachment of the mesentery is an oblique line starting 1 inch left from the midline and 1/2 inch below the transpyloric plane (above), and extending upto the right sacroiliac joint (below) for 6 inches.
5. *Pseudopancreatic cyst:* The smooth and round cyst has no mobility and often feels very firm rather than cystic one. Fluctuation may be absent. It is usually placed centrally above the umbilicus. Past history of trauma or acute pain abdomen (i.e. acute pancreatitis) is very important clue to diagnosis.
6. Hepatic (hydatid) cyst: The mass is present predominantly in the right hypochondrium. There may be presence of **'hydatid thrill'** (place three fingers firmly over the swelling and percuss the middle finger, when an 'after-thrill' produced by displacement of daughter cysts is felt by the index and ring fingers).
7. Renal cyst and hydronephrosis: The swelling is bimanually palpable and ballottable.
8. Splenic cyst: Should be differentiated from left-sided renal lump (read the section on 'Hepato-splenomegaly'); rarely bimanually palpable.
9. Choledochal cyst: Infant or an adult patient; commonly suffers from intermittent jaundice, fever and colicky pain in right upper abdomen. The mass feels cystic and is located in right hypochondrium.
10. Hydramnios: Associated with pregnancy.

Q. Other important physical examination in 'lump abdomen':

1. Anaemia.
2. Jaundice.
3. Assessment of nutrition.
4. Lymph nodes (especially Virchow's gland).
5. Pedal oedema. Any free fluid present in abdomen?
6. Temperature.
7. Examination of testes (one should not forget to palpate both testes).
8. Auscultation of the abdomen for signs of intestinal obstruction.
9. Palpation of other abdominal viscera.
10. Examination of CVS, respiratory, nervous and renal system.
11. P/R or P/V examinations.

Q. Mass in the epigastrium:

1. Carcinoma of the stomach.
2. Carcinoma of the head of pancreas.
3. ↑ of left lobe of liver (hepatoma, abscess).
4. Growth in transverse colon.
5. Pseudopancreatic cyst.
6. Omental mass, aortic aneurysm.
7. Epigastric hernia.

Q. Mass in the right hypochondrium:

1. Hepatic mass (hepatoma, abscess, cyst).
2. Gallbladder lump (carcinoma or mucocele).
3. Colonic mass.
4. Carcinoma of the head of pancreas.
5. Renal lump (right).
6. Omental mass.
7. Sausage-shaped mass (intussusception).

Q. Mass in the hypogastrium (or suprapubic region):

Full bladder, gravid uterus, ovarian cyst, uterine tumour and omental mass.

Q. Mass in the mid-abdomen:

1. Abdominal tuberculosis.
2. Lymphoma.
3. Pregnancy.
4. Mesenteric cyst/lymphadenitis.
5. Full bladder.
6. Ovarian cyst.

7. Retroperitoneal growth.
8. Omental mass.

Q. Palpable swelling in the groin:

1. Inguinal hernia.
2. Femoral hernia.
3. Inguinal lymphadenopathy (*see* page 210).
4. Lipoma, cyst (sebaceous).
5. Saphena varix.
6. Femoral artery aneurysm.
7. Undescended testis.
8. Psoas abscess.

Q. Mass or lump in the right iliac fossa:

1. Ileocaecal tuberculosis.
2. Amoebic typhlitis (inflammation of caecum).
3. Appendicular lump.
4. Carcinoma of caecum or ascending colon.
5. Tubo-ovarian mass.
6. Crohn's disease.
7. Impaction of roundworms.
8. Intussusception.
9. Dropped or unascended right kidney.
10. Lymphoma.
11. Carcinoid syndrome.
12. Iliac aneurysm.
13. Malignant undescended testicle.
14. Psoas abscess.
15. Transplanted kidney.

Q. Mass or lump in the left iliac fossa:

1. Amoebic colitis.
2. Carcinoma of colon.
3. Diverticulitis.
4. Tubo-ovarian mass.
5. Colon loaded with stool (pits on pressure).
6. Dropped or unascended left kidney.
7. Lymphoma, psoas abscess.

Q. Discharging 'fistula' over abdomen:

1. Faecal fistula (postoperative).
2. Tuberculosis of the intestine.
3. Intra-abdominal malignancy.
4. Crohn's disease (Fig. 2.14).
5. Scrofuloderma or trauma.
6. Actinomycosis.

- **Skin nodules over abdomen**—neurofibroma, lipoma, malignant deposits (e.g. Sister Marie Joseph's nodule around umbilicus), calcinosis, sarcoidosis.

Q. Classification of abdominal tuberculosis:

1. Tuberculosis of gastro-intestinal tract:
   a. Ulcerative type (produces malabsorption).

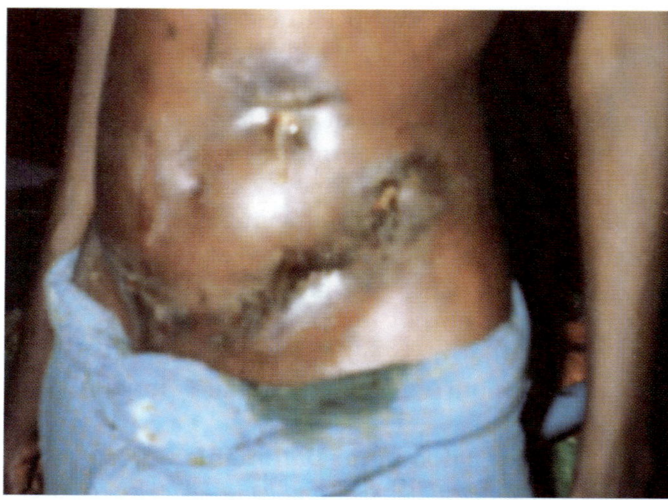

Fig. 2.14: **Multiple discharging fistula** in lower abdomen in Crohn's disease

   b. Hyperplastic type (produces gut obstruction).
   c. Ulcero-hyperplastic type.
2. Mesenteric lymph node tuberculosis (± tuberculosis of the mesentery).
3. Tuberculous peritonitis:
   a. Plastic type.
   b. Ascitic or exudative type; or encysted ascitic type (loculated).
   c. Fibrous or adhesive type.

[4. Tuberculosis of other abdominal solid organs like liver, pancreas, spleen, etc.].

- When the exudate is small and more fibrinous, it binds the intestine, mesentery with or without involvement of lymph nodes, and is known as **'tabes mesenterica'**; the lymph nodes may be palpable as rounded masses.
- Abdomen feels doughy and tender in tuberculous peritonitis. Special investigations like ascitic fluid study, barium follow through with 'spot film' of ileocaecal region, CT scan of whole abdomen, colonoscopy with ileoscopy, stool GeneXpert assay and laparoscopy with peritoneal biopsy are performed to diagnose suspected intestinal tuberculosis.

Q. 'Lymph node lumps' in the abdomen: possibilities?

These lumps feel variegated (firm to hard), surface may be nodular (due to individual large lymph nodes), occasionally tender (haemorrhage within) and may be present anywhere in the abdomen but in majority of cases they are present in epigastrium, umbilical area and right iliac fossa. They show restricted movement with respiration and there is absence of mobility. The common causes are:

1. Lymphoma (commonly pre- and para-aortic nodes).
2. Mesenteric lymph node tuberculosis.
3. Metastasis from carcinoma of neighbouring organs.
4. Metastasis from carcinoma of testes (always palpate the testes).
5. Filariasis (causes retroperitoneal lymphadenitis): Rare.

Q. Cystic swelling in hypogastrium: is it urinary bladder ?

Following points should be noted carefully in a full bladder:

a. Inspection: Midline oval swelling above symphysis pubis which may reach up to umbilicus.
b. Palpation: Normally the urinary bladder is not palpable. It feels firm or elastic in retention of urine. Application of pressure induces pain and discomfort, and desire for micturition. Side-to-side movement of the mass is not possible. In distension, upper and lateral borders are palpable but the lower border of the swelling cannot be reached.
c. Percussion: It is done from above downwards and the swelling is dull on percussion.
d. Confirmation: When a simple rubber catheter is introduced through the urethra, urine comes out and the swelling disappears.

Clinical Wisdom

D/D of full bladder are gravid uterus (firm, side to side mobility, vaginal signs +), ovarian cyst (not truely midline, right- or left-sided), and fibroid uterus (firmer, often knobbly, vaginal signs +).

Q. How to palpate the kidneys (Fig. 2.15)?

The lower pole of right kidney is commonly palpable in thin patients for obvious reasons. The right kidney is palpated from right side though the left kidney may be palpated from either side. The method of palpation goes like:

1. Preliminary preparations of the patient are the same as done during palpation of liver. Always sit on a stool for palpation of kidneys.
2. To palpate the right kidney, place the right hand horizontally in the right lumbar region anteriorly just lateral to rectus muscle, and the left hand is placed posteriorly in the right loin region to trap the kidney bimanually with inspiration **(bimanual palpation)**.
3. Push the right hand in a backward, upward and inward direction, and ask the patient to take deep inspiration. A firm mass may be felt in between the two hands (if kidney is enlarged).
4. Next, a sharp tap is given by the left hand placed in the loin region. The anteriorly placed right hand now feels the kidney, and the kidney then falls back (by gravity) on the posterior abdominal wall which is felt again by the left hand. This is **'ballottement'** (*confirmatory for kidney lump*). Ballottement demonstrates the mobility of the kidney.
5. The left kidney is then palpated by placing the right hand anteriorly in the left lumbar region and the left hand posteriorly in the left loin (from right side); one may place left hand anteriorly and right hand posteriorly in palpation of left kidney from left side.

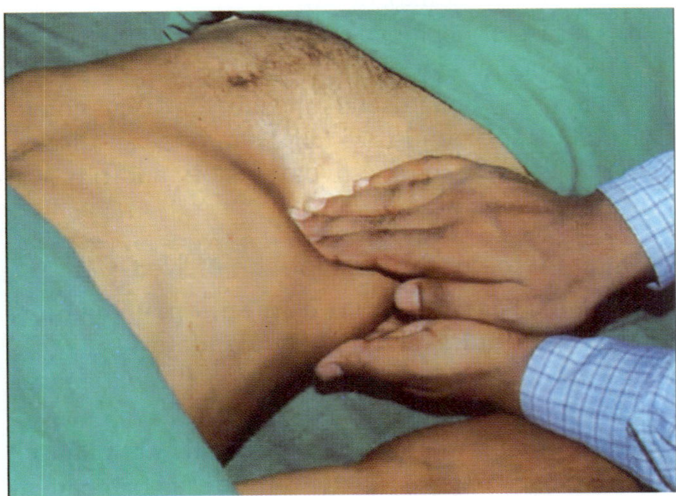

Fig. 2.15: Bimanual **palpation** of right **kidney**

Q. Common causes of palpable kidney:

A. Unilateral:

1. Dropped kidney (can be pushed to its normal position).
2. Hydro- or pyonephrosis (unilateral).
3. Wilms' tumour.
4. Hypernephroma.
5. Large cyst (solitary) in kidney.
6. Compensatory hypertrophy (other kidney damaged).
7. Perinephric abscess.

B. Bilateral:

1. Polycystic kidney (irregular surface).
2. Bilateral hydronephrosis.
3. Bilateral dropped kidney.
4. Diabetic nephropathy in early stage.
5. Amyloidosis.
6. Scleroderma.
7. Acromegaly.
8. Lymphoma.
9. Leukaemias.

Q. Points to note in a renal lump:

1. Site.
2. Size.
3. Shape (ovoid normally).
4. Consistency (resilient or firm in feel).
5. Margins (rounded).
6. Surface (normally smooth surface; irregular in polycystic kidney).
7. Tenderness.
8. Movement with respiration (kidney shows slight movement up to 3 cm with respiration).
9. Whether bimanually palpable and ballottable.
10. *Tenderness over the renal angle* (Fig. 2.16): Patient will be seated, and the angle formed by the lower border of 12th rib and lateral border of erector spinae muscle is pressed by the ball of the thumb or thrust given by ulnar aspect of closed fist: "Murphy's kidney punch". The test is done on both sides.
11. In left-sided renal lump: Examine for band of colonic resonance over the lump (by percussion).

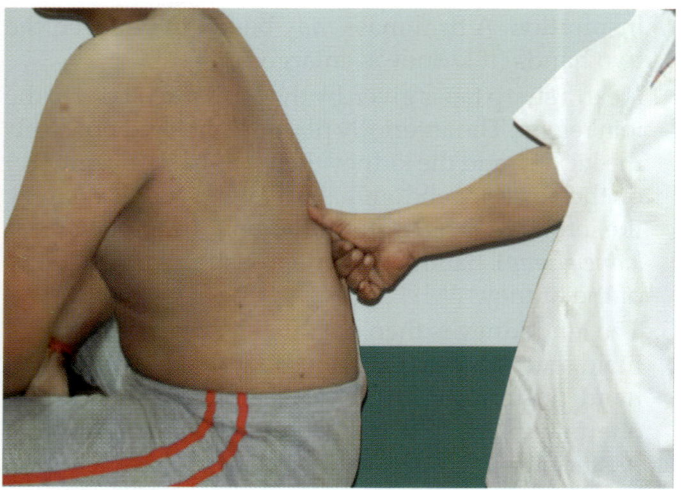

Fig. 2.16: Eliciting **"Murphy's kidney punch"** to demonstrate tenderness in renal angle

- **Renal angle** is tender in acute pyelonephritis, perinephric abscess, acute urinary obstruction, nephrolithiasis, tuberculosis of the kidney or following renal biopsy. Remember, *a kidney lump is bimanually palpable and ballottable*. The kidney is ballottable because it is a posterior abdominal organ.
- A transplanted kidney is diagnosed by a) (transplanted) kidney in right or left illac fossa, b) arteriovenous fistula in forearm (i.e. vascular access for haemodialysis), and c) laparotomy scar.

Q. D/D of renal lump:

1. Enlarged spleen.
2. Carcinoma of the bowel.
3. Carcinoma or cyst of the pancreas.
4. Riedel's lobe of liver.
5. Retroperitoneal tumour.
6. Gallbladder swelling.

Q. How to palpate the gallbladder?

The gallbladder is palpated in the same way as the palpation of liver, i.e. start palpation from right iliac fossa and move towards right hypochondrium. The normal gallbladder is not palpable. In pathological conditions, it is palpable just lateral to right rectus abdominis muscle near the tip of ninth costal cartilage. When palpable, it feels firm, smooth and globular; it moves freely with respiration. When there is hepatomegaly, an enlarged gallbladder may be palpable in right lumbar or right iliac fossa. The comparative mobility on respiration and the globular shape differentiate it from right kidney lump.

Q. Causes of palpable gallbladder:

The gallbladder is not palpable in health. If palpable, think of:

1. Mucocele/empyema of the gallbladder (firm, smooth and regular swelling).
2. Carcinoma of the head of pancreas (firm and globular swelling).
3. Carcinoma of the gallbladder (stony hard, irregular swelling).
4. Carcinoma of the common bile duct (firm and globular swelling).
5. Calculus obstructing cystic duct (firm and globular swelling).

- With jaundice: 2, 3 and 4, without jaundice: 1 and 5.

Q. D/D of gallbladder lump:

1. Hepatomegaly (especially Riedel's lobe of liver).
2. Right-sided kidney lump or suprarenal tumour.
3. Carcinoma of the hepatic flexure of colon.
4. Carcinoma of the pyloric region of stomach.

HEPATOSPLENOMEGALY — CASE 33

Q. Common causes of hepatosplenomegaly (i.e. enlargement of liver and spleen):

1. Chronic malaria.
2. Chronic kala-azar.
3. Haemolytic anaemia (congenital).
4. Cirrhosis of liver.
5. Chronic myeloid leukaemia.
6. Lymphoma.
7. Acute viral hepatitis.
8. Enteric fever.
9. Polycythemia vera.
10. Collagen vascular diseases like SLE.
11. Tropical splenomegaly syndrome.
12. Myelofibrosis or myelosclerosis.
13. Felty's syndrome.
14. Millary tuberculosis or disseminated tuberculosis.
15. Amyloidosis.

- ALL, AML, chronic lymphocytic leukaemia, sarcoidosis, brucellosis, storage disorders (Gaucher's disease and glycogen storage disease) and polycystic disease are other important causes.

Q. What is your diagnosis?

1. Give the provisional diagnosis (aetiological, e.g. it is a case of lymphoma), or say,
2. It is a case of hepatosplenomegaly probably due to chronic malaria, or say,
3. It is a case of hepatosplenomegaly for discussion (if aetiological diagnosis is not clear, one can discuss the D/D in the perspective of history and physical examination).

Q. Different methods for palpation of liver:

During palpation of abdomen, 'preliminary preparations' must be followed (mandatory):

1. Always stand on the right side of the patient (as mostly we are right-handed).
2. Flex the thighs (to relax the abdominal musculature).
3. Turn the patient's face to the left side (so that patient cannot breathe on examiner's face).

4. Ask the patient to breathe deeply but regularly with open mouth (liver, spleen, gallbladder and kidneys move with respiration).
5. Hands of the patient will lie by the side of his/her trunk (help to relax the abdomen).

Remember, the patient should lie flat comfortably on his back, on a firm mattress with the head supported by a pillow (to relax the abdomen); an extra pillow is needed for a patient in a special situation (e.g. dyspnoea or kyphosis). There should be good light for the purpose of examination. In the winter season, the hands of the examiner should be made warm by rubbing together vigorously. The patient should be relaxed and reassured, and should be explained briefly what you are going to do while taking permission to do so. A gentle and unhurried palpation with care of the painful sites gain confidence of the patient and helps in extraction of maximal information.

Exposure of abdomen from the xiphisternum to symphysis pubis is usually carried out in **inspection** of abdomen, leaving the chest and legs covered. Inspection of groins and genitalia should not be neglected and should be carried out with proper explanations to the patient.

Exposure of abdomen (for **palpation**):
- Above: The xiphisternum.
- Below: Just above the inguinal ligament (do not embarrass the patient by exposing genitalia).

There are three techniques for palpation of liver. *Most of the clinicians in India are well conversant with the conventional method*.

I. **Conventional or traditional method** (Fig. 2.17): Place the flat of right palm firmly over the *right iliac fossa* and press the hand inwards and upwards. *The hand is placed parallel to the arbitrary lower border of liver* (or the right subcostal margin) lateral to the right rectus abdominis muscle. At the height of inspiration press the fingers firmly inwards and upwards when the radial border of the right index finger will slip over the lower border of the liver, if it is palpable. At the phase of expiration, place the right palm on a higher level, by 1 cm at a time, over the anterior abdominal wall until you reach the right lower costal margin or detect the edge of liver. *Now palpate the epigastrium for the left lobe of liver* (move the hand from right hypochondrium to midline).

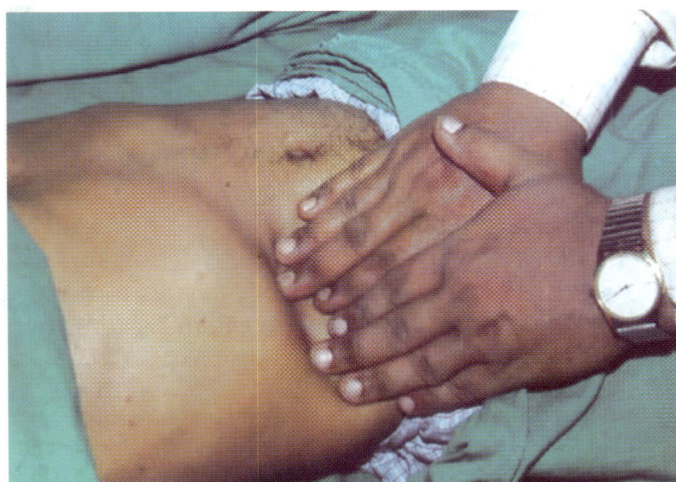

Fig. 2.18: Palpation of **liver (preferred method)**

II. **Preferred method (according to few clinicians)** (Fig. 2.18): Place *both hands* side by side flat on the anterior abdominal wall in the *right hypochondriac region* lateral to the right rectus abdominis muscle with the fingers pointing upwards. If any resistance is felt, *move the hands further downwards until the resistance disappears*. The patient is then asked to inspire deeply, and at the height of inspiration press the fingers upwards and inwards to confirm the edge of liver. The manoeuvre is repeated from lateral to medial side in search of the lower border of liver. When the hand is moved downwards, the loss of resistance demarcates the lower border of liver.

III. **Alternative method (according to few clinicians)** (Fig. 2.19): The right hand is placed flat in the *right iliac fossa with the fingers directing upwards*, lateral to

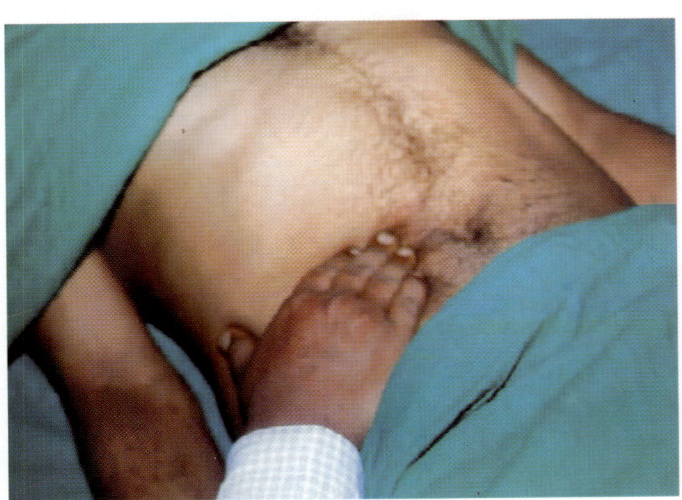

Fig. 2.17: Palpation of **liver (conventional method)**

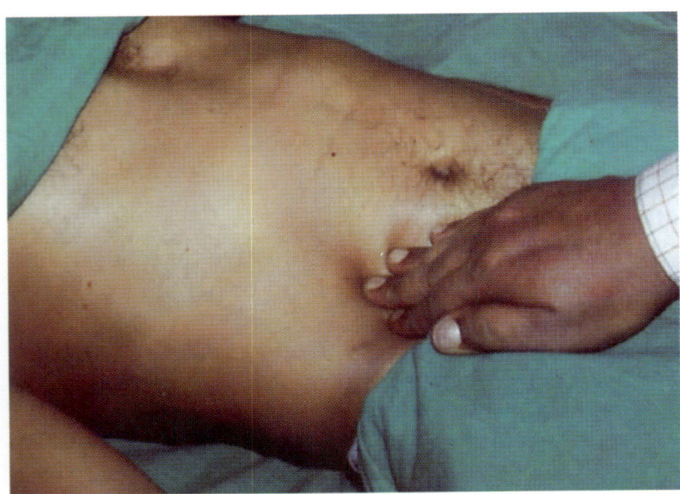

Fig. 2.19: Palpation of **liver (alternative method)**

the right rectus abdominis muscle (the finger tips lie parallel to rectus sheath). Now press the hand firmly upwards and inwards (index and middle one are the sensing fingers). At the height of inspiration, try to release the inward pressure while maintaing the upward pressure; with the inspiration, the tips of fingers will slip over the margin of the liver, if palpable. Now palpate the liver for surface, margin, tendemess, consistency, etc. as a routine. This manoeuvre is less sensitive than previous two methods.

- **Dipping method** is always applied in the presence of ascites.
- During palpation of liver, don't press patient's shoulder or bed by your left hand (a common mistake). Let your left hand hang normally by the side of your body.

Q. Points to note if liver is palpable:

1. Degree of enlargement: Expressed by centimetres/inches (preferable) or in number of examiner's fingers (preferably avoid) placed between the right costal margin and the lower border of the palpable liver at right MCL. Measurement is taken during natural expiration, preferably by a ruler. Some clinicians prefer to describe 'liver span' in this heading (*see* page 266).
2. Consistency: Soft, firm or hard. A normal liver is soft in feel.
3. Tenderness: Tender or non-tender.
4. Surface: Smooth or irregular (finely irregular or coarsely irregular).
5. Margin or border: Whether sharp or rounded. Usually a soft liver has rounded margin, and firm or hard liver has a sharp margin. The margin may be irregular in cirrhosis of liver.
6. Movement with respiration: Liver always moves 1–3 cm downwards with deep inspiration.
7. Left lobe enlarged or not (examine in the midline in the epigastrium between xiphoid process and umbilicus, and measure in mid-sternal line).
8. Any pulsation: Pulsatile or not (see below).
9. Upper border of liver dullness (normal or shifted): Percuss the right side of chest from above downwards along the right MCL. Normally the upper border of liver dullness is found in right 5th ICS at right MCL. For further details read the section on 'Hydropneumothorax'.
10. Palpable hepatic rub.
11. Place the stethoscope over the liver and auscultate carefully for any hepatic bruit or hepatic rub.

- In health, a liver is non-palpable in an adult. It is soft, non-tender, moves with respiration, with smooth surface and rounded margin, and without any pulsation or rub.
- *Right lobe* of the liver is palpated by keeping the hand lateral to the right rectus abdominis muscle while the *left lobe* is examined in the midline. *Caudate lobe* enlargement (e.g. in Budd-Chiari syndrome) is also appreciated in epigastrium. In infants, liver is palpable in health.
- During palpation, observe the facial grimace of the patient (for tenderness or any discomfort).

Q. How to examine for pulsatile liver (Fig. 2.20)?

1. Stand on the right side of the patient. While the patient is sitting in a chair (preferably), place your right palm over the liver (or right hypochondrium) and the left palm over the back, just opposite to the right palm (bimanual palpation).
2 Ask the patient to hold his breath after taking deep inspiration. Inspiration helps in descent of liver and increases venous return to right heart.
3. Look from the side and observe the separation of the hands along with expansile pulsation of the liver, if there is any, and appreciate the pulsation.

- Few clinicians prefer to examine pulsatile liver in supine position of the patient.
- Remember, the most common cause of pulsatile liver is CCF (produces functional tricuspid incompetence—TI). Thus, while examining the pulsatile liver, always look for engorged and pulsatile neck veins, tenderness in liver and bipedal oedema (indirect evidence of CCF). Common causes of pulsatile liver are:
  1. CCF (functional TI).
  2. Organic TI (systolic pulsation or systolic expansile liver).
  3. Tricuspid stenosis (presystolic pulsation).
  4. Haemangioma of liver or arteriovenous fistula in liver.
  5. Transmitted epigastric pulsation from RVH.

Q. Causes of tender liver:

1. Acute viral (or alcoholic) hepatitis.
2. Congestive cardiac failure.
3. Carcinoma of liver.
4. Pyogenic or amoebic liver abscess.
5. Drug-induced hepatitis.
6. Infected hydatid cyst of liver.

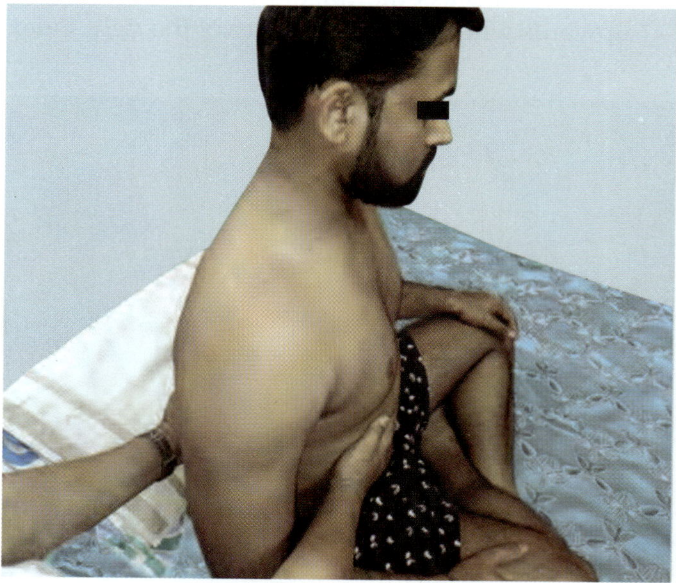

Fig. 2.20: Detection of **pulsatile liver**

7. Budd-Chiari syndrome (acute).
8. Acute cholangio-hepatitis.

- Inflammation (perihepatitis) or stretching of the Glisson's capsule makes the liver painful and tender.
- **'Congestive hepatomegaly'** due to any cause makes the liver tender. Congestive hepatomegaly is commonly found in CCF, constrictive pericarditis, dilated (congestive) cardiomyopathy and Budd-Chiari syndrome.

Q. In an enlarged and tender liver, what else you will examine?

1. Jaundice (acute viral hepatitis, carcinoma of liver) with clinical type (e.g. obstructive jaundice).
2. Engorged and pulsatile neck veins, dependent bipedal oedema and CVS (for CCF).
3. Intercostal oedema as well as tenderness in right lower chest (liver abscess).
4. Hard supraclavicular lymph nodes (carcinoma of the liver).

Q. Causes of left lobe enlargement of liver:

1. Amoebic liver abscess.
2. Hepatoma.
3. Metastasis in liver.
4. Gumma of liver (very rare): Hepar lobatum.

Q. Causes of soft, firm and hard liver (alteration in consistency):

A. Soft liver (feels like lips)

1. **Congestive cardiac failue.**
2. Acute viral hepatitis.
3. Fatty liver.
4. Acute malaria.
5. Visceroptotic normal liver.
6. Extrahepatic obstruction (EHO).

B. Firm liver (feels like tip of the nose)

1. **Cirrhosis of liver.**
2. Chronic malaria.
3. Chronic kala-azar.
4. Hepatic amoebiasis.
5. Lymphoma.
6. Chronic CCF (nutmeg liver).

C. Hard liver (feels like forehead)

1. **Hepatoma (hepato-cellular carcinoma).** } Rock-hard liver
2. **Metastasis in liver.** } Rock-hard liver
3. Chronic myeloid leukaemia.

Q. Liver enlargement with irregular surface:

a. **Finely irregular** (granular surface): Portal cirrhosis.
b. **Grossly or coarsely irregular** (nodular liver):
   1. Postnecrotic cirrhosis (macronodular).
   2. Metastasis in liver (large nodules with umbilication due to central softening).
   3. Hepatoma.
   4. Hepatic cysts (congenital, hydatid).
   5. Multiple liver abscess.
   6. Gumma or tertiary syphilis of liver (hepar lobatum—not seen nowadays).

- No. 1, 2, 4 and 5 produce 'knobbly liver'.

Q. Causes of hepatic bruit:

1. Hepato-cellular carcinoma (hepatoma).
2. Acute alcoholic hepatitis.
3. Haemangioma of liver.
4. Arteriovenous fistula in liver.

Q. Causes of hepatic rub:

1. After recent biopsy of liver (transient).
2. Carcinoma of liver (secondary or primary).
3. Perihepatitis (e.g. gonococcal).
4. Hepatic infarction.

Q. Degrees of enlargement of liver:

Enlargement of liver is expressed as:

- Mild enlargement (1–2 fingers or <4 cm).
- Moderate enlargement (2–5 fingers or 4–8 cm).
- Massive enlargement (>5 fingers or >8 cm).

Q. Causes of huge (massive) hepatomegaly:

1. Metastasis in liver or hepatoma.
2. Polycystic disease of liver.
3. Gross fatty change (i.e. fatty liver).
4. Amoebic liver abscess.
5. Chronic malaria or chronic kala-azar.
6. Amyloidosis of liver.

- **Mild-to-moderate hepatomegaly** occurs in malaria, kala-azar, enteric fever, miliary tuberculosis, leukaemias, fatty liver, cirrhosis (postnecrotic), congestive hepatomegaly, haemolytic anaemia, hepatic carcinoma, haemangioma of liver and storage disorders (Gaucher's disease).

Q. Hepatomegaly with jaundice:

1. Acute viral hepatitis.
2. Haemolytic anaemia.
3. Carcinoma of liver (secondary).
4. Cirrhosis of liver.
5. Weil's disease.
6. Lymphoma.
7. Rarely, amyloidosis.

Q. Hepatomegaly with heart failure:

1. Right ventricular failure (CCF).
2. Constrictive pericarditis.
3. Haemochromatosis.
4. Alcoholic liver disease with cardiomyopathy.
5. Acute cholangio-hepatitis.

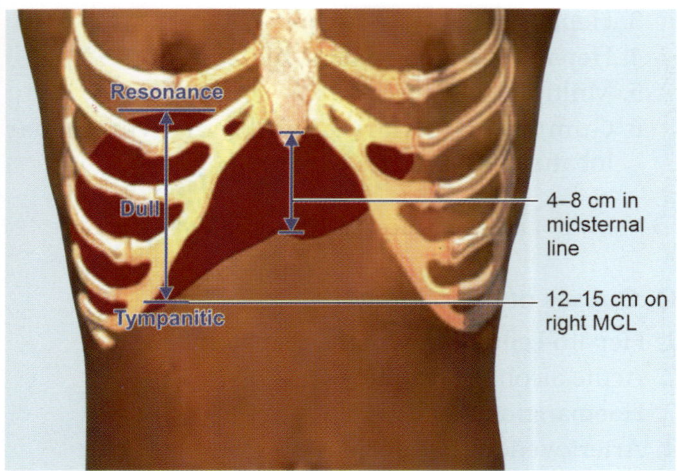

Fig. 2.21: Measurement of **liver span**

Q. What is the 'liver span' (Fig. 2.21)?

It is the vertical distance between the uppermost and lowermost points of hepatic dullness. It is detected by percussing the upper, and percussing or palpating the lower border of liver at the right MCL. The anterior liver span is usually 12–15 cm in an adult in the right MCL and is related to patient's age, sex, body mass, height, etc. (females having liver span less than males). Serial measurement is helpful to detect shrinkage or enlargement. Liver span in children is much smaller.

- Liver span is increased in true enlargement of liver, and not when it is displaced (e.g. palpable liver in downward displacement in emphysema). It is decreased in shrunken liver as in cirrhosis.

Q. Causes of rapid change in size of liver:

a. Rapid enlargement

1. Carcinoma of liver.
2. Amoebic liver abscess.

b. Rapid diminution

1. Fulminant hepatic failure.
2. Correction of CCF.
3. Cirrhosis of liver.
4. Relief of cholestatic jaundice.

Q. Conditions erroneously suggest upward hepatic enlargement:

1. Pleural effusion (right).
2. Basal pneumonia (right).
3. Subdiaphragmatic effusion (right).
4. Subdiaphramatic abscess (right).

Q. D/D of hepatomegaly:

1. Carcinoma of the stomach.
2. Malignancy in right kidney.
3. Carcinoma of the hepatic flexure of colon.
4. Omental mass (from tuberculosis or malignancy).
5. Large gallbladder lump.

Q. What is Riedel's lobe of liver?

It is a downward tongue-like projection and a congenital variation of the right lobe of liver, which is commonly found in females. It moves with respiration. It is usually mistaken with gallbladder or right kidney. It lacks the spherical contour of the distended gallbladder and always remains asymptomatic. Often ultrasonography is done for differentiation.

- *Caudate lobe* arises from the postero-superior surface of the right lobe of liver and is hypertrophied in Budd-Chiari syndrome.

Clinical Wisdom

Palpable liver may be due to downward displacement of the liver without any enlargement and may be seen in conditions like right-sided pleural effusion, emphysema, in normal children, tall and lean persons, visceroptosis, or in severe thoracic deformity. *So, a palpable liver may not be an enlarged liver.* Never forget to palpate the left lobe of liver, to percuss the upper border of liver dullness and to palpate bimanually for hepatic pulsation.

Auscultation over the liver (for hepatic bruit and rub) is optional and should be done if you are asked to 'examine the liver'.

Q. Different methods for palpation of spleen:

There are several methods for palpation of spleen. **'Preliminary preparations' of the patient** are the same as done during palpation of liver.

i. Standing on the right side of the patient, **place the flat of the left palm firmly over the left costal margin** posterolaterally and press it forward and medially, so as to enable a slightly enlarged soft spleen closer to the palpating right hand. Ask the patient to breathe in deeply and start palpating the spleen with the right hand. **Starting from the right iliac fossa**, move upwards and laterally towards the left hypochondrium, 1 cm at a time between each breath. If the spleen is not palpable, move the right hand more upwards with each inspiration until the fingertips reach under the left costal margin. Start well out to the left of costal margin and gradually move more medially. It is better to palpate the spleen with the fingertips but few clinicians prefer to use the radial border of right index finger (Fig. 2.22).

ii. If spleen is not palpable (or in a just palpable spleen) by the method mentioned above, turn the patient to **right lateral decubitus position** and palpate the spleen by hooked fingers of right hand placed under the left costal arch (especially in obese patient) or by the same palpatory method mentioned above (palm lying flat), beginning palpation close to the left costal margin while the patient is breathing in and out deeply. Patient will flex his left hip and knee while in right lateral decubitus position. The examiner's left hand should remain over the lowermost rib cage posterolaterally on the left side as before (Fig. 2.23).

iii. In case of a just palpable spleen, finally stand on the left side of the supine patient near his shoulder,

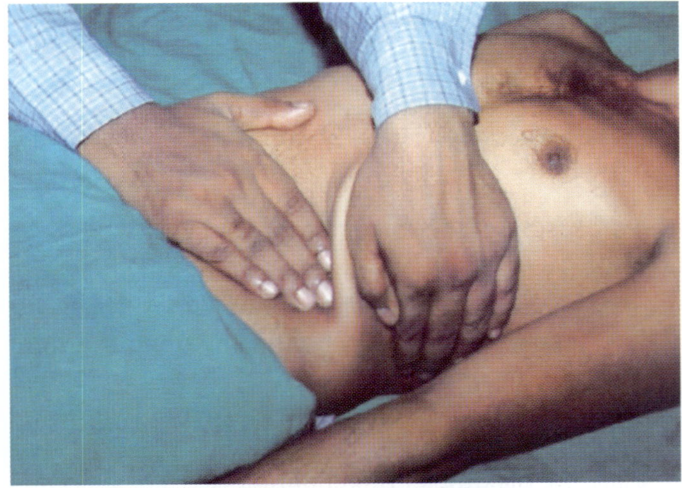

Fig. 2.22: **Palpation of spleen**

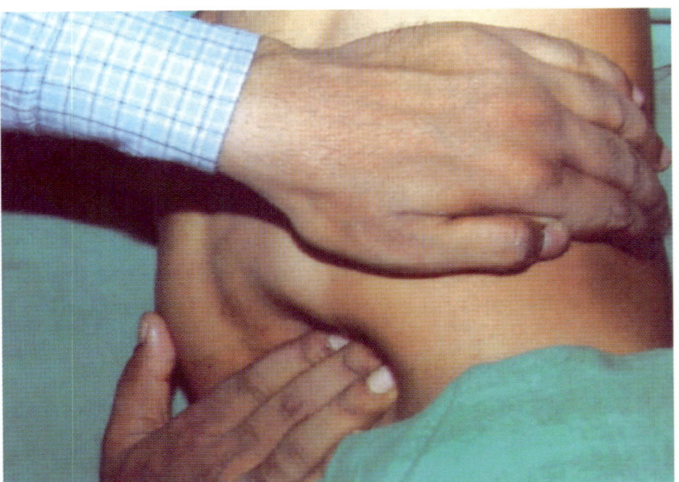

Fig. 2.23: Palpation of **spleen (just palpable)** in right lateral position

facing the foot end of the bed. Palpate the spleen by **hooked fingers of left hand** below the left costal margin while the patient breathes in and out deeply (classical hooking method); if fingers of the examiner's both hands are curled under the left costal margin, it is known as *Middleton's manoeuvre*. Hooking method may be done from the left side in sitting position of the patient (Fig. 2.24).

Clinical Wisdom

If the spleen is not palpable by method I, go for method II and then, for method III. Phases of respiration are very important in palpation of spleen. While palpating spleen, do not be hasty and rash (remember, spleen may be fragile in infectious mononucleosis and may be injured in aggressive palpation): rather show endurance—a just palpable spleen will definitely touch your fingers at the height of inspiration. Method I and II may be called bimanual palpation.

- Dipping method is always applied in the presence of ascites.

Q. Different methods for palpation of abdominal viscera:

There are four methods:

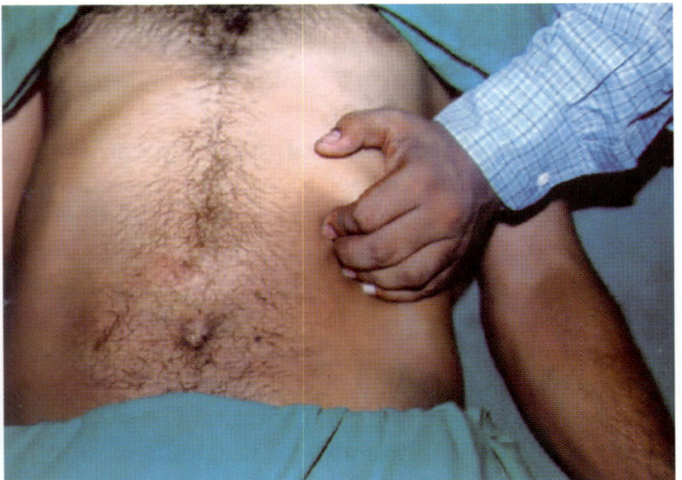

Fig. 2.24: Palpation of **spleen (just palpable) by hooking** from left side by left hand

1. Conventional, direct or classical method, e.g. palpation of liver.
2. Hooking method: Classically used in palpation of spleen.
3. Dipping method: Palpation in the presence of ascites.
4. Bimanual palpation: Classically for the palpation of kidneys.

Q. What is dipping method?

It is difficult to palpate the abdominal viscera by direct method in the presence of significant ascites. While performing dipping method, mould the palpating right hand to the shape of the abdomen, and then tap the abdomen sharply and quickly. The sudden and rapid displacement of fluid gives a tapping sensation over the surface of the enlarged liver or spleen which is comparable to patellar tap. The right hand is placed flat over the abdomen and a **sharp tap is given by flexing the metacarpophalangeal joints suddenly**. One or two sudden thrust displaces the fluid and the displaced fluid pushes the organ forward towards the palpating fingers. Many a time full description of an organ is not possible by dipping method (one can appreciate up to palpable or not, tender or non-tender, small or big lump). Preliminary preparations of the patient are the same as done during palpation of liver. It is better to start palpation from right iliac fossa by dipping method and proceeding anti-clockwise.

While palpating the spleen by dipping method, it is better to place the left palm over the left costal margin as done in the conventional method. Do not place both hands one over the other while palpating by dipping method.

Q. How to percuss for splenic dullness?

The anatomical position of the spleen is behind and below the left 9th, 10th and 11th rib, and its **long axis is lying along the direction of the left 10th rib.** Its antero-inferior end extends maximally upto the midaxillary line and the postero-superior end lies 4 cm lateral to the

T_{10} spine. The upper border of normal splenic dullness is present in left 9th rib and for this reason the 8th ICS (space above the 9th rib) in left midaxillary line is always resonant on percussion.

Percuss the left axilla from above downwards along the midaxillary line (either the patient lies supine or being seated while keeping the left hand over the head to expose the axilla) in the search of upper border of spleen.

If the same percussion, as described above, is done in lowest intercostal spaces (like 8th or 9th ICS) along the anterior axillary line and the spaces reveal dull percussion note, even on full inspiration, it is said that possible splenomegaly is present **(Castell's method)**.

Percussion for splenic dullness is carried with any of the three methods described below like:

1. Castell's method (see above) **(Fig. 2.25)**: A very sensitive clinical sign (sensitivity 82%, specificity 83%).
2. Percussion of Traube's semilunar space by Barkun's method (pages 80–81) (*see* **Fig. 1.32**).
3. Nixon's method **(Fig. 2.26)**: The patient is placed in right lateral position in bed. Percussion starts from midpoint of left costal margin (i.e. in the posterior axillary line) and is continued upwards, perpendicular to the left costal margin. The upper border of dullness, in health, is usually 6–8 cm above the left costal margin. If the dullness is >8 cm in an adult, it is presumed that splenomegaly is present.

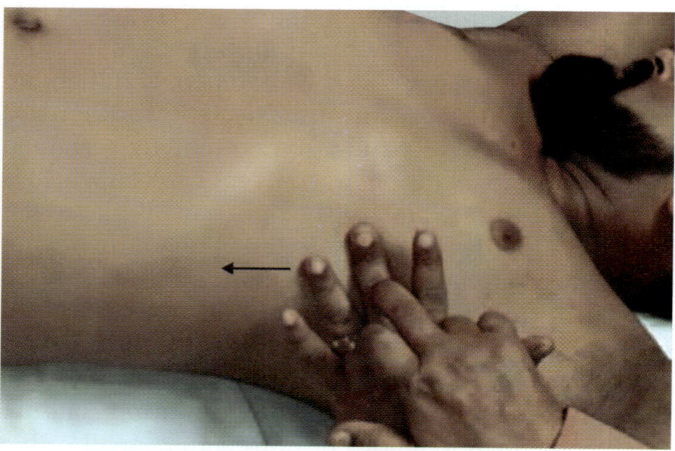

Fig. 2.25: Eliciting **splenic dullness–Castell's method**

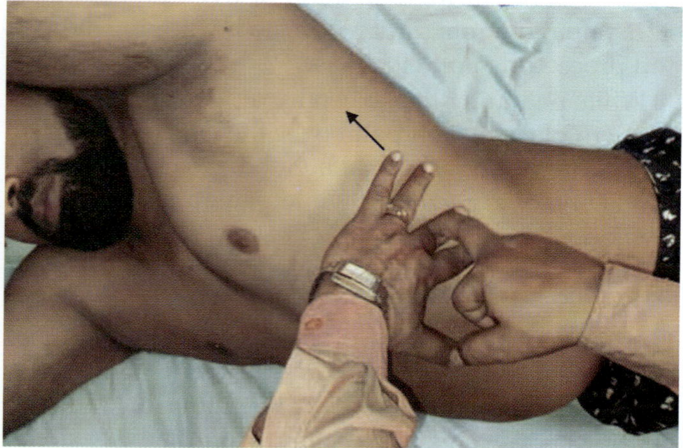

Fig. 2.26: Eliciting **splenic dullness—Nixon's method**

- Remember, splenic enlargement first takes place in superior and posterior direction before it becomes palpable per abdomen (i.e. subcostally)

Q. Percussion of the lower border of liver:

Always try to percuss from resonant to dull area:

1. Start percussion from below upwards, i.e. from right iliac fossa to right hypochondrium along the right MCL.
2. It is a *light percussion* (as lower border of liver is not covered by any organ).
3. Place the pleximeter finger parallel to right subcostal margin and the line of percussion will be perpendicular to that margin.

Q. Percussion of the upper border of liver:

1. Start percussion from above downwards in the right chest along the right MCL.
2. It is a *heavy percussion* (as upper border of liver lies under cover of the right lung).
3. Place the pleximeter finger in the right 2nd ICS parallel to arbitrary upper border of liver and the line of percussion will be perpendicular to that border.

Q. Percussion of the lower border of right lung:

1. Start percussion from above downwards in the right chest along the right MCL.
2. It is a *light percussion* (as it is a superficial organ).
3. Place the pleximeter finger in the right 2nd ICS (parallel to arbitrary lower border of lung) and the line of percussion will be perpendicular to that border.

Q. Points to note if spleen is palpable:

1. Degree of enlargement: Expressed by centimetres/ inches (preferable) or in number of examiner's fingers (preferably avoid) placed below the left costal margin upto the most distal point of spleen, along the splenic axis (spleen becomes just palpable when it is enlarged to 2–3 times more than its normal size. **Spleen usually enlarges towards the right iliac fossa.** In children, spleen may enlarge vertically towards the left iliac fossa). The measurement is taken along the splenic axis from a point on left costal margin (where crossed by left MCL) to the furthest extent of the spleen. Measurement is taken during natural expiration, preferably by a ruler.
2. Splenic notch: Very characteristic and felt on its anterior end of superior border.
3. Margin: Usually the margin is sharp.
4. Consistency: Soft, firm or hard.
5. Tenderness: Tender or non-tender.
6. Surface: Smooth or irregular.
7. Movement with respiration: Spleen always moves downwards and medially with respiration.

8. Fingers cannot be insinuated between the left costal arch and the enlarged spleen. Spleen has a tendency to bulge forward.
9. Palpable splenic rub: Present or not (for its detection, the patient must breathe in and out deeply).
10. Auscultation of splenic rub.
11. Upper border of splenic dullness.

Clinical Wisdom

No. 10 and 11 are optional and should be done if you are asked to 'examine the spleen'. Some clinicians prefer that a student should always percuss the spleen (D/D with left renal swelling) for any band of colonic resonance, at the time of palpation of spleen **(Table 2.4)**.

- Rule of odds in spleen: 1" thick, 3" broad, 5" long, 7 ounces weight and underlies 9–11 ribs.
- It is not clearly known, why the spleen in children enlarges vertically towards the left iliac fossa. Probably, it may be one of the reason that in a child other organs are not much enlarged (in comparison to adults) and thus the spleen makes its room vertically downwards towards the left iliac fossa.
- In the examination, do not delineate borders of spleen/liver by pen or pencil over patient's body.

Q. D/D of splenomegaly:

1. Enlaged lett kidney.
2. Enlarged left lobe of liver.
3. Carcinoma of the stomach.
4. Carcinoma of the splenic flexure of colon.
5. Omental mass (from tuberculosis or malignancy).
6. Malignancy of the tail of pancreas.

Q. Different degrees of enlargement of spleen:

a. Mild (up to 2 fingers, or 1–2 cm) or just palpable spleen ('spleen tip')

1. Acute malaria.
2. Acute kala-azar.
3. Enteric fever.
4. Acute viral hepatitis.
5. Subacute bacterial endocarditis (SBE).
6. Miliary tuberculosis.
7. Acute leukaemias.
8. Haemolytic anaemia.
9. Immune thrombocytopenic purpura (ITP).
10. Felty's syndrome.
11. Infectious mononucleosis.
12. Well's disease.

b. Moderate (2–5 fingers, or 3–7 cm, or up to the umbilicus)

1. Chronic malaria.
2. Chronic kala-azar.
3. Portal hypertension (e.g. cirrhosis).
4. Lymphoma.
5. Chronic lymphocytic leukaemia.
6. Collagen vascular diseases like SLE.
7. Congenital haemolytic anaemia (thalassaemia).
8. Chronic (active) hepatitis.

c. Huge or massive (>5 fingers, or >7 cm, or when the spleen crosses the umbilicus)

1. Chronic kala-azar or chronic malaria.
2. Thalassaemia major.
3. Chronic myeloid leukaemia (and also in hairy cell leukaemia).
4. Tropical splenomegaly syndrome.
5. Polycythemia vera.
6. Portal hypertension with hypersplenism (e.g. in cirrhosis).
7. Extrahepatic portal vein obstruction (EHO).
8. Myelofibrosis or myelosclerosis.
9. Storage disorders (Gaucher's disease), amyloidosis.
10. Splenic cyst, tumour or abscess.

- Normal spleen weighs <250 g; in massive splenomegaly, it weighs >1000 g in adults.
- Remember all the causes of massive splenomegaly were mild to moderate splenomegaly one day, and all moderate splenomegaly were mild in nature to start with.

Table 2.4: Differentiation between enlarged spleen and renal lump

Spleen (Fig. 2.22)	Left kidney
1. Spleen enlarges downwards, forwards and towards the right iliac fossa, and moves well with respiration	1. Kidney enlarges towards the left iliac fossa and having restricted movement with respiration
2. *Notch felt in superior border*	2. No notch felt
3. Sharp margin	3. Rounded margin
4. It is neither bimanually palpable nor ballottable	4. *Bimanually palpable and ballottable*
5. *Fingers cannot be insinuated between left costal margin and the enlarged spleen*	5. Fingers can be insinuated between left costal margin and the kidney
6. Percussion note is always dull over spleen	6. *Band of colonic resonance* anterior to enlarged left kidney may be elicited
7. *Tendency to bulge forward*	7. Tendency to bulge into the loin
8. Renal angle is non-tender	8. Renal angle may be tender
9. Cannot 'get above the swelling'	9. May 'get above the swelling' (e.g. in dropped kidney)
10. Felt superficial in the abdomen	10. Felt deep in the abdomen
11. Can cross midline	11. Does not cross midline

- A massive splenomegaly may be bimanually palpable but is never ballottable.

Clinical Wisdom

Spleen may be palpable without having actual enlargement in tall and lean persons, left-sided pleural effusion, emphysema (hyperinflated lung pushes spleen), visceroptosis, accessory spleen and sometimes in children.

Q. When do you search for splenic rub?

Splenic rub is heard in the situations where the patient complains of acute colicky pain in left upper quadrant of abdomen (often with radiation of pain to the tip of left shoulder) due to splenic infarction resulting in perisplenitis (with acute splenic tenderness). It is produced in conditions like:

1. Subacute bacterial endocarditis (SBE).
2. Chronic myeloid leukaemia.
3. After splenic puncture (e.g. in diagnosis of chronic kala-azar).
4. Sickle cell anaemia.
5. Vasculitis.
6. Splenic abscess.
7. Splenic torsion.
8. Severe septicaemia.

Clinical Wisdom

The characteristics of splenic rub are:

1. It is a coarse, scratchy to-and-fro sound heard with respiration, i.e. during movement of the spleen.
2. If the patient holds his breath, the rub stops.
3. The diaphragm of stethoscope should be placed over the spleen or left lower chest.

It should be differentiated from left-sided pleural rub (spleen is always tender in splenic rub) which is often very difficult. Treatment is by rest and analgesia. Repeated splenic infarction may be an indication for splenectomy.

- Acute splenic tenderness indicates splenic infarction, rupture or abscess (e.g. tuberculosis, HIV) formation.
- Always auscultate for spelnic rub over a hugely enlarged spleen. Splenic rub may be palpable.
- Spleen may be mildly tender in acute malaria, infectious mononucleosis, SBE and enteric fever.
- **Splenosis:** Peritoneal seeding of splenic rupture (traumatic) fragments not connected to portal circulation, and giving rise to abdominal pain later (like endometriosis).
- **Splenunculi:** Single or multiple accessory spleens.

Q. What do you mean by hypersplenism?

It is the splenic hyperactivity with increased blood cell destruction. Diagnostic criteria are:

1. Splenomegaly (of any size).
2. Pancytopenia (anaemia, leucopenia and/or thrombocytopenia).
3. Normal or hypercellular bone marrow.
4. Reversibility by splenectomy.

Causes: Either primary (no underlying disease) or secondary hypersplenism (connective tissue disorders, lymphoma, myeloproliferative disorders, cirrhosis of liver or congestive splenomegaly).

Q. Causes of 'hyposplenism':

It means absence of spleen or non-functioning spleen. It is usually associated with:

1. Dextrocardia (spleen is absent congenitally or asplenia).
2. Sickle cell disease (repeated splenic infarction leading to autosplenectomy).
3. Coeliac disease.
4. Dermatitis herpetiformis with enteropathy.
5. Fanconi's anaemia (aplastic anaemia with hypoplasia of spleen, kidney, thumb, or radii).
6. Surgical removal.

- Splenectomised or hyposplenic patients are prone to be infected with capsulated organisms like *Pneumococcus*, *Meningococcus*, *H. influenzae* or *E. coli*, and thus vaccination against these organisms is recommended to them. Parasitic infection babesiosis is also common in these patients.

Q. Myeloproliferative disorders:

Here, there is uncontrolled clonal proliferation of one or more of the cell lines in the bone marrow, and are classified as:

1. Chronic myeloid leukaemia.
2. Polycythemia vera.
3. Essential thrombocythemia.
4. Myelofibrosis (myeloid metaplasia).

Q. Hepatosplenomegaly with ascites:

1. Cirrhosis with portal hypertension.
2. Lymphoma.
3. Disseminated tuberculosis.
4. Acute leukaemia.
5. Viral hepatitis with hepato-cellular failure.
6. Congestive cardiac failure (CCF).
7. Systemic lupus erythematosus (SLE).

Q. Splenomegaly with jaundice:

1. Cirrhosis of liver (decompensated).
2. Acute malaria (*P. falciparum* commonly).
3. Haemolytic anaemia (e.g. thalassaemia).
4. Lymphoma.
5. Acute viral hepatitis.
6. Miliary tuberculosis.

Q. Splenomegaly with purpura or petechiae:

1. Acute leukaemias.
2. SLE.
3. Blast crisis of CML and CLL, lymphoma.
4. SBE.
5. ITP (splenomegaly in 10% cases).
6. Felty's syndrome, septicaemia.

Q. Hepatosplenomegaly with lymphadenopathy:

1. Lymphoma.
2. Leukaemia (ALL and CLL).

3. Disseminated tuberculosis.
4. SLE.
5. Sarcoidosis.
6. Felty's syndrome.
7. Infectious mononucleosis.
8. AIDS.
9. Toxoplasmosis, CMV infection.
10. CML with blast crisis.
11. Amyloidosis.
12. Kala-azar (African variety).

Q. Hepatosplenomegaly with pyrexia:

1. Malaria (acute).
2. Kala-azar (acute or chronic).
3. Enteric fever.
4. SBE.
5. Miliary tuberculosis.
6. Acute viral hepatitis.
7. Acute leukaemias, CML.
8. Lymphoma.
9. Collagen vascular diseases.
10. Brucellosis.
11. Still's disease

Q. Hepatosplenomegaly with anaemia:

1. Chronic malaria.
2. Chronic kala-azar.
3. Haematological malignancies, e.g. lymphoma and leukaemias.
4. Cirrhosis of liver.
5. Haemolytic anaemia (e.g. thalassaemia).
6. Severe iron deficiency anaemia.
7. Hypersplenism.
8. SBE.
9. SLE.
10. Still's disease.

Q. Reliable methods for measuring actual splenic size:

These are imaging procedures like:

1. Radionuclide scan.
2. Ultrasonography (USG).
3. Computed tomography (CT), and
4. Nuclear magnetic resonance imaging (MRI).

If a maximal craniocaudal diameter of spleen by these techniques (especially USG) crosses 13 cm, spleen is said to be enlarged.

Q. Causes of rupture of spleen:

1. Trauma in *normal spleen*.
2. By trivial trauma in a *diseased spleen*. The pathological conditions responsible are infectious mononucleosis, acute and chronic leukaemias, myelofibrosis, congestive splenomegaly (portal hypertension due to cirrhosis of liver or Budd-Chiari syndrome).

Q. Important physical signs in hepatosplenomegaly:

1. Anaemia (cirrhosis of liver, thalassaemia).
2. Jaundice (cirrhosis of liver, thalassaemia).
3. Facies: Mongoloid (thalassaemia) or hepatic facies (cirrhosis), butterfly rash in SLE.
4. Polycythemia (i.e. plethoric appearance with suffused conjunctiva).
5. Lymphadenopathy (lymphoma, lymphocytic leukaemia, infectious mononucleosis).
6. Spider naevi and palmar erythema (hepato-cellular failure from cirrhosis of liver).
7. Kayser-Fleischer ring in cornea (Wilson's disease).
8. Tremor (Wilson's disease).
9. Pigmentation (haemochromatosis).
10. Leg ulcers (congenital haemolytic anaemia).
11. Sternal tenderness (acute leukaemias and CML).
12. Haemorrhagic spots (acute leukaemias. SBE).
13. Changing murmur or appearance of new murmur—SBE.
14. Fundoscopy: Roth spots (SBE), choroidal tubercle (miliary tuberculosis).

Q. Investigations you like to perform in a case of hepatosplenomegaly:

A. Blood: Hb, TC, DC, ESR and some special tests:
   a. Leucocytosis: Pyogenic infections, polycythemia, leukaemia.
   b. Leucopenia: Malaria, kala-azar, enteric fever, Felty's syndrome.
   c. Pancytosis: Polycythemia.
   d. Pancytopenia: Hypersplenism.
   e. Reticulocytosis: Haemolytic anaemias.
   f. Thrombocytopenia: Leukaemia, hypersplenism.
   g. ESR: Increased in infective aetiologies, SLE, lymphoma, severe anaemia due to any cause; diminished in polycythemia and congestive cardiac failure.
   h. Blood culture: Often informative in SBE, enteric fever.
   i. Blood smear: For the diagnosis of malaria, kala-azar (buffy coat preparation), leukaemia (acute and chronic), hereditary spherocytosis, thalassaemia.
   j. Special tests: (i) Paul-Bunnell test for infectious mononucleosis, (ii) Serum iron—increased in thalassaemia, haemochromatosis, (iii) Serum copper—low in Wilson's disease, (iv) Serum bilirubin—high in cirrhosis with hepato-cellular failure, haemolytic anaemias, malaria, viral hepatitis, (v) Haemoglobin electrophoresis—increased HbF in thalassaemia, (vi) Congo red test for amyloidosis. (vii) Aldehyde test for chronic kala-azar, (viii) LE cell and phenomenon—collagen vascular disease (not done routinely), (ix) Red cell survival time—decreased in hereditary spherocytosis. (x) Antinuclear factor—positive in SLE, (xi) Rose-Waaler test (rheumatoid factor)—positive in Felty's

syndrome. (xii) Serum proteins—high globulin with low albumin is observed in cirrhosis of liver, chronic kala-azar, disseminated lupus. (xiii) Blood for HB_SAg, (xiv) Serum angiotensin-converting enzyme (SACE)—elevated in sarcoidosis, (xv) Serology: For HCV, CMV, EBV, HIV, and VDRL test for syphilis.

B. X-ray or radiology:
   a. Chest (PA view): For miliary tuberculosis (miliary mottling), lymphoma or sarcoidosis (mediastinal widening), extramedullary haematopoiesis (paravertebral shadow) in thalassaemia.
   b. Bones:
      i. Mosaic-pattern seen in small bones of hand in patients with thalassaemia.
      ii. Increased bone density in myelofibrosis or myelosclerosis.
      iii. Expansion of lower end of long bones (Erlenmeyer flask): Seen in Gaucher's disease.
   c. Skull: 'Hair on end' appearance in thalassaemia.
   d. Straight X-ray of abdomen: Not informative.

C. Lymph node biopsy (excission biopsy is always preferred to FNAC because it delivers more tissue for diagnosis): May be of value in tuberculosis, sarcoidosis, CLL and lymphoma.

D. USG of liver, spleen, free fluid in abdomen and for any mass (e.g. pre- and para-aortic lymph nodes):
   a. Hepatosplenomegaly is confirmed.
   b. Ascites may be present in portal hypertension, tuberculosis or lymphoma.
   c. Heterogenous echopattern of liver with splenomegaly and ascites: Portal hypertension due to cirrhosis.
   d. Enlarged abdominal lymph nodes: Lymphoma or tuberculosis.

E. Liver biopsy: May be of value in cirrhosis of liver, lymphoma, haemochromatosis or amyloidosis.

F. Bone marrow examination: For leukaemia, lymphoma, hypersplenism, Gaucher's disease, etc.

G. Skin test:
   i. Mantoux test: For tuberculosis (may be negative in lymphoma).
   ii. Kveim test: For sarcoidosis (not done nowadays).

H. Investigations for portal hypertension—*See* the section on 'Cirrhosis of liver'.

I. Splenic puncture: For the diagnosis of chronic kala-azar.

J. CT scan of whole abdomen may be done, if USG of abdomen is inconclusive.

K. Lymphangiography: For lymphoma (for demonstration of involvement of retroperitoneal nodes).

Q. D/D of hepatosplenomegaly:

A summary of the common causes of hepatosplenomegaly is presented as follows:

I. Chronic malaria:

a. Patient comes from an endemic zone with high rise of temperature associated with chill and rigor. Fever may come on alternate days periodically.
b. Severe anaemia, mild jaundice may be present.
c. Spleen: Moderate-to-massive enlargement, firm to hard and non-tender.
d. Diagnosis is confirmed by demonstration of malaria parasites in the peripheral blood.

II. Chronic kala-azar:

a. Patient comes from an kala-azar endemic zone.
b. Double rise of temperature (double quotidian) in 24 hours may be present (20% cases).
c. Appetite is preserved inspite of fever and loss of body weight.
d. Spleen: Massively enlarged, soft to firm (often a doughy feel) and non-tender (spleen of chronic kala-azar is softer than chronic malarial spleen).
e. Liver: Moderate enlargement, firm and non-tender. Ratio of liver and spleen is 2:5.
f. Alopecia, pigmentation.
g. Diagnosis is made by neutropenia, positive aldehyde test, direct agglutination test (DAT), or by demonstration of LD bodies in buffy coat preparation of blood, bone marrow smear or splenic puncture.

III. Thalassaemia (Cooley's anaemia) (*see* **Fig. 1.66A**)*:*

a. The patient is usually a child or young adult with positive family history.
b. Stunted growth, typical mongoloid facies, massive splenomegaly with moderate hepatomegaly, severe anaemia, mild jaundice, leg ulcers over malleoli of foot.
c. Diagnosis is done by:
   i. Microcytic hypochromic anaemia, reticulocytosis, anisocytosis, poikilocytosis, target cells.
   ii. Haemoglobin electrophoresis (HbF >2%).
   iii. Radiological study of skull and small bones of hand.

- Acquired haemolytic anaemia (e.g. autoimmune) may produce hepatosplenomegaly.

IV. Cirrhosis of liver (postnecrotic):

a. Features of chronic liver disease, e.g. dyspepsia, malaise, wasting, severe weakness. There may be past H/o jaundice.
b. Symptoms and signs of hepato-cellular failure (e.g. jaundice, spider naevi, palmar erythema).
c. Features of portal hypertension: Haematemesis, melaena, splenomegaly, venous prominences over abdomen, ascites.
d. Mild-to-moderate hepatomegaly with moderate splenomegaly. Both are firm and non-tender.
e. Presence of other stigmata of cirrhosis of liver.
f. Diagnosis is done by demonstration of oesophageal varices, splenoportalvenography, liver biopsy.

V. Chronic myeloid leukaemia:

a. The patient, around 30–80 years (peak: 55 years), presents with fever, dragging pain in the left hypochondrium and profound weakness. Weight loss and sweating are due to increased metabolic rate.
b. Anaemia: Mild.
c. Sternal tenderness: Present.
d. Spleen: Hugely enlarged, hard with occasional splenic rub (may be tender).
e. Liver: Mild-to-moderate enlargement.
f. Diagnosis is confirmed by 1.5–2.5 lac WBC/mm^3 with myelocytes, metamyelocytes, promyelocytes and few myeloblasts.

Clinical Wisdom

AML-mild splenomegaly, ALL-moderate splenomegaly, CML-huge splenomegaly, CLL-moderate splenomegaly.

VI. Lymphoma:

a. Progressive painless enlargement of cervical, axillary or inguinal lymph nodes, fever, loss of weight, pruritus, weakness, drenching night sweats.
b. Superior mediastinal syndrome may be present: Dyspnoea, engorged non-pulsatile neck vein, swelling of face, tortuous veins over chest wall.
c. Spleen: Moderately enlarged, non-tender.
d. Liver: Moderate enlargement.
e. Anaemia, eosinophilia in blood may be present. The lymph node biopsy is confirmatory.

VII. Acute viral hepatitis:

a. H/o jaundice preceded by anorexia, profound nausea, fever and occasional vomiting. Urine is yellow and stool may be of white coloured (in cholestasis).
b. There may be urticarial rash, arthralgia.
c. Hepatosplenomegaly: Mild to moderate, tender hepatomegaly with mild splenomegaly (soft).
d. Diagnosis is done by:
   i. High serum bilirubin, high SGPT (ALT), alkaline phosphatase (slight rise), prothrombin time estimation (may rise).
   ii. HB_SAg, I_gM anti-HAV or anti-HEV, anti-HCV in blood.

VIII. Enteric fever:

a. H/o rise of temperature in step-ladder pattern, frontal headache, constipation, epistaxis, rose spots in skin, relative bradycardia.
b. Tongue: Red margins with central coating (angry-looking tongue).
c. Spleen: Soft and tender, just palpable spleen at the end of first week.
d. Liver: Soft, non-tender, mild enlargement.
e. Diagnosis is done by neutropenia, blood culture and Widal test; rapid diagnosis by Typhidot (IgM) test.

IX. Polycythemia vera:

a. Symptoms like headache, fullness in head, pruritus, peripheral vessel thrombosis (due to increased viscosity of blood), visual disturbances commonly in a middle aged male patient.
b. Epistaxis, haematemesis or melaena, pruritus, peptic ulcer, peripheral vascular bleeding.
c. Face is plethoric, conjunctivas are congested and palms are red.
d. Spleen is enlarged in 75% cases and may be massive; hepatomegaly in 30% cases.
e. Diagnosis is made by raised haematocrit, low ESR, hyperplasia of all marrow elements in bone marrow examination. Erythropoietin level is decreased.
f. Treatment is done by venesection (300–500 mL), hydroxyurea, interferon α-2b (in failure of hydroxyurea), allopurinol (to treat hyperuricaemia following chemotherapy), and radioactive phosphorus ^{32}P.

X. Collagen vascular diseases (SLE):

a. Mostly a woman with fever, arthralgia, alopecia, oral ulcer, skin rash or lymphadenopathy.
b. Renal, lung or cardiac involvement: Oliguria, pleurisy, pericarditis, dyspnoea (i.e. multisystem disease).
c. Spleen: Usually there is moderately enlarged, firm, non-tender spleen.
d. Diagnosed by high ESR, positive antinuclear factor (ANF), antibody to double-stranded DNA and anti-Sm antibody (SLE), renal biopsy, etc.

XI. Tropical splenomegaly syndrome (previously known as Banti's syndrome):

a. The patient comes from a hyperendemic area with an exaggerated immune response to malarial antigen. The disease is common in females, and has familial and racial predisposition. Adults have high malarial antibody titres with low parasitaemia. Malaria parasites are not seen on R/E.
b. Spleen: Massive splenomegaly, liver: Mild-to-moderate enlargement.
c. Signs of portal hypertension may be present without any evidence of cirrhosis of liver (due to increased portal blood flow).
d. Chronic low grade haemolytic anaemia may be seen; low grade pyrexia.
e. Diagnosed by increased level of IgM, 'sinusoidal lymphocytosis' in liver biopsy (diagnostic).
f. Treated with proguanil which leads to regression of splenic size.

- The modern nomenclature of the disease is *'hyperreactive malarial splenomegaly'*.

XII. Myelofibrosis or myelosclerosis:

a. This may be primary, or develops from toxins, malignancy, lymphoma, irradiation (secondary).
b. Spleen: Massive, tender spleen; splenic rub may be present.
c. Hepatomegaly: Mild-to-moderate enlargement.
d. Leucoerythroblastic blood picture with high platelet count.

e. Bone marrow examination may not yield any result (dry tap) and often trephine biopsy is needed to demonstrate the fibrotic changes. X-ray shows ground-glass appearance (osteosclerosis) of all bones of axial skeleton.
f. There may be signs of haemorrhage into the skin.

XIII. Felty's syndrome:

a. It is a subgroup of rheumatoid arthritis with splenomegaly and neutropenia.
b. Age of onset is around 50–70 years and more common in females.
c. Features like weight loss, joint pain with deformity, lymphadenopathy, pigmentation, leg ulcers, vasculitis, chest infection, keratoconjunctivitis sicca, rheumatoid nodules may be present.
d. Spleen: Mild splenomegaly.
e. Diagnosis is done by anaemia, neutropenia, thrombocytopenia, and strongly positive rheumatoid factor.

XIV. Miliary tuberculosis (or disseminated tuberculosis):

a. Gradual onset with vague ill-health, high fever with drenching sweats, pallor, loss of weight.
b. Children or young adult; cough, breathlessness, anorexia, headache may be present.
c. Tachycardia, paucity of signs in the chest (few crepitations in late stages).
d. Mild, non-tender hepatomegaly with small palpable spleen.
e. Signs of meningeal irritation may be found.
f. Choroidal tubercles (unilateral or bilateral) may be visible (25%) on ophthalmoscopy (diagnostic). Chest X-ray shows miliary mottling bilaterally. Leucocytosis is usually absent. Mantoux test may be negative. Sputum examination may or may not demonstrate AFB.

XV. Amyloidosis (Fig. 2.27)*:*

a. Here, clumps of abnormal protein, i.e. 'amyloid' deposits in tissues and organs. It is of two types: Primary and secondary. Secondary variety occurs from presence of long-standing suppurative focus in the form of lung abscess, bronchiectasis, chronic osteomyelitis or may develop from rheumatoid arthritis (commonest), tuberculosis, Crohn's disease, multiple myeloma, lymphoma or leprosy.

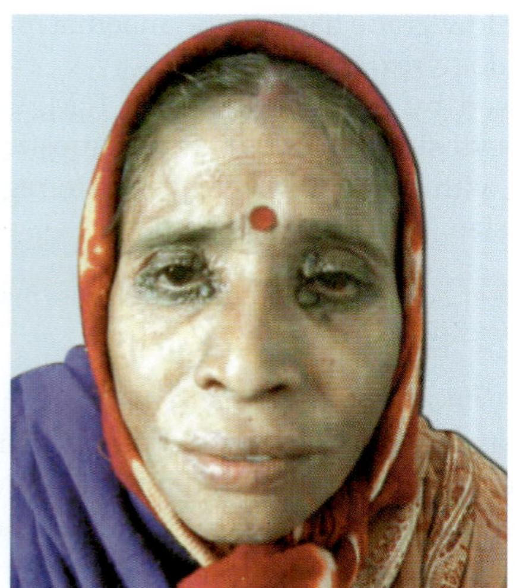

Fig. 2.27: Amyloidosis: Clustered waxy papules around the eyes with periorbital ecchymoses ('raccoon eyes'). She also had macroglossia

b. Wax-coloured papules/nodules around the face, shoulder-pad sign (prominent bilateral anterior deltoid area).
c. Visceromegaly: Macroglossia (tongue becomes stiff and firm to palpation), hepatosplenomegaly.
d. Evidence of nephrotic syndrome: Albuminuria, hypoproteinaemia, anasarca and hypercholesterolaemia.
e. Malabsorption, lymphadenopathy, peripheral neuropathy, cardiomyopathy may be present.
f. Liver, gingival, abdominal fat or rectal biopsy is done, which gives positive Congo red test.

Q. Differential diagnosis of hepatosplenomegaly in children:

1. Thalassaemia major.
2. Acute leukaemias (ALL > AML).
3. Indian childhood cirrhosis.
4. Acute viral hepatitis.
5. Enteric fever.
6. Disseminated tuberculosis.
7. Chronic malaria, chronic kala-azar.
8. Wilson's disease.
9. Storage disorders like Gaucher's disease, glycogen storage disease.
10. Still's disease
11. Sepsis.

Clinical Wisdom

Always try to say that liver and spleen are 'palpable' below the costal margin. If you say they are enlarged, it means that the upper border of liver and splenic dullness are in normal position. If you detect the upper borders in normal position, you may say 'they are enlarged'.

There may be scar marks (rounded) present in the right and/or left hypochondrium in a chronic patient of hepatosplenomegaly due to application of counterirritants by the quack doctors (used in remote villages) in a false attempt to reduce the size of liver and spleen (*see* Fig. 1.42).

CEREBELLAR DISORDER — CASE 34

Q. Functions of cerebellum:

Cerebellum has ipsilateral control over body, and

1. Regulates the rate, rhythm, range and force of muscular contraction.
2. Controls facilitatory action on tone and reflex activity of the body.
3. Maintains posture and equilibrium.
4. Integrates the voluntary and automatic movements—'coordination'.

Q. Morphological and functional division of cerebellum:

1. Archicerebellum (oldest part): Maintains locomotion and equilibrium (vestibular).
2. Palaeocerebellum (old part): Maintains the muscle tone and posture (spinocerebellar).
3. Neocerebellum (youngest part): Integration and coordination of fine muscular movements (corticocerebellar).

Q. Bedside assessment of the cerebellar function:

A cerebellar hemispheric lesion will produce ipsilateral signs. Cerebellar function is assesed from 'head to foot' by:

1. Titubation: Nodding of head either in antero-posterior ('yes-yes') or side to side ('no-no') direction. Sometimes, there is 'head tilt' towards the side of lesion. The patient may not sit or stand properly and may fall backwards.

- **Head-nodding** may also be seen in aortic regurgitation (syphilitic), parkinsonism, mannerisms, anticonvulsants-induced, patients with pendular nystagmus and mental retardation.
- **Head tilt** is also found in spasmodic torticollis (to any side), congenital ptosis (tilted backwards) and IVth cranial nerve palsy (tilted to opposite side).

2. Nystagmus: Horizontal, jerky nystagmus is present and the direction of nystagmus (fast component) is towards the side of lesion.

3. Speech (dysarthria): Dysarthria of staccato (incoordination of larynx) or scanning (incoordination of tongue) type. The speech is usually slow, slurred and irregular, and expressed with varying force. Often the patient scans the speech, i.e. he speaks syllable by syllable with undue emphasis on a particular syllable. Ask him to say 'artillery' or 'Motiur Rahaman': he will pronounce it as ar-til-ler-y or Mot-i-ur-Ra-ha-man (i.e. definite pauses between each syllable). Ideally, he is asked to repeat 'British Constitution' or 'Hippopotamus' to test articulation.

4. Hypotonia: Elicit the tone of the muscle, which will be flaccid both at rest (floppy limbs) and on passive movements of the parts.

5. Intention tremor: When tremor appears at the goal-point of an action, it is known as intention tremor. Ask the patient to hold a glass which is kept on the table or to hold your index finger which is kept away from him. The movements will be clumsy as he approaches the object. Finger-nose test also elicits intention tremor.

6. Dysmetria: It means inability to arrest the movements at desired point (i.e. inability to judge distance, speed and power of movement) and is elicited by *'finger-nose test'* **(Fig. 2.28A and B)**. The patient is asked to touch the tip of his nose with the tip of his index finger, first with eyes open and then with eyes closed (stand face to face infront of the standing patient, or sit in front of the sitting patient). At the beginning of the test, the patient is directed to outstretch or abduct his arm horizontally and then to bring the index finger towards the tip of his nose in a target to touch it. Instruct him to look straight ahead and not to focus on the index finger. Ask the patient to repeat the test as quickly as possible (first with eyes open and then eyes closed). This test can be modified by asking the patient to touch your index finger after touching his nose (finger-nose-finger test, which helps to detect milder type of incoordination). To make the test more difficult, the examiner's finger may be moved from place to place. First do the test on one side, then examine the other. The index finger of the patient may 'falls short' (hypometria) or 'overshoot' (hypermetria or past pointing) his nose. By this simple test one can assess the presence of:

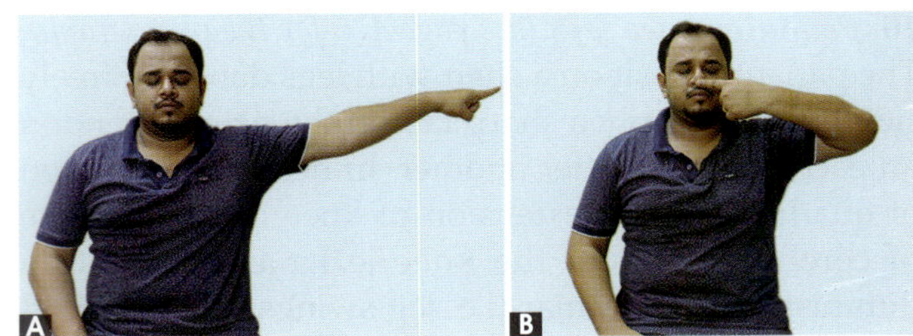

Figs 2.28A and B: Finger-nose test (A) and (B)

i. Intention tremor,
ii. Coordination, and
iii. Side of lesion (by seeing the past pointing).

7. Dyssynergia: It is the inability to perform complex movements as a coordinated temporal sequences when the movements may be broken down into their component parts (decomposition of movements) producing small, jerky and clumsy movements (like the modern break-dance or robot dance). The patient feels difficulty in performing complex movements.

8. Dysdiadochokinesia: The patient cannot execute rapid, repeated and alternating movements smoothly. He is asked to flex his elbows at right angle, and then pronate and supinate his forearm very rapidly 'as though screwing in a light bulb'. It can also be tested by asking the patient to supinate and pronate his right hand over the left palm very rapidly, and then the left hand over the right palm in the same way. In cerebellar lesion the movements are slow, clumsy, awkward, incomplete and often stops after few attempts (on the side of cerebellar lesion).

9. Rebound phenomenon: It is the inability to stop the movement of a body part when released suddenly after applying active resistance. Ask the patient to flex his elbow against resistance offered by you. As soon as you withdraw the resistance suddenly, the patient's hand tends to strike his face (because the antagonistic muscle like triceps cannot contract promptly). This is due to muscular hypotonia.

10. Pendular knee jerk *(see page 475 for the photograph)*: The patient will sit on a chair with legs dangling freely side by side. Apply a sharp tap on the patellar tendon on each side, one after another. In health, contraction of quadriceps with extension of knee occurs. In case of cerebellar lesion, the knee jerks are very often diminished or pendular (i.e. leg swings forwards and backwards several times) in nature. The first movement is followed by a series of diminishing oscillations (pendular) before the leg finally comes to rest. According to some clinicians, at least 4, to and fro movements in the leg are known as 'pendular'. If no response occurs, never forget to do the reinforcement test. Pendular knee jerk happens to be due to hypotonia.

11. Romberg's sign: Actually it a test of sensory ataxia. The test is negative in cerebellar disease (see below).

12. Gait:

a. This is a 'reeling', 'drunken' or 'lurching' gait due to presence of truncal 'ataxia'. The patient walks on a broad base, the feet being placed widely apart and irregularly; at times, the head is tilted towards the side of lesion (try in those patients, who are able to walk).
b. Next the patient is asked to walk along a straight line (cracks already present in the floor or you draw a line there). The patient sways and often falls towards the side of lesion during walking.
c. Tandem gait (heel to toe gait): The patient is asked to walk along a straight line with the heel of one foot touching the toes of the one behind. The patient is then told to turn backwards quickly. It is very difficult for a patient with cerebellar lesion to walk steadily by tandem gait. This gait is a sensitive test of early ataxia (a test of vermis of cerebellum).

Q. Presentation with cerebellar lesion:

Connections: Afferent fibres reach the cerebellum from spinal cord, vestibular system, basal ganglia and cerebrum. Cerebellum influences the LMN through its connections with the basal ganglia and cerebral cortex, via the thalamus. The common presentations are:

a. Hemispherical lesion: **Paralysis is not a feature of cerebellar disease** rather the patient presents with ipsilateral hypotonia (weakness), incoordination (ataxia), and difficulty in walking or swaying while walking.
b. Lesion at vermis: Produces truncal ataxia and the patient feels difficulty in sitting up or standing. Lesion at flocculonodular region produces vertigo, vomiting and gait ataxia, if they extend to the roof of 4th ventricle.

- The classical triad of cerebellar disease is '3A', e.g. ataxia, atonia and asthenia.

Q. Features of lesion at vermis (midline lesion):

In a midline cerebellar lesion there is little or no incoordination, no nystagmus and no hypotonia. But there are presence of:

i. Titubation (head-nodding).
ii. Truncal ataxia (ataxia of the body).
iii. Positive 'heel to toe' gait (tandem gait), and

(i–iii: 3'T')

iv. Difficulty in sitting, standing and unassisted walking (swaying and unsteadiness).

- Truncal ataxia is examined by observing the oscillation of the body while sitting without support.

Q. What is sensory ataxia (Table 2.5)?

For the production of a purposeful coordinated movement the cortex, the cerebellum, the reflex arc, impulses from eyes, labyrinth and cervical spine are required to function together. If such coordination is imperfect, motor performance becomes difficult. **Clumsiness of the movement (clinically manifested by unsteady gait) is known as ataxia provided, there is no motor and sensory deficit.** Ataxia is mainly of four types:

a. Cerebellar: Vascular lesion, cerebellar tumour, cerebellitis, cerebellar degeneration, hereditary ataxias, alcohol or phenytoin-induced.
b. Sensory: Peripheral neuropathy, tabes dorsalis.
c. Labyrinthine: Acute labyrinthitis, streptomycin-induced, Ménière's disease.
d. Central: Affection of vestibular nucleus as a result of vascular lesion in the medulla.
e. Miscellaneous: Optic ataxia, frontal lobe ataxia, severe muscular weakness, hypotonia, alcoholism.

Sensory ataxia results from defective proprioception (due to posterior column involvement) and can sometimes be alleviated with the help of vision. Thus sensory ataxia is increased when the eyes are closed in contrast to cerebellar ataxia which is not affected by vision. Tabes dorsalis is a classical example of sensory ataxia.

Sensory ataxia is usually due to affection of:

a. Peripheral sensory nerves: Peripheral neuropathy (e.g. leprosy, diabetes mellitus).
b. Posterior nerve roots: Tabes dorsalis, disc prolapse.
c. Posterior column: Multiple sclerosis, syringomyelia.
d. Post-central convolution: Diseases of parietal lobe (vascular, SOL).

- [**Apraxia:** Inability to perform certain purposive well-organized voluntary movement in the absence of motor weakness, sensory loss, cerebellar or extrapyramidal impairment, or ataxia. It develops in frontal and parietal lobe lesions. Ask the patient to light a cigerette with a matchstick, or copy a simple diagram. It seems, in apraxia, the person has forgotten to perform the motor act. Different types of apraxia are ideomotor, ideational, dressing, gait and constructional apraxia.
- **Agnosia:** Inability to recognise the nature of sensory input in spite of intact sensory, visual and auditory pathways, e.g. visual agnosia, tactile agnosia and auditory agnosia.]

Table 2.5: Differentiation between cerebellar and sensory ataxia

Features	Cerebellar ataxia	Sensory ataxia
1. Power of muscles	Normal	May be diminished (rarely)
2. Jerk (deep reflexes)	Pendular	Lost
3. Proprioceptive sensations	Present	Lost
4. Charcot joint and trophic changes	Absent	Present
5. Cerebellar signs	Present	Absent
6. Romberg's sign	Negative	Positive
7. Gait; H/o fall	Reeling gait; +	Stamping gait; +++
8. Postural instability	+	+++
9. Examples	Friedreich's ataxia, multiple sclerosis	Tabes dorsalis, peripheral neuropathy

Q. What is Romberg's sign?

It is important to remember that conventionally **it is a sign of sensory ataxia** (i.e. a test of posterior column function) and *not a test for cerebellar function*.

The patient is asked to stand with his feet close together (convergent heels with divergent toes). If he can do this, instruct him to close his eyes. Romberg's sign is said to be positive when the patient begins to sway or about to fall as soon as he closes his eyes. **The cardinal feature of this sign is that 'the patient is more unsteady standing with his eyes closed than when the eyes are kept open'.** A patient with cerebellar ataxia or labyrinthine lesion shows little or no increase in instability after closing the eyes (though the patient may show some unsteadiness with a tendency to fall at the beginning of the test with open eyes). False-positive Romberg's sign is observed in hysteria (hips sway more in comparison to ankles).

Prerequisites:

1. Patient will stand bare-footed.
2. Feet placed close to each other.
3. The examiner will stand very close to the patient and assure the patient of his safety.

Q. Diseases involving the posterior column:

Tabes dorsalis, subacute combined degeneration, cervical spondylosis, compressive myelopathy (posteriorly located), acute transverse myelitis, etc.

Q. Features of posterior column lesion:

Sensations conveyed by posterior column are described in page 164.

1. Motor functions:
   a. Nutrition: Mild wasting.
   b. Tone: Diminished.
   c. Power: Normal (i.e. preserved).
   d. Involuntary movements: Absent, rarely pseudo-athetotic movements are seen.
   e. Coordination: Usually normal.
2. Sensory functions:
   a. Touch (crude), pain and temperature: Unaffected.
   b. Deep sensations (joint, position, vibration sense) with fine touch: Lost. Abadie's sign is present.
   c. Girdle-like sensation at the level of compression: Present.
   d. Cortical sensations: Lost.
   e. Lhermitte's sign: Momentary electric shock-like sensation on the back (the spine and into the legs) evoked by neck flexion, and is also known as "Barber's chair sign" (causes of Lhermitte's sign are multiple sclerosis, cervical spondylosis, subacute combined degeneration, cervical cord tumour and syringomyelia). It indicates cervical cord compression.
3. Reflexes:
   a. Superficial: Normal.
   b. Deep reflexes or jerks: Diminished or may remain normal.
   c. Plantar response: Flexor.
   d. Bladder and bowel: Usually normal (urinary incontinence may be present).
4. Trophic changes: May be present (e.g. Charcot joint).
5. Romberg's sign: Present. Sensory ataxia and stamping gait.

- Loss of proprioception = 'Rombergism'.

Q. How to test for coordination:

It is the ability to perform complex movements smoothly and efficiently, and is assessed by:

A. In the upper limbs:

1. Watch the patient while dressing or undressing, picking up pins from the table, combing, etc.
2. Threading a needle.
3. Finger-nose test.
4. Dysdiadochokinesia.

B. In the lower limbs:

1. To make a large circle in the air with the foot while in lying down position.
2. Stance; walking along a straight line and tandem gait.
3. Heel-to-shin test.
4. Romberg's sign.

Clinical Wisdom

Remember, muscular weakness (developed from any disorder) may be accompanied by clumsiness of movement which may pose difficulty in interpretation of coordination.

Q. What is heel-to-shin (older term heel-knee) test (Fig. 2.29)?

The patient lies in bed (the eyes may remain open). Ask him to raise one leg high in the air and then place the heel of that flexed leg on the opposite knee and to then slide the heel down the anterior surface of leg (shin) towards the ankle up to the great toe. Before doing the test, demonstrate it clearly to the patient. Now ask the patient to do the test on the other side. In health, the movement of the heel is smooth and uniform throughout. In cerebellar disorder, the test becomes irregular with errors in the direction and speed of movement.

Q. Enumerate causes of 'recurrent fall':

1. Uneven or slippery floor.
2. Extreme weakness.
3. Vision loss.
4. Problem in balance.
5. Postural hypotension.
6. Dementia or impairment in cognition.
7. Disorder in gait or mobility limitation.
8. Functional disability (i.e. difficulty in performing basic day-to-day tasks).

Q. Common cerebeller disorders:

1. Cerebellar neoplasm (medulloblastoma, haemangioblastoma).
2. Multiple sclerosis.
3. Viral cerebellitis (e.g. post chickenpox cerebellitis).
4. Cerebellar abscess.
5. Hereditary ataxias (e.g. spinocerebellar ataxia, Friedreich ataxia).
6. Other spinocerebellar degeneration (signs of pyramidal tract lesion along with cerebellar signs).
7. Vascular: Thrombosis of the posterior inferior cerebellar artery, cerebellar haemorrhage.
8. Cerebello-pontine angle tumours.
9. Paraneoplastic syndrome from bronchogenic carcinoma.
10. Chiari malformations.
11. Cerebellar degeneration (*see* below).

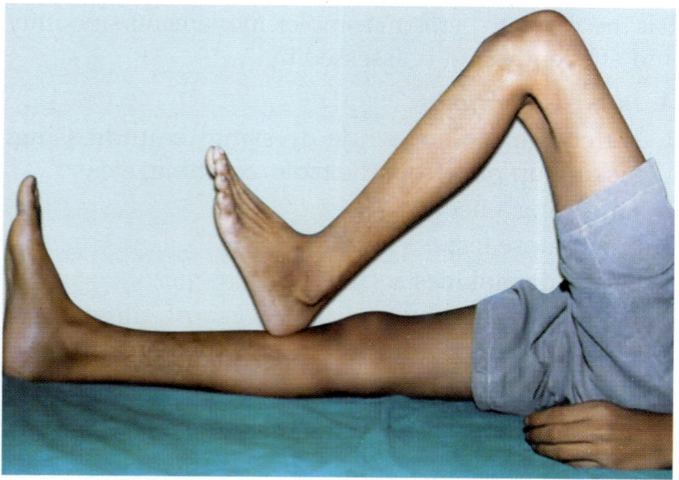

Fig. 2.29: Demonstration of **heel-to-shin test**

Q. Acquired causes of cerebellar degeneration:

1. Myxoedema.
2. Phenytoin or lithium toxicity.
3. Alcoholic degeneration (chronic alcoholism).
4. Neoplasm anywhere in the body, e.g. bronchogenic carcinoma (paraneoplastic syndrome).
5. Infection (HIV, abscess).
6. *Others:* Multiple sclerosis, haemorrhagic stroke, Creutzfeldt-Jakob (Prion) disease, autoimmune diseases.

- MRI of cerebellum is investigation of choice in cerebellar disorders.

BULBAR PALSY — CASE 35

Q. What is bulbar palsy?

It is the paralysis or loss of function of the muscles supplied by the cranial nerves arising from the bulb (old name for medulla oblongata), i.e. it is a palato-labio-glosso-pharyngo-laryngeal paralysis. Truely speaking, the motor nuclei of the IXth, Xth, XIth and XIIth cranial nerves are affected in bulbar palsy. So it is a **LMN type of paralysis**.

Q. What are the major symptoms?

1. Dysarthria (slurring of speech).
2. Dysphonia or nasal intonation.
3. Dysphagia.
4. Nasal regurgitation.
5. Dribbling of saliva.
6. Choking.

- 3'D's (i.e. 1, 2, 3 above) are major symptoms.

Q. What is pseudobulbar palsy?

It is the bulbar paralysis due to involvement of bilateral pyramidal tracts in the brainstem or above. So in this **UMN type of lesion**, the voluntary control of the muscles supplied by the IXth, Xth, XIth and XIIth cranial nerves is impaired.

Clinical Wisdom

12 cranial nerves can be divided into:
I. Pure motor: III, IV, VI, XI and XIIth.
II. Pure sensory: I, II and VIIIth.
III. Mixed: V, VII, IX and Xth.

Q. Clinical features of IXth, Xth, XIth and XIIth cranial nerves palsy (Table 2.6):

'The rule of three':

Table 2.6: Differentiation between pseudobulbar and bulbar palsy

Features	Pseudobulbar palsy	Bulbar palsy
1. Age	1. Usually above 60 years	1. Depends on the aetiology (usually middle aged)
2. Site of lesion	2. Cortex and subcortex	2. Medulla
3. Type of lesion	3. UMN type	3. LMN type
4. Onset	4. Always gradual	4. Acute or gradual
5. Memory loss and emotional instability	5. Present (labile)*	5. Absent
6. Blood pressure	6. May be high	6. Often normal
7. Facies	7. Masked facies	7. Nothing suggestive
8. Speech	8. Spastic dysarthria**	8. Flaccid dysarthria
9. **Tongue**	9. 'Spastic' and firm with pointed tip, there is neither wasting nor any fasciculation seen; small tongue	9. 'Flaccid', wasted, flabby with rounded tip, movements grossly diminished (may occupy one corner of the mouth); fasciculation+
10. **Jaw jerk**	10. Brisk	10. Absent
11. **Plantar response**	11. **Extensor**	11. **Flexor** or extensor (depends on aetiology)
12. Bulbar muscle involvement	12. Milder degree	12. Moderate to severe involvement

- Inappropriate and involuntary uncontrollable crying or laughter.* *Emotional lability* is not uncommon in Alzheimer's disease, dementia, traumatic injury of brain or multiple sclerosis.
- Donald Duck or hot potato dysarthria due to immobile and tight tongue.**

A. Glossopharyngeal nerve

1. Loss of sensation over the mucous membrane of pharynx.
2. Loss of taste sensation in the posterior 1/3rd of the tongue.
3. Do the 'gag reflex' (the afferent fibres are carried through IXth and the efferent through Xth cranial nerve; centre for the reflex lies in medulla) and examine for taste sensation in the posterior 1/3rd of the tongue.

   Gag reflex (Fig. 2.30): Depress the tongue with a spatula. Tickle the posterior wall of pharynx (pharyngeal reflex) or soft palate (palatal reflex) by a piece of cotton wrapped in a broom-stick and note its reflex contracion. Normally there is bilaterally symmetrical contraction of posterior pharyngeal wall and fauces of mouth (Xth cranial nerve). Test each side seperately, and ask for appreciation of touch sensation (IXth cranial nerve). This reflex is lost in bulbar palsy.

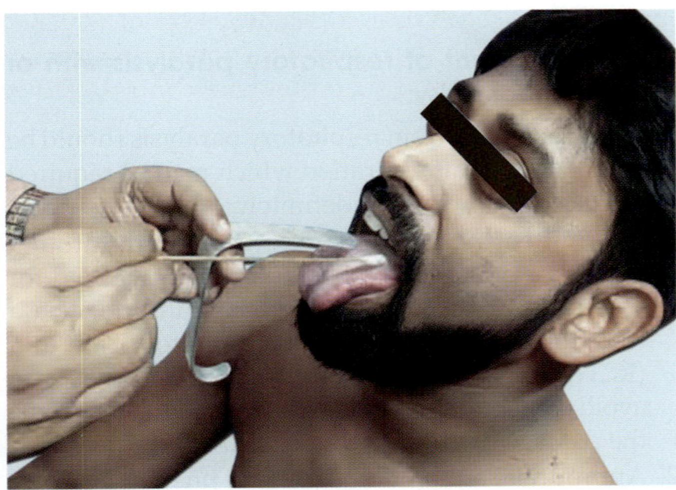

Fig. 2.30: Eliciting **Gag reflex**

B. Vagus nerve

a. Soft palate:
   1. Ask the patient for nasal intonation (twang) and hoarseness of voice. In nasal intonation, 'egg' is pronounced as 'eng'.
   2. Ask the patient for nasal regurgitation of liquids.
   3. Ask the patient to say 'Aaah'! and observe the soft palate with a torch whether both the sides of the palate arch upwards or not; or the soft palate is pulled to the normal side on saying 'Aaah'.

b. Pharynx:
   1. Dysphagia: Maximum to liquid and minimum to semisolid food, in contrast to mechanical dysphagia where dysphagia is maximum with solid food (liquid food needs immediate muscular contraction to swallow and this is why neurogenic dysphagia occurs earlier with liquid food).

      Moreover, pooling of secretions in the posterior pharynx is noted with drooling of saliva; there may be sensation of choking.
   2. Nocturnal cough: During sleep, saliva goes into the respiratory tract (i.e. aspiration) and may precipitate death due to pneumonia.
   3. Test the 'gag reflex' (lost in vagus nerve lesion).

c. Larynx:
   1. Hoarseness of voice (adduction of vocal cord is not possible); bovine cough.
   2. Inspiratory dyspnoea (abduction of vocal cord is not possible).
   3. Examine the vocal cord by indirect laryngoscopy.

C. Spinal accessory nerve

1. In bilateral paralysis of sternomastoid muscle, there is diminished ability to rotate neck and the head tends to fall back.
2. Test the power of sternomastoids from front.
3. Test the power of trapezius from behind.
   Read the section on 'Myotonia' for proper testing of these muscles.

D. Hypoglossal nerve

1. Ask the patient to protrude the tongue: Look for any deviation (deviated to the side of paralysis due to unopposed action of genioglossus of healthy side). The patient may not be able to protrude the tongue much beyond the teeth in bilateral XIIth nerve palsy.
2. Ask the patient to curl his tongue up and down, and sideways. Test the power of the tongue muscles (ask the patient to bulge his cheeks with the tongue against resistance offered by the examiner from outside).
3. While the tongue is kept within the oral cavity, observe for wasting and fasciculation.

Q. Causes of pseudobulbar and bulbar palsy:

A. Pseudobulbar palsy

1. Diffuse cerebral ischaemia (multi-infarct dementia): Multiple lacunar infarction.
2. Diffuse atherosclerosis (cerebral atrophy).
3. Chronic motor neurone disease (MND).
4. Sometimes in multiple sclerosis (a late event).
5. Cerebral vasculitis.
6. Following severe brain injury.

B. Bulbar palsy

a. Acute:
   1. Poliomyelitis (bulbar variety).
   2. Diphtheria.
   3. GB syndrome.
   4. Rabies.
   5. Organophosphorus poisoning.
   6. Encephalitis.
   7. Snake bite (Elapidae).
   8. Botulism.
   9. Myasthenic crisis.
   10. Medullary infarction.

b. Chronic:
   1. Chronic motor neurone disease (MND).
   2. Syringobulbia.
   3. Neoplasm in the medulla or pontine glioma.
   4. Basal meningitis.
   5. Fracture of the posterior cranial fossa.
   6. Multiple metastases involving lower cranial nerves.
   7. Neurosarcoid.
   8. Neurosyphilis.
   9. Multiple sclerosis (rare).

- Intermittent bulbar palsy: May be seen in myasthenia gravis and multiple sclerosis.
- **MND can develop into both pseudobulbar (UMN) and bulbar (LMN) palsy.**

Other features to note in bulbar palsy:

The features developing due to involvement of vital centres in the medulla should be carefully monitored (mainly in acute variety).

1. Cardiac centre: Tachycardia, different arrhythmias.
2. Respiratory centre: Tachypnoea, ataxic breathing, respiratory failure.
3. Vasomotor centre: Hypotension or hypertension.

There may be damage to fibre tracts like pyramidal tract (crossed hemiplegia or decerebrate rigidity), sympathetic trunk (ipsilateral Horner's syndrome), spinothalamic tract (loss of touch, pain, temperature sensation on the opposite side), medial lemniscus (ipsilateral loss of proprioception), vestibulospinal tracts (vertigo), descending tract and nucleus of the Vth cranial nerve (ipsilateral touch, pain and loss of temperature sensation in the face), and nystagmus.

Q. Reflexes in pseudobulbar and bulbar palsy:

1. *Superficial reflex*, i.e. plantar response is always extensor in pseudobulbar palsy and usually flexor in bulbar palsy (may be extensor rarely, depending on the aetiology, e.g. in motor neurone disease).
2. *Deep reflex*, i.e. Jaw jerk is brisk in pseudobulbar palsy and absent in bulbar palsy (a very important sign for differentiation at bedside).

Q. Disease with combined bulbar and pseudobulbar palsy—features:

Chronic motor neurone disease (amyotrophic lateral sclerosis) may have combined palsy and is characterised by wasted tongue with brisk jaw jerk.

Q. Management of respiratory paralysis with or without bulbar palsy:

A patient suffering from respiratory paralysis should be treated by artificial respiration which may be required for weeks or months, or indefinitely:

1. Intermittent positive pressure ventilation through a nasal or oral endotracheal tube (when needed for 2–3 days) or through a cuffed tube inserted via a tracheostomy, preferably in a respiratory care unit (RCU) with regular monitoring of blood gases to avoid over- or underventilation. Cuffed tube prevents the passage of pharyngeal secretions into the lungs.
2. Appropriate antibiotics to prevent pneumonia.
3. Care of the skin, bladder and bowel.

❍ **Treatment of bulbar palsy** requires the following:

4. Nasogastric suction by mechanical sucker.
5. Postural drainage: Foot end of the bed should be raised and the patient is turned in the semiprone position.
6. Proper fluid balance.
7. Chest physiotherapy.
8. Speech therapy.
9. Barium swallow with videofluoroscopy helps to 'visualise' swallowing.

Q. Causes of nasal regurgitation of fluid:

1. Paralysis of vagus nerve.
2. Bulbar and pseudobulbar palsy.
3. Polymyositis or dermatomyositis.
4. Myopathy.
5. Cleft palate.
6. Perforation or destruction of palate (leprosy, tuberculosis, irradiation, syphilis).
7. Malignant disease of nasopharynx (Fig. 2.31).

❍ Common causes of bulbar palsy: GB syndrome, MND, snake bite, diphtheria and poliomyelitis.

❍ Other symptoms of bulbar palsy are: difficulty in chewing, hoarseness of voice and stridor. D/D of bulbar palsy is pseudobulbar palsy.

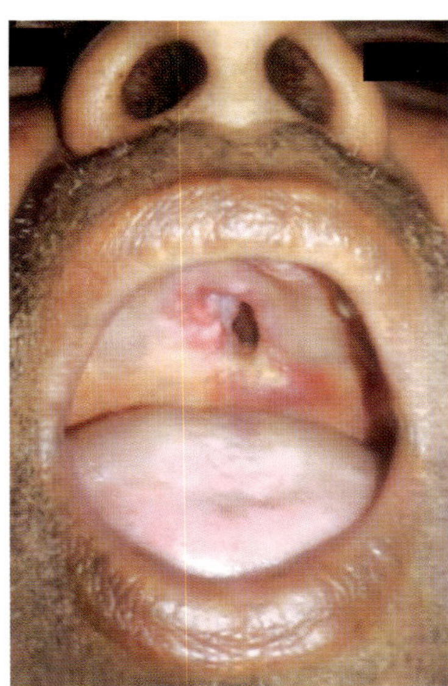

Fig. 2.31: Perforated palate due to malignancy of the nasopharynx

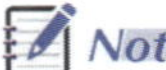

Clinical Wisdom

The gag and palatal reflexes are preserved (or exaggerated) in pseudobulbar palsy.

Note

Each of the long cases, e.g. valvular heart diseases, pleural diseases, parkinsonism, diabetic foot, lymphoma, thalassaemia, etc. may be treated as short cases.

Chapter

3

Spot Cases (Spotters)

"For one mistake made for not knowing, ten mistakes are made for not looking"

—**JA Lindsay** (1856–1931), a brilliant clinician and an author who was famous for his clinical axioms and aphorisms

ANAEMIA CASE 36

Q. Definition:

It is defined as the qualitative or quantitative diminution of RBC and/or haemoglobin concentration in relation to standard age and sex, and is clinically manifested by pallor. The cardinal sign of anaemia is pallor. It is not a disease but denotes manifestation of some disease, and thus a cause must be searched for.

Anaemia is commonly associated with various haematological and systemic disorders.

Q. Where will you look for anaemia?

Sites (examined in good natural light):

1. Lower palpebral conjunctiva (retract the lower eyelids downwards and ask the patient to look upwards—both eyes at a time). In health, palpebral conjunctiva is red, which appears pale pink in anaemia (experience teaches to differentiate normal from abnormal) **(Fig. 3.1)**.

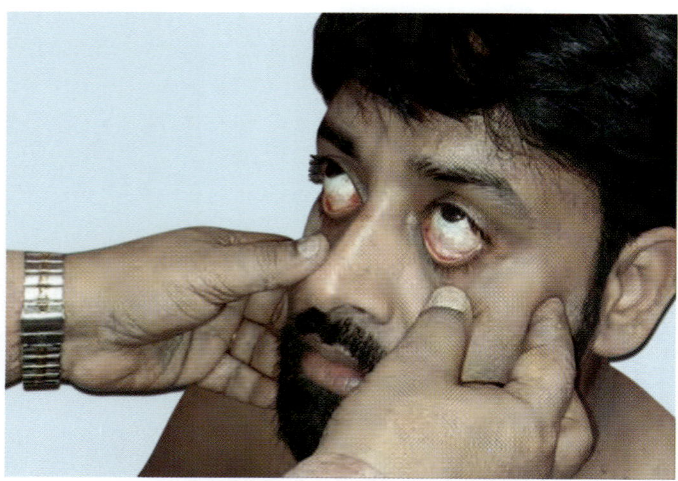

Fig. 3.1: Clinical demonstration of **anaemia**

2. Tongue, especially the tip and the dorsum.
3. Mucous membrane of palate (especially the soft palate).
4. Nail-beds (press the pulp to see the redness of nail-bed).
5. Palms, soles and general skin surfaces.

- Nail-beds are the windows of the cutaneous capillary network. Earliest anaemia is noticed in soft palate.
- Other areas like rectal or vaginal mucosa may be examined for anaemia (not practised).

Q. Clinical types of anaemia and its bedside assessment:

Anaemia is clinically classified as mild, moderate and severe types. It is totally a clinical assessment (highly subjective sign) and may not correspond with laboratory findings. Clinically we see the paleness of the skin/mucous membrane, or pallor. The colour of the tongue as well as the conjunctiva are more reliable than other sites in this respect (in adults). In children, palms and soles are to be especially looked for.

Q. Clinical classification (grading):

- Mild anaemia: 60–80% of Hb (9–12 g/dL).
- Moderate anaemia: 40–60% of Hb (6–9 g/dL).
- Severe anaemia: <40% of Hb (<6 g/dL) **(Fig. 3.2)**.

The normal haemoglobin concentrations in case of males and females are: Males: 13–17 g/dL, and females: 12–15 g/dL.

- Clinically, 15 g/dL may be taken as 100% haemoglobin.
- **According to WHO, anaemia in male is Hb <13 g/dL, and that of female is <12/dL.**

Q. Causes of 'pallor without anaemia':

See the section on 'Myxoedema'.

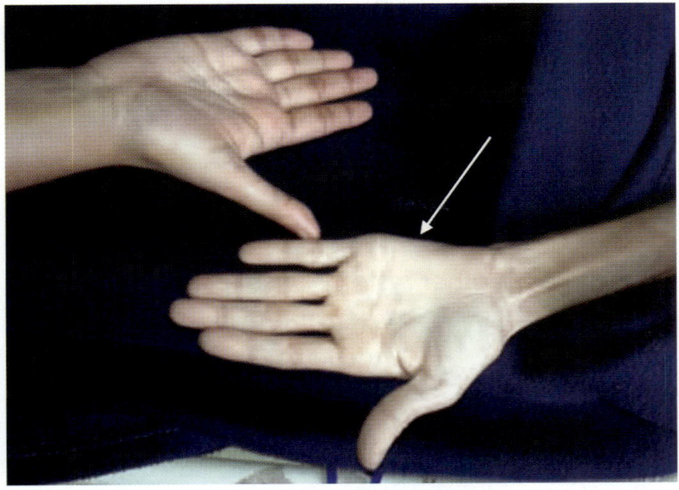

Fig. 3.2: **Severe anaemia** (compared with a normal hand)

- **Pallor** (paleness) is the waxy appearance of skin and mucous membrane (*see* **Fig. 1.40**). It depends on thickness and quality of skin, and quality and amount of blood in the capillaries. Thus, pallor and anaemia are not interchangeable terms. *There are many causes of pallor, and anaemia is commonest of them.* Pallor of mucous membrane is commonly due to anaemia; very often generalised pallor is attributed to severe anaemia. It is difficult to detect pallor in deeply pigmented individuals. The opposite term for pallor is plethora (e.g. ruddy complexion in polycythemia).
- Anaemia is a pathological condition while pallor is a clinical entity. A person without losing a drop of blood may become deadly pale (shock and collapse), and similarly a person looking severely pale may not be grossly anaemic (Sheehan's syndrome)
- Facial pallor is commonly seen in vasoconstriction, shock and low cardiac outputs state.
- Pallor > anaemia is common in myxedema, CRF and panhypopituitarism.

Clinical Wisdom

In general survey, one may write pallor (probably a better terminology) instead of anaemia.

Q. Differential diagnosis of anaemia:

Enumerate different causes of pallor (without anaemia): Vide page 392.

Q. Examination of the hands in anaemia:

1. Colour of nail-beds and palms gives an indication of presence of anaemia.
2. Koilonychia gives a clue to the type of anaemia, such as iron deficiency anaemia.
3. In severe anaemia, there may be visible capillary pulsation in nail-bed.
4. Presence of splinter haemorrhage or Osler's node points towards SBE.
5. Presence of ecchymosis (bruise) indicates acute leukaemia or aplastic anaemia.
6. Anaemia with finger deformities may indicate long-continued rheumatoid arthritis.
7. Lemon-yellow pallor suggests advanced pernicious anaemia.
8. Kunckle-pad hyperpigmentation indicates megaloblastic anaemia.
9. Yellowish discolouration of palm in myxoedema (i.e. carotenaemia).
10. Colour of palmar creases gives a clue to the degree of anaemia. When they are as pale as the surrounding skin, the patient usually has haemoglobin level <7 g/dL

- In ophthalmoscopy if the retina seems very pale, the haemoglobin concentration is usually <4 g/dL.
- Jaundice associated with anaemia points towards haemolytic anaemia.

Q. Haemoglobin concentration is 81–99%—is it anaemia?

Yes, it is anaemia but the pallor may not be clinically appreciated (so this group is not included in the clinical classification of anaemia).

Q. Symptoms referable to anaemia:

The symptoms and signs depend on severity of anaemia. The **common symptoms** are weakness, fatigue, lassitude, light-headedness, giddiness, fainting or syncope, anorexia, palpitations, breathlessness, anginal pain, insomnia, tinnitus, lack of concentration, intermittent claudication, tingling sensation in the extremities and menstrual irregularities. In anaemia, there is inadequate delivery of O_2 to peripheral tissues.

Q. Importance of 'history taking' in a patient of anaemia:

1. Present history: Commonly complaining of easy fatigability, shortness of breath and decreased effort intolerance.
2. Past history: H/o bleeding (e.g. haematemesis, melaena, epistaxis, menorrhagia or haemorrhoids), H/o blood transfusion in the past, or diarrhoea (tropical sprue). Any H/o chronic diseases (RA, CRF)?
3. Personal history: Alcohol consumption, walking barefooted (e.g. hookworm infestation).
4. Family history: Similar type of illness in the family suggests genetic inheritance, e.g. thalassaemia, HbE disease, haemophilia.
5. Dietary history: Should be taken to diagnose nutritional anaemia (e.g. pure vegetarians may suffer from vitamin B_{12} deficiency anaemia); less intake due to anorexia, dysphagia or poverty.
6. Treatment history: Bone marrow suppressant drugs, haemolysis (G_6PD deficiency with antimalarials), NSAID-intake or H/o radiation, previous surgery like gastrectomy or ileal surgery may lead to anaemia.
7. Menstrual history: Full menstrual history with amount of blood loss should be asked for.
8. Occupational history: H/o exposure to chemical solvents, lead, benzene, insecticides should be taken;

a cultivator working bare-footed may suffer from hookworm infestation.

9. Geographic background and ethnic origin: Important to diagnose thalassaemia, sickle cell anaemia, G_6PD deficiency.

Q. Important history to evaluate anaemia:

H/o chronic blood loss (bleeding peptic ulcer, haemorrhoids, menorrhagia), malabsorption (diarrhoea/steatorrhoea), nutritional intake, worm infestations, exposure to drugs/chemicals/radiation, bleeding tendencies, bowel habits, anorexia and loss of weight.

Q. Common causes of severe anaemia in a city hospital:

1. Nutritional.
2. Haematemesis and melaena.
3. Chronic bleeding haemorrhoids.
4. Uraemia.
5. Menorrhagia.
6. Thalassaemia.
7. Acute leukaemias.
8. Hookworm infestation.
9. Aplastic anaemia.
10. Carcinoma of stomach, lung, colon.

Q. Importance of stool examination in anaemia:

1. Presence of occult blood.
2. To diagnose hookworm ova.
3. Ova/parasite of *Giardia lamblia*.

Q. Classify anaemia (working classification):

A. *Based on morphology:* Normocytic (aplastic anaemia), microcytic (iron deficiency), macrocytic (megaloblastic anaemia).

B. *Based on aetiology:*
   a. Blood loss, which may be either acute or chronic.
   b. Inadequate production of RBC.
   c. Excessive destruction of RBC.

- It seems anaemia may result from nutritional deficiency, haemorrhage, haemolysis or hypoplasia of the bone marrow.

Q. Cardiovascular (CVS) features in severe anaemia:

1. Tachycardia.
2. Capillary pulsation.
3. BP: High systolic and normal (low) diastolic BP.
4. Water-hammer pulse.
5. Cervical venous hum.
6. Cardiomegaly (cardiac dilatation) and later, signs of heart failure.
7. Hyperdynamic apex beat.
8. Mitral systolic murmur due to functional MI (ring dilatation).
9. Haemic murmur over the aortic and pulmonary area.
10. Rarely mid-diastolic (non-rumbling) murmur in mitral area may be auscultated (due to relative stenosis at mitral valve) secondary to increased blood flow.

- No. 1, 4, 6 and 9 are most important. Oedema in general survey is a clinical clue at bedside.

Q. Features in other systems in severe anaemia:

1. General survey	a) Pallor, b) Dyspnoea, c) Ankle oedema or anasarca.
2. CVS	Already described above.
3. GI tract	Hepatosplenomegaly may be present.
4. Respiratory system	Basal crepitations.
5. Nervous system	Features of polyneuropathy, sometimes, there is papilloedema.
6. Lymphoreticular system	There may be presence of sternal tenderness (rare).

Q. Ankle oedema in anaemia:

1. Severe anaemia *per se* (renal retention of salt and water).
2. Congestive cardiac failure may be associated with.
3. Associated renal or hepatic disorders, hypoalbuminaemia, myxoedema.

Q. Common causes of anaemia in this part of world (e.g. India):

1. Nutritional anaemia (so, dietary history is important).
2. Hookworm infestation.
3. Chronic malaria, chronic kala-azar, tuberculosis.
4. Thalassaemia.
5. Tropical sprue.

Clinical Wisdom

Transfusion is usually required when Hb level goes below 7 g/dL. One unit (2 units in India) of packed red cells elevate the haemoglobin by approximately 1 g/dL. Life span of RBC is approximately 120 days.

- Globally, 'chronic blood loss' (from chronic duodenal ulcer, haemorrhoids, or fibroid in females) is probably the commonest cause of anaemia.

Q. Common causes of iron deficiency anaemia:

1. Nutritional deficiency.
2. Bleeding peptic ulcer.
3. Gastric erosion by NSAID.
4. Bleeding haemorrhoids.
5. Hookworm infestation.
6. Malabsorption syndrome.
7. Menorrhagia.
8. Pregnancy, lactation, adolescence.

- This is why stool is examined for ova/parasite/cyst/occult blood, upper and lower GI endoscopy are performed with barium study, and gynaecological evaluation are done for 'chronic blood loss'.
- Exclusively breast-fed children may develop iron deficiency anaemia as breast milk contains little iron.

Q. Clinical diagnosis of iron deficiency anemia:

1. H/o 'pica' (perverted appetite with compulsive eating of strange non-nutrient items such as clay—geophagia, ice—pagophagia, cornstarch—amylophagia, or coal) or chronic blood loss from GI tract.
2. Pallor (pearly white sclera).
3. Glossitis (bald or depapillated tongue).
4. Angular stomatitis, cheilosis.
5. Brittle finger nails, flat nails (platonychia) or even koilonychia.
6. Brittle hairs.
7. Dysphagia (Plummer-Vinson syndrome or Paterson-Kelly syndrome) as a result of post-cricoid web which can be demonstrated endoscopically or by barium swallow.
8. Restless leg syndrome and other 'symptoms referable to anaemia' (*see* page 283).
9. Mild splenomegaly, rarely.

- 'Pica' is also observed in pregnancy and some psychiatric disorder.

Q. Causes of glossitis and angular stomatitis:

A. Glossitis (inflammation with red and sore tongue):

a. Riboflavin deficiency: Magenta-coloured tongue.
b. Iron deficiency anaemia.
c. Nicotinic acid or vitamin B_{12} deficiency: The tongue is red, swollen, painful and is known as 'raw-beefy tongue'.
d. Folic acid deficiency.
e. *Bald tongue* (complete atrophy of papillae): Found in severe iron deficiency anaemia, tropical sprue, pernicious anaemia, pellagra and syphilis.
f. Median rhomboid glossitis: A lozenge-shaped denuded area in the middle of the tongue posteriorly. It is a congenital abnormality and as it feels nodular, it should be differentiated from carcinoma of the tongue.
g. Miscellaneous: Cirrhosis of liver, tuberculosis, chronic alcoholism, Sjögren's syndrome.

B. Angular stomatitis (inflammation or cracking of the epithelium at the angle or corner of the mouth):

a. Excessive use of tobacco, alcohol or betel-leaf.
b. Improperly-fitted denture.
c. Iron deficiency anaemia.
d. Riboflavin, nicotinic acid, folic acid and pyridoxine deficiency (Fig. 3.3).
e. Starvation or malnutrition.

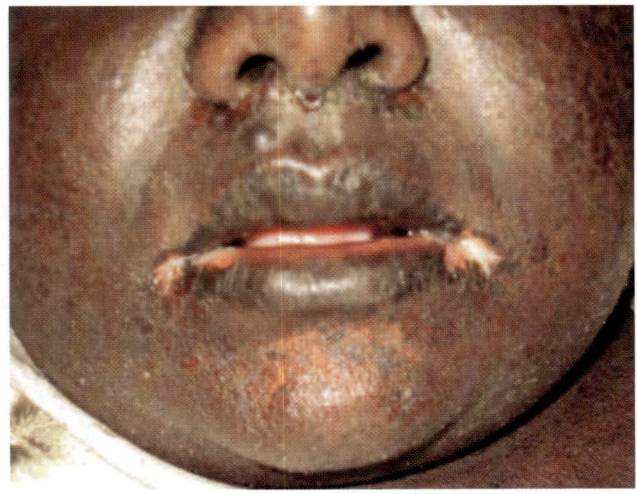

Fig. 3.3: **Angular stomatitis** due to vitamin B-complex and iron deficiency in a chronic debilitated patient; excoriation and crusting of skin around nostrils are seen

f. Herpes labialis, candidosis or streptococcal infection at the angle of mouth.
g. 'Perleche' (i.e. angular cheilitis) in children, are infective in origin.

Q. Causes of dimorphic anaemia:

When two distinct forms of RBC (i.e. microcytes and macrocytes) are circulating, it is called dimorphic anaemia. The causes are combined iron and vitamin B_{12}/folic acid deficiency, pregnancy, and hookworm anaemia with nutritional deficiency.

- Spurious anaemia: In pregnancy when plasma volume is ↑, Hb is relatively ↓, it is called spurious anaemia.

Q. Causes of haemolytic anaemia:

See the sections on 'Jaundice' and 'Thalassaemia'.

Q. How do you diagnose hookworm infestation?

1. Occupation, e.g. patients working in tea-garden, coal mines or a farmer who walks bare-footed.
2. Presence of ground itch at the site of entry in the skin.
3. Perversion of taste sensation with 'pica' (often they eat earth, mud or lime).
4. Blotting paper like tongue (very pale tongue) with puffy face and swelling of lower eyelids. Koilonychia and pedal oedema are frequently observed. There is lustreless hair with protuberant abdomen. Other features of iron deficiency anaemia may be present.
5. Pain in the epigastrium mimicking chronic duodenal ulcer.
6. Steatorrhoea or fatty diarrhoea.
7. Passage of small worms in stool.

Q. Causes of anaemia due to 'chronic systemic diseases':

A. Anaemia of chronic diseases (AOCD):
   a. Infection: SBE, lung abscess, tuberculosis, osteomyelitis, pyelonephritis.

b. Collagen vascular disorders: SLE.

c. Malignancy.

d. Rheumatoid arthritis.

B. Uraemia.

C. Endocrine disorders: Myxoedema, Addison's disease, panhypopituitarism.

D. Liver disease: Especially in alcoholics.

The whole spectrum is associated with normocytic normochromic anaemia. Group (A) may have microcytic anaemia, Group (B) may have Burr cells, and Group (C) and (D) may show macrocytic RBCs.

Clinical Wisdom

The total group will have low serum iron, low TIBC, and normal or elevated serum ferritin level.

Q. Outline of investigations in anaemia:

The investigations are directed to see the type and aetiology of anaemia:

A. The **type of anaemia** is ascertained by peripheral blood smear, blood indices and serum values:
   a. Peripheral blood smear: Hb content, RBC morphology, reticulocytes, malaria parasite.
   b. Blood indices: MCV, MCH, MCHC.
   c. Serum values: Serum iron concentration, TIBC, serum ferritin.

B. The **cause of anaemia** is determined by meticulous history taking, clinical examination, haematological tests (described above, along with full blood count), examination of stool/urine, chest X-ray, study of the GI system, renal and liver function tests, special haematological tests (Coombs' test, osmotic fragility test, Hb-electrophoresis, etc.), and in selective cases by bone marrow study and cytogenetic tests.

- RDW or 'red cell distribution width' test measures the differences in the volume and size of RBCs. High (major variations) or low (very little variations) RDW often indicates some specific anaemia.

Q. What is 'leucoerythroblastic' blood picture?

When normoblasts and myelocytes both are seen in the peripheral blood of patients suffering from *myelophthisic anaemia* (infiltration of bone marrow by tumour or granuloma), M_6 variety of AML, myelofibrosis or myelosclerosis, it is said that leucoerythroblastic blood picture is present.

Q. How do you examine a patient for polycythemia ('ruddy cyanosis')?

Polycythemia is the increase in red blood cells above normal.

It is examined in the same way as done for the clinical detection of anaemia, i.e. look for the lower palpebral conjunctiva, tongue, soft palate, nail-beds, palms and soles, and general skin surfaces (Fig. 3.4). The colour of the mucous membrane turns dusky-red.

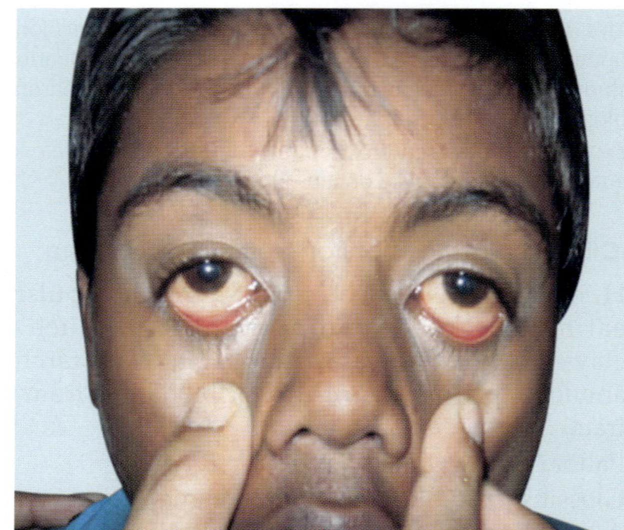

Fig. 3.4: Suffused bulbar conjunctiva and increased redness of lower palpebral conjunctiva in **polycythemia** from cyanotic congenital heart disease

Patients of polycythemia usually have facial plethora, suffused conjunctiva, red nose and ear lobes, cherry-red tongue, increased redness of lower palpebral conjunctiva and palmar erythema.

Q. Common causes of polycythemia in tertiary care hospitals:

1. COPD.
2. Cyanotic congenital heart diseases, e.g. Fallot's tetralogy (Figs 2.1 and 3.4).
3. Right-to-left shunt in the heart.
4. Polycythemia vera (or erythremia).

- High altitude and severe dehydration (relative polycythemia) are also common causes of polycythemia. Thrombosis, peptic ulceration (often with bleeding) and hyperuricaemia are noted complications of polycythemia vera. In polycythemia vera RBC, WBC, platelet count and absolute basophil count are increased along with splenomegaly; erythropoietin (EPO) level remains low (EPO level is increased in secondary polycythemia); **in polycythemia, Hb in male is >18 g/dL and in female it is >16 g/dL.**

Q. Anaemia and polycythemia in a single patient—is it possible?

Sometimes it is seen in Fallot's tetralogy where anaemia (iron deficiency) is not clinically evident in the presence of polycythemia. If Hb% is <18 g/dL, PCV is <55%, and MCHC is <28 g/dL, one should be suspicious about anaemia in the presence of polycythemia in a case of Fallot's tetralogy.

Q. Normal reticulocyte count, reticulocyte index and red cell mass (volume):

A. Reticulocyte count: 0.2–2% of RBCs (increased in haemolytic anaemia).

B. Reticulocyte index:

$$\text{Reticulocyte \%} \times \frac{\text{Patient's PCV}}{\text{Normal PCV}}$$

C. Red cell mass:
   i. Male: 30 mL/kg of body weight.
   ii. Female: 25 mL/kg of body weight (increased in polycythemia vera).

 *Conclusion*

Always examine both the lower palpebral conjunctiva because the presence of conjunctivitis in one eye (i.e. increased redness) may interfere with the interpretation of anaemia if anyone examines the infected eye only. While examining the tongue for anaemia, very often magenta-coloured tongue (riboflavin deficiency) misguides a clinician. By retracting the lower eyelids downwards, one can diagnose two other conditions, e.g. polycythemia (increased redness of both conjunctivae) and scleroderma (increased tightness of the skin during retraction). Do not examine the eyes for anaemia if it is rubbed or washed just before testing.

Pallor may be misleading and requires laboratory measurement of Hb concentration to diagnose anaemia.

Earliest sign of acute blood loss is tachycardia and postural hypotension, and not anaemia because haemodilution (resulting anaemia) is completed in 24–36 hours.

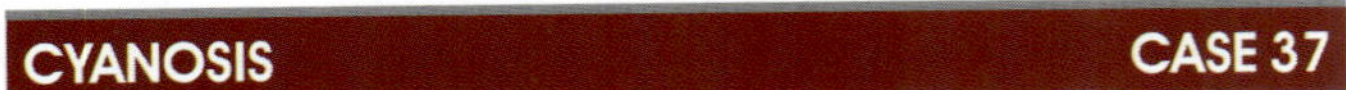

CYANOSIS — CASE 37

Q. What is cyanosis?

It is defined as bluish discolouration of the skin and mucous membrane due to presence of increased amount of reduced haemoglobin (>5 g/dL), or of haemoglobin derivatives (e.g. sulphaemoglobin and methaemoglobin) in the capillary blood (Fig. 3.5). Absolute concentration of reduced haemoglobin above 5 g/dL in the capillaries makes the blood dark and gives the tissue a bluish hue (in Greek words, *'kyanos'* means dark blue colour and *'osis'* means condition). According to few clinicians, >4 g/dL of reduced (desaturated) haemoglobin in the capillary blood produces cyanosis (recent view).

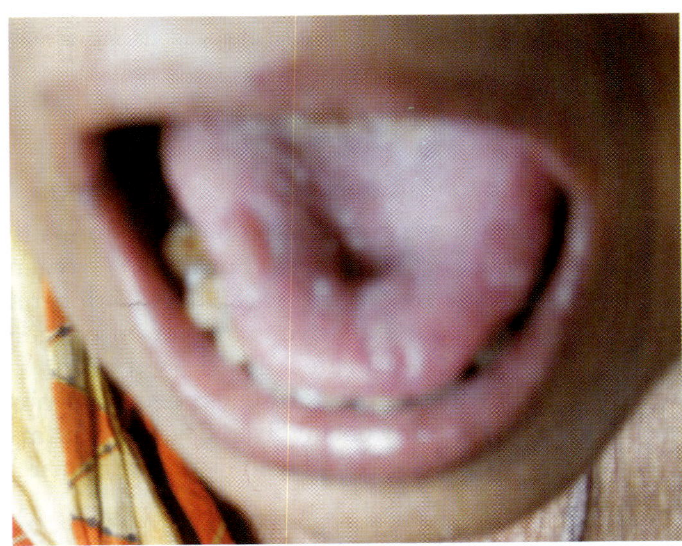

Fig. 3.5: **Central cyanosis** in acute severe asthma

Cyanosis (central) is a grave sign and needs immediate evaluation as well as intervention.

Q. Types of cyanosis (Table 3.1):

It is **principally of two types: Central and peripheral cyanosis**.

Table 3.1: Bedside differentiation between central and peripheral cyanosis

Features	Central cyanosis	Peripheral cyanosis
1. Sites	1. As described above. Commonly seen in warm mucous membranes like **tongue** and oral cavity	1. As described above. Tongue remains unaffected
2. Handshake	2. Hand feels warm (due to increased blood flow)	2. Hand feels cold (due to diminished blood flow)
3. Application of warmth and cold	3. No change	3. Warmth—cyanosis decreased Cold—cyanosis increased
4. Application of pure oxygen for 10 minutes	4. Cyanosis may improve (except in AV shunt)	4. No response
5. Exercise	5. May aggravate	5. May improve
6. **Clubbing** and polycythemia	6. Usually present	6. Absent
7. Pulse volume	7. Normal or high (due to arteriovenous shunt)	7. Usually low volume due to circulatory stasis
8. **Dyspnoea**	8. Patient is often breathless	8. No respiratory distress

- Application of warmth (Lewis test): by rubbing two palms, and cold: by adding ice over palms.
- It very difficult to diagnose cyanosis in the presence of polycythemia.
- Clubbing is absent in peripheral cyanosis and acutely developing central cyanosis.

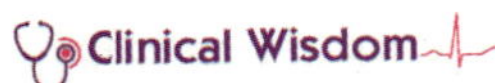

Clinical Wisdom

Pathology: Central cyanosis—Heart-lung unit, peripheral cyanosis—Local.

- Other clinical types of cyanosis are: Enterogenous, mixed and differential cyanosis.
- Cyanosis is more easily revealed in fluorescent light than in daylight.

Q. Peripheral cyanosis and sites to be examined:

In peripheral cyanosis, the arterial blood is normally saturated (*arterial PaO_2 is normal*) but there is oxygen unsaturation at the venous end of capillary. Peripheral cyanosis results from excessive extraction of oxygen from the normally saturated arterial blood. It is rarely a life-threatening medical emergency; mucous membranes are generally not involved. The mechanisms (i.e. microcirculation defect) play in its production are:

a. Reduced cardiac output.
b. Peripheral vasoconstriction.
c. Slow speed of circulation in the extremities.

Sites to be looked for (in good natural light):

1. Tip of the nose.
2. Ear lobules.
3. Outer aspect of lips, chin and cheeks.
4. Tip of fingers and toes.
5. Nail-bed of fingers and toes.
6. Palms and soles.

- Tongue remains unaffected. Mechanism: Stagnant as well as overutilisation hypoxia.

Q. Causes of peripheral cyanosis:

1. Shock or peripheral circulatory failure due to any cause.
2. Congestive cardiac failure (reduced cardiac output).
3. Exposure to cold air or cold water (possibly the most common cause worldwide).
4. Raynaud's phenomenon (read the section on 'Scleroderma'): Only seen in fingers and toes.
5. Frost bite.
6. Arterial obstruction, e.g. peripheral vascular disease (atherosclerosis, Buerger's disease, atheroembolism).
7. Venous obstruction: Produces local cyanosis (e.g. SVC syndrome, DVT).
8. Hyperviscosity syndrome (e.g. multiple myeloma, polycythemia, macroglobulinaemia).
9. Cryoglobulinaemia (immunoglobulins which precipitate at low temperature, e.g. lymphoma).
10. Mitral stenosis (lips, tip of the nose and cheeks may be cyanosed in mitral facies).
11. Septicaemia (gram-negative organisms commonly).

Q. Central cyanosis and sites to be examined:

There is decreased arterial oxygen saturation as a result of marked reduction in oxygen tension in the arterial blood (*arterial PaO_2 is reduced*) either due to imperfect oxygenation of blood in lung, or admixture of venous and arterial blood. This is usually detected when the oxygen saturation of arterial blood goes below 85%.

Sites to be looked for (in good natural light):

1. Tongue (mainly the margins as well as the undersurface) (**Fig. 3.5**).
2. Inner aspect of lips.
3. Mucous membrane of gum, soft palate, cheeks.
4. Lower palpebral conjunctiva.
5. **Plus,** the sites mentioned in the peripheral cyanosis (one must examine these sites)—As same deoxygenated blood circulates everywhere in the body, i.e. *patients with central cyanosis will also be cyanosed peripherally*.

- Mechanism: Hypoxic hypoxia.
- In dark-skinned persons, examination of oral mucous membrane and conjunctiva are more helpful.

Q. Causes of central cyanosis:

1. Cyanotic congenital heart diseases, e.g. Fallot's tetralogy (*see* **Fig. 2.1**), transposition of great vessels.
2. Acute pulmonary oedema (due to left-sided heart failure): Most common 'cardiac' cause.
3. Eisenmenger's syndrome (ASD, VSD or PDA with reversal of shunt): Tardive cyanosis.
4. Acute severe asthma.
5. COPD, cor pulmonale, respiratory failure, ARDS; respiratory depression (e.g. opium poisoning).
6. Lobar pneumonia.
7. Fibrosing alveolitis.
8. Tension pneumothorax.
9. Acute pulmonary thromboembolism.
10. Acute laryngeal oedema.
11. Pulmonary arteriovenous shunt (congenital, or acquired due to cirrhosis of liver).
12. Absolute increase in desaturated haemoglobin, e.g. polycythemia (red cyanosis).

- Never forget, *high altitude* (usually at a height of 13000 ft, due to low partial pressure of O_2) as a cause of central cyanosis.
- In arterial blood, 95% of Hb is saturated with O_2 (i.e. only 5% reduced) whereas in venous blood the O_2 saturation is 70% (i.e. 30% reduced). Hence normally a mean of the two (5% to 30%, i.e. 0.75 g/dL to 5 g/dL reduced Hb) is present in the capillaries, and skin and mucous membrane remain pink. If the level crosses >5 g/dL, the skin becomes blue or dusky.

Clinical Wisdom

Non-specific clinical signs of hypoxaemia like tachycardia, tachypnoea, agitation or confusion may be present with central cyanosis. Cyanosis is a subjective sign and thus pulse oximetry should be done to corroborate the objective assessment of SaO_2 (i.e. percentage of O_2 saturation in arterial blood).

Q. What is 'enterogenous cyanosis' or pigment cyanosis?

When cyanosis is produced due to the presence of excessive sulphaemoglobin (>0.5 g/dL) or methaemoglobin (>1.5 g/dL) in the blood, it is known as enterogenous cyanosis. Few clinicians include it within

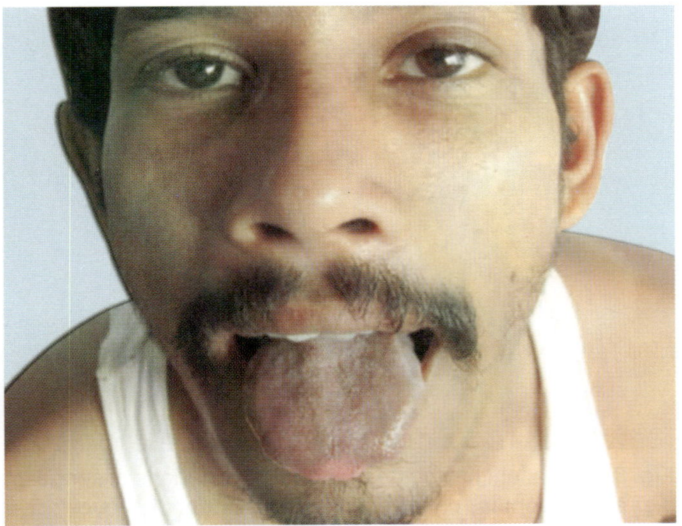

Fig. 3.6: Bluish-black tongue in **methaemoglobinaemia**

central cyanosis. The PaO_2 remains normal and thus it is called spurious cyanosis. The causes are:

1. Hereditary haemoglobin M disease (Fig. 3.6).
2. Poisoning by aniline dyes (often added in sweets).
3. Drugs like nitrates and nitrites (nitroglycerin, sodium nitroprusside, amyl nitrite), phenacetin, sulphonamides, dapsone; nitrite may be present in well-water.
4. Carboxyhaemoglobinaemia (a cherry-red flush common in smokers; not true cyanosis).

❍ Diagnosis is confirmed by spectroscopic examination of the blood.

Q. Differential diagnosis of bluish discolouration of body:

1. Cyanosis.
2. Carbon monoxide poisoning: Actually it is a cherry-red flush due to carboxyhaemoglobin. Carboxyhaemoglobin prevents the reduction of oxyhaemoglobin, and thus there is no cyanosis.
3. Argyria: Deposition of silver salts in the skin due to silver poisoning. The skin does not blanch on pressure (cyanosed skin blanches on application of pressure). It gives a slatey-grey hue.
4. Osteogenesis imperfecta (Fig. 3.7): Only the sclera is blue. Due to thinness of the sclera, the choroid with its vessels give rise to blue tinge in the eyes. Cardinal features of this disease are fragile bones with multiple fractures, blue sclera, loose-jointedness and deafness.
5. Drug like amiodarone (used in ventricular arrhythmias) may produce bluish hue in the skin (ceruloderma). Blue colour induced by metals (silver, gold, lead) and drugs (amiodarone, minocycline) is known as pseudocyanosis.

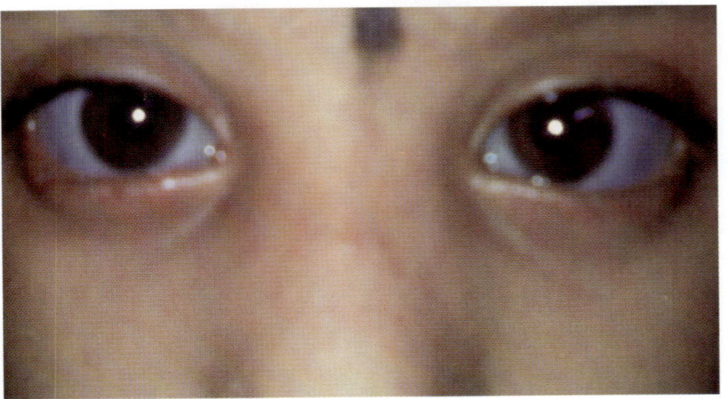

Fig. 3.7: **Blue sclera** in osteogenesis imperfecta

Q. Common aetiology of cyanosis at different ages:

- At birth: Transposition of great vessels.
- At 1 year of age: Tetralogy of Fallot (TOF).
- Middle age: VSD or ASD with Eisenmenger's syndrome, COPD.
- Old age: Chronic cor pulmonale.

Q. Central plus peripheral (mixed) cyanosis occurring in a single patient:

In mixed cyanosis, both arterial hypoxaemia and sluggish circulation are present.

1. CCF due to left-sided heart failure.
2. Acute myocardial infarction (cardiogenic shock) with acute LVF.
3. Rarely in polycythemia (red cyanosis).

❍ Remember, all causes of central cyanosis can also cause peripheral cyanosis as well.

Q. What is differential cyanosis?

1. Hands red (i.e. less blue) and feet blue: Seen in PDA with reversal of shunt (differential cyanosis).
2. Hands blue and feet red (i.e. less blue): Seen in transposition of great vessels with PDA (reverse differential cyanosis).

❍ Intermittent cyanosis is seen in Ebstein's anomaly. Cyclical cyanosis is characteristic of bilateral choanal atresia.

Q. What is orthocyanosis?

It is the development of cyanosis only in upright position due to hypoxia occurring in erect posture as a result of associated pulmonary arteriovenous malformations.

Q. What is acrocyanosis?

It is the persistent, painless bluish discolouration of the extremities, commonly affecting the hands. It is due to vasospasm in the cutaneous arteries and arterioles. It is common in newborns, emotional stress, anorexia nervosa and in some psychiatric illnesses.

Q. Facts to be remembered:

- Cyanosis with clubbing: Cyanotic congenital heart diseases, pulmonary arteriovenous fistula, fibrosing alveolitis, extensive bronchiectasis, cystic fibrosis.
- Cyanosis without clubbing: Peripheral cyanosis and acutely developing central cyanosis.
- Clubbing without cyanosis: SBE, ulcerative colitis, bronchogenic carcinoma, etc.

Q. How to diagnose enterogenous cyanosis?

1. H/o ingestion of blue sweets or drugs (mentioned earlier).
2. Skin and mucous membrane (tongue) are blue but the patient is not breathless.

Q. You are allowed to see only one site in cyanosis: what to do?

One should examine the tongue. **If the tougue is blue, the cyanosis must be central** but if the fingertips are blue, it may be either of central or peripheral in type.

Q. Other sites may be examined for central cyanosis (though not practised):

1. Nasal mucous membrane examined by nasal speculum.
2. Rectal mucous membrane seen by proctoscopy.
3. Retina examined by ophthalmoscopy.

Q. Both cyanosis and polycythemia are commonly present in:

1. Cyanotic congenital heart diseases, and
2. COPD.

- Physiological cyanosis may be seen in patients with polycythemia.

Q. How hypoxia and cyanosis are related?

- Hypoxaemia without cyanosis: Severe anaemia (Hb <5 g/dL), carbon monoxide poisoning.
- Cyanosis with hypoxaemia: If reduced Hb is >5 g/dL.
- Cyanosis without hypoxaemia: Polycythemia vera (red cyanosis).

Clinical Wisdom

After examination of the patient for cyanosis, one should examine for the presence of dyspnoea and clubbing. It should be remembered that a severely anaemic patient (Hb level <5g/dL) is possibly not cyanosed (though there is decreased arterial O_2 saturation). For cyanosis to become clinically evident, there must be a minimum quantity of reduced Hb (at least 5 g/dL) in the blood perfusing the skin.

Cyanosis is mostly seen in areas with rich blood supply along with thin epidermis (e.g. lips, ears or cheeks).

JAUNDICE — CASE 38

Q. Definition:

It is defined as yellowish discolouration of the skin and mucous membrane due to excess amount of bilirubin present in the blood (Fig. 3.8). Icterus is the technical term for jaundice.

Q. What is latent jaundice?

The normal serum bilirubin level is 0.3–1.0 mg/dL. *Clinical jaundice is evident when serum bilirubin crosses 3 mg/dL*. Jaundice is latent, i.e. clinically not appreciated

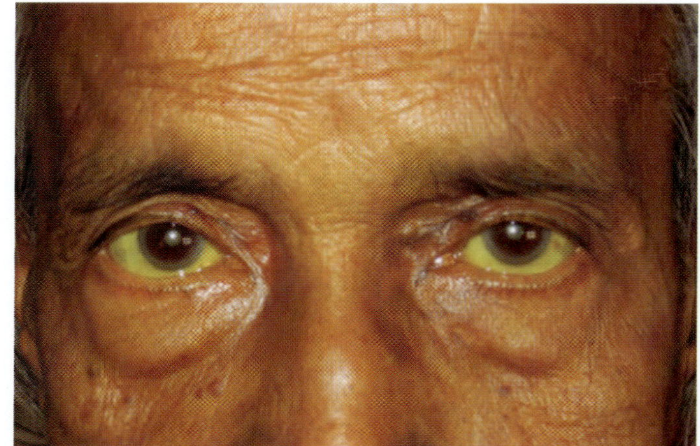

Fig. 3.8: A patient having **deep jaundice** with signs of senilities, e.g. **arcus senilis,** cataract and **'bags under the eyes'**; few seborrhoeic warts are seen around the eyes

(only detected by serum analysis) when the serum bilirubin level is in-between 1 and 3 mg/dL. Scleral icterus means serum bilirubin >3 mg/dL.

Q. Sites to be examined in a patient of jaundice:

Jaundice is always seen in bright natural daylight as it is not possible to detect light yellow colour in the presence of artificial or fluorescent light. **Take the patient in front of an open window** (never put a lighted torch) and look for:

1. Upper bulbar conjunctiva (sclera is examined by retracting the upper eyelids upwards and asking the patient to look downwards—both eyes at a time) (Fig. 3.9).
2. Undersurface of the tongue (sublingual mucosa).
3. Mucous membrane of palate (especially the soft palate).
4. Palms and soles.
5. General skin surfaces.

- Early staining by bilirubin occurs at periphery of sclera.

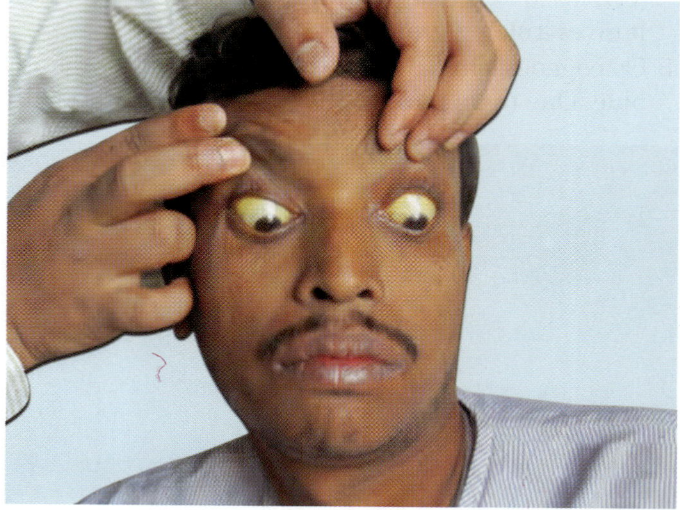

Fig. 3.9: Clinical demonstration of **jaundice**

Q. Why the upper bulbar conjunctiva is selected for examination?

1. Sclera contains a lot of elastin (bilirubin has a strong affinity for elastic tissue), and
2. A white background is formed by sclera.

Q. Differential diagnosis of jaundice (icterus):

1. Carotenaemia (carotenoderma): Skin is yellow (mainly the palms and soles, forehead and nasolabial folds) but the sclera and mucous membrane are unaffected. The serum is also yellow in colour; the stool and urine are of normal colour.
2. Quinacrine or mepacrine toxicity (previously used in malaria and tapeworm infestations): Skin, urine and eyes (only the regions of the sclera exposed to light) are yellow.
3. Diffuse xanthomatosis: Skin takes a yellowish-orange tinge.
4. Muddy sclera: Exposed part of sclera looks dirty yellow; non-pathological.
5. Old subconjunctival haemorrhage makes the conjunctiva yellowish.
6. Acriflavin and picric acid ingestion (skin yellow, sclera normal).

Q. Body secretions where bilirubin is found (in jaundice):

1. Found in body fluids like CSF, joint fluid, cysts.
2. Absent from true secretions like tears, saliva, pancreatic juice.

- Scar tissue is rarely bilirubin-stained. Bilirubin has a strong affinity for elastic tissue (sclera, skin), nervous tissue (basal ganglia) and as it binds with proteins, it is more evident in exudates. Bilirubin and biliverdin are main bile pigments.

Q. What is unilateral jaundice?

1. In patients with hemiplegia.
2. In the presence of unilateral oedema.
   Paralysed extremity and oedematous areas tend to remain less coloured as good circulation is necessary to stain the tissues.
3. Rarely, yellowish discolouration is seen in one eye when the other eye is 'artificial'.

- Right palm may look yellowish in health, who cooks at home (after using turmeric, especially in females).
- 'Artificial eye' or 'glass eye' is usually implanted due to trauma in childhood or as a result of ocular melanoma. There is no vision in that eye, no ocular movement and light reflex is absent. The eye does not glisen (dry) **(Fig. 3.10)**.

Q. Clinical classification of jaundice:

1. Haemolytic (excessive production of bilirubin due to breakdown of RBC).
2. Hepato-cellular (↓ uptake, and conjugation of bilirubin), and

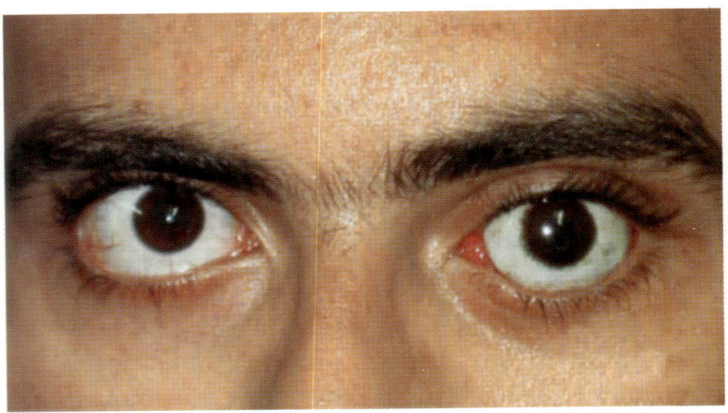

Fig. 3.10: Dry and lustreless artificial left eye (glass eye). There is absence of blood vessels and pupillary reactions

3. Obstructive (impaired excretion of bilirubin):
   a. Intrahepatic (medical).
   b. Extrahepatic (surgical).

- Jaundice is described clinically as mild(<6 mg/dL), moderate (6–15 mg/dL) and severe (>15 mg/dL).
- Jaundice may also be classified by chemical nature of bilirubin: conjugated and unconjugated hyperbilirubinaemia.
- Jaundice may be prehepatic (haemolytic), hepatic and posthepatic (obstructive).

Clinical Wisdom

Inflamed and swollen hepatocytes in acute viral hepatitis or chronic hepatitis may block biliary canaliculi, and give rise to intrahepatic obstruction.

Q. Features of haemolytic jaundice:

1. Urine: Freshly passed urine is of normal colour as there is absence of bilirubin in urine (unconjugated bilirubin is not water-soluble) but if the urine sample is kept for sometime, it turns dark yellow due to conversion of urobilinogen to urobilin (by oxidation)—**acholuric jaundice**.
2. Stool: High-coloured due to excess amount of stercobilinogen and stercobilin.
3. Jaundice: Usually mild and there is **lemon-yellow tinge** of bulbar conjunctiva. Serum bilirubin is usually less than 6 mg/dL and predominantly of unconjugated variety.
4. Anaemia (mild, moderate or severe, according to the degree of haemolytic process).
5. Splenomegaly: Very characteristic (spleen is the slaughterhouse of RBC in haemolysis).
6. The patient may have typical facies (e.g. chipmunk facies in thalassaemia).
7. Reticulocytosis in peripheral blood examination.

- In health, bilirubin cannot be detected in urine. *Urochrome and uroerythrin are the pigments which give normal urine its characteristic straw-yellow colour.* In health, urinary urobilinogen (detected by Ehrlich's aldehyde test) and fecal stercobilinogen excretion per day are 1–3.5 mg and 40–280 mg, respectively.

Q. Features of obstructive jaundice:

1. Urine: Deep yellow or mustard oil-like colour (due to presence of conjugated bilirubin).
2. Stool: Pale or clay coloured (china-clay) with steatorrhoea (steatorrhoea means frothy, bulky, pale, offensive, soft, greasy stool which floats on the water of the toilet pan, and is difficult to flush from the toilet pan) due to absence of bile pigment in the stool.
3. Jaundice: Usually deep jaundice and the bulbar conjunctiva turns **greenish-yellow** due to oxidation of bilirubin to biliverdin (green). Jaundice is gradually progressive (carcinoma of the head of pancreas) or fluctuating (stone in CBD). Serum bilirubin is usually very high and predominantly of conjugated variety **(Table 3.2)**.
4. Generalised pruritus with scratch marks in skin and shiny nails (bile salts irritate the free nerve endings; recent view is that pruritus is due to upregulation of opioid receptors and ↑ level of endogenous opioids).
5. Sinus bradycardia: Probably bile salts directly inhibit the sinoatrial (SA) node.
6. Xanthelasma around the eyes or xanthoma in the knees, buttocks may be seen due to hypercholesterolaemia (in prolonged cholestasis). Clubbing may be evident (e.g. primary biliary cirrhosis).
7. Bleeding manifestations like petechiae, purpura or ecchymosis are seen due to vitamin K deficiency (lack of bile salts produces vitamin K malabsorption as it is a fat-soluble vitamin).
8. Gallbladder: May be palpable. This indicates the site of obstruction in the bile duct and is usually due to carcinoma of the head of pancreas (not due to choledocholithiasis)—according to *Courvoisier's law*.
9. Prolonged obstructive jaundice may produce osteomalacia, bone pain, bone fracture, or night blindness due to vitamin D, or A deficiency, respectively (due to malabsorption or steatorrhoea) These type of bony changes in obstructive jaundice is known as 'hepatic osteodystrophy'.
10. Rarely, there may be hepatosplenomegaly. History of fever with chill and rigor, and pain abdomen may be present due to cholangitis. There may be abdominal pain (biliary colic) in choledocholithiasis.

- Features of *chronic cholestasis* are pruritus with scratch marks, xanthoma, bruising and bone pain.
- 'Pruritus' is an unpleasant sensation of the skin that provokes intense urge to scratch.

Table 3.2: Differentiation between surgical and medical jaundice

Features	Extrahepatic (surgical) obstruction	Intrahepatic (medical) obstruction
A. History:		
i. Age	i. Middle aged or old	i. Usually young
ii. Antecedent history	ii. Previous attack, dyspepsia	ii. History of contacts, injections or blood transfusion
iii. Rate of development of jaundice	iii. Slow	iii. Rapid
iv. Pain	iv. Common (H/o colic)	iv. Uncommon (usually ache over liver)
v. Type of jaundice	v. Fluctuates or persistent	v. Acute onset, slow fall with recovery
vi. Pruritus	vi. Characteristically prominent feature	vi. Often transient
vii. Anorexia	vii. Present but not so prominent	vii. A prominent feature
B. Examination:		
i. Splenomegaly	i. Rare	i. May be present
ii. Hepatomegaly	ii. Slightly tender hepatomegaly	ii. Markedly tender hepatomegaly
iii. Palpable gallbladder	iii. May be palpable due to carcinoma of the head of pancreas	iii. Not palpable
iv. Ascites	iv. Usually absent	iv. May be present in severe and prolonged obstruction
v. Temperature	v. May be raised (due to cholangitis)	v. Raised initially
vi. Anaemia	vi. May be present	vi. Usually absent
C. Laboratory investigations:		
i. WBC count in blood	i. Increased or normal	i. Diminished or normal
ii. Differential count of WBC	ii. Neutrophilia	ii. Increase in lymphocytes or eosinophils (in drug-induced hepatitis)
iii. Serum bilirubin	iii. Usually 3-10 mg/dL; may be more	iii. Varies with severity
iv. AST and ALT	iv. <5 times of normal	iv. >5 times of normal
v. Alkaline phosphatase	v. >3 times of normal	v. <3 times of normal
vi. Ultrasonography or CT scan	vi. May diagnose stones in CBD or carcinoma of the head of pancreas	vi. Splenomegaly
D. Therapeutic trial:		
'Prednisolone white wash' test	No response	Often +ve

Q. Features of hepato-cellular jaundice:

1. Urine: Yellowish.
2. Stool: High-coloured, and becomes pale if there is intrahepatic cholestasis.
3. Jaundice: **Orange-yellow tinge** of the bulbar conjunctiva (conjugated > unconjugated bilirubin). There is acute onset of jaundice and it is a moderate jaundice.
4. Anorexia, nausea, vomiting, fever with chill and rigor may be present before the appearance of jaundice (e.g. in viral hepatitis); may have relative bradycardia in viral hepatitis.
5. Tender hepatomegaly is frequent.
6. Variable pruritus.
7. There may be bleeding manifestations as a result of hepato-cellular failure.
8. H/o affection of other members of the family or locality (viral hepatitis), drug intake (rifampicin) or poisoning (copper sulphate), or cirrhosis of liver.

Q. Bilirubin and hepatic enzymes in different types of jaundice:

1. Haemolytic: Increase in unconjugated bilirubin along with increased urobilinogen in urine (with reticulocytosis in blood).
2. Obstructive: Increase in conjugated bilirubin along with increase in alkaline phosphatase (with pale stools).
3. Hepato-cellular: Increase in both type of bilirubin (conjugated > unconjugated) along with increased AST and ALT.

Q. Importance of 'history taking' in a patient of jaundice:

- Duration.
- Appetite, nausea, weight loss.
- H/o contact with jaundiced patient (Hep A) or recent outbreak in the community (Hep A).
- Colour of urine and stool.
- Pruritus, fever or rigor (e.g. cholangitis).
- GI bleeding (e.g. chronic liver disease).
- H/o pain abdomen (biliary colic).
- Travel history (Hep A).
- Tattooing, IV drug abuser, blood transfusion (Hep B or C).
- Drugs (e.g. rifampicin), alcohol.
- Man having sex with man, or female sex worker.
- Past H/o jaundice (recurrent), biliary surgery (recent) or pancreatitis.
- Family H/o jaundice, e.g. Wilson's disease, hereditary spherocytosis.

Q. Jaundice in CVS and respiratory disorders:

a. CVS: Infective endocarditis, severe CCF (due to congestion in liver), recent cardiac surgery (infective hepatitis), prosthetic valve-induced microangiopathic haemolysis, and hypertension being treated by methyl dopa.
b. Respiratory system: Pulmonary thromboembolism, consolidation, and amyloidosis (as a complication of bronchiectasis).

Q. Different bile salts and bile acids:

A. Bile salts: Sodium taurocholate and sodium glycocholate.
B. Bile acids:
   a. Primary: Cholic acid and chenodeoxycholic acid.
   b. Secondary: Deoxycholic and lithocholic acid.
   c. Tertiary: Ursodeoxycholic acid.

Q. What is Murphy's sign?

Ask the patient of *acute cholecystitis* to breathe in deeply, and now try to palpate the gallbladder in sitting position. There is tenderness and catch in the breath (i.e. arrested breath) at the height of inspiration with a mass felt there. This sign is not found in chronic cholecystitis. When the examination is performed with the patient lying, it is known as Moynihan's method.

Q. What is Courvoisier's law?

Palpable, non-tender, smooth gallbladder in a patient of obstructive jaundice is due to neoplastic obstruction (usually due to carcinoma of the head of pancreas) of the common bile duct (CBD), and not due to impacted stone in the CBD. In case of choledocholithiasis, the gallbladder is usually small and contracted, and thus non-palpable due to repeated cholecystitis.

Q. Common examples of different types of jaundice in city hospitals:

A. Haemolytic:

1. Thalassaemia (i.e. haemoglobinopathies).
2. Mismatched blood transfusion.
3. Snake bite (Viperidae group).
4. Malaria (especially falciparum malaria).
5. Rh incompatibility.
6. Primaquine or sulphonamide-induced (in G_6PD deficiency).

B. Obstructive:

a. Intrahepatic (medical) cholestasis:
   1. Cholestatic viral hepatitis.
   2. Chronic active hepatitis.
   3. Cirrhosis of liver (especially primary biliary cirrhosis).
   4. Lymphoma or tuberculosis.
   5. Pregnancy in last trimester (recurrent cholestasis).
   6. Drugs: Chlorpromazine, chlorpropamide, oral contraceptives, erythromycin estolate, methimazole, methyl testosterone, anabolic steroids.

7. Secondary carcinoma of liver (jaundice is rarely seen in hepatoma).
8. Dubin-Johnson syndrome.

b. Extrahepatic (surgical) cholestasis:
1. Gallstone impaction in CBD.
2. Carcinoma of the head of pancreas, periampullary carcinoma.
3. Carcinoma of the gallbladder.
4. Enlarged glands at porta hepatis.
5. Stricture of CBD.
6. Sclerosing cholangitis (from inflammatory bowel disease), cholangiocarcinoma.

C. Hepato-cellular:

1. Viral hepatitis (type A, B, C and E commonly).
2. Drugs: Rifampicin, INH, after halothane anaesthesia, paracetamol overdose.
3. Poisons: Copper sulphate.
4. Pregnancy: Acute fatty liver of pregnancy.
5. Alcoholic hepatitis, chronic hepatitis, cirrhosis of liver.
6. Weil's disease, septicaemia.
7. Right-sided heart failure.
8. Wilson's disease.

- A young person with jaundice is more likely to have viral hepatitis (take H/o travel, alcohol abuse, male homosexuality, female prostitution, blood transfusion, tattooing) whereas an elderly person with jaundice and weight loss is more likely to suffer from carcinoma of the hepatobiliary tract.
- **The causes of haemolytic jaundice are same as that of haemolytic anaemia** (*see* page 196).

Q. Diseases present as latent jaundice:

1. Mitral stenosis (i.e. passive venous congestion of liver).
2. Congestive cardiac failure.
3. Acute myocardial infarction.
4. Acute pulmonary thromboembolism.
5. Cirrhosis of liver.
6. Pernicious anaemia.
7. Acute pancreatitis.

Q. Fluctuating or intermittent jaundice:

1. Gilbert's syndrome.
2. Stone impaction in CBD (Charcot's biliary triad).
3. Periampullary carcinoma.
4. Haemolytic anaemias.
5. Chronic hepatitis.
6. Spasm of bile duct.
7. Recurrent pancreatitis.

Q. What is 'prednisolone white wash' test?

If 30 mg of prednisolone (reduces cellular oedema) is given daily for 5 days to a patient of hepato-cellular jaundice with features of obstruction (e.g. cholestatic viral hepatitis), there is a 40% fall in serum bilirubin. This test differentiates between medical and surgical obstructive jaundice (in a desperate situation) and gives positive result in medical jaundice. The test should not be used routinely. Before doing the test, hepatitis B and C markers must be negative.

Q. Fractionation of normal bilirubin:

Normal serum bilirubin level is 0.3–1.0 mg/dL.

i. Conjugated fraction is 0.1–0.3 mg/dL, and
ii. Unconjugated fraction is 0.2–0.7 mg/dL.

Q. Differences between conjugated and unconjugated bilirubin:

	Unconjugated	Conjugated
1. Water solubility	0	+
2. Affinity for lipids	+	0
3. Renal excretion	0	+
4. van den Bergh reaction	Indirect	Direct

Q. Familial non-haemolytic hyperbilirubinaemias:

Unconjugated hyperbilirubinaemia:

1. Gilbert's syndrome.
2. Crigler-Najjar syndrome (types I and II).

Conjugated hyperbilirubinaemia:

1. Dubin-Johnson syndrome.
2. Rotor syndrome.

- In Dubin-Johnson syndrome, the liver is stained by melanin in the centrilobular zone.

Q. Predominantly conjugated and unconjugated hyperbilirubinaemias:

A. Conjugated hyperbilirubinaemia (with >50% conjugated fraction):

i. Viral or drug-induced hepatitis.
ii. Drug-induced cholestasis.
iii. Cholestatic jaundice of pregnancy.
iv. Cirrhosis of liver.
v. Extrahepatic biliary obstruction (stone in CBD).
vi. Dubin-Johnson syndrome.
vii. Rotor syndrome.
viii. Secondary carcinoma of liver.

- Among steps of bilirubin metabolism (uptake, conjugation and excretion), excretion is the rate-limiting step and is usually affected most. Thus, conjugated hyperbilirubinaemia predominates in hepato-cellular diseases.

B. Unconjugated hyperbilirubinaemia (usually with >80% unconjugated fraction):

i. Haemolysis.
ii. Ineffective erythropoiesis.
iii. Prolonged fasting (<300 cal/day).
iv. Sepsis.
v. Gilbert's syndrome and rarely, Crigler-Najjar syndrome.
vi. Neonatal jaundice.

Q. Hepatic disorders uncommonly associated with jaundice:

1. Hepato-cellular carcinoma (hepatoma).
2. Amoebic liver abscess.
3. Cystic disease of liver.

Q. Both jaundice and anaemia seen in a patient:

1. Haemolytic anaemia (i.e. thalassaemia, sickle cell anaemia).
2. Vitamin B_{12} deficiency.

Q. Can you detect jaundice at night?

As previously discussed, jaundice should always be seen in broad daylight. But in a desperate situation, one has to examine the patient for jaundice at night remembering that in the presence of artificial light:

- Mild jaundice may be missed.
- Severely anaemic patient seems to have mild jaundice.
- Fluorescent or tube light gives yellow reflection in normal eye mimicking jaundice.

Q. Medical causes of extrahepatic obstruction:

1. Sclerosing cholangitis in ulcerative colitis.
2. Obstruction by round worm in CBD.
3. Enlarged lymph nodes at porta hepatis in lymphoma.

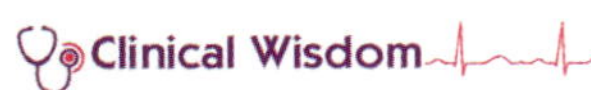

Never put lighted torch inside the oral cavity to diagnose anaemia, cyanosis or jaundice.

- Highest level of bilirubin is observed in hepato-cellular jaundice (may be >50 mg/dL). In cholestatic (obstructive) jaundice, bilirubin may reach up to 40 mg/dL and then remains around 30–40 mg/dL as a result of balance between renal excretion and conversion of bilirubin to other metabolites. In hepato-cellular jaundice, this balance is not seen rather high level of bilirubin may be explained by concomitant haemolysis and renal insufficiency.

PULSE — CASE 39

Q. Definition:

It is the expansion and elongation of the arterial wall imparted by the column of blood, and is passively produced by the pressure changes during ventricular systole and diastole. Commonly we examine the pulse in the radial artery in hand, which is one of the most accessible peripheral artery. Moreover, as soon as the hand (radial artery) of a patient is touched, it builds the doctor-patient relationship.

Pulse, blood pressure, respiration and temperature are regarded as **'vital signs'** in clinical medicine. O_2 saturation in peripheral capillaries (SpO_2) is regarded as 5th vital sign by some clinicians.

Q. Points to note in examination of pulse:

1. Rate.
2. Rhythm.
3. Volume.
4. Condition of the arterial wall.
5. Comparison between two radial pulses.
6. Radio-femoral delay.
7. Any special character.
8. Palpation of other peripheral arteries.

Clinical Wisdom

Pulse should always be described under these eight points. 'Tension' is the indirect estimation of blood pressure. Estimation of tension by palpation is totally unreliable and thus, it is not included within the points under examination of pulse. Tension (i.e. blood pressure) should be accurately measured by sphygmomanometer.

Q. How to examine the pulse (Fig. 3.11)?

The radial pulse at the right wrist of the patient (present lateral to the flexor carpi radialis tendon) is generally examined with the pulp of three fingers (index, middle and ring finger) by compressing the artery against head of the radius; the ring finger blocks the retrograde flow, index finger stabilises (holds steady) the artery over the bone, and middle finger perceives the waveforms and counts the pulse—'the **trisection method**'. The patient's forearm will be semipronated and the wrist slightly flexed during examination of radial pulse.

The rate and rhythm are better palpated in the radial artery. To note the volume and character of the arterial pulse, one should examine the carotid artery (it is the nearest pulse to the aorta). Pulsus alternans, pulsus paradoxus and collapsing pulse are better felt in radial artery. Brachial artery is felt for pulsus bisferiens and also to record blood pressure.

Q. How to count the rate?

Always count the beats for 15 seconds and multiply by four to get the pulse rate but it is worthwhile to remember that in a patient with arrhythmia (also in bradycardia and tachycardia), one must count the beats for at least one minute.

Q. What are the variations in pulse rate?

Definition of rate: Number of beats per minute. Normally it ranges between 60 and 100 beats per minute

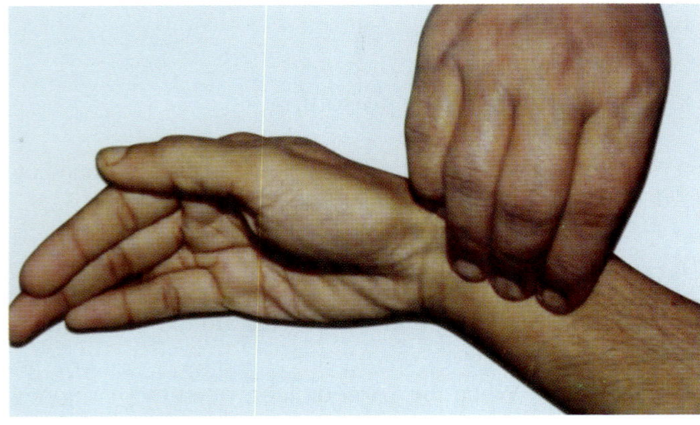

Fig. 3.11: Palpation of **radial artery** ('the pulse')

(average 72 beats per minute in an adult). Usually it remains 140 beats per minute at birth. SA node is the natural pacemaker of the heart (i.e. the normal cardiac rhythm is **'sinus rhythm'**—72 beats/minute).

A. Tachycardia: Pulse rate is above 100 per minute. Normally it is found in children.

a. Sinus tachycardia: Pulse rate is above 100 per minute where the impulse is originating from the SA node. The heart rate in sinus tachycardia varies between 100 and 160 per minute. The common causes are:
   i. Exercise, emotion, excitement, smoking, intense pain, anxiety, and in children.
   ii. Heart failure.
   iii. Thyrotoxicosis.
   iv. Severe anaemia.
   v. Pyrexia.
   vi. Shock (e.g. acute myocardial infarction).
   vii. Myocarditis.
   viii. Acute haemorrhage.
   ix. Pregnancy.
   x. Hypoxia.
   xi. Drugs like salbutamol, nifedipine or atropine.
b. Relative tachycardia: Read the section on 'Abnormal temperature'.
c. Paroxysmal tachycardia: Pulse rate is above 160 beats per minute. It is divided into two types:
   1. Supraventricular (PSVT) [i.e. atrial (PAT) or nodal (PNT)].
   2. Ventricular (VT).

Common causes of paroxysmal tachycardia are rheumatic carditis, ischaemic heart disease (IHD), thyrotoxicosis, hypertensive heart disease, cardiomyopathy, WPW syndrome.

B. Bradycardia: Pulse rate is below 60 per minute. It is commonly found in:

i. Athletes, yoga, meditation or during deep sleep.
ii. Myxoedema.
iii. Obstructive jaundice.
iv. Increased intracranial tension.
v. Drugs like β-blockers or digitalis.
vi. Hypothermia.
vii. 2° heart blook, complete heart block (CHB).
viii. Sick sinus syndrome (sino-atrial disease).
ix. Vasovagal attacks.
x. Severe hypoxia.
xi. Organophosphorus poisoning.

- Athletes, yoga and meditation develop a high vagal tone but during sleep the sympathetic activity is reduced.

Clinical Wisdom

Regular athletic training and myxoedema are the commonest causes of bradycardia.

Nodal rhythm: When the SA node fails, often the AV node originates impulse at the rate of 40–60 per minute resulting in a pulse rate of 40–60 per minute; **Idioventricular rhythm**: When cardiac impulse arises from the ventricular walls at the rate of 36 per minute, the pulse rate at ventricular rhythm will be 36 (30–40) per minute, and is known as idioventricular rhythm.

a. Sinus bradycardia: Pulse rate is below 60 per minute where the impulse is originating from the SA node. The common causes are: All the causes mentioned above in 'bradycardia' except complete heart block (in CHB, idioventricular rhythm occurs at the rate of 36 per minute; it is not sinus rhythm).
b. Relative bradycardia: Read the section on 'Abnormal temperature'.

- Tachycardia (Greek takhus = swift, kardia = heart); Bradycardia (Greek bradus = slow, kardia = heart).

Q. Bradycardia associated with convulsions:

1. Complete heart block (Stokes-Adams syndrome).
2. Increased intracranial tension due to meningo-encephalitis, brain tumour, CVA.
3. Prior to development of coma in myxoedema.

Q. Disproportionately rapid pulse in shock:

1. Acute myocardial infarction.
2. Septic shock.
3. Myocarditis.
4. Tachyarrhythmias.

Q. Possible causes of increased sleeping pulse rate:

1. Thyrotoxicosis.
2. Rheumatic carditis.
3. Atrial fibrillation.
4. Atropinised patient.
5. Myocarditis due to any cause.
6. Fever due to any cause; sometimes in REM sleep.

Q. What is pulse deficit (i.e. apex-pulse deficit)?

Definition: It is the difference between the heart rate (ventricular rate) and the pulse rate. It is commonly found in atrial fibrillation and multiple ectopic beats. The methods of detection of pulse deficit are:

1. First count the heart rate for one minute and then the pulse rate for next one minute (examination in two different cardiac cycles): Commonly practised method, or
2. One examiner counts the heart rate and the other examiner counts the pulse rate at the same time (using single cardiac cycle) for one minute (best method) **(Fig. 3.12)**, or
3. One may put his stethoscope at the apex and simultaneously count the dropped beats in the pulse (using single cardiac cycle) for one minute.

- Pulse deficit is obtained in atrial fibrillation (>10/min) and multiple ectopics (<10/min), and is due to the fact that some weak hearbeats are not transmitted to the peripheral arteries.

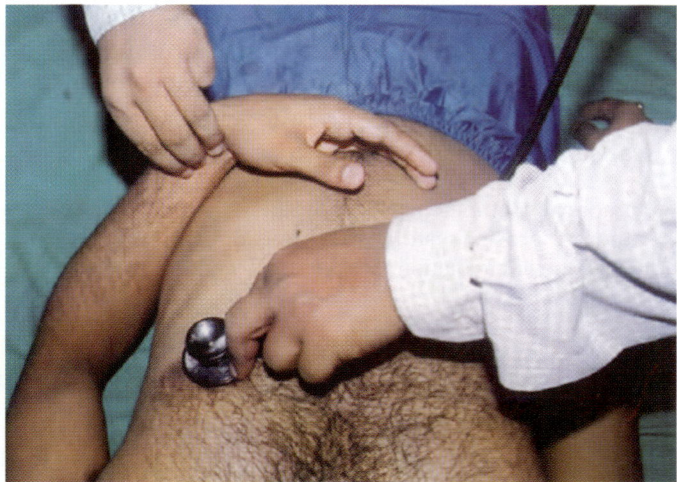

Fig. 3.12: Examining **'pulse deficit'** simultaneously by two examiners

Q. What is an ectopic beat?

In ectopic rhythm, the impulse arises from sites other than the SA node, and may arise from the atrial wall, AV node or ventricular wall. The ectopic beat is small, occurs prematurely and is followed by a compensatory pause. The compensatory pause results in a 'missed' or 'dropped' beat in pulse.

Pulse felt at the wrist (cadence): Small pause followed by small beat (i.e. the ectopic), big pause followed by big beat.

Causes: Overindulgence of tea, coffee, cigarettes, alcohol; anxiety, dyspepsia; rheumatic, ischaemic, hypertensive, thyrotoxic and cardiomyopathic heart diseases, digitalis overdose.

Synonym of ectopic beat: Premature beat, extrasystoles.

- Ectopic beats occur as occasional or repeated irregularities superimposed on a regular pulse rhythm.

Q. How can you modify ectopics (supraventricular) in a patient?

Ectopics can be abolished by vagotonic procedures, and vagolytic procedures increase the ectopics. When ectopic pace-maker is situated in the atrium (producing paroxysmal atrial tachycardia), vagotonic procedures often terminate the attack. Vagotonic procedures have no effect on ventricular tachycardia.

Vagotonic procedures: Mechanical measures like *carotid sinus massage* (the patient lies flat with extended neck. Exclude occlusive carotid disease, i.e. there should not be any carotid bruit. Now put your left thumb first on the right side of the neck at the level of the upper border of thyroid cartilage and massage for 3–5 seconds at a time; next try on the left side with right thumb), self-induced gagging or vomiting, pressure over the eyeballs, valsalva manoeuvre, coughing as well as breath holding, 'duck-diving reflex' (i.e. ice water splashed over face), head lowering between the knees, stretching the arms and body; drug like digitalis.

Vagolytic procedures: Exercise; drugs like atropine and amyl nitrite.

- Exercise increases supraventricular ectopics and diminishes ventricular ectopics.

Q. Irregularities in the rhythm:

Rhythm is the spacing of successive beats (pulse wave) in time. Normal pulse is regular in rhythm and is known as **sinus rhythm**, because it is generated by the SA node. Irregularities (i.e. *arrhythmia*) are of two types:

1. **Regularly irregular**, i.e. irregularity comes at regular interval and is seen in extrasystoles, 2° heart block, sinus arrhythmia, pulsus bigeminus, etc.
2. **Irregularly irregular** or completely irregular, i.e. irregularity between two pulse beats in every aspect (rate, rhythm, volume, etc., i.e. totally chaotic). It is commonly seen in atrial fibrillation, multiple ventricular extrasystoles, atrial flutter with varying degrees of heart block, etc.

Q. What is sinus arrhythmia?

Definition: It is the increase in pulse rate with inspiration and decrease in pulse rate with expiration. It is a physiological phenomenon, which is commonly observed in children and athletes.

Mechanism: The increased amount of blood which comes in the left ventricle in expiration increases the stroke volume. This event immediately stimulates the baroreceptors (i.e. vagal stimulation) leading to slowing of the heart rate.

- Sinus arrhythmia may be absent in CCF and autonomic neuropathy.

Q. Differentiation between multiple (ventricular) ectopics and atrial fibrillation (AF):

Both the conditions present as irregularly irregular pulse. So, they have to be differentiated:

1. First count the pulse rate. If it is >100 per minute, it is AF but if the pulse rate is <100 per minute, it may be multiple ectopics or digitalised AF (treated case of AF).
2. The ectopic beat is a small one and occurs prematurely. So one may get the typical cadence of: Small pause followed by small beat, big pause (compensatory pause) followed by big beat. If this typical cadence is felt, it is ectopic and not a case of atrial fibrillation (totally chaotic).
3. Now **count the pulse deficit**. If it is >10, it is AF. If the pulse deficit is <10, again it may be multiple ectopios or digitalised AF. To differentiate between the last two, following measures are adopted.
4. The patient is allowed to do **mild exercise** (if the condition permits). He will sit from lying down position and touch the toes with his fingers, and will lie down again. This is done for 5–6 times

successively. It is known that the heart of AF becomes more irregular after exercise. If after exercise the pulse deficit goes above 10, it is a case of digitalised AF and if the pulse deficit remains same (below 10) or diminished, the diagnosis of multiple ectopics becomes obvious.

5. Next the patient is examined for:
   a. JVP: a-wave is absent in AF; a-wave is present in multiple ectopics.
   b. S_1: Varying intensity of S_1 in AF; no change in multiple ectopics.
   c. Auscultation of the apex: If MS is the aetiology of AF, presystolic component of the murmur will disappear; no change of murmur in multiple ectopics.
6. ECG: 'P' waves will be replaced by 'f' waves in AF; ectopics are easily diagnosed by ECG.
7. Fluoroscopy: Definite contraction of atria is absent in AF. Atria contracts normally in ectopics.

Q. Irregular rhythm with normal heart rate:

1. Multiple extrasystoles, 2. Digitalised AF, 3. Sinus arrhythmia.

- Arrhythmias with regular rhythm: 1° heart block, atrial flutter, ventricular tachycardia.

Q. What is volume of the pulse?

It is the amplitude of the pulse wave, or the excursion/uplift felt at the wrist, and usually **reflects the width of pulse pressure** (systolic BP minus diastolic BP), which depends on two factors:

i. Stroke volume, and
ii. Compliance of the arteries.

The carotid, brachial or femoral arteries are more useful for assessing pulse volume and character than the radial pulse. Normal pulse pressure is 30–60 mm of Hg (i.e. normal pulse volume).

Q. What are the changes in the pulse volume?

A. High volume pulse (pulsus magnus; pulse pressure >60 mm of Hg):

1. Hyperkinetic circulatory states like:
   i. After exercise.
   ii. Severe anaemia.
   iii. Pyrexia.
   iv. Pregnancy.
   v. Aortic incompetence.
   vi. Thyrotoxicosis.
   vii. Arteriovenous communications like PDA, Paget's disease, etc.
   viii. Chronic cor pulmonale.
   ix. Hepato-cellular failure.
   x. Hypercarbia.
   xi. Beriberi.
2. Atherosclerosis (the arteries are rigid, i.e. less compliant; so there is wide pulse pressure as the systolic BP is high) or systemic hypertension.
3. Complete heart block or bradycardia due to any cause.

- In aortic incompetence: Systolic BP ↑ and diastolic BP ↓; atherosclerosis: systolic BP ↑ and diastolic BP normal; hyperkinetic circulation: Systolic BP ↑ and diastolic BP near normal.

B. Low volume pulse (pulsus parvus; pulse pressure <30 mm of Hg):

1. Shock due to any cause, e.g. acute myocardial infarction, massive haemorrhage, hypovolaemia or septicaemic shook (as a result of poor vascular tone), cardiogenic shock.
2. Severe aortic stenosis or tight mitral stenosis.
3. Peripheral arterial disease.
4. Congestive cardiac failure.
5. Pericardial effusion.
6. Constrictive pericarditis.

- Varying volume of pulse (a combination of high, low and normal volume) is common in atrial fibrillation, ventricular tachycardia and Takayasu's arteritis.

Q. What is a thready pulse?

This is a low volume pulse with rapid pulse rate. This type of pulse is seen in peripheral circulatory failure, e.g. cardiogenic shock, haemorrhage or dehydration.

- 'Jerky pulse' (spike and dome waveform pattern) is felt in idiopathic hypertrophic subaortic stenosis (IHSS).

Q. What is a bounding pulse?

It is commonly seen in hyperkinetic circulatory states where the pulse volume is high (due to high pulse pressure) with increased blood flow.

Q. How to assess the condition of the arterial wall?

Normally the arterial wall is impalpable and *may be palpable in old age due to arteriosclerosis*. The artery becomes tortuous, thickened and feels like a cord in arteriosclerosis which is known as "Monckeberg's medial sclerosis" or Osler's sign (calcification of the medial coat of large arteries). This is an age-related change; remember, atherosclerosis occurs in intima, having no tortuosity and is often associated with occlusive arterial disease. In the presence of thickened and tortuous artery, one may observe locomotor brachialis. Condition of the arterial wall is assessed by:

a. Compress the brachial artery above the elbow by ball of the left thumb (i.e. making a bloodless column) and now roll the radial artery over radius by index and middle fingers of the right hand, or
b. First place the index and middle fingers of both the left and right hand over the radial artery side by

side and exsanguinate the artery by moving the two middle fingers in opposite direction. The radial artery is now rolled over the radius by two index fingers.

Q. Causes of absent radial pulse:

1. Anatomical abnormality (aberrant radial artery or congenital anomaly).
2. Severe atherosclerosis.
3. Takayasu's disease.
4. Embolism into the radial artery.
5. [Death].

- Raynaud's disease does not affect the peripheral pulse because it is a disease of arterioles.

Q. Inequality between two radial pulses (radio-radial delay):

Simultaneously palpate both the radial arteries of the patient by both of your hands, using your left hand for patient's right hand and *vice-versa* for the other hand. **In health, there is no radio-radial delay**. The causes of inequality or radio-radial delay are:

1. Normal anatomical variations.
2. Thoracic inlet syndrome, e.g. cervical rib.
3. Aneurysm of the arch of aorta.
4. Pre-subclavian coarctation.
5. Supravalvular aortic stenosis (congenital).
6. Pulseless disease (Takayasu's arteritis).
7. Peripheral embolism or atheromatous plaque.
8. Atherosclerosis of aorta.
9. Pressure over axillary artery by lymph nodes.
10. Iatrogenic: Blalock-Taussig shunt operation in Tetralogy of Fallot.

Q. Causes of radio-femoral delay:

For detection of radio-femoral delay, standing on the right side of the patient, one should palpate the radial artery with the left hand and femoral artery with the right hand simultaneously (Fig. 3.13). **Normally, in health, there is no radio-femoral delay** (in health, radial and femoral pulsations are felt equally and synchronously) but it should be remembered that the pulsation of arteria dorsalis pedis comes 0.02 to 0.03 seconds later than the radial artery. In radio-femoral delay, the femoral pulse is of small volume and occurs after the radial pulse. Causes of radio-femoral delay are:

1. Coarctation of aorta (important bedside diagnostic clue in a young hypertensive).
2. Atherosclerosis of aorta.
3. Thrombosis or embolism of aorta.
4. Aortoarteritis.

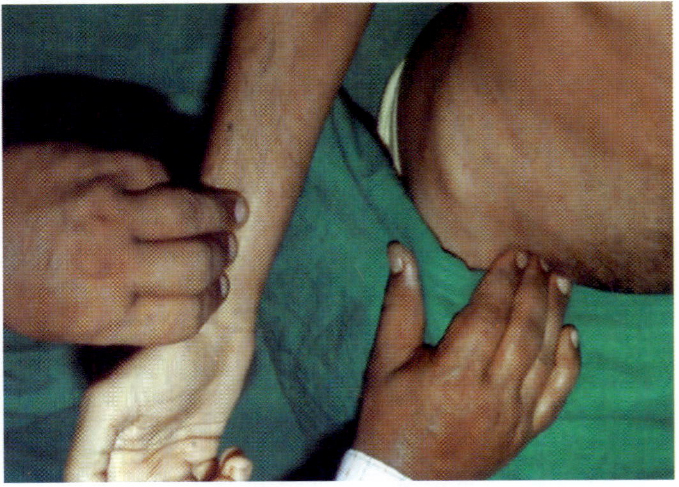

Fig. 3.13: Examination for **radio-femoral delay**

Q. Basic bedside features and common investigations of coarctation of aorta:

1. Commonly a young male patient with hypertension, headache, epistaxis, intermittent claudication, palpitations, anginal pain or cold extremities.
2. The upper extremity and thorax may be well-developed in comparison to lower extremities.
3. Upper extremity pulses are normal. Palpation of pulses may reveal **radio-femoral dealy** (symmetrical reduction and delay of femoral pulses in comparison to radial pulses). All the pulses like radial, carotid, brachial, femoral, popliteal and *arteria dorsalis pedis* should be examined on both sides in details. Pulsation of arteria dorsalis pedis may be absent.
4. Prominent suprasternal and carotid pulsation.
5. Collateral pulsations are present (seen as well as felt) in axilla, trunk and infrascapular area (Suzman's sign). Suzman's sign (dilated, tortuous and pulsatile arteries) is best elicited when the patient stands and bends forward with arms hanging down at sides.
6. **Systemic hypertension** (upper extremity high BP with low or normal BP in lower extremity).
7. Bruit over the collaterals.
8. Left ventricular type of cardiac enlargement (heaving apical impulse); a systolic murmur may be heard over the anterior chest and back. Continuous murmur may be present over collaterals.
9. Clinical associations: Bicuspid aortic valve, PDA, VSD, berry aneurysm of circle of Willis, polycystic kidneys, Turner's syndrome.
10. Fundoscopy: Retinal arteries are tortuous with frequent 'U'-turn (cork-screw appearance). Curiously, hypertensive retinopathy is rare.
11. Rib notching from 3rd to 8th rib in chest X-ray due to dilated collaterals—Known as *Dock's sign*. Also there are poorly developed aortic knuckle and cardiomegaly.
12. Barium swallow of oesophagus shows double indentations due to pre- and post-coarctation dilatation: '3 sign' or 'reverse E sign'.
13. ECG: LVH.
14. Complications: Severe hypertension leading to complications like stroke, subarachnoid haemorrhage (due to ruptured berry aneurysm), premature CAD and LVH, infective endocarditis.

15. Confirmation: CT and CMR (cardiac magnetic resonance) angiography are confirmatory. Echocardiography and aortography may be done.
16. Management: Treatment of hypertension and LVH; balloon dilatation with stent insertion, or surgery with end-to-end anastomosis by Dacron or Teflon graft.

- Post-subclavian type is the commonest variety of coarctaion of aorta.
- Reverse coarctation (pulse absent in upper limbs but present in lower limbs) is seen in Takayasu's disease.

Q. Examination of other peripheral pulses (Fig. 3.14):

1. Ulnar artery: At the wrist on medial side where it crosses the distal end of radius.
2. Brachial artery: Palpated by the thumb (left thumb for left arm and *vice versa* for right arm) at or just above the elbow (in the antecubital fossa, just medial to the tendon of biceps muscle).
3. Subclavian artery: Ask the patient to shrug his shoulders. The artery is felt from behind by pressing the index finger downwards, from above the middle of the clavicle.
4. Carotid artery (Fig. 3.15): Palpated with the thumb (left thumb for right carotid and *vice versa*), medial to sternomastoid, and at or just below the level of thyroid cartilage. Pressure over the carotid sinus may sometimes induce syncope and this is why carotid artery should always be palpated one by one with the patient lying in bed. Dancing carotids in AI, slow upstroke in AS and jerky carotids are characteristic of HOCM.
5. Femoral artery (*see* Fig. 3.13 where the right hand is palpating femoral artery): Lies midway between anterior superior illac spine and pubic tubercle (i.e. mid-inguinal point), at the level of the groin or inguinal ligament. Femoral artery his lateral to femoral vein.

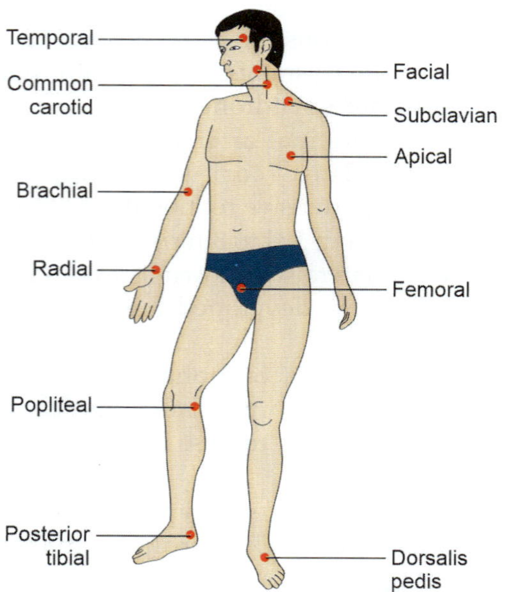

Fig. 3.14: Different **peripheral pulses**

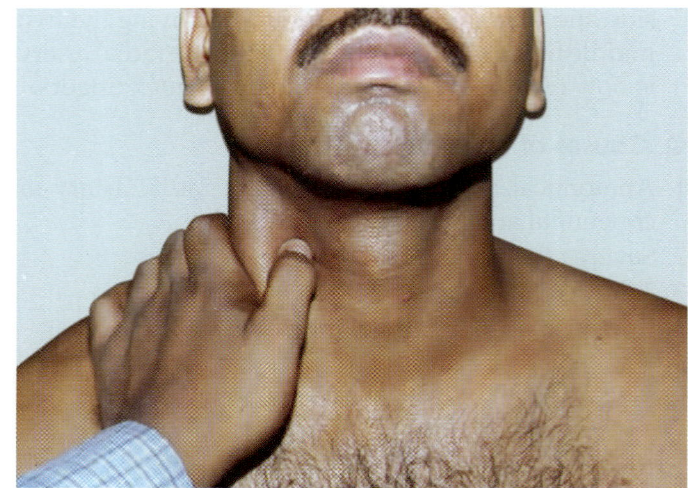

Fig. 3.15: Palpation of **carotid artery** (carotid pulse)

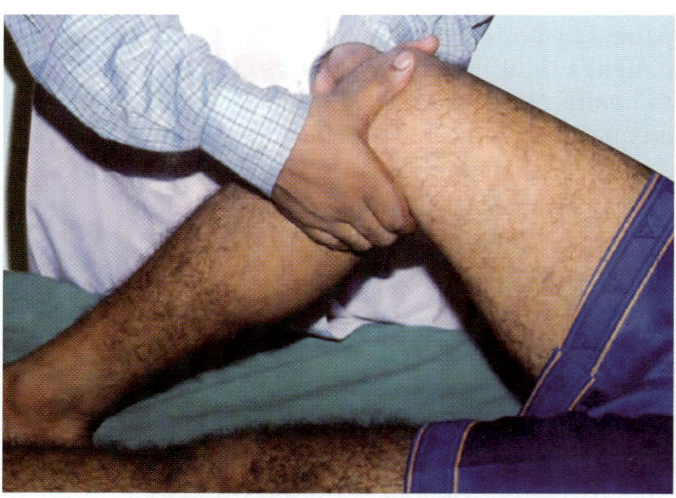

Fig. 3.16: Examination of **popliteal artery**

6. Popliteal artery (Fig. 3.16): The patient lies supine with semiflexed knee at 45°. The fingertips of both hands are pressed in the middle of the popliteal fossa (i.e. knee crease) while both thumbs rest on tibial tuberosity. It may be palpated in prone position with knee partly flexed.
7. Posterior tibial artery (Fig. 3.17): Lies approximately in the midway between the medial malleolus and heel; better palpated after inversion of the foot as it causes relaxation of the flexor retinaculum.
8. Arteria dorsalis pedis (Fig. 3.18): Palpated lateral to the extensor hallucis longus tendon on the 'proximal' part of dorsum of the foot; it may be absent in about 10% normal subject. Before palpation, make the extensor hallucis longus tendon prominent by asking the patient to extend his great toe against resistance (Fig. 3.19).

Clinical Wisdom

Duration at which pulse wave arrives in different arteries after systole is—carotid artery: 30 msec, brachial artery: 60 msec, femoral artery: 75 msec and radial artery: 80 msec.

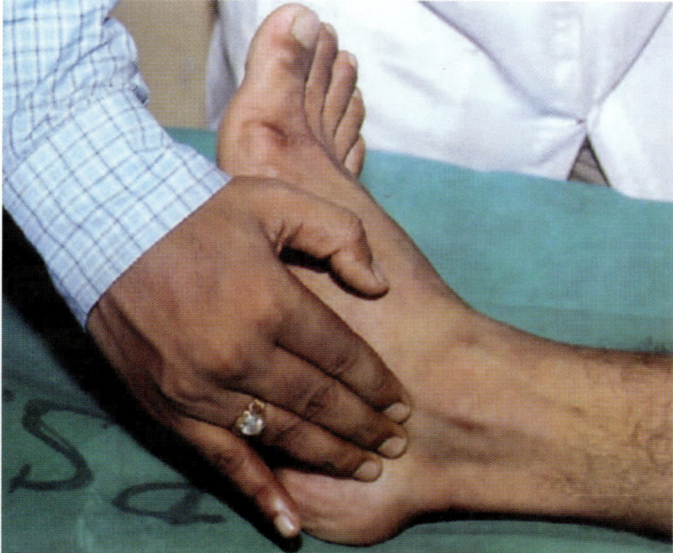

Fig. 3.17: Palpation of **posterior tibial artery**

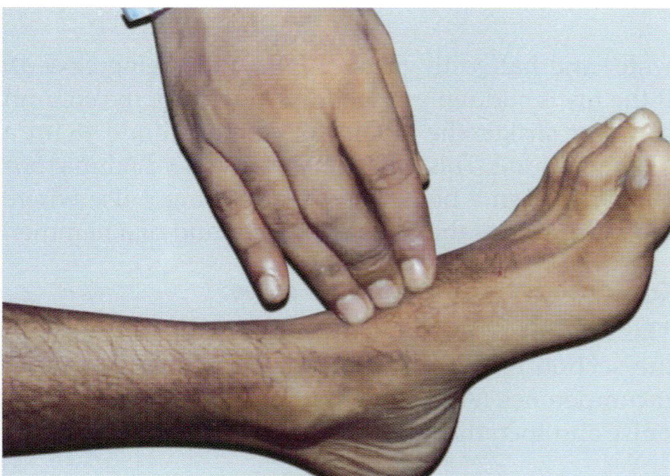

Fig. 3.18: Palpation of **arteria dorsalis pedis** (pedal pulse)

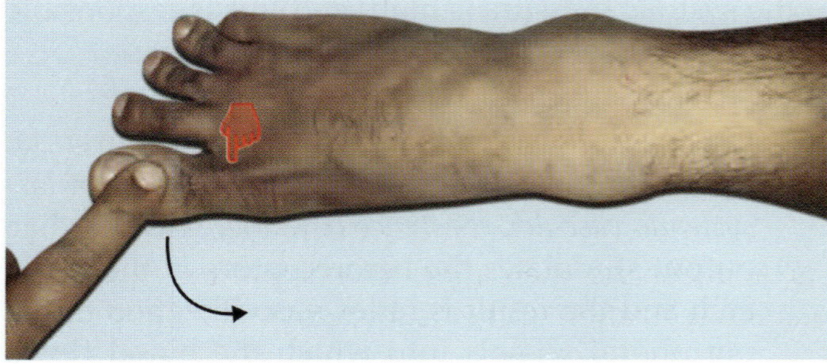

Fig. 3.19: Muscle power testing of **extensor hallucis longus**

Q. Describe the normal arterial pulse (adult):

The rate is 72 per minute. The beats are regular in rhythm, and normal as well as equal in volume. There is no inequality between the two upper limbs, and the upper and the lower limbs. The condition of the arterial wall is normal (neither thickened nor tortuous, i.e. the vessel wall is soft) and the pulses are of normal **character (catacrotic pulse)**. All the peripheral pulses are symmetrically palpable.

- Character of pulse is described in the section on 'Water-hammer pulse'. Throbbing carotids in aortic incompetence is known as "Corrigan's pulse".
- Examination of the pulse is one of the most ancient and time-honoured practice of the medical profession. Try to **comment on pulse deficit** while describing the pulse of atrial fibrillation.
- Pulse becomes faster (rapid) after a meal, after smoking, during menstruation and in the evening.

WATER-HAMMER PULSE — CASE 40

Q. Define 'character' of pulse:

The volume, waveform and some special features (e.g. collapsing nature) altogether give rise to character of the pulse, which is often helpful to clinical diagnosis of specific diseases or disorders.

Q. Different 'characters' of pulse (Fig. 3.20):

1. Anacrotic pulse.
2. Dicrotic pulse.
3. Water-hammer pulse.
4. Pulsus bisferiens.
5. Pulsus alternans.
6. Pulsus bigeminus.
7. Pulsus paradoxus.
8. Thready pulse, jerky pulse, bounding pulse.

Q. What is catacrotic pulse (Fig. 3.20)?

The normal arterial pulse is known as catacrotic pulse which is described in the section on 'Pulse'. It has following waves:

- Percussion wave (P, the rapid upstroke in pulse, and is produced by ejected blood in arterial system).

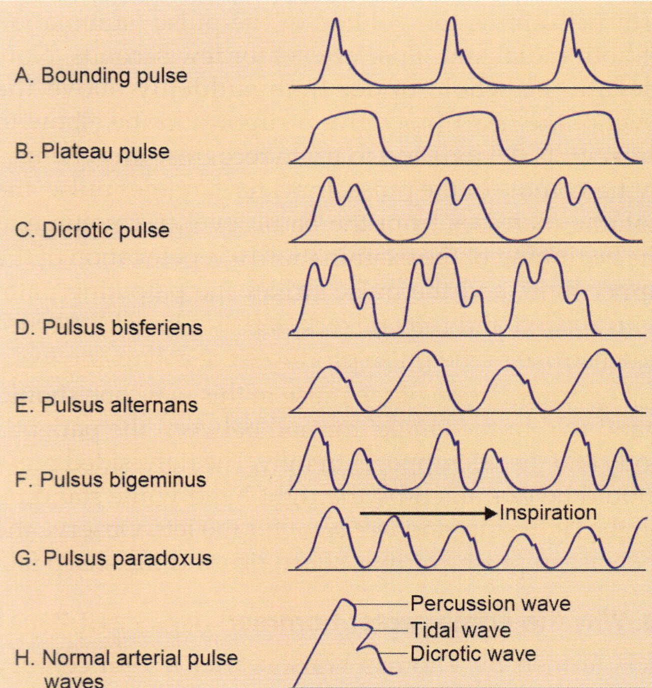

Fig. 3.20: Different **pulse waves**

- Tidal wave (T, the second small upstroke, and is generated along the arterial wall).
- Dicrotic notch and dicrotic wave (in downstroke of pulse; due to elastic recoil of the vessel).

The wavy patttern in pulse is not felt in health since it is obliterated by normal vascular tone.

Q. What is pulse pressure and mean arterial pressure?

Pulse pressure is the difference between systolic and diastolic BP (roughly reflects the volume of the pulse). Mean arterial pressure is approximately the arithmetic mean of diastolic and systolic pressure, and is calculated by diastolic pressure plus 1/3rd of pulse pressure.

Q. What is water-hammer pulse (or high volume collapsing pulse):

This is characterised by:

1. High volume pulse.
2. Sharp rise (i.e. percussion wave).
3. Ill-sustained, and
4. Sharp fall (i.e. collapse).

A high volume pulse gives the water-hammer character when the pulse pressure is at least above 60 mm of Hg. A **collapsing pulse** occurs where there is rapid run-off of blood from the aorta or the arterial system. The collapsing nature (pulse disappears fast from palpating hand) is often reliably detected by palpation of the carotid artery.

> ❍ All collapsing pulses are of high volume but all high volume pulses are not necessarily collapsing.

Q. Demonstration of water-hammer pulse (Fig. 3.21A):

Palpate the wrist in such a way that your webs fall on the radial artery and rest of the palm lies over the ulnar artery. Examine the volume of the pulse (summation of both radial and ulnar artery) for few seconds. Now elevate the whole upper limb suddenly above the level of the heart (may give a support in the elbow to prevent its flexion) and to try to recognise any changes in the volume of the pulse. In water-hammer pulse, the volume increases from the basal level (i.e. volume at the beginning of the examination) after elevation of the upper limb, and the pulse strikes the palpating palm with a rapid and forceful jerk (felt as a knock). Abrupt downstroke of the pulse produces the collapsing feel.

For examination of the pulse in this way, one should stand within the 'angle' formed between the patient's body and the said upper extremity. The right-sided pulse should be examined by the right hand while standing on the right side, and *vice versa* for the left. Observe the increase in pulse volume, sharp rise and the sharp fall.

Q. Why the name 'water-hammer' (Fig. 3.21B)?

It is termed by Thomas Watson after a 19th century victorian toy called 'water-hammer'. This is a peculiar toy where a sealed glass cylinder is half-filled with

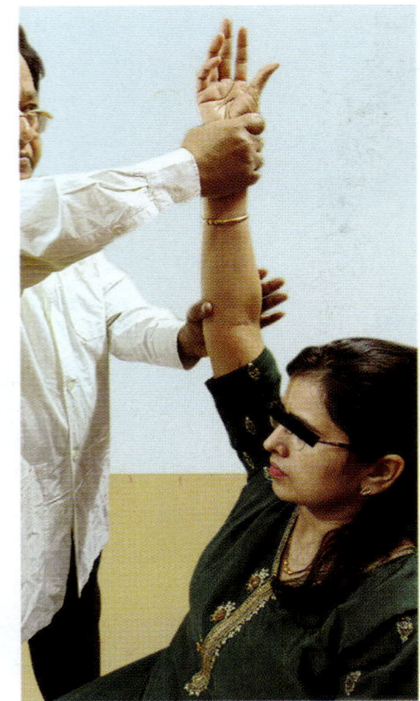

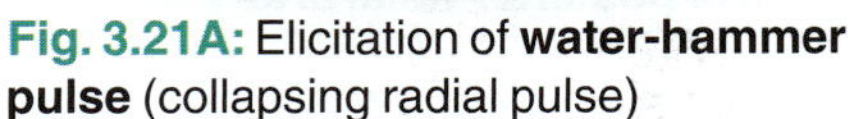

Fig. 3.21A: Elicitation of **water-hammer pulse** (collapsing radial pulse)

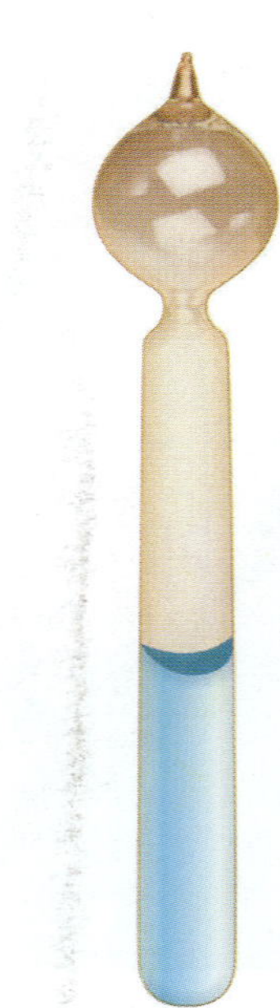

Fig. 3.21B: Water-hammer **toy**

water and half with vacuum (two ends being closed). If the toy is suddenly placed upside down, the column of water strikes the other end of the cylinder with a blowing sound. This is why the term water-hammer has been coined in a high volume collapsing pulse where the pulse strikes the fingers like the thud of a hammer.

Q. Causes of water-hammer pulse:

The causes are mentioned in 'high volume pulse' in the section on 'Pulse'. One should remember **aortic incompetence** (AI) as the first cause of water-hammer pulse and then the others.

Q. Why this type of pulse is seen in aortic incompetence (AI)?

A. In AI, the left ventricular stroke volume is high (so the systolic pressure is high) and this is responsible for 'sharp rise' or rapid upstroke in the pulse.

B. The collapsing character is due to:
   1. Diastolic leak back into the left ventricle from aorta.
   2. Rapid run-off to the periphery as a result of *low systemic vascular resistance* (the increased cardiac output stimulates the baroreceptors in the aortic arch and the result is reflex vasodilatation of the peripheral vessels into which the blood flows rapidly).

Clinical Wisdom

> No. 1 and 2 of (B) are responsible for low diastolic pressure and thus in AI, there is a high pulse pressure. These factors are responsible for 'sharp fall' too.

Q. Why do you elevate the arm?

Mechanisms of action:

1. Aided by the gravity (after elevation of the arm), there is fall of blood column (resulting in vasodilatation)

and thus, it helps to reduce the diastolic pressure more. So the pulse pressure widens, or

2. It may be so that the artery palpated at wrist becomes more in the line of aorta after elevation of the arm, and thus allows direct systolic ejection and diastolic backward flow.

Q. Other parts to be examined in a patient with water-hammer pulse:

1. Count the pulse rate (bradycardia in complete heart block, tachycardia in thyrotoxicosis).
2. Examine the condition of the arterial wall (for arteriosclerosis).
3. See the facies for exophthalmos or examine for tremor (thyrotoxicosis).
4. Record the surface temperature (pyrexia).
5. Examine for anaemia (severe anaemia).
6. Examine for jaundice (cirrhosis with hepato-cellular failure).
7. Examine the chest for emphysema (chronic cor pulmonale).
8. One should not forget to auscultate the aortic and neoaortic area for an early diastolic murmur (AI).

Lastly, one should examine the patient for capillary pulsation, digital pulsation, carotid dance, pistol shot sound which are usually associated features of water-hammer pulse.

Q. Anacrotic pulse:

It is a *low volume pulse* with an upstroke felt in the ascending limb. Anacrotic pulse is found in severe valvular aortic stenosis (AS). Typically the pulse in aortic stenosis is known as pulsus **'parvus et tardus'** (slow rising low volume pulse)—'parvus' means low volume and 'tardus' means slow or late. One may feel carotid shudder in the presence of anacrotic pulse. Pulse of AS is also known as 'plateau pulse'.

Q. Dicrotic pulse:

When an upstroke is felt in the descending limb of the pulse wave, it is known as dicrotic pulse. The first wave is percussion wave while the second wave is exaggerated dicrotic wave. The dicrotic wave is felt due to hypotonia of the vessel wall. This is also a *low volume pulse* due to very low stroke volume with decreased peripheral resistance, and is found in:

a. Second week of typhoid fever (possibly related to circulating vasculotoxins).
b. Endotoxic shock.
c. Hypovolaemic shock.
d. Diffuse myocardial disease.

Q. What is pulsus bisferiens?

1. It is a *high volume double-beating pulse* (single pulse wave with two peaks in systole).
2. Method of palpation: **Best palpated in big arteries like brachial and carotid arteries.** Try to press and occulde the brachial artery—now, slowly release the pressure and feel the double-beating nature of the pulse.
3. The first lift is due to 'percussion wave' (P) and the second lift is due to 'tidal wave' (T). It is said that if P>T, then Al>AS; and if T>P, usually AS>AI. Thus, we can determine the dominant lesion.
4. It is commonly found in:
   a. Combined AS and AI (commonest).
   b. Isolated severe AI, and
   c. Hypertrophic obstructive cardiomyopathy (HOCM).
5. Pathophysiology:
   a. Due to 'ventury effect' within the left ventricle.
   b. Another view explains that the 'dip' in the pulse is felt due to energy dissipation in the production of a loud systolic murmur of AS (Bernoulli effect).
   c. The first component is due to large volume of blood ejected in systole and the second component is due to elastic recoil in the arteries (best reasoning).

- Three different causes of **double-beating pulse** are: (i) bisferiens, (ii) anacrotic, and (iii) dicrotic pulse.

Q. Pulsus alternans:

This is rarely found. When the alternate pulse waves are weak, i.e. of low volume *(the rhythm remains regular in contrast to ectopics)* in a patient with acute left ventricular failure, pulsus alternans is said to be present. It is **better demonstrated in radial arteries**. In a patient with LVF (severe myocardial failure), some ventricular muscle fibres are healthy and some are degenerated and thus, produces normal and weak beat respectively (defective electromechanical coupling). One should search for gallop rhythm and basal crepitations when pulsus alternans is felt (features of LVF). It is due to prolonged recovery time of damaged myocardium and indicates a poor prognosis.

The compensatory pause of ectopics are absent here.

Q. Pulsus bigeminus:

Clinically, two beats and a pause thereafter recur repeatedly in a regular fashion (bigeminy means twins). The second beat is an ectopic and thus, there is a pause after it. It is commonly found in digitalis toxicity and 3:2 heart block. In pulsus trigeminus, three beats and a pause recur in a regular fashion.

Q. Pulsus paradoxus:

Here, the pulse volume decreases with inspiration and increases with expiration (not truely the opposite of sinus arrhythmia which denotes the changes in pulse rate only). The **'paradox'** is that the heart sounds may still be audible on auscultation over the apex at a time when no pulse (pulse wave may totally disappear in inspiration) is palpable at the radial artery. It is commonly seen in:

1. Acute severe asthma.
2. Cardiac tamponade.
3. Chronic constrictive pericarditis.
4. Chronic obstructive pulmonary disease (COPD).
5. Sometimes, in SVC syndrome.
6. Restrictive cardiomyopathy.

The probable mechanisms are:

1. Intrapericardial pressure rises more during inspiration (as a result of traction on the pericardium) which in turn diminishes cardiac output by causing obstruction in venous return (in cardiac tamponade). Increased intrapericardial pressure in cardiac tamponade also impedes diastolic filling.
2. Anti-Bernheim effect: During inspiration, more blood comes in the right ventricle which pushes the interventricular septum to the left side and thereby diminishing the left ventricular cavity, and resulting in low cardiac output. During acute severe asthma and other causes mentioned above, the degree of negative pressure generated during inspiration is exaggerated. So, more blood is sucked in the right heart, resulting in pulsus paradoxus.

- Pulsus paradoxus is a misnomer and is actually an exaggeration of normal physiological phenomenon. In health, there is a fall in systolic BP in inspiration which is <10 mm of Hg (so, not detectable normally) but in pulsus paradoxus, there is an exaggerated inspiratory fall in systolic BP >10 mm of Hg.

Q. Pulses confirmed by sphygmomanometer:

1. Pulsus paradoxus: Systolic BP is more in expiration than in inspiration by >10 mm of Hg.
2. Water-hammer pulse: Pulse pressure is usually greater than at least 60 mm of Hg.
3. Pulsus alternans: When the strong beats (Korotkoff sounds) are heard during measurement of systolic BP (initial part of measurement), the pulse rate remains half of the actual rate (as weak beats do not reach the radial artery). With gradual lowering of the mercury column, the weak beats are also heard and thus, the pulse rate doubles, i.e. returns to the actual pulse rate (Gallavardin sign).

Q. Other uses of sphygmomanometer:

1. To measure the blood pressure (principal use of the instrument).
2. Hess' capillary fragility test: See the section on 'Haemorrhagic spots'.
3. Latent tetany: When the pressure is raised above the systolic BP for 3 minutes, typical carpal spasm appears (main d'accoucheur) and is known as Trousseau's sign.
4. To assess the respiratory reserve: Blow the mercury column (by placing the mouth to the inlet tube) up to 40–50 mm of Hg and to try to hold it at this level.
5. Diagnosis from recording of BP of lower limb: Lower limb systolic BP > upper limb systolic BP and if the difference is above 20 mm of Hg, it is known as Hill's sign, which is diagnostic of AI. Lower limb systolic BP < upper limb systolic BP happens to occur in coarctation of aorta.
6. To draw venous blood.
7. Previously used as a rotating tourniquet in a patient of LVF (for reduction of venous return): Keep the cuff inflated in all the limbs at 80 mm of Hg (i.e. at diastolic pressure) for 15 minutes.
8. To draw blood during blood donation.

Q. Describe the pulse in complete heart black (CHB):

The pulse of CHB has some special characters like:

1. Rate 36–40 per minute (bradycardia).
2. Rhythm: Regular.
3. Volume: High.
4. Condition of the arterial wall: May be thickened (as the patients are of advanced age).
5. Neither radio-radial nor any radio-femoral delay.
6. Character: May have water-hammer character.
7. All the peripheral pulses are palpable.
8. Special character: It is a 'fixed' pulse, i.e. no alteration in pulse rate after exercise, pyrexia or injection of atropine.

In CHB, carotid artery shows carotid dance at the rate of 36–40 per minute (ventricular rate), and internal jugular veins reflect atrial pulsation at the rate of 72 per minute with cannon waves appearing from time to time. There is beat to beat variation in the BP (fluctuating BP). BP is of high systolic and normal diastolic pressure. There is varying intensity of S_1 (cannon sound); rarely a mid-diastolic murmur may be audible (Rytand's murmur).

ABNORMAL TEMPERATURE — CASE 41

Q. Normal body temperature and its variations:

Fever is both a symptom and sign, which alerts the physician to the underlying abnormality.

1. **Normal (euthermia):** 98°F–99°F (with a diurnal variation of 1.5°F: the temperature is lowest in the morning and is highest in between 4–6 PM—this circadian rhythm is controlled by hypothalamus).
2. **Subnormal:** Below 98°F.
3. **Pyrexia or febrile:** Above 99°F.
4. **Hypothermia:** Below 95°F.
5. **Hyperpyrexia:** Above 106.7°F.

- Though varies from person to person, recent studies reveal that oral AM temperature of >98.9°F or an oral PM temperature of >99.9°F would define a 'fever' or 'pyrexia'. The term pyrexia comes from the Greek word 'pyro' (fire).

Q. Methods of taking body temperature:

1. **Oral:** The thermometer is placed under the tongue and the patient breathes through the nose with lips firmly closed. It reflects the body-core temperature.

2. **Axillary** or groin: Very convenient, placed in the armpit or folded groin; generally 0.5-1°F lower than oral temperature. Axilla, groin and natal cleft should preferably be avoided in adults.
3. **Rectal:** Most reliable as well as accurate, and it is 0.5–1°F higher than oral temperature.
4. **Temporal:** Electronic thermometer placed on skin of forehead; 0.5–1°F lower than oral temperature.

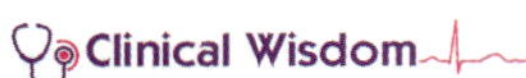

Thermometer is kept at least for 2 minutes in all the sites and the rectal > oral > axillary temperature.

- Recently, a **tympanic membrane thermometer** (i.e. electronic thermometer used in the ear measuring infrared heat waves from tympanic membrane) is used for fast and accurate reading of core temperature.

Q. Which site will you prefer in infants?

The axilla, or groin with thigh flexed over the abdomen (also convenient in an unconscious patient).

Q. If not mentioned, which site is preferred for recording of temperature?

Oral temperature commonly and if the oral temperature crosses 99°F, the patient is declared febrile. In axilla, when the temperature is above 98.6°F or 37°C (the arrow is marked here in the clinical thermometer), it is said that the patient is running temperature. Oral temperature does not change with sweating or vasoconstriction (axillary temperature may change). Majority of common people are well conversant with Fahrenheit (F) scale though temperature is nowadays recorded in centigrade or Celsius (C) scale, and the conversion formula is:

$$\frac{C}{5} = \frac{F - 32}{9}$$

Back of examiner's hand (more sensitive than thicker palm) is best suited to notify patient's temperature.

Q. Features associated with fever:

Common constitutional symptoms are headache, anorexia, myalgia, chill, rigor, shivering, furring of tongue, sudaminal rash (sweat-retention rash), herpes labialis, febrile rash, febrile convulsions, confusion, and delirium. Common signs are fever, flushing of face, tachypnoea, relative brady- or tachycardia and dehydration.

Q. Common causes of pyrexia:

1. Different infections (bacterial, viral, fungal).
2. Autoimmune (e.g. SLE) and autoinflammatory disorders (e.g. familial Mediterranean fever).
3. Neoplastic (e.g. hypernephroma).
4. Endocrine (e.g. thyrotoxicosis), haematological (e.g. sickle cell crisis), metabolic (e.g. gout), traumatic (e.g. crush injury), vascular (e.g. AMI), and by physical agents (e.g. heat stroke).
5. Miscellaneous: Drug fever, factitious fever, habitual hyperthermia.
6. Undiagnosed fever: In spite of repeated investigations, the aetiology is not revealed.

Q. Contraindications of taking oral temperature:

1. Infants and children.
2. Mentally dull persons, e.g. Down syndrome.
3. During convulsions or H/o recurrent fits; H/o repeated sneezing.
4. Immediately after taking hot tea, hot coffee, chewing tobacco or smoking.
5. Inflammation within the oral cavity, e.g. stomatitis, ulcer in the mouth, impacted wisdom teeth.
6. During severe dyspnoea.
7. Unconscious or restless patients.
8. Trismus (tetanus, tetany).
9. Paralysis of the tongue; Bell's palsy.
10. In mouth breathers.

Q. Different causes of hypothermia:

1. Myxoedema coma.
2. Prolonged exposure to cold (in street beggars, accidental in elderly, or in mountaineering).
3. Peripheral circulatory failure due to any cause.
4. Enteric fever if associated with haemorrhage or perforation (commonly in the 3rd week).
5. Hypoglycaemia.
6. Panhypopituitarism; adrenal insufficiency.
7. Artificial hypothermia induced in open heart surgery.
8. Near-drowning.
9. Alcohol intoxication; sedatives and hypnotics overdose.
10. Autonomic dysfunction.

- Always confirm hypothermia with rectal temperature. Hypothermia in a septic patient is prognostically worse than high fever. Sepsis in elderly may not have fever—'the older is colder'.

Q. Causes of hyperpyrexia:

In hyperpyrexia, hypothalamas changes the normal body temperature set point.

1. Malaria.
2. Septicaemia.
3. Encephalitis.
4. Pontine haemorrhage.
5. Lobar pneumonia.
6. Heat stroke.
7. Malignant hyperthermia (haloperidol-induced).
8. Thyroid storm.
9. Neuroleptic malignant syndrome (halothane-induced).
10. Dhatura poisoning.
11. Rabies; pyogenic meningitis.

12. Serotonin syndrome (SSRI or MAO inhibitors-induced).
13. Drug-induced (e.g. amphetamines).

- 'Low grade fever': Temperature present daily, especially in the evening, for several days and is around 100°F. It is commonly found in tuberculosis, UTI or autoimmune diseases.
- **Hyperthermia:** Very high temperature without change in hypothalamic set point. Here, the uncontrolled rise in very high temperature beats the body's ability to dissipate heat.

Q. Fever with disturbed consciousness (or fever with delirium):

1. Encephalitis.
2. Cerebral malaria.
3. Meningitis.
4. Pyrexia complicated by metabolic disorders, e.g. hypoglycaemia.
5. Typhoid state.
6. Brain abscess.
7. CVA with fever (e.g. chest infection).
8. Rarely in dhatura poisoning.
9. Septicaemia.

Q. Causes of 'aseptic fever' (fever without infection):

1. Heat stroke.
2. Lymphoma, leukaemias or disseminated malignancy.
3. Collagen vascular disease, e.g. SLE.
4. Pontine haemorrhage.
5. Thyroid storm.
6. Drug fever, e.g. rifampicin or sulphonamides.
7. Acute myocardial infarction (AMI).
8. Gout.
9. Porphyria.
10. Crush injury.
11. Radiation sickness.
12. Over-atropinisation.

- **Fever with leucocytosis but there is no infection:** Acute pancreatitis, AMI, diabetic ketoacidosis and gout.

Q. What is 'hectic' temperature?

There is a big swing in the temperature which rises with chill and rigor, often with facial flushes, persists for few hours and suddenly falls with profuse sweating. The common causes are:

1. *Pent-up pus anywhere in the body* (lung abscess, liver abscess, empyema thoracis, empyema of the gallbladder, subdiaphragmatic abscess).
2. Septicaemia or pyaemia.
3. Encephalitis.
4. Rarely in advanced tuberculosis.

Q. Causes of fever with chill and rigor:

1. Malaria.
2. Urinary tract infection (UTI).
3. Pent-up pus anywhere in the body (e.g. lung abscess).
4. Septicaemia or pyaemia.
5. Cholangitis.
6. Subacute bacterial endocarditis (SBE).
7. Thrombophlebitis.
8. Acute pyelitis or acute pyelonephritis.
9. Acute lobar pneumonia (e.g. pneumococcal).
10. Agranulocytosis.
11. Pyrogen reaction after fluid infusion or blood transfusion.
12. Filariasis.

Q. Pathogenesis of chill and rigor:

It should be looked upon in the setting of 'thermostat'. When the temperature is rising to a higher level, heat is being conserved, the cutaneous vessels are constricted (so the patient feels cold) and the patient may even shiver violently. The shivering is known as 'rigor', which may be associated with piloerection and teeth chattering. When the higher temperature is reached, heat loss starts and the cutaneous vessels dilate for dissipation of heat. The patient feels hot and sweating starts.

Normal temperature is maintained in health by regulating a balance between heat gain and heat loss, governed by the hypothalamus.

Q. What is meant by 'fall by crisis or lysis'?

Fall of temperature is also known as defervescence. They are:

Fall by crisis: When the raised temperature falls to normal or subnormal level very quickly within 6–12 hours and is associated with severe sweating, it is known as fall by crisis. This is usually seen in:

1. Acute lobar pneumonia.
2. Enteric fever complicated by intestinal haemorrhage or perforation.
3. Adrenal crisis (seen in meningococcal meningitis).
4. Septicaemic shock.
5. Dengue.

Fall by lysis: When the temperature falls gradually in steps over several days, it is known as fall by lysis. It is usually seen in:

1. Uncomplicated enteric fever.
2. Rheumatic fever.
3. Acute bronchopneumonia.

Clinical Wisdom

Most of the raised temperature falls by lysis. Use of antipyretics may precipitate fall by crisis.

Q. What do you mean by 'periodic fever'?

It is the periodic attacks of pyrexia alternating with a period of apyrexia, and is commonly seen in:

1. Hodgkin's disease (Pel-Ebstein fever).

2. Brucellosis.
3. Relapsing fever (*Borrelia*-induced).
4. Malaria.
5. Rat bite fever.
6. Dengue (saddle-back fever).

- Blackwater fever (malaria), black fever (kala-azar), Q fever (*Coxiella burnetii*), glandular fever (Epstein-Barr virus), 7-day fever (leptospirosis) and pretibial fever are special forms of fever.

Q. What is 'recurrent fever syndrome'?

Most of these conditios (previously known as periodic fever syndrome) are hereditary and result from a gene mutation. The syndromes are basically autoinflammatory diseases. These non-infectious causes of fever mainly affect children. They are familial Mediterranean fever (FMF), tumour necrosis factor receptor-associated periodic syndrome (TRAPS), neonatal-onset multisystem inflammatory disease (NOMID), hyperimmunoglobin D syndrome (HIDS), etc. FMF is the commonest variety.

Q. Diagnostic clues in fever:

A meticulous clinical examination gives a lot of clues in diagnosis of fever.

- Toxic look: Typhoid, septicaemia, miliary tuberculosis, typhus.
- Marked perspiration: Septicaemia, rheumatic fever, amoebic liver abscess, brucellosis.
- Severe myalgia: Influenza, dengue, chikungunya, leptospirosis.
- Purpura: Acute leukaemias, septicaemia, meningococcaemia.
- Convulsions: Febrile (in children), meningitis, cerebral abscess, tuberculoma.
- Lymphadenopathy: Tuberculosis, lymphoma, leukaemia, secondary syphilis (rare), SLE, AIDS.

Q. What is pyrexia of unknown origin (PUO) or fever of unknown origin (FUO)?

Definition (by Petersdorf and Beeson, 1961):

1. Fever higher than 101°F on several occasions.
2. A duration of fever for more than 3 weeks.
3. Failure to reach a provisional diagnosis after one week of inpatient investigations.

Diseases which may initially present as PUO:

1. Lymphomas, leukaemias, multiple myeloma and carcinoma (especially of lung, liver and kidney).
2. Collagen vascular diseases, e.g. SLE, rheumatoid arthritis, Still's disease, polyarteritis nodosa.
3. Tuberculosis, SBE, subphrenic abscess, liver abscess, brucellosis, fungal infection, AIDS.
4. Factitious fever, drug fever, habitual hyperthermia, use of immunosuppressive drugs.

Afterwards, PUO has been classified into 4 different types (Durack and Street, 1991):

1. Classic PUO (as previous one, except the time frame which is 3 outpatient visits or 3 days in hospital without determining the cause, or one week of 'intelligent and invasive' ambulatory investigations), e.g. hidden infection, obscure malignancy, collagen vascular diseases, autoinflammatory diseases.
2. Nosocomial PUO (hospital-acquired), e.g. septic thrombophlebitis.
3. Neutropenic PUO (when neutrophil count is $\leq$500/mm^3), e.g. perianal infection, candidosis.
4. HIV-associated PUO (e.g. tuberculosis, NHL, drug fever).

The most recent classification of PUO has been further modified as:

1. Fever >101°F on at least two occasions.
2. Duration of illness ≥3 weeks.
3. No known immunocompromised state.
4. Diagnosis still remains uncertain after a thorough history taking, physical examination, and some obligatory investigations like ESR, CRP, platelet count, TC/DC, Hb%, electrolytes, creatinine, AST, ALT, alkaline phosphatase, LDH, CK, ANF, RF, chest X-ray, urine analysis, blood culture, abdominal USG, Mantoux test, etc.

Clinical Wisdom

Diagnosis of PUO requires 'repeated' physical examination, intelligent interviewing the patient and specific investigations.

Fever persisting for >2 weeks in loosely termed as 'prolonged fever'.

Q. When the recording of rectal temperature is preferred?

1. Possible hypothermia.
2. In collapsed, comatosed or elderly patients.
3. Invalid patients.
4. Cholera patients (surface temperature is subnormal but rectal temperature is raised), and
5. In algid malaria.

Clinical Wisdom

The rectal temperature is recorded with a special 'low-reading' thermometer. It is stouter than the clinical thermometer, with a rounded bulb (to reduce the risk of injury) and is graduated up to 90°F.

Q. Relative bradycardia and relative tachycardia:

It is known that with per degree (°F) rise of temperature in an adult, the pulse rate is increased by 10 beats/minute. In children, the rise may be up to 12–15 beats/minute. **Pulse-temperature dissociation** is manifested by relative brady- and tachycardia.

A. **Relative bradycardia:** Here, the increase in pulse rate is less than 10 beats/minute with per degree (°F) rise of temperature. For example, the pulse rate in relative bradycardia will be about 80/minute, when the temperature is increased by 2°F (actually it should be 92/minute). It is seen in:

i. Any viral fever (e.g. in yellow fever: Known as Faget's sign).
ii. First week of enteric fever.
iii. Sometimes in pyogenic meningitis.
iv. Brucellosis, dengue, psittacosis, Weil's disease, drug fever.

B. **Relative tachycardia:** Here, the increase in pulse rate is more than 10 beats/minute with per degree (°F) rise of temperature. For example, the pulse rate will be about 120/minute, when the temperature is increased by 3°F (actually it should be 102/minute). It is seen in:

i. Acute rheumatic carditis.
ii. Diphtheritic myocarditis.
iii. Tuberculosis.
iv. Polyarteritis nodosa.

Q. Types of fever:

There are three classical types of fever:

I. Intermittent: Fever is present only for several hours and **always touches the baseline** sometime during the day. It has three subdivisions:

i. Quotidian: The paroxysm of fever occurs daily (i.e. daily rise and daily fall). The examples are:
   a. Double infection of *P. vivax*.
   b. Pent-up pus anywhere in the body.
   c. Tuberculosis.
   d. Urinary tract infection.
   e. Septicaemia.
   f. Amoebic liver abscess.
ii. Tertian:The paroxysm occurs on alternate days, which is found in,
   a. Benign tertian malaria (commonly by *P. vivax* and rarely by *P. ovale*).
   b. Malignant tertian malaria (*P. falciparum*).
iii. Quartan: When two days intervene between consecutive paroxysmal atacks, it is quartan pyrexia and is found in quartan malaria (*P. malariae*) which is rare in India.

II. Continued (or continuous): Fever does not fluctuate more than 1°C (1.5°F) during the 24 hours period and **never touches the baseline**. The examples are:

a. Lobar pneumonia.
b. Second week of enteric fever.
c. Miliary tuberculosis.
d. Meningococcal meningitis.
e. Acute rheumatic fever.
f. Collagen vascular diseases, e.g. SLE.

III. Remittent: Daily fluctuation of fever is more than 2°C (3°F) during the 24 hours period and it **never touches the baseline**. The common examples are:

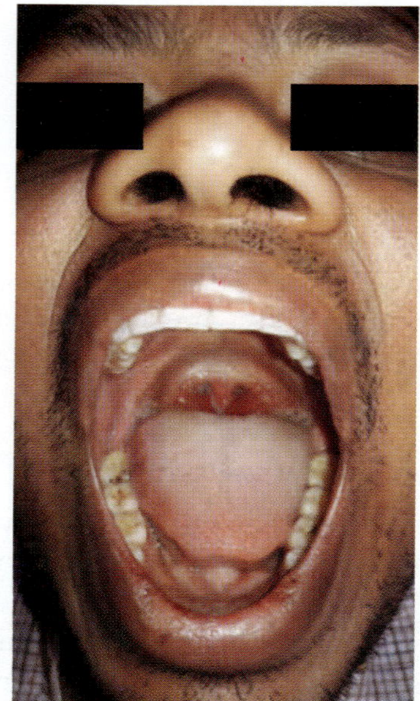

Fig. 3.22: Acute tonsillitis presenting with sore throat and pyrexia

a. Amoebic liver abscess.
b. Sometimes in urinary tract infection.
c. Third week of enteric fever.
d. Acute bronchopneumonia.
e. Acute tonsillitis (Fig. 3.22).
f. Bacteraemia, septicaemia, pyaemia.

- In the present era of antipyretics and antibiotics, classical typing is rarely possible.

Q. What is double quotidian fever (camel hump fever)?

It is the double fever spike in a single day and is seen in:

1. Kala-azar (classical example).
2. Gonococcal perihepatitis or endocarditis.
3. Sometimes in acute bacterial endocarditis.

Q. Appearance of rash in a febrile patient (i.e. fever with rash):

The mnemonic: 'very sick person must take double tea' for appearance of rash in exanthematous fever.

1st day	Varicella, i.e. chickenpox (mainly in trunk; all forms seen at a time, no umbilication of vesicle).
2nd day	Scarlet fever (over chest, neck, scapula; mainly macular).
3rd day	Pox (smallpox), not seen nowadays as it has been eradicated globally (peripheral distribution, rashes come in a sequence; monomorphic, umbilication of vesicle).
4th day	Measles (maculo-papular; over forehead, hairline near ears, face and trunk).
5th day	Typhus (macular; over shoulders, chest, extremities, palms and soles) (Fig. 3.23).
6th day	Dengue (morbilliform; over dorsum of hands and feet, trunk) (Fig. 3.24).

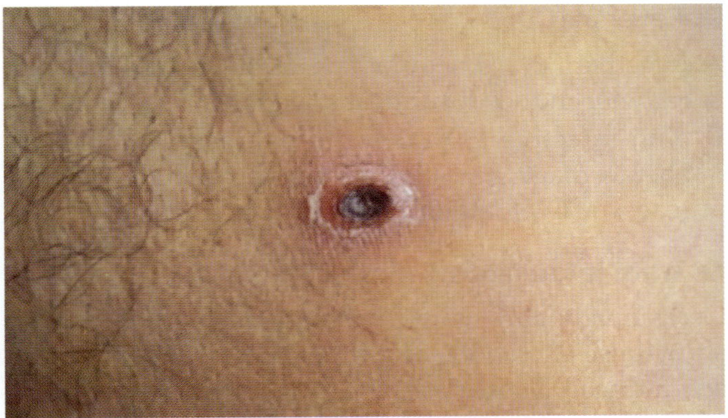

Fig. 3.23: Typical **eschar** formation in **scrub typhus**

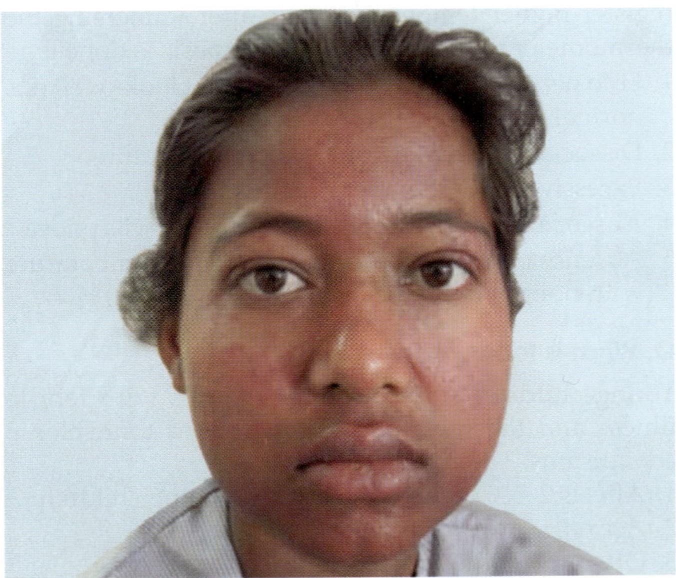

Fig. 3.24: Erythematous **rash in dengue** fever

7th day Typhoid fever (rose spots over abdomen, flanks and back; pale-pink; fades on pressure).

- There are many other infections and diseases with rash: rubella, *Meningococcus*, *Rickettsia*, parvovirus, echovirus, HIV, Still's disease and vasculitis.
- Never forget 'drug rash' which may appear at any time or any day during fever.

Q. Features of enteric fever in its first week:

1. Step-ladder pattern of pyrexia.
2. Frontal headache.
3. Constipation (diarrhoea, vomiting and pain abdomen may be seen in children).
4. Anorexia, nausea, cough and epistaxis.
5. Flushed face with toxic look.
6. Angry looking tongue: Central coating with red tip and margins.
7. Caecal gurgling (due to presence of fluid feces and air)—palpate right iliac fossa.
8. Relative bradycardia and rarely diorotic pulse.
9. Rose spots appearing on the 7th day (usually appears on 7th–10th day).
10. There may be just palpable, soft and tender spleen at the end of first week.

Q. What is typhoid state?

Usually the untreated enteric fever patient enters into this toxaemic stage along with high rise of temperature at the onset of 3rd week of illness and is manifested by some neurological (encephalitis-like) features such as:

a. Semiconsciousness or unconsciousness.
b. Low muttering delirium.
c. Coma vigil: Patient lies with half-open eyes but ignorant of his surroundings (staring stupor).
d. Subsultus tendinum: Involuntary movements of fingers and wrists due to muscular twitching.
e. Carphology: Agitated plucking of the bed sheets, and
f. Convulsions rarely.

- This moribund situation should be tackled urgently. Meningism may be present.

Q. What is pulse-respiration ratio?

It is seen that with per degree (°F) rise of temperature, there is an increase in respiratory rate by 2–3/minute. The pulse-respiration ratio goes like this:

a. Normal pulse: respiration = 4 : 1 (72 : 18).
b. Increased pulse respiration, e.g. 12 : 1 (72 : 6) is seen in narcotic poisoning.
c. Decreased pulse: respiration, e.g. 2 : 1 (112 : 56) is seen in acute lobar pneumonia.

Q. Herpes labialis ('fever blisters' or 'cold sore') with pyrexia (Fig. 3.25):

These are painful and tender vesicles on the outer surface of lips, and is commonly observed in:

1. Acute lobar pneumonia.
2. Influenza.
3. Malaria.
4. Meningococcal meningitis.
5. Weil's disease.
6. *Mycoplasma pneumoniae* infection.
7. AIDS.
8. Physiological—sunlight, menstruation.

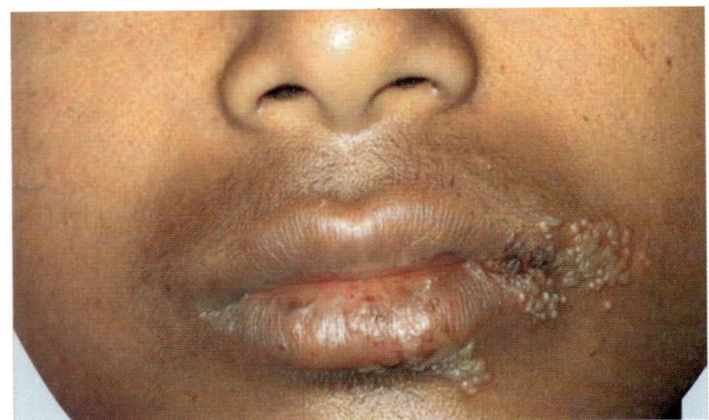

Fig. 3.25: Herpes simplex virus infection **(herpes labialis)** leading to ulcerative stomatitis, in a patient recovering from meningitis

Clinical Wisdom

Herpes labialis is due to activation of herpes simplex virus, type 1 infection with elevated body temperature. In lobar pneumonia, herpes labialis often gives clue to the side affected in lung (i.e. herpes on the side of consolidation) and stages of pneumonia.

Q. Fever with patch or membrane seen in the throat:

1. Acute follicular tonsillitis (*see* **Fig. 3.22**).
2. Faucal diphtheria.
3. Infectious mononucleosis.
4. Candidiasis (candidosis) or thrush.
5. Agranulocytosis.
6. Vincent's angina.
7. Acute lymphoblastic leukaemia.
8. Tonsil stones.

Q. What are the 'benefits' of fever?

There is release of endogenous pyrogen with rise of temperature and this leads to activation of T-lymphocytes and thus, it enhances the host defence mechanism. Fever is sometimes beneficial in:

1. Neurosyphilis.
2. Chronic arthritis (rheumatoid arthritis).
3. Widespread carcinomatosis.
4. Uveitis.

- Ill-effects of fever are epileptiform fits (i.e. damage of brain), loss of weight (anorexia, ↑ BMR, ↑ protein catabolism, water loss), and sweating-induced salt and water depletion.
- Blunting of pyrexial response may occur in old age, CRF and immunocompromised patients.

Q. Physiologic events on body temperature:

A. Diminished temperature: On rising in the morning (lowest), old age.

B. Increased temperature: Exercise, in the evening, ovulation and smoking.

Q. Agents causing 'drug fever':

1. Sulphonamides.
2. Iodides, bromides.
3. Thiouracils.
4. Barbiturates.
5. Penicillin.
6. Salicylates.
7. Rifampicin ('flu syndrome').
8. Phenolphthalein (used in laxatives).
9. Ecstasy (recreational drug).
10. Phenytoin, quinidine.

- The underlying mechanism is hypersensitivity and 50% patients have eosinophilia **(remember, the usual response in fever is eosinopenia)**. There may be rash, chills, fatigue and relative bradycardia. Drug fever disappears after discontinuation of the offending drug.
- DRESS: Drug reaction with eosinophilia and systemic symptoms. It is a severe adverse drug reaction.

Q. Fever in ICU:

A. Infective (70%): Pneumonia, UTI, sinusitis, diarrhoea, catheter-induced, surgical infections.

B. Non-infective (30%): Acute pancreatitis, cerebral haemorrhage, transfusion reaction, haematoma, drug reaction, DVT, autoimmune and neoplastic.

Q. What is factitious or fraudulent fever?

Occasionally patients purposefully (i.e. manipulating) show false elevations of temperature which are often self-induced. These patients are usually young women, often attached to health professionals. They may infect themselves with bacteria, ingest thyroxine or falsely register higher temperature (e.g. after immersing the thermometer in hot water). The diagnosis is done by:

1. H/o personality disorder. The patient looks well (i.e. normal or non-toxic).
2. Dissociation between pulse and temperature.
3. Excessively high temperature (e.g. 106°F).
4. Absence of chills, sweats, tachycardia, tachypnoea.
5. Absence of normal diurnal variation in temperature with normal ESR and CRP.

Q. What is febrile convulsions?

Young children often develop seizures with febrile illness and these are short, generalised tonic-clonic convulsions. The characteristics are:

1. Affects 2–5% of the population of young children.
2. *Age range is from 6 months to 5 years.*
3. Often there is a positive family history.
4. Convulsions are not related to the degree of elevation of temperature as they may occur even with moderate fever.
5. Seizures last for less than 5 minutes and is generalised.
6. There is no recurrence in majority.
7. It is not associated with interictal EEG abnormalities or any neurodeficit.

Management is done by tepid sponge bathing, antipyretics and inj. diazepam (0.2–0.5 mg/kg, per dose, shot push IV). Predictive factors for recurrence are: young age of onset, low fever, family H/o febrile convulsions and short duration of fever before convulsions.

Epilepsy may develop in less than 3% of all children with febrile convulsions. Predictive factors for future development of epilepsy are: partial onset, prolonged seizure (>10 min), more than one seizure in 24 hours and family H/o epilepsy.

Q. Invasive methods of recording core temperature:

A catheter to measure pulmonary artery temperature, temperature-sensing indwelling urinary catheter, rectal/oesophageal temperature transducers (probes) or temperature assessment by extracorporeal membrane oxygenation (ECMO)—record more accurate temperature though with higher risks. These methods are often used in critical care units.

Q. Why there is a kink in the clinical thermometer?

It prevents the return of the mercury column when the thermometer is taken out of the body.

Q. Why the thermometer is triangular in cross-section?

It magnifies the mercury-line into a wider strip to help in easy reading.

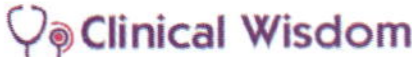

Clinical Wisdom

One should always try to record oral temperature in the long and short cases.

OEDEMA — CASE 42

Q. What is oedema?

Oedema is accumulation of excessive amount of tissue fluid in the subcutaneous tissue (or serous sacs) due to increase in extravascular (interstitial) component of the extracellular fluid volume resulting in swelling of tissue. That is to say, *clinically apparent increase in interstitial fluid volume is oedema*. A weight gain of several kilograms commonly precedes overt manifestation of oedema.

Clinical Wisdom

Total body water (60-65% of body weight in kg) is distributed as 2/3 ICF and 1/3 ECF; of the ECF, the distribution is 2/3 IF and 1/3 plasma. So in a person weighing 70 kg, intracellular fluid is 28 litres, while 9.4 litres is interstitial fluid, and 4.6 litres is the blood volume (totally having 42 litre of water). ICF = Intracellular fluid, ECF = Extracellular fluid, IF = Interstitial fluid.

Q. How to demonstrate oedema clinically?

Examination sequence (by digital pressure method):

1. First inspect the legs for any swelling.
2. Apply firm pressure for few seconds (at least 15 seconds to maximally upto 30 seconds) sequentially *over the medial malleolus, 2–3 cm above the medial malleolus, lower end of tibia (medial surface) and the upper part of shin bone by tip of the right thumb, i.e. press over a bony background*. Now inspect and palpate the area for any dimple or pitting (i.e. indentation). If it is seen that the dorsum of the foot is swollen, now one should press there. Do the same manoeuvre on the opposite side.
   In oedema-forming states, **ambulatory patients** develop oedema on the dependent parts, i.e. the ankle (or pedal oedema). 'Pitting' (i.e. the skin is indented) is the cardinal sign of subcutaneous oedema, which gradually fills in by redistribution of the displaced fluid. Pitting oedema reflects increased interstitial fluid while non-pitting oedema may reflect protein deposition (*see* Fig. 1.9).
3. Now examine the 'BACK', i.e. turn the patient into prone position and press by tip of the right thumb over sacrum. Sacral oedema is found in **patients confined to bed** for prolonged period (Fig. 3.26). *Sacrum must be examined in all patients with oedema.*

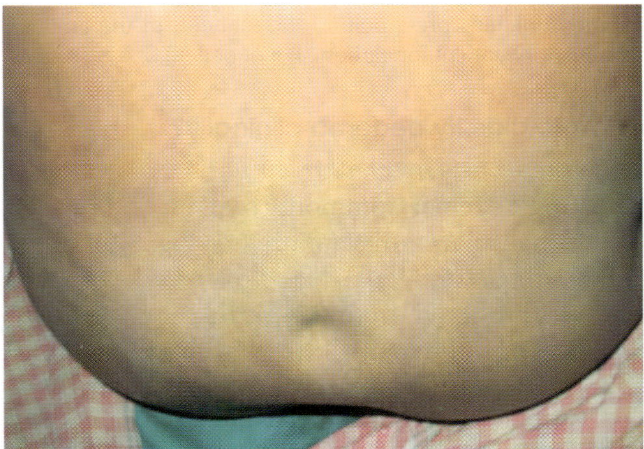

Fig. 3.26: **Sacral oedema** in a patient of congestive cardiac failure with prolonged recumbency. Here, the patient is sitting in the bed.

4. Then examine for 'parietal oedema' (Fig. 3.27): Press the chest piece of stethoscope or the tips of the five fingers of right hand, over the abdominal parietis or thigh for few seconds. Look for pitting oedema there. Oedema of the parietis (e.g. abdominal wall) may also be assessed by pinching the skin with thumb and index finger for few seconds (at least 5 seconds).

Clinical Wisdom

Observe carefully for puffy face, puffy lower eyelids and scrotal oedema. It is said that oedema is also recognised by pallid and glossy appearance of the skin with less prominent superficial veins, and at times by its doughy feel—actually **non-pitting oedema may be recognised at the bedside in this way**. Oedema may be seen in the genitalia, trunk, face, upper extremity, over sternum, vertebra and forehead in a case of anasarca.

- Apply the pressure by your tip of the thumb so that there is blanching of thumbnail (to detect pitting).
- If *upper part of body is involved* press over wrist, lateral epicondyle at elbow, sternum, vertebra and forehead for demonstration of oedema.

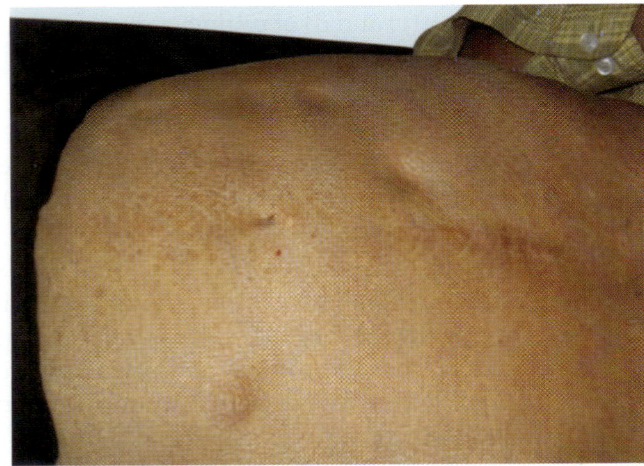

Fig. 3.27: **Parietal oedema** demonstrated by pressing the tips of the five fingers of right hand over the abdomen. Ascites and scar of past abdominal operation are also evident. Here, the patient is lying supine in bed

- Some clinicians press behind the malleoli in the ankles in ambulatory patient for earliest sign of oedema.

Q. How to classify oedema clinically?

A. Whether it pits on pressure or not:

I. **Pitting oedema:** Commonly seen in:
   a. Congestive cardiac failure (*see* **Fig. 1.9**).
   b. Cirrhosis of liver.
   c. Nephrotic syndrome.
   d. Hypoproteinaemia with severe anaemia, e.g. in protein-losing enteropathy, starvation, kwashiorkor (nutritional oedema).
   e. Pericardial effusion.
   f. Constrictive pericarditis.
   g. Drugs: Amlodipine (i.e. vasodilators), liquorice, NSAIDs, corticosteroid, oestrogens.
   h. Venous obstruction.
   i. Neurogenic oedema (due to autonomic dysfunction).
   j. Beriberi, epidemic dropsy.

II. **Non-pitting oedema** or 'solid oedema': Commonly seen in:
   a. Myxoedema (usually it is infiltrative oedema due to deposition of mucinous material).
   b. Lymphatic oedema (late stage), e.g. filariasis (due to organisation of protein-rich fluid) (*see* **Fig. 1.77**), malignant infiltration or radiation injury.
   c. Angioneurotic oedema.
   d. Chronic venous insufficiency (with darkened and discoloured skin due to haemosiderin).
   e. Pretibial myxoedema in Graves' disease.
   f. Scleredema (post-streptococcal, self-limited, painless oedematous induration of face, scalp, neck, trunk and upper extremities) or initial stage of scleroderma.

B. According to distribution of oedema:

I. **Generalised:** It is known as **'anasarca'** (oedema was previously known as 'dropsy') and the causes are the same as, a) b) c) and d) of pitting oedema. Points e) and f) too may develop into anasarca.

II. **Localised:** The common causes are:
   a. Venous obstruction: Pregnancy, SVC syndrome, IVC syndrome, varicose veins in legs, prolonged recumbency, deep venous thrombosis (DVT), immobilised or paralysed limb.
   b. Lymphatic obstruction (lymphoedema): Filariasis (and even elephantiasis), tuberculosis, trauma, carcinoma of the breast, following radical mastectomy, radiation injury, Milroy's disease (congenital hypoplasia of lymph vessels, benign disorder affecting young girls) (**Fig. 3.28**).
   c. Allergic cause: Angioneurotic oedema, acute anaphylaxis.
   d. Inflammatory: Caused by insect bite, snake bite, trauma, ischaemia or infections, vasculitis, severe septicaemia, and is probably due to liberation of histamine and other factors (increases capillary permeability).
   e. Miscellaneous: Bruises, sprains, cellulitis, fracture, gout.

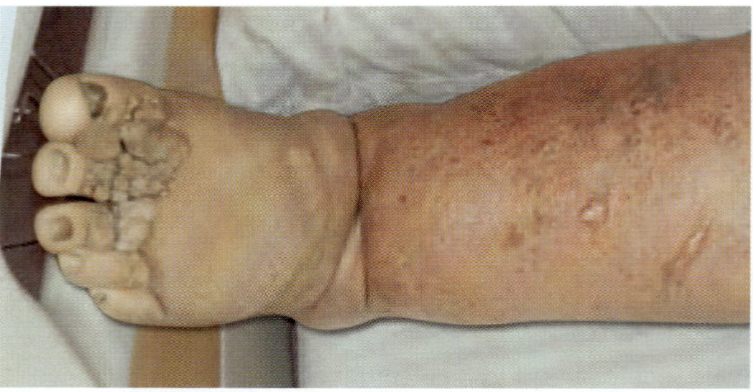

Fig. 3.28: **Milroy's disease** (congenital **lymphoedema**) with non-pitting oedema

- Localised causes may present as **unilateral oedema**; cyclical oedema may be unilateral.
- Oedema may be restricted to limited region like pedal, sacral, facial, genital or becomes generalised.
- In the early stage, lymphatic oedema is soft and pits easily on pressure.
- Oedema may be 'postural', especially in the lower limbs (e.g. prolonged bus journey) and is due to failure of muscle movement.

Clinical Wisdom

'Slow' pitting oedema (>40 seconds) is found in CCF in comparison to 'fast' pitting oedema (<40 seconds) observed in hypoproteinaemia, i.e. nephrotic syndrome. This division is done arbitrarily by obliteration of pitting by slow return or rapid return of displaced fluid, respectively.

Q. Grading of oedema (pitting)—a rough clinical assessment:

A. Based on pitting depth and duration of the indentation:

Grades	Pitting depth	Duration of indentation
1	≤2 mm	Disappears immediately
2	2–4 mm	Disappears in 10–15 seconds
3	4–6 mm	May last for 30 seconds
4	6–8 mm or more	May last for >30 seconds

B. Severity of oedema (pitting):

Grades	Areas of involvement
Mild	Both feet/ankles
Moderate	Both feet + lower legs, hands or lower arms
Severe	Generalised bilateral pitting oedema, including both feet, legs, arms and face

Q. What is angioneurotic oedema (Quincke's oedema) (Fig. 3.29)?

This is the swelling of dermis and subcutaneous tissue, and is of two types: hereditary and acquired.

1. It is a specific form of allergic oedema which results from hypersensitivity.

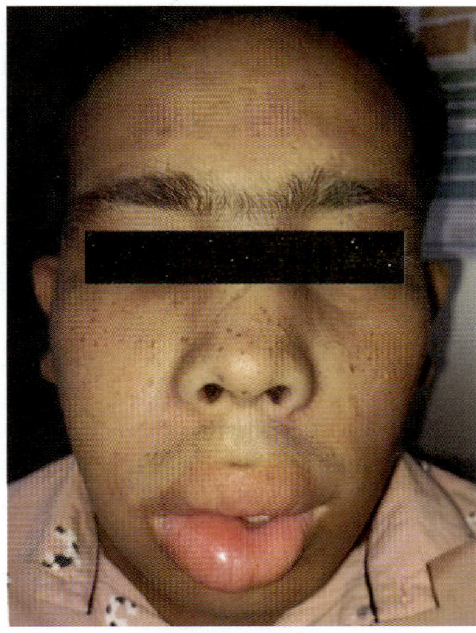

Fig. 3.29: **Angio-oedema** of lips

2. It is a solid oedema; involves deeper layer of skin; usually lasts for a few hours. Resolves slowly.
3. Commonly localised in tongue, lips, uvula, face, eyelids, etc. Usually patchy involvement.
4. The swelling develops rapidly, and is pale or faintly pink in colour.
5. Associated with itching; may be ACE inhibitor induced (acquired).
6. Congenital (hereditary) variety is due to C_1 esterase inhibitor deficiency (without itching).
7. It can involve GI tract leading to cyclic abdominal pain.
8. May threaten life by suffocation, if larynx or tongue is affected.

Q. Symptoms of oedema:

Localised swelling (feet, ankles, hands) or swelling of the whole body, facial puffiness, bloating, rapid weight gain, pain and tightness of the affected part, breathlessness or development of indentation when pressed by finger. Onset, duration, progression, aggravating and relieving factors should be asked for.

Q. How much body weight is to be increased for development of pitting oedema?

Minimally 10–15% increase in body weight (i.e. 5–6 litres of fluid) is necessary for demonstration of pitting oedema. It is also seen that pitting oedema occurs when the circumference of the limb is increased by 10%.

Q. Why lymphatic oedema is intractable?

Lymphoedema is also known as 'brawny' oedema where the skin feels indurated and thickened with peau d'orange appearance of the skin (i.e. orange peel skin) (*see* **Fig. 1.74**).

It is known that restriction of lymphatic flow results in increased protein concentration in the interstitial fluid (water and solutes are reabsorbed in capillaries), a situation which severely impedes removal of retained fluid.

Q. Most reliable index of progress to treatment in a case of oedema:

Day to day alteration in body weight.

Q. How cardiac oedema differs from renal oedema?

A. Congestive cardiac failure:

1. Patients will be dyspnoeic.
2. Engorged and pulsatile neck vein with soft, tender, mild hepatomegaly.
3. Sometimes associated with right ventricular gallop rhythm.
4. Evidence of heart disease, i.e. cardiomegaly may be present.
5. Oedema **starts in the dependent part (around the ankles and pretibial region)** and then **ascends** progressively; pitting oedema. It is also present over the sacrum in a patient who is largely bed-bound. Oedema is initially noticed at the end of day's work (shoes become tighter in the evening) (*see* **Fig. 1.9**).

B. Nephrotic syndrome:

1. A history of previous renal disease may or may not be elicited.
2. Oedema **starts in the face (mainly periorbital)**, arms and then **descends**. Oedema is usually noticed in the early morning. Swelling of scrotal sacs and lower eyelids (due to low tissue tension) are classical (*see* **Figs 1.57 and 1.58**), pitting oedema; sacral oedema in non-ambulatory patients.
3. Evidences of massive proteinuria, severe hypoproteinaemia and hypercholesterolaemia.

- Periorbital and scrotal loose subcutaneous tissue favour accumulation of oedema fluid there (in nephrotic syndrome).
- In CRF, oedema may be either due to renal insufficiency or cardiac failure secondary to hypertension.

Q. Evolution of oedema in different systemic diseases:

1. Congestive cardiac failure: Legs → face → ascites.
2. Nephrotic syndrome: Face (periorbital puffiness) → legs → ascites (with scrotal swelling).
3. Cirrhosis of liver: Ascites → legs → face (rarely involved).
4. Nutritional oedema: Oedema feet with puffiness of face → ascites.

Q. Common causes of pedal oedema:

Pedal oedema may be unilateral or bilateral (*see* below).

1. Congestive cardiac failure.
2. Nutritional oedema, protein-losing enteropathy, hypoalbuminaemia due to any cause.
3. Cirrhosis of liver.
4. Varicose veins, deep vein thrombosis (DVT); abdominal mass (tumour, cyst, pregnancy).
5. Filariasis or chronic lymphatic obstruction, Milroy's disease (**Fig. 3.28**).
6. Nephrotic syndrome.

7. Cyclical oedema (female > male, pitting oedema, temporal relationship with menstrual cycle).
8. Drug-induced: Nifedipine or amlodipine, fludrocortisone, NSAIDs, oestrogens, corticosteroids.
9. Miscellaneous: Pericardial effusion, constrictive pericarditis, immobility (e.g. hemiplegia), postural (inactive persons or prolonged immobilisation), cellulitis, over inflamed joint, lipaedema (abnormal fat deposition in the hips, thighs and legs sparing feet; only in women), irradiation.

- **Unilateral:** Deep vein thrombosis, cellulitis, angioneurotic oedema, ruptured Baker's cyst, diabetic foot, filariasis (early stage), hermiplegic side and trauma; **Bilateral:** Other causes mentioned in the question above.
- In oedema of legs, try to determine its upper level (e.g. oedema up to mid-thigh, etc.)
- Possible aetiology of **acutely swollen leg:** DVT, cellulitis, trauma or fracture, arterial occlusion, arthritis or insect bite.

Q. Common causes of facial puffiness:

1. Familial: facial cellulitis.
2. Hypoproteinaemia (nephrotic syndrome, acute nephritis, severe anaemia, protein-energy malnutrition).
3. Congestive cardiac failure, pericardial effusion, constrictive pericarditis.
4. Myxoedema.
5. SVC syndrome.
6. Cushing's syndrome.
7. Angioneurotic oedema.
8. Trichinosis as a result of infected pork ingestion.

- **'Conjunctival oedema'** is common in hypoalbuminaemia, Weil's disease, Graves' disease, fluid overload and SVC syndrome.
- **'Periorbital oedema (or puffiness)'** is found in nephrotic syndrome, acute glomerulonephritis, myxoedema, angioneurotic oedema, heart failure, dermatomyositis, trichinosis, excessive crying, orbital cellulitis, allergic eye disease and thyroid eye disease. Loose subcutaneous tissue favours accumulation of fluid around the eyes.

Q. Different mechanisms of oedema formation:

The four main factors are:

1. Low plasma oncotic pressure, e.g. hypoproteinaemia (in cirrhosis of liver).
2. High capillary hydrostatic pressure, e.g. congestive cardiac failure, DVT.
3. Increased capillary permeability, e.g. acute inflammation, amlodipine-induced.
4. Obstructed lymphatic drainage, e.g. filariasis, radiation.

Q. Why there is oedema in heart failure?

1. Impairment of renal blood flow results in more salt and water resorption.
2. Increase in venous pressure (thus, in right-sided heart failure there is venous congestion in systemic circulation, i.e. there is development of oedema, and in left-sided heart failure there is pulmonary venous congestion).
3. Secondary hyperaldosteronism.
4. Increased level of ADH.
5. Some lymphatic factors may play a role.
6. Chronic passive venous congestion of liver from heart diseases (produces hypoalbuminaemia).

- In lipodermatosclerosis (the skin is teethered and cannot expand to accommodate oedema fluid), ankle may be spared in early oedema. Usually a female patient presents with painful areas of inflammation with induration. It may produce non-pitting oedema.
- Be careful in examining a patient of anasarca as the patient may have bilateral hydrothorax, ascites, hydrocele (with or without scrotal oedema) and rarely, pericardial effusion. Oedema restricted only in the upper half of the body is commonly due to SVC syndrome.
- **Filariasis** may be given as a spot case (*see* **Fig. 1.77**).

Clinical Wisdom

Examination by the **tip of the thumb:** Oedema is demonstrated; painful pressure over root of the nose (supraorbital pressure) or sternum for sense of arousal in coma or hysteria is exerted by tip of the thumb.

Examination by the **ball of the thumb**: a) Sternal tenderness, b) Murphy's kidney punch, c) Carotid massage, and d) Air sinus tenderness are demonstrated clinically.

CLUBBING — CASE 43

Q. What is clubbing?

This is the bulbous swelling of the terminal part of the fingers and the toes with an increase in the soft tissue mass (particularly on the dorsal surface), and increased antero-posterior as well as transverse diameter of the nails due to proliferation of subungual connective tissue, interstitial oedema, and dilatation of arterioles and capillaries (**Fig. 3.30**). Clubbing is also known

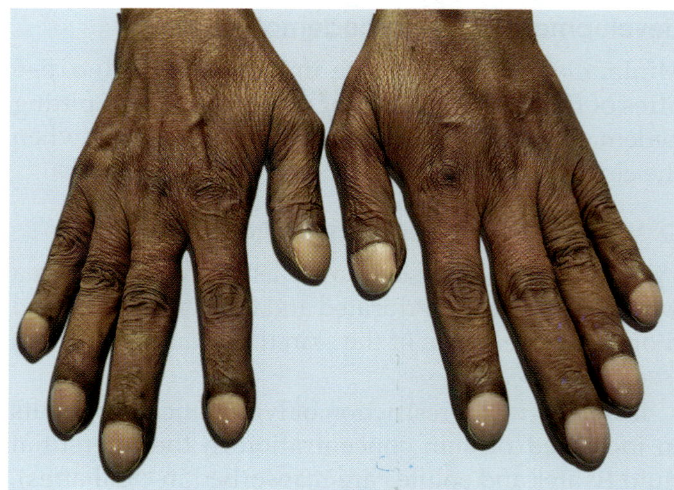

Fig. 3.30: Pandigital **clubbing** seen in cyanotic congenital heart disease

as Hippocratic fingers; clubbing was first described by Hippocrates in a patient of empyema thoracis approximately 2400 years ago. It is a window in clinical medicine and is usually a valuable clue to an underlying disease.

Q. What is onychodermal angle?

It is the angle formed between the nail and the nail-bed. It is also known as **Lovibond's angle** ('profile sign'). The normal angle is approximately 160°. Clinically it is judged by the angle formed between the nail and the adjacent skin-fold. Thus, the other name for clubbing is Lovibond's sign.

Q. How will you examine for clubbing?

a. **First step:** Bring the patient's fingers at your eye level and look tangentially. Observe the onychodermal angle. If the angle is 180° or more, it is said that clubbing is present (Fig. 3.31).
b. **Second step:** Very early clubbing can be detected by increase in fluctuation of the nail-bed (due to softening of the nail-bed). To elicit 'fluctuation', the patient's finger (say the middle finger) is placed on the pulp of examiner's two thumbs and held in this position by gentle pressure with the tips of examiner's middle fingers applied on the patient's proximal interphalangeal joint. The patient's finger is now palpated over the base of the nail by the tips of examiner's index fingers (Fig. 3.32). There is always some amount of fluctuation present in normal fingers (a very subjective sign). When fluctuation is obvious (due to clubbing), nail matrix gives a spongy feel and palpation of the nail-bed may give the impression that the nail is floating on its bed.

- For detection of clubbing, first examine the onychodermal angle and then for fluctuation.

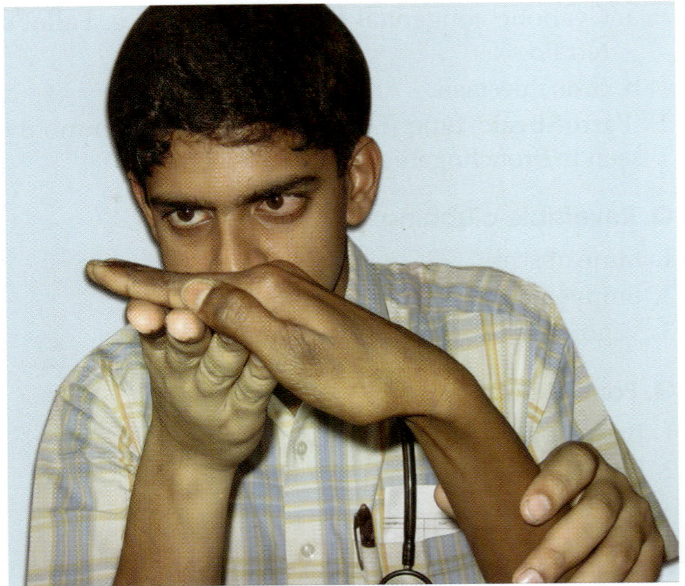

Fig. 3.31: **Detection of clubbing** by bringing patient's fingers at eye level and looking tangentially (profile sign)

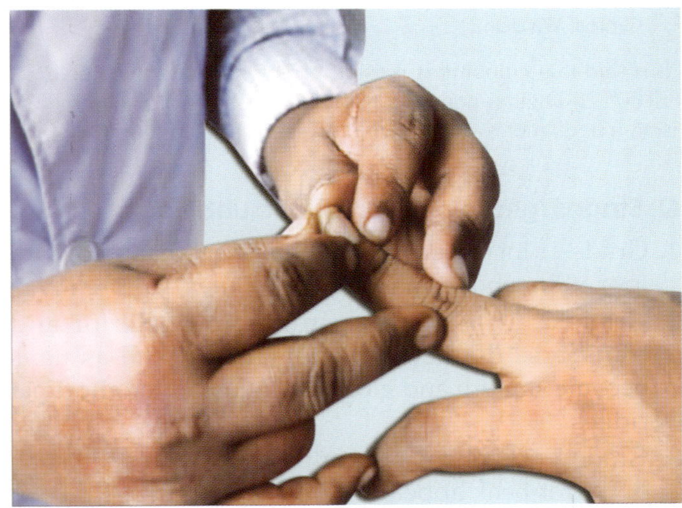

Fig. 3.32: Examination for **'fluctuation'** at nail-bed

Q. Alternative methods for detection of clubbing:

Few clinicians prefer this method. Place the nails of two fingers of two hands (preferably the thumbs or ring fingers of both hands are taken for examination) face to face and look for the diamond-shaped area formed between the two nails and the proximal nail-folds. The normally formed diamond-shaped area is obliterated in the presence of clubbing. This is known as **window sign** or **Schamroth's sign** (Fig. 3.33).

- [**Shadowgraphy:** Magnified shadow images of right index finger, and **thermography:** Where an infra-red camera is used to detect increased temperature in distal digits in clubbing, can help in diagnosis].

Q. Digital Index:

It is an objective measurement (or numerical assessment) of clubbing. For individual finger, the circumference at nail-bed (i.e. at the site of onychodermal junction) is divided by the circumference at the distal interphalangeal joint. The individual digit ratio of 10 fingers are added. The final value is now divided by 10, and if it is found to be >1, clubbing is said to be present. Digital index in health is <1.

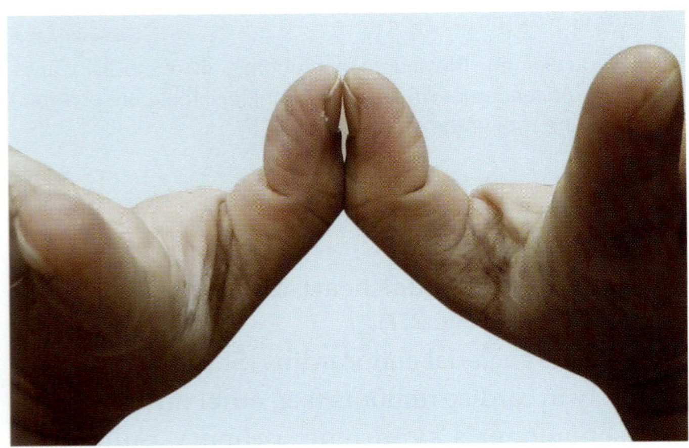

Fig. 3.33: Demonstration of **Schamroth's sign**

Clinical Wisdom

It is said that **clubbing is present** if: 1) Onychodermal angle is >180°, 2) Digital index is >1, and 3) Presence of Schamroth's sign (i.e. diamond-shaped window gap is obliterated).

Q. Stages (grade or degree) of clubbing:

1. Grade 1: Increased fluctuation of the nail-bed with loss of onychodermal angle.
2. Grade 2: 1° + increase in antero-posterior and transverse diameter of the nails as well as nails become smooth and glossy with loss of longitudinal ridges.
3. Grade 3: 2° + increased pulp tissue (with drumstick or parrot-beak appearance).
4. Grade 4: 3° + wrist and ankle swelling due to HOA (hypertrophic osteoarthropathy).

Clinical Wisdom

The severity is classified as mild, moderate and gross. Affection of 20 digits (10 fingers plus 10 toes) is known as **pandigital clubbing,** while according to few clinicians: 1° and 2° are designated as **mild clubbing**, and 3° and 4° as **severe clubbing.**

Q. What is HPOA?

It is known as hypertrophic pulmonary osteoarthropathy (HPOA) where there is 'subperiosteal new bone formation' with periosteal thickening (in a patient of clubbing) at the lower end of radius, ulna, tibia and fibula, and the patient complains of swelling as well as pain in the wrist (most common) and ankle; the elbow and knee joint may be affected. The joints become swollen and tender on palpation. Ultimately other bones like ribs, clavicle, scapula may be affected. HPOA is commonly seen in bronchogenic carcinoma (usually from squamous cell variety) and that is why the term 'pulmonary' is added, and is probably due to release of vascular endothelial growth factor (VEGF) in the circulation. It is diagnosed by X-ray; isotope bone scanning may reveal increased periosteal activity. HOA may be **familial** (pachydermoperiostitis; autosomal dominant inheritance) or idiopathic.

Clinical Wisdom

When you examine the patient for clubbing, always look for any swelling and tenderness in the wrist or ankle. If these are present, the clubbing is of grade 4 or 4°.

Q. Causes of clubbing:

A. Cardiac causes:

1. Cyanotic congenital heart diseases like Fallot's tetralogy (see Fig. 2.1).
2. Subacute bacterial endocarditis (SBE).
3. Rarely in cardiac tumours (e.g. atrial myxoma).
4. Eisenmenger's syndrome, primary pulmonary hypertension, etc.

B. Lung and pleural causes:

1. Bronchietasis.
2. Lung abscess.
3. Bronchogenic carcinoma.
4. Empyema thoracis.
5. Fibrosing alveolitis (ILD).
6. Pleural mesothelioma.
7. Pulmonary arteriovenous fistula.
8. Cystic fibrosis.
9. Rarely in long-standing extensive fibrocaseous tuberculosis.

C. Ulcerative colitis.

D. Billary cirrhosis, sometimes in hepato-pulmonary syndrome.

E. Intestinal causes:

1. Malabsorption syndrome.
2. Crohn's disease.
3. Polyposis coli.
4. Coeliac disease.

F. Normal: Found normally in some people (idiopathic) or neurological (e.g. syringomyelia)

G. Genetic: May be a familial condition (rare).

- Remember the mnemonic 'Clubing' to remember the causes. Majority of the causes of clubbing remain within the CVS and respiratory system. Uncomplicated *COPD does not give rise to clubbing*.
- Clubbing may be primary (idiopathic, hereditary) and secondary (acquired).
- The commonest cause in young is bronchiectasis and that in elderly is bronchogenic carcinoma.

Q. Different types of clubbing:

1. **'Drumstick'** type (i.e. bulbous terminal part) is seen in:
   a. Cyanotic congenital heart diseases, e.g. Fallot's tetralogy.
   b. Bronchiectasis.
2. **'Parrot-beak'** type (i.e. biconvex nail): Commonly seen in bronchogenic carcinoma.

Q. Reversible clubbing:

1. Lung abscess.
2. Empyema thoracis.
3. Vagotomy in bronchogenic carcinoma.

Q. Painful clubbing:

1. Bronchogenic carcinoma.
2. SBE.
3. Lung abscess.

Q. Clubbing limited to upper extremity:

Chronic obstructive phlebitis of upper extremity as a result of chronic IV drug addiction (e.g. heroin).

Q. Clubbing limited to lower extremity (differential clubbing):

In infected abdominal aortic aneurysm; sometimes in PDA with reversal of shunt (with cyanosis).

Q. Unilateral clubbing:

1. Presubclavian coarctation of aorta (left-sided clubbing).
2. Bronchogenic carcinoma (commonly apical).
3. Cervical rib; long-continued hemiplegia.
4. Aneurysm of subclavian or axillary artery.
5. Erythromelalgia.
6. Arteriovenous fistula of brachial vessels.

Q. Unidigital clubbing:

1. Hereditary (if bilateral).
2. Repeated local trauma.
3. Rarely from median nerve injury or deposition of tophi (gout).
4. Sarcoidosis.
5. Thyrotoxicosis.
6. Digital mucoid cyst.

Q. What is 'acute' clubbing?

When the clubbing develops very rapidly, e.g. in lung abscess and empyema thoracis, it may evolve as early as 10–14 days after the onset of illness, and is known as 'acute' clubbing.

Q. Why the pulp tissue is increased in clubbing?

This is due to:
1. Proliferation of subungual connective tissue.
2. Interstitial oedema.
3. Dilatation of arterioles and capillaries, or opening of anastomosing channels at nail-bed.

Q. Most 'reliable' early sign of clubbing:

It is the loss of normal onychodermal angle. One of the earliest sign is increased fluctuation of the nail-bed, though not always reliable.

Q. Causes of 'pseudoclubbing':

This is due to subperiosteal bone resorption of terminal phalanges (there is absence of soft tissue proliferation and increased curvature of nails) and is seen in:
1. Scleroderma.
2. Acromegaly.
3. Hyperparathyroidism.
4. Leprosy.
5. People working with vinyl chloride (acroosteolysis).

Q. Which finger is usually affected first in clubbing?

Usually the index finger.

Q. Points to note when clubbing is detected:

1. Unilateral or bilateral.
2. The degree of clubbing.
3. Duration of clubbing.
4. Painful or not.
5. Presence or absence of central cyanosis.
6. Presence or absence of dyspnoea.

Q. Possible mechanisms of clubbing:

The different hypothesis are:
1. Anoxic (arterial hypoxaemia): This is the most important theory which leads to 'opening up of deep arteriovenous anastomotic channels' of the terminal phalanges resulting in overgrowth of soft tissues; example: Fallot's tetralogy.
2. Toxic: The example is SBE.
3. Reflex (neurogenic): Vagotomy often improves the clubbing in bronchogenic carcinoma.
4. Metabolic: The example is thyrotoxicosis.
5. Humoral: Increased growth hormone, parathormone, bradykinin, e.g. in acromegaly.
6. Pressure changes between the radial and the digital arteries.
7. Reduced ferritin (ferritin may escape oxidation in lungs and leads to dilatation of arteriovenous anastomosis by entering into systemic circulation) may play an important role (recent view).

Q. Pathogenesis of clubbing:

1. Hereditary predisposition: An autosomal dominant gene of variable penetrance has been detected.
2. Vasodilators, e.g. growth hormone, parathormone, prostaglandins, bradykinins, 5-HT and adenine nucleotides may be responsible for the development of clubbing. In bronchogenic carcinoma, vasodilator substances normally detoxified by lungs enter into systemic circulation unaltered.
3. There is trapping of megakaryocytes and platelet clumps with local release of platelet-derived growth factor (PDGF), VEGF and other cytokines (TNF-α), which increase the capillary permeability and accentuate proliferation of connective tissue **(latest and most acceptable theory)**.

Q. Some other uncommon causes of clubbing:

1. Thyrotoxicosis (part of thyroid acropachy).
2. Asbestosis.
3. Occupational, i.e. in jackhammer operators.
4. Sarcoidosis.
5. Amoebic liver abscess.
6. Portal cirrhosis.
7. Syringomyelia.
8. Palmoplantar keratoderma.

Q. What is koilonychia?

It is the 'spoon-shaped deformity' of the nail usually found in chronic iron deficiency anaemia **(Fig. 3.34)**. Koilonychia develops as a result of retarded growth of the nail plate. '*Koilos*' means hollow and '*onikh*' means nail. Toe nails are affected earlier than the finger nails.

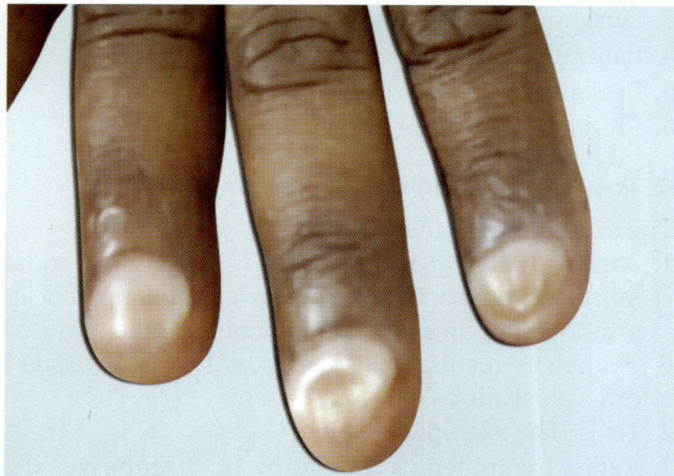

Fig. 3.34: **Koilonychia** (concave nails) is seen in index and middle fingers in chronic iron deficiency anaemia from bleeding haemorrhoids

Q. How to examine for koilonychia?

Bring the patient's fingers at your eye level and look tangentially (same as clubbing). Observe as well as palpate the nail plates for any flattening or spooning.

Q. Stages of koilonychia:

There are three stages:

a. First stage: 'Stage of brittleness', where the nail becomes brittle and rough.
b. Second stage: 'Stage of flattening' (platonychia); the nail is thin, flat and without longitudinal ridges.
c. Third stage: 'Stage of spooning', where the nail becomes concave.

- In the third stage, the indentation may be deep enough to hold a drop of water on the nail.

Q. Causes of koilonychia:

1. Long-standing iron deficiency anaemia (commonest).
2. Idiopathic or familial (autosomal dominant).
3. Onycholysis due to any cause (e.g. onychomycosis) may give rise to spooning of nails.
4. Overuse of solvent (e.g. nail varnish remover) or detergents.

[5. Very rarely in thyrotoxicosis or myxoedema.]

Clinical Wisdom

After examination of one hand for clubbing, examine the other hand and next examine the toes.

MOON FACE — CASE 44

Q. Describe the face:

The face looks bloated and rounded (like the full moon) (Fig. 3.35).

Q. Common causes of moon face:

1. Cushing's syndrome (and Cushing's disease): With hirsutism and facial plethora.

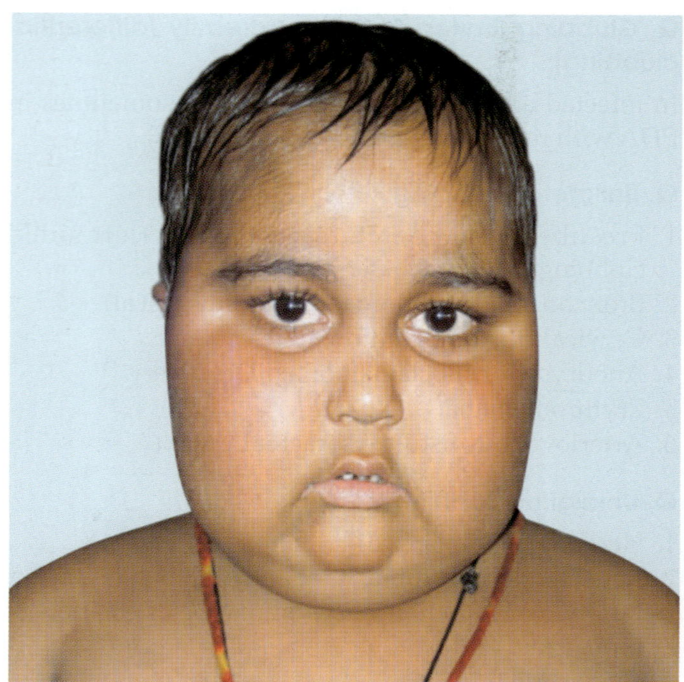

Fig. 3.35: **Moon face** with facial plethora, excessive hair growth in forehead, double chin and obesity—an effect of long-continued steroid therapy

2. Nephrotic syndrome (marked periorbital oedema; with baggy lower eyelids) (*see* Fig. 1.57).
3. Acute glomerulonephritis (periorbital oedema with narrowing of palpebral fissure).
4. Prolonged steroid therapy (often with hirsutism and facial plethora) (Fig. 3.35).
5. Myxoedema (with baggy lower eyelids, fall of lateral eyebrows).
6. Superior mediastinal syndrome (with prominent veins in forehead and temple region) (*see* Fig. 2.2).
7. Angioneurotic oedema of face (lips may be swollen, patchy involvement) (*see* Fig. 3.29).
8. Subcutaneous emphysema of face, extending from chest (asymmetrical swelling).
9. Rarely, advanced stage of CCF, severe hypoproteinaemia and alcoholism (puffy face).
10. Simple obesity.

- Read individual section for description.

Q. 'Check list' prior to corticosteroid therapy:

1. H/o diabetes mellitus.
2. Pyogenic infection anywhere in the body.
3. Presence of active tuberculosis.
4. Peptic ulcer, gastritis or +ve occult blood in stool.
5. Uncontrolled hypertension.
6. Evidence of osteoporosis.
7. Bleeding tendencies.
8. Previous H/o any psychological disorder.
9. Pregnancy and lactation.

Q. Common indications for corticosteroid therapy:

1. Addison's disease; Sheehan's syndrome.
2. Anaphylactic shock.
3. Acute severe asthma.
4. Circulatory shock.
5. Acute lymphoblastic leukaemia.
6. SLE and other collagen diseases.
7. Rheumatoid arthritis.
8. Nephrotic syndrome.
9. Acute rheumatic carditis.
10. Increased intracranial tension.
11. Interstitial lung disease (ILD).
12. In organ transplants to prevent rejection.
13. Lymphoma.
14. Giant cell arteritis.
15. Vasculitides.
16. Pemphigus vulgaris.

Q. How to reduce the side effects of corticosteroid?

The chance of systemic effects, osteoporosis are increased, if the daily dose of prednisolone is >7.5 mg. So, give steroids only in established indications with lowest possible dose, single dose, alternate days therapy than daily dosing, morning dose with minimal possible duration; curtail sodium and calorie intake, supplement with calcium and/or vitamin D, and bisphosphonates (if steroid used for >3 months), add H_2RA/PPI, avoid smoking and alcohol consumption, start aerobic exercise—may minimize the side effects on prolonged use.

Q. Side effects of prolonged corticosteroid therapy:

a. Metabolic effects: More or less identical to those seen in Cushing's syndrome, e.g. hyperglycaemia, hypokalaemia, hypochloraemia, alkalosis, sodium and fluid retention, osteoporosis, etc **(Table 3.3)**.
b. Suppression of hypothalamo-pituitary-adrenal (HPA) axis: In a patient with suppressed HPA axis, it may take months or years to recover fully. The dosage of steroid given only in the morning, or on alternate days, or gradual withdrawal of the drug will produce less suppression of HPA axis. Treatment for 3 weeks or less with prednisolone <5 mg/day will not suppress adrenal axis significantly.
c. Features like Cushing's syndrome: Moon face, truncal obesity, growth retardation, acne, hirsutism, purple striae, easy bruising, osteoporosis, avascular necrosis of bone, peptic ulcer, pancreatitis, hypertension, diabetes mellitus, glaucoma, cataract, CCF, psychosis, myopathy and impotence.

Table 3.3: Differences between ACTH and corticosteroid therapy

Features	ACTH	Corticosteroid
1. Administration	Parenteral	Oral and parenteral
2. Sodium retention	More marked	Less marked
3. Adrenal androgen	Increased	No rise
4. Adrenal atrophy	Absent	Present
5. Acne	More	Less than ACTH

- Morning cortisol level in serum is low in iatrogenic Cushing's syndrome (i.e. steroid-induced) in comparison to true Cushing's syndrome where the level is high.

Q. Effects of sudden withdrawal of corticosteroid therapy:

The patients should be advised to avoid sudden drug withdrawal as it may produce:

1. Suppression of HPA axis.
2. Acute adrenal insufficiency.
3. Pseudotumour cerebri (especially affecting young and obese women; there is headache, papilloedema, constricted visual field with absent neurological signs, dilated ventricles on CT scan; idiopathic condition, may be treated with steroid or ventriculo-peritoneal shunt).

Q. What is 'Facies'?

It is the 'expressions in the face' of the patient, and very often these facial signs collectively lead to prompt aetiological diagnosis of a disease. The facies may be anxious, sad, calm, happy, expressionless, pyrexial, toxic, dehydrated, puffy or may show some specific characteristics of a particular disease, e.g. parkinsonism, thyrotoxicosis or acromegaly. As face is known as 'mirror of the mind', reading of face is very important in clinical medicine.

Q. Identification points (moon face):

a. Rounded and bloated face: Moon face.
b. With obesity: Cushing's syndrome, prolonged steroid therapy, myxoedema, simple obesity.
c. With engorged neck veins: SVC syndrome, acute glomerulonephritis.
d. Expressionless face: Myxoedema.
e. Malar flush or plethora of face: Myxoedema or Cushing's syndrome.
f. With hirsutism: Cushing's syndrome or prolonged steroid therapy.
g. With breathlessness: SVC syndrome or receiving steroid for bronchial asthma.
h. With anasarca: Nephrotic syndrome.
i. With pallor: Nephrotic syndrome, myxoedema, SVC syndrome.

Clinical Wisdom

If after careful and meticulous **examination of face** (in any patient), no diagnosis (of any 'specific facies') is reached, always try to look for:

1) Tongue (cyanosis, severe anaemia), 2) Pseudoptosis or partial ptosis, 3) Mild exophthalmos or enophthalmos, 4) Malar flush, 5) Masked facies, 6) Artificial eye, 7) goitre (though not a structure within the face), and 8) Ask the patient to show the upper teeth (facial palsy).

DWARFISM (SHORT STATURE) CASE 45

Q. What is dwarfism?

Dwarfism or short stature is a condition where the height of a person is much below in relation to chronological age and sex of that person as compared to a normal individual.

Q. Common causes of dwarfism or 'short stature':

1. Heredofamilial.
2. Constitutional (delayed growth and puberty): The commonest cause.
3. Protein-energy malnutrition (PEM), e.g. marasmus and kwashiorkor.
4. Rickets.
5. Cretinism (hypothyroidism).
6. Pituitary dwarf (hypopituitarism).
7. Achondroplasia, mucopolysaccharidosis; progeria.
8. Cyanotic congenital heart diseases, e.g. Fallot's tetralogy.
9. Gross kyphoscoliosis; collapse of vertebra due to osteoporosis (↓height in elderly).
10. Down syndrome, Turner's syndrome (Fig. 3.36), Cushing's syndrome, Noonan's syndrome.
11. Pseudohypoparathyroidism.
12. Cystic fibrosis, bronchiectasis, thalassaemia major, coeliac disease, osteogenesis imperfecta, renal tubular acidosis, uncontrolled type 1 diabetes mellitus, intrauterine growth retardation.

Q. What is cretinism?

Cretinism—hypothyroidism since birth due to partial or complete failure of thyroid gland (commonly due to thyroidal agenesis).

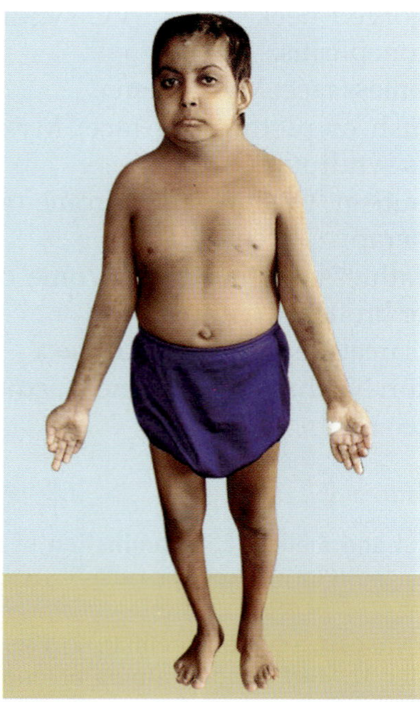

Fig. 3.36: Short stature, webbed neck, low hair line, low set ear, 'shield-like' chest with mild mental subnormality in **Turner's syndrome** (girl aged 18 years)

Juvenile myxoedema—onset of hypothyroidism since childhood but develops before puberty (commonly due to dyshormonogenesis).

Myxoedema—onset of hypothyroidism after puberty (probably Hashimoto's thyroiditis is the commonest cause).

Q. Describe the facies in cretinism (Fig. 3.37):

The facies resembles an old man's face:

1. Appearance is dull, expressionless and idiotic; large head with sparse scalp hair.
2. Depressed bridge of the nose, broad flat nose with big nostrils.
3. Hypertelorism (widely set eyes) with wrinkling of eyebrows, narrow palpebral fissures.
4. Sparse, coarse and brittle hair with dry skin.
5. Lips are thick and everted with big, fissured, protruded tongue (macroglossia).
6. Delayed dentition with hoarse voice.

Q. Other morphologic characteristics of cretin (Fig. 3.38A):

1. Short stature but maintains the infantile proportion, i.e. upper segment > lower segment.
2. The patient is lethargic and apathetic.
3. Markedly retarded intelligence. Memory is grossly impaired.
4. Skin is dry, scaly, rough and cold; skin looks pale yellow (i.e. carotenaemia).
5. Thick and short neck with presence of supraclavicular pad of fat.
6. Pot-bellied abdomen with umbilical hernia.
7. Flaccid muscles with marked hypotonia.

Q. Features of hypothyroidism in neonatal period:

1. Prolonged physiological jaundice.
2. Hoarse cry.
3. Somnolence.

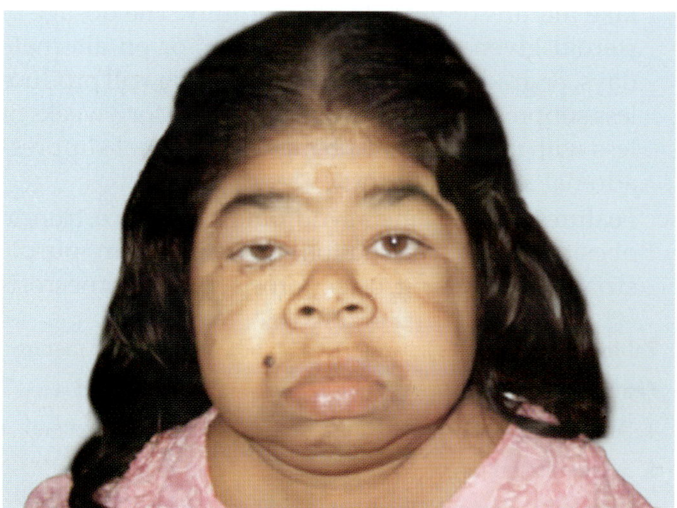

Fig. 3.37: Cretinism showing dwarfism, depressed bridge of the nose, broad flat nose with big nostrils, thick lips with a dull, idiotic and expressionless puffy face

4. Feeding problem (difficulty in sucking).
5. Constipation, and
6. Delayed milestones of development (later months).

Q. How to differentiate between cretin and pituitary dwarf?

The characteristics of cretin **(thyroid dwarf)** are (Fig. 3.38A):

a. Depressed bridge of the nose; coarse facies.
b. Lack of intelligence, and
c. More or less, normal genial development.

The characteristics of **pituitary dwarf** are (Fig. 3.38B):

a. 'Juvenile' facies; characteristically 'chubby'.
b. Normal intelligence, and
c. Sexual infantilism.

Q. Laboratory diagnosis of cretinism:

A. Blood:

a. High serum cholesterol.
b. Low radioactive I^{131} uptake.
c. T_4 level is low with high TSH level.

- In neonates, heel-prick blood sample is used.

B. ECG: Low voltage.

C. Skeletal X-ray (of long bones and pelvis):

a. Delayed closure of epiphysis (i.e. bone age is less than that of chronological age).
b. Delayed dentition.
c. **Epiphyseal dysgenesis**: Instead of one epiphysis, there are multiple epiphyses (diagnostic).

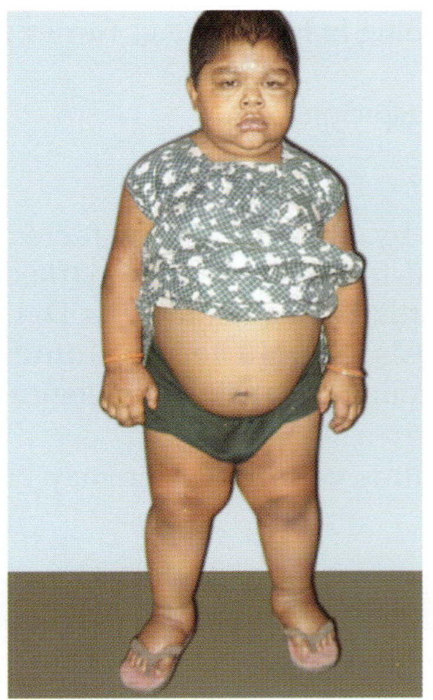

Fig. 3.38A: A **cretin** aged 16 years presented with short stature, coarse facies like depressed bridge of the nose, thick lips, broad flat nose and an idiotic look, and **pot-bellied abdomen with umbilical hernia**

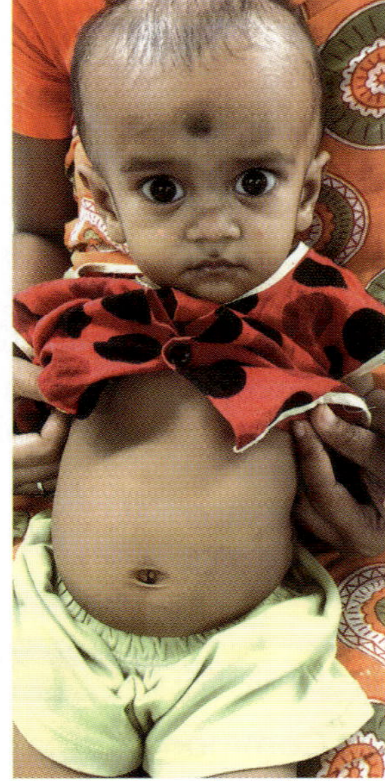

Fig. 3.38B: **Pituitary dwarf**–Juvenile facies, thick, short and plump (chubby) with normal intelligence; a boy aged 5 years

Q. Treatment of cretinism:

1. Very small dosage of L-thyroxine is needed. Initial dose is 10–25 μg, and the dose is adjusted according to clinical improvement and biochemical findings.
2. Rehabilitation.

Q. Differentiation of dwarfism (short stature) by body ratio:

A. Upper segment = Lower segment is seen in:

a. Heredofamilial.
b. Constitutional, and
c. Pituitary dwarf.

B. Upper segment > Lower segment is seen in:

a. Achondroplasia.
b. Rickets.
c. Cretinism, and
d. Juvenile myxoedema.

C. Upper segment < Lower segment is seen in: Spinal deformities, post-menopausal osteoporosis of spine.

- Remember, short stature may be associated with features of delayed puberty.

Q. Characteristics of Turner's syndrome (gonadal dysgenesis) (Figs 3.36 and 3.39):

The genetic constitution is 45, XO (karyotype); usually recognised at puberty in girls by short stature, webbed neck (i.e. a fan-like fold of skin extending from shoulders to neck), low hair line over back of the neck, 'shield-like' chest, widely spaced nipples, cubitus valgus (i.e. increased carrying angle) and mild mental retardation. Primary amenorrhoea, failure of development of secondary sexual characters, streak gonads, sterility, peripheral lymphoedema, short 4th metacarpals and coarctation of aorta may be associated features.

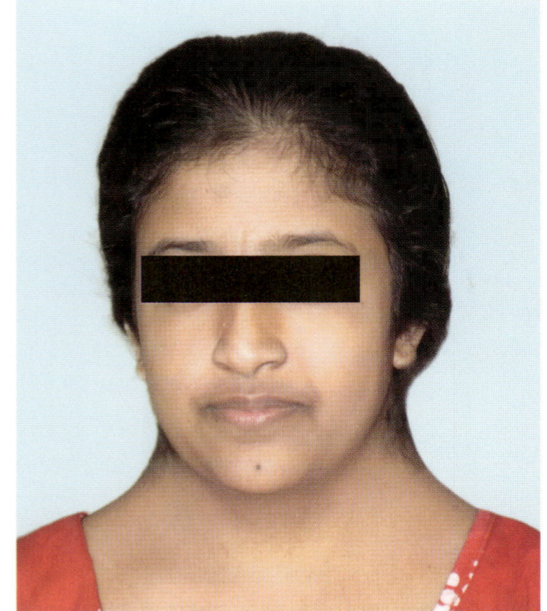

Fig. 3.39: **Turner's syndrome** with webbed neck and low hair line

Q. What is achondroplasia (Fig. 3.40)?

Dwarfism in achondroplasia results from decrease in the proliferation of cartilage present in growth plate (due to a defect in the fibroblast growth factor receptor-3 gene). It is an autosomal dominant disease and is usually recognised at birth. The dwarf jokers in the circus are usually achondroplasia patients. The characteristics are:

a. Dwarfism.
b. Normal mental (intelligence), dental, endocrine and sexual development; normal trunk.
c. Short limbs.
d. Large head with saddle nose.
e. Increased lumbar lordosis; kyphoscoliosis.

Q. What is pseudohypoparathyroidism?

In this condition, the secretion of parathormone (PTH) is increased but due to end organ resistance, there is no response to PTH hormone and thereby, resulting in clinical features of hypoparathyroidism. It is a hereditary disorder with distinctive skeletal and developmental defects. These patients have elevated levels of serum PTH. The common features are:

a. Short height with stocky built.
b. Round face with short neck.
c. Mental retardation.
d. Epileptic convulsions.
e. Short 4th and 5th metacarpals and metatarsals (Fig. 3.41).
f. Basal ganglia calcification.

Q. What is progeria?

It is the 'premature ageing' mimicking senile appearance of a person. This very rare disease is manifested by accelerated atherosclerosis, atrophy of subcutaneous fat, alopecia, dwarfism, mild mental retardation and skeletal hypoplasia, and is followed by angina, myocardial infarction and systemic hypertension. Death usually occurs before the age 20.

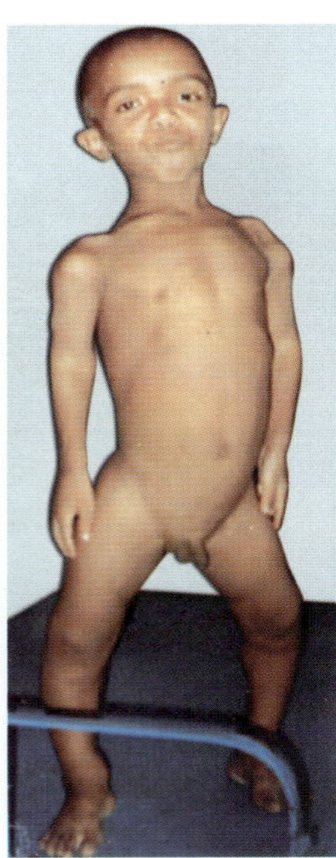

Fig. 3.40: **Achondroplasia** characterized by dwarfism with short limbs and a relatively large head. Normal development of external genitalia is seen

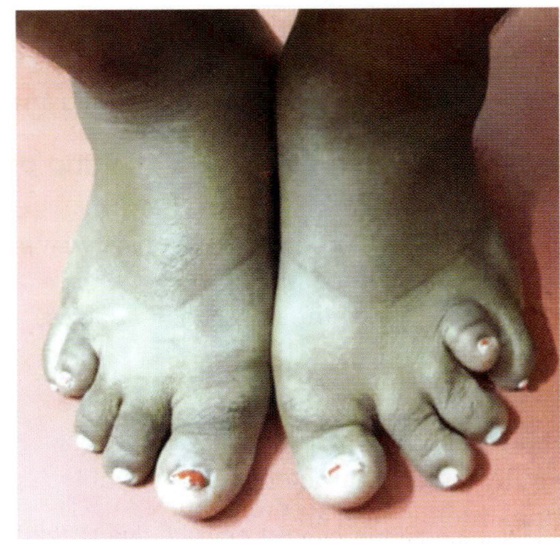

Fig. 3.41: **Pseudohypoparathyroidism** with short 4th metatarsals

Q. Basic investigations performed in dwarfism:

1. History: Natal history (prenatal, intranatal and postnatal), family and personal history.
2. Physical examination: Height, weight, arm-span, secondary sexual character, evidence of systemic disease.
3. Thyroid function tests.
4. Growth hormone assay (blood level of IGF-1 may be done).
5. Assessment of bone age (non-dominant hand and wrist are used for radiology).
6. Chromosomal karyotyping in females (e.g. Turner's syndrome).
7. Others: According to suspicion.

Q. Identification points:

Cretins are diagnosed by typical 'coarse facies' and other morphological features (there is marked physical and mental retardation; sometimes, its D/D is mucopolysaccharidosis, i.e. Hurler or Hunter syndrome). Cretins look younger to their chronological age.

If the height of an adult is <4 feet, he/she may be called a dwarf.

TALL STATURE — CASE 46

Q. Common causes of 'tall stature':

1. Constitutional (idiopathic): The commonest cause.
2. Racial, or familial.
3. Marfan's syndrome.
4. Gigantism (cerebral) and acromegaly.
5. Hypogonadism.
6. Klinefelter's syndrome.

7. Homocystinuria (inherited disorder of amino acid metabolism).
8. Supermales (XYY) and superfemales (XXX).

Q. What is 'build' or 'built'?

It is the 'skeletal framework' of a person in relation to his/her age and sex as compared to a normal person. Build is classified into two groups:
1. Short stature, and
2. Tall stature (less common than short stature).

- Short stature: Below 3rd percentile for height of normal population of same age and sex.
  Tall stature: Above 97th percentile for height of normal population of same age and sex.
- **Stature** is the total height measured from crown to heel. 'Build' is important in clinical practice due to the fact that some diseases are prevalent in tall stature while some are in short stature.
- **Body constitution (somatotypes)** differs from person to person. They are divided into:
  a. Normosthenic: With normal body build.
  b. Asthenic: Lean bodies, narrow shoulders, thin limbs and flat chest. They are prone to visceroptosis and neurasthenia.
  c. Sthenic: Thick trunk, short neck, broad shoulders, and thick and short limbs. They are more likely to develop hypertension and ischaemic heart disease.

Q. Differentiate tall stature by body ratio:

The skeletal height of a person is measured from crown to heel when he/she stands erect against the wall to which a vertical scale is attached.

Upper segment (crown to pubis): Lower segment (pubis to heel) ratio of our body is approximately 1.8:1 at birth; by the age of 10 years the ratio becomes 1:1, and it is approximately 0.9 : 1 in adults because the legs grow more rapidly than the trunk. Hence, in tall stature:

A. Upper segment = Lower segment is seen in:
a. Constitutional, and
b. Pituitary causes (i.e. hyperpituitarism).

B. Upper segment > Lower segment is seen in:
a. Precocious puberty, and
b. Adrenal cortical tumour.

C. Upper segment < Lower segment is seen in:
a. Marfan's syndrome.
b. Klinefelter's syndrome.
c. Hypogonadism (e.g. eunuchoidism), and
d. Homocystinuria.

Q. Clinical features of Marfan's syndrome:

Martan's syndrome is characterised by triad of symptoms (A, B and C described below).

A. Skeletal abnormalities like:
1. Crown to heel height is above average (i.e. tall stature; usually attains >6 feet) with thin built (asthenic).
2. Lower segment > Upper segment of body.
3. Arm-span> height.
4. Hyperextensible joints (Steinberg's sign or *thumb sign*—in which the thumb, when opposed across the palm inside the clenched hand, extends beyond the ulnar border of the palm) (Fig. 3.42).
5. Kyphoscoliosis, straight back syndrome.
6. Anterior chest wall deformity (pectus excavatum and pectus carinatum).
7. High arched palate.
8. Long slender fingers and toes (arachnodactyly, i.e. 'spider fingers') (Fig. 3.43).
9. Metacarpal index >8.4 (the length of each of the last four metacarpal bones is divided by the width at its midpoint, and the values are averaged).

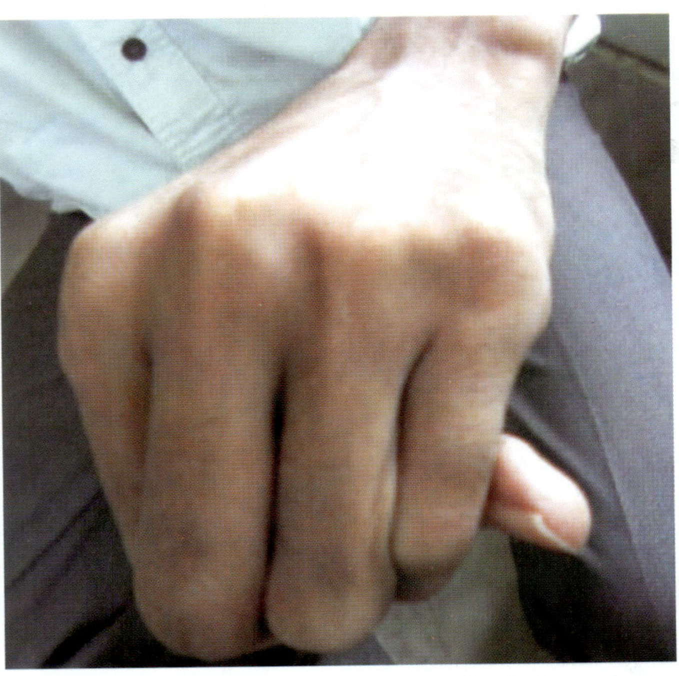

Fig. 3.42: **Steinberg's sign** or thumb sign in **Marfan's syndrome**

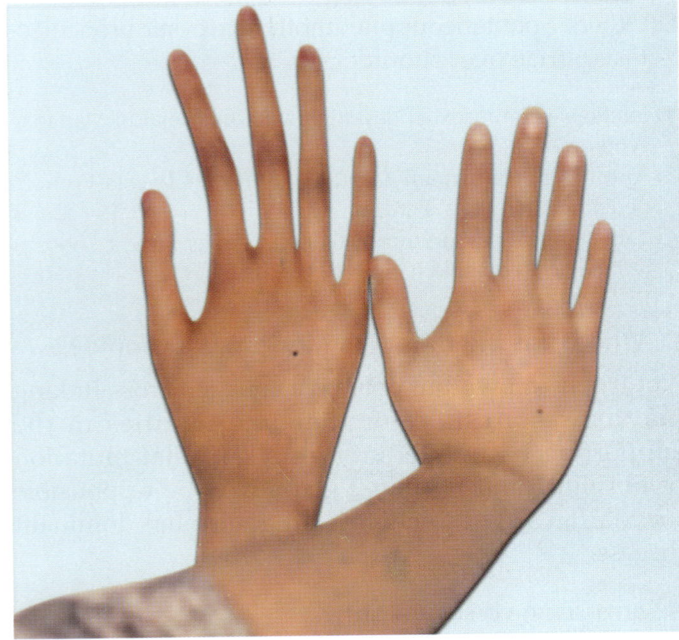

Fig. 3.43: **Arachnodactyly**—long and slender fingers, compared with a normal-sized hand in **Marfan's syndrome**

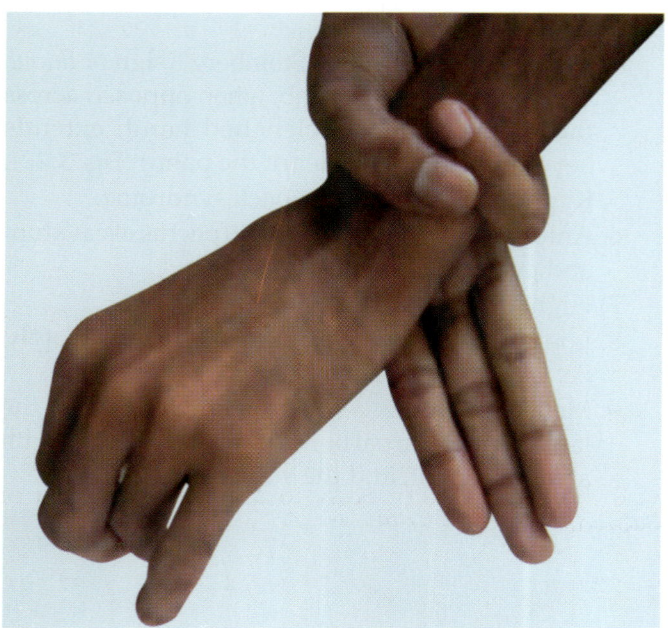

Fig. 3.44: **Wrist sign** in **Marfan's syndrome**

10. *Wrist sign* (Walker-Murdoch sign) (Fig. 3.44)—in which the patient can enclose his wrist with the thumb and little finger of other hand, and the digits overlap each other by at least 1 cm (normal subjects can not do this).
11. Loose-jointedness, pes planus (flat feet) commonly, or pes cavus.
12. Long and narrow facies (dolicocephalus).

B. Subluxation or dislocation of lens upwards (look for iridodonesis). Myopia, retinal detachment and blue sclera may be seen.

C. CVS (CVS abnormalities are major cause of morbidity and mortality):
1. Aortic incompetence.
2. Dissecting aneurysm of ascending aorta.
3. Mitral valve prolapse.

D. Others: Spontaneous pneumothorax, cystic bronchiectasis, striae over shoulders.

- Intelligence and sexual development are normal in Marfan's syndrome.
- Antoine Bernard-Jean Marfan (1858–1942) was French pediatrician in Paris, France.
- Tall, lean and thin persons with long, slender fingers: Loosely termed as 'Marfanoid habitus'.

Q. Where lies the defect in Marfan's syndrome?

Not truely known but defective collagen cross-linking may be responsible for the abnormalities in the supporting tissue. Recently it is said that mutation of fibrillin-1 and fibrillin-2 genes may be responsible for Marfan's syndrome. It is an autosomal dominant disease.

Q. Arm-span versus height:

Normally, the arm-span (i.e. distance between fingertips of middle fingers when hands are outstretched at right angles to the body, and with elbow and wrist extended horizontally parallel to the ground) is, more or less, equal to the height of a person. Arm-span becomes greater than height in conditions where lower segment > upper segment of the body (see above for body ratio). Height is greater than arm-span in hyperpituitarism, precocious puberty and adrenal cortical tumour.

Abnormally short arm-span is characteristic of cretinism and achondroplasia.

Q. Diagnostic points in Klinefelter's syndrome:

1. Tall stature (due to hypogonadism) with eunuchoid body proportions in a male; obese.
2. Lower segment > upper segment of the body. Crown to pubis length < pubis to heel.
3. Gynaecomastia with loss of secondary sexual characters.
4. Phenotypically male with small, firm testis; small penis; male psychosexual orientation.
5. Mental subnormality (mild) with infertility.
6. Azoospermia (sterility) with elevated levels of plasma and urinary gonadotropins.
7. Chromatin (Barr) body is present (chromosomal pattern is 47, XXY) in buccal smear preparation.

- Eunuchoidism, gynaecomastia and hypogonadism are triad for Klinefelter's syndrome.
- Harry F. Klinefelter, Jr. (1912–1990) was an American physician at Johns Hopkins Hospital, Baltimore.

Q. Features of homocystinuria:

1. It is due to reduced activity of the enzyme cystathionine β-synthase.
2. Present between 3 and 5 years. Mental retardation; tall stature with autosomal recessive inheritance.
3. Displacement of lens downwards; Marfanoid habitus.
4. Life-threatening thrombotic episodes may occur.
5. Elevated plasma methionine and homocystine levels.

Q. What is meant by eunuchoidism?

In a general sense, androgen loss reflects eunuchoidism. If testicular failure occurs before puberty it results in hypogonadism, lack of sexual maturation and tall stature with long legs—collectively known as **eunuchoidism**.

Q. Why there is tall stature in hypogonadism?

Testosterone accelerates epiphyseal ossification and fusion. When there is lack of testosterone in human body, there is uninhibited longitudinal growth. **Hypogonadism** is assessed by axillary or public hair, testicular volume, breast or stretched penile length and Tanner stage (a scale of physical development by sexual maturity rating).

Q. Clinical associations in 'tall stature':

Accident-proneness, isolated signs of virilism, signs of early puberty (Fig. 3.45) and rarely, symptoms of hyperthyroidism.

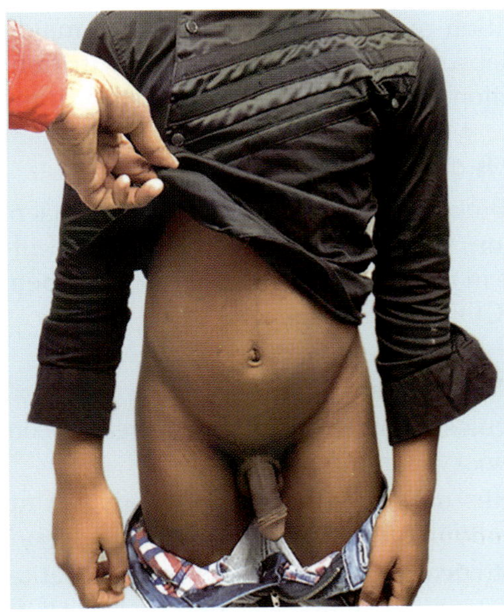

Fig. 3.45: **Precocious puberty** in a boy aged 7 years

Clinical Wisdom

One should always examine the testes, palate (high arched), fingers, spine and CVS (for AI) in tall patients.

EMACIATION — CASE 47

Q. What is emaciation (*see* Figs 1.39 and 3.46)?

Generalised undernutrition, i.e. loss of total body fat and diminution of muscle bulk.

Q. How do you assess nutrition at the bedside?

Nutrition is the 'nourishment' of the body. It is clinically assessed by (semi-quantitatively):

1. Subcutaneous fat: Assessed by picking up 'skinfold' between the index finger and thumb. Actually, it should be measured by a special caliper (Harpenden or Schofield's caliper).
2. Bulk of muscle mass: Measure the mid-arm circumference or mid-thigh circumference by a tape from the elbow joint or knee joint, respectively (i.e. from a fixed point).
3. Signs of vitamins, minerals and nutrients deficiency: Assessed by the presence of glossitis, cheilosis, angular stomatitis, xerophthalmia, Bitot's spot, koilonychia, etc.

Remember, even the presence of mild oedema (as a result of hypoproteinaemia), anaemia, or koilonychia indicates malnutrition. For the assessment of subcutaneous fat and muscle bulk, always compare with the other side of body to diagnose localised or generalised nature of the disease process.

- In the presence of anasarca, nutrition cannot be properly assessed. **Skinfold thickness** in the mid-triceps region (midway between acromion and olecranon process on extensor surface of arm, when the arms are hanging by the side of the body) is the most commonly used site; other sites assessed are biceps (flexor surface of mid-arm), infrascapular and suprailiac region (Fig. 3.47). **Mid-arm circumferance** is measured between acromion and olecranon process, usually of the non-dominant arm (*see* Figs 1.50A and 3.48).
- To assess the nutritional state, clinical history including dietary history and physical examination, along with anthropometric measurement are necessary.

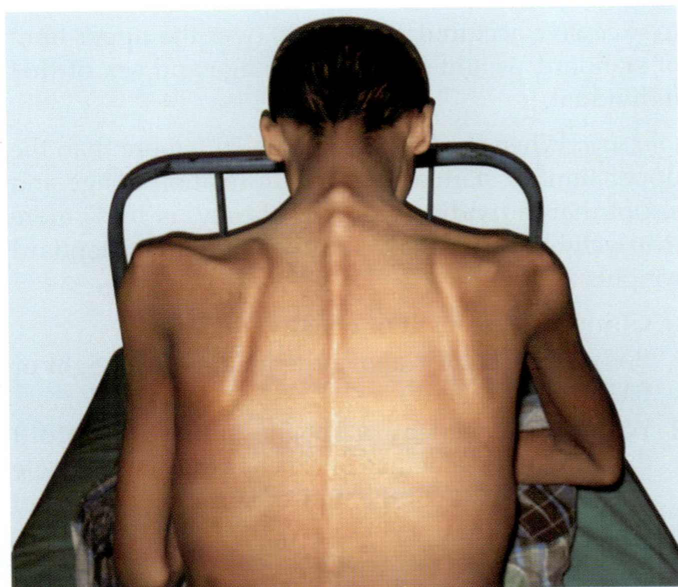

Fig. 3.46: **Emaciation** evidenced by wasting (e.g. supraspinatus), winging of the scapulae (prominent medial border) and vertebral prominence in pulmonary tuberculosis

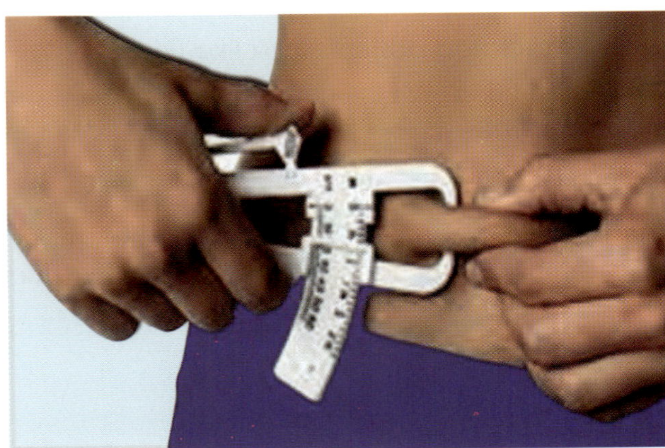

Fig. 3.47: Method of measuring **skinfold thickness**

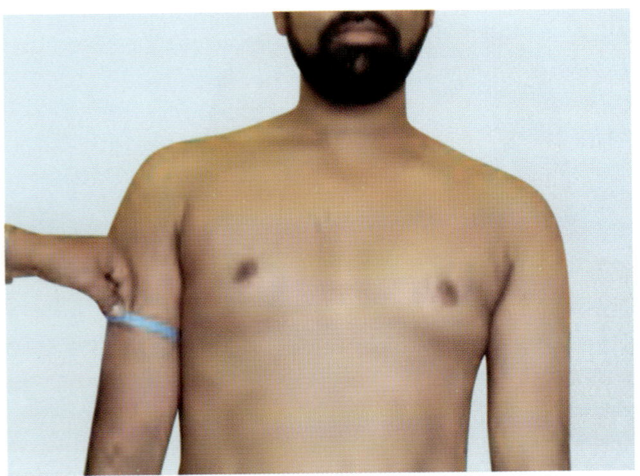

Fig. 3.48: Measuring **mid-arm circumference**

Clinical Wisdom

Average adult triceps skinfold thickness: Males 12.5 mm, females 16.5 mm.
Average adult left mid-arm circumferance: Males 25.5 cm, females 23 cm (Table 3.4).

Table 3.4: Indicators of nutritional depletion

Anthropometric	Chemical	Others
1. % of weight loss (>10%) (sub- or undernutrition)	1. Serum albumin (<35 g/L)	1. Skin anergy
2. Mid-arm circumference (M <23 cm, F <22 cm)	2. Serum transferrin (<2 g/L)	2. Lympho-cytopenia
3. Triceps skinfold thickness (M<10 mm, F <13 mm)	—	—

- Hb%, serum haematinics (iron, TIBC, ferritin, B_{12} and red cell folate) and prothrombin time are also indices of nutrition.

Q. How the 'nourishment' of the body is divided?

- Normal.
- Underweight (e.g. malnutrition, emaciation and cachexia).
- Overweight.
- Obese.

Q. How emaciated patients look like (Fig. 3.49)?

'All skin and bone'. All the bony prominences become more prominent.

Q. What is malnutrition?

Undernutrition with signs of vitamin, mineral and essential amino acid deficiency is known as malnutrition.

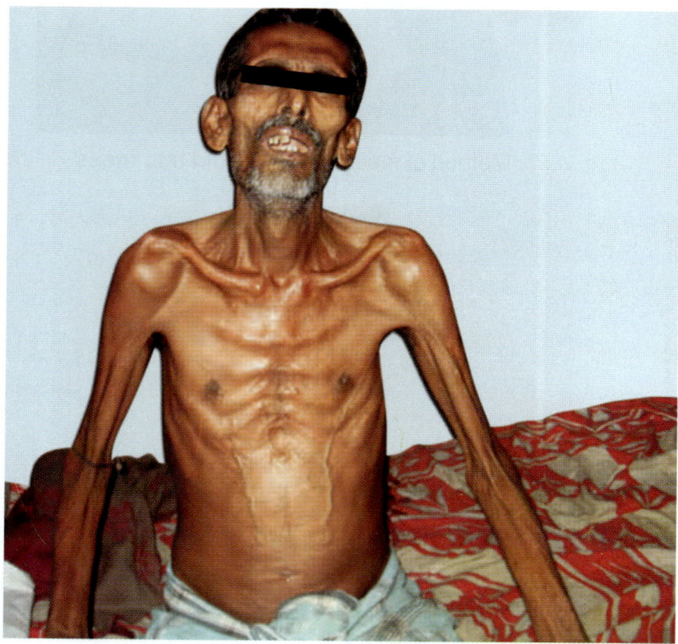

Fig. 3.49: **Cachexia** (anaemia plus emaciation) with **sarcopenia** (decrease in muscle mass)—all skin and bone condition

Malnutrition may be due to starvation, maldigestion and malabsorption. Remember, overnutrition is also malnutrition. So, a complete dietary history is important.

Q. What is cachexia (Fig. 3.49)?

It is combined manifestations of anorexia, anaemia plus emaciation, i.e. a profound state of general ill-health. Decrease in muscle mass is known as **'sarcopenia'** (e.g. old age, COPD patients).

Q. Common causes of emaciation:

1. Tuberculosis (long-standing and untreated, commonly pulmonary; common in India).
2. Diabetes mellitus (in spite of increased appetite; especially in type 1 DM).
3. Thyrotoxicosis (in spite of increased appetite).
4. Disseminated malignancy (commonly malignancy of colon, lung, pancreas, stomach).
5. Acquired immune deficiency syndrome (AIDS—slim disease).
6. Anorexia nervosa (psychogenic): Rare.

- Other causes of 'wasting' or **'weight loss'** are malabsorption, malnutrition (e.g. kwashiorkor or marasmus), cirrhosis of liver, Addison's disease, motor neurone disease, Sheehan's syndrome. Voluntary weight loss occurs in treatment of obesity, by anorexic drugs, models and gymnasts. Unexplained and unintentional weight loss of >3 kg in previous 6 months is known as **'significant'**. A calorie deficit of 1000 Kcal/day will give rise to a weight loss of near about 1 kg/week, i.e. 7000 Kcal is equivalent to 1 kg of fat.
- Localised muscle wasting is characteristic of disuse atrophy, poliomyelitis, motor neurone disease, muscular dystrophy, peripheral neuropathy, cord lesions and local nerve injuries.

Q. How to diagnose obesity clinically?

Overweight: When the body weight is 10% excess (due to excessive accumulation of fat) over the upper limit of standard weight in relation to age and sex of that individual.

Obesity: When the body weight is 20% more than the upper limit of standard weight in relation to age and sex of that individual. 'Morbid obesity' is 100% more overweight (BMI >40) over the upper limit of standard weight.

Clinical assessment of obesity:

1. Body weight >20% above the ideal body weight or BMI >30 (see below).
2. When measured by a special caliper, a fatfold thickness of greater than one inch in the inferior angle of scapula (male) or the mid-triceps region (female) is known as obesity.
3. Ponderal index >17

$$\text{Ponderal index} = \frac{\text{Weight in kilograms}}{\text{Height in meters}^3}$$

4. Waist-hip ratio (*see* later).

- Obesity can be quantified by anthropometry (i.e. skinfold thickness), densitometry (underwater weight), CT or MRI scan (measures mesenteric fat).

Q. How do you classify obesity clinically?

Obesity is divided into peripheral (android, gynoid and truncal) and central (abdominal or visceral) obesity.

1. Android: Excessive fat deposition at waist (predominant in men).
2. Gynoid: Excessive deposition of fat at hip or thigh (predominant in women).
3. Truncal: Excessive fat deposition on face, neck and upper trunk (e.g. Cushing's syndrome).

- Abdominal obesity: There is deposition of fat in the abdominal viscera and omentum (so, called visceral obesity). 'Apple-shaped obesity' (more fat in abdomen) is more harmful than 'pear-shaped obesity' (more fat in hips and thighs). 'Apple-shaped obesity' is linked with DM, IHD, ↑ lipids, hypertension and insulin resistance (see below).

Q. How can you assess obesity by body mass index (BMI) or Quetelet index?

BMI (a measure of generalised obesity) is obtained by calculating a person's weight in kilograms and dividing it by the person's height in metres squared (kg/m^2). For example, an adult male weighing 60 kg with a height of 1.70 metres has a BMI of $60/1.70^2 = 20.7$; BMI is height-dependent and thus short and tall persons of similar proportions have a similar BMI. BMI in children is less reliable than adults as an indicator of excess body fat. WHO classification of BMI is:

Category	BMI range (non-Asian)
Underweight	<18.5
Healthy weight	18.5–24.9
Overweight	25.0–29.9
Moderately obese	30.0–34.9
Severely obese	35.0–39.9
Morbidly obese	≥40

- BMI range for Asian: Underweight <18.5, normal 18.5–22.9, overweight 23–24.9, obese 25–29.9, and morbidly obese ≥30.

Abdominal (central or visceral) obesity can be clinically measured by **'waist–hip ratio'** at the bedside **(Fig. 3.50)**. The ratio is measured by dividing the waist circumference in centimetres by the hip circumference in centimetres. The waist is usually measured at its narrowest point whereas the hips are measured at the fullest point around the buttocks, in erect position of the patient; make sure that tape is horizontal around the waist and hip. Abdominal obesity is important (especially the mesenteric fat) because it is more atherogenic than peripheral fat, and is strongly correlated with insulin resistance. *In a true sense, waist circumferance is a strong predictor of abdominal obesity.*

Waist circumference: It is measured mid-way between the superior iliac crest and the lower costal margin.

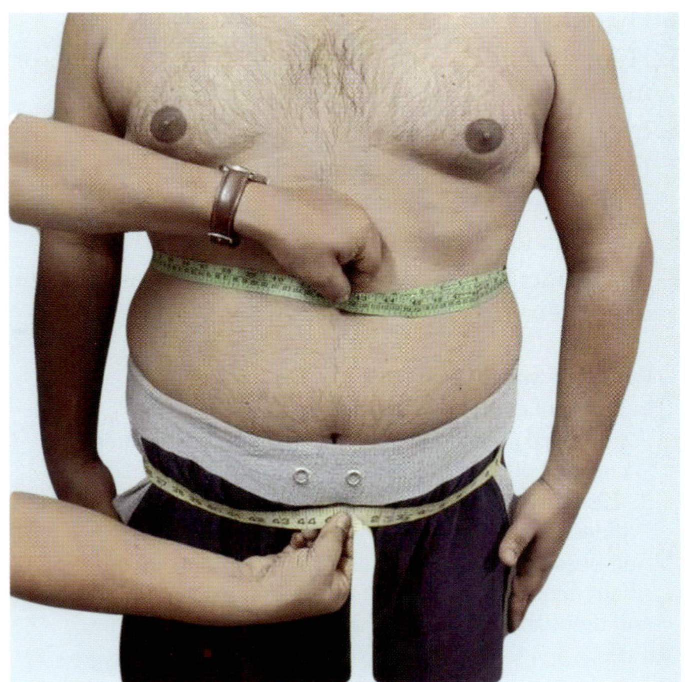

Fig. 3.50: Measuring **waist-hip ratio**

Substantially increased waist measurement in males >102 cm and in females >88 cm (it is in Europids; in South Asians, it is >90 and >80, respectively) indicate high-risk abdominal obesity associated with cardiovascular risk and metabolic complications.

Hip circumference: It is measured at 1/3rd the distance between anterior superior iliac spine and the patella, or from greater trochanter of one side to greater trochanter of other.

Systemic hypertension, diabetes mellitus, ischaemic heart disease, hyperlipidaemia and insulin resistance may be associated with abdominal obesity, and the morbidity and mortality risks are increased if the waist-hip ratio is found to be >0.90 in males or >0.85 in females (indicates obesity).

The BMI is useful in the assessment of both obesity and malnutrition.

Q. Enumerate the tools to assess nutrition:

The commonly used tool is Subjective Global Assessment (SGA), which includes:

a. Medical history: H/o weight loss, dietary history, gastrointestinal and functional impairment.
b. Physical examination: Loss of subcutaneous fat, wasting of muscles, ankle or sacral oedema, signs of vitamins/minerals deficiency (e.g. macrocytic anaemia, night blindness) assessed by skinfold thickness, mid-arm circumferance, BMI and waist-hip ratio.

Q. Common causes of obesity:

1. Idiopathic (simple obesity).
2. Physical inactivity (sedentary habit).
3. Cushing's syndrome.

4. Hypothyroidism (primary).
5. Hypothalamic disorders (Fröhlich's syndrome, or injury).
6. Insulinoma.
7. Laurence-Moon-Biedl syndrome, Prader-Willi syndrome, Pickwickian syndrome.
8. Leptin deficiency.
9. Iatrogenic: Prolonged therapy with corticosteroid or oestrogen.

- Causes of **'weight gain'** are:
  1. Different causes of obesity.
  2. Increased fluid retention due to nephrotic syndrome, CCF, cirrhosis of liver, pregnancy.
  3. Less physical activity, overeating, familial, psychiatric illness, e.g. depression.
- Anti-obesity drugs are phentermine (anorexiant, not used now), sibutramine, orlistat, liraglutide and rimonabant. Sibutramine and rimonabant have been withheld in some countries.

Q. Essential amino acids:

a. Essential (cannot be synthesised in humans but are indispensable for synthesis of some important proteins): Nine in number, i.e. tryptophan, histidine, methionine, threonine, isoleucine, valine, phenylalanine, lysine and leucine.

b. Conditionally essential (if there is adequate dietary supply, they can be synthesised from other essential amino acids). Five in number, i.e. cyteine, tyrosine, arginine, proline and glycine.

Q. Features of hypoalbuminaemia:

a. Causes: PEM, chronic liver disease (e.g. cirrhosis of liver), protein-losing enteropathy, nephrotic syndrome, burns, trauma with sepsis (hypercatabolic states).

b. Normal serum level: 3.5–5.5 g/dL (usually <2.5 g/dL have serious hypoalbuminaemic features).

c. Features: Weakness, dependent oedema, anasarca, conjunctival oedema with oedema of the eyelids, polyserositis, ascites, leuconychia and increased susceptibility to infection.

Q. Types of vitamins:

- Fat-soluble: Vitamins A, D, E and K
- Water-soluble: Vitamin B-complex and vitamin C

Vitamin B-complex are thiamin (B_1), riboflavin (B_2), niacin or nicotinic acid (B_3), panthothenic acid (B_5), pyridoxine (B_6), biotin (B_7 or vitamin H), Folate (B_9) and cobalamin (B_{12}).

Q. Signs of vitamin A deficiency:

1. Toad's skin: Follicular hyperkeratosis (phrenoderma).
2. Xerosis of the conjunctiva, Bitot's spot, xerophthalmia and keratomalacia.
3. Recurrent respiratory and gastrointestinal infection.

Clinical Wisdom

Most important symptom of vitamin A deficiency is night blindness (other causes of *night blindness or nyctalopia* are retinitis pigmentosa, peripheral chorioretinitis, retinal detachment, zinc-deficiency and malingering). **Bitot's spot** is whitish, raised, foamy and triangular spot with its base towards limbus; it is present on the bulbar conjunctiva, a little away from the limbus.

- Essential fatty acid (linoleic acid, linolenic acid and arachidonic acid) deficiency also cause phrenoderma.
- Other causes of **xerophthalmia** in clinical practice are Sjögren's syndrome, chronic conjunctivitis, anaesthetic cornea, Stevens-Johnson syndrome, burns, lid scarring and pemphigold.

Q. Signs of riboflavin (vitamin B_2) deficiency:

1. Magenta-coloured tongue (glossitis) (Fig. 3.51).
2. Cheilosis (cracks and fissures at mucocutaneous junction of the lip), angular stomatitis.
3. Keratitis, vascularisation of cornea, corneal opacity, angular blepharitis.
4. Seborrhoeic dermatitis (face, scrotum) with loss of hair; fissures in the nasal orifice.
5. Anaemia.
6. Polyneuropathy.

Q. Signs of nicotinic acid (vitamin B_3) deficiency:

1. Cheilosis, angular stomatitis.
2. Raw-beefy tongue: Red, swollen and painful tongue.
3. Dermatitis (pellagra): Especially seen on the exposed part of the body with erythema, cracking, desquamation and exudation in acute cases. There may be roughening and pigmentation of skin. Dermatitis in the neck (Casal's collar) is pathognomonic.
4. Dementia and delirium (acute form).
5. Diarrhoea.

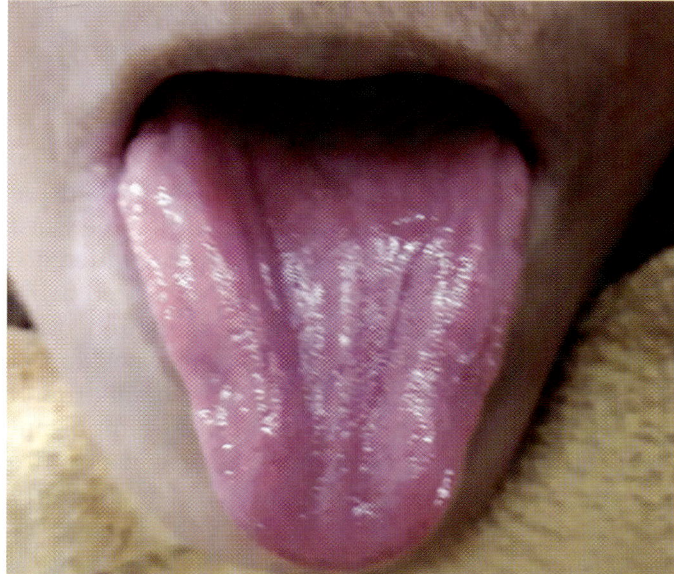

Fig. 3.51: **Magenta-coloured tongue** (pink tongue with glossitis) in riboflavin deficiency

Common causes of **cheilosis** are:

a. Iron deficiency anaemia.

b. Deficiency of riboflavin, nicotinic acid, folic acid and vitamin B_{12}.

c. Exposure to cold weather (cracked lip—in the middle of lower lip).

Q. Signs of pyridoxine (vitamin B_6) deficiency:

Though vitamin B_6 deficiency is rare, it may produce: 1. Polyneuropathy, 2. Mild depression (in women taking oral contraceptive pills), 3. Hypochromic anaemia, 4. Convulsions, and 5. Cheilosis, glossitis, seborrhoea.

- **Uses of pyridoxine** in clinical practice are:
  a. Along with INH (to prevent peripheral neuropathy), penicillamine, L-dopa and cycloserine therapy (these drugs are pyridoxine-antagonist and may produce convulsions).
  b. Sideroblastic anaemia.
  c. Neonatal convulsions.
  d. Vomiting of pregnancy.
  e. Rare diseases like xanthurenic aciduria, cystathioninuria, oxaluria.
  f. High doses of vitamin B_6 is beneficial in carpal tunnel syndrome, diabetic neuropathy, autism, schizophrenia and premenstrual syndrome.
- Increased homocysteine level in plasma is associated with acute myocardial infarction and stroke. Folate (low dose), vitamin B_{12} and B_6 supplementation reduce the homocysteine level in plasma efficiently.

Q. Signs of dehydration:

Dehydration is common in severe vomiting, diarrhoea, insufficient fluid consumption or in diuretic overdose.

1. Face is drawn (facies Hippocraticus).
2. Shrunken eyes.
3. Pinched-up nose.
4. Parched lips.
5. Hollowness of temporal fossa.
6. Depressed anterior fontanelle (infants).
7. Tongue is dry and coated.
8. Skin is dry and wrinkled, subcutaneous tissue feels lax.
9. The sign of ridge (Fig. 3.52): If the skin is pinched up by index finger and thumb, and then released, a ridge is formed which subsides slowly (in severe dehydration) instead of it springing back with normal elasticity, i.e. there is loss of elasticity of skin (i.e. loss of skin turgor).
10. The eyeballs are soft due to lowering of intraocular tension.
11. Hypotension with weak pulse; collapse of jugular veins.
12. Scanty, dark, concentrated urine of high specific gravity.

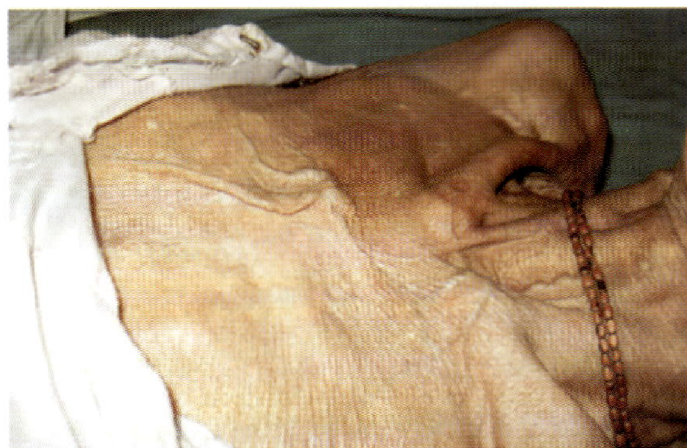

Fig. 3.52: Loss of elasticity of skin in severe dehydration—**'the sign of ridge'**, usually tested over the sternal area

- Features of **shock** are: Cold and clammy extremities, tachycardia with thready pulse, hypotension (systolic BP <90 mm of Hg), tachypnoea and urine output <30 mL/hour.

Clinical Wisdom

Assess **'hydration status'** by seeing skin turgor, moistness of the tongue, postural hypotension, intraocular tension, peripheral oedema (ankle and sacral), ascites and JVP. Remember, in health, skin elasticity is lost in old age and tongue remains dry in mouth breathers.

EXAMINATION OF NECK VEINS — CASE 48

Q. Internal or external jugular vein?

Always examine the internal jugular vein; external jugular vein is less reliable because it is:

1. Superficial and prone to kinking.
2. Does not directly drain into SVC.
3. May have valves, may pierce fascia.
4. Engorged, if patient wears a tight collar, and
5. Not a direct reflector of central venous pressure (CVP).

- Internal jugular vein is in direct continuity with the right atrium and reflects the pressure changes in the right atrium as well as CVP. As it is deeply situated, the internal jugular vein is difficult to visualise (many a time only a diffuse pulsation is visible when the CVP is raised). JVP measures the volume status at the bedside.

Clinical Wisdom

Recent view is that both external and internal jugular veins have valves and as internal jugular vein is difficult to visualise, the external jugular vein is gaining importance. A non-obstructive external jugular vein can be assessed for JVP in a desparate situation.

Q. Prerequisites for accurate assessment of neck veins (Fig. 3.53) (Table 3.5):

1. The patient should be reclining supine at 45° (angle formed by trunk and the level of the bed at waist is 45°).
2. Neck muscles should be 'relaxed' properly (examination is done with a 'back-rest' or properly adjusted pillows; if 'back-rest' is not available, patient's body can be lifted and supported on examiner's left arm

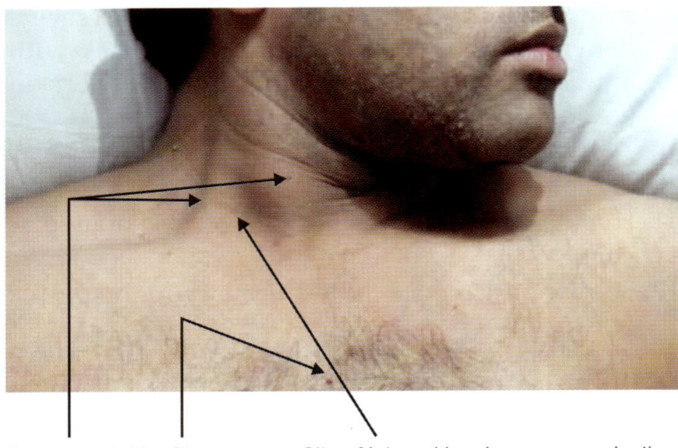

Fig. 3.53: Site for **jugular venous pulse examination** at 45° semi-reclined position

to make an angle of 45° but proper relaxation of neck muscles is not achieved by this method).

3. Good light is necessary for visualisation of neck veins. A light source, e.g. a torch illuminated from behind (tangential application) helps to visulaise the waves in a better way.
4. It is better to observe the right internal jugular vein (the innominate vein may be compressed by the aortic knob which damps and elevates the venous pressure in the left jugular vein).
5. It is better to stand on the right side with patient's face slightly turned to the left for observation of right-sided neck vein.
6. One should look in-between the two heads of sternomastoid muscle and if it seems full, observe the uppermost point of distension (one may identify the internal jugular pulsation with the help of hepato-jugular reflux, or by occluding it with gentle digital pressure above the clavicle).

Clinical Wisdom

If in the sitting position neck veins are fully engorged, it is not necessary to examine the patient at 45°, and in that situation measure venous pressure in sitting position. Similarly, the patient may have to lie flat if the jugular venous pressure (JVP) is very low.

Q. Causes of increased jugular venous pressure (JVP) (see Fig. 1.8):

A. Engorged and pulsatile neck vein:

1. **Congestive cardiac failure (commonest cause of raised JVP).**
2. Chronic constrictive pericarditis.
3. Cardiac tamponade.
4. Tricuspid incompetence (prominent 'v' wave) and tricuspid stenosis (prominent 'a' wave).
5. Restrictive cardiomyopathy.
6. Chronic cor pulmonale.
7. Pulmonary thromboembolism.
8. Circulatory overload: After massive fluid infusion or blood transfusion, pregnancy, cirrhosis of liver or acute nephritis (i.e. salt and water retention).
9. Complete heart block (from time to time cannon waves are seen).

- ↑ JVP is the first sign to appear and last sign to disappear in CCF or right heart failure.
- JVP is increased in cardiogenic shock.

B. Engorged and non-pulsatile neck vein:

1. **Superior mediastinal syndrome (commonest).**
2. Rarely in chronic constrictive pericarditis (advanced stage).
3. Valsalva manoeuvre.

- 'Unilateral' non-pulsatile ↑ JVP is seen in innominate vein thrombosis.

Q. Low jugular venous pressure (JVP):

1. Dehydration (commonest).
2. After haemorrhage (hypovolaemia) or patient in hypovolaemic shock.
3. After massive diuretic therapy.

Table 3.5: Bedside differentiation between venous and arterial pulsation in neck

Venous pulsation	Arterial pulsation
1. Wavy or undulating; laterally placed	1. Jerky or abrupt; medially placed
2. Better seen than felt	2. Better felt than seen
3. Becomes prominent on expiration	3. No change
4. Becomes prominent on lying down	4. No change
5. Becomes prominent an application of abdominal pressure (hepato-jugular reflux)	5. No change
6. Prominent movement is inward	6. Prominent movement is outward
7. Can be abolished by gentle digital pressure applied above the clavicle (important point of differentiation at the bedside)	7. Does not affect arterial pulsation
8. Two positive waves are seen (when in sinus rhythm)	8. One positive wave is seen (when in sinus rhythm)
9. It has a definite upper level	9. No such level is seen
10. Pulsatile displacement of the ear lobes in high CVP	10. Absent in arterial pulsation
11. Becomes prominent on Valsalva manoeuvre	11. No change

Q. Points observed in neck vein at the bedside:

A. Engorged or not.
B. If engorged:
   a. Pressure,
   b. Pulsation (waveforms), and
   c. Hepato-jugular reflux.

Q. Importance of hepato-jugular reflux (Fig. 3.54):

When firm pressure is applied by right hand on any part of the abdomen for at least 10 seconds, especially over the right hypochondrium, there is 'transient' rise in JVP as the hepatic venous reservoir is compressed (the patient reclining at 45°). This is hepato-jugular reflux (often called abdomino-jugular reflux).

In health, significant alteration of JVP does not occur by this manoeuvre. A positive hepato-jugular reflux is defined by a sustained rise of >3 cm in JVP for at least 15 seconds after release of the hand. The commonest cause of a positive reflux is right-sided heart failure. Its importance lies in:

1. To diagnose impending, incipient (early stage) or overt right heart failure (CCF).
2. To differentiate between arterial and venous pulsation, and
3. To differentiate between obstructive and non-obstructive causes of engorged neck vein (absent or negative hepato-jugular reflux is seen in SVC syndrome and Budd-Chiari syndrome).

Q. Waves seen in neck vein:

Positive waves—a, c and v; actually, there are two positive waves (a and v) seen clinically as c-wave is small and rarely appreciated at the bedside. Negative troughs (waves)—x and y. In diseased states, like:

- a-wave is absent in atrial fibrillation.
- v-wave [so called 'systolic wave' or 'cv' wave (Lancisi sign), which may oscillate the ear lobule] becomes very prominent in TI.

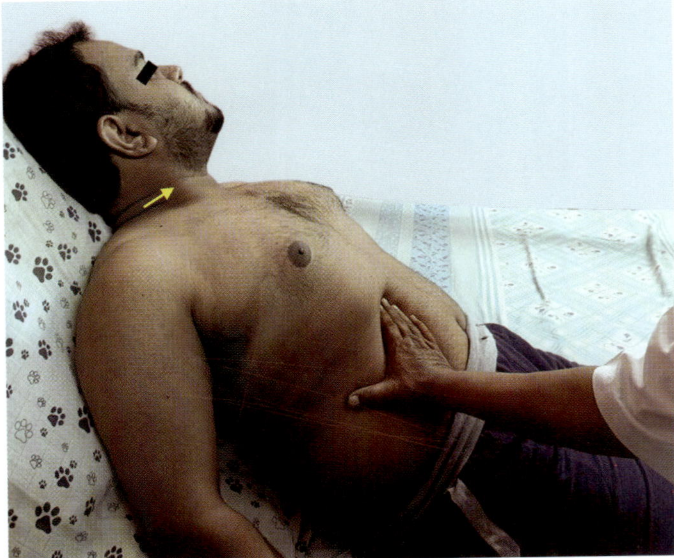

Fig. 3.54: Elicitation of **hepato-jugular reflux**

- Small x-descent in TI, and prominent x-descent in cardiac tamponade.
- Slow y-descent in TS, and sharp y-descent is found in constrictive pericarditis.

Q. Mechanism for production of different waves in neck vein:

'a' wave	Right atrial contraction. It is the most dominant wave in JVP.
'c' wave	Closure and bulging of tricuspid valve towards the right atrium (according to few clinicians, it is due to transmitted carotid impulse).
'x' descent	Righ atrial relaxation with downward descent of tricuspid valve.
'v' wave	Passive right atrial filling against closed tricuspid valve during ventricular systole.
'y' descent	Right ventricular filling with atrial emptying into the ventricles.

- a-wave coincides with S_1, v-wave with S_2. x-descent follows S_1, y-descent follows S_2.
- **Sequence of events in JVP:** a wave (first positive wave) → c-wave (second positive wave) → x-wave (first negative wave) → v-wave (third positive wave) → y-wave (second negative wave) (Fig. 3.55A).

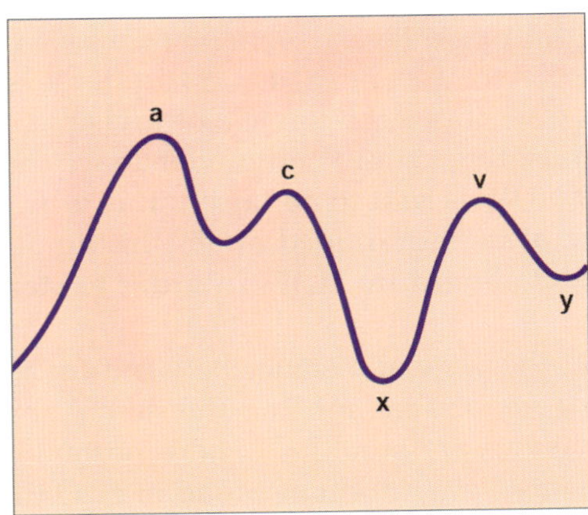

Fig. 3.55A: Different **waves of neck veins** in health

Q. What is giant a-wave (venous Corrigan)?

When the right atrium contracts against outflow tract obstruction, giant a-wave is produced, e.g. in:

1. Tricuspid stenosis.
2. Pulmonary hypertension, and
3. Pulmonary stenosis.

- Exaggerated a-waves are the hallmark of right atrial hypertrophy.

Q. Cannon wave:

Huge pathological (i.e. very large) a-wave is known as cannon wave. It is seen when the right atrium contracts against closed AV valve (i.e. tricuspid valve). It is commonly found in:

1. Regular: Nodal tachycardia, junctional rhythm.
2. Irregular: Complete heart block, classic AV dissociation with ventricular tachycardia.

Q. Kussmaul's sign:

In normal healthy persons, the neck venous pressure falls (so, the height lessens) on deep inspiration due to sucking of blood into the right atrium. Reverse happens after deep expiration.

But in patients with constrictive pericarditis, severe right-sided heart failure, right ventricular infarction (produces decreased right ventricular compliance), restrictive cardiomyopathy, massive pulmonary thromboembolism and cardiac tamponade (less common), there is paradoxical rise in JVP after deep inspiration due to non-accommodation of increased venous return to right side of the heart. This is Kussmaul's sign and is also known as venous pulsus paradoxus.

- Adolph Kussmaul (1822–1902) was a German physician and Professor of Medicine. He also coined the term 'polyarteritis nodosa'. Acidotic breathing is labelled after his name as "Kussmaul's breathing".

Q. Why the neck vein is examined at 45° (Fig. 3.55B)?

Regardless of body position, the centre of the right atrium lies 5 cm below the sternal angle (the 'reference point'). When a person is lying flat, the jugular veins are seen distended in the neck. If he/she is at 90° (sitting), the upper level of vein is never seen normally. But if the person reclines at 45°, the upper level of vein is just visible above the clavicle or invisible. So, if we see the pulsating venous column far above the clavicle at 45°, the JVP is said to be raised. It is why the neck veins are always examined at 45°. In the other way, **the patient should lie at 45° in order to standardise reading**.

At 45°, the vertical distance between the top of the oscillating venous column and the sternal angle is the jugular venous pressure (JVP) and is normally 3–4 cm. Thus, 4 cm + 5 cm = **9 cm of blood or H_2O (or <7 mm of Hg) is the normal venous pressure, right atrial pressure, JVP or CVP** (1 mm of Hg = 1.36 mm of blood or H_2O).

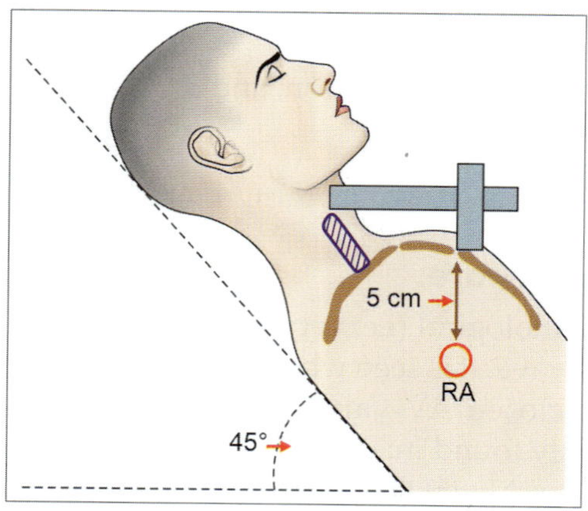

Fig. 3.55B: Examination of **jugular venous pressure (JVP)** in health

Q. How venous pressure is measured at bedside (Fig. 3.56)?

It is measured by the vertical height of internal jugular vein above the sternal angle. Clinically, it is done with the help of two postcards (rulers or scales); one postcard is placed vertically over the sternal angle and the other is placed horizontally from the top of the oscillating venous column up to the first postcard when the patient is reclined at 45°. The junctional point between the two postcards is marked and the vertical distance from this point to the sternal angle is measured, e.g. if it is seen to be 6 cm in a patient of CCF, the JVP of that patient will be 6 cm + 5 cm = 11 cm of blood, i.e. JVP is raised.

Q. What is Anthem sign (Fig. 3.57)?

This newly described non-invasive bedside assessment of CVP may be of value for early learners and obese patients (not for examination hall). In 'supine position' of the patient, he/she is asked to put the right hand over anterior chest at the sternal level mimicking the hand position during observation of national anthem

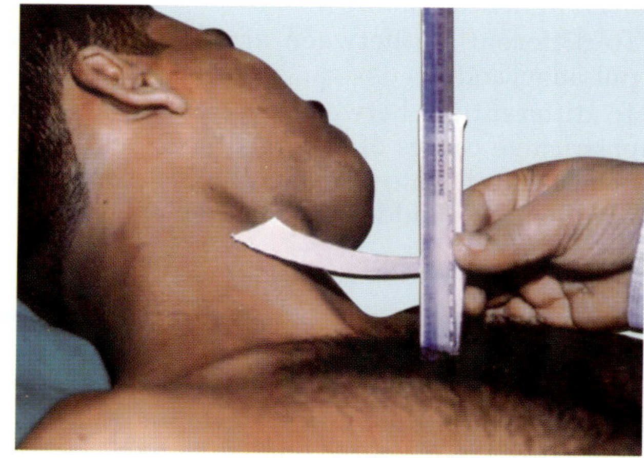

Fig. 3.56: **Measurement** of jugular **venous pressure (JVP)**

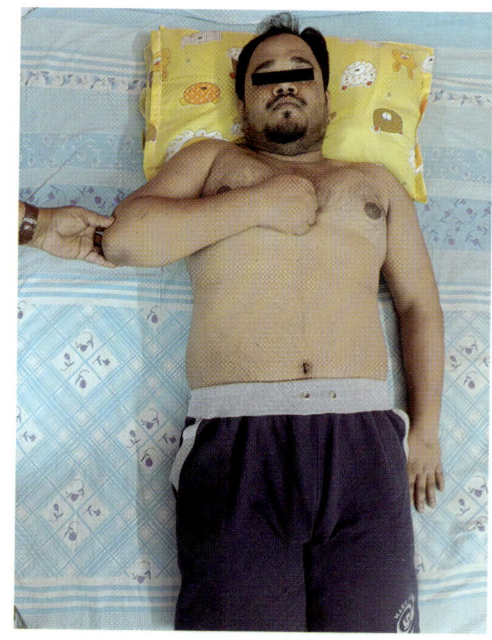

Fig. 3.57: **Anthem sign**

(i.e. hand is folded at elbow with keeping the right fist over sternum). CVP is considered to be elevated if any venous engorgement is found in the right hand, as the hand lies above the level of right atrium.

Q. Describe the neck vein in CCF:

a. Engorged and pulsalite.
b. JVP is raised (measure, if possible).
c. Waves are seen.
d. Hepato-jugular reflux is present.

- ↑JVP is a manifestation of abnormal right heart dynamics.
- During elicitation of hepato-jugular reflux in a suspected patient of CCF, patient will C/o pain (as the liver is tender on palpation due to congestive hepatomegaly). Also look for bipedal oedema. These are Indirect evidences in the examination hall.

Q. What is Friedreich's sign?

It is the rapid y-descent in the venous pulse seen in constrictive pericarditis and is due to rapid inflow of blood into the right ventricle as soon as the tricuspid valve opens.

Q. Bedside diagnosis of constrictive pericarditis:

When acute fibrinous or serofibrinous pericarditis (i.e. from tuberculosis, bacterial infection, haemopericardium or neoplastic infiltrations) heals and leads to obliteration of pericardial sac by granulation tissue, thick and fibrous pericardium encase the heart and the disorder is known as chronic constrictive pericarditis. It is full of 'bedside signs' and is diagnosed by:

1. Fatigue, dyspnoea on exertion, orthopnoea, loss of weight (symptoms).
2. Protuberant abdomen (ascites).
3. Peripheral oedema and systemic venous congestion.
4. Rapid, low volume pulse and pulsus paradoxus.
5. Elevated CVP with Friedreich's sign (sharp y-descent).
6. Kussmaul's sign.
7. Invisible or feeble apex beat with normal-sized heart; distant (or quiet) heart sounds.
8. Pericardial knock heard at lower left sternal border.
9. Congestive hepatomegaly with ascites; ascites > peripheral oedema.
10. Splenomegaly.

- The **pathophysiology of clinical features in constrictive pericarditis** are:
  - ↓Ventricular filling (just like cardiac tamponade): Kussmaul's sign, Friedreich's sign, pulsus paradoxus.
  - Systemic venous congestion: ↑JVP, oedema, ascites and hepatomegaly.
  - Pulmonary venous congestion: Dyspnoea, orthopnoea (rare).
  - ↓Cardiac output: Fatigue, low volume pulse.
- One of the common D/D of constrictive pericarditis at the bedside is cirrhosis of liver.
- Constrictive pericarditis is a potentially curable cause of diastolic heart failure, which is full of clinical signs.

Clinical Wisdom

Pericardial knock: This is a low frequency extra sound in early diastole and is probably due to restrictive effect of adherent pericardium on diastolic expansion of the ventricle. It comes earlier than S_3.

Conclusion

During examination of the neck veins in the examination hall, always ask for 'back-rest'. If not supplied, support the patient's trunk on your left arm to make an angle of 45°.

Although the neck veins are engorged and pulsatile in biventricular failure, it is primarily a sign of right ventricular failure.

SPIDER NAEVI — CASE 49

Q. What are these?

These are telangiectases that consist of a **centrally dilated arteriole** from which numerous small vessels radiate resembling the legs of a spider **(Fig. 3.58)**. Usually it is a sign of hepato-cellular failure.

Q. Common sites:

In the upper half of thorax **(necklace area)** and back of upper chest commonly; face, forearms and dorsum of hands. Rarely, they are seen in mucous membrane of oral cavity and nose.

Q. Method of demonstration:

The central arteriole (central prominence) is occluded by giving pressure with a pinhead or glass slide (diascopy), and the response is **immediate blanching of the whole naevus**. If the pressure is released, the naevus goes back to its original shape and colour, which shows *filling from the centre to the periphery*.

Q. Size of spiders:

From a pinhead to 0.5 cm in diameter. When it attains large size, it may be seen or felt to pulsate.

Q. Other names of spider naevi:

Arterial spider, spider telangiectasis, spider angioma, vascular spider, naevus araneus.

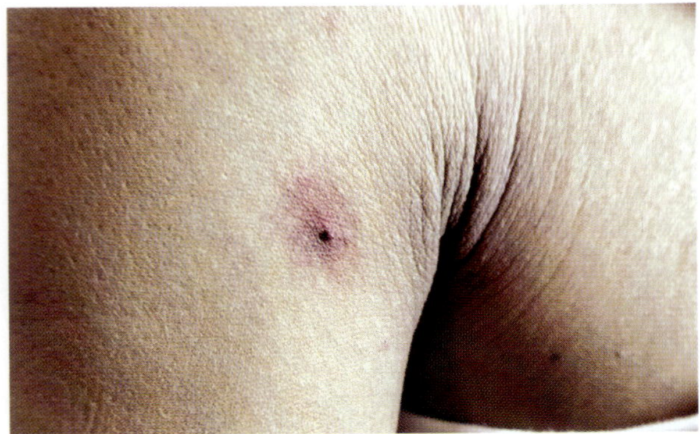

Fig. 3.58: Spider naevi at upper arm in cirrhosis of liver

Q. Clinical associations:

1. Cirrhosis of liver, especially in alcoholics.
2. Viral hepatitis (transient).
3. During third trimester of pregnancy.
4. Occasionally, in children.
5. Sometimes, in thyrotoxicosis.
6. In some healthy persons (2%)–≤3 in number, F > M.
7. Oestrogen therapy.

Q. Aetiopathogenesis:

Spiders are formed due to hyperoestrogenaemia in cirrhosis of liver (diminished hepatic clearance of precursor androstenedione results in increased peripheral conversion to oestrogen). It is known that oestrogen has a dilating effect on spiral arteries of endometrium and such a mechanism may be responsible for the development of cutaneous spiders. Nowadays, it is said that the ratio of (high) oestrogen and (low) testosterone level is the main factor for production of spiders. Various VEGFs may also play a role.

Q. Differential diagnosis:

1. Mosquito bite: The 'fresh' mosquito bite marks blanch like spiders. H/o using mosquito nets at night should be taken. Mosquito bite marks may be present anywhere in the body.
2. Hereditary haemorrhagic telangiectasis (HHT): *'Telangiectasia'* are cluster of dilated capillaries and venules which may be visible on the skin surface, particularly on the lips and usually blanch on pressure. The common sites of HHT are mucosal surfaces like tongue, lips, nose, palate, pharynx, oesophagus and stomach. It is generally connected with a single vessel. Telangiectasis may be seen in CREST syndrome.
3. Haemorrhagic spots: Petechiae and purpura never blanch on pressure.
4. Venous star (Fig. 3.59): It is seen in persons with elevated venous pressure, which never blanches on external pressure. The common sites are back, legs, lower part of anterior chest wall and dorsum of foot. Here, *the blood flows from the periphery to the central part* in contrast to vascular spiders where blood flows from the centre to the periphery. It is usually 2–3 cm in diameter.
5. Campbell de Morgan's spots (cherry angioma): These spots are very common in aged persons (size: 1–2 mm in diameter), and are commonly seen in anterior abdominal wall and front of the chest. They do not blanch on pressure and are usually elevated from the skin surface.
6. Rose spots: Seen in enteric fever, especially over abdominal skin; blanch on pressure.

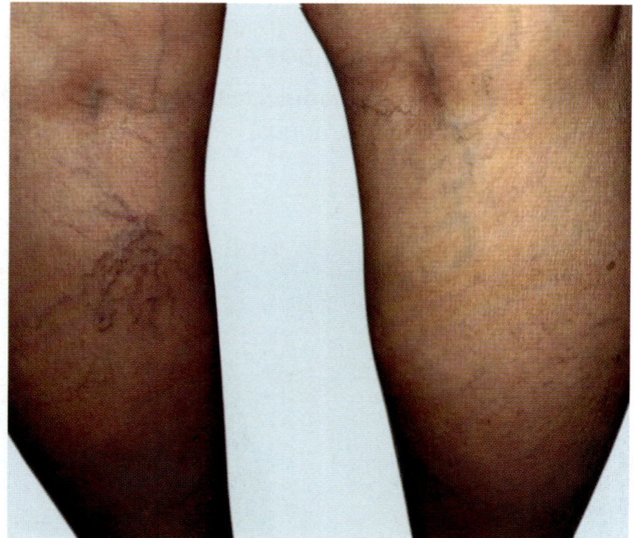

Fig. 3.59: Venous star at back of leg

Q. Why the spiders are mostly seen in necklace area?

It is said that spiders are seen in the area drained by superior vena cava (above the line joining both nipples). Actually, the basic cause is not clearly understood but it is expected that exposure of the necklace area to sunlight may damage the skin in such a way that appropriate internal stimulus may provoke the development of spiders in the said area. Experiment shows that people in the nudist colony having cirrhosis of liver show spiders distributed all over the body.

Q. Draw inference it a previously seen spider disappears:

1. The hepato-cellular failure is corrected (good prognosis), or
2. The fall of blood pressure in a case of hepato-cellular failure (commonly due to fresh haematemesis or melaena) may be responsible for the disappearance of spiders (bad prognosis).

Conclusion

One should search spiders meticulously in its specified area of distribution. **Spider naevi, a sign of hepato-cellular failure, is seen in decompensated cirrhosis of liver.** Spiders are very often missed, if not carefully searched. Confirm it by 'blanching response' after application of pressure by a pinhead or glass slide.

PALMAR ERYTHEMA — CASE 50

Q. What is this?

It is **commonly seen** that **in a setting of hepato-cellular failure**, the palms become bright red in colour (and also warm). Thus, other name of palmar erythema is 'liver palms'. The soles of the feet may be similarly involved.

Q. Sites affected within the palm (Fig. 3.60A):

1. Thenar eminence.
2. Hypothenar eminence.
3. Pulp of the fingers, and
4. Bases of the fingers.

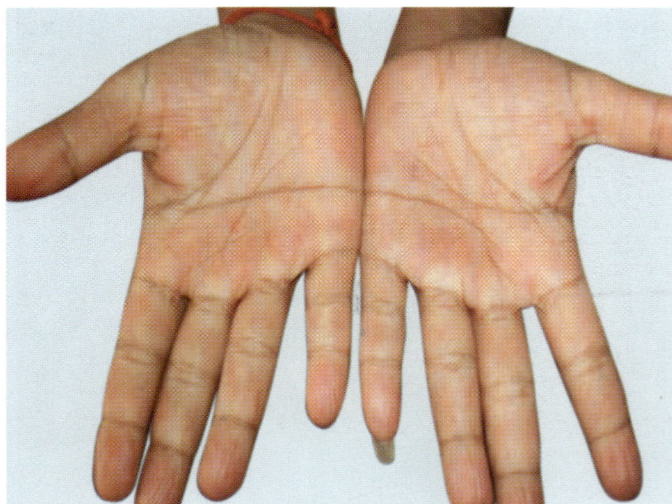

Fig. 3.60A: Classical **palmar erythema** involving thenar and hypothenar eminences, webs and pulps of the fingers in cirrhosis of liver

Q. Method of demonstration:

Like the spider naevi, **palmar erythema blanches on pressure**. Here, a glass slide is used for application of pressure when the erythema vanishes, while the redness of palm reappears rapidly after release of pressure (Fig. 3.60B). In the absence of glass slide, press the patient's palm with your thumb.

- At times, the palm flushes synchronously with the pulse rate after being pressed by a glass slide. The patient may complain of throbbing or tingling sensation in palms.

Q. Clinical associations:

1. Cirrhosis of liver.
2. In alcoholics.
3. Long-standing rheumatoid arthritis.
4. Pregnancy.

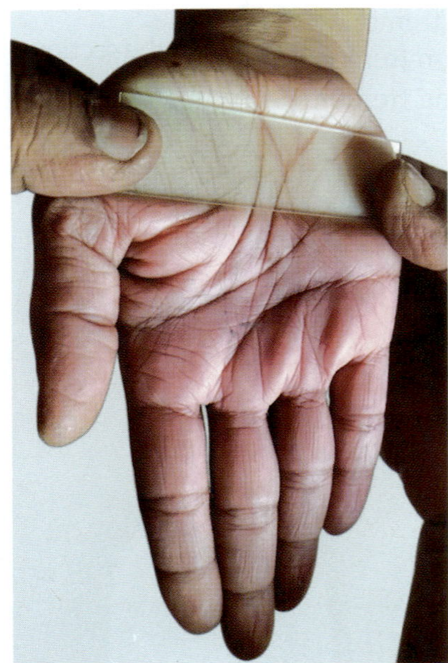

Fig. 3.60B: **Demonstration of palmar erythema** by a glass slide. Spider naevi is also examined in this way

5. Thyrotoxicosis.
6. Chronic leukaemias.
7. Rarely, in some normal persons (familial).
8. Hyperdynamic circulation, e.g. high fever.

- Remember, *polycythemia* causes redness of the palm and sole; so, search for plethoric face, dusky-red oral mucous membrane, cherry-red tongue and suffused conjunctiva.

Q. Aetiopathogenesis:

Same as spider naevi, or a non-specific change indicative of hyperdynamic circulation.

Q. Skin and appendicular changes in hepato-cellular failure:

1. Spider naevi.
2. Palmar erythema.
3. Bleeding manifestations: Due to coagulation disorder (hypoprothrombinaemia) and defects in the platelet (number and functional abnormalities) petechiae, purpura or ecchymosis may be seen.
4. 'Paper money' skin: It is usually seen in upper arms and is also observed in the common sites for spider naevi. These are nothing but small blood vessels and resemble silk threads in United States' dollar bills.
5. White spots: In arms and buttocks (demonstrated after cooling the skin); forerunners of a spider.
6. White nails (leuconychia): This is due to opacity of the nail-bed. All the fingers may be affected but thumb and index fingers are especially involved. Hypoalbuminaemia is thought to be responsible for production of white nails.
7. Gynaecomastia: May be unilateral and is developed as a result of hyperoestrogenaemia. It is said that spironolactone therapy is the commonest cause of gynaecomastia in a patient of cirrhosis of liver.
8. Clubbing: Especially seen in biliary cirrhosis.
9. Jaundice: In case of severe jaundice, skin may become yellow. Jaundice gives some guide to the severity of hepato-cellular failure.
10. Diffuse pigmentation of the body, particularly over the face.
11. Dupuytren's contracture, especially in alcoholics.
12. Scanty pubic and axillary hair; frequency of shaving is less in males.
13. Xanthoma (in palmar creases) or xanthelasma (around eyes) are seen in primary biliary cirrhosis.

EXAMINATION OF THE HANDS — CASE 51

Q. Points to note in hands:

Examine the hands in the sequential order as described below:

A. **Shake hands** with the patient (to assess surface temperature, skin and the grip strength) may reveal:
   a. Warm and moist hand: Thyrotoxicosis, type II respiratory failure, pyrexia (only warm).

b. Warm and blue hands: Central cyanosis, and cold and blue hands—peripheral cyanosis.
c. Cold and moist hand: Anxiety neurosis; moist and doughy handshake—acromegaly; cold and clammy hand with peripheral cyanosis—shock.
d. Cold and dry hand: Myxoedema; only cold hand—low cardiac output (e.g. heart failure), hypothermia, Raynaud's phenomenon.
e. Patient cannot relax his hand after handshake: Myotonia.
f. Weak grip strength: Weakness of the small muscles of hands or weakness of flexor muscles.
g. Rough, thick palm: Phrenoderma (vitamin A or essential fatty acid deficiency), arsenic poisoning **(Fig. 3.61A)**, tylosis (hyperkeratosis of palm often associated with oesophageal carcinoma), psoriasis, verruca vulgaris, multiple corn or callosities.
h. Shaking hand producing pain: Rheumatoid arthritis.

B. Colour changes:

a. Anaemia or pallor (the palmar creases become pale when the Hb level is <7 g/dL).
b. Jaundice: Mainly the palms, dorsum rarely.
c. Cyanosis: Tips of fingers, nail-beds and palm.
d. Palmar erythema.
e. Janeway's lesion (non-tender maculopapular lesion present in thenar eminence in SBE).
f. Carotenaemia (orange-yellow or lemon-yellow colour of palm).

C. Finger deformities:

a. Arachnodactyly (long slender, spider-like fingers) (*see* **Fig. 3.43**): Marfan's syndrome, hypogonadism.
b. Polydactyly (extra finger) **(Fig. 3.61B)**: Laurence-Moon-Biedl syndrome, Turner's syndrome, associated with VSD.
c. Syndactyly (joined fingers): Poland's syndrome, underlying congenital heart disease.
d. Clinodactyly (incurved finger): Commonly affects the little finger in Down syndrome.
e. Sclerodactyly (tight skin over the phalanges): Scleroderma.

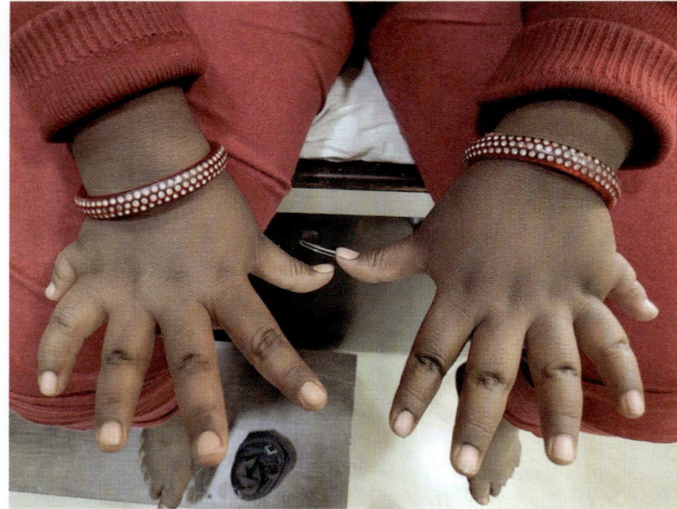

Fig. 3.61B: Polydactyly in hands in LMB syndrome

f. Broad hand with thick, large, square-tip fingers (spade-shaped hand): Acromegaly.
g. Brachydactyly (short fingers) **(Fig. 3.62A)**: Down syndrome, Turner's syndrome, mucopolysaccharidosis.
h. Fingerisation of thumb: Holt-Oram syndrome.

D. Clubbing: Vide page 314.

E. Wasting of the small muscles of hands (vide page 342)**:** Leprosy, MND, syringomyelia, rheumatoid arthritis, etc.

F. Pulsation:

a. Capillary pulsation (*see* the section on 'Aortic incompetence').
b. Digital artery pulsation (*see* the section on 'Aortic incompetence').
c. Pulse: Give the classical description (some clinicians may not like to include 'examination of pulse' under examination of the hand).

G. Tremor:

a. Static tremor.
b. Action tremor.
c. Intention tremor.
d. Flapping tremor.

} Read the section on 'Tremor'

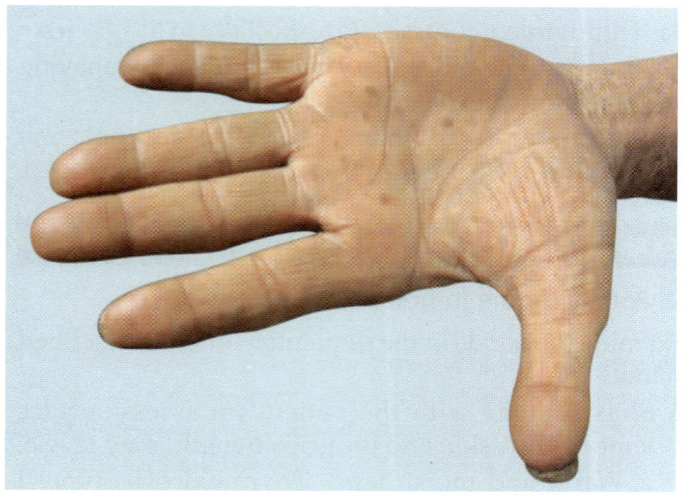

Fig. 3.61A: Palmar hyperkeratosis in arsenic toxicity

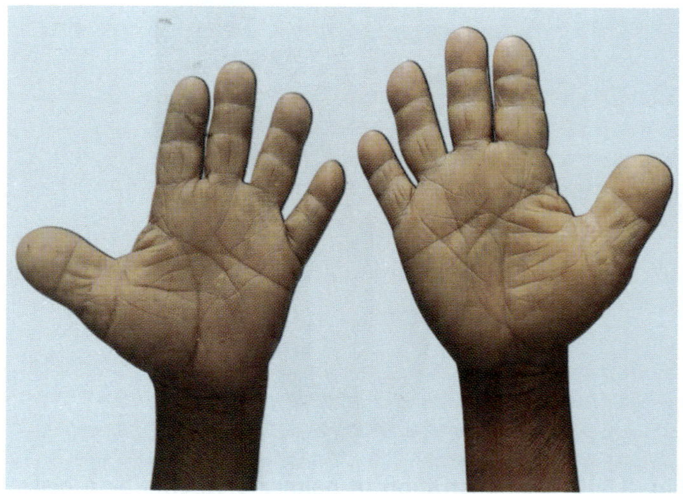

Fig. 3.62A: Brachydactyly in Down syndrome

H. Swellings:

a. Osler's node (tender papule mainly in the pulp of fingers): Seen in SBE.

b. Heberden's node (Fig. 3.62B): Hard bony nodules seen at the dorsal aspect of DIP joints in osteoarthritis (OA).

c. Bouchard's node: Hard bony nodules seen at the dorsal aspect of PIP joints in osteoarthritis (OA).

d. Rarely, rheumatoid nodules, or nodule formation in leprosy.

e. Gouty tophi: Over dorsal aspect of PIP and DIP joints.

f. Calcinosis: Scleroderma.

g. Oedema over dorsum of the hand. Ganglion, neurofibroma, lipoma are of surgical interest.

I. Hand deformities:

a. Spindle-shaped fingers (due to swelling of PIP joints): Rheumatoid arthritis, scleroderma.

b. Swan neck deformity (hyperextended PIP joints and flexed DIP joints) (Fig. 3.63): Rheumatoid arthritis.

c. 'Boutonniere' or button-hole deformity (flexed PIP joints and hyperextended DIP joints): Rheumatoid arthritis, and is just reverse of swan neck deformity.

d. Volar subluxation with radial deviation at wrist and ulnar deviation of digits: Rheumatoid arthritis.

e. Z-deformity of thumb (hitch-hiker's thumb): Rheumatoid arthritis.

f. Swelling of DIP joints only: Osteoarthritis, psoriatic arthropathy or scleroderma. In psoriasis, 'telescoped' phalanges may produce shortening of fingers with gross impairment of function.

g. Dupuytren's contracture (painless flexion contracture of ring and little fingers due to thickening, fibrosis and shortening of ulnar side of palmar fascia) (Fig. 3.64). Puckering of palmar skin is characteristic. It is common in males and may be uni- or bilateral. The causes are:

i. Repeated trauma to palm.
ii. Alcoholic cirrhosis.
iii. Phenytoin sodium therapy in epileptics.
iv. Working with vibrating tools.
v. Manual workers (e.g. gardener).
vi. Diabetes mellitus.
vii. Peyronie's disease.
viii. Chronic alcoholism.
ix. Idiopathic.
x. Familial (autosomal dominant).

h. Surgical deformities like club hand, Madelung's deformity, mallet finger, etc.

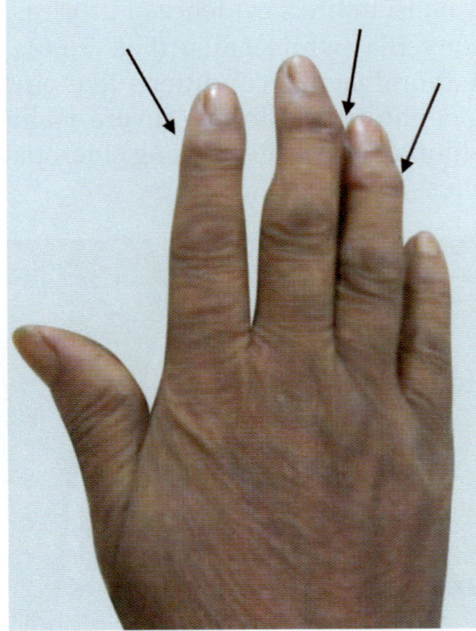

Fig. 3.62B: Hard bony nodules **(Heberden's nodes)** seen over dorsal aspect of DIP joints in **osteoarthritis**. 1st carpometacarpal joint is affected here (thumb is opposed). MCP joints are not involved

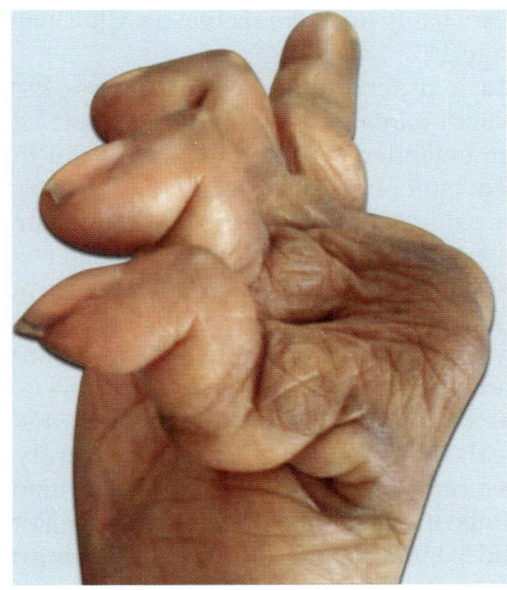

Fig. 3.63: Swan neck **deformity in rheumatoid arthritis**: PIP joints are hyperextended while DIP joints are flexed

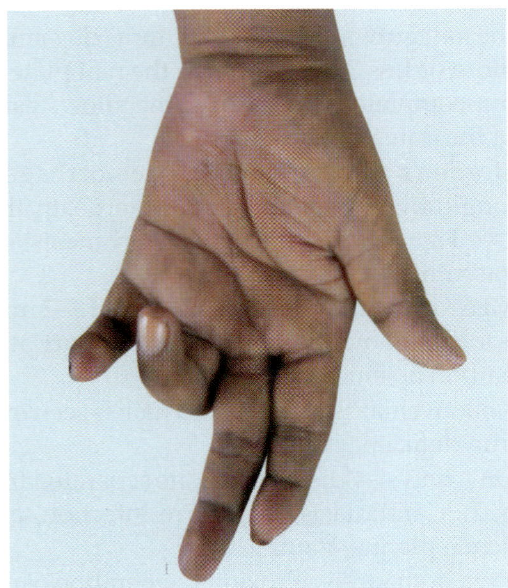

Fig. 3.64: **Dupuytren's contracture** in an alcoholic cirrhosis of liver

i. Claw hand: Read the section on 'Claw hand' (vide page 345).

j. Main d'accoucheur: Metacarpophalangeal (MCP) joints are flexed, the PIP and DIP joints are extended with opposition of the thumb. It is commonly seen in tetany and also known as carpal spasm. The method of demonstration of carpal spasm by sphygmomanometer is known as Trousseau's sign. [There is another Trousseau's sign in internal medicine which is characterised by migratory thrombophlebitis in a patient with carcinoma of the pancreas].

k. Jaccoud's arthritis: Rheumatic arthritis usually heals without deformity; very rarely, minor deformity of hand (marked ulnar deviation of MCP joints due to subluxation) may persist. Rarely, SLE and Sjögren's syndrome may develop into this type of deformity.

l. Short 4th and 5th metacarpals in pseudohypoparathyroidism ('dimpling sign' or Archibald's sign).

m. Wrist drop: Radial nerve palsy.

n. Hemiplegic hand: Flexed fingers and even may have flexion contracture.

o. Mutilated or deformed hand: See page 371.

p. Hypermobile joints: Ehlers-Danlos syndrome, Marfan's syndrome.

q. Ape hand: Median nerve damage with difficulty to oppose the thumb.

❍ Armand Trousseau (1801–1867) was Physician, Paris, France who actually died from gastric carcinoma.

J. Nail changes:

a. Pitting (thimble) nails: Psoriasis, atopic eczema, alopecia areata, trauma, etc.

b. Beau's line (Fig. 3.65): Transverse ridges develop during recovery from any febrile illness due to temporary alteration of nail growth rate. In health, the nail grows at a rate of 0.1 mm/day and it takes more or less 3–4 months for the nail plate to grow out completely. So, Beau's line allows estimation of the date of illness.

c. Horder's line or splinter haemorrhage (linear longitudinal haemorrhage underneath the nails) (*see* Fig. 1.20): SBE, trauma, trichinosis, systemic vasculitis, etc.

d. Mees' line: Transverse white stria of 1–2 mm width appears above lunula (the white part at base of nail) in arsenic poisoning.

e. Koilonychia: 'Spoon-shaped nail' is seen in chronic iron deficiency anaemia.

f. Onycholysis ('distal' nail plate separated from nail-bed): Candidiasis, ringworm infection, psoriasis, lichen planus, trauma, etc.

g. Onychomadesis: 'Proximal' seperation of nail plate from nail-bed in trauma, pemphigus and poor nutrition.

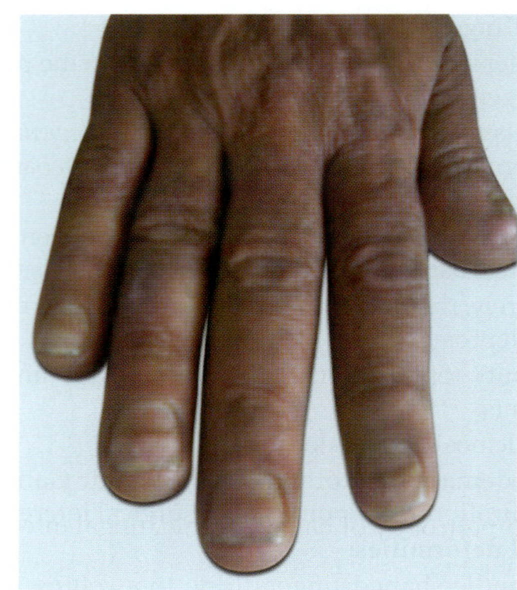

Fig. 3.65: **Beau's line** in nails—transverse ridges developed during recovery from febrile illness

h. Nail-fold thrombi: Scleroderma and other collagen vascular diseases (vasculitis).

i. Green nail: Severe *Pseudomonas* infection.

j. Blue lunula (azure arcs): $CuSO_4$ poisoning, Wilson's disease, zidovudine therapy, argyria (silver deposition), cyanosis and ochronosis. Bluish-red discolouration of nail is common in polycythemia.

k. Red lunula: Seen in congestive cardiac failure.

l. Black nail: Hair dyes, Peutz-Jeghers syndrome.

m. Brown nail: Hydroquinone-induced.

n. Grey-black nail: Melanoma.

o. Bitten nails: Persons with anxious personality.

p. Fungal infection of nails (onychomycosis): Candidiasis, ringworm (tinea unguium).

q. Shiny nails: Indirect evidence of pruritus.

r. Leuconychia (white nails) (Fig. 3.66): Seen in hypoalbuminaemic conditions like cirrhosis of liver, nephrotic syndrome, severe malnutrition, kwashiorkor and protein-losing enteropathy; also known as *Terry's nail*.

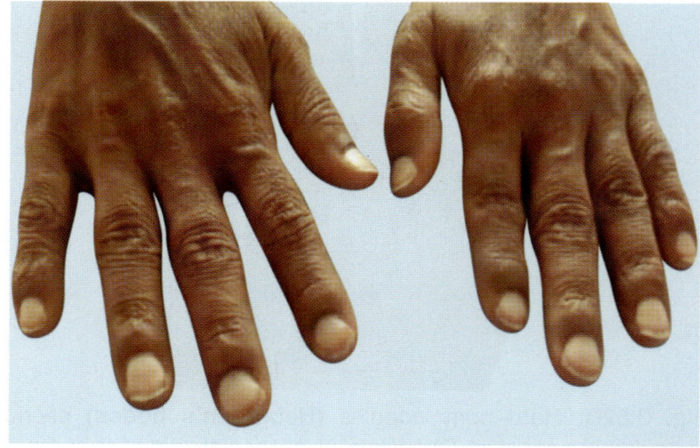

Fig. 3.66: **White nails** found in hypoalbuminaemia (e.g. cirrhosis of liver)

s. Yellow nails in 'yellow nail syndrome'; other components of the syndrome are lymphoedema of the extremities and pleural effusion.
t. Half-and-half nail (proximal half is white and distal half is pink with a distinct transverse line of seperation): Seen in uraemia, also known as *Lindsay nail*.
u. Platonychia (flat nails): Hereditary, iron deficiency anaemia.
v. Pterygium unguis (growth of the cuticle onto the nail plate): Seen in lichen planus.
w. Paronychia or whitlow (i.e. swollen and inflamed nail-bed): Working in wet conditions, diabetes, repeated trauma.
x. Hypertrophy of nails: Chronic fungal infection.
y. Absence or atrophy: Nail-patella syndrome, congenital ectodermal defect.
z. Subungual fibroma (Koenen's tumour): Observed in tuberous sclerosis.
α. Brittle nail (onychorrhexis): Fungal infection, iron deficiency anaemia, psoriasis, peripheral vascular disease.
β. Missing nail in nail-patella syndrome: Presents with (hereditary) nephrotic syndrome.
γ. Muehrcke's lines: A pair of white transverse lines which disappears on pressure; seen in hypoalbuminaemia.
δ. Plummer's nail: Seperation of distal margin of nail from nail-bed in Graves' disease.
ε. Wider nail: Acromegaly.
ζ. Long narrow nail: Hypopituitarism, hypogonadism.
η. Convex nail: Clubbing.
θ. Chromonychia (coloured nail) (Fig. 3.67): Congenital, infections (fungal, *Pseudomonas*), drug-induced.
ι. Pale nails: Anaemia, shock.

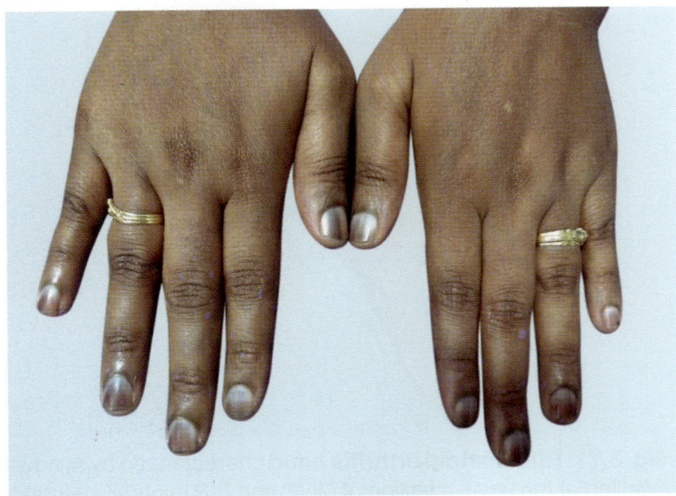

Fig. 3.67: Chromonychia (coloured nails) as a result of repeated fungal infection

K. Skin changes (mainly dorsum of the hand):

a. Hyperpigmentation (e.g. knuckles hyperpigmentation in megaloblastic anaemia).
b. Hypopigmentation.
c. Ichthyosis (fish skin) (Fig. 3.68); tripe palms (velvety palms) indicate internal malignancy.
d. Palmar xanthoma: Seen in familial hyperlipidaemia.
e. Lilac-coloured knuckles in dermatomyositis (Gottron's sign) (Fig. 3.69).
f. Petechiae, purpura, ecchymosis.
g. Rash (from diseases or drugs).
h. Scabies infestation in webs of fingers.

L. Miscellaneous:

a. Nicotine staining in right index and middle fingers in chronic smoker (Fig. 3.70).
b. Single palmar crease (simian crease) in Down syndrome.

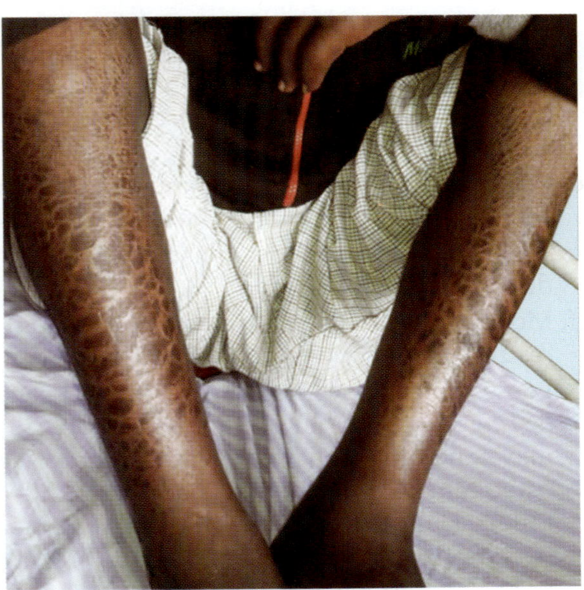

Fig. 3.68: Ichthyosis over legs

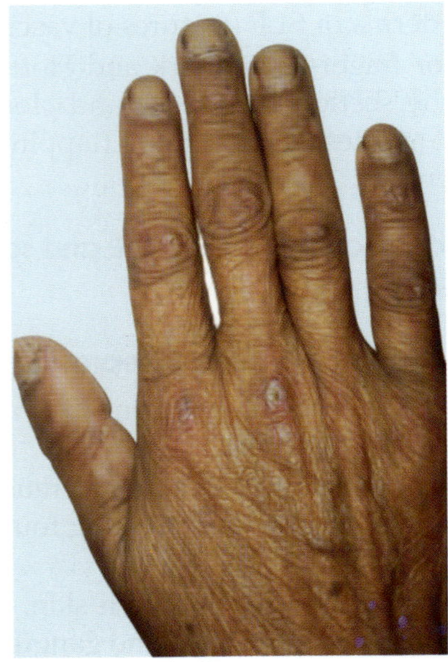

Fig. 3.69: Gottron's papules over knuckles and PIPs in dermatomyositis

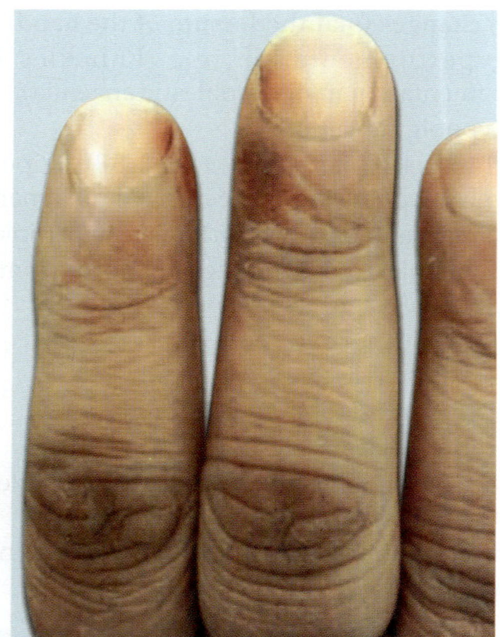

Fig. 3.70: Nicotine stain in fingers of a chronic smoker

c. Involuntary movements like chorea, athetosis, minipolymyoclonus, etc.
d. Power of individual small muscles should be tested; sensory loss, if any, should be detected.
e. Trophic ulcers: Leprosy, vasculitis, Raynaud's disease, syringomyelia.
f. Movement at different joints: To find out any restriction of movement.
g. Loose-jointedness: Tested by passive hyperextension of fingers, and even the hyperextended fingers may touch the forearm. It is commonly seen in osteogenesis imperfecta, Marfan's syndrome, Ehlers-Danlos syndrome and in some normal persons.
h. Pulp atrophy, telangiectasia, digital infarction, digital ulceration, digital gangrene, triphasic colour response of Raynaud's phenomenon: In scleroderma or SLE (features of vasculitis).
i. Test for finger-flexion jerk and Hoffmann's sign (see the sections on 'Jerks and clonus'), grasp reflex, and test for myotonia (tapping the thenar eminence).

Q. Examination of the hand in SLE and scleroderma:

Read the individual sections.

Q. Examination of the hand in leprosy:

1. Read the skin changes in TT and LL varieties from the section on 'Leprosy'.
2. Claw hand with wasting of the small muscles of hand (commonly ulnar clawing affecting fourth and fifth fingers), and
3. Trophic changes: Dry and rough skin, brittle nails, loss of hair, digital ulceration and gangrene, tapering and conical fingertips with trophic ulcers, and loss of distal digits.

Q. Examination of the hand in rheumatoid arthritis:

1. Spindle-shaped fingers (swelling of PIP joints, DIP joints unaffected).
2. Swelling of the wrist and different joints (MCP and PIP) in the hand: No swelling at DIP joints.
3. Swan neck deformity (described earlier): Due to disruption of the volar plate of PIP joints, often with associated rupture of the insertion of flexor sublimis.
4. 'Boutonniere' or button-hole deformity (described earlier): Chronic synovitis of PIP joints lead to rupture of central slip of extensor tendon (looks like gap of button hole) allowing protrusion of joint between two lateral slips of extensor tendon.
5. Volar subluxation with radial deviation at wrist and ulnar deviation of digits ('zigzag' deformity) **(Fig. 3.71)**: Due to bowstring action of displaced extensor tendons.
6. Z-deformity of thumb: Due to muscle wasting, rupture of tendon and weakened joint capsule.
7. Opera glass hand appearance: Mutilating arthropathy.
8. Dorsal subluxation of lower end of ulna (piano sign).
9. Palmar erythema (seen in long-standing rheumatoid arthritis).
10. Joint movements are painful and restricted.
11. Grip-strength is poor.
12. Wasting of the small muscles of hand: Chiefly due to disuse atrophy; carpal tunnel syndrome, vasculitis, mononeuritis multiplex or rarely prolonged use of corticosteroids may be attributed.
13. Digital infarction, digital gangrene, splinter haemorrhage, nail-fold thrombi.
14. Tenosynovitis.
15. Carpal tunnel syndrome (with evidence of wasting of thenar muscles).

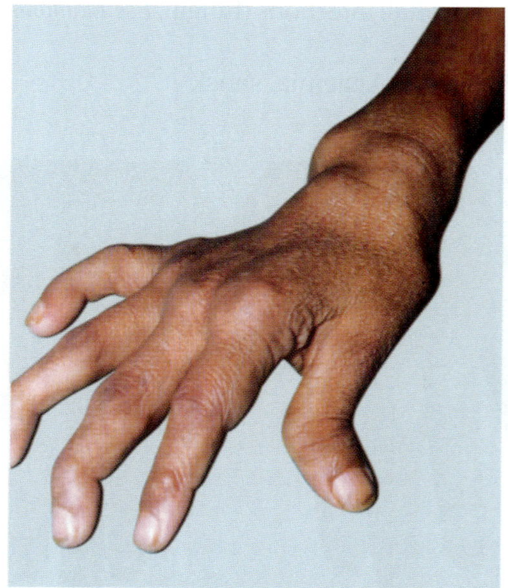

Fig. 3.71: Rheumatoid arthritis hand characterized by synovial swelling at the wrist, swelling of MCP and PIP joints, Z-deformity of thumb, and swan neck deformity of fingers with mild ulnar deviation of hand

16. Rheumatoid nodule (may be seen over knuckles in dorsum of hands).
17. Trigger finger (flexion deformity from which the finger can be extended only by force).
18. Rupture of the extensor tendons of ring and little fingers resulting in 'dropped finger' (rare).
19. Purpuric rash (thrombocytopenia due to Felty's syndrome or methotrexate theapy).
20. Raynaud's phenomenon.
21. Pallor (anaemia) in severe active deforming disease.

Q. 'Vasculitis' and its characteristic skin changes:

Vasculitis is the necrotising inflammation of blood vessels. Endothelial oedema, and proliferation with haemorrhage contribute to the occlusion of the vascular lumen and subsequent ischaemic changes along with organ damage. Vasculitis is commonly due to infections, immunological disorders (e.g. SLE), drugs (e.g. allopurinol), and malignant diseases. It is classified according to the size of vessel involved [Chapel Hill Consensus Conference (CHCC) classification, 1994].

Classification:

a. Large-vessel vasculitis: Giant cell arteritis (temporal arteritis) (Fig. 3.72) and Takayasu's arteritis (aortic arch syndrome or pulseless disease).
b. Medium-sized vessel vasculitis: Classical polyarteritis nodosa and Kawasaki disease (mucocutaneous lymph node syndrome).
c. Small-vessel vasculitis of arterioles, capillaries and venules: Wegener's granulomatosis (granulomatosis with polyangiitis) (Fig. 3.73), microscopic polyangiitis, Churg-Strauss syndrome (eosinophilic granulomatosis with polyangiitis), cutaneous leucocytoclastic vasculitis (hypersensitivity vasculitis), Henoch-Schönlein purpura (IgA vasculitis) and essential mixed cryoglobulinaemia.

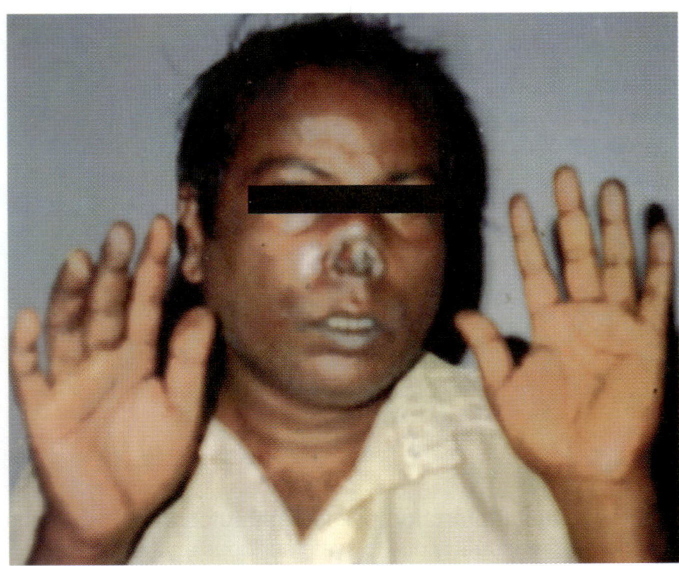

Fig. 3.73: **Vasculitis** (Wegener's granulomatosis). Raynaud's phenomenon (colour changes in the tip of the fingers) with destruction of nose and nasal septum is seen. Hands are very cold on palpation

- SLE, Behcet's disease, scleroderma, polymyositis or dermatomyositis, SBE, rheumatoid arthritis and paraneoplastic syndromes are also associated with vasculitis.
- **ANCA-associated vasculitis** are Wegener's granulomatosis, Churg-Strauss syndrome, IgA vasculitis and microscopic polyangiitis. ANCA stands for antineutrophil cytoplasmic antibody.
- CHCC classification has been revised in 2012 to improve the existing nomenclature (with inclusion of vasculitis due to HBV, HCV, lupus, sarcoid, RA, etc.).
- **Dermatological manifestations of vasculitis:**
  1. Large arteries (Fig. 3.74): Digital gangrene.
  2. Small arteries:
     a. Palpable purpura.
     b. Urticarial rashes (tender).

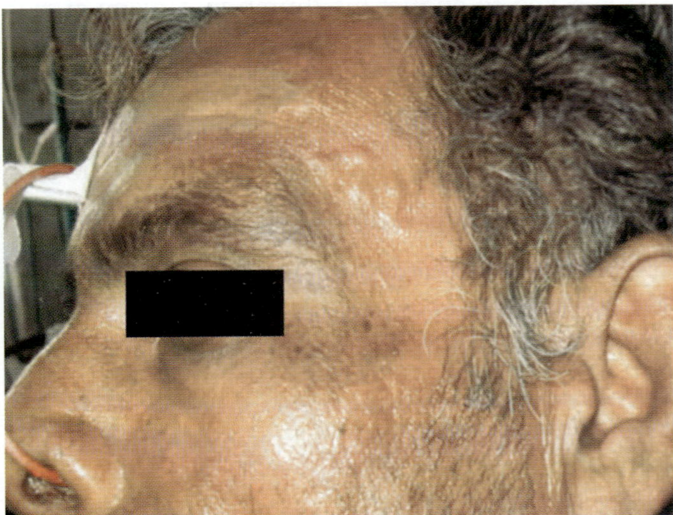

Fig. 3.72: Visible, inflamed and tender temporal artery in temporal arteritis **(giant cell arteritis)**; the patient presented with severe headache and claudication of the jaw

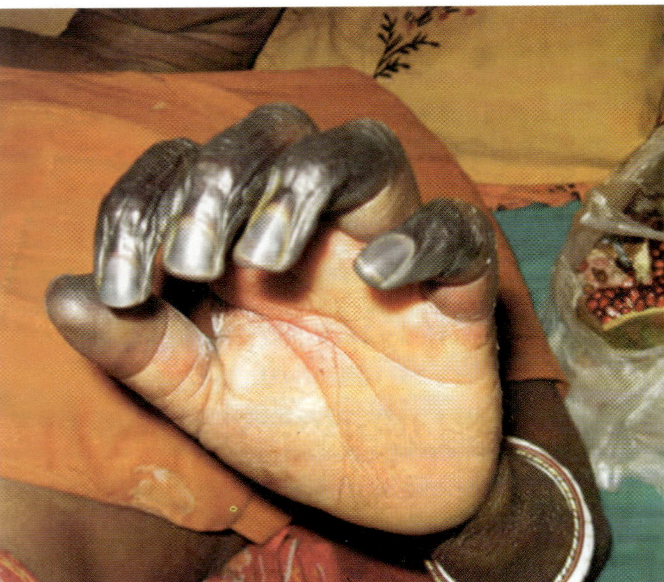

Fig. 3.74: Dry **gangrene of the digits**. This patient of septicaemia had gangrene of all the digits of four limbs–'symmetrical peripheral gangrene'

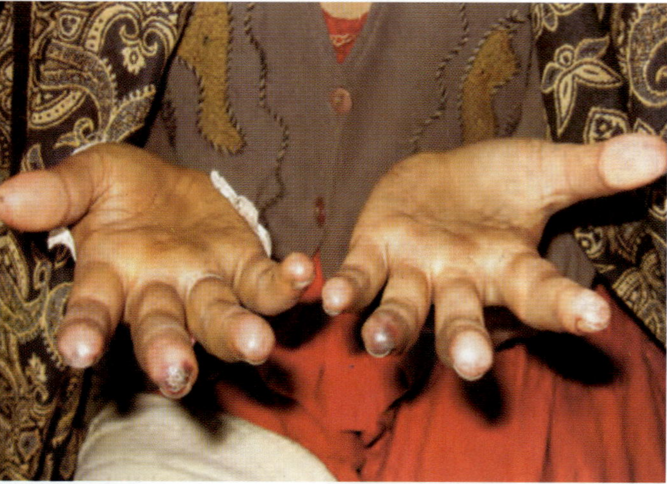

Fig. 3.75: **Digital infarction**, painful **digital ulceration**, periungual erythema in **vasculitis** due to systemic lupus erythematosus

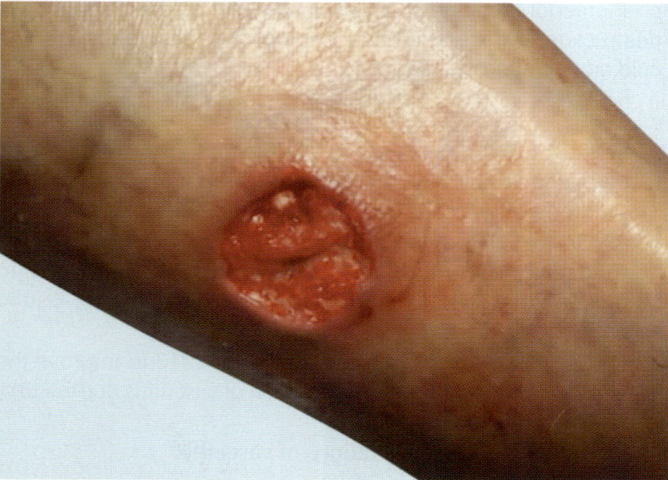

Fig. 3.76: **Punched-out ulcer** due to **systemic vasculitis**

c. Morbilliform eruptions (look like measles rashes).
d. Maculopapular eruptions.

3. Arterioles and very small arteries (Fig. 3.75).
   a. Digital infarction (pitted scars).
   b. Digital ulceration.
   c. Nail-fold thrombi.
   d. Vesicular or bullous lesion.
   e. Splinter haemorrhage.
   f. Raynaud's phenomenon.
   g. Pulp atrophy.
   h. Necrotic ulcer (Fig. 3.76).

- Vasculitis in collagen vascular diseases is responsible for these characteristic skin lesions in hands.

WASTING OF THE SMALL MUSCLES OF HANDS: CASE 52

Q. How to diagnose wasting of the small muscles of hands?

1. Flattening of palm due to wasting of thenar and hypothenar muscles.
2. Prominent knuckles and other bony prominences.
3. Flexor-extensor tendons will stand out.
4. The interosseous space in the dorsum of hand will be hollowed or depressed due to wasting of interossei and lumbricals.

Q. What are the smalll muscles of hand?

A. **Thenar muscles:**
   1. Abductor pollicis brevis,
   2. Flexor pollicis brevis, and
   3. Opponens pollicis.

B. **Hypothener muscles:**
   1. Abductor digiti minimi,
   2. Flexor digiti minimi, and
   3. Opponens digiti minimi.

C. Adductor pollicis.
D. Palmaris brevis (superficial muscle of hand).
E. Palmar and dorsal interossei.
F. Lumbricals.

Clinical Wisdom

Ulnar nerve supplies all the small muscles of hands except the thenar muscles and the two lateral lumbricals, which are supplied by median nerve. The first muscle involved in injury of:
a. Median nerve: Abductor pollicis brevis.
b. Ulnar nerve: Abductor digiti minimi.

Q. Test of interossei and lumbricals:

Test the patient's ability to flex all of his MCP joints and to extend all the DIP joints of hand (Fig. 3.77). Remember, the palmar interossei are also adductors and dorsal interossei are abductors of fingers (Fig. 3.78A adn B).

Test of 1st dorsal interosseous: Place the flat of the hand with seperated fingers over a table and ask the patient to abduct his index finger against your resistance. The muscle can be seen and felt to contract in the space between thumb and index finger (Fig. 3.78B).

Q. How to test these small muscles of hands?

I. Abductor pollicis brevis (Fig. 3.79): The patient is asked to abduct his thumb in a plane at right angles to the palmar aspect of index finger, against resistance offered by your index finger. The muscle

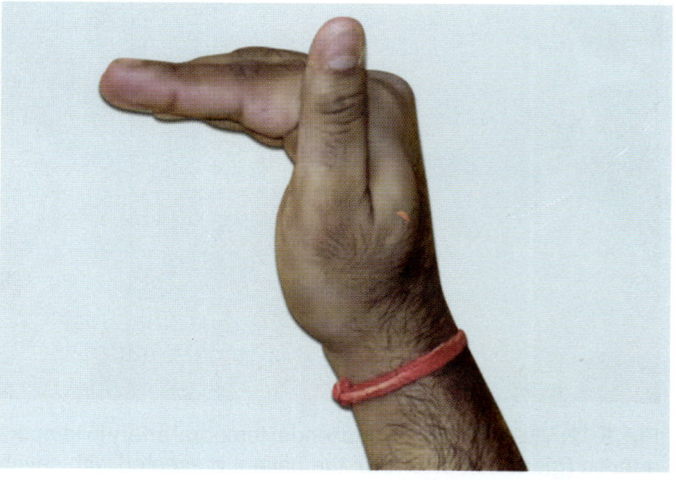

Fig. 3.77: Testing **lumbricals (and interossei)**

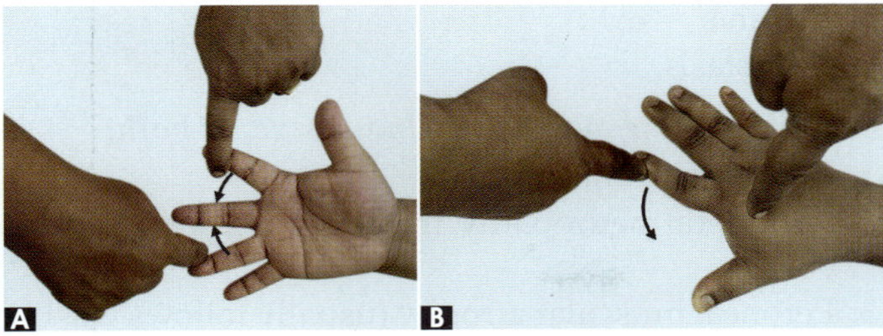

Fig. 3.78A and B: Testing (A) **palmar** and (B) first **dorsal interossei**

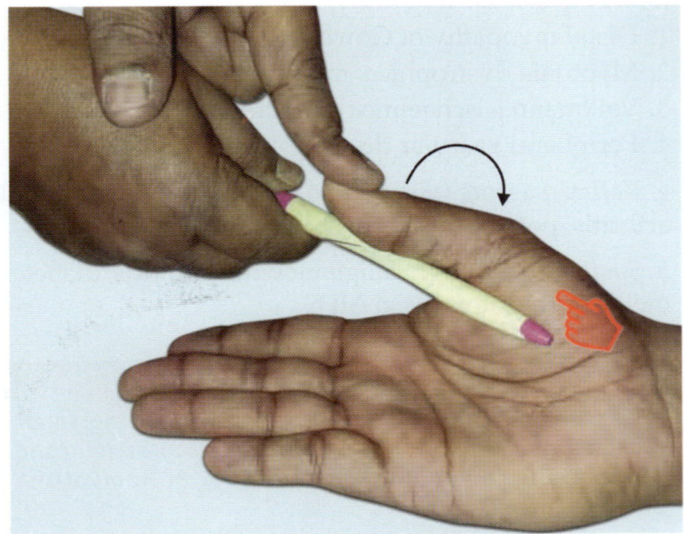

Fig. 3.79: Testing **abductor pollicis brevis**

can be seen and felt to contract. This muscle is affected first in carpal tunnel syndrome.

II. Adductor pollicis: Give the patient a book ('book test') and ask him to grasp it firmly between the thumb and other fingers of both hands (Fig. 3.80). In health, the thumbs remain straight whereas in lesions of the ulnar nerve, the terminal phalanx of the thumb of the affected hand will be flexed (Froment's sign).

III. Opponens pollicis: Ask the patient to touch the tip of all the fingers with his thumb. You can oppose the movement with your thumb or index finger, or you can ask the patient to swing the thumb across the palm (Fig. 3.81). See the different thumb movements in Fig. 3.82.

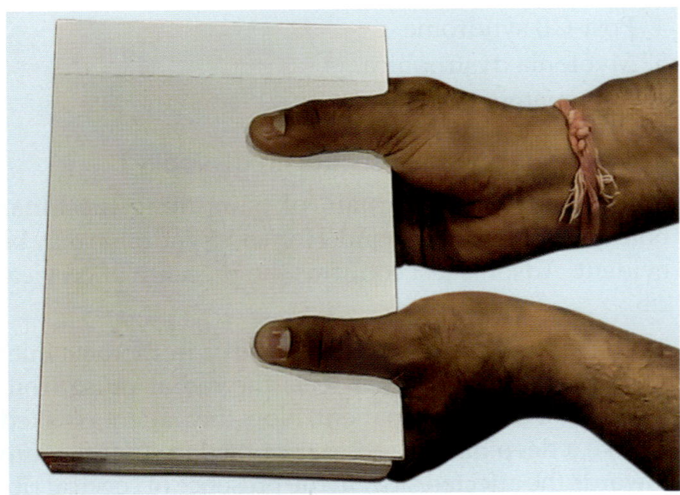

Fig. 3.80: Testing the function of **adductor pollicis**

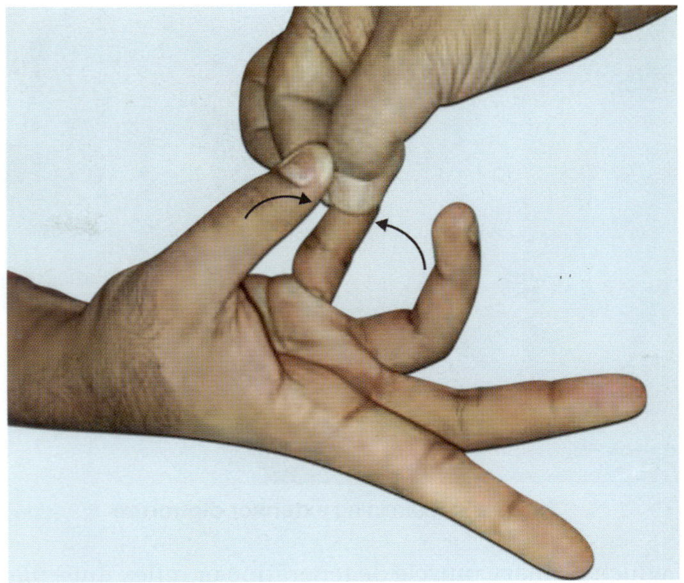

Fig. 3.81: Testing **opponens pollicis**

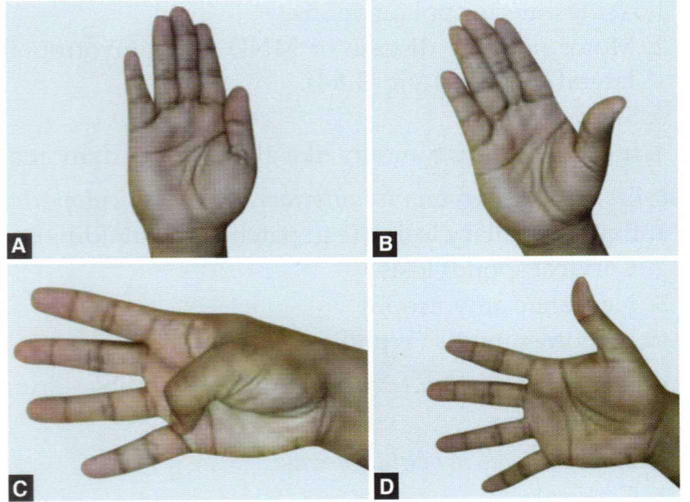

Fig. 3.82: Range of thumb movements. (A) Adduction; (B) Abduction; (C) Flexion; (D) Extension

- In wasting of the small muscles of hands the patient cannot open and close the hands as quickly as possible, cannot squeeze examiner's fingers; neither can hold a paper between two fingers firmly (weakness of palmar interossei), nor between thumb and index finger (weakness of adductor pollicis).
- Test the **extensor digitorum muscle:** The examiner tries to flex the patient's extended fingers at MCP joints, while the patient attempts to extend it (Fig. 3.83).

Q. Common causes of wasting of the small muscles of hand (bilateral):

The small muscles of the hand are supplied by C_8 and T_1 segments of the spinal cord. The causes of wasting, therefore, include lesions in the lower motor neurones at any point between these spinal segments and the muscles, together with certain other conditions in

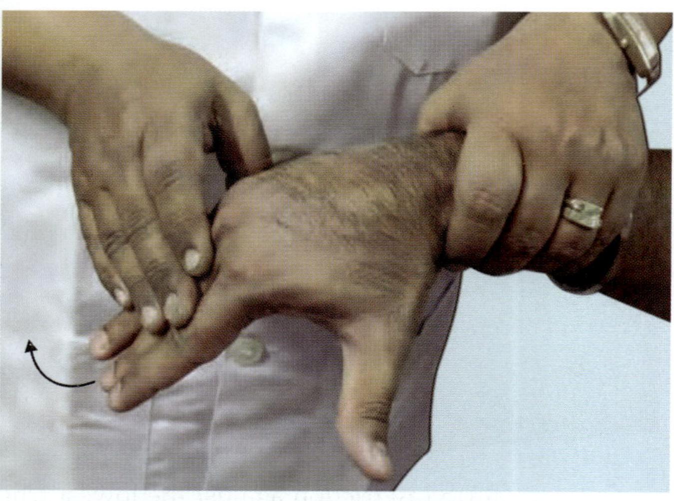

Fig. 3.83: Examining **extensor digitorum**

which primary muscle degeneration or reflex muscular wasting occurs.

a. Lesion in the anterior horn cells:
1. Acute anterior poliomyelitis.
2. Motor neurone disease or MND (e.g. amyotrophic lateral sclerosis) (Fig. 3.84).
3. Syringomyelia.
4. Intramedullary tumours like glioma, ependymoma.

b. Lesion in the nerve roots (anterior roots) or radiculopathy:
1. Extramedullary lesion (e.g. patchy arachnoiditis).
2. Cervical spondylosis.
3. Neuralgic amyotrophy.
4. Leptomeningitis (syphilitic): Rare.

c. Lesion in the spinal nerve: Klumpke's paralysis from birth injury.

d. Lesion in the brachial plexus:
1. Cervical rib.
2. Thoracic inlet syndrome.
3. Trauma.
4. Metastasis.

e. Lesion in the median or ulnar nerve, or both:
1. Injury or trauma.
2. Peripheral neuropathy from leprosy, lead neuritis, etc.
3. Peroneal muscular atrophy (usually follows wasting of legs and feet).
4. Carpal tunnel syndrome.

f. Muscle disease and others:
1. Distal myopathy of Gowers.
2. Myotonia dystrophica, rarely.
3. Volkmann's ischaemic contracture.
4. Peripheral vascular disease.

g. Reflex wasting (due to disuse atrophy): Rheumatoid arthritis, post-paralytic, post-fracture.

h. Systemic wasting: Malignancy, tuberculosis, diabetes mellitus, thyrotoxicosis, AIDS.

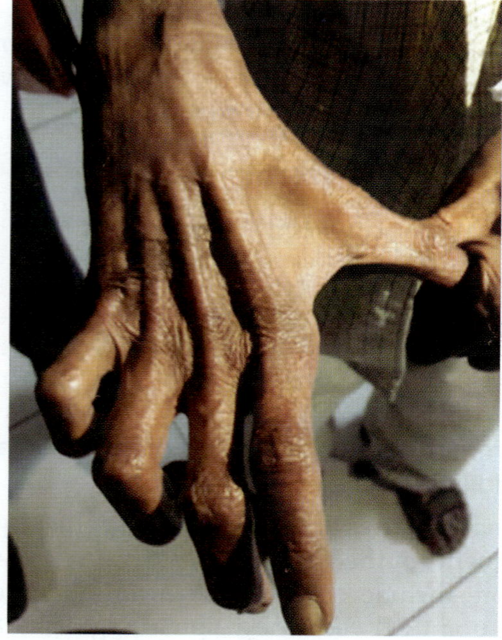

Fig. 3.84: **Small muscle wasting** in motor neurone disease

Clinical Wisdom

Five common causes of bilateral wasting of the small muscles of hands are: 1. Leprosy, 2. Motor neurone disease, 3. Rheumatoid arthritis, 4. Poliomyelitis, 5. Syringomyelia.

Q. Wasting of small muscles in one hand (i.e. unilateral):

1. Trauma to median or ulnar nerve.
2. Cervical cord compression.
3. Old poliomyelitis.
4. Leprosy.
5. Lesion in brachial plexus (trauma/tumour).
6. Pancoast's tumour (apical lung carcinoma).

Q. Wasting of small muscles of both upper and lower extremities:

1. Peroneal muscular atrophy.
2. Distal myopathy of Gower's.
3. Distal spinal muscular atrophy.
4. Post-GB syndrome.
5. Myotonia dystrophica.
6. Rheumatoid arthritis.

Q. How to diagnose cervical rib clinically?

The patient may complain of pain along the ulnar border of forearm and hand. Horner's syndrome may be evident. Adson's test confirms the presence of cervical rib.

Adson's test: This test is also positive in thoracic inlet syndrome. The examiner feels the radial pulse from the back of the sitting patient. Now the patient is asked to take a deep breath and to turn the face (not flexion) towards the affected side. In the presence of cervical rib, there will be obliteration or diminution of pulse.

Q. Identification points for an aetiological diagnosis:

1. History from childhood:
   a. Poliomyelitis.
   b. Klumpke's paralysis.
2. If complains of neck pain:
   a. Cervical spondylosis.
   b. Intra- or extramedullary tumour.
   c. Cervical rib (may be associated with bony lump in neck).
3. If associated with fasciculation and brisk tendon reflexes in upper extremities: Amyotrophic lateral sclerosis.
4. Associated with painful swelling of joints: Rheumatoid arthritis.
5. If there are **trophic changes** in hand:
   a. Leprosy.
   b. Syringomyelia.
   c. Cervical rib.
6. Examine the elbow for signs of old injuries like excessive callus, cubitus valgus deformity (for nerve injury) or for **thickened ulnar nerve** (leprosy).
7. If there is:
   a. No sensory loss: MND.
   b. Dissociation of sensory loss: Syringomyelia.
   c. Sensory loss: Peripheral neuropathy, leprosy, cervical cord compression.

CLAW HAND — CASE 53

Q. Describe the claw hand deformity:

Claw hand or 'main-en-griffe' is a condition where the metacarpophalangeal (MCP) joints are hyperextended, and the PIP and DIP joints are flexed (Fig. 3.85).

We know that the lumbricals are the main flexors of the first phalanx and the interossei are the sole extensors of the middle and distal phalanges. When the lumbricals are paralysed, there is hyperextension at MCP joints (by unopposed action of extensor digitorum) and when the interossei are paralysed, the PIP and DIP joints are flexed. So **claw hand is produced by the paralysis of interossei and lumbricals.**

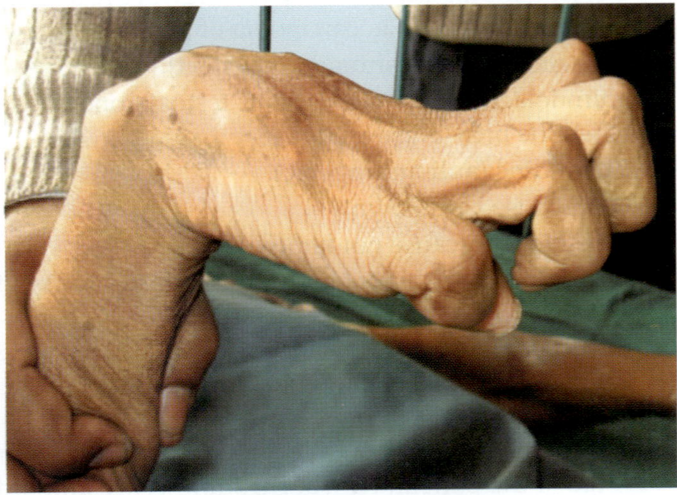

Fig. 3.85: **Claw hand** deformity

Q. Enumerate the common causes of claw hand:

The interossei and lumbricals are supplied by the C_8 and T_1 segments of the spinal cord through the ulnar and median nerves. So any lesion of the segments or nerves will produce the claw hand deformity.

1. **True claw hand:**
   a. Combined lesion of ulnar and median nerves by injury or leprosy (tuberculoid variety) will produce claw hand. It is obvious that only ulnar nerve affection will produce ulnar claw hand.
   b. Cervical spondylosis.
   c. Cervical rib (by friction against the lowest trunk of the brachial plexus) or thoracic inlet syndrome.
   d. Klumpke's paralysis.
   e. Motor neurone disease (progressive muscular atrophy, amyotrophic lateral sclerosis), syringomyelia, intramedullary tumours, etc.
2. **Mimicking (pseudo) claw hand:** These are basically surgical conditions like:
   a. Dupuytren's contracture.
   b. Volkmann's ischaemic contracture.
   c. Post-burn contracture.

Clinical Wisdom

The diseases which produce wasting of the small muscles of hands may show some degree of claw deformity.

Q. Aetiological differentiation by sensory functions:

1. Motor neurone disease, either amyotrophic lateral sclerosis or progressive muscular atrophy: No sensory loss.
2. Injury to the ulnar and median nerve:
   a. Practically, all modalities of sensation in the palm and the dorsum of hand are lost.
   b. In the dorsum of hand, a small area escapes sensory loss (over the base of thumb and the first interosseous space) as it is supplied by radial nerve.
3. Leprosy: Patchy and distal sensory involvement (peripheral neuropathy).
4. Syringomyelia: Dissociated sensory loss, i.e. loss of pain and temperature sensation with preservation of fine touch sensation.

Q. Hand feels very cold: what will you think?

It is due to vasomotor insufficiency produced by the presence of cervical rib, thoracic inlet syndrome or as a result of severe form of vasculitis (e.g. Raynaud's phenomenon) (Fig. 3.73). The affected hand feels colder than the normal side, and becomes pale (and painful) when elevated and blue when dependent for some time.

Q. What is wrist drop (*see* Fig. 1.53)?

A. Definition: It is due to paralysis of the extensors of wrist. There will be difficulty in extension of wrist and fingers (finger drop). In an attempted extension of fingers, there will be flexion of MCP joints and extension of interphalangeal joints due to unopposed action of lumbricals and interossei, respectively.

B. Method of testing: Ask the patient to make a fist and try to flex the wrist forcibly against patient's effort to maintain the posture. Normally, it is almost impossible to flex the wrist overcoming the patient's wrist extensors. But in wrist drop, patient's wrist will be very easily flexed by the examiner.

C. Aetiology:

1. Radial nerve palsy (trauma, saturday night palsy or compression at axilla).
2. Chronic lead poisoning, and
3. Other peripheral neuropathies (including mononeuritis multiplex).

Q. Identification points for an aetiological diagnosis:

Same as described in the section on 'Wasting of the small muscles of hands'.

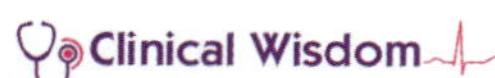
Clinical Wisdom

Never forget to palpate the ulnar nerve in the elbow (e.g. leprosy) and to examine for trophic changes in the fingers in a patient with claw hand or wasting of the small muscles of hands.

GYNAECOMASTIA — CASE 54

Q. What is gynaecomastia (Fig. 3.86)?

This is a condition where the male breast looks like that of a female (often called 'man boobs'). On inspection, even the nipple and areola assume a feminine appearance. Early gynaecomastia is characterised by proliferation of both the fibroblastic stroma (glandular breast tissue) and the duct system; eventually the number of ducts decrease. It is usually painless but elderly person with gynaecomastia may have little pain. Gynaecomastia results from an increase in the oestrogen/androgen ratio.

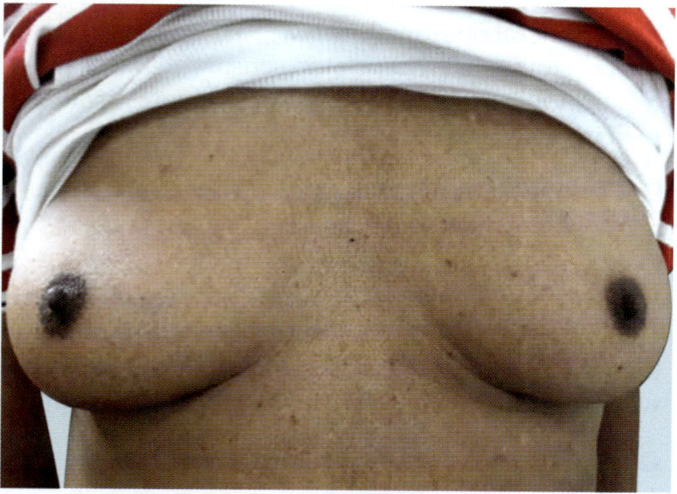

Fig. 3.86: Gynaecomastia following anti-androgen therapy in carcinoma of the prostate

Gynaecomastia (gynaecomazia) is the benign enlargement of male breast tissue, which is >2 cm palpable, firm, subareolar gland and ductal tissue.

Q. What is lipomastia?

Lipomastia or 'false' enlargement of breast (found in obesity) is best palpated with flat of the palm while gynaecomastia is best appreciated with fingers. In lipomastia, no glandular breast tissue is there but only mammary fat is present. One should remember that no breast tissue is palpable in normal man.

- **Pseudogynaecomastia** is found in lipomastia (i.e. obesity), neurofibromatosis, cold abscess, and malignant or leukaemic deposits.
- **Painful gynaecomastia:** Puberty or adolescence, drug-induced (e.g. spironolactone), hepatoma and cirrhosis of liver.

Q. Examination of the patient for gynaecomastia:

1. Examine the breast tissue first with flat of the palm, then with fingers to confirm the glandular tissue. Tenderness indicates rapid growth.
2. Age of the patient.
3. Unilateral or bilateral.
4. **Stature** of the patient, and signs of eunuchoidism or feminisation.
5. H/o taking drugs (produce gynaecomastia) or alcoholism.
6. H/o mumps or castration.
7. See the **face** carefully; examine both the **testes**.
8. Examine the **liver, spleen,** and search for any hepato-celullar failure.
9. Look for the signs of carcinoma of the lung in the form of SVC obstruction, collapse of the lung.
10. Examine the spine for any tenderness or gibbus (caries spine → cold abscess underneath breast).
11. Signs of leprosy: Nodules, hypopigmented spots in skin or thickened peripheral nerves, etc.
12. P/R examination to exclude carcinoma of the prostrate for which diethylstilbestrol is advised.

Q. Drugs producing gynaecomastia:

1. Oestrogens or anti-androgen (e.g. cyproterone) therapy in males (e.g. carcinoma of prostate).
2. Digitalis (due to oestrogen-like effect).
3. Spironolactone (reduces serum testosterone level): Often the breasts are tender.
4. Cimetidine (anti-androgenic).
5. INH (cause not known).
6. Methyl dopa (cause not known).
7. Marijuana, cannabis or heroin abuse (associated with high oestrogen and low testosterone).
8. Busulfan, phenothiazines, tricyclic antidepressants, ketoconazole, diazepam, phenytoin.

Q. Explanation of your method of examination:

1. Age of the patient: Newborn, adolescence and old age may have physiological gynaecomastia.

2. Stature of the patient: Klinefelter's syndrome and hypogonadism may have tall stature.
3. Drugs, mumps orchitis, castration: All produce gynaecomastia.
4. Examination of testes:
   a. Testicular tumour: Asymmetry of testes, smooth or lobulated (e.g. Leydig cell tumour).
   b. Klinefelter's syndrome: Small and firm testes.
   c. Cirrhosis of liver with hepato-cellular failure or haemochromatosis: Small and soft testes.
   d. Lepromatous leprosy: Atrophied small and soft testes.

❍ By Prader orchidometer (to measure testicular volume), testicular size <3 cm indicates atrophy (normal adult size is 4–7 cm, and volume 15–25 mL). Pre-pubertal males have small and rubbery testes.

5. Examination for hepatosplenomegaly:
   a. Cirrhosis of liver.
   b. Leprosy.
   c. Acute leukaemia (leukaemic deposits in breast may mimic gynaecomastia).
6. Facies:
   a. Puffy, bloated and congested: SVC obstruction due to carcinoma of the lung.
   b. Leonine facies: Lepromatous leprosy.
   c. Hepatic facies: Cirrhosis of liver with hepato-cellular failure.
   d. Rarely in true hermaphroditism.
7. Spine: Cold abscess may form behind the breast tissue in a patient suffering from caries spine (from the back, abscess coming in front through muscle plane). It is not true gynaecomastia and usually produces unilateral painless swelling of the breast.
8. Examination of the skin is done for hypopigmented anaesthetic spots, fall of body hairs and eyebrows, and subcutaneous nodules for lepromatous leprosy which causes gynaecomastia.
   Sparse pubic hair is common in hypogonadism.
9. P/R examination: If the patient gives history of taking anti-androgen drugs (probably suffering from carcinoma of the prostrate), a P/R examination should be done.
10. Unilateral or bilateral: Gynaecomastia may be unilateral to start with. Klinefelter's syndrome and physiological gynaecomastia are bilateral.

Q. Common causes of gynaecomastia:

1. Physiological: Newborn, adolescence and old age.
2. Klinefelter's syndrome (47, XXY).
3. Hepato-cellular failure commonly from alcoholic cirrhosis; hepatoma.
4. Drug-induced.
5. Bronchogenic carcinoma.
6. Lepromatous leprosy.
7. Starvation; recovery from wasting diseases (refeeding gynaecomastia).
8. Hypogonadism due to any cause (secondary testicular failure from orchitis, malignancy or castration).
9. Oestrogen-secreting testicular (Sertoli cell tumour) or adrenal tumours.
10. Hyperthyroidism, renal failure, hyperprolactinaemia, carcinoma of the breast, local trauma.

Q. How to proceed for diagnostic evaluation?

After proper clinical evaluation:
1. A careful drug history is taken.
2. Measurement and examination of testis (if both are small and firm, a karyotype is indicated; it testes are asymmetric, an evaluation for testicular tumour is warranted).
3. Liver function tests.
4. Blood for testosterone, LH, FSH, oestradiol, prolactin and hCG estimation.
5. 24-hours urinary 17-ketosteroid estimation.

Explanation: If there is:
- LH ↑ and tesosterone ↓ = testicular failure.
- LH ↓ and testosterone ↓ = most likely there is increased primary oestrogen production (e.g. Sertoli cell tumour of the testis).
- LH ↑ and testosterone ↑ = androgen resistance or gonadotropin-secreting tumour.
- ↑ Urinary 17-ketosteroid = feminising adrenal tumour.

Work up is necessary where:
a. Drug history is negative.
b. Breast is tender with rapid growth.
c. Breast mass >4 cm in diameter.

Q. How do you like to treat your patient?

1. Reassurance for pubertal gynaecomastia (may presist for 2–3 years).
2. Treatment of the cause like leprosy, hepato-cellular failure, withdrawing the offending drug, etc.
3. Painful gynaecomastia who are not candidates for other therapy: Treatment with anti-oestrogens, e.g. tamoxifen (20 mg/day) or raloxifen (60 mg/day) should be tried. Aromatase inhibitors (testolactone) or androgens (e.g. danazol, 200 mg twice daily) can be effective. Patients with testicular insufficiency may be benefited by androgen replacement therapy.
4. Indication for surgery (simple mastectomy or liposuction):
   i. Severe psychological problem.
   ii. Continued growth or tenderness.
   iii. Cosmetic problem.
   iv. Suspicion of malignancy.

❍ In gynaecomastia, the risk of developing carcinoma of the breast is very very rare.

Q. Common causes of hyperpigmentation:

1. Familial, racial.
2. Sunburn or sun tan.
3. Addison's disease.
4. Haemochromatosis.
5. Peutz-Jeghers syndrome.
6. Chronic kala-azar.
7. Cirrhosis of liver.
8. Uraemia.
9. Drug-induced.
10. Pellagra.
11. Facial pigmentation in chloasma.
12. Porphyria (cutanea tarda).
13. Freckles, lentigo (post-sun exposure).
14. Urticaria pigmentosa.
15. Acanthosis nigricans.
16. Melanoma.
17. Scleroderma.
18. Paraneoplastic syndrome.
19. Chronic arsenical poisoning (arsenicosis).
20. Malnutrition, starvation.
21. SLE.
22. Alkaptonuria.
23. Primary biliary cirrhosis.
24. Nelson's syndrome.

- Drug-induced: Clofazimine (reddish-brown), busulfan, hydroxychloroquine, oral contraceptive pills, bleomycin, phenothiazines, heavy metals (arsenic, gold), tetracycline, amiodarone, minocycline, psoralens.
- Abnormal increased pigmentation is known as **hyperpigmentation** which may be localised (commonly due to dermatological disorders) or generalised (commonly due to systemic diseases).

Q. Causes of hypopigmentation:

Read the section on 'Pityriasis versicolor'.

Q. Sites examined for increased pigmentation at the bedside:

1. Face.
2. Inside the oral cavity, especially buccal mucosa (commonly seen in Addison's disease, malabsorption syndrome, chronic cachexia, Peutz-Jeghers syndrome and haemochromatosis), palate and tongue.
3. Palmar creases.
4. General skin surface (pressure points; normally pigmented areas like areola, genitalia, axilla, knuckles, sun-exposed areas; recent scars); palms and soles.

Q. Pigments commonly responsible for pigmentary disorders in humans:

1. Melanin: Hyperpigmentation and hypopigmentation.
2. Carotene: Carotenaemia.
3. Bilirubin: Jaundice.
4. Iron: Haemochromatosis and haemosiderosis.
5. Silver: Slatey-grey hue (argyria).

Q. Pigmentation in chronic kala-azar:

Due to increased black pigmentation, the disease is known as kala-azar (the Hindi version of 'black' is '*kala*'). Hyperpigmentation occurs as a result of disturbance in melanin metabolism. Pigmentation is commonly seen **around the mouth, on the temple and forehead**.

Q. Pigmentation in Addison's disease (Fig. 3.87):

Pigmentation in Addison's disease is due to increased pituitary MSH and ACTH secretions. At first, tanning is noticed following sun exposure. Afterwards, there is increased pigmentation **at pressure points** (elbow), in the **areas normally pigmented** (areola, genitals, knuckles, axilla, palmar creases, old and new scars) and also in the **mucous membranes** (mouth and genitals). Rarely, there may be areas of vitiligo.

Q. Features of Addison's disease:

Commonly the patient is a female and suffers from:

1. Asthenia (glucocorticoid ↓).
2. Hypotension (mineralocorticoid ↓).
3. Hyperpigmentation (ACTH ↑).
   Cardinal manifestations (No. 1–3)
4. Anorexia, malaise, weight loss.
5. Decreased body hairs.
6. Hyperkalaemia.
7. Hypoglycaemia.
8. Nausea, vomiting.
9. Chronic fatigue syndrome.
10. Acute adrenal crisis.

- Thomas Addison (1793–1860) was an English physician in Guy's Hospital, London, UK.

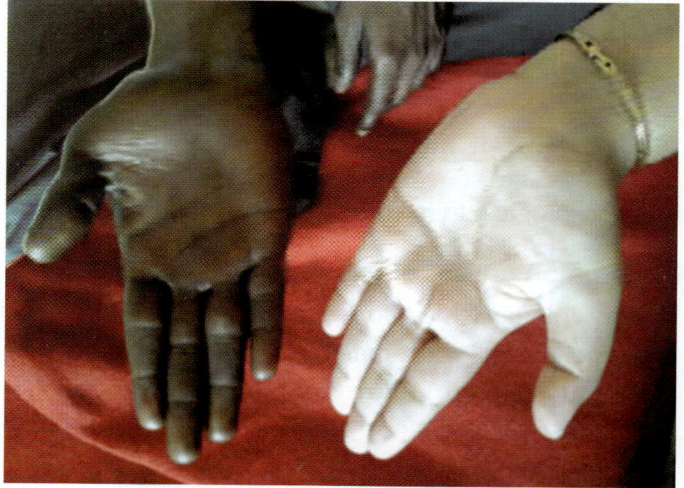

Fig. 3.87: **Black palm** with blackish palmar creases in **Addison's disease,** compared with a normal hand

Q. Differentiation between primary and secondary adrenocortical hypofunction:

Glucocorticoids, mineralocorticoids and androgens are low in both the conditions. In primary (Addison's disease) cases, there are features of:

1. Presence of pigmentation.
2. Absence of hypothyroidism and hypogonadism, and
3. High plasma ACTH level.

In secondary hypofunction (in involvement of pituitary or hypothalamus), there are:

1. Absence of pigmentation.
2. Presence of hypothyroidism and hypogonadism, and
3. Low plasma ACTH level.

Q. What is haemochromatosis?

It is an iron-storage disorder with inappropriate increase in intestinal iron absorption. There is deposition of iron in parenchymal cells with eventual tissue damage. The disease is clinically manifested by:

1. Excessive generalised skin pigmentation (due to increased melanin and iron deposition; melanin gives the typical bronzing or slatey-grey hue of the skin).
2. Diabetes mellitus (*bronze diabetes*).
3. Arthropathy (arthritis and chondrocalcinosis).
4. Cardiac involvement: CCF, cardiomyopathy, arrhythmia.
5. Hepatic involvement (cirrhosis or hepato-cellular carcinoma) with hepato-cellular failure.
6. Loss of libido and testicular atrophy (hypogonadism).

- The **pigmentation is more pronounced** on face, neck, lower forearms, dorsa of hands, lower legs, genitals and in scars.

Q. Treatment of haemochromatosis:

1. Phlebotomy.
2. Iron chelation by desferrioxamine.
3. Treatment of CCF, hepato-cellular failure, diabetes mellitus, etc.

- There is ↑ serum iron, ↑ serum transferrin saturation, ↑ serum ferritin and ↑ hepatic iron content (estimated by liver biopsy or high-intensity MRI).

Q. How a haemochromatosis patient dies?

1. CCF.
2. Hepato-cellular failure.
3. Hepato-cellular carcinoma (in treated cases).

Q. What is Peutz-Jeghers syndrome (Fig. 3.88A)?

In this syndrome, there are numerous polyps seen in small and large intestine. The polyps show features of hamartoma on histological section. Chance of malignant transformation is very rare. The syndrome is associated with mucocutaneous pigmentation and rarely, germinal cell tumour of ovary. Commonly it gives rise to **perioral and lip pigmentation**.

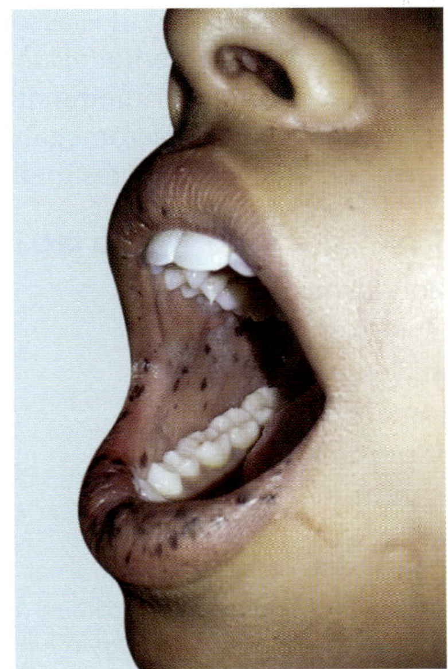

Fig. 3.88A: **Peutz-Jeghers syndrome** with **perioral pigmentation**

Q. What is chloasma or melasma?

A common hypermelanosis of young females (very rare in males) frequently precipitated by pregnancy (chloasma gravidarum) or by prolonged use of oral contraceptive pills (also known as 'mask of pregnancy'). The pigmentation is generally seen on malar prominences and bridge of the nose (bilateral and frequently symmetrical); also seen in forehead and moustache area. It is a benign condition.

Q. What is acanthosis nigricans (Fig. 3.88B)?

It is a thickened, velvety hyperpigmentation predominantly of the flexures of the body (e.g. sides of

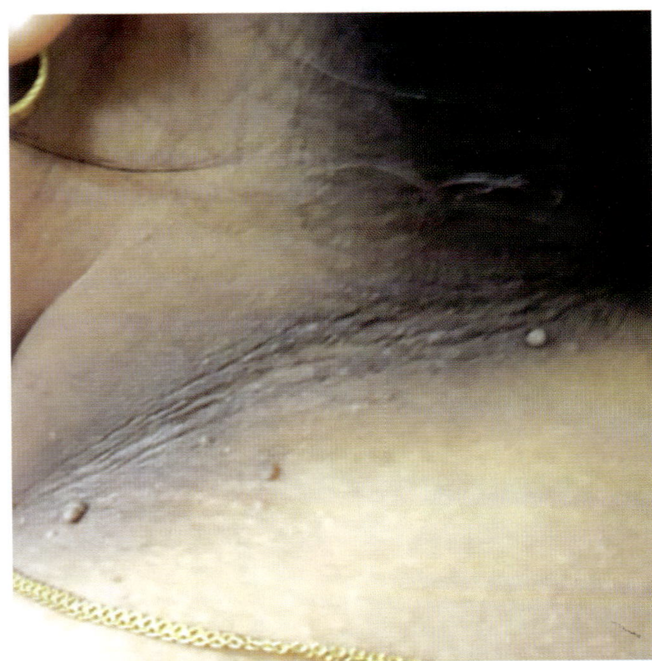

Fig. 3.88B: **Acanthosis nigricans**—brown to black, poorly defined, velvety hyperpigmentation of the skin of neck in type 2 diabetes mellitus (indicating insulin resistance) with skin tags (acrochordons)

neck, axilla and groin). In majority, it is associated with *obesity* who is also having underlying *insulin resistance*. It can be a reflection of internal malignancy (e.g. GI tract), or endocrinopathy such as acromegaly, Cushing's syndrome or insulin-resistant diabetes mellitus.

Q. Causes of 'plethoric face' (with a red hue):

1. Chronic alcoholism.
2. Cushing's syndrome.
3. Polycythemia (*see* **Fig. 3.4**).
4. SVC syndrome.
5. Chronic cor pulmonale.
6. Carcinoid syndrome.

- See the section on 'Mitral stenosis' for causes of 'malar flush'
- **'Oral pigmentation'** (i.e. pigmentation within oral cavity) is characterisitic of malabsorption syndrome, Addison's disease, haemochromatosis, heavy metal exposure (e.g. Hg, bismuth), use of drugs (e.g. busulfan), pregnancy and the 'black hairy tongue' (vide page 429).

SCABIES — CASE 56

Q. Aetiology and transmission:

This contagious disease is caused by the mite *Sarcoptes scabiei* contracted through close personal contact or contaminated clothings. After copulation the fertilised female mite excavates a burrow in the stratum corneum. From egg → nymphs hatch out → mature in 2 weeks into adult males and females on the surface of the skin → they mate, and reinvade the skin of same or other person. The incubation period of scabies is 3 weeks.

Doctors, paramedicals and inmates of mental hospitals are at particular risk to acquire scabies.

Q. Characteristic distribution of scabies (Fig. 3.89A):

1. Webs of fingers, wrist, ulnar border of forearm and arm, anterior axillary folds.
2. Front of chest, areola in female breast, umbilical and periumbilical region, belt line and lower abdomen.
3. Shaft of penis, scrotum, vulva, folds of buttock, groin, medial aspect of thigh, knee, front of ankle, webs of toes.

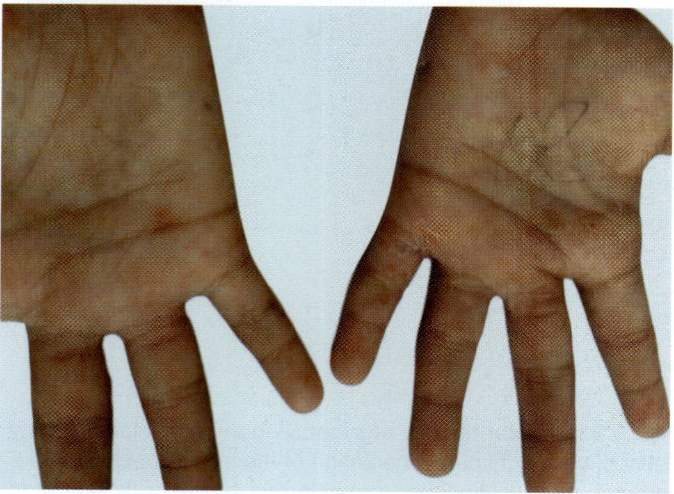

Fig. 3.89A: Scabies seen in different parts of palm and fingers

- **Spread** is by prolonged close contact, sharing of clothings and beddings, and by sexual exposure.
- An imaginary circle intersecting the main sites of involvement of both sides—Finger webs, wrist, axilla, areola, umbilicus, lower abdomen, genitalia and buttocks has long been called the 'circle of Hebra'.

Q. Which part of body is usually spared in scabies?

Face and scalp (face and scalp may be affected in infants).

Q. How to diagnose scabies?

Scabies is usually diagnosed by history and clinical examination:

1. Specific lesion with typical distribution.
2. Burrow.
3. **Nocturnal pruritus** (intractable).
4. H/o affection of several members of the family at a time (as scabies is highly contagious).
5. Demonstration of mite *Sarcoptes scabiei* from the burrow (confirmation of diagnosis).

Q. Most pathognomonic lesion of scabies:

Burrow or tunnel (linear or curved) is the most pathognomonic and characteristic lesion.

This is an irregular or linear skin-coloured ridge caused by tunneling of the mite in the stratum corneum layer of skin. It is seen in areas mentioned under distribution of lesion. The burrow can be identified by 'ink method' (touched with a drop of ink) when the burrow absorbs the ink and is highlighted as a dark line (may be up to 15 mm).

Q. Commonest lesion in scabies:

Papulo-vesicles.

Q. Describe the different lesions:

1. Papules (itchy and red).
2. Vesicles.
3. Pustules.
4. Impetigo.
5. Burrow, and
6. Indurated nodules.

Q. Mode of spread:

1. Very close and intimate contact with scabies patient (e.g. sharing the bed).
2. Overcrowding.
3. Poverty.
4. Poor hygiene.
5. Sexual promiscuity (considered a STD).

Q. Why there is nocturnal itch?

When the patient retires in warm bed, the mites start moving within the burrow.

Q. Non-itchy scabies:

1. Norwegian scabies, or
2. Scabies with psychiatric illness.

Q. What is Norwegian (crusted) scabies?

Widespread hyperkeratotic and crusted lesions of scabies (extremely infectious) resulting from infestation with thousands or millions of mites, and are present in:

1. Mentally retarded patients (e.g. schizophrenia, Down syndrome).
2. Patients with poor cell-mediated immunity (e.g. lepromatous leprosy, AIDS).
3. Severely debilitated patient (e.g. severe malnutrition), and
4. Immunocompromised states e.g. diabetes mellitus, glucocorticoid therapy, organ transplantation.

- Initially described in Norwegian leprosy patients, and thus named so.

Q. Lesions present in face:

1. Neonates.
2. Norwegian scabies.

Q. D/D of scabies:

1. Pediculosis corporis.
2. Atopic dermatitis.
3. Papular urticaria.
4. Dermatitis herpetiformis.

Q. Mention some itchy lesions in skin (dermatological causes of pruritus):

1. Scabies (nocturnal; after hot bath).
2. Dermatitis herpetiformis.
3. Urticaria.
4. Lichen planus (Fig. 3.89B).

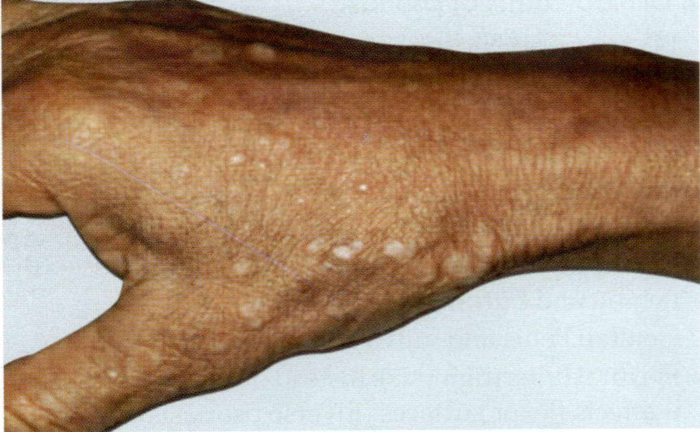

Fig. 3.89B: **Lichen planus**—Pruritic, purplish, plane-topped, polygonal papules and plaques (6 'P's); look for Koebner's phenomenon, Wickham striae

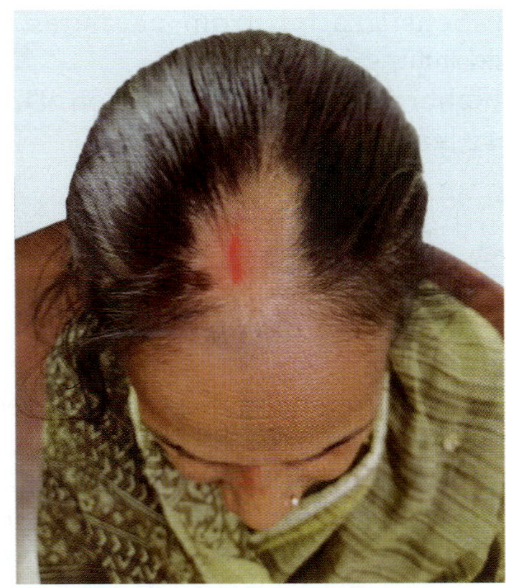

Fig. 3.89C: Bindi dermatitis—a form of contact dermatitis

5. Insect bite.
6. Psoriasis.
7. Eczematous and atopic dermatitis.
8. Pediculosis.
9. Ringworm.
10. Seborrhoeic dermatitis.
11. Drug eruption.
12. Allergic contact dermatitis (Fig. 3.89C).
13. Xerosis (dry skin).

Q. Medical (systemic) causes of generalised pruritus:

1. Obstructive jaundice (medical or surgical).
2. Diabetes mellitus.
3. Chronic renal failure.
4. Polycythemia vera (especially after a hot bath).
5. Systemic mastocytosis.
6. Lymphoma (Hodgkin's disease commonly).
7. Carcinoid syndrome.
8. Leukaemias.
9. Multiple myeloma.
10. Primary biliary cirrhosis.
11. Thryotoxicosis.
12. Drugs like cocaine, morphine.
13. Drug reaction; pregnancy (last trimester).
14. HIV infection.
15. Neurosis.
16. Old age, especially in winter; dry skin.
17. Malignancy (internal).
18. Psychogenic.

- Pruritus (severe) may be complicated by lichen simplex chronicus (local skin thickening due to scratching), local infections and prurigo nodularis (nodules developing at the site of itching).

Q. Complications of scabies:

1. Pyoderma, especially impetigo and ecthyma.
2. Acute glomerulonephritis (AGN): Due to sensitisation by nephritogenic strains of streptococci (most dangerous).

3. Eczema: Sensitization from parasites or from prolonged itching.
4. Rarely, sulphur dermatitis after initiation of treatment.
5. Secondary lymphadenitis.

Clinical Wisdom

Always search for signs of scabies infection in a patient with acute glomerulonephritis.

Q. Management:

1. At first, the treatment of secondary infection is done by antibiotics. Patient should cut his nails short and his daily used articles (towel, pillow, bed-sheet) should be kept separate and laundered properly. Antihistaminics and calamine lotion may be necessary to control itching. Pre-application with keratolytic agents like 6% salicylic acid is helpful in crusted scabies. Asymptomatic family members (close contacts) should be treated simultaneously as scabies is highly contagious.
2. Instructions to the patient: May start with a warm bath and dry thoroughly afterwards. Apply the medicine thinly but thoroughly over the whole body from chin downwards (both involved and uninvolved areas). It is better to rub the medicine into the skin. Treatment is best done at night before going to bed. Avoid touching mouth or eyes with hands. Change the undergarments and bed-sheets on the next day and launder them. The patient may take a bath in the morning with soap and water.
   Topical and oral treatment are available. A single overnight application with permethrin is sufficient. In pregnant women and infants, sulphur ointment, permethrin and crotamiton are preferred. Benzyl benzoate needs 3 applications at 12-hourly interval without intervening bath. Sulphur ointment is used once daily for consecutive 3 days. Do not repeat the drugs unless instructed.
3. Medicines used:
   a. Benzyl benzoate lotion (25%) or emulsion (children and young adult 12.5%).
   b. Unguentum sulphur (adult 10%, child 5%).
   c. Gamma benzene hexachloride or Lindane (1%) as lotion, cream or shampoo.
   d. Crotamiton (10%) as lotion or cream.
   e. Mitigal: 10% solution in liquid paraffin.
   f. Monosulfiram (25%; tetmosol): Used as soap or lotion.
   g. Topical thiabendazole.
   h. *Permethrin (5%)*: Used as cream; single application, may be repeated after 1 week.
   i. Malathion (0.5%) lotion.
   j. Esdepallethrine 0.63% aerosol: May be tried.
   k. *Ivermectin* (200 µg/kg, orally in single dose; adult dose is 12 mg) effectively treat scabies. Two doses at 1–2 weeks apart are required for crusted scabies. Even lotion ivermectin (0.5%) can be used.

- *Itching in scabies* is probably due to development of sensitisation to some of the products (e.g. saliva-scabin) of the mite.

Q. How to diagnose (confirm) scabies under the microscope?

A selected lesion is scraped by sterile needle or scalpel 6–7 times and the scrapings are transferred to a glass slide on which 10% KOH solution has already been kept. The slide is then examined with low power magnification for mites, eggs or fecal pellets.

PSORIASIS — CASE 57

Q. Describe the lesion:

Psoriasis is a chronic dermatogical condition caused by an overactive immune system. The lesions are:

1. Red, scaly papules or plaques.
2. Sharply defined.
3. Covered with varying amount of loosely adherent silvery-white scales.
4. Present over knees, elbows, hands, lumbosacral region, scalp, rarely in palms and soles *(i.e. mainly over the extensor surfaces)*.
5. The lesions are pruritic.
6. Localised lesion to sites of trauma, e.g. scratching **[Koebner's (isomorphic) phenomenon]**.
7. Scraping the scales leaves behind punctate bleeding spots **(Auspitz's sign)**: *Diagnostic*.

- Usually in young adults, both sexes with genetic predisposition; unpredictable course with relapses and remissions, worse in winter season; no available test to predict outcome. It is characterised by increased epidermal proliferation due to excessive division of cells in stratum basale.
- Psoriasis may be a presenting sign of HIV infection.
- Exacerbating factors in psoriasis, if any:
  1. Psychological factors.
  2. Drugs: β-blockers, ACE inhibitors, antimalarials, alcohol.
  3. Infections like β-haemolytic *streptococci*, HIV.
  4. Sunburn or mechanical injury.

Q. Clinical forms of psoriasis:

1. Plaque psoriasis: Commonest lesion; coin shaped (numular) **(Fig. 3.90A)**.
2. Guttate: Raindrop-like, small-sized, shiny scales **(Fig. 3.90B)**.
3. Pustular: Often with sterile pus in palms and soles, or involving total body folds; may have fever.
4. Erythrodermic form: Exfoliative dermatitis with itching and burning; may be fatal.
5. Genital: Penis and vulva affected.
6. Flexural (intertriginous): Instead of extensor surfaces, it affects flexor surfaces (inverse psoriasis).
7. Rupioid: Hyperkeratotic, cone-shaped **(Fig. 3.90C)**.
8. Scalp psoriasis: Fairly common; not associated with alopecia.

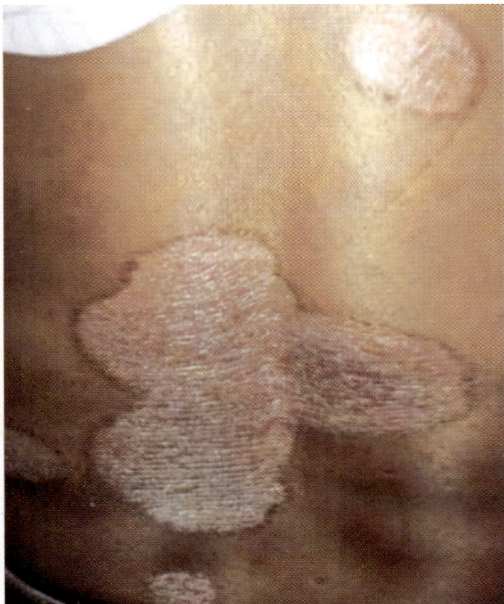

Fig. 3.90A: Erythematous, sharply-defined, **plaque-like**, scaly lesions of **psoriasis** in back of a young male

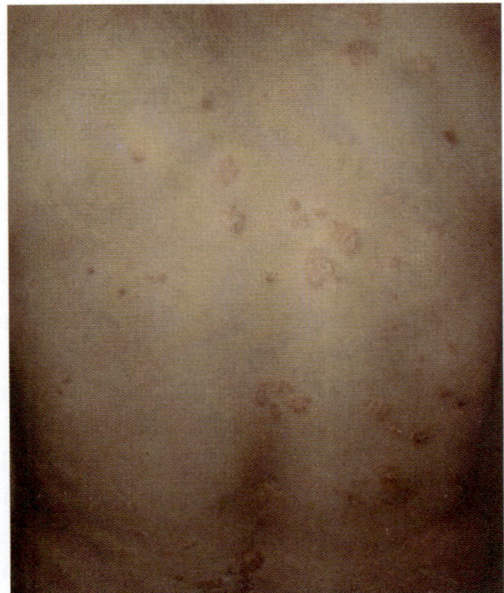

Fig. 3.90B: Small-sized scaly lesions of **guttate psoriais**

9. Generalised pustular: Known as 'von Zumbusch' psoriasis; rare but very serious.

- *Exfoliative dermatitis* **(erythroderma)** is common in psoriasis, contact dermatitis, atopic dermatitis, pityriasis rubra pilaris, drug-induced (e.g. suphonamides, dapsone) and systemic diseases (lymphoma/carcinoma (Fig. 3.91A)/mutiple myeloma/ HIV infection).

Q. Describe the nail changes in psoriasis:

Nail changes are often associated with arthropathy and may reflect the severity of the disease.

1. Pitting (thimble pitting).
2. Subungual hyperkeratosis.
3. Destruction of nail plates and thickening of nail (onychodystrophy).
4. Discolouration (yellow-brown) of nail plates ('oil drop' sign), and

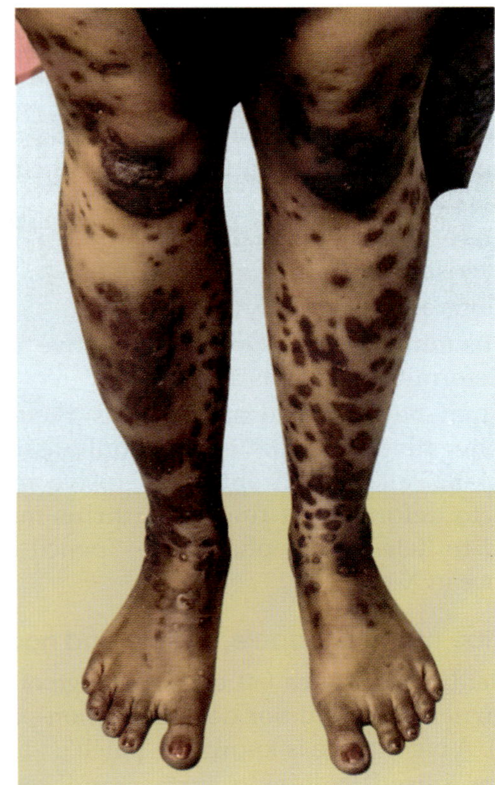

Fig. 3.90C: Thick, keratotic lesions of **rupioid psoriasis**

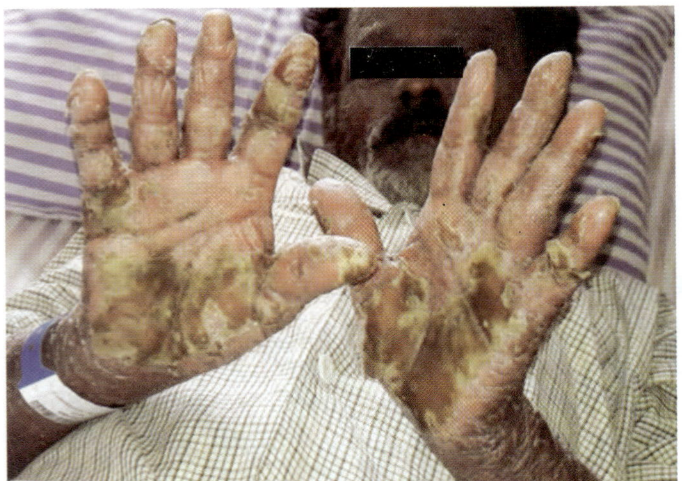

Fig. 3.91A: **Exfoliative dermatitis** (erythroderma) from internal malignancy

5. Onycholysis (separation of nail from nail-bed) and horizontal ridging.

- **Onycholysis** is the most characteristic nail lesion in psoriasis.

Q. Causes of pitting nail:

1. Psoriasis.
2. Eczema.
3. Alopecia areata.

Q. Diseases with Koebner's phenomenon:

1. Psoriasis.
2. Lichen planus.
3. Viral wart.

Q. What is psoriatic arthropathy (Fig. 3.91B)?

Arthritis occurs in 5–10% patients of psoriasis. The five distinct clinical forms of arthritis are:

1. Asymmetrical oligoarthritis (40%).
2. Symmetrical seronegative arthritis (25%): Rheumatoid arthritis pattern.
3. Arthritis of **distal interphalangeal joint** (15%): Most characteristic.
4. Sacroiliitis and/or spondylitis (15%).
5. Arthritis mutilans (5%): Severe destructive arthritis with deformities of hands and feet.

There may be associated nail changes; rheumatoid factor is negative. Arthritis is commonly associated with HLA-B27 allele. Arthropathy is erosive and may progress to deformity of fingers (arthritis mutilans may lead to 'telescoped' phalanges—'pencil-in-cup' appearance in X-ray).

Q. Describe macule, papule, vesicle and nodule:

A. **Macule:** Localised area (<1 cm) of change of colour in skin, neither raised nor depressed (non-palpable lesion). A big macule is known as 'patch' (>1 cm).

B. **Papule:** Raised from skin surface and generally <5 mm in size; a big papule is known as 'plaque' (>5 mm).

- **Vesicle** is small (<5 mm), usually clear fluid-containing elevated lesion whereas **bulla** is large vesicle (>5 mm). **Nodules** are solid elevations in skin of >5 mm in diameter.
- *Scale* means excess of loose, normal and abnormal horny layer; *crust* means dried-up exudate; *excoriation* means loss of skin by scratching; *lichenification* is thickening of epidermis with exaggerated skin margin.

Q. Histology of skin lesion in psoriasis:

1. Parakeratosis (immature cells in stratum corneum).
2. Acanthosis (hyperplasia of stratum malpighii).
   (1 and 2 reflecting increase in skin turnover)
3. Loss of granular cell layer.
4. Dilated and tortuous blood vessels in dermal papillae.
5. Rarely, neutrophilic abscesses (microabscesses of Munro) in the horny layer.

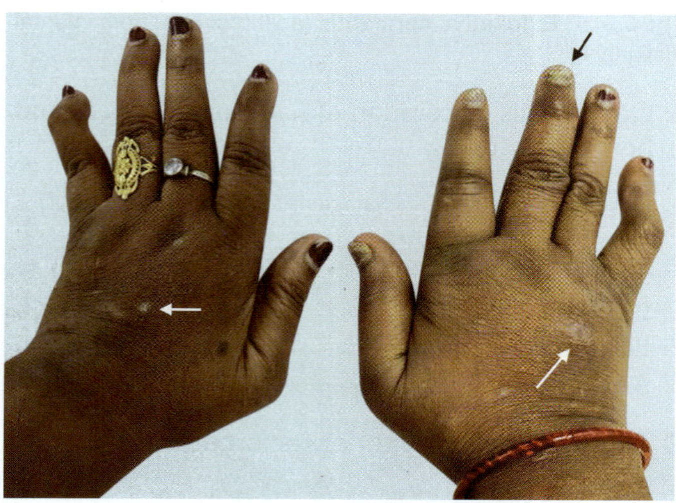

Fig. 3.91B: Deformed hand in **psoriatic arthropathy** with skin and nail changes

Q. Investigations you like to perform:

1. Blood for TC, DC to exclude superadded infections.
2. Skin scrapings and nail clippings may be examined for tinea (for differential diagnosis from fungal infection).
3. Rheumatoid factor: Negative (for differential diagnosis of arthropathy).
4. X-ray of affected joints may show 'pencil-in-cup' deformity: Arthritis mutilans.
5. Skin biopsy may be done (seldom necessary because the **clinical picture is very characteristic**).

Q. Management:

The treatment is concerned with control rather than cure, and is divided into four categories:

- Topical agents (emollients): 'Weak' tar, corticosteroids, vitamin D_3 agonists or dithranol preparations.
- PUVA or PUVB therapy.
- Systemic agent: Retinoids (tazarotene), immuno-suppresive drugs (cyclosporin A) or newer biological agents (infliximab).
- Intensive treatment with topical agents and UV-rays under medical supervision (No. 6 below).
- **Psoriasis is treated by:**
  1. Coal-tar preparations with keratolytics (salicylic acid 3–5%) as an ointment.
  2. Dithranol (0–1%) cream: Used locally; it inhibits DNA synthesis.
  3. Corticosteroid ointment may be used locally (systemic corticosteroid is strictly contraindicated).
  4. PUVA therapy (photochemotherapy): 'P' stands for Psoralen taken orally and UVA stands for ultra-violet light-A, i.e. of long-wavelength (320–400 nm). Oral psoralen is followed 2 hours later by UVA therapy; 2–5 sittings/week are necessary (total 10–20 sittings). UVB is helpful in winter season.
  5. Topical preparations of retinoic acid derivatives (0.05–0-1%) may be tried in localised plaques.
  6. Tropical therapy with ultraviolet rays:
     a. Goeckerman regimen: Crude coal tar plus UVB.
     b. Ingram regimen: Dithranol (anthralin) plus UVB.
  7. Methotrexate: Used in severe erythrodermic form, arthropathy or resistant cases. Methotrexate is used once weekly in a dose of 5 mg BDPC (used over 24 hours), and is supplemented by folic acid therapy (5 mg, once weekly except the day of methotrexate).
  8. Calcipotriol (vitamin D_3 analogue): Applied twice daily, not exceeding 100 g/week. Calcitriol and tacalcitol are other vitamin D_3 analogues.

9. NSAID for arthropathy.
10. Nail dystrophy is resistant to treatment.

- Oral corticosteroid may be used judiciously in refractory psoriasis, psoriatic arthropathy and erythrodermic form. Flexural psoriasis is treated with calcitriol (vitamin D_3 analogue) and 0.1% tacrolimus ointment. Resistant cases may be treated with cyclosporin A, mycophenolate, hydroxycarbamide, acitretin or hydroxyurea. TNF-α blockers or biologics (infliximab, etanercept, adalimumab, golimumab, ustekinumab) are now being tried with success in severe disease. Newer JAK-inhibitor like tofacitinib (oral) is a hopeful choice.
- **Division of UV rays:** UVC: Wavelength 10–290 nm (does not reach earth), UVB: 290–320 nm, UVA: 320–400 nm, visible white light we see: 400–700 nm, infrared rays (primarily evoke heat) >700 nm.

Q. Brief outline of common dermatological disorders:

A. **Impetigo:** It is a highly infectious superficial pyogenic infection of the skin. The infected areas, commonly around the mouth and nose, look like as inflamed plaques with a crusted surface. It is of two types like, a) Bullous impetigo—seen in newborn and is caused by *Staphylococcus aureus*, b) Non-bullous impetigo—encountered in young children and is due to *Staphylococcus aureus* or *Streptococcus pyogens*.

B. **Pemphigus** (Figs 3.92 and 3.93)**:** It is an autoimmune blistering disorder of skin and mucous membrane characterised by loss of cohesion between epidermal cells (i.e. acantholysis). This rare and potentially life-threatening disease has different types like:

a. Pemphigus vulgaris: Typically begins in mucosal surface which may progress to involve the skin to give rise to intraepidermal thin-walled, flaccid, fragile bullae. These bullae may rupture with extensive denudation of skin and mucous membrane with less tendency to heal. The scalp, face, mouth, neck, axilla, groin and trunk are typically involved sites. **Nikolsky's sign** (extension of blister on application of pressure to the affected skin) is positive.

b. Pemphigus foliaceus: It is the superficial form of pemphigus in contrast to pemphigus vulgaris, where the blisters occur in deeper epidermis.

c. Paraneoplastic pemphigus: Results as a complication of carcinoma and lymphoma.

d. Pemphigus vegetans: Here, blisters appear on groin, under the arms, mouth and on the feet.

e. Pemphigus erythematosus: An overlap syndrome with features of SLE and localised form of pemphigus folicaceus.

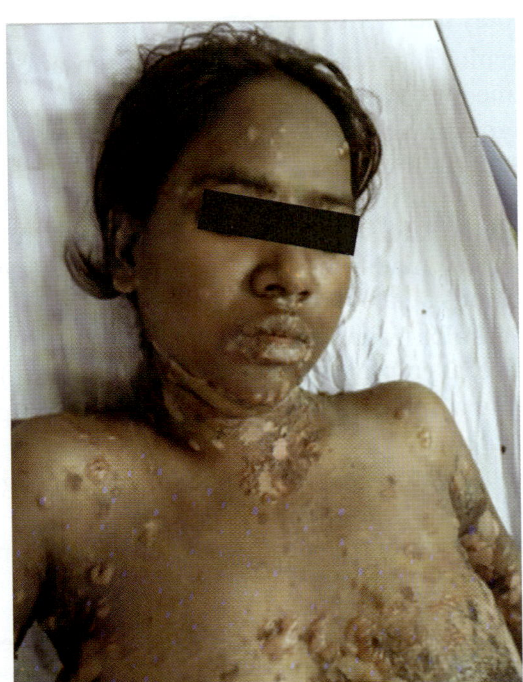

Fig. 3.92: Flaccid bullae of **pemphigus**; rupture of blisters/bullae resulted in denuded areas in places

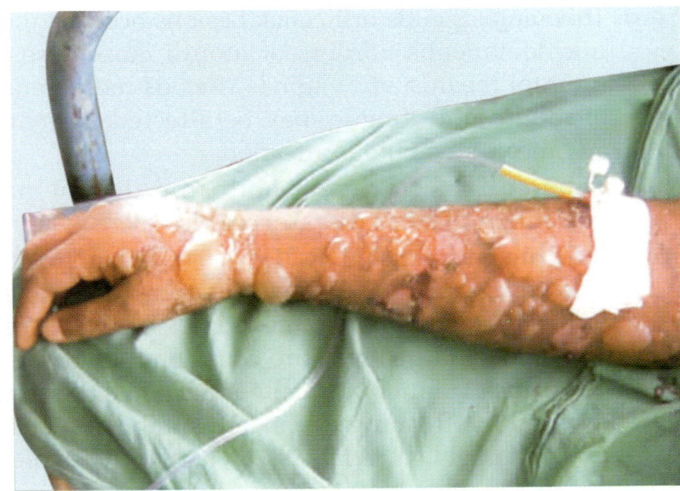

Fig. 3.93: Thin-walled, **flaccid**, easily-ruptured **bullae in pemphigus**; may affect mucous membrane (pemphigoid has tense bullae with rare involvement of mucosa)

- Scarring does not occur in pemphigus unless the lesions are secondarily infected.

C. **Pemphigoid:** Subepidermal tense bullae with less chance of rupture, and a positive tendency to heal without scarring. Typically involves trunk, limbs and flexures of the body. Mucosa of mouth are rarely involved. It is a relatively benign condition though it may be associated with (occult) lymphoma. Nikolsky's sign in negative.

D. **Dermatological manifestations of tuberculosis:**

a. **Lupus vulgaris:** Most common cutaneous tuberculosis as a result of post-primary infection. Red-brown nodules appear which look like apple-jelly when pressed with a glass slide (i.e. diascopy). Erythema, scaling and scarring plaques are common. Lupus means 'wolf', as in severe lupus vulgaris, the involved site mimicks bitten.

b. Tuberculosis verrucosa cutis: Warty lesion on a erythematous base.

c. Scrofuloderma: Associated with an infected discharging lymph node with ulceration on scarring.

d. Tuberculosis cutis orificialis: Lesions occur at the mucocutaneous borders of mouth, nose, anus, urethral meatus and vagina. Mucous membrane of mouth and tongue may be affected. It is an advanced tuberculous affection.

Tuberculids, erythema nodosum, erythema induration (Bazin's disease) are also there.

E. **Fixed-drug eruptions (FDR)** (Fig. 3.94): The inflamed patches (drug eruptions) *recur at the same site* each time if the drug is taken again for next time. Sites like face (lips), hands and genitalia are commonly involved. FDR are due to immunologically-mediated reactions. The common offending agents are sulphonamides, phenolphthalein, NSAIDs, salicylates ornidazole, ciprofloxacin, phenytoin, etc.

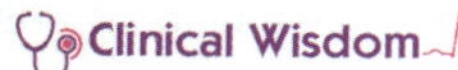

Clinical Wisdom

Always examine the nails and joints in a patient of psoriasis. Psoriasis does not affect the mucous membrane. Never forget to examine the back of elbows, front of knees, back of the trunk and scalp.

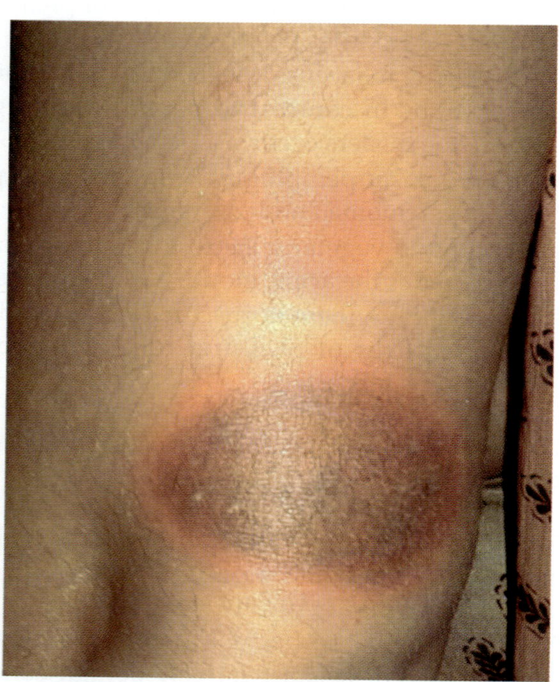

Fig. 3.94: **Fixed-drug eruptions** (FDR) at the back of arm with co-trimoxazole in *Pneumocystis jiroveci* pneumonia in an adult patient with AIDS

PITYRIASIS VERSICOLOR — CASE 58

Q. Characteristics (Fig. 3.95):

1. Caused by *Malassezia furfur* (*M. furfur* is possibly the parasitic form of a common saprophytic yeast, often called *Pityrosporum orbiculare*).
2. Occurs in warm and humid climates; a relatively common condition affecting young adults.
3. Well-defined, hypopigmented small macules with fine branny scales (the lesion is of various size, shape and colour).

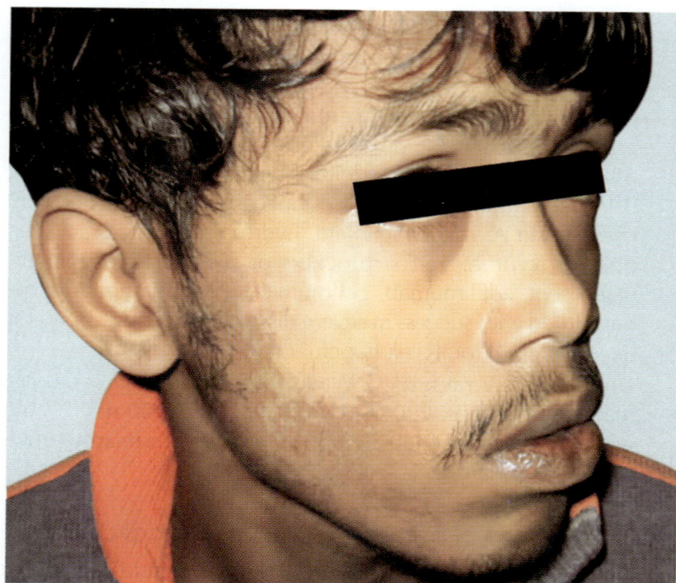

Fig. 3.95: **Pityriasis versicolor (tinea versicolor)**—manifested by hypopigmented macules in right side of the face

4. Generally non-itchy.
5. Many small spots may coalesce and form a large depigmented spot.
6. Classical sites are front of the chest, back of the chest, sides of neck, upper arm and face.
7. Sweating aggravates the condition; diabetes mellitus and pregnancy may be predisposing factors.
8. Asymptomatic except the cosmetic problem.

- The fungal hyphae and budding yeast may be seen in the scrapped scales when treated with 10% KOH solution and is seen by light miscroscopy; on inspection under Wood's lamp, it gives yellow fluorescence.

Q. D/D of hypopigmented (hypomelanotic i.e. loss of skin colour) spots or hypopigmentation:

1. Tuberculoid leprosy (test for touch sensation and examine for thickened nerve).
2. **Vitiligo** (may be idiopathic, sometimes associated with autoimmune diseases. Vitiligo is commonly associated with systemic disorders like Hashimoto's thyroiditis, Addison's disease, diabetes mellitus and pernicious anaemia. White hairs may be seen in vitiliginous areas) (Fig. 3.96).
3. Pityriasis alba (found on the face of children; probably infective; asymptomatic, remits spontaneously).
4. Post-burn (past H/o burn) (Fig. 3.97) or post-inflammatory.
5. Tuberous sclerosis (H/o convulsions, low intelligence and adenoma sebaceum in face).
6. Prolonged chloroquine therapy (H/o prolonged intake, e.g. rheumatoid arthritis, SLE).

- **Others:** Pityriasis versicolor, psoriasis, DLE, albinism (inherited disorder of lack of melanin in skin), phenylketonuria, naevus depigmentosus, piebaldism (manifested by a white forelock) and idiopathic guttate hypomelanosis.

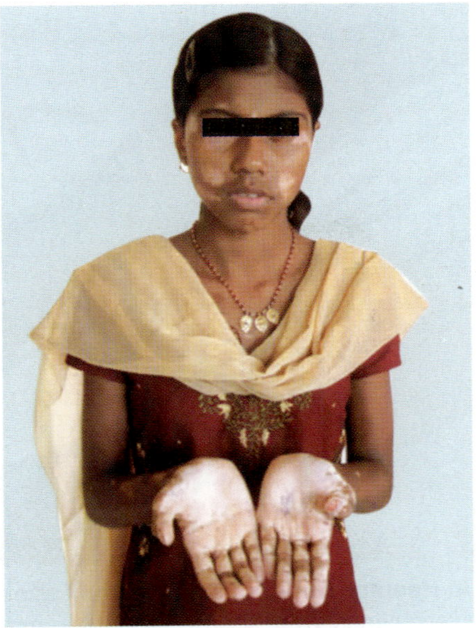

Fig. 3.96: **Vitiligo** seen in palm, forearm and face

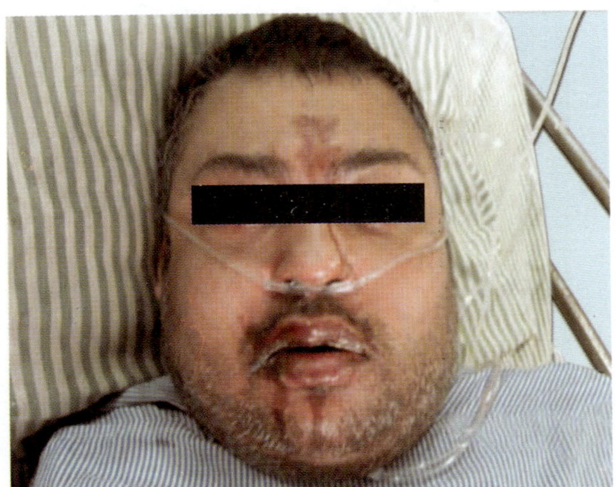

Fig. 3.97: **Acid burn** (recent) over forehead, lips and chin in suicidal acid ingestion, and is not a skin disease

Q. Common scaly lesions in skin:

1. Psoriasis.
2. Pityriasis rosea.
3. Seborrhoeic dermatitis.
4. Lichen planus (*see* **Fig. 3.89B**).
5. Certain eczema.
6. Exfoliative dermatitis (erythroderma) (*see* **Fig. 3.91A**).
7. Ringworm.
8. Ichthyosis (*see* **Fig. 3.68**).

Q. What is ringworm (Fig. 3.98)?

Skin infection in ringworm is caused by different dermatophytes (fungi) like *Trichophyton, Epidermophyton* or *Microsporum*. The lesion may be single or multiple, small or large, usually circular (ring-like, hence known as ringworm) with papulo-vesicular scaly active barder, itchy with central clearing, spread peripherally and heals with hyperpigmentation. The prefix **tinea** (which indicates ringworm) follows the affected region of the body like tinea corporis (body), tinea cruris (thigh and buttocks), tinea capitis (scalp), tinea pedis (feet), tinea manuum (hand), tinea barbae (beard) and tinea unguium (nail).

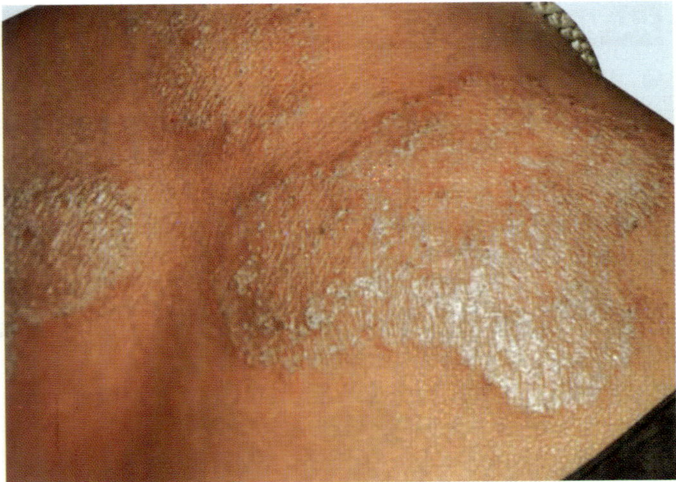

Fig. 3.98: **Ringworm** over upper part of back **(tinea corporis)**—dry scaly plaque with polycyclic irregular borders and relative central clearing

Diagnosis is done by demonstration of hyphae on examination of skin scrapings, hairs or nail clippings after dissolving in a drop of 10–20% KOH solution for several hours, and examined under light microscope. Treatment is done by local application of antifungal agents (miconazole, econazole, clotrimazole, tolnaftate, Whitfield ointment, etc.); lotions and powders are preferred for intertriginous and hairy (scalp) areas to be applied for 2–4 weeks. Systemic antifungal antibiotic like griseofulvin (10 mg/kg/day, after meals in twice daily dose for several weeks) is used in extensive lesion and in affection of scalp, nail (most resistant to treatment) and bearded area. Griseofulvin-resistant cases may be treated by oral ketokonazole (200 mg once or twice daily). Itraconazole (100–200 mg/day), fluconazole (150 mg/week) or terbinafine (250 mg/day) orally may be given for 4–8 weeks.

- Tinea pedis = athlete's foot, and tinea cruris = 'Dhobi' itch.

Q. Treatment of pityriasis versicolor:

1. Maintenance of good personal hygiene.
2. Sodium thiosulphate (25% aqueous solution) once daily for 3 weeks used locally.
3. Selenium sulphide (2.5%): Apply at night and wash-off in the following morning, for 4 weeks.
4. Topical tolnaftate (1%), clotrimazole, miconazole (2%), econazole, ketoconazole (2%) may be tried: Apply twice daily for 10 days.
5. Retinoic acid (0.025%) cream may be of some help.
6. Azoles: Oral ketoconazole 200 mg OD/BD, or oral itraconazole 100 mg, BD is used for 1 week in resistant cases. Ketoconazole shampoo (2%) may be tried.

Clinical Wisdom

Mention the finding of pityriasis versicolor in long/short case, if present in your patient.

HAEMORRHAGIC SPOTS CASE 59

Q. What are these?

These are red, blue or black spots in the skin deep to the epidermis. As they contain extravasated blood, they do not disappear on application of pressure by a pinhead, glass slide (diascopy) or on stretching the skin of the affected areas.

Q. How to classify haemorrhagic spots?

The arbitrary classification goes like:

1. **Petechiae:** 1–2 mm in diameter (i.e. pinhead-size, punctate or tiny) (Fig. 3.99A).
2. **Purpura:** A bit larger, 3–5 mm in diameter (Fig. 3.99B).
3. **Ecchymosis (bruise):** Large confluent (>5 mm) purpuric lesions (Figs 3.100A and B).
4. **Haematoma:** Large haemorrhages in the skin with surface elevation (fluctuant collection) (Fig. 3.101).

- Petechiae and purpura are collectively known as '**purpuric spots'**. Day by day, there is progressive colour changes (red → bluish → black) in haemorrhagic spots. Perifollicular haemorrhage is seen in scurvy.

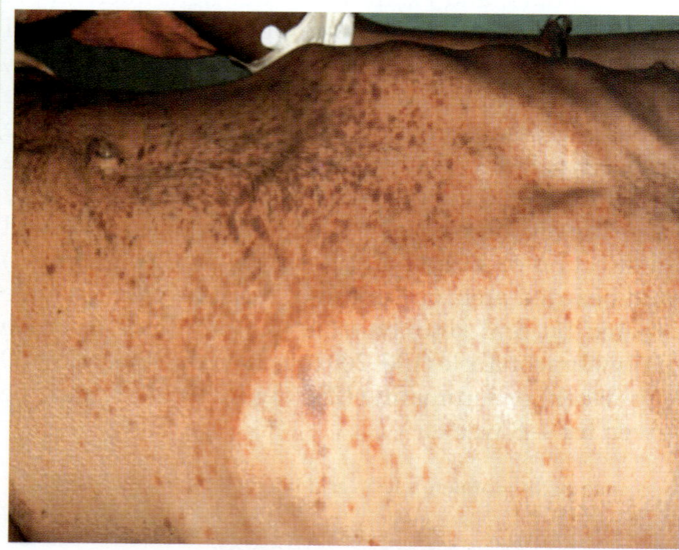

Fig. 3.99A: Haemorrhagic spots like **petechiae and purpura** are visible over anterior chest and abdomen in septicaemia

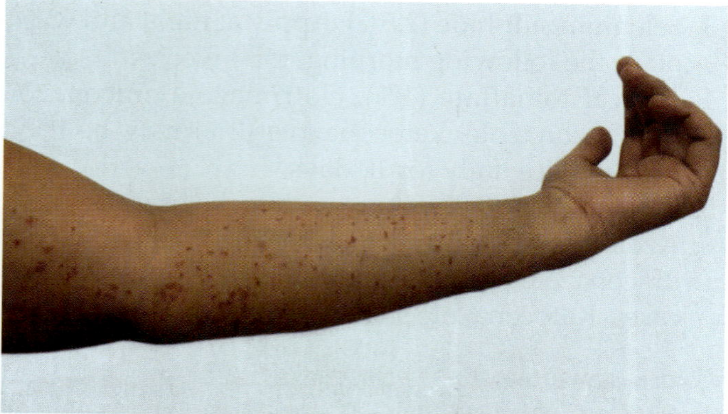

Fig. 3.99B: Purpuric rashes in HSP (IgA vasculitis) in upper extremity (though common in buttock and lower extremity)

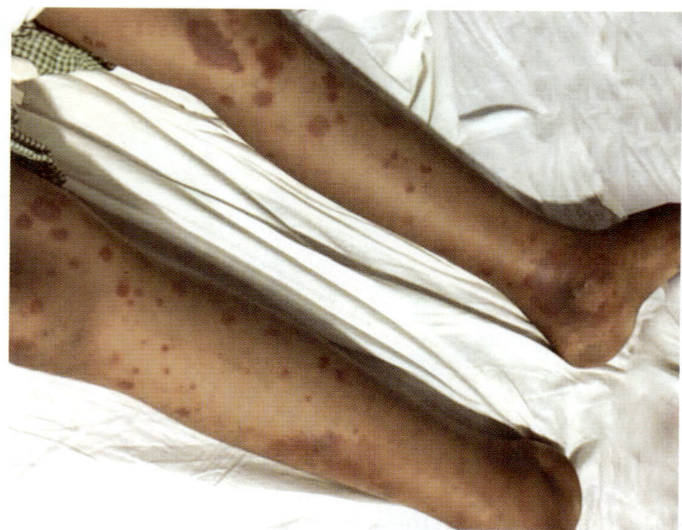

Fig. 3.100A: Haemorrhagic spots of different sizes (petechiae, purpura and ecchymosis) are seen in dengue haemorrhagic fever

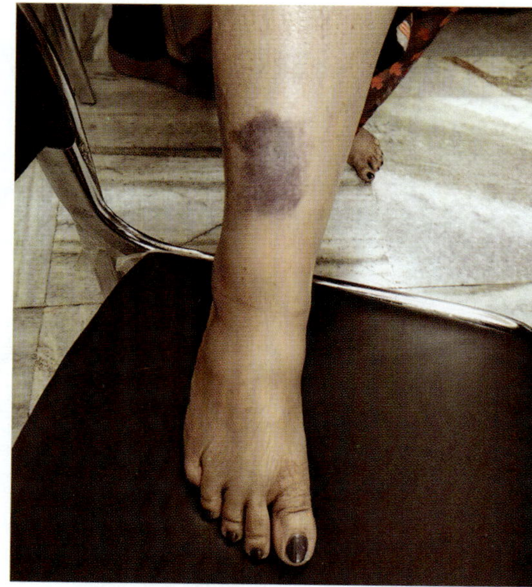

Fig. 3.100B: Ecchymosis with clopidogrel therapy taken for IHD

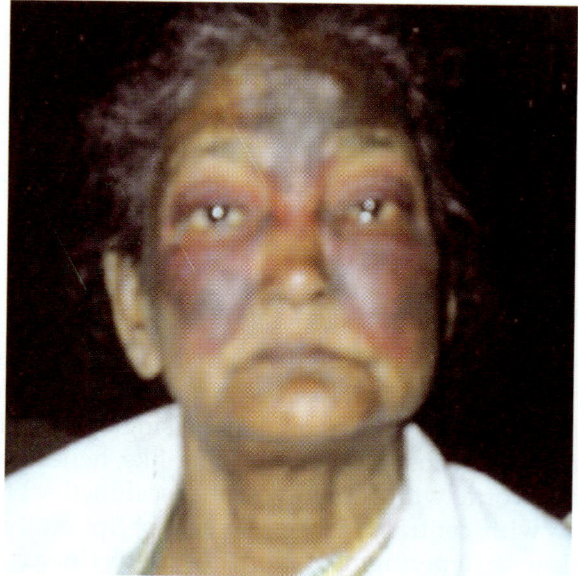

Fig. 3.101: Facial haematoma, mild periorbital haematoma **(raccoon eyes)** and blood collection in forehead in a case of head injury

Q. Differential diagnosis:

1. **Telangiectasia:** Small, dilated blood vessels visible on skin surface, especially on the lips.
2. Mosquito bite marks.
3. Spider naevi.
4. Very small panniculitis or erythema nodosum.
5. Cherry angioma or Campbell de Morgan's spot.
6. Drug rash (H/o offending drug intake, often blanches, may be itchy).

Q. How to differentiate haemorrhagic spots from others?

Telangiectasia, spiders, fresh mosquito bite marks blanch on application of pressure given by a pinhead or glass slide (diascopy), and the colour returns on releasing the pressure. **Haemorrhagic spots (or purpuric spots) never blanch on compression (identification point).**

Q. Significance of haemorrhagic spots:

Haemorrhagic spots may be due to (A) and/or (B) and/or (C) mentioned below:

a. Thrombocytopenia (quantitative defect): Either due to diminished production or increased destruction of platelet [e.g. idiopathic thrombocytopenic purpura or immune thrombocytopenic purpura (ITP), drug-induced, infections, aplastic anaemia, etc.].
b. Vessel wall abnormalities, vasculitis or increased capillary fragility: Seen in Henoch-Schönlein purpura (HSP), scurvy, uraemia, ageing, etc.
c. Platelet functional (qualitative) defect: Thrombasthenia or Glanzmann's disease (defect in platelet aggregation), after use of drugs like aspirin or phenylbutazone.

Q. Causes of non-thrombocytopenic purpura:

A. Vessel wall abnormalities, e.g.
   1. Infection: *Meningococcus*, viral infection, septicaemia.
   2. Henoch-Schönlein purpura (HSP) or allergic purpura.
   3. Hereditary haemorrhagic telangiectasis (HHT) or Rendu-Weber-Osler disease.
   4. Drugs: Penicillin, sulphonamides, corticosteroids.
   5. Senile purpura.
   6. Purpura simplex (devil's pinches).
   7. Cushing's syndrome.
   8. Scurvy.
   9. Paraproteinaemias.
   10. Vasculitis.
   11. Uraemia.
   12. Purpura fulminans (with life-threatening endovascular thrombosis and DIC).
   13. 'Easy bruising syndrome' (benign disorder).

B. Platelet functional defects (defects in platelet adhesion, aggregation or granule release).

- In (A): BT—Normal or increased; platelet count—Normal.
- In (B): BT—Increased; platelet count—Normal.

Q. Diagnosis of thrombocytopenia from history:

Clinical features: Apart from easy bruisability and haemorrhagic spots in the skin (petechiae, purpura or ecchymosis), the patient gives H/o spontaneous bleeding from nose (epistaxis) and gums (mucous membrane), haematuria, melaena or menorrhagia. Petechiae are the hallmark of platelet-related bleeding.

Management: Platelet transfusion is required to treat patients with severe thrombocytopenia associated with bleeding. In a moribund patient, other supportive measures like high dose IV immunoglobulin, a brief course of corticosteroid, or even plasmapheresis is recommended.

Q. Importance of splenomegaly with purpuric spots:

1. Acute leukaemias.
2. SLE.
3. Lymphomas.
4. Blast crisis of CML and CLL.
5. SBE.
6. ITP (splenomegaly in 10% cases only).
7. Myelofibrosis.
8. Hypersplenism due to any cause.

- Splenomegaly does not favour the diagnosis of ITP.

Q. Laboratory tests of ITP:

1. Low total platelet count (normal platelet count is 1.5 lac–4 lac/mm^3). Peripheral blood smear may show large platelets.
2. *Prolonged bleeding time (BT) with normal coagulation time (CT).*
3. Antiplatelet antibodies may be found in blood.
4. To evaluate the secondary causes of ITP: Serology for hepatitis C, HIV infection, and ANF for SLE.
5. Bone marrow examination reveals megakaryocytes in normal or increased numbers with normal morphology in a hypercellular marrow. Sometimes, there are increased vacuolisation and diminished number of granules in the megakaryocytes.

- Normal BT is 2.5–10 minutes (Ivy) and normal CT is 9–15 minutes (glass tubes).
- Bleeding time (BT) is a sensitive measure of platelet number as well as function.

Q. Characteristics of HSP (IgA vasculitis or anaphylactoid purpura) (Fig. 3.99B):

1. A self-limiting small-vessel vasculitis which often occurs after upper respiratory tract infection. It usually affects children and young adults.
2. The purpuric rashes are urticarial (palpable and itchy) and at times bilaterally symmetrical.

3. The rashes are usually present in buttocks, extensor surfaces of arms and lower legs; face and trunk spared—some purpuric rash coalesce and become necrotic.
4. HSP is often associated with heamaturia and proteinuria (focal segmental proliferative glomerulonephritis), arthralgia or arthritis, and colicky abdominal pain (may have intussusception).
5. The coagulation profile (BT and CT) remains normal. Serum IgA level is increased in 50%.

- EH Henoch (1820–1910) and his teacher JL Schönlein (1793–1864) described the disease in 1860. Purpura and arthritis were associated by Schönlein, while purpura and GI involvement by Henoch.
- Thrombocytopenia = flat purpura, and vasculitis = raised purpura.

Q. Probable causes of palpable purpura:

A. Vasculitis due to any cause: HSP, polyarteritis nodosa, leucocytoclastic vasculitis, etc.
B. Infective emboli: Meningococcaemia, disseminated gonococcal infection, measles, septicaemia.

- Palpable purpura are raised from surface, present in buttocks and extensor surfaces bilaterally, and are often pruritic.

Q. Demonstration of Hess' capillary fragility test:

It is a test for diagnosis of increased capillary fragility (e.g. dengue haemorrhgic fever) or immune thrombocytopenic purpura (ITP). The procedure goes like this:

1. Blood pressure cuff is wrapped in upper arm and pressure is raised. The pressure is maintained halfway between systolic and diastolic BP for 5 minutes.
2. 1″ below the elbow joint, a circle of 1″ diameter is drawn on the anterior aspect of upper forearm. The haemorrhagic spots already present within the circle are noted.
3. Normally after application of pressure by BP cuff, up to 10 new haemorrhagic spots may appear. But in pathological states (mentioned above), more than 20 new spots (diagnostic) may appear within the circle after deflation of BP cuff.

This test may be negative in mild to moderate thrombocytopenia but is positive in severe thrombocytopenia (ITP). This test is also known as **Tourniquet test** (or Rumpel-Leede capillary fragility test).

Q. Cause of sudden death in thrombocytopenia:

Sudden massive haemorrhage in any vital organ like intracerebral haemorrhage may be fatal in a patient of thrombocytopenia.

Q. Thrombocytosis and thrombocythemia:

a. **Thrombocytosis:** Platelet 4 lac/mm^3 which is a temporary elevation, e.g. post-splenectomy, severe bleeding, etc. Thrombocytosis is regarded as part of acute phase reaction.
b. **Thrombocythemia:** Platelet 8 lac/mm^3 which is a sustained elevation. It is regarded as a myeloproliferative disorder.

- Platelet count <1 lac/mm^3 is known as thrombocytopenia.
- 1 unit of platelet transfusion raises the count by 10000/mm^3.

Q. Purpura in young and elderly:

a. Young: ITP, HSP, SLE, drug-induced, acute leukaemias, infections (e.g. *Meningococcus*).
b. Elderly: Senile purpura, leukaemia, drug-induced, scurvy, paraproteinaemias.

Q. Drugs causing thrombocytopenia:

1. Sulphonamides.
2. Penicillin.
3. Cyclophosphamide.
4. Thiazides.
5. Quinine.
6. Carbamazepine.
7. Aspirin.
8. Heparin.

Q. Common medical causes of purpura:

1. Thrombocytopenia (e.g. ITP).
2. Acute leukaemias.
3. Aplastic anaemia (no splenomegaly).
4. Drugs (no splenomegaly).
5. SLE.
6. Lymphoma.
7. Hepato-cellular failure.
8. SBE.

Q. Causes of gum bleeding (Fig. 3.102):

1. Gingivitis.
2. Thrombocytopenia (e.g. ITP).
3. Acute leukaemias.
4. Aplastic anaemia.
5. Scurvy (spongy and friable gum).
6. Haemophilia.
7. Anticoagulant therapy.
8. Vincent's infection.
9. Viperidae snake bite (Fig. 3.103).

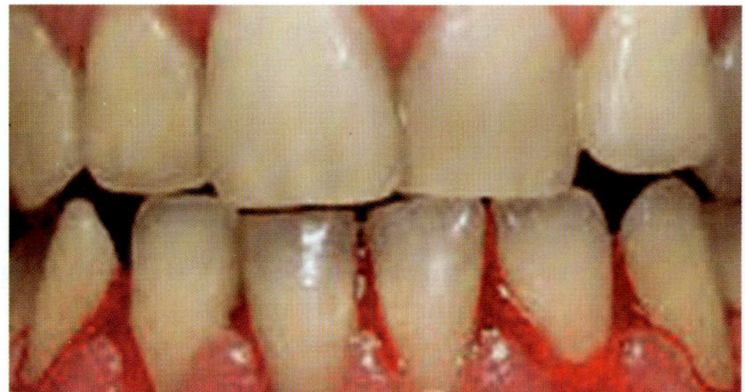

Fig. 3.102: **Gum bleeding** in aplastic anaemia

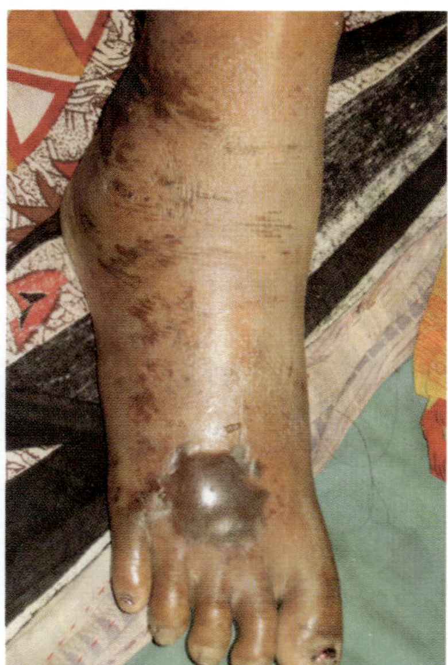

Fig. 3.103: Viperidae **snake bite** with cellulitis, oedema and haemorrhagic blister formation in and around the site of bite

Q. Causes of gum hypertrophy (Fig. 3.104):

1. Poor oral hygiene.
2. Phenytoin therapy in epileptics.
3. Pregnancy.
4. Scurvy.
5. Acute monocytic leukaemia.
6. Idiopathic familial fibromatosis.
7. Nifedipine or amlodipine therapy.
8. Histiocytosis X disease.
9. Wegener's granulomatosis.

- Spongy and bluish gums are commonly seen in cyanotic congenital heart diseases.

Q. Medical causes of epistaxis:

1. Systemic hypertension.
2. Bleeding disorders (ITP, haemophilia)/anticoagulant therapy/DIC; acute leukaemias.
3. Vasculitis.
4. High altitude.
5. Rendu-Weber-Osler disease (hereditary haemorrhagic telangiectasis).
6. Uraemia, aplastic anaemia.
7. Kala-azar, malaria, enteric fever, measles, infectious mononucleosis, rheumatic fever, diphtheria.

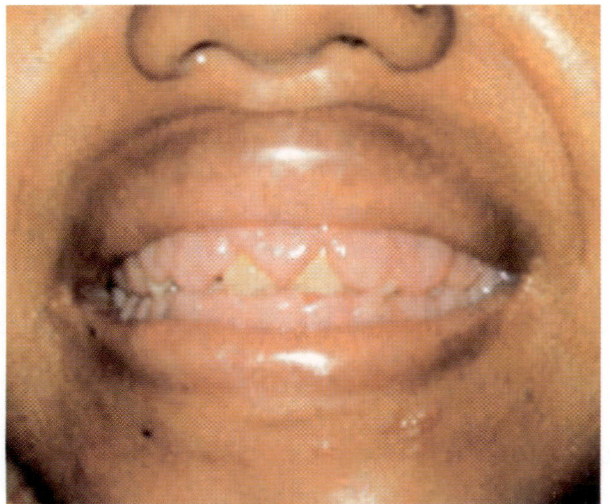

Fig. 3.104: **Gum hypertrophy** in acute myeloid leukaemia

Q. Safe analgesics in purpura:

Codeine and paracetamol have no effect on platelet number and function.

Q. Purpuric eruption with pyrexia:

1. Dengue.
2. Infective endocarditis.
3. Meningococcaemia.
4. Purpura fulminans.
5. Viral haemorrhagic fever.
6. Gram-negative septicaemia.
7. Rocky Mountain spotted fever.
8. Disseminated gonococcal infection.
9. Cutaneous small-vessel vasculitis.
10. Rat-bite fever.

Q. Critical platelet count:

It is 20000/mm^3. Below this level, spontaneous haemorrhage in any vital organ (e.g. intracerebral haemorrhage) or anywhere in the body may endanger the life of the patient. These patients require immediate temporary support with platelet or fresh blood transfusion. Recently, haematologists opined that the level may be near about 10000/mm^3 to have risk of internal bleeding.

Q. Sites and organs to be examined in a case of purpura:

Read the 'Scheme of examination' from 'Lymphoreticular system'.

Q. What do you mean by 'bleeding disorders'?

Bleeding disorders are usually due to one of the following abnormalities:

a. Coagulation disorders.
b. Platelet disorders (number and/or function defect) or von Willebrand factor defects, and
c. Vessel wall abnormalties.

A detailed history, meticulous physical examination and few initial screening tests are required to evaluate bleeding disorders. They are summarised below:

A. **Coagulation disorders** (e.g. haemophilia, Christmas disease): Only in males (e.g. haemophilia), family history +ve (due to X-linked inheritance, there is oblique transmission, i.e. uncles and nephews may be the sufferer), life-long history, spontaneous bleeding into viscera, retroperitoneum, muscles (calf, psoas, tongue) and joints (e.g. knee haemarthrosis) are characteristic (*see* Fig. 1.62); purpura is rare, bleeding from nose, mouth, GI tract, urinary tract, wounds or in the subcutaneous tissue may occur. Bleeding starts several hours after trauma or surgery (H/o induced and prolonged bleeding), and is notorious for persistence (not profuseness); local pressure is ineffective; absence of splenomegaly, normal BT with prolonged CT, while platelet count remains normal. Acquired coagulation disorder may result from vitamin K deficiency or oral anticoagulant therapy.

B. **Platelet disorders:** H/o drug intake (especially aspirin), or past H/o ITP. Bleeding occurs characteristically from mucous membrane (gum), nose (epistaxis), skin (petechiae, purpura, bruises), buccal mucosa, and per vaginum; bleeding may occur from GI tract, CNS or superficial wounds; bleeding happens to occur immediately after trauma or surgery (e.g. tooth extraction), and local pressure is effective to stop bleeding; may have splenomegaly, increased BT with normal CT, while low platelets in thromocytopenia and normal plalelets count in thrombasthenia. Qualitative disorders of platelet are adhesion defect (von Willebrand's disease, Bernard-Soulier syndrome) and aggregation defect (Glanzmann's thrombasthenia, uraemia, aspirin therapy).

C. **Vessel wall abnormalities:** Consider age of the patient (common in old age), petechiae/purpura, recurrent bleeding at a single site, bleeding occurs immediately after trauma or surgery, and local pressure is effective. There is absence of splenomegaly, normal or elevated BT with normal CT, and normal platelet count. See page 359 for causes of vessel wall abnormalities.

- (B) and (C) are commonly characterised by easy bruising and spontaneous bleeding.
- Investigations done are full blood count and blood film, coagulation screen (PT, PTT, thrombin time, platelet count, bleeding time), coagulation factor assays, fibrinogen and FDPs estimation, vWF antigen and activity, platelet function and fibrinolysis assays.

Clinical Wisdom

In the presence of purpuric spots, one should examine the patient for 'blanching reaction' which is always absent here. Always perform the Hess' capillary fragility test in a suspected patient of ITP.

LEPROSY — CASE 60

Q. Definition:

This is a chronic granulomatous disease caused by *Mycobacterium leprae* (a gram-positive, acid- and alcohol-fast bacillus) which principally attacks the skin, peripheral nerves and nasal mucosa. It is also known as **Hansen's disease** (Fig. 3.105).

Mycobacteria are so called because they resist discolourisation with acid-alcohol due to their complex cell wall.

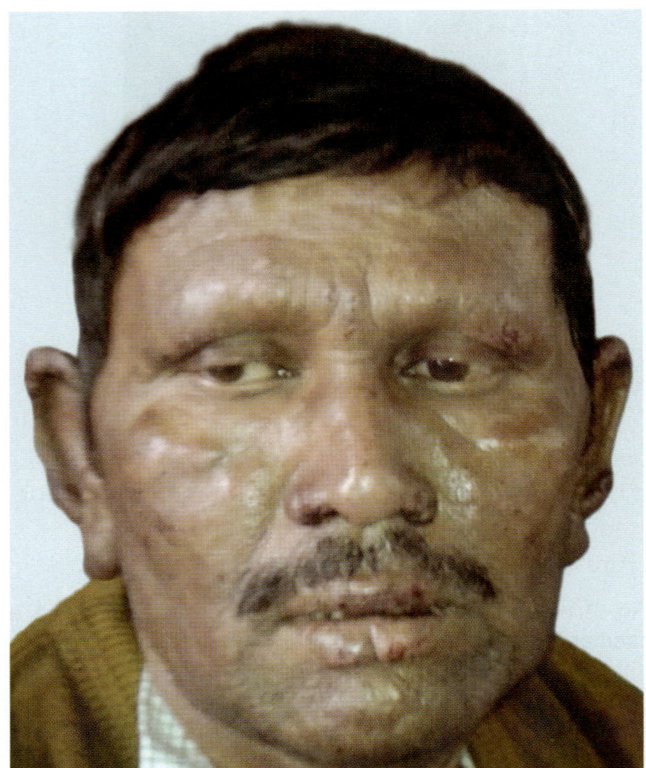

Fig. 3.105: Leonine face (lion-like) of Hansen's disease

Q. What are the different forms?

1. Two polar forms are:
   - i. Lepromatous (LL), and
   - ii. Tuberculoid (TT).
2. Borderline or dimorphous leprosy:
   - i. Borderline tuberculoid (BT).
   - ii. Borderline (BB).
   - iii. Borderline lepromatous (BL).
3. Indeterminate leprosy (I)
   - i. Non-classifiable early lesion.
   - ii. Transforms into any polar form, or
   - iii. May spontaneously remit.

- Principally, there are two main forms: Polar forms and borderline leprosy.

Q. What do you mean by LL and TT forms?

A. Lepromatous leprosy (LL) means:

- i. Highly bacillated (multibacillary or MB),
- ii. Low resistance (impaired cell-mediated immunity), and
- iii. Systemic infectious form.

B. Tuberculoid leprosy (TT) means:

- i. Non-infectious (paucibacillary or PB),
- ii. High resistance (i.e. high cell-mediated immunity), and
- iii. Localised disease.

Q. Muitibacillary or paucibacillary?

a. Multibacillary: BB, BL and LL.
b. Paucibacillary: I, BT and TT.

- Multibacillary (MB): Has 6 or more skin lesions which may have bacilli.
  Paucibacillary (PB): Has 5 or less skin lesions with no bacilli.
- WHO classification: MB or PB.
  Different forms: 1 and 2 (of previous question), i.e. LL, TT, BT, BB, BL.
  [Indeterminate leprosy: not in any classification].

Q. Describe the skin lesion of TT variety:

1. Solitary lesion or a couple of lesions.
2. Macular or raised as plaques, or as rings with flat centre (central healing).
3. Sharply defined or circumscribed.
4. *Hypopigmented*, dry, scaly lesion.
5. *Hypoaesthetic*, hypohydrotic (diminished sweating) and hypotrichotic (loss of hair).
6. Present anywhere in the body, especially in arms, buttocks, legs and face.

PLUS

The nerve twig or the peripheral nerve supplying the skin lesion may be thickened, e.g.

a. Great auricular nerve across the sternomastoid muscle (in the posterior triangle) at neck.
b. Ulnar nerve at elbow (behind medical epicondyle in olecranon groove) (Fig. 3.106A).
c. Median nerve at wrist (against carpal bones).
d. Radial cutaneous nerve at wrist.
e. Common peroneal nerve at the neck of fibula (Fig. 3.106B).
f. Posterior tibial nerve around medial malleolus.
g. Sural nerve at the lateral part of ankle.

Clinical Wisdom

It is compulsory to *test the touch sensation* in the skin lesion in all suspected patient of TT variety. Always palpate the nerves proximal to the skin lesion. One should look for the great auricular nerve in the neck (by turning the head to the opposite side, the nerve stands out), the ulnar nerve in the funny bone or the common peroneal nerve at the neck of fibula. *Test the nerves for thickening, nodularity and tenderness, and its motor as well as sensory functions.*

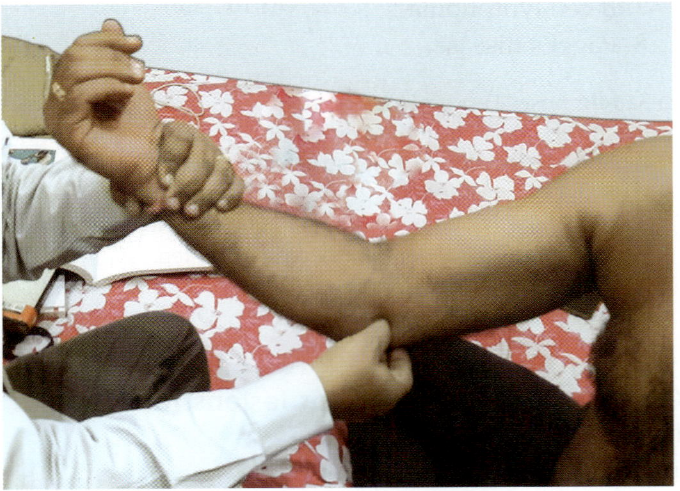

Fig. 3.106A: Palpation of **ulnar nerve**

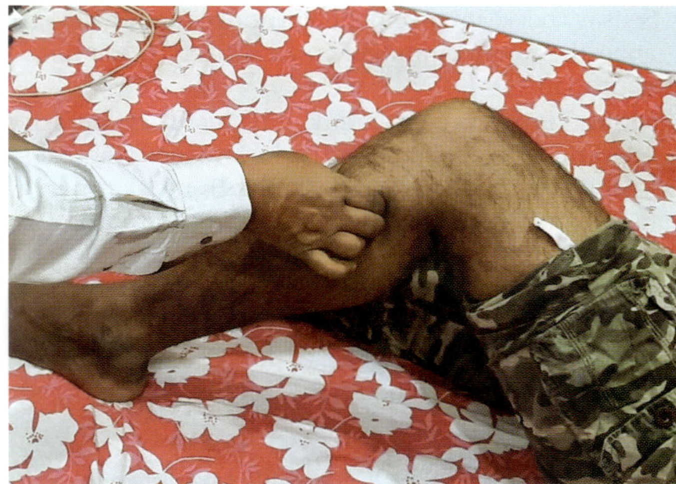

Fig. 3.106B: Palpation of **common peroneal nerve**

- In leprosy, pain and temperature sensations are lost earlier than touch sensation.

Q. Describe the skin lesion of LL variety:

1. Hypopigmented macules, plaques or *nodules* (may be bilaterally symmetrical) widely scattered in the body. *Gradually the skin becomes infiltrated and thickened.*
2. Ill-defined (with margins that merge imperceptibly with normal skin).
3. The surface of the lesion is smooth, shiny but without any central healing (inverted-saucer).
4. If the lesion advances, 'leonine facies' (Fig. 3.105) may be seen.
5. Both the loss of cutaneous sensation and nerve involvement are late features.

PLUS

a. Lymphadenopathy (painless).
b. Hepatosplenomegaly.
c. Peripheral neuropathy with trophic changes (watch the sole of the feet for trophic ulcer).
d. Testicular atrophy (with impotence) and gynaecomastia; pedal oedema.
e. Ocular lesions: Keratitis, iridocyclitis, etc.
f. Miscellaneous: Anaemia, nephrotic syndrome, nasal collapse.

Clinical Wisdom

In a suspected patient of LL variety, one should examine the eyes (e.g. corneal anaesthesia or ulcer), palpate the liver, spleen and testes, test for peripheral neuropathy, search for lymphadenopathy and neurotrophic atrophy of digits, and gynaecomastia. Look at the face carefully and never forget to test the touch sensation in the skin lesion. Palpate the nerves proximal to the skin lesion (though a late and non-prominent feature).

Q. Different types of nerve involvement in leprosy:

a. Nerve thickening: Classical description given in TT variety (*see* above).

b. Sensory nerve involvement with gloves and stockings anaesthesia is commoner in LL variety (peripheral neuropathy).

c. Motor nerve involvement may result in muscle weakness, wasting, paralysis and contractures lately. The ulnar nerve (claw hand), median nerve (ape hand), common peroneal nerve (foot drop) or posterior tibial nerve (claw toes) may be affected, which are common in TT variety.

d. Cranial nerve involvement: Facial (often bilateral) (Fig. 3.107) or trigeminal nerve (loss of corneal reflex); sometimes, multiple cranial nerves are involved (polyneuritis cranialis multiplex).

- Always consider leprosy as a possible cause of peripheral neuropathy in India. Central nervous system is not affected in leprosy. Ulnar nerve abscess with adjacent cellulitis in skin is common in BT variety.

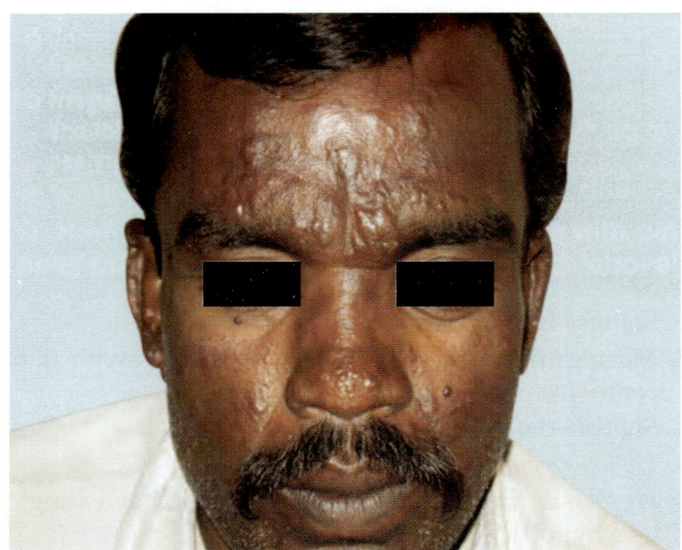

Fig. 3.108: A **leprosy** patient showing thickened skin of face and forehead, especially the infiltrated earlobes

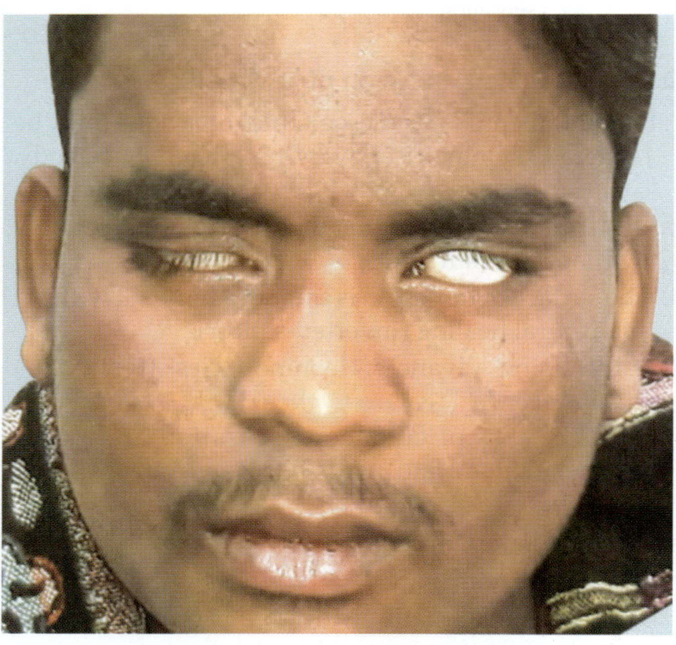

Fig. 3.107: **Bilateral facial palsy** in leprosy who is being treated by clofazimine (reflected by pinkish-brown discolouration of skin)

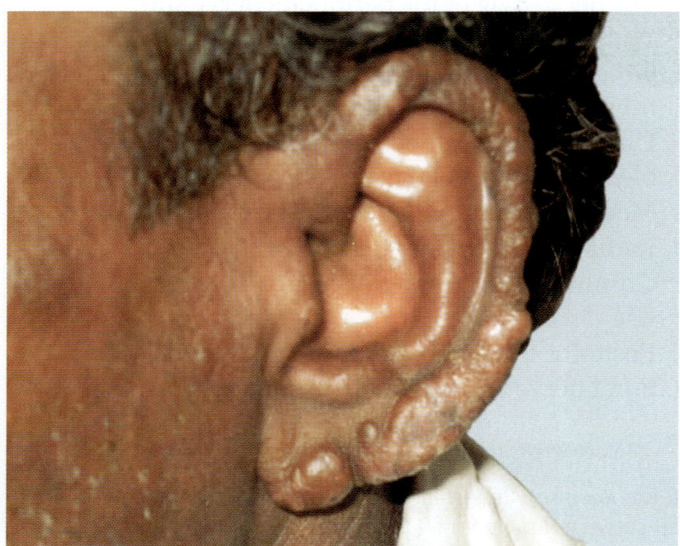

Fig. 3.109: Infiltrated ear in **lepromatous leprosy**

Q. Describe the leonine face:

A. Description (Figs 3.105 and 3.108):

1. Lines on the forehead become deeper as well as the upper central incisor teeth loosen or fall out.
2. Loss of hair in the lateral part of eyebrows (madarosis) and thick eyebrows.
3. Depressed bridge of the nose, broad nose with nasal collapse (saddle nose).
4. Thickened skin of face and forehead, especially the infiltrated earlobes (Fig. 3.109).
5. There may be perforated nasal septum; hoarse voice.

B. Causes (actually, No. 2–8 mimic leonine face):

1. Leprosy (lepromatous): Classical leonine facies.
2. Albright's disease (fibrous dysplasia of bone).
3. Carcinoid syndrome.
4. Cleidocranial dysostosis.
5. Primary hypertrophic osteoarthropathy.
6. Amyloidosis.
7. B-cell lymphoma.
8. Paget's disease.

- **Saddle nose:** Lepromatous leprosy, ectodermal dysplasia, fractured nasal bone, achondroplasia and congenital syphilis; **destruction of nasal structures:** lepromatous leprosy (Fig. 3.110), Wegener's granulomatosis (*see* Fig. 3.73), relapsing polychondritis, midline granuloma and lupus vulgaris.
- **Perforation of nasal septum:** Lepromatous leprosy, syphilis (posterior perforation), Wegener's granulomatosis, intranasal trauma, tuberculosis (anterior perforation) and workers involved in chromium plating.

Q. D/D of multiple nodular lesions (or irregular thickening) in face:

1. Leprosy (lepromatous).
2. Post kala-azar dermal leishmaniasis (PKDL).

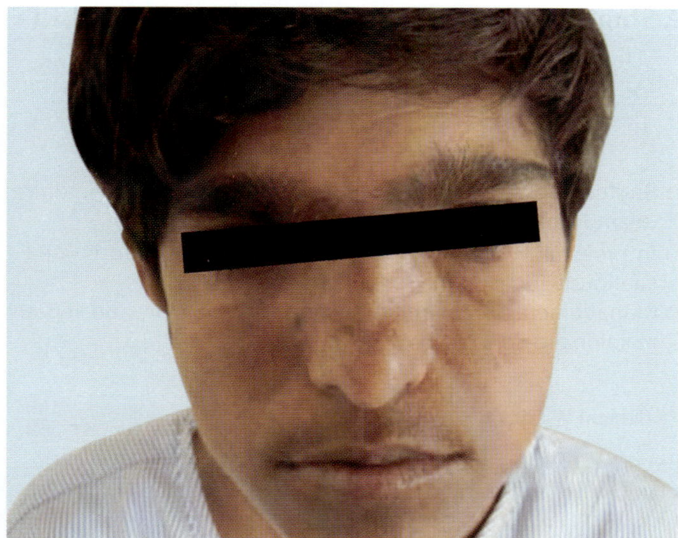

Fig. 3.110: Destruction of nasal structures in a suspected case of lepromatous leprosy

3. Sarcoidosis.
4. Acne rosacea.
5. Non-Hodgkin's lymphoma.
6. Amyloidosis (*see* **Fig. 2.27**).
7. Rhinophyma.
8. Secondary syphilis.

Q. Do you know any other variety of leprosy?

1. Histoid leprosy: Succulent cutaneous nodules and a variant of LL variety.
2. Neuritic leprosy: Thickened peripheral nerves without any skin lesion, probably of TT type; common in India.

Q. Describe the hand of a leprosy patient:

Read the section on 'Examination of the hands'.

Q. Causes of thickened peripheral nerves:

1. Leprosy.
2. Multiple neurofibromatosis.
3. Acromegaly.
4. Amyloidosis (primary).
5. Charcot-Marie-Tooth disease (juvenile).
6. Sarcoidosis.
7. Chronic Guillain-Barré syndrome (CIDP).
8. Dejerine-Sottas type neuropathy.
9. Refsum's disease.
10. Repeated injury to the nerve.
11. Idiopathic hypertrophic neuropathy.

Q. Complications of leprosy:

1. Crippling of hands.
2. Blindness (due to corneal anaesthesia).
3. Tuberculosis (one of the major cause of death).
4. Amyloidosis (secondary).
5. Lepra reactions.
6. Social outcast.

Q. Lepromin skin test in all the varieties of leprosy:

It depends on the cellular immunity or resistance of the patient though it has no value in diagnosing leprosy (as it may be positive in normal people). In Lepromin test, suspension of dead bacilli (*M. leprae*) is injected intradermally, and the findings read after 4 weeks. *It helps in classifying the disease.*

- TT: Strongly positive.
- LL: Negative.
- BT: Positive.
- BB: Negative or weakly positive.
- BL: Negative.

Q. Reactions (lepra reactions) in leprosy:

A. **Type I** (reversal reaction): Existing skin lesions may develop erythema and swelling, peripheral nerves become tender and painful, with sudden loss of nerve function (e.g. foot drop). Common in BL, BT and BB variety. It is a type IV delayed hypersensitivity reaction and is being treated by aspirin, corticosteroid and chloroquine, with continued antimycobacterial treatment.

B. **Type II** or erythema nodosum leprosum (ENL): Common in LL or BL variety. It occurs in patients in their second year of treatment. Acute crops of painful, tender nodules develop with pain in the nerves, fever, arthritis, glomerulonephritis, lymphadenopathy, iridocyclitis, bone pain and epididymo-orchitis. ENL is treated by analgesics, antipyretics, chloroquine, thalidomide or prednisolone, and increasing the dose of clofazimine, with continued antimycobacterial treatment. ENL develops due to immune complex-mediated vasculitis. Eye care is done by hydrocortisone or atropine drop.

C. Lucio phenomenon: Rare, occurs in diffuse non-nodular LL variety (develops angular ulcer).

Q. Incubation period of leprosy and portal of entry of *M. leprae*:

Incubation period: Generally 2–6 years, may be more; 2–5 years for TT and 8–12 years for LL variety (as *M. leprae* has doubling time of 12 days, i.e. very slow multiplication time).

Portal of entry: Through nasal mucosa or by inoculation through skin (needs prolonged close contact). Droplets from the sneezes of a lepromatous patient is highly infectious. Untreated patients (man is the only reservoir) with smear-positive extensive disease are potential source of infection.

Q. What are the differential diagnosis of leprosy?

A. Skin lesions:

1. Hypopigmented lesions like vitiligo, psoriasis, pityriasis versicolor.
2. SLE.
3. Lupus vulgaris (tuberculosis of skin).

4. Yaws.
5. Dermal leishmaniasis.
6. Sarcoidosis.

B. Claw hand: Read the section on 'Claw hand'.
C. Peripheral neuropathy: Read the section on 'Peripheral neuropathy'.
D. Peripheral nerve thickening: Read the causes of 'Thickened peripheral nerves' discussed above.

Q. Cardinal features of leprosy:

- Hypopigmented, anaesthetic patches in skin.
- Thickened peripheral nerves.
- AFB seen on slit-skin smear or biopsy.

Q. How to establish your diagnosis?

The diagnosis is essentially clinical. The investigations performed are:

A. By slit-skin smear method: Principally the multibacillary disease (BB, BL and LL) is diagnosed by this method and it is less informative in paucibacillary (I, BT and TT) variety. The pinched skin between thumb and forefinger is incised by a scalpel and the exposed area is scrapped. The juice is then stained by Ziehl-Neelsen's method (to find out acid-fast bacilli) and put under the microscope. Now the bacterial index (BI) i.e. the number of bacilli living or dead are calculated and scored on a logarithmic scale. Typical histology after skin biopsy also helps in diagnosis.
Other sites of incision: Skin lesions (nodules), earlobes, dorsum of the middle or ring finger, nasal mucous membrane.
B. Biopsy of lymph nodes, nerves, liver may demonstrate the bacilli (rarely required).
C. Serology or PCR testing for *M. leprae* DNA—neither sensitive nor specific for diagnosis.
Associated features: Mild anaemia, high ESR and hyperglobulinaemia (may give false-positive serological tests like VDRL, rheumatoid factor and ANF in LL variety).

Q. How are you going to treat a leprosy patient?

Recommended treatment regimens in leprosy for adults (modified WHO guidelines):

A. Paucibacillary disease (I, BT and TT)

i. Rifampicin—600 mg, once monthly (single supervised dose).
ii. Dapsone—100 mg daily (self-administered dose).
Duration—6 months.

B. Multibacillary disease (BB, BL and LL)

i. Rifampicin—600 mg, once monthly (single supervised dose).
ii. Clofazimine—300 mg once monthly (single supervised dose).

PLUS

iii. Daily dose of clofazimine (50 mg) and dapsone (100 mg)—both self-administered dose.
Duration—12 months.

C. Single lesion paucibacillary disease (I, BT and TT)

i. Rifampicin 600 mg
ii. Ofloxacin 400 mg
iii. Minocycline 100 mg
} as a single dose

- Bacteriostatic: Dapsone and clofazimine; Bactericidal: Rifampicin.
- In pregnancy: Clofazimine is not used, rifampicain is used cautiously in first trimester but dapsone is safe.
- Management of anaemia, secondary infection and lepra reaction are done accordingly.

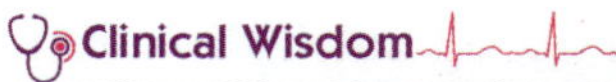

Because of long generation time of the bacillus, low dose rifampicin is sufficient (once monthly use).

Q. Side effects of clofazimine and dapsone:

A. Clofazimine (Fig. 3.107):
1. Skin pigmentation (red colouration of skin, urine and body secretions).
2. Abdominal pain.
3. Pruritus and ichthyosis.
4. Anorexia, nausea and vomiting.
5. Diarrhoea.

B. Dapsone (diaminodiphenyl sulphone/DDS):
1. Exfoliative dermatitis.
2. Haemolytic anaemia.
3. Agranulocytosis.
4. Methaemoglobinaemia.
5. Avoided in G_6PD deficiency.
6. Psychosis.
7. Hepatitis.
8. Hypoproteinaemia.

Q. Use of rifampicin in internal medicine:

1. Tuberculosis and in non-tuberculous mycobacteria.
2. Leprosy.
3. Chemoprophylaxis of persons at risk of developing meningococcal meningitis.
4. Legionnaires' disease.
5. Brucellosis (with co-trimoxazole or tetracycline-streptomycin combination).
6. Eradication of chronic carrier state in enteric fever (with co-trimoxazole).
7. Endocarditis due to *Staphylococcus epidermidis* or *Corynebacterium spp.* (often with vancomycin).
8. Anthrax.
9. Anaplasmosis.
10. Primary amoebic meningoencephalitis (caused by *Naegleria fowleri*).
11. Pruritus (may be used in pruritus associated with cholestasis).
12. Bartonellosis (chronic).
13. Cat-scratch disease.
14. Prevention of *Haemophilus influenzae*.

15. In Q fever (*Coxiella burnetii* infection) with doxycycline or ciprofloxacin.
16. In selective cases of chronic reactive arthritis.

- The rifamycins include rifampicin (most commonly used), rifabutin and rifapentine.

Q. Other drugs (other than dapsone) used in leprosy:

1. Acedapsone (DADDS).
2. Ethionamide.
3. Thiacetazone.
4. Prothionamide.
5. Thiambutosine.
6. Minocycline.
7. Ofloxacin, moxifloxacin.
8. Clarithromycin.
9. Streptomycin/kanamycin.
10. Corticosteroid (in lepra reactions).

- Vaccination by BCG with heat-killed *M. leprae* is being tried for prevention of leprosy.

Q. Other modalities of treatment in leprosy:

1. Education of the patient. Paralysis from reactional neuritis: Splinting of the limb.
2. Tarsorrhaphy for corneal anaesthesia.
3. Trophic ulcer in feet: Rest, self-care, use of crutches, walking plaster.
4. Infection: Appropriate antibiotic.
5. Special protective footwear for anaesthetic feet.
6. Plastic surgery in face or reconstructive surgery in limbs.
7. Haematinics and multivitamins.
8. Physiotherapy to prevent contracture and muscle atrophy.
9. Rehabilitation.

- Hypopigmentation in leprosy is due to: 1. Direct invasion at melanocyte level, 2. Defective transfer of melanin into keratinocytes, and 3. Vascular changes leading to atrophy of melanocytes.

NEUROFIBROMATOSIS — CASE 61

Q. What is neurofibroma (Fig. 3.111A)?

These are benign, soft, rubbery, non-tender papules or nodules varying in size from a pea to a cricket ball which develops from the Schwann cells and fibroblasts of the neurilemmal sheath of the peripheral nerve (a form of hamartoma). Majority are symptomless but occasionally there is paraesthesia. **The mass may be moved from side to side only** but is otherwise fixed by the nerve from which it arises.

Q. What is neurofibromatosis?

It is also known as "von Recklinghausen's disease" and has an autosomal dominant inheritance (Fig. 3.111B).

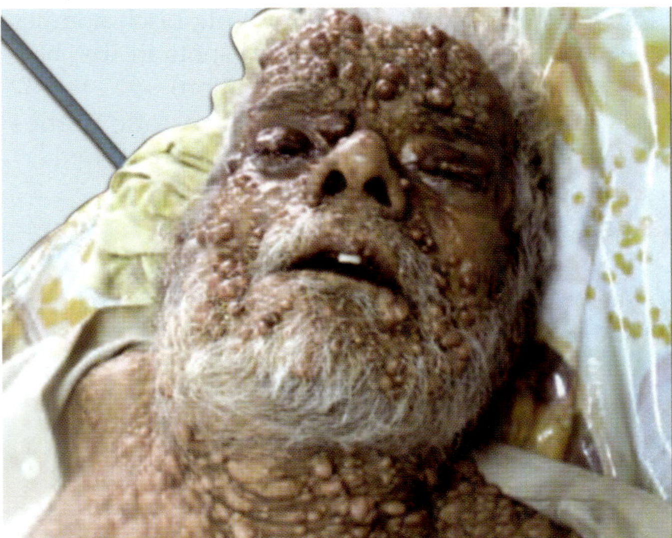

Fig. 3.111A: Multiple **neurofibroma**

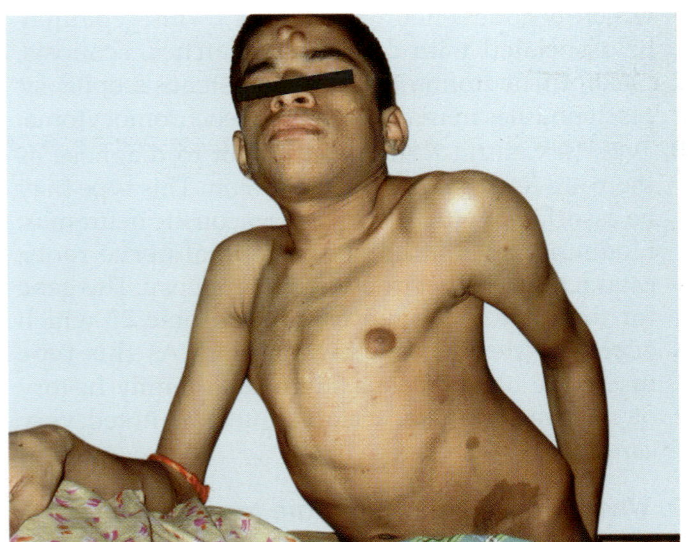

Fig. 3.111B: von Recklinghausen's disease—neurofibroma at forehead, cafe-au-lait spots in abdomen, pectus carinatum and kyphoscoliosis are present

Here, multiple neurofibroma are associated with cafe-au-lait spots and axillary freckling. Cafe-au-lait (colour of white coffee or coffee in milk) spots are round to ovoid, pale yellow-brown macules that vary in diameter from 1–2 mm to more than 15 cm and is usually present on the trunk, and also in buttocks and lower extremites. Solitary spots are 'common birthmarks'. Smooth bordered (coast of California) cafe-au-lait spots are common in neurofibromatosis whereas jagged borders (coast of Maine) is commonly seen in McCune-Albright syndrome.

- Friedrich Daniel von Recklinghausen (1833–1910) was Professor of Pathology, Strasbourg, France.

Q. Conditions associated with cafe-au-lait spots:

1. Neurofibromatosis which is characterised by:
   - i. Six or more spots.
   - ii. Uniformly hypomelanotic, circumscribed.

iii. Diameter >1.5 cm with multiple Lisch nodules in iris (1 mm yellow-brown spots in iris, best revealed by slit-lamp examination).

2. McCune-Albright syndrome (polyostotic fibrous dysplasia): Larger and more irregular than No. 1.
3. Occasionally in normal population.
4. Multiple endocrine neoplasia-type III.
5. Tuberous sclerosis.
6. Watson's syndrome (neurofibroma with pulmonary stenosis).
7. Ataxia-telangiectasia.
8. Bloom syndrome.

Q. What are the types of neurofibromatosis?

A. Type I (von Recklinghausen's disease): Peripheral form (found in >70% cases) and thus, readily recognized by the cutaneous lesions. It is due to an abnormal gene carried on chromosome 17 which encodes 'neurofibromin-1'. This type may be associated with cafe-au-lait patches, scoliosis, plexiform neurofibroma, aqueduct stenosis, epilepsy, Lisch nodules in iris and rarely pheochromocytoma.

B. Type II: Central form and difficult to diagnose as there are few or no cutaneous lesion. This type may be associated with optic glioma, acoustic neuromas, meningiomas, entrapment of spinal nerve roots, cataract, mental retardation and epilepsy. The gene for this type is located on chromosome 22 which encodes 'Merlin' or Schwannomin. As this type may have no cutaneous stigmata, a family history of cerebral or spinal lesion should be noted very carefully.

Q. Where the neurofibromas are mostly found?

Mainly they are present by the sides of the neck and in the extremities (cafe-au-lait spots are primarily present on the trunk). The tumours are felt as movable, bead-like nodules. Rarely, they are painful and tender on pressure.

Q. When to investigate neurofibromatosis?

In the presence of:

1. Symptoms of cerebral or spinal involvement (acoustic neuroma may present as cerebello-pontine angle tumour, and spinal involvement may present as paraplegia), and
2. Malignant change (sarcomatous change may occur in few cases).

Q. What is plexiform neurofibroma (Fig. 3.111C)?

This is diffuse neurofibromatosis with an overgrowth of the skin and subcutaneous tissue. In this way large hanging folds of skin may be formed. The commonest sites are temple (in connection with branches of trigeminal nerve), the upper eyelid and the back of the neck. The severe form of this variety is known as 'elephantiasis neuromatosa' (usually involves the lower limb).

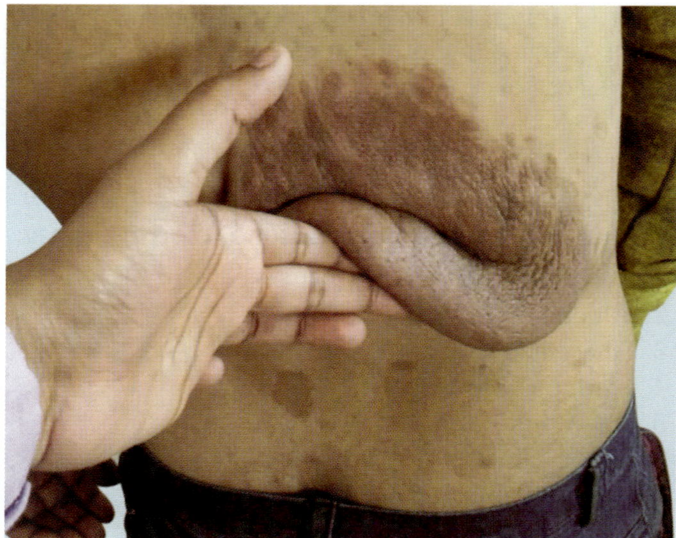

Fig. 3.111C: Plexiform nerofibroma

Q. What is pachydermatocele?

It is a very rare variety of neurofibromatosis in which coils of soft tissues hang around the neck.

Q. What is phakomatosis?

These are a unique group of diseases in which neurological abnormalities are combined with congenital defects in skin, retina and other organs. The causes of phakomatosis are neurofibromatosis (types I and II), tuberous sclerosis (Fig. 3.112), von Hippel-Lindau syndrome, Klippel-Trénaunay syndrome and Sturge-Weber syndrome (Fig. 3.113). These are also known as 'congenital neurocutaneous syndrome' (i.e. involvement of skin and nervous system).

'Phakoma' (collection of abnormal neuroglial tissue) is seen in the retina by ophthalmoscopy (greyish circular mass about the size of half the optic disc).

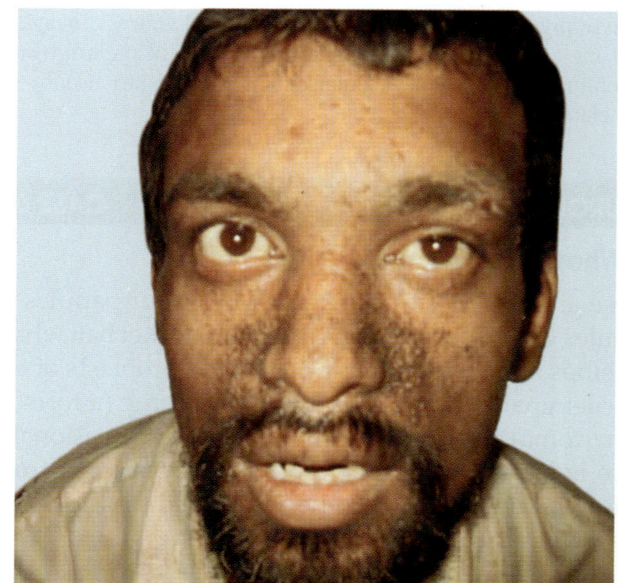

Fig. 3.112: Adenoma sebaceum, low intelligence and H/o epilepsy (injury in left eyebrow due to fall from convulsions) – classical triad in **tuberous sclerosis**

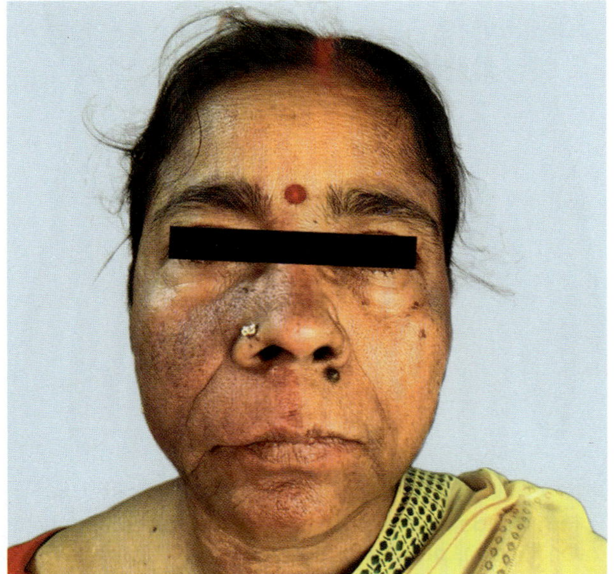

Fig. 3.113: **Sturge-Weber syndrome** with port-wine stain in right face. She had H/o convulsions

Clinical Wisdom

If you see a patient with neurofibroma, always search for: 1. Scoliosis, 2. Cafe-au-lait spots, and 3. Axillary freckles.

- Biopsy is usually contraindicated in neurofibroma as it may change into neurofibrosarcoma. Surgery may be considered for cosmetic reason, pain or pressure symptoms.
- CO_2 laser treatment have been used to remove neurofibromas (equal to or better than excision).

SCLERODERMA — CASE 62

Q. Describe the face of the patient (Fig. 3.114):

The term scleroderma (henceforth called systemic sclerosis—SSc) refers to thickening or hardening of skin due to abnormal collagen deposition in dermis. The typical 'facies' goes like this:

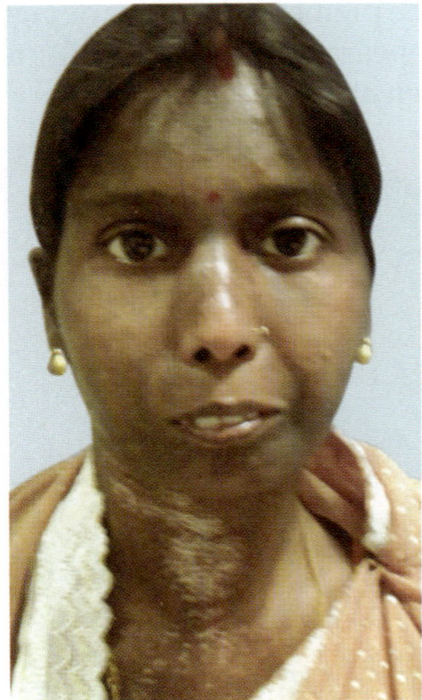

Fig. 3.114: **Scleroderma** showing mask-like facies, pinched up nose, taut and shiny skin over the face, and salt-pepper appearance in neck

1. *Mask-like facies* (loss of facial expression)—reduced mobility of eyelid, cheek and mouth.
2. Absence of normal skin wrinkling in face and forehead ('ironed out' skin folds).
3. Pinched-up nose or beaking of the nose.
4. Difficulty to open the mouth fully—small mouth (*microstomia*) with radial furrows around the lips on closing (tobacco-pouch, fish-mouth or crow-feet appearance). Oral hygiene is poor.
5. Skin over the face seems taut and shiny.
6. Pigmentation and depigmentation.
7. Telangiectasia over face and lips.

- The typical facies is known as 'mauskopf' (mouse head) appearance.

Q. Common causes of masked facies:

Poverty of expression in face (hypomimia) is seen in:

1. Parkinsonism.
2. Scleroderma.
3. Hypothyroidism (myxoedema).
4. Bilateral UMN type of facial nerve palsy.
5. Depression.
6. Myasthenia gravis and facial myopathies.
7. Dementia.
8. Sometimes in pseudobulbar palsy.

- 'Masked facies' is a window in clinical medicine.

Q. Types and subtypes of systemic sclerosis:

A. Systemic sclerosis (SSc) is a multisystem disorder of unknown aetiology affecting skin (*scleroderma*), CVS, GI tract, kidneys, musculoskeletal system, lungs and vasculature. Localised form without systemic involvement is known as *localised scleroderma*.

B. SSc is divided into two subgroups: *Limited* cutaneous scleroderma (LcSSc; 70%) and *diffuse* cutaneous scleroderma (DcSSc; 30%). GI tract, lung, kidney and heart are involved in both the groups. LcSSc → indolent onset with slow progression; skin involvement over sites restricted distal to elbow or knee. Face is always involved. LcSSc is now synonymous with CREST syndrome (*see* afterwards), and in DcSSc → rapid onset with rapid progression; involvement of skin of fingers which rapidly involves the whole body, trunk and face.

C. Localised scleroderma is again divided into two subgroups: *Morphoea* and *linear scleroderma*.

D. *Scleroderma sine scleroderma* (2%): Systemic features without any skin involvement.

Q. Initial suspicion of scleroderma in a patient:

1. While examining the patient for anaemia, i.e. when the lower eyelids are retracted downwards, it seems

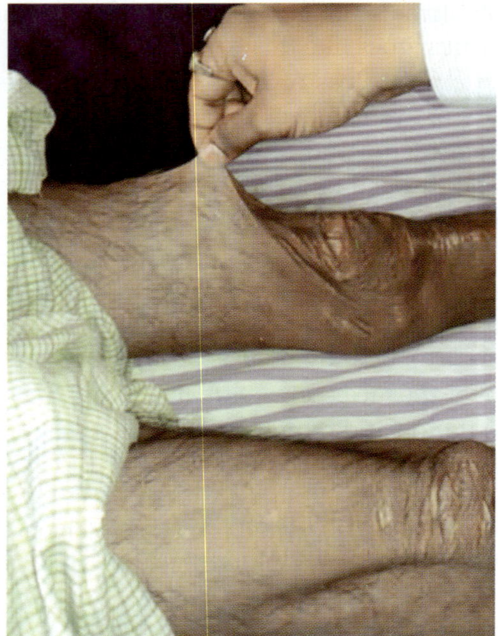

Fig. 3.115: **Stretchy skin** with loose joints in **Ehlers-Danlos syndrome**

very tight and the lower palpebral conjunctiva is not exposed fully.

2. Characteristic facies, especially in a middle-aged female patient (30–50 years).

- Loose, thin and stretchy skin is seen in Ehlers-Danlos syndrome and cutis laxa (Fig. 3.115).

Q. Stages of scleroderma:

There are three stages:

1. Oedematous stage (non-pitting oedema).
2. Indurated stage.
3. Atrophic stage.

Q. How the patients present themselves?

Very often the first symptom is Raynaud's phenomenon, or symmetrical swelling or stiffness of the fingers. Otherwise, it depends on which stage (see above) the patient presents.

Q. Examine the hand of your patient (scleroderma) (Fig. 3.116):

1. Skin is very taut, smooth and shiny, firm and thick, and the skin of the fingers cannot be pinched-up (sclerodactyly) as it is tightly bound to underlying subcutaneous tissue.
2. Raynaud's phenomenon (Fig. 3.117A).
3. Symmetrical swelling (puffiness) of fingers. The MCP and IP joints may be swollen.
4. Limitation of full extension and flexion of fingers (flexion contracture).
5. Pulp atrophy (soft tissue at fingertips is lost): Acroosteolysis.
6. Dermal sclerosis may lead to decreased sweating, dry skin and loss of hair.

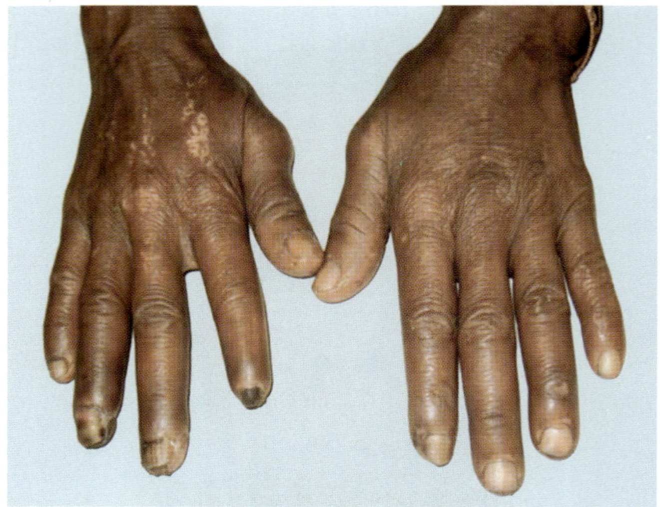

Fig. 3.116: **Hands in scleroderma** showing **sclerodactyly** (tight skin over fingers), **pulp atrophy** (acroosteolysis in right index finger), digital infarction, nail changes, salt-pepper skin and H/o Raynaud's phenomenon

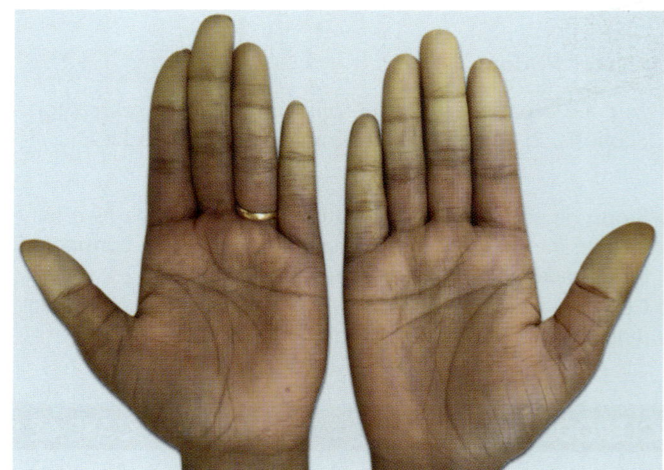

Fig. 3.117A: 'Triphasic colour response' in the hands in a patient of scleroderma—the **Raynaud's phenomenon**; numbness, burning and pain in the fingers are associated with

7. Skin may be pigmented and/or depigmented (salt-pepper appearance) (Fig. 3.117B); telangiectasia may be seen at the base of nails.

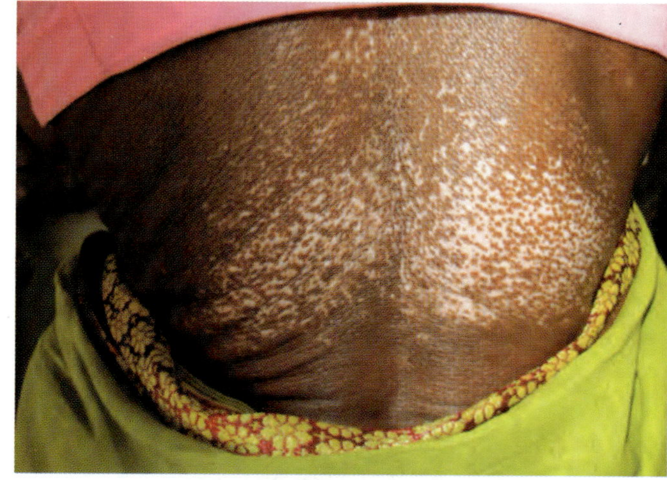

Fig. 3.117B: **Salt-pepper appearance** in skin of lower back [depigmentation (white-like salt) and pigmentation (black-like pepper)] in scleroderma

8. Nail-fold thrombi, dilated nail-fold capillary loops, digital infarcts, painful digital ulceration and rarely digital gangrene. Pitted scars, especially on the tips of the fingers.
9. Pseudoclubbing may be present (due to resorption of bone of terminal phalanx).
10. Calcific deposits (calcinosis cutis) in the subcutaneous tissue (sometimes skin may break down with discharge of calcific material) **(Fig. 3.117C)**.

- The changes in the nail-fold capillaries are best examined clinically by an ophthalmoscope or capillary microscope. Skin thickness is assessed by 'modified Rodnan skin score'.

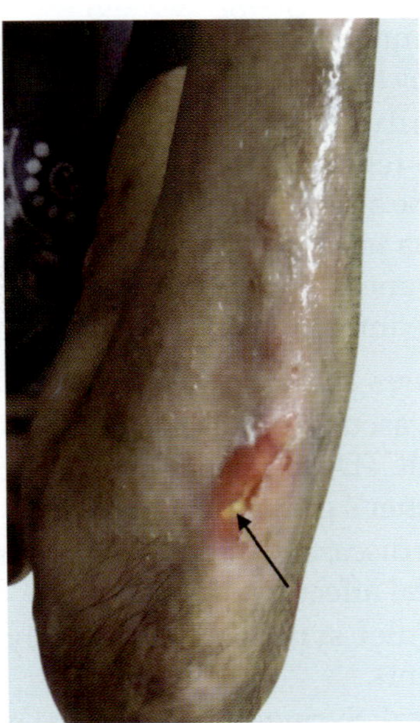

Fig. 3.117C: Calcinosis cutis. Calcium salts deposited in skin are seen

Q. Causes of deformed/mutilated fingers/toes:

1. Leprosy.
2. Scleroderma.
3. Buerger's disease.
4. Congenital defect.
5. Frost bite.
6. Diabetic foot.
7. Syringomyelia.
8. Vasculitis.
9. Atherothrombosis.
10. Antiphospholipid syndrome.
11. Arthritis mutilans (psoriasis).
12. Trauma.
13. Porphyria.
14. Amyloid neuropathy.
15. Lesch-Nyhan syndrome.
16. Mononeuritis multiplex.

Q. Respiratory system involvement in SSc:

Respiratory system involvement is the major cause of morbidity and mortality in SSC.

1. Aspiration pneumonia (due to dysphagia).
2. Interstitial lung disease ('honeycomb lung' in chest X-ray; there is absence of clubbing).
3. Pulmonary arterial hypertension (10–15%)—Common in long-standing disease.
4. Chronic cor pulmonale.
5. Malignant alveolar or bronchiolar cell neoplasm.
6. Pleurisy, rarely.
7. Restriction of chest movement (due to very tight skin mimicking Roman breast plate)—'hidebound chest'.

Q. CVS involvement in SSc:

1. Pericarditis.
2. Heart block (conduction defects).
3. Arrhythmia.
4. Restrictive cardiomyopathy (myocardial fibrosis).
5. Heart failure (right heart failure from cor pulmonale, and left heart failure from cardiomyopathy).
6. Systemic hypertension.

Q. Gastrointestinal tract involvement in SSc:

1. Heartburn, regurgitation of gastric contents due to reflux oesophagitis (symptoms are more when the patient lies flat).
2. Dilatation and atony of distal oesophagus: Peptic oesophagitis.
3. Dysphagia, especially to solid foods (manometry shows ↓ amplitude or disappearance of peristaltic waves in lower 2/3rd of the oesophagus) due to oesophageal hypomotility; odynophagia may occur.
4. Delayed gastric emptying due to atony and dilatation.
5. Recurrent occult upper GI bleeding indicates 'watermelon stomach', i.e. antral vascular ectasia.
6. Malabsorption syndrome (due to bacterial overgrowth).
7. Chronic constipation, distension and sometimes intestinal pseudo-obstruction (due to atony).
8. Pneumatosis cystoides intestinalis (radiolucent cysts within the wall of small intestine).

- Dysphagia is a very important symptom of SSc.

Q. Musculoskeletal manifestations of SSc:

1. Symmetrical polyarthritis (like rheumatoid arthritis).
2. Restriction of hand movement (mostly due to stiffness of skin).
3. Leathery crepitations can be palpated over tendon sheaths or moving joints (especially knee joints) in an advanced disease.
4. Carpal tunnel syndrome.
5. Resorption of terminal phalanges resulting in pseudoclubbing.
6. Proximal muscle weakness, wasting (due to disuse) and low grade myositis.

Q. Renal involvement in SSc:

1. Hypertension.
2. Non-progressive proteinuria.

3. 'Scleroderma renal crisis' (10–15%): It is due to obliterative vasculopathy of renal cortical arteries and is one of the commonest cause of death.

Q. How to assess the severity of scleroderma at the bedside?

Normally in health, a person's 4 fingers (excluding thumb) easily enter within his oral cavity when placed side by side. In scleroderma, as the mouth becomes smaller, all the four fingers may not enter within the oral cavity. Observe the number of patient's fingers entering within the oral cavity with ease and clinically guess the severity.

Q. What are the differential diagnosis?

1. Causes of Raynaud's phenomenon (*see* below).
2. CREST syndrome (calcinosis, Raynaud's phenomenon, oesophageal dysmotility, sclerodactyly and telangiectasia). This is synonymous with a subset of limited cutaneous scleroderma.
3. Eosinophilic fasciitis.
4. Pseudo-scleroderma (amyloidosis, scleredema, acromegaly and scleromyxoedema).

Q. Drugs or toxins producing scleroderma-like lesion:

1. Vinyl chloride.
2. Pentazocine.
3. Bleomycin.
4. Epoxy resins and aromatic hydrocarbon.

- Silica dust, cocaine or adulterated rapeseed oil are also blamed.

Q. How to confirm your diagnosis?

Antinuclear factor (ANF) is present in 95% cases. Antinuclear antibodies to anti-topoisomerase I (also called anti-Scl-70) is found in 30% patients of diffuse cutaneous variety; anti-centromere antibodies are found in 70% cases of limited cutaneous variety (e.g. CREST syndrome). Rheumatoid factor is positive in 30%.

Chest X-ray (to see cardiomegaly), urine for R/E (proteinuria), X-ray of hands (acroosteolysis or calcinosis), barium swallow or motility study of oesophagus (confirms oesophageal hypomotility) and CT scan of thorax (to demonstrate interstitial lung disease) also help in diagnosis. Skin biopsy is not so important in diagnosis.

Q. What is mixed connective tissue disease (MCTD)?

It is an overlap syndrome characterised by the combination of SLE, scleroderma, polymyositis and rheumatoid arthritis. It is associated with unusually high titres of circulating antibody to a nuclear ribonucleoprotein (U1-RNP). Renal and neurological features are uncommon but pulmonary fibrosis and secondary pulmonary hypertension may be lethal.

Q. What is Raynaud's phenomenon?

Definition: It is a vasospastic disorder (intense vasospasm of peripheral arteries), manifested clinically by the classical 'triphasic colour response' which is sequential development of digital blanching (*pallor* due to vasospasm of arteries), cyanosis (*blue* due to sluggish blood flow and accumulation of deoxygenated blood following ischaemia) and rubor (*redness* due to vasodilatation and reactive hyperaemia) of the fingers and toes bilaterally following cold exposure and subsequent rewarming (Fig. 3.117A). The changes in the fingers and toes are often diagnosed by nail-fold capillography. The fingers are affected more than toes. Numbness, tingling, burning and severe pain in digits are common features. *Usually cold and stress are precipitating factors*.

It is usually a cold-induced digital ischaemia secondary to reflex sympathetic vasoconstriction. The duration of the attack is variable and may last for hours. Some patients may experience bicolour response (e.g. pallor and cyanosis). In chronic and severe cases, there may be tissue infarction and loss of digits.

Common causes are:

1. Collagen vascular diseases (Fig. 3.73) like systemic sclerosis, MCTD, dermatomyositis, CREST syndrome, SLE, Wegener's granulomatosis.
2. Raynaud's disease (women of late teens, bilateral and symmetrical affection of hands).
3. Thoracic inlet syndrome (especially in unilateral involvement).
4. Neurological: Syringomyelia, spinal cord tumours.
5. Trauma: Vibration injury, use of pneumatic drills, cold injury, typing.
6. Blood dyscrasias: Myeloproliferative disorders, hyperviscosity syndrome, cryoglobulinaemia.
7. Drugs: Ergot derivatives, β-blockers, methysergide.
8. Arterial disease: When affected by microemboli, e.g. atherosclerosis, Buerger's disease.

Clinical Wisdom

Nowadays Raynaud's phenomenon is broadly divided into two categories:

a. The idiopathic variety called Raynaud's disease (No. 2), and
b. The secondary variety described above (No.1 to 8 except No. 2).

- D/D of Raynand's phenomenon are acrocyanosis, erythromelalgia, chilblains, cold aglutinin disease.
- AG Maurice Raynaud (1834–1881) was a physician in Paris and described the sign in 1862.

Q. D/D of hardness (or thickening) of skin:

1. Morphoea (localised scleroderma): Presents as solitary or multiple patches of thickened skin.
2. Lymphoedema.
3. Vascular insufficiencies (chronic).

4. Recurrent cellulitis with venous stasis.
5. Lipoid proteinosis.
6. Carcinoid syndrome.
7. Scirrhous carcinoma (hardening of skin of chest).
8. Porphyria cutanea tarda.
9. Chronic graft-versus-host disease.
10. Toxic oil syndrome (linked to consumption of contaminated rapeseed oil).
11. Eosinophilia-myalgia syndrome (due to consumption of L-tryptophan).
12. Nephrogenic systemic fibrosis (uraemic patients on haemodialysis—gadolinium-induced by MRI).
13. Diabetic cheiroarthropathy.
14. Pseudo-scleroderma (vide above).

Q. Treatment modalities used in SSc:

Virtually no agent has been shown to arrest skin changes. The treatment modalities used are:

1. Patient's education, counselling and family support are mandatory. Previously used drugs like D-penicillamine (↓ collagen cross linkage and ↓ skin thickening) and colchicine (↓ procollagen to collagen conversion) are no longer used now.
2. Treatment of reflux oesophagitis (by PPI and prokinetics), blind loop syndrome (by anibiotics), myositis (by glucocorticoids), articular symptoms (by NSAIDs and weekly methotrexate), respiratory tract infection (by antibiotics), interstitial lung disease (by glucocorticoids and immunosuppressants like rituximab; pirfenidone and nintedanib are promicing drugs), pulmonary hypertension (by diuretics, oral anticoagulation, digoxin, bosentan, sildenafil, IV epoprostenol or treprostinil, or iloprost by inhalation), CVS involvement (pericarditis by glucocorticoids) and hypertension (ACE inhibitors) due to renal involvement are done accordingly.
3. 'Scleroderma renal crisis' is a medical emergency, and requires intensive control of hypertension and use of ACE inhibitors. High dose corticosteroid (>10 mg/day) may precipitate this condition.
4. IFN-α, IFN-γ and human recombinant relaxin therapy are being tried with mixed results.
5. Clinical trials of immunosuppressive drugs (methotrexate, mycophenolate mofetil, cyclosporine, azathioprine) are underway.
6. **Raynaud's phenomenon** patients should wear gloves and woolen mittens, minimise cold exposure, protect the body with warm clothings and abstain from tobacco smoking. Drugs used are calcium-channel blockers (nifedipine, amlodipine or diltiazem), prazocin, losartan, 5-phosphodiesterase intibitors (sildenafil; tadalafil works better), topical nitroglycerine, IV prostaglandins, low-dose aspirin/dipyridamole (to prevent platelet aggregation), endothelin-1 receptor antagonist (bosentan, especially in digital ulcers; costly), naftidrofuryl oxalate, calcitonin gene-related peptides and statins (empirical use). One should avoid β-blockers, ergotamine, sympathomimetics and OC pills. Digital sympathectomy may be effective in some patients; local injections of botulinum type A into the digits are applied in severe ischaemia.
7. Regular exercise and skin lubricants help in maintaining flexibility of limbs and pliability of skin.

Q. Clinical use of colchicine:

1. Acute gout, pseudogout.
2. Scleroderma (not used now).
3. Primary biliary cirrhosis.
4. Amyloidosis.
5. Familial Mediterranean fever.
6. Study of chromosomes (colchicine arrests cell division at the metaphase).
7. Psoriasis.
8. Behcet's syndrome.
9. Myelofibrosis.
10. Erytherna nodosum.
11. Sarcoid arthritis.
12. Recurrent oral ulcers/pericarditis.
13. Osteoarthritis.

SYSTEMIC LUPUS ERYTHEMATOSUS (SLE) CASE 63

Q. Describe the face of the patient:

1. Classical photosensitive **'butterfly' rash** over the malar areas and bridge of the nose (never involves the nasolabial folds)—slightly raised erythema, may be scaly.
2. The lesion consists of erythema and oedema in acute phase, atrophy and telangiectasia in chronic phase.
3. Patchy alopecia.
4. 'Lupus hairs'—short, broken hairs seen above the forehead.
5. Ulcers within the oral cavity (palatal ulcer especially, usually painless and recurrent) **(Fig. 3.118)** and nasal mucous membrane (seen after opening the mouth or careful examination of the nose).

Clinical Wisdom

The face with the 'butterfly' rash looks like the face of wolves ('lupus' is Latin for 'wolf'). The patient is commonly a female one (F: M = 9: 1) in her second or third decade of life. Butterfly rash in SLE is due to apoptosis of keratinised layer of skin exposed to sunlight/UV light.

- **Alopecia** is loss of hair in the scalp, and is of two types: *Cicatricial* (DLE, scleroderma, lichen planus, pseudopelade, burn, bacterial folliculitis) **(Fig. 3.119)** and *non-cicatricial* [alopecia areata **(Fig. 3.120)**, SLE, telogen effluvium, bullous pemphigoid, tinea capitis, ectodermal dysplasia **(Fig. 3.121)**] **(Fig. 3.122)**.

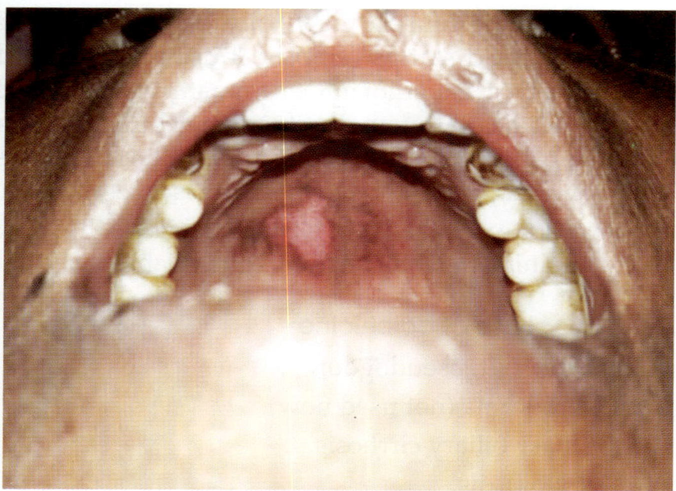

Fig. 3.118: Painless **oral (palatal) ulcer** in systemic lupus erythematosus

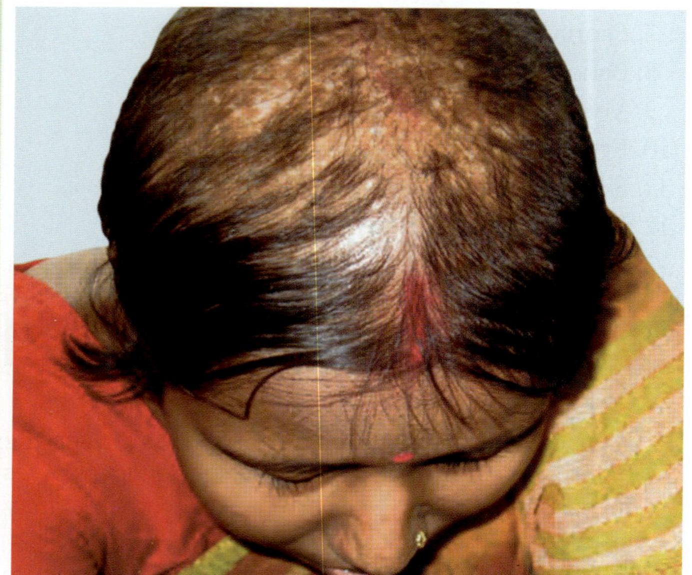

Fig. 3.119: **Scarring alopecia** following bacterial folliculitis (inflammatory)

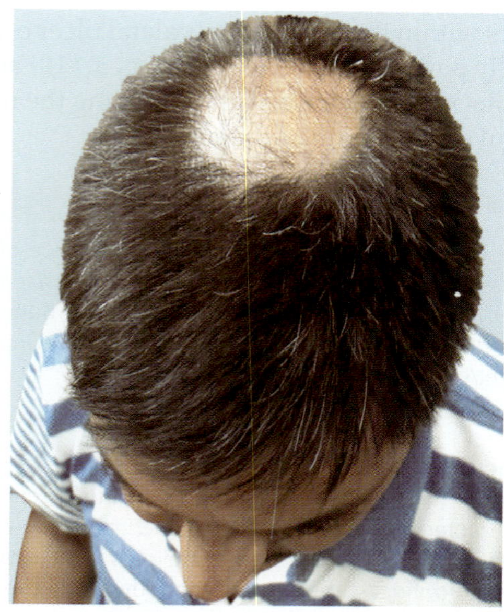

Fig. 3.120: **Alopecia areata** in scalp

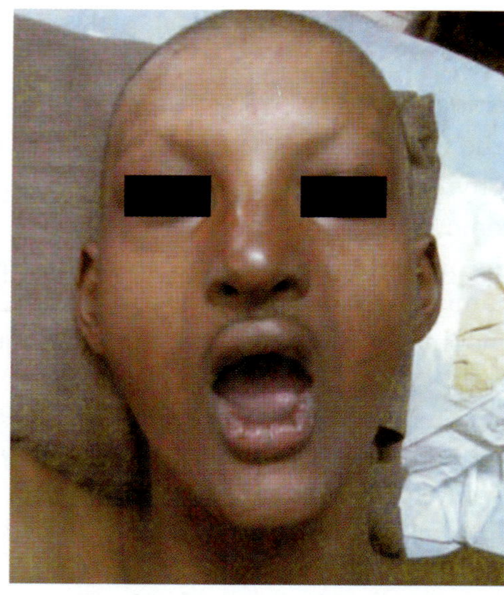

Fig. 3.121: Abnormalities of ectodermal structures such as hair, teeth, nails, sweat glands are seen in **ectodermal dysplasia**. This patient is lacking in scalp hair, eyebrows, moustache, beard, teeth and sweat glands

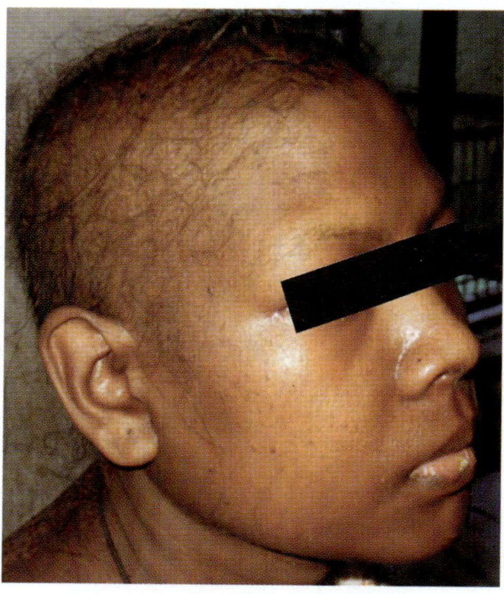

Fig. 3.122: Chemotherapy-induced **non-scarring alopecia**

Q. Causes of erythematous butterfly-like lesion in face (Fig. 3.123):

1. SLE.
2. Rosacea (due to vasodilatation and telangiectasia, there are red patches with acneiform papules and pustules with nose disfigurement, or rhinophyma of nose; blushing of face ↑ after taking tea, coffee, etc.) (Fig. 3.124A).
3. Discoid lupus erythematosus (DLE) or mixed connective tissue disease (MCTD).
4. Lupus vulgaris (commonest form of skin tuberculosis).
5. Photosensitive reaction (after ingestion of drugs like tetracycline or phenothiazines).
6. Chloasma or melasma.
7. Leprosy (lepromatous).

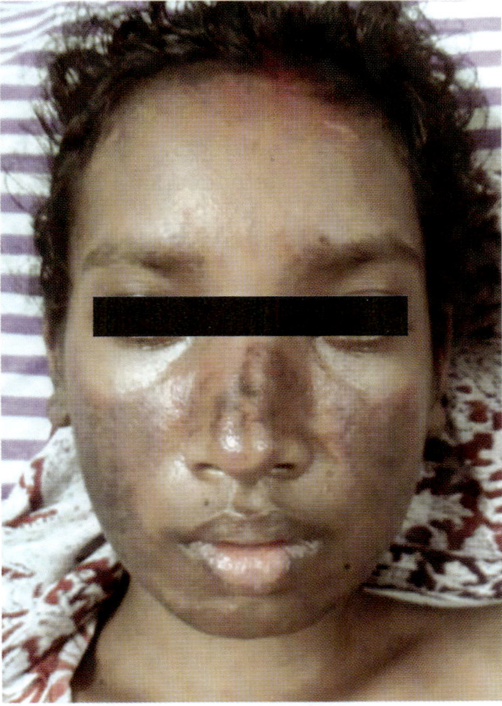

Fig. 3.123: Systemic lupus erythematosus (SLE) with classical **'butterfly' rash** in the face

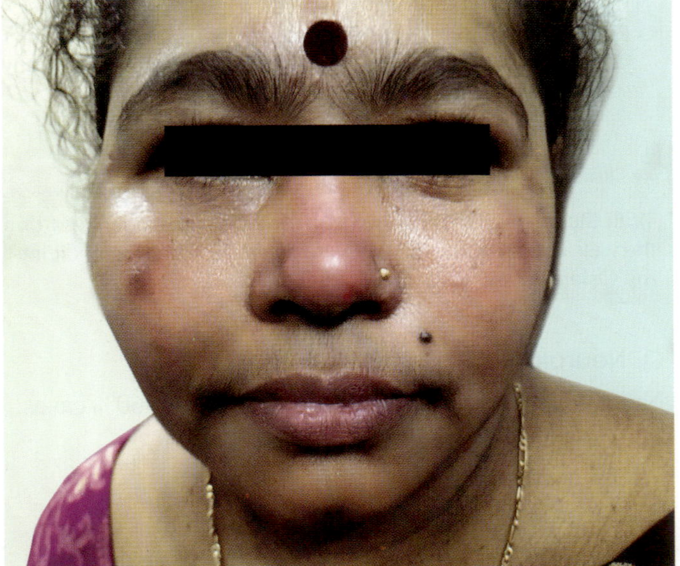

Fig. 3.124A: Rosacea, which commonly affects 30–50 years old females

8. Dermatomyositis (purple or lilac-coloured heliotrope rash, especially the juvenile variety) (Fig. 3.124B).
9. Post kala-azar dermal leishmaniasis (PKDL).
10. Pemphigus erythematosus (an uncommon variant of pemphigus).
11. Polymorphous light eruption.
12. Sarcoidosis (lupus pernio).

- **Dermatomyositis** is diagnosed by heliotrope rash (eyelid and face), V-sign (rash in anterior chest), shawl sign (rash over upper back), Gottron's sign (rash over knuckles of hands) (*see* Fig. 3.69) and mechanic's hand (cracked fingers).

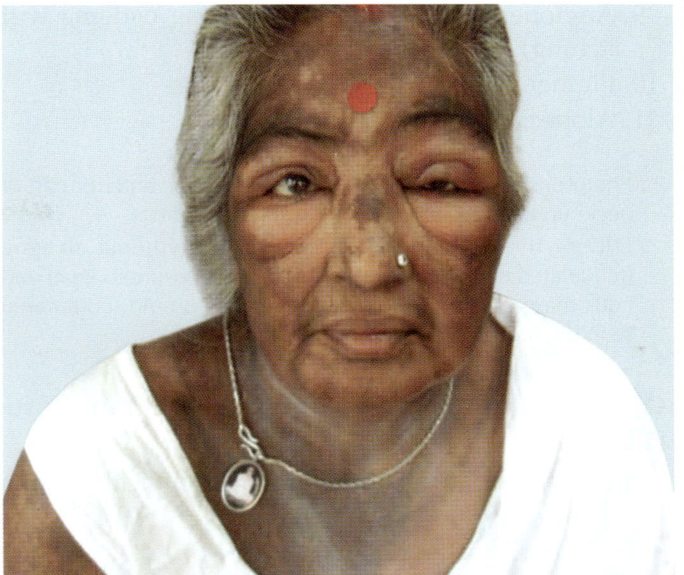

Fig. 3.124B: Dermatomyositis with heliotrope (lilac-coloured) rash in eyelids, periorbital oedema, and purple pigmentation in forehead, nose, chest and upper arm

Q. Other skin lesions in SLE (*see* Fig. 3.75):

The skin is affected in 85% patients of SLE:

1. Ill-defined, erythematous macular or maculopapular rash with fine scaling (particularly in sun-exposed areas); photosensitivity—worsening of rash often indicates 'flare'.
2. Vasculitic lesions on the fingertips and around the nail folds, purpura.
3. Bullous lesion, hives; recurrent urticaria; lichen planus-like dermatitis.
4. Panniculitis (lupus profundus).
5. Periungual erythema.
6. Digital infarcts (watch the tips and pulps of fingers for any tiny cicatrical depression).
7. Livedo reticularis (cyanotic mottling of skin with fishnet or reticulated appearance) (Fig. 3.125).
8. Raynaud's phenomenon.

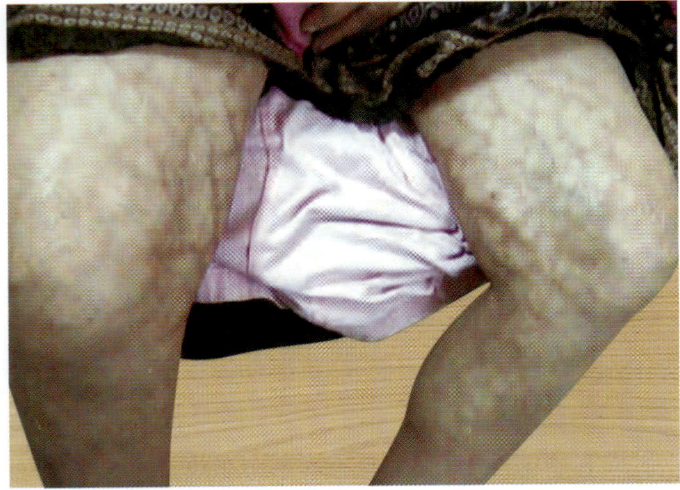

Fig. 3.125: Livedo reticularis–cyanotic mottling of skin with fishnet appearance in SLE with antiphospholipid syndrome

9. Angioneurotic oedema (non-pitting oedema with itching).
10. Pigmentation.
11. Alopecia.

- Photosensitive rash occurs in face, ears, chin, anterior part of neck, upper back and extensor surfaces of arms.
- D/D of livedo reticularis in skin are erythema ab igne (reticulated erythema due to prolonged exposure to heat) and cutis marmorata (physiological reaction to cold, commonly seen in children).

Q. What is chronic discoid lupus erythematosus (CDLE)?

Lupus erythematosus (LE) has three clinical variants like:

- Systemic lupus erythematosus (SLE).
- Chronic discoid lupus erythematosus (CDLE).
- Subacute cutaneous lupus erythematosus (SCLE).

CDLE is a chronic skin ailment which is commoner than SLE. The skin lesions heal with scarring, and the other characteristic features are (Fig. 3.126):

1. Photosensitivity and erythema.
2. Scaling with atrophy.
3. Telangiectasia.
4. Hypopigmentation and keratotic plugging.
   Sites: Face, arms, neck, scalp, ears.

- It is seen that 5–10% patients with DLE progress to SLE, while DLE is present in approximately 20% of patients with SLE. DLE is associated with positive ANF (30%) and normal complement level.

Q. Causes of telangiectasias:

These are clusture of small, dilated blood vessels visible on skin surface; they blanch on application of pressure given by a pinhead.

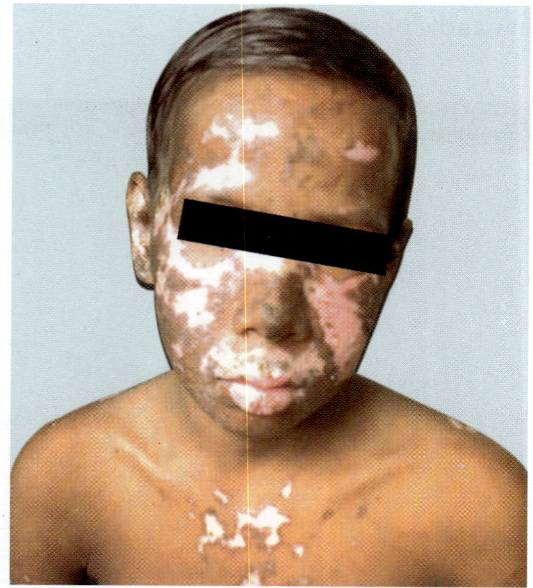

Fig. 3.126: Discoid lupus erythematosus (DLE) with hypopigmentation and atrophy seen in face and upper chest

a. Systemic diseases: SLE, scleroderma, dermatomyositis, hereditary haemorrhagic telangiectasis, ataxia-telangiectasia, carcinoid syndrome, spider naevi in cirrhosis of liver.

b. Primary cutaneous disorder: Acne rosacea, ionising radiation, actinically damaged skin.

Q. Common clinical features of SLE:

SLE is a multisystem disease. The common clinical features are:

1. Arthritis and arthralgia (commonest).
2. Malaise and tiredness.
3. Fever (presents as PUO).
4. Skin eruptions.
5. Anorexia, nausea and vomiting.
6. Myalgia.
7. Pleurisy.
8. CNS abnormalities.
9. Lymphadenopathy.
10. Renal involvement.

- Splenomegaly occurs in 20–30% and hepatomegaly in 25% patients of SLE.
- Arthritis is non-erosive and non-deforming (rarely deformity with Jaccoud's arthritis).
- Read the Systemic Lupus International Collaborating Clinics (SLICC) criteria for classification and diagnosis of SLE from any standard textbook of medicine.

Clinical Wisdom

With the passage of time the name of the disease changes from the well-known quote 'he who knows syphilis, knows medicine' (by Osler)...diabetes...AIDS...to SLE (in modern era).

Q. Neurological manifestations of SLE:

Neurological involvement occurs in up to 60% cases.

1. Cognitive dysfunction.
2. Convulsions.
3. Depression.
4. Organic psychosis.
5. Cranial nerve involvement.
6. Transverse myelitis.
7. Aseptic meningitis.
8. Organic brain syndrome (psychosis, seizure).
9. Migraine.
10. Chorea.
11. Cerebellar ataxia.
12. Rarely, peripheral neuropathy.
13. Cerebrovascular accidents.

- Fundoscopy may reveal white, hard exudate called 'cytoid body'.
- **Ocular manifestations** are sicca syndrome, conjunctivitis, episcleritis and vasculitis.

Q. Cardiopulmonary involvement in SLE:

1. Pericarditis, myocarditis, non-bacterial verrucous endocarditis involving the mitral and aortic valve (known as Libman-Sacks endocarditis, which may produce a murmur).
2. Heart block and arrhythmia may occur.
3. Ischaemic heart disease (due to premature narrowing of coronary arteries).
4. Recurrent pleurisy and pleural effusion (exudate; bilateral).
5. Lupus pneumonitis (pulmonary infection is very common).
6. 'Shrinking lung syndrome' (X-ray shows elevation of diaphragm and liner scars from recurrent pulmonary infarction).
7. Fibrosing alveolitis.
8. Intrapulmonary haemorrhage (from vasculitis), pulmonary hypertension, ARDS.

- **GI involvement** is painless mouth ulcer, mesenteric vasculitis and pancreatitis (rare).

Q. What is drug-induced SLE:

1. Drugs with positive ANF: INH, phenytoin, phenothiazines, α-methyl dopa and levodopa.
2. Drugs associated with exacerbations of SLE: Sulphonamides, penicillin and oral contraceptives.
3. Drugs producing syndrome similar to SLE: Hydralazine and procainamide.

Clinical Wisdom

ANF and anti-histone antibody (70%) are positive in drug-induced SLE. Renal and neurological manifestations are uncommon, and the main presentations are fever, arthralgia or arthritis and serositis. Complement levels are normal.

Q. Renal manifestations of SLE:

It carries the worst prognosis. Renal biopsy is an important guide to prognosis in SLE.

1. Minimal proteinuria, haematuria, cellular casts (so regularly screen urine for protein and blood).
2. Nephrotic syndrome (minimal change to crescentic glomerulonephritis).
3. Chronic renal failure.
4. Urinary tract infections.

Q. Classification of 'lupus nephritis':

It is done by International Society of Nephrology and Renal Pathology Society (2003, mild revision done in 2016). Clinical renal involvement occurs in approximately 30% cases, of which 25% will develop ESRD within 10 years. There are six classes:

Class I	Minimal mesangial lupus nephritis (LN).
Class II	Mesangial proliferative LN.
Class III	Focal LN.
Class IV	Diffuse LN.
Class V	Membranous LN.
Class VI	Advanced sclerotic LN.

Q. Causes of pain abdomen in SLE:

1. Peritonitis.
2. Pancreatitis.
3. Perisplenitis.
4. Mesenteric vasculitis.
5. Complication of corticosteroid therapy (peptic ulcer).
6. Gallbladder perforation from necrotising arteritis.

- **Death in SLE** usually results from infections, neurological complications or renal failure.

Q. How to establish the diagnosis of SLE?

1. Blood examination reveals normocytic normochromic anaemia or immune haemolytic anaemia, leucopenia, lymphocytopenia, thrombocytopenia, clotting factor defect (due to antibodies formed against factor VII, IX and X). ESR tends to be high with active disease.
2. Urine analysis: Proteinuria (may be in nephrotic range), haematuria, RBC casts.
3. LE cell: Phenomenon may be positive (not done nowadays).
4. Coombs' test and rheumatoid factor (30%) may be positive.
5. False positive serological test for syphilis, positive lupus anticoagulant (LA).
6. Blood urea and creatinine may be high in renal involvement.
7. **Antinuclear factor (ANF) is present in 98% cases. Antibodies against native double-stranded DNA (anti-ds DNA, 70%) is highly specific for SLE.** Anti-Sm antibody (Smith, 25%) is specific for SLE.
8. Hypocomplementaemia C_3 (i.e. C_3 <5.5 mg/dL).
9. Skin biopsy taken from uninvolved sun-hidden part shows deposits of immunoglobulins and complement components at epidermal and dermal junction [called 'lupus band test' (60%)].
10. Renal biopsy.

- It is to be remembered that *C-reactive protein (CRP) is normal* in SLE unless and otherwise there is superadded infection, pleurisy or arthritis (high CRP). Anticardiolipin antibody should be done to diagnose secondary antiphospholipid antibody syndrome. Presence of anti-Ro antibody in a pregnant SLE increases chance of neonatal lupus with complete heart block.
- **Renal involvement:** 24-hour urinary protein, serum urea and creatinine, urine for R/E and renal biopsy.
- Neurolupus: EEG, CT or MRI done.

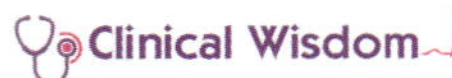

↑ ESR, ↑ anti ds-DNA and ↓ C_3 may indicate disease 'flare'.

Q. Autoantibody associations in different subsets of SLE:

Autoantibodies are immunoglobulins which bind to antigens within autologous (self) tissue. Antinuclear antibody (ANA) or factor (ANF) are antibodies produced against nuclear component of a cell. ANA is detected by indirect immunofluorescence (IIF) assay using HEp-2 cells. The different components are:

1. Anti-ds DNA: Nephritis, serositis, vasculitis.
2. Anti-Sm: Specific for SLE.
3. Anti-Ro/La: Photosensitivity, neonatal lupus.
4. Antiphospholipid antibody/lupus anticoagulant: Coagulopathy, abortion, thrombocytopenia.
5. Anti-U1-RNP (nuclear ribonucleoprotein): Mixed connective tissue disease (MCTD).
6. Anti-histone: Drug-induced lupus (e.g. hydralazine or procainamide-induced).
7. Anti-ribosomal P antibody: CNS lupus (psychosis, depression).
8. C_{1q} autoantibody: Having prognostic significance in lupus nephritis.

Other autoantibodies in different connective tissue diseases are:

- Anti-centromere: CREST syndrome.
- Anti-SSA (anti-Ro)/SSB (anti-La): Sjögren's syndrome.
- Anti-topoisomerase I (anti-Scl-70): Diffuse cutaneous scleroderma.
- ANCA:
  c-ANCA (anti-proteinase-3): Wegener's granulomatosis.
  p-ANCA (anti-myeloperoxidase): Systemic vasculitis, microscopic polyangiitis.
- Anti Jo-1: Polymyositis, dermatomyositis with lung involvement.

Q. How will you manage this patient?

There is no cure for SLE. The aim of treatment is to maintain remission and control acute 'flares'.

1. Patient's education regarding the disease, reassurance and psychological support. Avoidance of ultraviolet light exposure with use of sunscreen cream. Restful life.
2. NSAID: For arthritis, arthralgia, myalgia, pleurisy, fatigue, fever, etc.
3. Hydroxychloroquine 400 mg/day (ophthalmological examination at least once a year should be done and the patient should avoid ultraviolet light) for skin lesions and arthritis.
4. Low dose corticosteroid in debilitaling skin lesion. Corticosteroid is also indicated (60 mg/day of prednisolone) in cardio-pulmonary, CNS and haematologial involvement. Gradually, the dose is tapered after two weeks and the patient is maintained on 10 mg prednisolone/day. Anticonvulsants are needed to control seizures.
5. Renal lesions need special mention. ACE inhibitors, ARBs and diuretic are used from time to time. Renal biopsy should be done prior to treatment. Focal lupus glomerulonephritis respond well to treatment with prednisolone (40–60 mg/day till symptoms disappear). However, diffuse and membranous lesions do not respond well and they need urgent therapy with 1 g of IV methyl prednisolone daily for 3 consecutive days followed by maintenance daily or alternate-day prednisolone (also used in organ damage in SLE). The widely accepted 'pulse' regimen goes like this: cyclophosphamide 500 mg/m^2, IV, monthly for 6 months → then 500 mg/m^2, IV, 3 monthly for 2 doses → mycophenolate mofetil (1 g BD/day) or azathioprine (1.5–3 mg/kg of body weight/day) for 2 years. Short-term studies show that mycophenolate is superior to cyclophosphamide in induction as well as maintenance phase. Other immunosuppressive drugs used are methotrexate, belimumab, tacrolimus, cyclosporin. Rituximab (anti-CD20) is used in refractory cases to reduce the level of antibodies.
6. Infection anywhere in the body is treated by proper antibiotic.
7. Skin rash may be treated by sunscreen cream, topical steroid, retinoids or dapsone.
8. Statins for hyperlipidaemia.
9. Plasmapheresis may be tried.
10. SLE with pregnancy is treated with lowest dose of prednisolone for the shortest period.
11. Antiphospholipid antibody syndrome needs low dose aspirin and anticoagulant therapy.

Clinical Wisdom

Treatment of renal lupus—Type I: follow-up, no treatment, Type II: may require steroid, Type III, IV, V: immunosuppressive therapy, Type VI: dialysis or renal transplantation. Symptomatic treatment for oedema and hypertension; rituximab and dialysis may be required in some patients.

Q. What is antiphospholipid antibody syndrome (APS) or Hughes syndrome?

In APS, there is persistently elevated levels of anti-phospholipid/anti-cardiolipin antibody/antibody to β_2 glycoprotein 1, and/or positive test for lupus anticoagulant, and the presence of one of the following, i.e. arterial or venous thrombosis, recurrent foetal loss and thrombocytopenia. APS is of two types: primary (no cause found) and secondary (with SLE, rheumatoid arthritis, systemic sclerosis, etc.).

Clinical features are recurrent arterial or venous thromboembolism, recurrent foetal loss, thrombocytopenia, livedo reticularis (Fig. 3.125), valvular heart disease, chorea/migraine/epilepsy or catastrophic occusion of blood vessels. APS is being treated with life-long anticoagulants (heparin), antiplatelets (aspirin), IVIG and immunosuppressants.

Q. Tests which are helpful in following the clinical course of SLE:

1. Titre of anti-ds DNA.
2. Serum C_3 level.
3. Haematocrit.
4. ESR.
5. WBC count.

6. Platelet count.
7. Urine analysis.
8. Serum creatinine.

Q. Indications for use of chloroquine in internal medicine:

1. Malaria.
2. Hepatic amoebiasis.
3. Rheumatoid arthritis.
4. SLE and DLE.
5. Sjögren's syndrome, Whipple's disease.
6. MCTD.
7. Lepra reaction (type 1).
8. Porphyria cutanea tarda.

ERYTHEMA NODOSUM — CASE 64

Q. Characteristic lesion (Fig. 3.127):

1. Single or multiple non-ulcerating, dusky bluish-red or erythematous nodular lesion, usually in children or young adults; F> M.
2. Generally present on the extensor sufaces; **shins are the usual site**, thigh, upper arm or forearm rarely.
3. Painful and tender; at times bilateral and symmetrical; non-itchy.
4. With mild constitutional symptoms like fever, chills, malaise, arthralgia; may be recurrent.
5. Lesion is generally self-limiting (2–6 weeks). They fade through bruishing and staining (erythema contusiformis); usually heal without scarring.

Q. Common causes of erythema nodosum:

1. Tuberculosis (especially primary)—so, a chest radiography is essential.
2. β-haemolytic streptococcal infection (commonly after streptococcal sore throat).
3. Sulphonamide therapy.
4. Leprosy (lepromatous).
5. Sarcoidosis.
6. Ulcerative colitis or Crohn's disease.
7. Other durgs like oral contraceptives, barbiturates, penicillins, iodides and bromides.
8. Histoplasmosis or coccidioidomycosis, Behcet's syndrome.
9. Brucellosis, psittacosis, tularaemia.
10. Rarely in rheumatic fever.
11. Bacterial gastroenteritis (*Salmonella, Shigella, Yersinia*); *Chlamydia infection*.
12. Idiopathic (unknown factor).

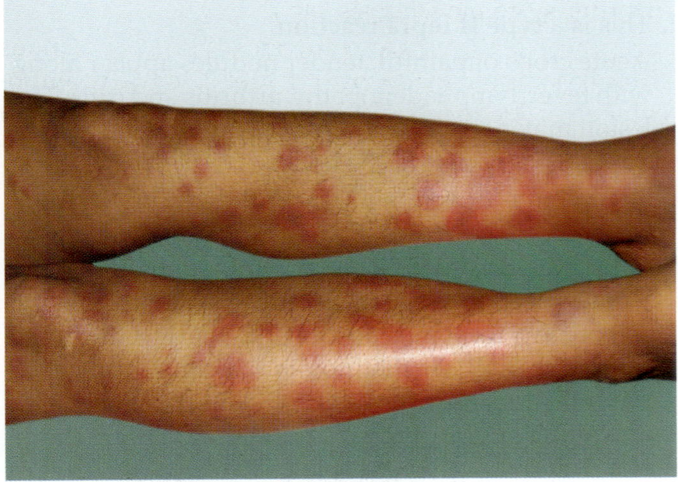

Fig. 3.127: Multiple **erythema nodosum** (septal panniculitis) in sarcoidosis

Q. Basic pathology of the lesion:

Actually, their appearance reflects patchy inflammation of subcutaneous fat (panniculitis) and small blood vessels (vasculitis). This is an example of type III (immune-complex) allergic reaction.

Foreign proteins and bacteria are slowly removed from the 'front of the legs' due to poor lymphatic drainage (as tibia splints the overlying tissue, the massage of the lymphatic channels is reduced)—this is why shins are the usual site.

Erythema nodosum is a septal panniculitis and is not of vasculitic in origin.

Q. Differential diagnosis:

1. Resolving bruises.
2. Thrombophlebitis.
3. Erythema induratum.
4. Erythema chronicum migrans (Lyme disease).
5. Erythema multiforme.
6. Cutaneous vasculitis or metastases.

Q. Different allergic reactions of primary pulmonary tuberculosis:

1. Erythema nodosum.
2. Phlyctenular keratoconjunctivitis.
3. Some cases of pleural effusion (not accepted by all), and
4. Sometimes, pneumonitis from exudative hypersensitivity lesion.

Q. Investigations performed in erythema nodosum:

1. Blood for TC, DC, ESR, CRP, serum angiotensin-converting enzyme (SACE).
2. Search for streptococcal infection: Throat swab culture for Gr. A *streptococci*, ASO titre.
3. Chest X-ray (PA view): To exclude pulmonary tuberculosis or sarcoidosis. CT scan of chest may be necessary in selected cases.
4. Mantoux test: Positive in tuberculosis and negative in sarcoidosis.
5. Stool examination to rule out gastrointestinal diseases.

- Tuberculosis is loosely termed as **'Koch's infection'** after Robert Koch, who identified *Mycobacterium tuberculosis* in 1882.

Q. Treatment:

1. Stoppage of the offending drug.
2. Treatment of the primary disease.
3. Analgesics (NSAID).
4. Lotio calamine paint over the lesion.
5. Prednisolone (up to 30 mg/day), potassium iodide orally (400–900 mg/day) for one month, dapsone (100 mg/day) or colchicine (0.5 mg BD) in stubborn cases.

Q. What is erythema multiforme (Fig. 3.128A and B)?

It is a cell-mediated hypersensitivity reaction to different immunological agents resulting in pleomorphic skin eruptions with macules, papules, bullae along with **target or iris lesion**. The target lesion consists of three concentric zone of colour changes (central cyanotic hue, a pale oedematous intermediate zone with a red periphery). The common aetiology are infections (herpes simplex, *Mycoplasma*), drugs (sulphonamides, penicillin, barbiturates, carbamazepine), collagen vascular diseases, malignancy (carcinomas and lymphomas) and idiopathic.

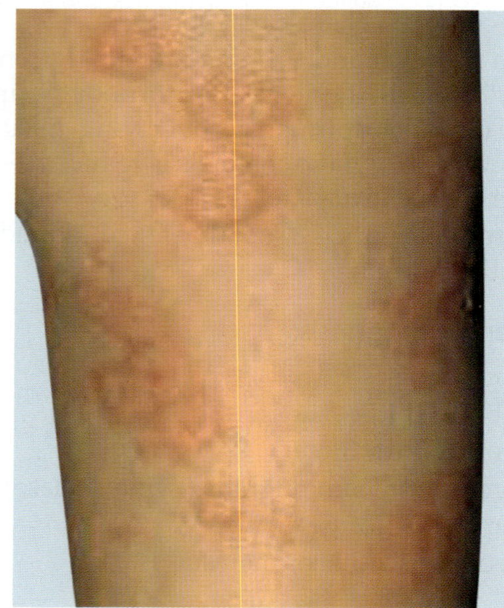

Fig. 3.128A: Target lesion in **erythema multiforme**

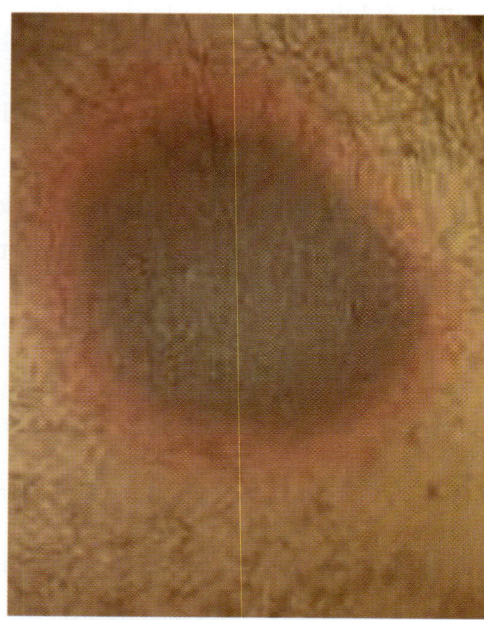

Fig. 3.128B: **Target lesion** (central blister, oedematous ring and erythematous border)—a close-up view

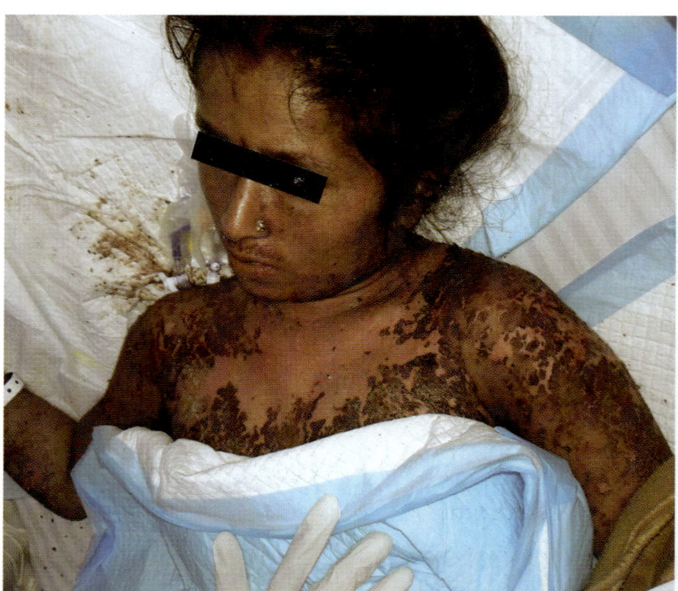

Fig. 3.129: Extensive skin lesions in **Stevens-Johnson syndrome** with signs of healing

Stevens-Johnson syndrome (SJS) is a variety of erythema multiforme where skin eruptions (erythematous or bullous lesion) are associated with mucous membrane involvement (oral cavity, eye, genital) and fever (Fig. 3.129).

SJS and toxic epidermal necrolysis (TEN) are diseases with blistering/epidermal detachment along with mucosal ulceration. Skin detachment in SJS is <10%, in SJS-TEN overlap 10–30%, and in TEN, it is >30%.

Q. What is erythema nodosum leprosum (ENL)?

1. Lepromatous leprosy (50%) and borderline lepromatous leprosy (25%) patients suffer from this type of skin reaction during the initiation of therapy (within 2 years).
2. This is a **type II lepra reaction**.
3. Acute crops of painful, tender nodules appear along with fever, lymphadenopathy, arthritis and iritis. The lesion may necrose and discharge sterile pus. It may appear in any part of the body.
4. Treatment is done mainly by thalidomide, 100 mg 3 times daily. The dose is gradually reduced over weeks or months. Thalidomide is strictly contraindicated in females of child bearing age due to its teratogenicity. According to some leprologist, thalidomide has no role in ENL. If thalidomide is contraindicated, prednisolone may be used. NSAIDs (as analgesic-antipyretic) are given, if necessary. The dose of clofazimine is increased to 200–300 mg daily for few weeks during the reaction period. Iritis is managed by local instillation of 1% atropine sulphate.

Q. Lesions characteristically found over the shin:

1. Erythema nodosum.
2. Pretibial myxoedema.
3. Necrobiosis lipoidica diabeticorum (NLD).
4. Lichen amyloidosis.

Q. Identification points:

Single or multiple bluish-red, tender, nodular lesion in anterior aspect of one or both legs, especially in younger patients.

SUBCUTANEOUS NODULES — CASE 65

Q. Differential diagnosis (Table 3.6):

1. Lipoma, fibroma.
2. Neurofibroma.
3. Rheumatoid nodule.
4. Rheumatic nodule.
5. Leprosy (*see* Fig. 3.109).
6. Calcinosis.
7. Cysticercosis.
8. Osler's node (*see* Fig. 1.20).
9. Tophi.
10. Xanthoma.
11. Metastatic carcinoma (deposits from carcinoma, lymphoma, leukaemias).
12. Panniculitis.
13. Heberden's and Bouchard's node (OA).

Q. Common sites for rheumatoid nodule (Fig. 3.130):

These nodules signify underlying vasculitis and active disease in rheumatoid arthritis. They are situated:

1. Most commonly over the extensor surface of elbows.
2. Back of the head.
3. Over the sacrum in bed-ridden patients.
4. Extensor tendons of fingers and toes.
5. Over the scapulae.
6. Achilles tendon.
7. Margins of patella.

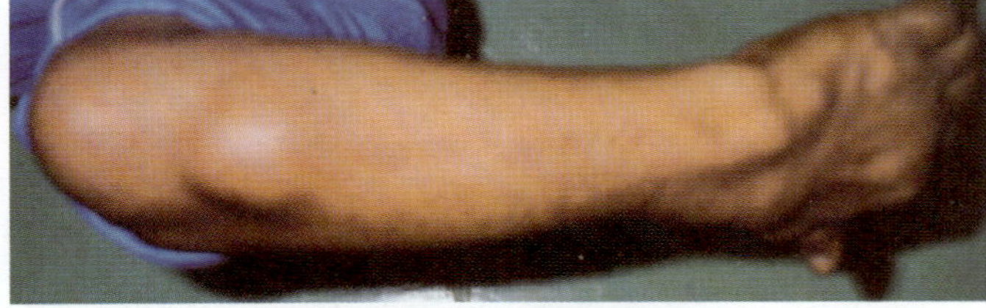

Fig. 3.130: **Rheumatoid nodule** on extensor surface of upper part of forearm

Q. Common sites for rheumatic nodule (Fig. 3.131):

The distribution is more or less like rheumatoid nodules, i.e. situated over the bony prominences or at the site of pressure points while lying in bed. The nodules are formed due to acute rheumatic fever.

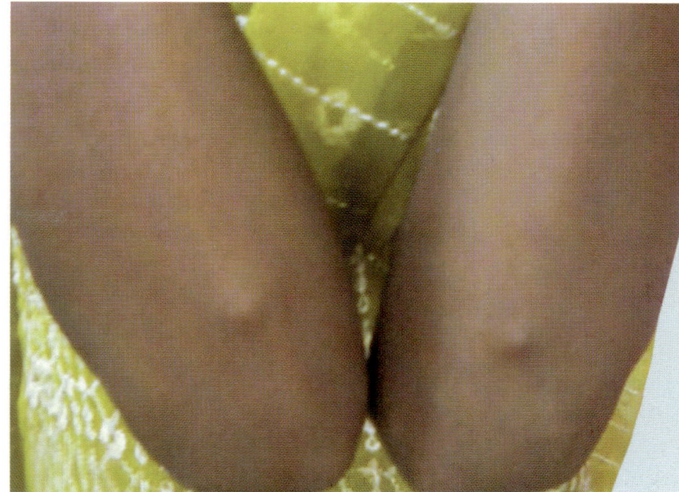

Fig. 3.131: **Rheumatic nodules**—small nodules over olecranon process of a young girl suffering from **acute rheumatic fever**

Q. Common sites for tophi formation (Fig. 3.132):

1. Helix and antihelix (Fig. 3.133).
2. Along ulnar surface of forearm.
3. Olecranon process.
4. Fingers and toes (dorsal aspects).
5. Achilles tendon, and
6. Other pressure points in the body.

Tophi signifies chronic gouty arthritis in a patient and often after ulceration, chalky or pasty material may come out from the nodule. Tophi are small, firm swellings in the subcutaneous tissue mostly around a joint and are nothing but aggregation of monosodium urate (MSU) crystals. Under polaroscopic microscope, urate crystals are needle-shaped and negatively birefringent.

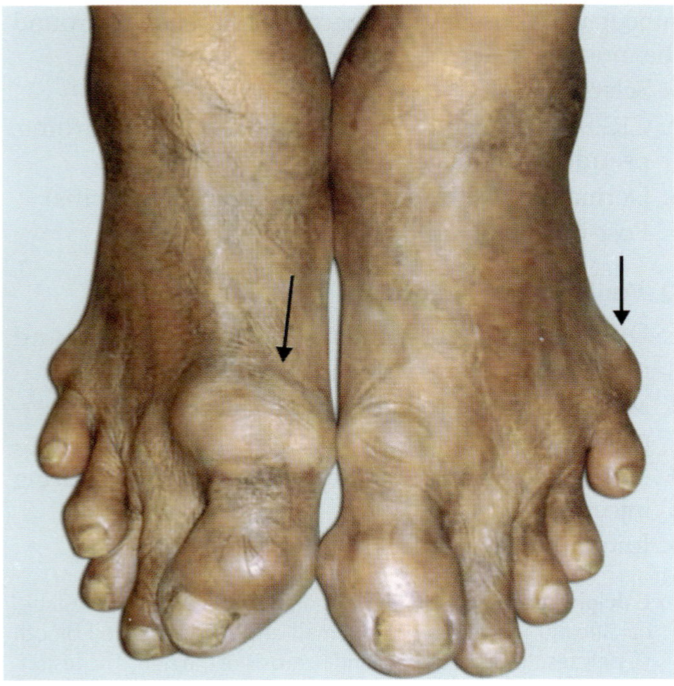

Fig. 3.132: **Chronic tophaceous gout** with tophi present over base of great toe and lateral part of feet

Table 3.6: Differentiation between rheumatoid and rheumatic nodules

Features	Rheumatoid nodule	Rheumatic nodule
1. Size	Big	Relatively smaller
2. Ulceration	Frequently occur	Does not ulcerate
3. Secondary infection	May occur	Not common
4 Tenderness	Non-tender	May be tender
5. Fixity to skin	Very often fixed	Skin is free
6. Incidence	20%	3–5% in India
7. Association	Indicates active disease with +ve RF	Associated with active rheumatic carditis

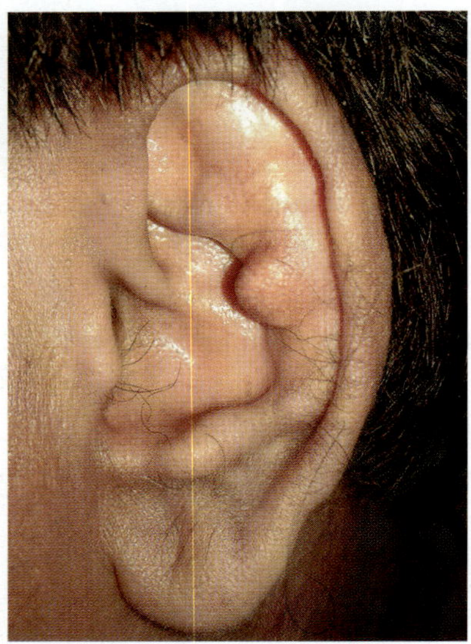

Fig. 3.133: Small **tophi in helix** of ear in chronic gout

- Patients of **pseudogout** have calcium pyrophosphate dihydrate (CPPD) crystals which are rhomboid-shaped and positively birefringent (weakly) under polaroscopic microscope. They do not produce tophi.

Q. What is calcinosis (Fig. 3.117C)?

It is the calcium deposition in the skin (as white papules), subcutaneous tissue or connective tissue sheaths around the muscles. The clinical associations are:

1. Scleroderma.
2. CREST syndrome, SLE, Ehlers-Danlos syndrome, pseudoxanthoma elasticum.
3. Dermatomyositis (especially childhood myositis).
4. Post-infective, tumour and trauma.

Q. Varieties of calcinosis:

1. Dystrophic (with normal serum calcium and phosphorus): Due to collagen vascular diseases.
2. Metastatic: Due to either hypercalcaemia or hyperphosphataemia.
3. Latrogenic: From extravasation of calcium salt during injection.
4. Idiopathic.

- **Calciphylaxis:** A poorly understood disorder where metastatic calcification in the media of small and medium-sized blood vessels results in ischaemia and necrosis of the skin. The lesion is plaque-like, dusky or purplish, extremely tender, which progresses to ulceration. Biopsy of the lesion confirms the diagnosis. A patient of uraemia on haemodialysis or having a kidney transplant may be complicated by calciphylaxis.

Q. Nodules formed by cysticercosis:

These are small firm subcutaneous nodules present in the skin or voluntary muscles anywhere in the body. One should palpate the tongue in search of such a nodule. These nodules contain calcified cyst of *Taenia solium*. Patients are commonly pork-eater and give features of neurocysticercosis (convulsions, behavioural changes, hydrocephalus). Calf muscles may be hypertrophied.

Q. Describe the nodules caused by xanthoma:

Mainly there are two varieties

1. Planous: Classical example is **xanthelasma around the eyes** (*see* Fig. 1.18). They are also seen in palmar creases, below the breast, chest or back, and are characteristically soft, yellowish plaque which are subcutaneous or intracutaneous tissue deposition of lipids.
2. Tuberous: Commonly seen in extensor surface of wrist, elbow, knee, ankle and **buttock** (Fig. 3.134). Xanthomas are seen in patients with prolonged cholestasis or familial hypercholesterolaemia.

Q. What is panniculitis?

These are tender nodules (0.5–10 cm) present in the subcutaneous fat either singly or in multiple crops. Panniculitis may or may not be associated with systemic disease (connective tissue disease, lymphoma, acute

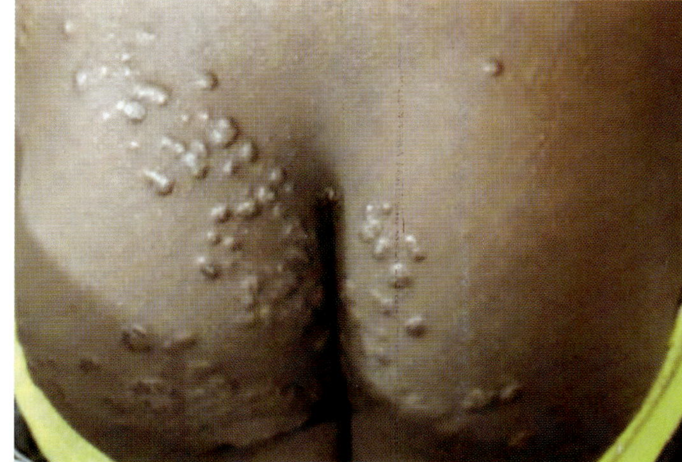

Fig. 3.134: **Xanthoma** over buttocks in familial hypercholesterolaemia

pancreatitis). The hallmarks of diagnosis are presence of fat-filled macrophages, fat cell necrosis and infiltration of inflammatory cells in histological picture. Erythema nodosum is a common example of panniculitis (septal) (Fig. 3.127).

Clinical Wisdom

Thus, subcutaneous nodules are diagnosed by proper history taking, sites of nodule formation, mobility of overlying skin, presence of tenderness and ulceration, arthritis, carditis or any murmur.

DOWN SYNDROME (MONGOLISM) CASE 66

Q. What is Down syndrome?

It is the commonest chromosomal disorder (1 in 700 newborns). Chromosome 21 is present in triplicate (i.e. total 47 chromosomes) as a result of non-disjunction during meiosis and is known as 'trisomy-21'.

Q. Describe the facies (mongol facies) (Fig. 3.135A):

1. Small, round and flat face, brachycephaly; with downy forehead and short, wide fleshy neck.
2. Upwards-slanting eyes (oblique orbital fissure) with epicanthic folds at inner angles.
3. Low set ears; ears are small and dysplastic.
4. Small nose with depressed bridge of the nose.
5. Hypertelorism (widely set eyes).
6. High arched palate with small teeth.
7. Open mouth with protruded and furrowed tongue (macroglossia), with
8. An idiotic look (cheerful idiot—an older terminology which is disheartening).

- There are Brushfield's spot on the iris and typical facial grimace on crying.

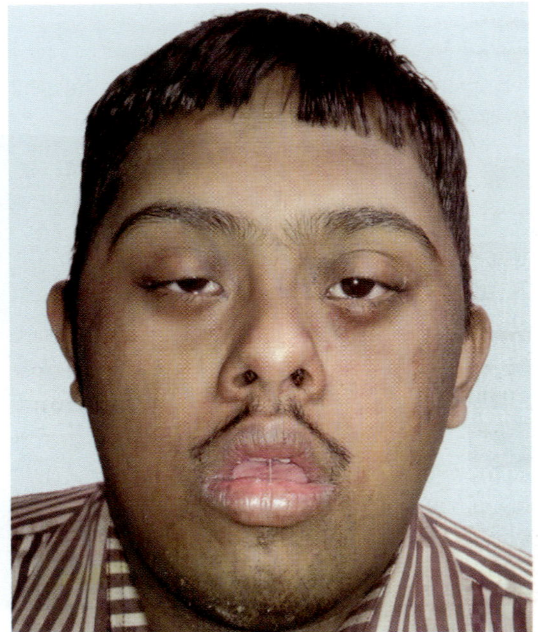

Fig. 3.135A: **Down syndrome** with characteristic facial features

- It is often said that the tongue is normal but it protrudes because of small size of the oral cavity.
- Epicanthic folds may also be seen in Turner's syndrome.

Clinical Wisdom

John Langdon Haydon Down (Langdon-Down) was Physician (1828-1896), the London Hospital, London who first described the syndrome in 1862.

Q. Features in different systems in Down syndrome:

a. CVS: Endocardial cushion defects, e.g. VSD, ASD, PDA.
b. Gastrointestinal system: Duodenal stenosis, biliary atresia, severe periodontal disease.
c. Haematopoietic: There is manyfold higher incidence of acute leukaemia (AML in the newborn and ALL in older children).
d. Neuromuscular: Hypotonia (poor Moro's reflex), floppiness in neonate, seizure disorder.
e. Skeletal: Short-height, joint hyperextensibility.
f. Personality: Very pleasant with clean habits, affectionate, friendly and **fond of music**.
g. Intelligence: IQ is generally low (from mild to severe) and often very much mentally retarded (average IQ 50, ranges 20–75). Speech and social developments are severely affected.

- Patients of Down syndrome may develop early Alzheimer's disease in the 3rd or 4th decade.
- Coeliac disease may be associated with Down syndrome. Sleep apnoea may pose a problem.
- **Breaking news:** Movie starring actor James Martin with Down syndrome won Oscar Award in 2023.

Q. Diagnostic points in hand, foot and eye:

A. Hand:

1. Short and broad hands (simian hand); short, stubby spatula-like fingers (Fig. 3.62A).
2. Single transverse palmar crease (simian crease) (Fig. 3.135B).
3. Clinodactyly (hypoplasia of middle phalanx of 5th finger produces 'incurving' little finger)—Siegert's sign.
4. Missing of one crease in little finger (cause same as point 3).
5. Characteristic dermal markings in fingers (dermatoglyphics): More than eight ulnar loops on fingers, and the ATD angle (distal axial triradii) becomes obtuse.

B. Foot:

1. Increased gap between first and second toe (sandal gap).
2. Sub-hallucial pad of fat.
3. Single, deep and longitudinal crease in the sole of feet.

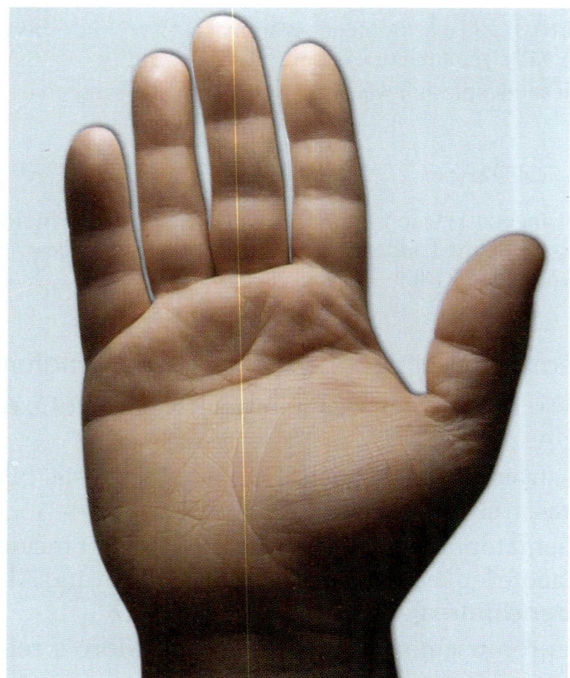

Fig. 3.135B: **Simian crease** in palm in mongolism

C. Eye:

1. Brushfield's spot (whitish speckling on the iris).
2. Sometimes, cataract is present.
3. Rarely, squint and high myopia may be observed.

Q. Cause of death:

1. Recurrent respiratory tract infections.
2. Septal defects in heart, or
3. Acute leukaemia (usually AML).

Q. Management:

There is no definite treatment for Down syndrome. Management is aimed at treatment of respiratory tract infections, acute leukaemia, VSD or proper rehabilitation. They are usually trainable children but may be educable rarely. Average life expectancy is 60 years.

- Down syndrome and Klinefelter's syndrome are associated with increased maternal age (>35 years) whereas, Marfan's syndrome and achondroplasia are seen with increased paternal age. Prenatal diagnosis of Down syndrome may be done by amniocentesis or chorionic villus biopsy.

Q. Identification points:

Typical facies, grimace and behaviour.

HYDROCEPHALUS — CASE 67

Q. What is hydrocephalus?

This is the dilatation of ventricles of brain due to increase in the volume of CSF within the ventricles resulting from a disturbance in the circulation (of CSF). It may be due to obstruction of CSF circulation or there may be failure of CSF absorption by the arachnoid villi.

- Hydrocephalus can occur at any age, but is most common in infants and adults >60 years and older.

Q. Diagnosis of a child with hydrocephalus:

1. Abnormal enlargement of head, especially the frontal area.
2. Sutural separation.
3. Bulging of the anterior fontanelle.
4. 'Setting sun' sign: The eyes appear to be pushed down and thus both the upper bulbar conjunctiva become visible (Fig. 3.136A).
5. Scalp veins are dilated, and the skin over the scalp is thin and shiny.
6. Macewen sign: Skull is resonant (cracked-pot) on percussion.
7. Shrill and high-pitched cry.
8. Irritability, seizures, vomiting, sleepiness, headache, difficulty in feeding, changes in personality.

Q. Circulation of CSF:

Choroid plexus of lateral ventricles (major source of CSF formation)—Foramen of Monro—Third ventricle—Aqueduct of Sylvius—Fourth ventricle in the medulla—Foramen of Magendie and Luschka—Cisterna magna and cisterna pontis—Subarachnoid space. CSF is absorbed into venous sinuses by arachnoid villi.

- Amount or volume of CSF: 100–150 mL. Daily formation of CSF is 1500 mL.

Q. Types of hydrocephalus:

A. **Compensatory:** Due to cerebral atrophy from any cause.

B. **Hypertensive:**
   a. Obstructive: If the circulation of CSF is obstructed within the ventricular system.

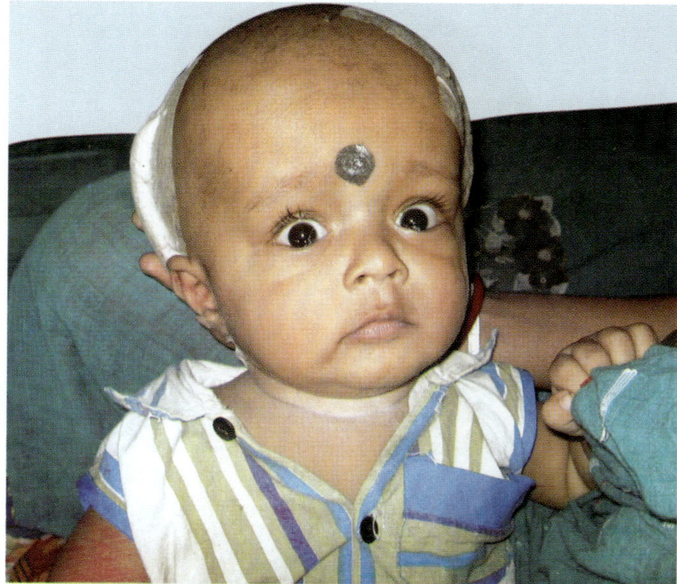

Fig. 3.136A: **Hydocephalus** with 'setting sun' sign. The baby had a recent shunt surgery

b. Non-obstructive or communicating (i.e. obstruction distal to fourth ventricle): Resulting from occlusion of the subarachnoid cisterns (due to arachnoiditis) or interference with the CSF absorption.

Q. Features of late-onset hydrocephalus:

1. Head size may not enlarge.
2. Sutural separation may not be evident.
3. Mental retardation.
4. Presence of papilloedema.
5. Spastic and ataxic child (legs are more involved).
6. Urinary incontinence.

Q. Aetiology of hydrocephalus:

1. Meningitis (bacterial or tuberculous).
2. Head injury.
3. Subarachnoid haemorrhage.
4. Sagittal sinus thrombosis.
5. Brain tumours (posterior fossa).
6. Cerebral haemorrhage.
7. Congenital, e.g. Arnold-Chiari malformation.
8. 'Normal pressure' hydrocephalus.
9. Cerebellar abscess or haemorrhage.
10. 3rd ventricle colloid cyst.

- Obstructive—5, 6, 7, 9 and 10; non-obstructive—1, 2, 3, 4 and 8; 1, 2 and 3 are responsible for majority of cases.

Q. Causes and features of acute hydrocephalus:

The causes are:

1. Head injury with its complications.
2. Subarachnoid haemorrhage.
3. Acute exudative meningitis.
4. Cranial surgery.

The features are:

1. Severe headache and vomiting.
2. Drowsiness, convulsions or coma.
3. Papilloedema may be evident.
4. 6th cranial nerve palsy (false localising sign).
5. Jerks: Brisk (may be lost).
6. Plantar response: Extensor.

Q. What is 'normal pressure' hydrocephalus (NPH)?

It is a misnomer. Initially there is increased pressure but ultimately CSF haemodynamics compromise (ventricles dilate) and it becomes normal or low pressure hydrocephalus. Actually, it is a variety of communicating hydrocephalus. This rare condition is predominantly seen in old age with the triad of symptoms such as **dementia, ataxia** and **urinary incontinence** (Hakim's or Adams triad). Though it may result from head injury, subarachnoid haemorrhage or meningitis, many a time no cause is identified.

- In adult and aged: Hydrocephalus ex-vacuo occurs when an injury or stroke damages the brain and consequently the brain matter shrinks. In Alzheimer's disease, the brain may shrink and CSF fills the extra space. In these situation, the ventricles are dilated and ICP remains normal.

Q. How to diagnose hydrocephalus very early?

By serial recording of head circumference of the child. An increase in the head circumference by more than 1 cm in every 2 weeks for the first 3 months of life, makes the pediatrician suspicious.

Q. What is normal intracranial pressure (ICP)?

It is 5–10 mm of Hg when measured indirectly. Nowadays, devices measure ICP directly by implanting intraventricular catheter into the lateral ventricles. When ICP is >15 mm of Hg, it is known as raised ICP.

Q. What is benign intracranial hypertension (BIH)?

Previously the term BIH was used synonymously with pseudotumour cerebri, meningeal hydrops or otitic hydrocephalus. It is a benign or idiopathic raised ICP developed as a result of diffuse swelling of brain with dilated ventricular system. The patient characteristically presents with headache, vomiting and papilloedema. **BIH commonly develops** from corticosteroid withdrawal, tetracycline or nalidixic acid therapy, hypervitaminosis A, Addison's disease, hypoparathyroidism, or COPD with type II respiratory failure. The CSF is under increased pressure but its analysis remains normal. CT scan of brain is within normal limit except the dilated ventricles. Acetazolamide or repeated lumbar puncture may be of some help.

Q. Diagnosis of hydrocephalus by investigations in children:

1. X-ray of skull:
   i. Enlargement of calvarium.
   ii. Sutural diastasis (separation).
   iii. Thinning of bone.
   iv. Silver-beaten appearance (chronic case).
   v. Erosion of posterior clinoid process.
   vi. Deepened sella turcica.
2. Ventriculography or cisternography by a suitable contrast medium (to see the site of obstruction).
3. Pneumoencephalography is tried to localise the site of obstruction: Not done nowadays.
4. CT or MRI scan (to show enlarged ventricles and cortical atrophy).
5. CSF flow studies may be done (CSF analysis is not informative).
6. Measurement of ICP: Diagnostic.

Q. Differential diagnosis of hydrocephalus:

1. Megalencephaly (with severe mental retardation, and absence of IIT).
2. Chronic subdural haematoma (mostly with enlargement of the parietal regions).

Q. Treatment of hydrocephalus:

It is important to treat the child before irreparable damage sets in:

a. Drug: Acetazolamide (50–75 mg/kg/day) or furosemide for reduction of CSF production.

b. Shunt surgery:
   i. Ventriculo-peritoneal (commonly used).
   ii. Ventriculo-atrial.
   iii. Ventriculo-caval (to jugular vein or superior vena cava).
   iv. Lateral ventricle to cisterna magna.
   v. Ventriculo-ureteric.

   Different varieties of silastic valves are used and the commonly used one is 'Spitz-Holter' valve.

c. Miscellaneous: Compressive head wrapping, repeated lumbar puncture (in acute hydrocephalus), different diuretics, steroid, isosorbide are tried. Neurosurgical removal of tumour, if necessary.

- For communicating variety: Drugs used; for obstructive variety: Shunt surgery done.

Q. Complications of 'shunt':

1. Shunt closure: Displacement, kinking or plugging of the shunt.
2. Ventriculitis (by *Staphylococcus albus*).
3. Bacterial colonisation of the shunt.
4. Shunt nephritis (acute glomerulonephritis).
5. SVC obstruction.

Q. How the head circumference of a child is measured?

Ideally by a steel tape. The tape is passed over the most prominent part of the occiput and the forehead above the supraorbital ridges.

- Always measure the head circumference in a child with apparent enlargement of head.

RICKETS — CASE 68

Q. Clinical manifestations:

A. Symptoms:

1. Fretful, irritable, pale child with flabby muscles in the age group of 4 months to 2 years.
2. Delayed development.
3. Failure to sit, crawl, stand and walk at the normal ages.
4. Recurrent respiratory and GI tract infections.
5. Rocking of head in pillows with sweating in forehead (during sleep).
6. Poor dentition with late eruption of teeth.
7. Manifestations of tetany may develop.

B. Signs:

a. Head:
   1. **Craniotabes** (thin and deformed skull)—*earliest manifestation of rickets*, when the occipital or parietal bone is compressed and released, there is feeling like compressing a ping pong ball (egg-shell crackling feeling). It is seen below the age of 1 year and is due to small islands of unossified area in the skull.
   2. Frontal and parietal bossing with large head (philosopher's head).
   3. Quadrate skull with 'hot-cross bun' appearance; skull is apparently larger than normal.
   4. Widening of sutures.
   5. Late appearance of temporary teeth.
   6. Delayed closure of anterior fontanelle.

- Other causes of *craniotabes* are hydrocephalus, congenital syphilis and osteogenesis imperfecta.

b. Chest:
   1. Pigeon chest (pectus carinatum).
   2. Rachitic rosary (swelling or beaded appearance of the costochondral junction).
   3. Harrison's sulcus (linear transverse depression by the side of xiphoid process).
   4. Kyphoscoliosis.

c. Abdomen:
   Pot-belly—due to multiple factors like weakness of abdominal muscles, gaseous distension, hepato-splenomegaly, visceroptosis or lumbar lordosis.

d. Extremities:
   1. Epiphyseal enlargement at wrists and ankles.
   2. 'Knock knee' or 'bow leg' (when the child starts walking and thus, unusual before 1 year).
   3. Genu valgum, varum or recurvatum (acrobatic rickets).
   4. Pelvic deformities (triradiate pelvis—occurs in later childhood and may produce difficulties during childbirth).

- **Rickets** develops as a result of vitamin D deficiency in growing children before the fusion of epiphysis, while vitamin D deficiency in adults after closure of epiphyseal growth plate is **osteomalacia**.

Q. Different range of ages in 'Pediatrics age group':

According to Indian Academy of Pediatrics (IAP), the 'pediatrics age group' of paients range from birth to 18 years of age. This group is subdivided according to period of life as:

- Neonate (newborn) : First 4 weeks after birth
- Infant : First year of life
- Toddler : 1–3 years
- Preschool child : 3–6 years
- School age child : 6–10 years (boys), 6–12 years (girls)
- Adolescent : 10–18 years

Q. How to diagnose rickets?

a. Classical clinical features.
b. Radiological changes (of upper extremity):
   1. Cupping, widening and fraying (saucer deformity) of lower end of radius and ulna.
   2. Diminution of bone density.
   3. Widening of wrist (soft issue shadow).
   4. Increased distance between the distal end of bones of forearm and metacarpal bones because of non-calcification of the rachitic metaphysis.
c. Biochemical changes:
   1. Plasma alkaline phosphatase is raised (of diagnostic value): Indicates osteoblastic activity.
   2. Low phosphorus (due to associated secondary hyperparathyroidism).
   3. Plasma calcium tends to fall from its normal value (usually remains normal).
   4. Plasma 25-hydroxyvitamin D_3 level is low in majority of patients (<10 ng/mL).

- Clinical rickets may occur with normal level of plasma calcium and phosphorus.
- Normal serum allkaline phosphatase level a) 2–4.5 Bodansky units, b) 4–13 King-Armstrong units , c) 35–130 International units/per liter.
- Remember, in health, alkaline phosphatase is elevated during skeletal growth.

Q. What are the early manifestations of rickets?

1. Irritability and restlessness.
2. Head rolling and sweating in forehead, especially during sleep.
3. Craniotabes.
4. Rachitic rosary.
5. Big anterior fontanelle.
6. Swelling of wrists.
7. Delayed dentition.

Q. Radiological evidences of 'healing rickets':

1. The density of metaphysis is increased and roughness is diminished.
2. Epiphyseal cartilage becomes horizontal.
3. Horizontal "Harrison's line" are seen in the lower end of diaphysis (initially near the epiphysis).

Q. Management of rickets:

1. Vitamin D: 1000–2000 IU orally daily, depending on the age of the child and severity of the disease, for 6–12 weeks followed by daily supplement of 400 IU of vitamin D **(standard daily requirement of vitamin D is 400 IU or 10 μg)**. Few clinicians prefer larger doses (up to 800 IU); 500–1000 mg calcium is prescribed daily. Therapeutic dose is continued so long the alkaline phosphatase level remains high (normalisation of alkaline phosphatase is a good indicator of healing).
2. Diet: Must be rich in vitamin D and calcium e.g. milk, cod liver oil, halibut liver oil, fatty fish, egg, liver, fortified margarine should be taken.
3. Calcium may be given in the form of lactate or gluconate.
4. Treatment of **tetany** is done by inj. calcium gluconate (10% solution) 20 mL in normal saline by IV route, slowly to run over 4–8 hours (inj. calcium chloride may be given). If tetany is not controlled by calcium, administration of IV magnesium may be necessary (in patients with malabsorption, magnesium depletion may be a contributing factor to tetany). Correction of alkalosis should also be done.
5. If after administration of vitamin D, no sign of radiological healing is seen within 4 weeks, the dose is increased to several thousand IU. If no healing is observed even after this larger dose, 'refractory rickets' should be considered.
6. The child should be encouraged to play outdoors for exposure to sunlight.

Q. What is 'refractory rickets'?

Definition: These patients develop rickets in spite of receiving the preventive daily dose (400 IU) of vitamin D and do not show signs of healing rickets in X-ray, obtained 2 weeks after the parenteral administration (deep IM) of 2 doses of 6 lakh IU of vitamin D given at 15 days interval. The causes are:

1. Renal:
   i. Renal tubular acidosis.
   ii. Fanconi's syndrome.
   iii. Familial hypophosphataemic rickets (X-linked dominant; with renal tubular loss of phosphate).
2. Malabsorption (e.g. coeliac disease).
3. Hepatic dysfunction: Impairs 25-hydroxylation of vitamin D.
4. Miscellaneous:
   i. Hypophosphatasia (deficiency of alkaline phosphatase).
   ii. Children on long-term antiepileptic drugs.
   iii. Certain tumours may secrete parathormone like substances.

- Alkaline phosphatase is low in one variety of rickets only: Rickets due to hypophosphatasia.
- For causes of rickets, read 'Bedside Clinics in Medicine, Part II'.

Q. Treatment of 'refractory rickets':

a. Large dose as much as 15 lakh IU of vitamin D, deep IM is administered daily and subsequently, 3 lakh IU of vitamin D is used daily as maintenance dose. In the presence of renal disease, 1 mg of 1α-hydroxycholecalciferol may be given daily, orally.
b. Administration of neutral phosphate salts, and
c. The treatment of the primary cause.

Q. What is vitamin D_2 and D_3?

Vitamin D_2 is ergocalciferol, and vitamin D_3 is cholecalciferol.

Q. Commonest cause of vitamin D deficiency in India:

Lack of exposure to sunlight.

Q. What is hypervitaminosis D?

Chronic oral intake of large dosage of vitamin D (50000–100000 IU daily) for months may give rise to hypotonia, anorexia, nausea, vomiting, irritability, constipation, abdominal pain, failure to thrive and pallor. Hypervitaminosis D is associated with high serum calcium level. Hypercalcaemia ultimately leads to renal damage and eventually metastatic calcification develops. The treatment is:

1. Administration of vitamin D is stopped immediately.
2. EDTA, sodium phytate may be used.

Q. Megavitamin question–vitamins responsible:

There may be **'hypervitaminosis'** with:

1. Vitamin A: Anorexia, nausea, vomiting, pain abdomen, bone pain, weight loss, cracked lips, benign intracranial hypertension, hyperostosis, hair loss and desquamation of skin. High doses of carotenoids are avoided in smokers due to an increased risk of lung cancer, and in hypothyroid patients who may develop carotenaemia.
2. Vitamin D: Mentioned above.
3. Vitamin C: Oxalate stone, scurvy in the offspring, increased intestinal absorption of iron.
4. Pyridoxine or vitamin B_6: Sensory polyneuropathy.
5. Vitamin K: Jaundice in newborn if given to pregnant women.
6. Vitamin E: Malaise, headache, GI ailments and reduced platelet aggregation.
7. Niacin: Flushing, pruritus, aggravation of asthma, gout and acanthosis nigricans.

Q. When the fontanelles close normally?

Anterior fontanelle closes by 10–24 months. Posterior fontanelle closes by 2–3 months after birth.

Q. Delayed closure of anterior fontanelle:

1. Malnutrition.
2. Rickets.
3. Congenital syphilis.
4. Cretinism.
5. Hydrocephalus.
6. Down syndrome.
7. Mucopolysaccharidosis.
8. Achondroplasia.

Q. Bulged anterior fontenelle:

1. Crying infant.
2. Increased intracranial tension (e.g. meningitis, encephalitis, brain tumour).
3. Hydrocephalus.
4. Benign intracranial hypertension (corticosteroid withdrawal, vitamin A overdose, tetracycline therapy).
5. Galactosaemia.

Q. High arched palate (Fig. 3.136B):

1. Down syndrome.
2. Marfan's syndrome.
3. Cyanotic congenital heart diseases.
4. Turner's syndrome.
5. Chronic thumb-sucking.
6. Crouzon syndrome.

- Keep the patient's mouth wide open and look for palate keeping the eyes at the level of patient's upper incisor teeth—If the roof of palate is not visible, it is known as high arched palate.

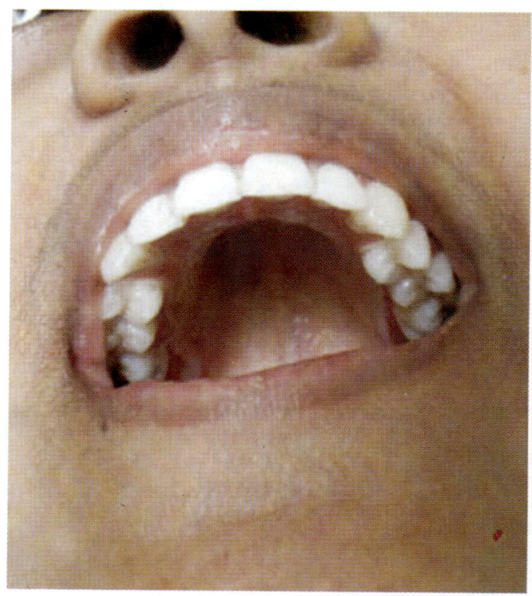

Fig. 3.136B: High arched palate

Q. Frontal bossing (prominence) of skull:

1. Thalassaemia major.
2. Rickets.
3. Congenital syphilis.
4. Hydrocephalus.
5. Achondroplasia.
6. Acromegaly.
7. Ectodermal dysplasia.
8. Ehlers-Danlos syndrome.

Q. Depressed bridge of the nose (Figs 1.66A, 3.37, and 3.105):

1. Racial
2. Cretinism.
3. Thalassaemia major.
4. Down syndrome.
5. Lepromatous leprosy.
6. Congenital syphilis.
7. Wegener's granulomatosis.

8. Ectodermal dysplasia.
9. Achondroplasia.
10. Osteopetrosis (marble bone disease).
11. Hurler syndrome.
12. Midline granuloma.

Q. Upwards-slanting (mongoloid) of eyes:

1. Racial.
2. Down syndrome.
3. Ectodermal dysplasia.
4. Prader-Willi syndrome.

Q. Anti-mongoloid slant of eyes:

1. Noonan's syndrome.
2. Apert's syndrome.
3. Turner's syndrome.
4. Alport syndrome.

Q. Hypertelorism (widely set eyes) (Fig. 3.137):

1. Racial.
2. Down syndrome.
3. Cretinism.
4. Thalassaemia major.
5. Craniostenosis (e.g. Crouzon syndrome).
6. Turner's sydrome.
7. Ehlers-Danlos syndrome.
8. Noonan's syndrome.

- **Hypertelorism** is diagnosed clinically by measuring inter inner-canthal distance between two eyes which is more than half of the inter-pupillary distance, or inter-pupillary distance >85 mm where the average normal value is 60 mm. Hyperplasia of lesser wing of sphenoid bone is usually responsible for hypertelorism (e.g. in thalassaemia).

Q. Hypotelorism:

It is the decreased distance between orbits, and is found in ethmocephaly, cebocephalia or Patau's syndrome.

Q. Sabre tibia (anterior tibial bowing) (Fig. 3.138):

1. Congenital syphilis.
2. Paget's disease (osteitis deformans).
3. Rickets.
4. Osteogenesis imperfecta.
5. Osteopetrosis.

- 'Sabre' literally means cavalry sword with curved blade.

Q. Prominent supraorbital ridges:

1. Racial.
2. Acromegaly.
3. Paget's disease.
4. Achondroplasia.
5. Hydrocephalus.
6. Thalassaemia.

Q. Low set ears:

1. Down syndrome (Fig. 3.135A).
2. Elfin facies.
3. Trisomy-13 (Patau's syndrome).
4. Trisomy-18 (Edwards syndrome).

- Normally, 1/3rd of the length of pinna is seen above an imaginary horizontal line, extending from outer canthus of eye to ipsilateral pinna. If <1/3rd of length of pinna is seen above that line, low set ears are said to be present.

Q. Deep ear lobe cleft (Frank's sign) (Fig. 3.139):

Though occasionally congenital, the prominent diagonal crease seen over the ear lobe is now well-recognised as strong and independent risk factor for coronary heart disease.

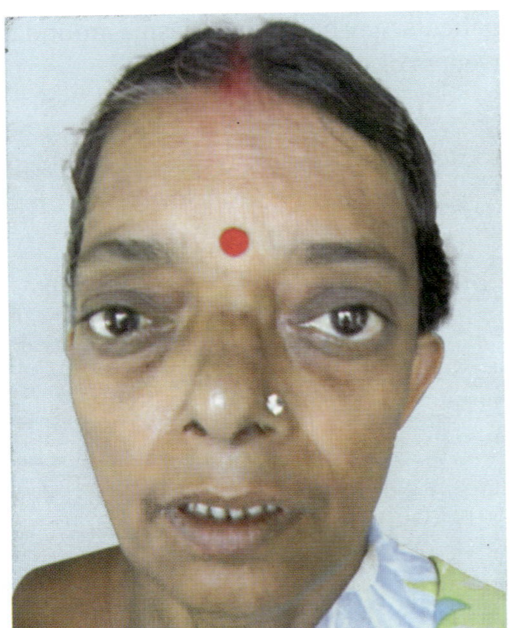

Fig. 3.137: Hypertelorism (widely set eyes) in craniostenosis

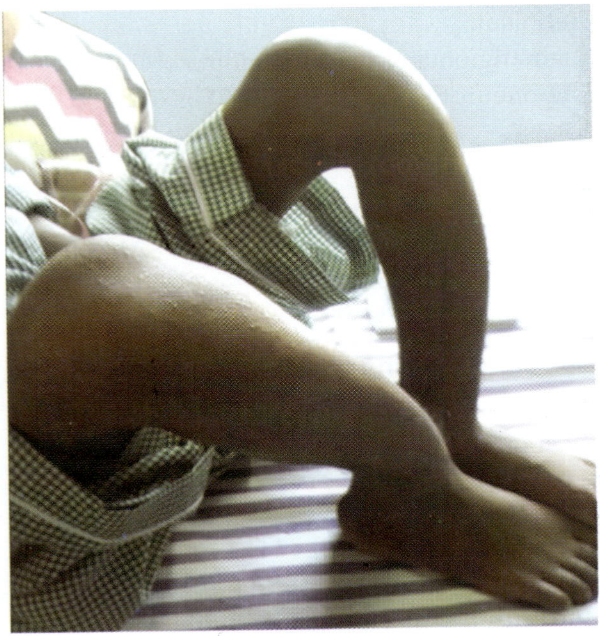

Fig. 3.138: Sabre tibia in rickets

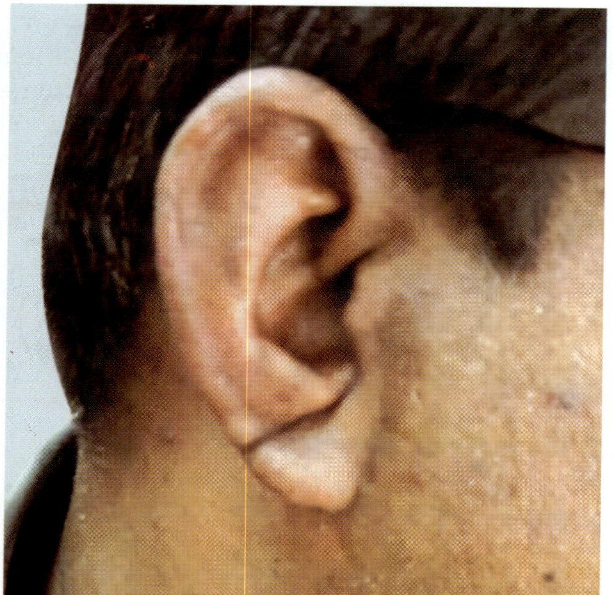

Fig. 3.139: **Diagonal ear lobe crease**—a strong morphological feature of coronary artery disease

Q. Short neck:

1. Cranio-vertebral anomalies.
2. Cretinism.
3. Down syndrome.
4. Turner's syndrome.
5. Hurler syndrome.
6. Noonan's syndrome.

Q. Low hairline (hairline below C_4 vertebra):

1. Klippel-Feil anomaly.
2. Turner's syndrome (Fig. 3.39).
3. Pseudohypoparathyroidism.
4. Noonan's syndrome.

Q. Big lips:

1. Acromegaly.
2. Cretinism.
3. Haemangioma or lymphangioma of lip.
4. Angioneurotic oedema of lips (Fig. 3.29).

Q. Small chin (micrognathia):

1. Turner's syndrome.
2. Treacher Collins syndrome.
3. William's syndrome.
4. Foetal alcohol syndrome.

Q. Blue sclera (as the choroid pigment is visible):

1. Osteogenesis imperfecta (Fig. 3.7).
2. Newborn baby.
3. Marfan's syndrome.
4. Ehlers-Danlos syndrome.

Q. Other bedside stigmata for clue to diagnosis:

- **Hutchinson's triad (congenital syphilis):** Hutchinson's teeth, interstitial keratitis, VIIIth nerve deafness.
- Monkey face: Marasmus, hypertrichosis lanuginosa.
- **Polydactyly (supernumerary fingers)** (Fig. 3.61B): Congenital, Laurence-Moon-Biedl (LMB) syndrome, associated with retinal degeneration/mental retardation/genital hypoplasia.
- Quadrate skull: Rickets, osteopetrosis.
- **Perforation of palate** (*see* Fig. 2.31): Leprosy, tuberculosis, malignancy, syphilis, congenital, irradiation.

Q. Identification points (rickets):

1. Fretful child.
2. Apparently large head.
3. Swelling of lower end of wrists and ankles.
4. Hypotonia.
5. Pot-bellied abdomen.
6. 'Knock knee' or 'bow leg'.

MYXOEDEMA — CASE 69

Q. What is myxoedema?

Myxoedema results from failure of the thyroid gland (primary disease of the thyroid) after puberty and is characterised by wide-spread deposition of mucinous material (mucopolysaccharides, hyaluronic acid and chondroitin sulphate) in different parts of the body, and is clinically manifested by poverty of physical, mental and metabolic activities

Q. Describe the facies in myxoedema (hypothyroidism) (Fig. 3.140):

1. Dull expressionless, puffy face (periorbital puffiness with baggy lower eyelids).
2. Coarse hair, fall of hair in scalp (patchy alopecia) and lateral 1/3rd of eyebrows (madarosis).
3. Dry, rough and coarse skin.
4. Facial pallor (sometimes, rose-purple malar flush is seen); thick lips and macroglossia may be present. The patients may have xanthelasma around the eyes.
5. Hoarseness of voice with bradylalia.

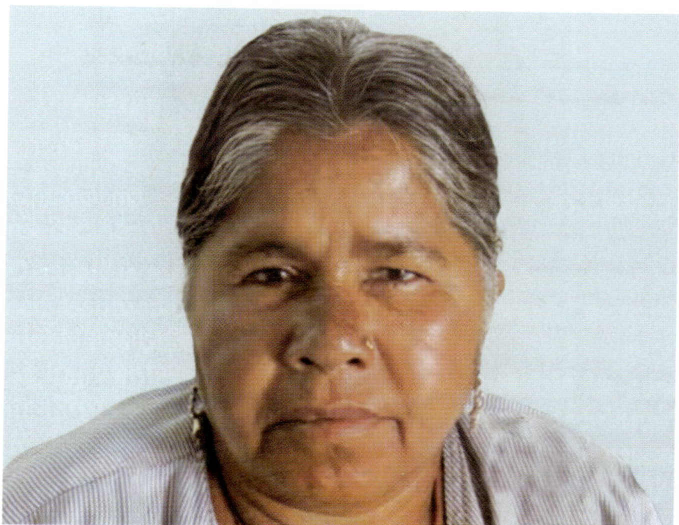

Fig. 3.140: Expressionless puffy face in **myxoedema**

- Always look at the swollen neck and fullness of the supraclavicular fossa or for any thyroidectomy scar during inspection of face. Myxoedema is one of the D/D of *moon face as well as masked face*.
- **'Bags under the eyes'** or **'baggy lower eyelids'** are often seen in insomnia, senility, chronic alcoholism, prolonged crying, nephrotic syndrome and myxoedema. It may not have any clinical significance (Figs 3.8 and 3.141).

Clinical Wisdom

Madarosis (Queen Anne's sign) is common in leprosy, myxoedema, overactive immune system, alopecia areata, amyloidosis and neurodermatitis (Fig. 3.142).

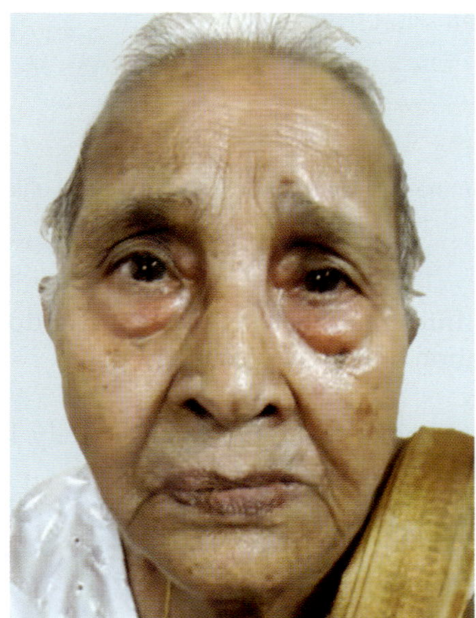

Fig. 3.141: **Baggy lower eyelids** due to senility

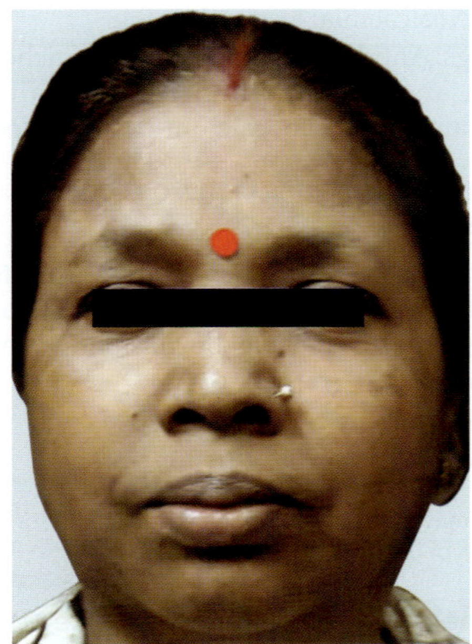

Fig. 3.142: **Madarosis**—loss of lateral third of eyebrows in myxoedema

Q. Is there any goitre?

Usually thyroid tissue is not readily palpable in myxoedema. If palpable, think of:

1. Hashimoto's thyroiditis.
2. Iodine deficiency (less common).
3. Use of antithyroid drugs (lithium, amiodarone, iodide), and
4. Malignancy of the thyroid gland.

Clinical Wisdom

Model case with diagnosis: It is a patient of myxoedema probably due to Hashimoto's thyroiditis.

Q. Why do you say myxoedema (Table 3.7)?

Myxoedema is common in females and there are presence of the following:

A. Common *symptoms* are (if you are allowed to take the history):
   i. Tiredness, lethargy, somnolence; hoarse voice.
   ii. Weight gain; non-pitting swelling of legs.
   iii. Cold intolerance; dryness of skin.
   iv. Constipation.
   v. Menorrhagia or irregular bleeding.
   vi. Effort angina.
   vii. Loss of libido.
   viii. Stiff and aching muscles, arthralgia.
   ix. Deafness.
   x. Repeated abortions in productive age.

B. The *signs* are:
   i. Classical 'facies' with physical sluggishness.
   ii. Dry, cold, rough or coarse skin with lustreless, brittle and scanty hairs. There may be lemon-yellow tint of the skin due to carotenaemia.
   iii. Moderate to severe anaemia.
   iv. Deep and hoarse voice (due to myxomatous infiltration of vocal cord); bradylalia; macroglossia
   v. Sinus bradycardia.
   vi. Obesity (mild) with non-pitting oedema or solid oedema of legs (supraclavicular fossa, neck and limbs are swollen more): Due to deposition of mucopolysaccharides substances.
   vii. Delayed relaxation of ankle jerk (it is better to demonstrate by 'special method' where the patient has to kneel-down on a chair).

- One must examine all the points. Weight gain occurs despite a poor appetite.
- *Bradylalia* is also seen in depression and parkinsonism.
- *Heat intolerance* is seen in hyperthyroidism and menopause.

Clinical Wisdom

Other common causes of **hoarse voice** are laryngitis, singer's nodule, voice-abuse, excessive use of tobacco, recurrent laryngeal nerve palsy (e.g. bronchogenic carcinoma), bulbar palsy and angioneurotic oedema.

Table 3.7: Differentiation between primary (myxoedema) and secondary hypothyroidism

Features	Primary	Secondary
1. Skin	Thick and without wrinkles	Thin with fine wrinkles
2. Hair	Coarse	Fine
3. Menstrual irregularities	Menorrhagia	Amenorrhoea
4. Secondary sexual characters	Normal	Poor
5. Heart size	May be enlarged	Small
6 Goitr	May be present	Absent
7. Soft tissue oedema	Marked	Absent
8. Blood pressure	Normal or high	Low
9. Cholesterol	Increased	Normal
10. TSH	High	Low
11. Plasma cortisol	Normal	Low
12. TRH stimulation test	Exaggerated response	No response
13. Thyroid autoantibodies	May be present	Absent

- Primary: Disease of the thyroid, secondary: Hypothalamic-pituitary disease.
- To diagnose primary and secondary hypothyroidism clinically, one should examine the skin, hairs, secondary sexual characters and soft tissue oedema.

Q. Why there is anaemia in myxoedema?

1. Lack of thyroxine: Normocytic normochromic type.
2. Menorrhagia: Iron deficiency anaemia.
3. Sometimes, myxoedema is associated with pernicious anaemia.

Q. Mention causes of 'pallor without anaemia':

1. Peripheral circulatory failure (e.g. low cardiac output in acute LVF) or shock (ashen-grey pallor with cold and clammy skin), or vasoconstriction due to any cause; syncope.
2. Acute myocardial infarction.
3. Very tight aortic stenosis or mitral stenosis.
4. Myxoedema (pallor > anaemia): Pallor is due to vasoconstriction plus lemon-yellow tint due to carotenaemia, plus anaemia.
5. Nephrotic syndrome.
6. Sheehan's syndrome or panhypopituitarism.
7. Vasovagal attack, fear, exposure to cold, intense emotion; increased carotenoid pigment.
8. Night workers.
9. Oedematous conditions, e.g. anasarca.
10. Thick skin (e.g. scleroderma).

- **Pallor** may be associated with or without anaemia:
  a. Pallor with anaemia: All types of severe anaemia, SBE, etc.
  b. Pallor without anaemia: Described above.

Q. Mention the causes of constipation in clinical practice:

Though difficult to **define**, constipation is the infrequent passage of hard stools which is very difficult to evacuate, or stool frequency <3 times/week (highly subjective).

A. Acute: Intestinal obstruction; acute abdomen (e.g. perforation of hollow viscus).

B. Chronic:

a. Faulty habits, lack of physical activity, less intake of fibre; less access to toilet facility.
b. Painful anal conditions, e.g. anal fissure, haemorrhoids, proctitis.
c. Obstructive lesions like rectal carcinoma or stricture.
d. Disturbed motility: Irritable bowel syndrome, systemic sclerosis, pregnancy, myopathy, Chagas disease, parkinsonism, spinal injury, atonic colon, chronic idiopathic constipation.
e. Metabolic: Hypothyroidism, hypokalaemia, hypercalcaemia; lead poisoning.
f. Drugs: Antidepressants, codeine, anticholinergics, iron and calcium supplements, aluminium containing antacid, calcium-channel blockers.

Q. Cardiovascular signs in myxoedema:

1. Pulse: Sinus bradycardia.
2. BP: Systolic pressure may be high due to hypercholesterolaemia and atherosclerosis (with or without xanthelasma). There may be diastolic hypertension.
3. Features of CCF (rare).
4. Cardiomyopathy.
5. Features of pericardial effusion, rarely.

- Patient may complain of anginal pain (IHD) or exertional shortness of breath.

Q. Why there is cardiomegaly in myxoedema?

1) Cardiac dilatation, 2) Pericardial effusion, or 3) Cardiomyopathy.

Q. Dermatological manifestations in myxoedema:

Non-pitting oedema of hands and feet, periorbital puffiness, dry and lustreless skin with alopecia, purplish lips, malar flush, xanthelasma, carotenaemia and occasionally erythema ab igne.

Q. Features in nervous system in myxoedema:

1. Higher function:
   i. Poor memory, delayed cerebration.
   ii. Psychosis (myxoedema madness).
   iii. Depression.
   iv. Myxoedema coma.
   v. Mental confusion, convulsions due to syndrome of inappropriate ADH secretion (SIADH): Rare.
2. Speech: Slow (bradylalia), sluggish and hoarse.
3. Cranial nerves: Nerve type of deafness.
4. Cerebellar ataxia.
5. Hypotonia; proximal muscle weakness.
6. **Ankle Jerk: Delayed relaxation** (myotonic reflex); at times there is 'hung-up reflex'.
7. Entrapment neuropathy: Carpal tunnel syndrome.
8. Myotonia (Hoffman's syndrome): Painful cramps in muscles.
9. Muscle stiffness, and aches and pains in muscle; percussion myoedema (a small ridge of temporary swelling at the point of stimulation by hammer).
10. Rarely, pseudomyotonia.
11. Peripheral neuropathy, rarely.
12. Unmasking of myasthenia gravis.
13. Hypokalaemic periodic paralysis.

Q. What is subclinical hypothyroidism?

The patient is asymptomatic (or with few symptoms) and clinically euthyroid but biochemically T_3 and T_4 are in the lower limit of normal with high TSH. These patients should be treated, if TSH is >10 µU/mL with the goal of normalising TSH.

Q. What is myxoedema coma?

It is a rare but dangerous presentation of myxoedema, seen usually in elderly during winter months, due to acute thyroid hormone deficiency and is characterised by:

1. Hypothermia (body is cold and dry without any shivering)—temperature as low as 80°F.
2. Hypotension.
3. Hyponatraemia.
4. Hypoventilation with CO_2 retention.
5. Hypoxia.
6. Hypoglycaemia.
7. Bradycardia.
8. Convulsions.
9. Unconsciousness.

There is very high mortality (50%), and the survival depends upon early recognition and treatment.

Q. Carotenaemia (carotenoderma) and its clinical associations:

Carotenaemia is the presence of increased amount of carotene within the body. It is seen in:

1. Eating large quantities of carrots, oranges, papaya, mango and other vegetables, e.g. squash.
2. Hypothyroid (due to impaired metabolism of carotene in the liver).
3. Diabetes mellitus.
4. Receiving β-carotene for the treatment of erythropoietic porphyria.
5. Anorexia nervosa.
6. Simmond's disease.
7. Castrated male.

It produces an orange-yellow or lemon-yellow colour of skin, especially of face (forehead and nasolabial folds), palms and soles. Sclera never turns yellow (D/D of jaundice).

Q. What is juvenile myxoedema?

In this condition, hypothyroidism starts during childhood and adolescence period (before puberty) but the thyroid function is normal at birth or infancy. There is delayed puberty, growth retardation with delayed bone age and galactorrhoea. See also page 320.

Q. How will you investigate the case?

1. Blood:
   a. Low Hb (usually normocytic normochromic, or macrocytic anaemia) and low RBC count.
   b. Cholesterol: High (>200 mg/dL).
2. Chest X-ray: Cardiac shadow may be enlarged (heart failure or pericardial effusion).
3. ECG:
   a. Low voltage (R-waves in limb leads are <5 mm and that in precordial leads are <10 mm).
   b. Sinus bradycardia.
   c. Non-specific ST-T changes.
4. Plasma TSH estimation: Elevated in myxoedema (normal value 0.3–5 µU/mL).
5. Plasma T_3 and T_4 estimation: Low in myxoedema (normal value of T_3 is 80–150 ng/100 mL and that of T_4 is 4–12 µg/100 mL).
6. Radioactive Iodine 131 uptake by the thyroid gland is reduced.
7. Photomotogram (instrumental recording of jerks): Delayed relaxation of ankle jerk; not used now.
8. Muscle enzymes: Elevated LDH, SGOT (AST) and CK.
9. FNAC and USG of thyroid gland in selective cases may be helpful.
10. Thyroid peroxidase (TPO) antibodies may be demonstrated in Hashimoto's thyroiditis.

- Serum T_3 does not discriminate reliably between euthyroid and hypothyroid patients, and ideally should not be measured in a case of myxoedema.
- Biochemical abnormatities: Hyperlipidaemia, hyponatraemia, ↑CK and LDH, hyperprolactinaemia.

Q. D/D of myxoedema:

1. Ageing.
2. Nephrotic syndrome.
3. Angioneurotic oedema.
4. Post-menopausal syndrome.

Q. How to treat this case?

An initial daily dose of 50 µg of L-thyroxine (i.e. T_4) is recommended, and can be increased by 25–50 µg increments at 2–3 weeks' interval until an euthyroid state is attained and the dose is then maintained. In majority, usually the maintenance dose is 100–150 µg/day. The drug is given as a single daily dose (before breakfast) because of its long half-life (7 days). Therapy should usually be uninterrupted and 'life-long'. Efficacy of replacement therapy is measured by serum TSH level.

If the patient suffers from angina pectoris, start the daily dose with 25 µg and increase by 25 µg at 4 weeks' interval with performing serial ECGs. Increased dose may precipitate anginal pain. During pregnancy, an increase in T_4 dosage about 25–50 µg is usually needed.

Q. How to treat myxoedema coma?

It is a medical emergency and should be treated promptly.

1. Triiodothyronine (T_3): 20 µg IV bolus is followed by 20 µg every 8 hourly, IV until there is sustained clinical improvement (thyroxine or T_4 is usually not available for parenteral use; if available, T_4 is given as IV bolus in a dose of 400–500 µg). If IV preparation of T_4 is unavailable, T_4 may be given 300 µg stat orally and followed by 100–300 µg daily.
2. Hydrocortisone hemisuccinate: 100 µg, IV, 8 hourly.
3. IV saline infusion: To combat hypotension; monitor cardiac output.
4. Support hypothermia: Slow rewarming of the patient by wrapping with a blanket in a warm room.
5. High-flow oxygen or assisted ventilation. Correct hypoglycaemia and electrolytes imbalance.
6. Treatment of arrhythmias and heart failure accordingly, preferably in an ICU.
7. Antibiotics, as infection is very often the precipitating factor.

Recovery within 24 hours is usual. Lifelong T_4 replacement is required after recovery.

Q. Identification points:

Usually a middle-aged overweight female patient having puffy, expressionless face with baggy lower eyelids and hoarse voice.

Clinical Wisdom

The **'endocrine system'** comprises of: 1. Hypothalamus and pituitary, 2. Thyroid gland, 3. Parathyroid glands, 4. Islets cells of pancreas (endocrine part of pancreas), 5. Adrenal glands, 6. Gonads (testes and ovaries), [and 7. Adipose tissue or mass (adipocyte is an endocrine cell)].

HYPERTHYROIDISM — CASE 70

Q. Common causes of hyperthyroidism (thyrotoxicosis):

1. Graves' disease (diffuse toxic goitre): Commonest cause of thyrotoxicosis.
2. Solitary toxic nodule (adenoma).
3. Toxic multinodular goitre.
4. Subacute thyroiditis.
5. TSH producing pituitary adenoma.

- The word goitre comes from Latin 'gutter' means throat. Goitre is the enlargement of the thyroid gland.

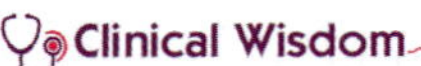
Clinical Wisdom

Model case with diagnosis: This is a patient of Graves' disease with exophthalmos and atrial fibrillation.

Q. Confirmation of the neck swelling as goitre (Fig. 3.143):

Ask the patient to swallow and note whether the swelling moves upwards on swallowing (because of its attachment to the larynx). *Neck swellings which move upwards on swallowing are* thyroid, thyroglossal cyst, subhyoid bursitis, pretracheal and prelaryngeal lymph nodes fixed to trachea and larynx respectively. Thyroglossal cyst also moves upwards with protrusion of the tongue.

- Mild thyromegaly is better seen than felt. Normal adult thyroid gland weighs 20–25 g.

Q. Examination of the thyroid gland:

A. *Inspection* (from the front): Note the position, diffuse or localised nature of swelling, extent, shape, size, overlying skin (dilated veins, thyroidectomy scar, local signs of inflammation) of the swelling present

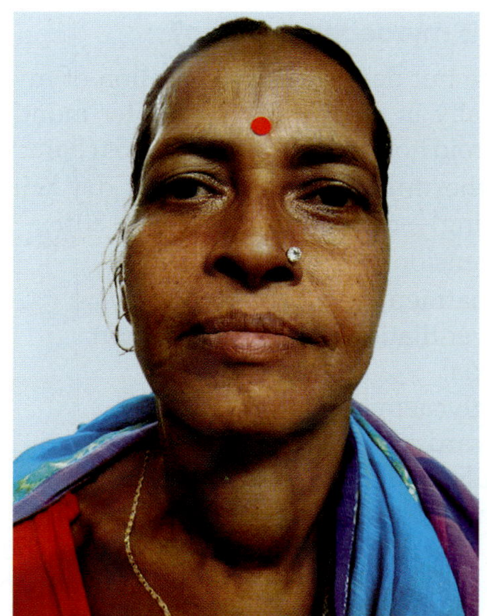

Fig. 3.143: Goitre (the neck swelling) moves upwards on swallowing. The eyes are normal here

in the neck; as thyroid swelling moves upwards on swallowing (spontaneous swallowing or may give a glass of water to swallow), look for the inferior border as soon as the gland moves up.

B. *Palpation* **from the behind: At first, palpation of the thyroid gland should always be done from the behind** on a sitting patient by using both hands (especially by the pulps of the fingers) with slight flexion of the neck (to relax the sternomastoid muscles), and thumbs placed over the nape of the neck. Note the size, shape, consistency, mobility, etc. Palpate the lateral lobes and isthmus.

C. *Palpation* **from the front:** Expose the neck properly and extend the neck slightly. Often each lobe of the thyroid gland is better palpated from the front by **Lahey's method**, e.g. for palpation of the right lobe, the gland is pushed to the right from the left side; the right lobe becomes more prominent and now palpated by the left hand. Henceforth, the following points are noted carefully:
   a. Size: Small or large.
   b. Shape: Localised or diffuse swelling, nodular (single or multiple) or not.
   c. Surface: Smooth or irregular.
   d. Consistency: The different consistency are soft (normal gland, Graves' disease), firm (simple goitre, Hashimoto's thyroiditis), hard (carcinoma of the thyroid) or woody feel (Reidel's thyroiditis); a cystic thyroid swelling may feel solid and a solid one cystic.
   e. Temperature: Warm to feel in Graves' disease.
   f. To get below the swelling: Ask the patient to swallow again (to test the possibility of retrosternal extension).
   g. Mobility: Fixed or mobile (the gland is moved horizontally and vertically). Mobility is lost in carcinoma of the thyroid with infiltration.
   h. Tenderness: Tender (thyroiditis, malignancy, bleeding within cyst) or non-tender.
   i. Relation with the neighbouring structures (pressure effect, fixity, etc.):
      i. Trachea: Deviated or not.
      ii. Carotid sheath: Carotid pulsation is increased in Graves' disease whereas the pulsation may not be felt in a patient with thyroid carcinoma.
      iii. Oesophagus: C/O dysphagia.
      iv. Recurrent layngeal nerve: May produce hoarseness of voice.
      v. Sympathetic trunk: Produces Horner's syndrome (pseudoptosis, miosis, anhidrosis of ipsilateral face, and enophthalmos).
      vi. Sternomastoid muscle (test the function, as malignancy may infiltrate the muscle).
      vii. Skin and subcutaneous tissue.
   j. Thrill: Present over the thyroid gland (present in Graves' disease due to increased vascularity).
   k. Palpate the cervical lymph nodes (from behind).

D. *Percussion:* Though not very helpful, percussion of the sternum may be done to detect the presence of retrosternal goitre (read the section on 'Percussion of the sternum or base of the heart'). Changing the percussion note from resonant to dull note indicates the possibility of retrosternal goitre.

E. *Auscultation:* Search for systolic bruit over the lateral lobes of thyroid gland (present in Graves' disease due to increased vascularity). Ask the patient to hold his breath and then auscultate. Presence of systolic bruit in the thyroid gland may be confused with carotid bruit or venous hum (*see* below).

F. *Measurement:* Measure the circumference of the neck by a tape at the most prominent part.

- The isthmus which lies in front of 2nd, 3rd and 4th tracheal rings, is better palpated from the front. From above downwards in the midline of neck there are thyroid cartilage, cricoid cartilage and isthmus.
- *Hyperthyroidism is often associated with goitre (diffuse or nodular).*
- Cervical lymph nodes should always be palpated to exclude metastasis from thyroid carcinoma.

Clinical Wisdom

Thyroid bruit: More prominent in upper part of neck than lower part (as superior thyroid artery arises from external carotid artery); **Carotid bruit:** Obviously more prominent in lower part of neck (over common carotid artery) than upper part; **Venous hum:** Disappears on gentle pressure applied over base of the neck.
A thyroid bruit is almost pathognomonic of Graves' disease.

Q. Pemberton's sign:

Ask the patient to raise both arms above the shoulders until they touch the ears and to keep them in that position for more than 1 minute. Facial congestion (plethora), central cyanosis, respiratory distress with stridor, and venous congestion of head and neck occurs in patient with retrosternal goitre or mediastinal mass, and is known as Pemberton's sign; it is due to obstruction of great vessels (by pressure effects of retrosternal goitre or mediastinal mass on arm raising) at thoracic inlet. This test should not be done routinely.

Q. Why do you say that it is Graves' disease?

As there is presence of exophthalmos and diffuse goitre, it is a patient of Graves' disease.

The **examination findings** (for example): Thyroid gland is diffusely enlarged, measuring 8.5 × 8.0 cm, left lobe is a bit larger than right; isthmus is not palpable. The gland is soft, non-tender; freely mobile with smooth surface, not fixed with underlying structures or overlying skin. There is no lymphadenopathy, no retrosternal extension but there is bruit audible over the left lobe.

Q. What is simple diffuse goitre?

It is goitre with no sign of toxicosis, and the causes are Iodine deficiency, puberty goitre and use of goitrogens (drugs like amiodarone, lithium, PAS and vegetables like cabbage, cauliflower, turnips).

Q. Features of ophthalmopathy and dermopathy:

Graves' disease is characterised by the **classical triad** of diffuse goitre, ophthalmopathy and dermopathy (pretibial myxoedema).

I. Ophthalmopathy: Read the section on 'Exophthalmos'.

II. Cutaneous manifestations (dermopathy) in Graves' disease:

1. Skin: Warm, hyperhidrotic and moist hand (due to cutaneous vasodilation); palmar erythema, rarely spider naevi, malar flush.
2. Hair: Friable, fine and silky; alopecia.
3. Nails: Separation of the distal margin of the nail from its nail-bed (Plummer's nail).
4. *Pretibial myxoedema:* The affected area (bilaterally over the shin) is raised, thickened, hyperpigmented and indurated plaque with "peau d'orange" appearance along with growth of coarse hair. There is non-pitting oedema over the shins.
5. Pigmentation: Hyper- and hypopigmentation (vitiligo) may be seen.
6. Thyroid acropachy: Clubbing and swollen fingers with bony changes resembling hypertrophic osteoarthropathy may accompany the dermal changes in distal extremities.

Q. Physical findings in CVS in Graves' disease:

1. Pulse:
   i. Tachycardia (persists even when the patient is sleeping, i.e. high sleeping pulse rate; *see* page 296).
   ii. High volume collapsing pulse which may be of water-hammer in character (due to wide pulse pressure), capillary pulsation.
   iii. Atrial fibrillation (irregularly irregular pulse), ectopics.
   iv. Carotid dance and suprasternal pulsation (due to hyperkinetic circulatory state).
   v. Other points in pulse: Usually within normal limit.
2. Signs of congestive cardiac failure (high output failure and often refractory) may be present. There may be worsening of angina or heart failure in the elderly due to high cardiac output.
3. Heart:
   i. Apex: Hyperdynamic and present in normal position.
   ii. S_1 and P_2 may be loud (due to tachycardia).
   iii. Murmur: Systolic murmur at the apex (due to increased blood flow).
   iv. Means-Lerman scratch: To-and-fro scratchy sound is heard in the pulmonary area or over the upper sternum in midsystole (possibly due to rubbing of pleura and pericardium as a result of hyperkinetic circulatory state mimicking pericardial rub). It is rarely found.

- Common symptoms related to CVS are (i) Palpitations with sweating, (ii) Angina pectoris, and (ii) Dyspnoea due to CCF. *Sleeping pulse rate is important to determine the severity of thyrotoxicosis.*

Q. Gastrointestinal manifestations in Graves' disease:

Loss of weight in spite of increased appetite, hyperdefecation (diarrhoea and steatorrhoea), vomiting.

Clinical Wisdom

The patient may present with weight loss, increased appetite, irritability, heat intolerance, tremor, hyperkinesia, palpitations, increased sweating or exophthalmos.

Q. Three cardinal signs of Graves' disease:

1. Tachycardia, 2. Tremor, and 3. Exophthalmos—always examine these signs in hyperthyroidism **(Table 3.8)**.

- Robert J. Graves (1796–1853) was an Irish surgeon, Meath Hospital, Dublin, Republic of Ireland.

Q. Facies in thyrotoxicosis (Fig. 3.144):

Better known as 'stare'; an anxious startled look due to lid retraction (agitated or terror face). Exophthalmos and other eye changes like infrequent blinking may be noted. Moist facial skin with a malar flush is sometimes seen and may be associated with a goitre in the neck.

Q. Clinical features regarding involvement of nervous system:

A. Symptoms:

1. Insomnia, nervousness, emotional lability or hyperirritability; perspiration.
2. Hyperkinesia, akathisia (i.e. feeling of inner restlessness).
3. Depression, mania or psychosis.
4. Difficulty in rising from squatting position or climbing upstairs (due to proximal muscle weakness).
5. Stupor or coma (thyroid storm).

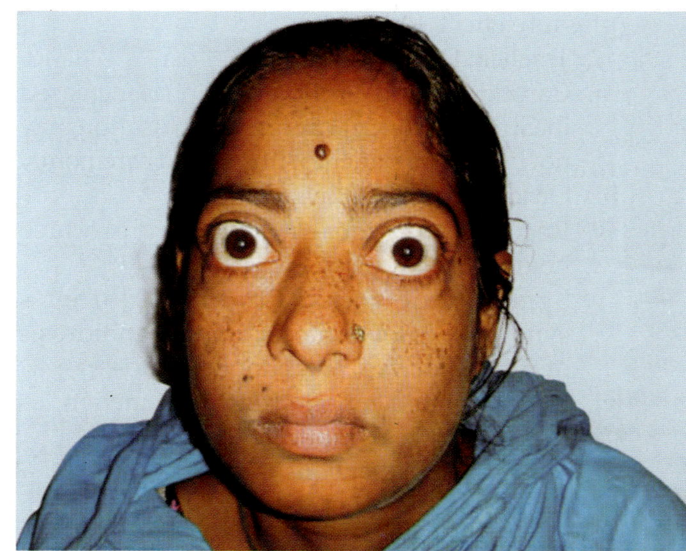

Fig. 3.144: Thyrotoxicosis with **exophthalmos** and staring look

B. Signs:

1. Fine tremor (most prominent feature): Tested in outstretched hands and protruded tongue. In severe cases, the whole body may be shaking and trembling.
2. Proximal muscular weakness and wasting: 'Thyroid myopathy'. Fasciculation may be seen.
3. Myasthenic syndrome and hypokalaemic periodic paralysis may occur.
4. Chorea.
5. Deep reflexes (jerks): Exaggerated.
6. Pseudoclonus or ill-sustained clonus.
7. Plantar response: Flexor.

- **Apathetic thyrotoxicosis:** Some elderly patients of thyrotoxicosis present with features more like hypothyroidism. They have very few signs like fatigue and weight loss. Diagnosis needs high index of suspicion.

Q. Differential diagnosis of thyrotoxicosis:

A. Anxiety neurosis is the commonest differential diagnosis (having tremor in both):

Anxiety neurosis:

1. Appetite—Diminished.
2. Hands—Cold and moist.
3. Sleeping pulse rate—Normal.
4. Pulse pressure—Normal
5. Goitre—Not present.
6. Eye signs—Absent.

Thyrotoxicosis:

1. Appetite—Increased (with weight loss).
2. Hands—Warm and moist.
3. Sleeping pulse rate—Raised.
4. Pulse pressure—Increased.
5. Goitre—Present.
6. Eye signs—Present.

B. Other conditions where there is rapid weight loss are:

1. Diabetes mellitus.
2. Pulmonary tuberculosis.
3. Malabsorption syndrome.
4. Malignancy.
5. Pheochromocytoma.
6. AIDS.

C. Chronic alcoholism: Tremor, tachycardia, sweating, emotional lability in alcoholism may resemble thyrotoxicosis.

Q. Examination of 'neck' in clinical medicine:

1. Swelling like branchial cyst, sternomastoid tumour, cystic hygroma, carotid body tumour, Ludwig's angina, dermoid cyst, etc. are of surgical interest.
2. Skin: Scar, old tracheostomy mark, signs of inflammation, fistula (branchial), sinus, actinomycosis (rare), pityriasis versicolor, Casal's collar, acanthosis nigricans (insulin resistance in diabetes), vitiligo (autoimmune disorder), scrofuloderma, acrochordons (skin tags), etc.
3. Enlargement of the thyroid gland (page 394).
4. Lymph nodes (page 207).
5. Salivary glands.
6. Neck vessels (page 329).
7. Examination of trachea (page 72); tracheal tug (page 47).
8. Neck rigidity (page 142).
9. Short neck (associated with low hair line) is found in cranio-vertebral anomaly, e.g. platybasia, Klippel-Feil anomaly (page 157).
10. Great auricular nerve: Thickened in tuberculoid leprosy (by turning the head to the opposite side, the nerve stands out).
11. Spasmodic torticollis (page 462) or other abnormal movements (e.g. tics).
12. Buffalo hump (Cushing's syndrome).
13. Suprasternal pulsation, carotid dance (pages 40 and 41) and other pulsations (page 330).
14. Webbing of neck in Turner's syndrome (page 321).
15. Swelling of neck in conditions like SVC obstruction, subcutaneous emphysema, bull-neck (malignant diphtheria).
16. Deglutition: Ask the patient to swallow (to confirm a thyroid swelling).
17. Power testing of neck muscles, e.g. sternomastoids (page 467); wasting of sternomastoid muscle in myotonic dystrophy.
18. Restriction of neck movement along with pain (flexion, extension, rotation, side-bending) occurs in cervical spondylosis, ankylosing spondylitis, atlanto-axial dislocation.
19. Ciliospinal reflex (page 443).
20. Auscultation: Thyroid bruit, carotid bruit and venous hum (page 395); auscultation over trachea.

- First palpate the back and sides of **neck**, which are better palpated from the front; then the patient is allowed to sit on a stool and the examination (i.e. palpation) is carried out from behind.

Q. Mention the investigations you like to perform In hyperthyroidism:

1. Serum T_3 and T_4 (free and total both) are increased. TSH is very low (<0.05 μU/mL or undetectable).
2. Radioactive Iodine (I^{131} or I^{132}) uptake (RAIU) is increased.
3. Resin T_3 uptake (RT_3U) is increased.
4. Free thyroxine index (FTI) is increased (FTI = serum $T_4 \times RT_3U$).
5. T_3 suppression test: After the administration of T_3, the iodine uptake is not suppressed.
6. Serum TSH level after TRH administration: Blunted response (very helpful test).
7. ECG: Shows sinus tachycardia, ectopics, and/or atrial fibrillation.

8. Thyroid (radionuclide) scan: Done by technetium 99m which shows localised or generalised increased uptake. It is useful in suspected cases of functioning thyroid nodule.
9. USG of neck to see single, multinodular or diffuse goitre.
10. Others:
    i. Anti-thyroglobulin antibodies: Raised (also elevated in Hashimoto's thyroiditis).
    ii. Basal metabolic rate (BMR) is increased (normal BMR in male is 40 calorie/m^2 of body surface/hour).
    iii. Serum PBI is increased (normal level is 3.6–8.5 µg/dL): Not used nowadays.
    iv. Low serum cholesterol.
    v. Serum LATS (long-acting thyroid stimulator) is increased: Not routinely used.
    vi. Antibodies against thyroid peroxidase (TPO) enzyme and thyroglobulin are present in most cases of Graves' disease.
    vii. Measurement of TSH receptor antibodies (TSHR-Ab), which are specific for Graves' disease.
    viii. Needle aspiration (FNAC) of thyroid nodule in selected cases.
    ix. High urinary as well as serum calcium and phosphate.
    x. Raised SGPT (ALT), alkaline phosphatase, bilirubin; glycosuria ('lag storage').

- In 5% patients of thyrotoxicosis (T_3 toxicosis) serum T_3 is much raised but T_4 remains in the upper limit of normal.
- Increased BMR is also characteristic of fever and pheochromocytoma.

Q. Outline of management of thyrotoxicosis:

1. **Antithyroid drugs:** Propylthiouracil (100–200 mg, 6–8 hourly), carbimazole, methimazole, iodide or potassium perchlorate is used; these drugs inhibit the formation of thyroid hormones. While diminishing the toxicity, these drugs increase the size and vascularity of the thyroid gland. Carbimazole is the commonly used drug.
2. **Radioactive Iodine (I^{131}):** Usually 370 MBq (10 mCi) to 555 MBq (15 mCi) of I^{131} is given orally; may be repeated at 12 weeks.

   Indications:
   a. All patients >40 years of age.
   b. Toxicity due to drugs or relapse after surgery.
   c. Thyrotoxic heart disease.

   Contraindications:
   a. During pregnancy and lactation (antithyroid drug is the best choice).
   b. In children.
3. Surgery (subtotal or near-total thyroidectomy)—in patients with relapse after drug therapy.
4. General measures:
    i. Good nutritious diet.
    ii. **Propranolol:** Dosage up to 160 mg/day, i.e. 20–40 mg, every 6 hourly (may need higher doses) may be given. Propranolol antagonises the sympathomimetic manifestations and thus, it alleviates palpitations, tremor, sweating and lid retraction. Propranolol is contraindicated in CCF, heart block, bronchial asthma, peripheral vascular disease and diabetes.
5. *For thyroid eye disease:*
    i. Low salt diet and diuretics, with elevation of the head end at night to reduce orbital oedema. Smoking should be stopped.
    ii. Tinted glass with side frames (to protect the eyes from sun, wind and dust) to reduce lacrimation. The eyelids can be taped at night.
    iii. 1% methyl cellulose and hypromellose eyedrops for lubrication.
    iv. Prednisolone: 30–120 mg/day with or without cyclosporine in malignant exophthalmos.
    v. External irradiation or lateral tarsorrhaphy to prevent exposure keratitis.
    vi. Orbital decompression or corrective eye muscle surgery, rarely.
6. For dermopathy (pretibial myxoedema):
    i. Hyaluronidase or triamcinolone (intralesional injection).
    ii. Topical high potency corticosteroids with occlusive dressing.
    iii. Compressive therapy; ultra-violet radiation.
    iv. Octreotide is being tried recently.

- Exophthalmos does not necessarily decrease after successful treatment of thyrotoxicosis.

Table 3.8: Clinical differentiation between Graves' disease and toxic nodular goitre

Features	**Graves' disease**	Toxic nodular goitre
1. Age	1. <35 years	1. >35 years
2. Goitre	2. Smooth, diffuse enlargement	2. Nodular
3. Onset of symptoms	3. With goitre	3. Goitre first, symptoms later
4. Eye signs	4. Present	4. Absent or rare
5. Cardiac symptoms	5. Slight	5. Severe
6. Neuromuscular symptoms	6. Prominent	6. Slight
7. Other autoimmune diseases	7. Common	7. Uncommon

Clinical Wisdom

Thyrotoxicosis with atrial fibrillation: more in elderly with toxic nodular goitre. Propranolol, amiodarone, antithyroid drug, anticoagulant and cardioversion (may be needed) are mode of therapy.

Q. How carbimazole is given?

The usual dose is 10–20 mg, orally 2–3 times daily till the patient becomes euthyroid. Usually the patient becomes euthyroid in 6–8 weeks and the maintenance dose is then started as 10–15 mg/day *for 12–18 months*. The maintenance dose is determined by the measurement of T_4 and TSH. Stop the treatment if patient remains euthyroid on 5 mg daily dose of carbimazole.

Side effects: Agranulocytosis (patient complains of sore throat or fever), drug rash, drug sensitivity, hepatitis, drug fever, arthralgia, etc.

- Leucopenia or agranulocytosis is the most dangerous complication of antithyroid drugs. If the absolute neutrophil count is <1500/mm^3 of blood, antithyroid medication should be discontinued.

Q. Use of beta-blockers in internal medicine:

Remember the indications from head to foot as:

1. Anxiety states.
2. Migraine (as prophylaxis).
3. Glaucoma (chronic open-angle).
4. Thyrotoxicosis.
5. Prevention of variceal haemorrhage (i.e. portal hypertension).
6. Cardiovascular system: Systemic hypertension, angina pectoris (stable and unstable), myocardial infarction, cardiac arrhythmias (especially tachyarrhythmias), hypertrophic obstructive cardiomyopathy (HOCM), mitral valve prolapse syndrome (MVPS), dissection of aorta, cyanotic spells of Fallot's tetralogy.
7. Essential tremor.
8. Pheochromocytoma.
9. Alcohol withdrawal syndrome.

Q. Thyroid storm or thyrotoxic crisis:

It is an extreme degree of hyperthyroid state precipitated by surgery, infection, severe stress, or develops spontaneously in patients with hyperthyroidism. The patient usually suffers from abrupt onset of restlessness, delusions, hyperpyrexia, delirium, tachyarrhythmias, hypotension, vomiting, diarrhoea and often coma, and may succumb from heart failure, arrhythmias and hyperpyrexia. It is managed urgently in ICU with IV sodium iodide or oral Lugol's iodine with oral propylthiouracil, dexamethasone, propranolol, and correction of water and electrolyte imbalance.

Q. Identification points (thyrotoxicosis):

1. Goitre with exophthalmos is the first clue—the patient looks anxious, restless and fidgety.
2. Now examine for tremor and tachycardia.
3. Never forget to examine the jerks.

Clinical Wisdom

If thyrotoxicosis is given as a long case, examine the patient in the following way:

A. General survey (especially nutrition, facies, neck glands, pulse, BP, skin and appendages).
B. Examination of the thyroid gland and eye.
C. Systemic examination:
   a. CVS,
   b. Nervous system,
   c. GI system,
   d. Respiratory system, and
   e. Reticulo-endothelial system.

- **Hyperthyroidism** indicates glandular hypertrophy of thyroid and **thyrotoxicosis** is increased circulating free thyroid hormones along with toxic features.
- Heat intolerance is a common general symptom of hyperthyroidism.
- **Endocrine emergencies** in clinical practice are thyroid storm, myxoedema coma, pituitary apoplexy, adrenal crisis, severe hypercalcaemia and Nelson's syndrome. Read the section on 'Diabetes mellitus' for diabetic emergencies (e.g. hypoglycaemia, DKA).

EXOPHTHALMOS — CASE 71

Q. What is exophthalmos (Fig. 3.144)?

It is the forward protrusion of the eyeball when a portion of the sclera is visible above and below the cornea. Previously, it was defined as the visibility of the *lower sclera* of more than 2 mm when the patient looks straight forward (few clinicians still believe this definition).

In exophthalmos (e.g. unilateral), the globes appear asymmetric.

Q. How the exophthalmos is tested at the bedside?

1. The patient is asked to look straight forward. The examiner stands **in front of the patient** and the visibility of the upper and lower sclera is noted. **The visibility of the lower sclera is more important** as in thyrotoxicosis, the presence of lid retraction (contraction of Muller's muscle), may give the false impression of exophthalmos.
2. The examiner stands **behind the patient**, tilts the patient's head backwards and looks vertically down the slanting forehead in the plane of superciliary ridges. Thus, one may be sure whether any part of the eyeball (globe) is visible (proptosis) or not. This is known as **Naffziger's sign**.

- *According to few clinicians, exophthalmos and proptosis carry the same message.*
- In health, one-third of the cornea is covered by the upper eyelid.

Q. What are the common causes of exophthalmos?

I. Unilateral:

1. Early thyrotoxicosis (Graves' disease).
2. Retro-orbital tumour.
3. Cavernous sinus thrombosis.
4. Chloroma (AML); malignant and lymphomatous deposits (Fig. 3.145).
5. Orbital 'pseudotumour'.
6. Varicosity of orbital vein, carotico-cavernous fistula, aneurysm of orbital vessels, superior orbital fissure syndrome, orbital haemorrhage.
7. Orbital cellulitis.
8. Sphenoid wing meningioma.

- So, both eyes are not necessarily affected simultaneously in exophthalmos.

II. Bilateral:

1. Thyrotoxicosis (Graves' disease).
2. Bronchial asthma (long standing).
3. SVC syndrome.
4. Cirrhosis of liver (few cases).
5. Cushing's syndrome.
6. Craniostenosis (e.g. oxycephaly).
7. Cavernous sinus thrombosis (bilateral).
8. Hand-Schuller-Christian disease, Wegener's granulomatosis, sarcoidosis, nasopharyngeal carcinoma affecting both the orbits.

Clinical Wisdom

Commonest cause of exophthalmos is thyrotoxicosis whether it is unilateral or bilateral; 2, 4 and 5 of (II) produce apparent exophthalmos due to lid retraction.

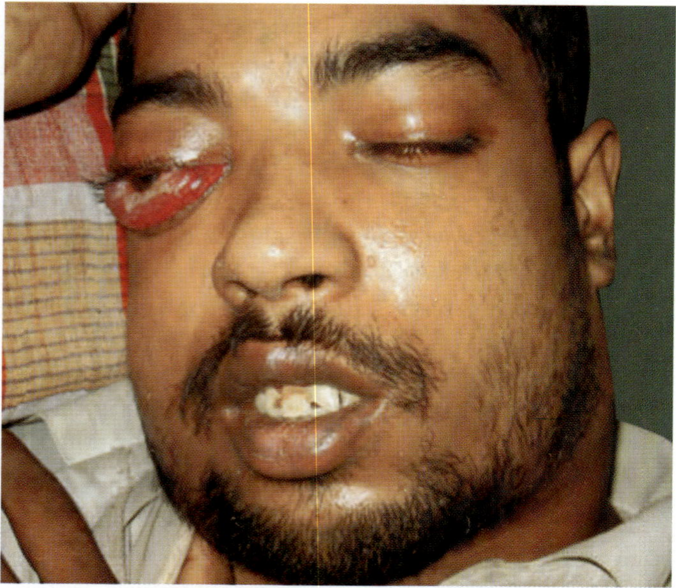

Fig. 3.145: A moribund patient showing **proptosis** due to involvement of the right eye from **lymphoma** (NHL); cervical adenopathy is also noted

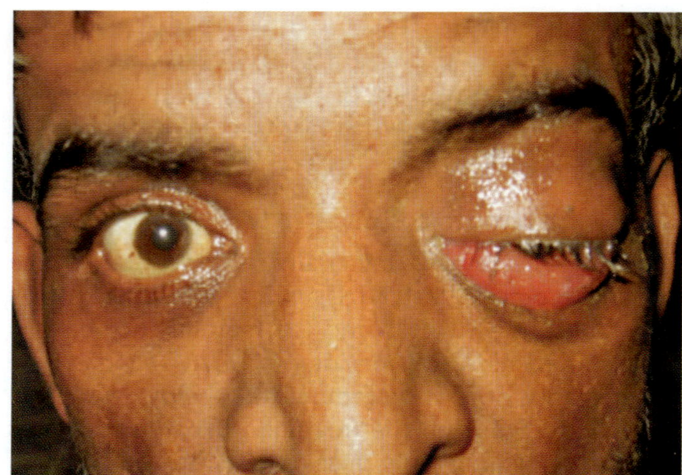

Fig. 3.146A: Cavernous sinus thrombosis in the left side resulting in proptosis, ptosis and ophthalmoplegia

- **Cavernous sinus thrombosis** (Fig. 3.146A) = chemosis of conjunctiva, exophthalmos, ptosis, ophthalmoplegia, papilloedema and reduced sensation in ophthalmic division of trigeminal nerve.
- Intermittent proptosis: Orbital varix, recurrent orbital haemorrhage, periodic orbital oedema.
- Pseudoproptosis: Shallow orbits, pathological myopia and contralateral enophthalmos.

Q. Other eye signs in thyrotoxicosis (Table 3.9):

Eye signs in Graves' disease are divided into two parts: A) Spastic (staring look, lid lag, lid retraction) and B) Mechanical (proptosis, ophthalmoplegia and congestive oculopathy). As a whole, they are:

1. Widening of the palpebral fissure.
2. **von Graefe's sign (lid lag):** When the patient is asked to look downwards suddenly, the upper eyelid lags behind (exposing the sclera between the upper eyelid and cornea).
3. **Joffroy's sign:** Absence of wrinkling on the forehead on looking upwards (head must be fixed).
4. **Möbius's sign:** Lack of convergence of the eyeball (the test for accommodation is done and Moebius's sign is elicited).
5. **Stellwag's sign (staring look):** Infrequent blinking.
6. **Dalrymple's sign** (lid retraction) This is equivalent to visibility of the upper sclera when the patient looks forward.
7. **Jendrassik's sign:** Paralysis of extraocular muscles.
8. **Gifford's sign:** Difficulty in everting upper eyelid.

- Bilaterally dilated pupil may be found as a result of sympathetic overactivity.
- Swollen extraocular muscles (typical of Graves' disease) and other features of thyroid eye disease are detected by orbital USG or CT scan. Unilateral proptosis usually implies a space-occupying lesion and warrants urgent CT scan or MRI of orbit (along with thyroid function test).

Table 3.9: Classification of eye changes in Graves' disease

Class	Mnemonics	Definition
0	(N)	No signs, no symptoms
1	(0)	Only signs (stare, lid retraction, lid lag), no symptoms
2	(S)	Soft tissue involvement (symptoms and signs)
3	(P)	Proptosis >22 mm (measured by Hertel exophthalmometer)
4	(E)	Extraocular muscle involvement (external ophthalmoplegia, e.g. having diplopia)
5	(C)	Corneal involvement (ulceration)
6	(S)	Sight loss (optic nerve involvement)

- This classification was done by American Thyroid Association. Remember the acronym 'NO SPECS'. The disease process passes through 6 stages.
- Extraocular muscles: Earliest affection—inferior rectus, least affection—lateral rectus.

Q. Ocular complaints in Graves' disease:

1. Bulging of the eyes.
2. Grittiness or pain in eyes.
3. Redness of the eye.
4. Photophobia.
5. Excessive lacrimation.
6. Ophthalmoplegia.
7. Squint.
8. Diplopia.
9. Difficulty in moving the eyes.
10. Loss of visual acuity.

Q. Causes of pulsating exophthalmos:

Carotico-cavernous fistula and saccular aneurysm of ophthalmic artery.

Q. Physical examination in exophthalmos (from thyrotoxicosis):

1. Warm and moist hand.
2. Puise rate: Whether tachycardia present or not.
3. Tremor: Ask the patient to stretch out the arms and to spread the fingers. Look for the presence of fine tremor. One may examine the protruding tongue for fine tremor.
4. Goitre present or not (also examine for the presence of systolic thrill and/or bruit present over thyroid).
5. CVS: See the section on 'Hyperthyroidism'.
6. Jerks: Exaggerated.

- One should examine these 6 points in all patients with exophthalmos. Features like warm and moist hand, tachycardia, tremor, exaggerated jerks and goitre are evident in Graves' disease.

Q. What is exophthalmic ophthalmoplegia?

It is the presence of exophthalmos, chemosis of conjunctiva (oedema of conjunctiva and injection of sclera) and weakness of extraocular muscles (sparing pupillary and ciliary muscles) leading to diplopia and squint (Table 3.9).

Pathophysiology: Cytokine-mediated proliferation of fibroblasts within the orbit → secretion of glycosaminoglycans (hydrophilic) → increase in interstitial fluid volume → associated infiltration of chronic inflammatory cells → swelling of the extraocular muscles → increase in retrobulbar pressure → proptosis → optic nerve compression in severe cases.

Q. What is malignant exophthalmos (Fig. 3.146B)?

Progressive (severe) bulging of the eyeballs, conjunctival oedema, exposure keratitis with corneal ulceration and visual loss (blindness) are features of malignant exophthalmos.

Q. What is enophthalmos?

In this condition, the eyeball is retracted inwards or recessed within the orbit. It is very rarely seen. The common causes are:

1. Phthisis bulbi (shrinkage of the eyeball from prolonged endophthalmitis) (Fig. 3.147) or microphthalmos.
2. Horner's syndrome.
3. Old age (due to atrophy of orbital fat)—physiological; trauma, emaciation.

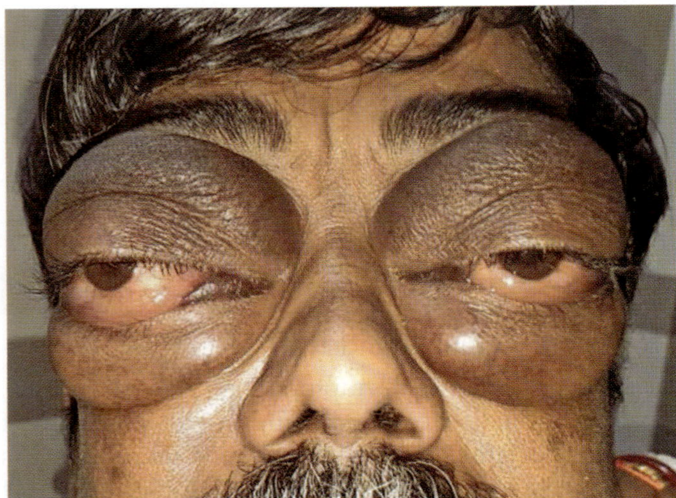

Fig. 3.146B: **Malignant exophthalmos** in a patient of thyrotoxicosis

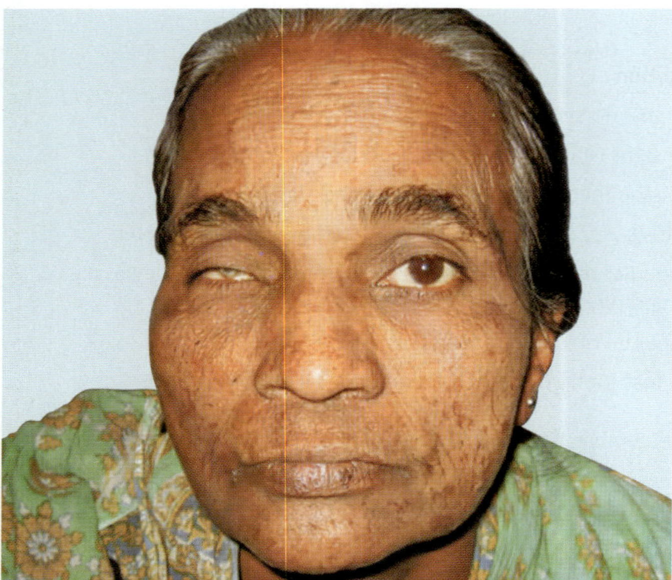

Fig. 3.147: **Enophthalmos** (right)—phthisis bulbi of the right eye resulting from smallpox in childhood

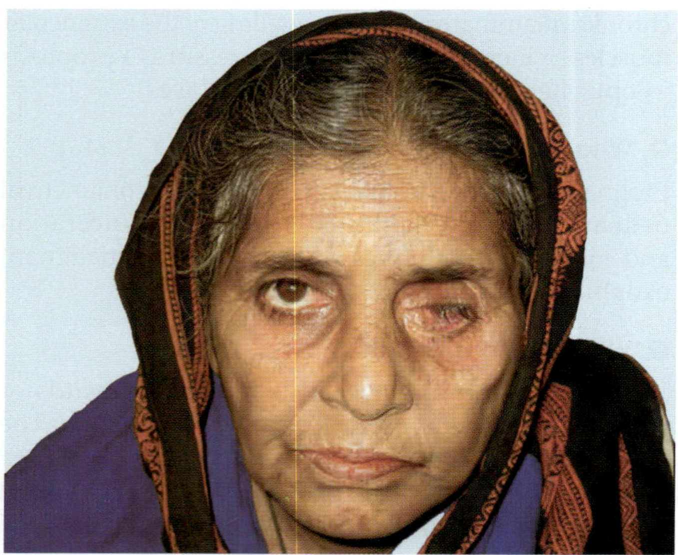

Fig. 3.148: **Enucleation** of the left eye

4. As a consequence of resolved orbital cellulitis or post-irradiation.
5. Severe dehydration (facies Hippocraticus).
6. Fracture of the orbital floor.
7. Enucleation of the eye with prosthesis **(Fig. 3.148)**.

- Management of thyroid ophthalmopathy has been described in the section on 'Hyperthyroidism'.

CUSHING'S SYNDROME — CASE 72

Q. What is Cushing's syndrome?

It is a syndrome with symptom complexes and signs, produced due to prolonged inappropriate elevation of free corticosteroid in the circulation. **Commonly** it is due to therapeutic administration of steroids or ACTH for long time (iatrogenic). Non-iatrogenic (i.e. Cushing's disease or adrenal adenoma) Cushing's syndrome is rare.

- Harvey Williams Cushing (1869-1939) was a neurosurgeon, Harvard University, Massachusetts, USA.

Q. Diagnosis of the case by inspection:

The disease is four times more common in women than men:

1. Moon face (dusky and plethoric too; excess hair in face) **(Figs 3.35 and 3.149)**.
2. Obesity (central obesity with thin limbs).
3. Buffalo hump.
4. Purple striae.
5. Proximal myopathy.
6. Hirsutism in females.

Q. Causes of Cushing's syndrome:

A. ACTH-dependent
- Pituitary tumour (Cushing's disease).
- Ectopic ACTH-secreting tumour (e.g. bronchogenic carcinoma).
- Iatrogenic (ACTH therapy).

B. Non-ACTH-dependent
- Iatrogenic (glucocorticoid therapy).
- Adrenal adenoma.
- Adrenal carcinoma.
- Pseudo-Cushing's syndrome.
- Others (e.g. macronodular adrenal hyperplasia).

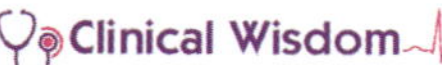

Model case with diagnosis: The patient is suffering from iatrogenic Cushing's syndrome.

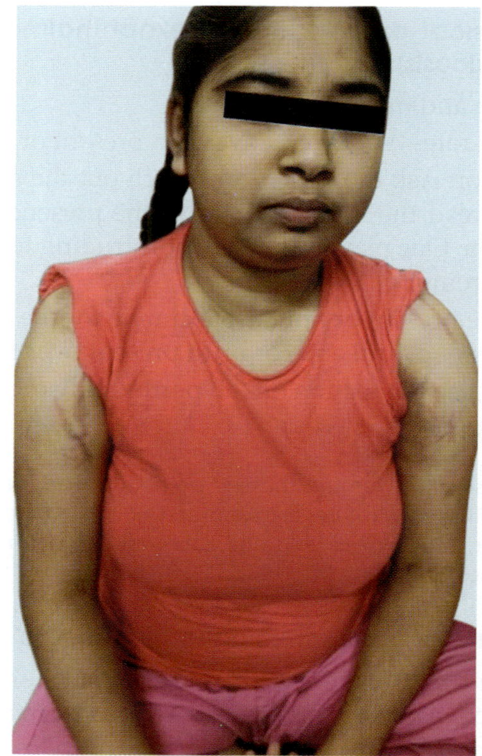

Fig. 3.149: 'Moon face' due to **Cushing's syndrome**. Purple striae are seen.

Q. Describe the clinical features of Cushing's syndrome:

A. Fat deposition:

a. Obesity: Weight gain is the commonest symptom and thus, obesity is the most frequent sign. There is centripetal (like a lemon on matchstick) deposition of adipose tissue though generalised obesity is not uncommon. Fat deposition in the mesenteric bed produces 'abdominal obesity', and over face and trunk develops into 'truncal obesity'. The fat deposition spares the extremities.

b. Moon facies: Due to fat deposition in the upper part of the face (supramalar region).

c. Buffalo hump: Due to deposition of fat in the interscapular area (upper part).

B. Skin and hair changes:

a. Plethoric appearance: Due to thinning of the skin and rarely due to associated polycythemia.

b. *Purple* striae (striae are linear, wrinkled, white or pink-coloured marks over the skin): Commonly seen over abdomen, buttocks, breast, thigh and arms (Fig. 3.149). This is produced due to break-down of collagen fibres in the dermis and thus, the vascularised subcutaneous tissues are exposed. These 'striae distensae' are often painful (*see* Fig. 2.11).

[*White* striae (striae albicantes) are usually observed following pregnancy, after paracentesis abdominis in ascites or when an obese person looses weight rapidly (due to rupture of elastic fibres of skin) (*see* Fig. 2.10); *pink* striae are common during pregnancy and in simple obesity with rapid increase in weight].

c. Easy bruisability and ecchymosis: Due to loss of perivascular supporting tissue (i.e. there is increased capillary fragility).

d. Hyperpigmentation: This is due to excess MSH secretion found in bilateral adrenal hyperplasia secondary to pituitary tumour or ectopic ACTH secretion from non-endocrine tumours like bronchogenic carcinoma. This is not a very common feature.

e. Thinning of hair. Frontal baldness in females.

f. Increased incidence of skin infection (e.g. tinea versicolor).

C. Myopathy: Loss of protein in muscle leads to proximal myopathy (difficulty in combing hairs or getting up from squatting position).

D. Bony changes: Osteoporosis is commonly seen in spine, ribs and femurs (due to loss of protein matrix of the bones); patient may present with backache (vertebral compression fracture); kyphosis.

E. Hypertension: It is due to the increased plasma volume and enhanced vascular response to catecholamines. This appears not to relate to sodium retention as previously believed. There may be ankle oedema or cardiomegaly.

F. Diabetes mellitus: Due to antagonistic action of cortisol on insulin.

G. Secondary sexual characters:

a. Female: Hirsutism, acne, oligomenorrhoea or amenorrhoea, recession of temporal hair, clitoromegaly.

b. Male: Loss of libido, impotence may be seen.

H. Psychiatric abnormality:

a. Depression.

b. Psychosis.

c. Emotional instability.

d. Irritability.

I. Growth:

a. Growth retardation is a rule in children.

b. Diminution of height in adult patients may occur due to collapse of the vertebrae (as a result of severe osteoporosis).

J. Miscellaneous:

a. Cataract.

b. Peptic ulcer.

c. Poor wound healing with little inflammatory response.

d. Mild bilateral exophthalmos.

e. Electrolyte disturbance (↑Na^+, ↓K^+, ↓Cl^-).

f. Avascular necrosis of bone.

g. Increased susceptibility to infections, e.g. tuberculosis and fungal infections.

Q. Causes of moon face:

Read the section on 'Moon face'.

Q. What is hirsutism, virilisation and defeminisation?

A. Hirsutism: It is the excessive growth of terminal hair in women in a pattern characteristic of men.

B. Virilisation (i.e. androgen excess in females): The characteristic features are:

i. Frontal baldness.

ii. Increase in size of shoulder girdle muscles.

iii. Coarsening of voice.

iv. Acne and seborrhoea.

v. Hirsutism.

vi. Clitoromegaly.

vii. Increased libido.

C. Defeminisation:

i. Reduction in breast size.

ii. Loss of female body contours.

iii. Loss of gynoid fat distribution.

Q. Causes of hirsutism:

Patients of hirsutism usually need full endocrinal assessment to evaluate the androgenaemia.

1. Familial.
2. Idiopathic or simple hirsutism.
3. Cushing's syndrome, virilising ovarian tumour (e.g. arrhenoblastoma) (Fig. 3.150).

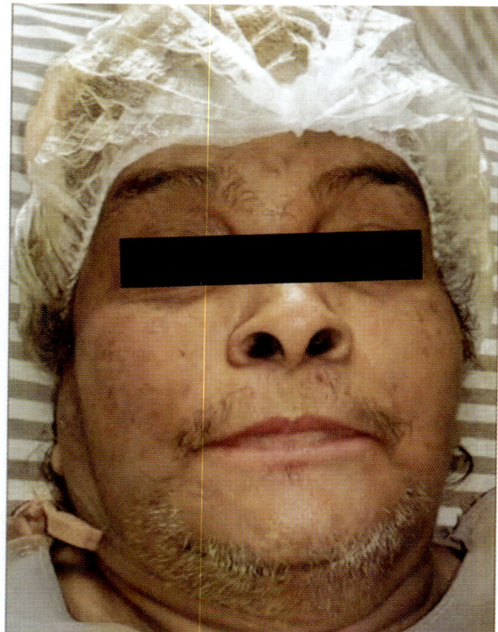

Fig. 3.150: **Hirsutism** in virilizing ovarian tumour

4. Polycystic ovarian disease (PCOD).
5. Adrenal androgen secreting tumour (adenoma, carcinoma), congenital adrenal hyperplasia.
6. Hyperprolactinaemia.
7. Acromegaly.
8. Drug-induced: Phenytoin, OC pills, corticosteroid or ACTH therapy, androgens, diazoxide, cyclosporin, psoralens, minoxidil.
9. Menopause.

- Hirsutism is divided into two groups (i) with virilisation (severe PCOD, congenital adrenal hyperplasia, virilising ovarian neoplasm), and (ii) without virilisation (other causes).
- Therapy is done by bleaching, waxing, electrolysis, laser, anti-androgens and treatment of cause.

Q. 'Hair-types' in both sex:

Adults have two types of hair, vellus and terminal. Vellus type is soft, fine, usually colourless, and mostly short. Terminal hair is long, dark, coarse, and sometimes curly. In women, vellus hair covers face/chest/back and gives the impression of 'hairless' skin; in most of the men, terminal hair covers face and body. Terminal hair covers scalp, pubic and armpit in both the sex. A mixture of vellus and terminal hair covers lower armpit and legs in men and women.

- **Greying or whiteness of hair (canities)** is common in ageing, hereditary, over vitiligo, pernicious anaemia, thyrotoxicosis, albinism and chloroquine toxicity.

Q. What is Cushing's disease?

It is the hypercortisolism producing bilateral adrenal hyperplasia due to excess ACTH secretion from the anterior pituitary gland while Cushing's syndrome is caused by excess glucocorticoid secretion from adrenal cortex.

Q. Hormones secreted from adrenal gland:

Adrenal glands comprise of an outer cortex and an inner medulla. The cortex is a part of hypothalamic-pituitary-adrenal axis, which sceretes cortisol and adrenal androgen after getting signal from above. The cortex is divided into 3 zones from outer to innermost as:

A. Cortex
- Zona glomerulosa—mainly secretes aldosterone (mineralocorticoids)
- Zona fasciculata—predominanly secretes cortisol (glucocorticoids)
- Zona reticularis—mainly secretes sex steroids (androgen, oestrogen and progesterone)

B. Medulla
- Produces catecholamines (adrenaline, noradrenaline and dopamine)

Q. How do you like to investigate your case?

1. Blood examination: Mild neutrophilic leucocytosis, eosinopenia and lymphocytopenia. Haematocrit may be high.
2. Electrolytes: Hypernatraemia, hypokalaemia, hypochloraemia, metabolic alkalosis.
3. Urine: Glucose may be present in urine and there is elevated urinary 17-hydroxycorticoids.
4. Glucose tolerance test: Impaired glucose tolerance. Diabetes is seen in <20% patients.
5. X-rays:
   a. Spine: Osteoporosis in spine produces cod-fish vertebra or fish-mouth like appearance of intervertebral space. Osteoporosis is also seen in pelvis and skull.
   b. Chest: There may be superior mediastinal widening due to:
      i. Bronchogenic carcinoma (produces ectopic ACTH) or bronchial carcinoid.
      ii. Fat accumulation, or
      iii. Tumour of thymus (may be associated with Cushing's syndrome).
   c. Skull: Enlargement of the pituitary fossa in Cushing's disease only.
6. CT or MRI scan of the abdomen (adrenal adenoma or carcinoma), brain (pituitary tumour) or chest. If no mass is seen in abdomen, adrenal vein sampling or adrenal scintigraphy may be done; in suspected Cushing's disease in the absence of pituitary mass, selective catheterisation of inferior petrosal sinus is done to measure ACTH.
7. Selective adrenal arteriography and venography: Not used nowadays.
8. 19-[^{131}I] iodocholesterol scanning: Differentiates adrenal tumours from bilateral adrenal hyperplasia.
9. Plasma cortisol level: The normal blood level is 5–25 µg/dL at 8 AM. Normally, the cortisol level is highest at 8 AM and lowest at 12 midnight but in Cushing's syndrome the level remains uniformly

elevated throughout the 24-hours period (loss of the circadian rhythm). In difficulty, midnight salivary cortisol is collected for measurement.

10. Plasma ACTH level (at 8 AM):
    i. Very high level (>300 ng/L): Ectopic ACTH secretion due to malignancy (from small-cell carcinoma of the bronchus).
    ii. Moderate level (80–300 ng/L): Ectopic ACTH secretion from bronchial carcinoid (benign tumour) or pituitary dependent disease.
    iii. Normal level (10–80 ng/L) or low level: Adrenal disease.
11. 48-hours low dose dexamethasone suppression test (dexamethasone does not cross-react in radioimmunoassay for cortisol): This test is done in two stages. There is failure of complete suppression of cortisol in Cushing's syndrome. This is a highly sensitive test.
12. Metyrapone test (exaggerated response is seen in Cushing's disease and the test is negative in Cushing's syndrome).
13. Insulin tolerance test: Insulin-induced hypoglycaemia does not stimulate the plasma cortisol level in Cushing's syndrome, which is a feature in normal healthy persons.
14. 24-hours urinary free cortisol excretion >250 µg/day is diagnostic (normal value <90 µg/day).
15. Demonstration of the adrenal tumour may be done by IVP, aortogram, retroperitoneal air insufflation (not practised nowadays).

- In pituitary tumour and ectopic ACTH syndrome: ↑ACTH and ↑cortisol. In adrenal tumour: ↓ or undetectable ACTH and ↑cortisol.

Clinical Wisdom

1. Adrenal hyperplasia and ectopic ACTH syndrome are ACTH-dependent.
2. Adrenal adenoma and carcinoma are not ACTH-dependent.

Q. Differentiation of Cushing's syndrome from ectopic ACTH syndrome:

Ectopic ACTH syndrome will have:

1. Sudden onset.
2. Hyperpigmentation.
3. Oedema (more common).
4. Hypertension (more common).
5. Hypokalaemic alkalosis (more common).
6. Markedly elevated ACTH level (>300 ng/L).

Q. What is "pseudo-Cushing's syndrome"?

These patients (excess cortisol as part of another illness) often physically mimic Cushing's syndrome (Cushingoid appearance) and may have high urinary output of 17-hydroxycorticoids. They are: 1. Primary obesity, 2. Chronic alcoholism, and 3. Severe depression.

Q. Management of your case:

I. Adrenal adenoma: Surgically removed via a loin approach and suboptimal replacement therapy with 0.5 mg of dexamethasone is started for a variable length of time.

II. Adrenal carcinoma: Resected as far as possible and the tumour bed is irradiated. Treatment with o, p'-DDD (3–6 g/day) is started immediately.

III. Cushing's disease:
   i. Trans-sphenoidal removal of the adenoma (treatment of choice).
   ii. Radical hypophysectomy: If no tumour is seen.
   iii. Bilateral adrenalectomy with pituitary irradiation with yttrium-90 implantation to prevent the development of Nelson's syndrome.

IV. Ectopic ACTH secretion:
   i. Surgical removal or therapy of primary tumour (small-cell carcinoma of lung; tumour of the pancreas, thymus, ovary; bronchial carcinoid, etc.)
   ii. '*Medical or chemical adrenalectomy*' is done by:
      a. Metyrapone (2–4 g/day).
      b. o, p'-DDD or mitotane (3–6 g/day).
      c. Aminoglutethimide (1 g/day), trilostane (200 mg–1 g/day), or cyproheptadine (24 mg/day).
      d. Ketoconazole (600–1200 mg/day).

V. Supportive therapy is done by:
   i. High protein intake.
   ii. Treatment of hypertension, diabetes mellitus, electrolyte imbalance, etc.
   iii. Psychiatric treatment.

- Causes of death are hypertension, myocardial infarction, heart failure and secondary infections.

Q. What is meant by primary adrenocortical deficiency?

It is known as **Addison's disease** (opposite to Cushing's syndrome) and is characterised by:

1. Asthenia, weakness and weight loss (glucocorticoid deficiency).
2. Hyperpigmentation of buccal mucous membrane, face, recent scars, palmar creases, pressure points (ACTH excess) **(Fig. 3.87)**—Dull, slate-coloured, and
3. Hypotension with postural drop (mineralocorticoid deficiency).

- ↓ Cortisol →↑ ACTH →↑ melanin → pigmentation; vitiligo (10–20%) may occur due to autoimmunity.

Q. What is 'adrenal crisis', 'Addisonian crisis' or acute hypoadrenalism?

A. It is a symptom complex of anorexia, nausea, vomiting, abdominal pain, fever, somnolence, hypovolaemic shock with low pulse volume and low BP, confusion or coma. Confirmation is done by ↓Na^+, ↑K^+, hypoglycaemia, lymphocytosis and eosinophilia. It is commonly precipitated by:

i. Infection or septicaemia.
ii. Surgical stress or trauma.
iii. Fluid loss (diarrhoea).
iv. Sudden withdrawal of long-term corticosteroid therapy.

B. It may be due to affection of the adrenal gland by:

i. Tuberculosis.
ii. Metastasis.
iii. Autoimmune damage, or
iv. Surgical destruction.

C. Treatment is done by (correct 3'S', i.e. salt, sugar and steroid):

i. Hydrocortisone hemisuccinate 100 mg, IV, 6 hourly for a few days. After recovery, oral prednisolone therapy is continued.
ii. Normal saline and 10% glucose drip: Several litres are required within the first few hours.
iii. Dopamine as a vasoconstrictive agent.
iv. Treatment of the precipitating cause, e.g. antibiotics for infection.
v. Mineralocorticoid replacement by fludrocortisone (0.1 mg, orally, daily) after stoppage of saline with liberal salt intake.

❍ Bilateral adrenal haemorrhage from meningococcaemia (Waterhouse-Friderichsen syndrome) is a known aetiology.

Q. What is Nelson's syndrome?

It is known that 10–20% patients of Cushing's syndrome undergoing bilateral adrenalectomy develop chromophobe adenomas with hyperpigmentation and erosion of the sella turcica in the subsequent years. The plasma ACTH level in these patients are extremely high. This syndrome does not occur if these patients are immediately treated with pituitary irradiation in addition to bilateral adrenalectomy. This condition is treated by surgery, radiotherapy and drugs (sodium valproate).

Q. Classification of different glucocorticoid preparations:

A. Short-acting (1/2 life is <12 hours):

i. Cortisol (hydrocortisone).
ii. Cortisone.

B. Intermediate-acting (1/2 life is 12–36 hours):

i. Prednisone.
ii. Prednisolone.
iii. Methylprednisolone.
iv. Triamcinolone.

C. Long-acting (1/2 life is >48 hours):

i. Paramethasone.
ii. Betamethasone.
iii. Dexamethasone.

Clinical Wisdom

If the potency of cortisol is taken as 1, the potency of prednisolone will be 4 and that of dexamethasone will be 30–40; so dexamethasone is 8–10 times more potent than prednisolone.

Q. Identification points (Cushing's syndrome):

1. Obesity.
2. Face: (i) Moon face, (ii) Dusky and plethoric, (iii) Hirsutism, and may have acne.

❍ Old photographs may be useful for clinical diagnosis.

ACROMEGALY — CASE 73

Q. How to diagnose acromegaly by inspection (Fig. 3.151)?

1. Prognathism (lantern jaw or bull-dog jaw): Lower incisors (mandible) protrude in front of the upper incisors (maxilla), and widened spaces between upper and lower teeth (also there is splaying of the teeth, i.e. interdental seperation); heavy chin.
2. Enlargement of the face as a whole with prominent supraorbital ridges as a result of enlargement of maxillary, frontal and ethmoid sinuses; frontal bossing.
3. Macroglossia with thick lips, large ears, and fleshy and stubby nose (tongue may show indentations from the teeth).
4. Thick skin with hypertrichosis (e.g. bushy eyebrows), hyperhidrosis and increased sebum production (greasy skin); exaggerated nasolabial folds.
5. Spade-shaped hand (broad hand with thick, large, square-tip fingers) with warm, sweaty and doughy feeling; there is increase in volume of the hands and feet. Broad toes.
6. Deep, husky and resonant voice due to inceased thickness of vocal cord.

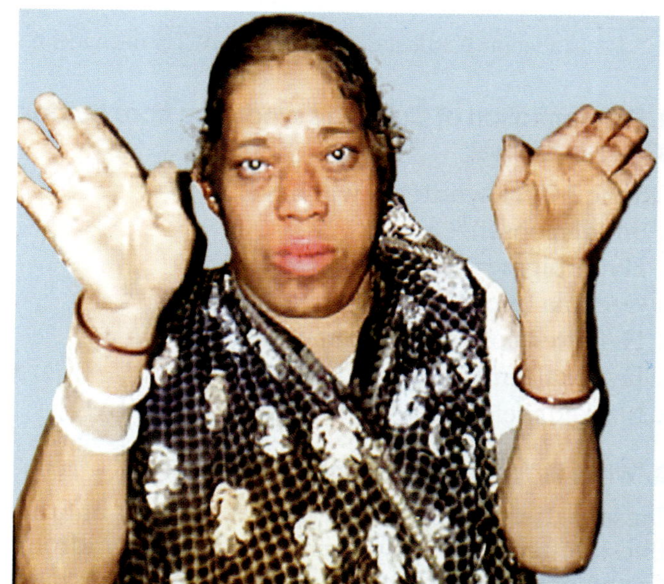

Fig. 3.151: Acromegaly characterized by prognathism, enlargement of face and 'spade-shaped' hands

- It is a disease of middle age. Common complaints are headache, changes in appearance, visual-field defects, soft tissue swelling and increased sweating.
- Larger ears and nose are due to cartilagenous overgrowth.
- Females may have a masculinised appearance with mild hirsutism.

Clinical Wisdom

Other causes of **prognathism** are: Fragile-X syndrome, osteopetrosis (certain variety) and nemaline myopathy. In prognathism, lower teeth overbites the upper teeth.

Q. Cranial nerve involvement in acromegaly:

1. Bitemporal hemianopia (pressure on optic chiasma)—Commonest.
2. Blindness due to optic atrophy (affection of optic nerve).
3. External ophthalmoplegia (paralysis of III, IV and VIth cranial nerves).
4. Deafness (VIIIth nerve palsy).

- So, visual field testing should be done in all cases of acromegaly.
- Other 'pressure effects' by the enlarged pituitary gland may be upward pressure to hypothalamus (polyphagia, polydipsia, thermal dysregulation), on temporal lobe (complex partial seizure), and features of raised intracranial tension.

Q. Metabolic and circulatory changes in acromegaly:

1. Glucose intolerance (25%).
2. Diabetes mellitus (10%), and
3. Hypertension (25%).

Q. Investigations you like to perform:

A. Hormone assay:

1. Radioimmunoassay shows increased basal level of GH (normal level <0.5 µg/L).
2. GH level fails to be suppressed <0.3 µg/L during an oral glucose tolerance test (GTT).
3. Estimation of plasma somatomedin level (i.e. IGF-1) by radioimmunoassay (almost always raised in acromegaly).

- Due to pulsatile nature of GH secretion, a single random GH level is not useful for diagnosis. In 30% patients, the serum prolactin level is elevated due to co-secretion by the tumour. In acromegaly, insulin-like growth factor-1 (IGF-1) levels are increased and the major biochemical effects of growth hormone (GH) is mediated by IGF-1. Thus, atheromatous disease, colon polyps and carcinoma of the colon may complicate acromegaly in the long run.

B. Visual field examination (perimetry): A common defect is bitemporal hemianopia.

C. Radiological changes:

1. Skull (lateral view):
   a. Enlargement of the pituitary fossa (i.e. enlarged sella turcica).
   b. Sometimes, there is double floor of pituitary fossa.
   c. Erosion of posterior clinoid process.
   d. Prominent supraorbital ridges and jaw.
   e. Enlargement of the frontal and maxillary sinuses.
2. Extremities:
   a. Tufting of the terminal phalanges, i.e. 'arrow-head appearance'.
   b. 'Heel-pad thickness' is increased, i.e. >23 mm suggests acromegaly.
3. Spine: There is evidences of kyphoscoliosis and osteoporosis.
4. Chest: Cardiomegaly.
5. Ultrasonography of abdomen: Organomegaly (especially hepatosplenomegaly).
6. CT or MRI scan of brain to visualise pituitary gland: Reveals pituitary (macro-) adenoma.

D. Biochemical:

1. Oral glucose tolerance test: Impaired.
2. Raised serum phosphorus and alkaline phosphatase level.
3. Elevated urinary calcium and hydroxyproline.
4. Pituitary function test: Partial or complete anterior hypopituitarism may be present.

- **'Heel-pad thickness'** is also increased in obesity and oedema-producing states.
- Enlarged sella turcica is also seen in pregnancy, primary hypothyroidism and empty sella syndrome.

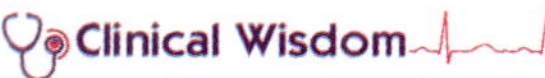

Model case with diagnosis: A patient of acromegaly due to anterior pituitary tumour with osteoarthritis of knee.

Q. Assessment of 'activity' in acromegaly:

1. Increasing size of gloves, rings, hats or shoes.
2. Ill-fitting previous dentures.
3. Excessive sebum secretion.
4. Excessive sweating.
5. Increasing headache.
6. Increasing visual field defect.
7. Facial and acral deformities.
8. Serial photography (gradually progressive macrosomia).
9. Rise in the plasma GH and IGF-1 levels.

Q. What is gigantism?

GH stimulates skeletal and soft tissue growth, and hypersecretion of GH before the fusion of epiphysis is known as *gigantism*. *Acromegaly* is hypersecretion of GH after the fusion of epiphysis and usually results from a pituitary macroadenoma (>10 mm).

Q. Why the nomenclature acromegaly?

'Acral' means peripheral (hands and feet), and 'megaly' means enlargement.

Q. What is the opposite terminology of 'prognathism'?

It is micrognathia (receding chin), which is found in temporo-mandibular (TM) joint ankylosis, Pierre Robin syndrome and Treacher Collins syndrome. JIA is an acquired cause of micrognathia.

Q. Commonest pituitary 'hormone producing' tumour:

Prolactinoma (usually microadenoma <10 mm).

Q. Features in respiratory and cardiovascular system of acromegaly:

- Respiratory system: Deep and husky voice, increased size of sinuses, obstructive sleep apnoea syndrome.
- CVS: Systemic hypertension, cardiomegaly, cardiomyopathy, CCF.

Q. Other features of acromegaly:

1. Headache.
2. Arthropathy.
3. Osteoarthritis.
4. Pseudogout.
5. Myopathy (proximal).
6. Peripheral neuropathy.
7. Carpal tunnel syndrome.
8. Visceromegaly (liver, kidney, heart, tongue).
9. ↑ Skin pigmentation; fibromata mollusca.
10. Acanthosis nigricans.
11. Galactorrhoea (in females).
12. ↓ Libido, oligomenorhoea, infertility.

Q. Causes of carpal tunnel syndrome (CTS):

'Carpal tunnel' is formed at wrist by carpal bones behind and flexor retinaculum in front. The causes of CTS are:

1. Rheumatoid arthritis.
2. Myxoedema.
3. Acromegaly.
4. Compression of median nerve by oedema, tenosynovitis, Colles' fracture, fibrosis or fasciitis.
5. Primary amyloidosis.
6. Pregnancy in the third trimester (due to oedema) or premenstrual oedema.
7. Osteoarthritis, rarely.
8. Exposure to vibration (drivers of tractor, mobile crane; workers involved in chipping, grinding or using drills), work-related (computer operators), eosinophilic fasciitis, systemic sclerosis.
9. Diabetes mellitus.
10. Obesity.
11. Patients on haemodialysis (due to deposition of β_2-microglobulin, which is an amyloid).
12. Idiopathic (probably the commonest cause): Comman in middle aged, obese female.

CTS is due to entrapment of median nerve while it passes through the carpal tunnel at wrist. Nocturnal

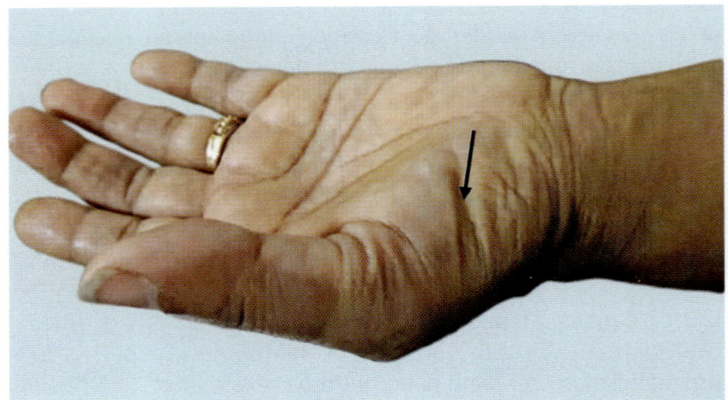

Fig. 3.152: **Carpal tunnel syndrome** (CTS) with wasting of abductor pollicis brevis muscle of left hand

pain, paraesthesia and numbness of radial three-and-a-half fingers are complained, commonly by a female patient. There may be weakness of the abductor pollicis brevis muscle (at thenar eminence) with or without wasting (Fig. 3.152). Tapping over the median nerve at carpal tunnel produces paraesthesia along the cutaneous distribution of the nerve (*Tinel's sign*); and the symptoms may be reproduced on passive maximal wrist flexion (*Phalen's test*); raising the BP above systolic pressure for 2 minutes produces paraesthesia (tourniquet test). *Nerve conduction study confirms the diagnosis.*

Avoiding precipitating activities, a wrist splint at night, local corticosteroid injection or surgical decompression (in prolonged latency on NCV) of the carpal tunnel are different modes of treatment in CTS.

Q. Different 'entrapment neuropathy' in clinical medicine:

Direct pressure on a nerve due to compression may involve:

- Median nerve (at wrist): Carpal tunnel syndrome.
- Ulnar nerve (at elbow in cubital tunnel).
- Radial nerve (at spiral groove of humerus after a fracture).
- Lateral femoral cutaneous nerve (trapped under inguinal ligament): Meralgia paraesthetica.
- Common peroneal nerve (at the neck of fibula).
- Posterior tibial nerve (at the flexor retinaculum at ankle joint): Tarsal tunnel syndrome.
- Suprascapular nerve (trapped in the spinoglenoid notch).

Q. What is Sheehan's syndrome?

It is a postpartum necrosis of anterior pituitary (hypopituitarism) with a positive H/o persistent prolonged bleeding following delivery. Ultimately there is failure of lactation, persistent amenorrhoea and reduction of secondary sexual characters (e.g. atrophy of breast, loss of axillary and pubic hair).

Q. Outline of management of acromegaly:

1. **Medical:** Bromocriptine (long-acting dopamine agonist)—usual dose is 10–60 mg daily in divided

doses. It is started in a low dose of 1.25–2.5 mg/day and the dose is gradually increased. Side effects are nausea, vomiting, dyskinesia, postural hypotension, constipation, etc. Bromocriptine is useful along with other modalities of therapy. Another **dopamine agonist** used is cabergoline (0.5 mg daily) which also shrinks tumours; quinagolide too may be used. Nowadays, **somatostatin analogues** (octreotide or lanreotide) are treatment of choice in resistant cases. The dose of octreotide is 50 µg tds/day (starting dose) to 1500 µg/day by SC injections, and that of lanreotide is 30–60 mg by deep SC injections given monthly. Growth hormone receptor antagonists (e.g. pegvisomant 10–20 mg, SC, daily) are most effective but costly drugs.

2. **Surgical:**
   a. Trans-sphenoidal (for small tumours) and trans-frontal surgery (for large tumours).
   b. Stereotaxic placement of probes (radio-surgery).
   c. Cryosurgery.
3. **Radiotherapy:**
   a. External gamma irradiation (total 4500 rads).
   b. Accelerated proton beam (total doses up to 10000 rads may be given).
   c. Local implantation of radioactive isotopes of yttrium or gold into the pituitary fossa via a transnasal stereotaxic operation.

- Surgery is usually required in visual field defect. Trans-sphenoidal approach is regarded as first line of treatment; external radiotherapy (gamma knife) is employed as second line of treatment if symptoms persist after surgery. Control of hypertension and diabetes is done accordingly.
- The target of treatment is to achieve a mean GH level <2.5 µg/L.

Q. Identification points:

1. Prognathism.
2. Enlargement of the face, and
3. 'Spade-shaped' hand.

PALPATION OF BASE OF THE HEART — CASE 74

Q. Method of palpation of base of the heart (Fig. 3.153):

The **patient will sit and lean forward** as base of the heart comes closure to chest wall in this position of the patient. Standing on the right side of the patient, put your right palm over the sternum transversely in such a way that your fingers lie over the *pulmonary area*, centre of the palm rests over the sternum, and thenar-hypothenar eminences lie over the *aortic area*.

- **'Base of the heart' includes aortic and pulmonary area.**
- Patient should take natural respiration. Events in pulmonary area are accentuated in inspiration and that of aortic area are augmented in expiration.

Q. What to palpate?

1. Pulsation.

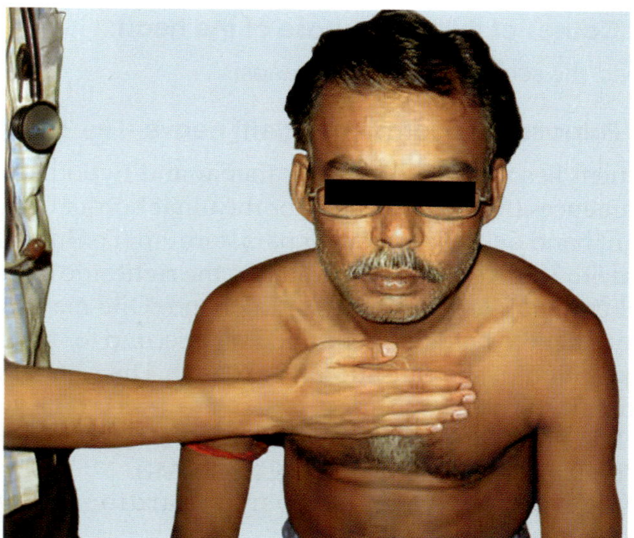

Fig. 3.153: Palpation of **base of the heart** (in sitting position)

2. Palpable heart sounds (P_2 or A_2), and
3. Thrill.

Q. Palpate aortic, pulmonary, mitral and tricuspid areas (*see* Fig. 1.4)**:**

a. Aortic area: Patient will sit and lean forward; put your right palm over right 2nd ICS.
b. Pulmonary area: Patient will sit and lean forward; put your right palm over left 2nd ICS.
c. Mitral area: Read the section on 'Mitral incompetence' (i.e. palpate the mitral area, i.e. page 27).
d. Tricuspid area: Patient will be lying in supine position. Put your right palm over left 4th ICS (close to the sternum).

Q. Causes of pulsation over the pulmonary and aortic area:

Read page 41, in the section on 'Aortic incompetence'.

Q. Causes of palpable heart sounds in precordium:

For palpation of heart sounds, use whole flat of the right palm.

a. Palpable S_1 (mitral area): Produces 'tapping' apex beat in MS.
b. Palpable S_2 (P_2): Best palpable in pulmonary area. Palpable S_2 (P_2) is found in pulmonary hypertension of any aetiology; palpable $S_2(A_2)$ in aortic area is common in systemic hypertension. Palpable P_2 or A_2 is known a 'diastolic shock' or 'diastolic knock'. Read the section on 'Mitral incompetence' for the causes of pulmonary hypertension.
c. Palpable S_3: In LVF (mitral area) or RVF (lower left parasternum).
d. Palpable S_4 (mitral area): Responsible for 'double' kicking apex beat in IHSS.

- *For demonstration of any event (palpation, percussion or auscultation) in aortic or pulmonary area, always ask the patient to sit and lean forward.*

Q. Causes of thrill in the base of the heart:

Read the section on 'Aortic stenosis'.

Q. Palpation for parasternal (left) heave (Fig. 3.154):

Patient lies supine. Place your thenar and hypothenar eminences (heel of the palm), or the ulnar border of the right hand over the lower left parasternum (i.e. 3rd, 4th and 5th ICS) vertically. Standing on the right side of the patient, look for any lifting of the hand. One may ask the patient to hold the respiration for a second for better perception of the pulsation (i.e. heave). The causes of left parasternal heave are:

1. **RVH due to any cause (commonest).**
2. Left atrial hypertrophy (rare; e.g. in MI).
3. ASD (left parasternal lift).
4. Aortic aneurysm.

- 'Heave' means the impulse is forceful and well sustained while 'lift' means the impulse is forceful but it is ill sustained.

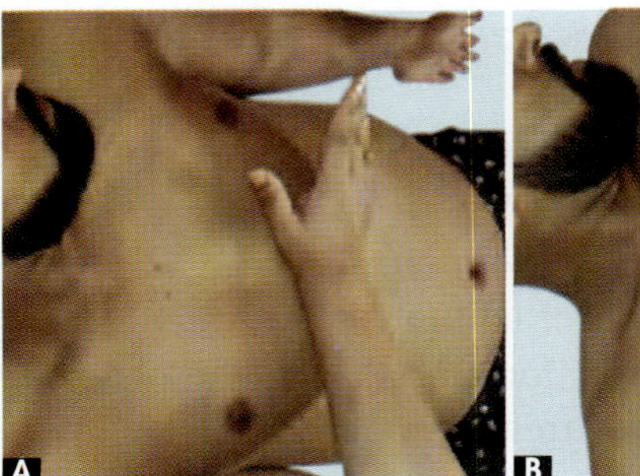

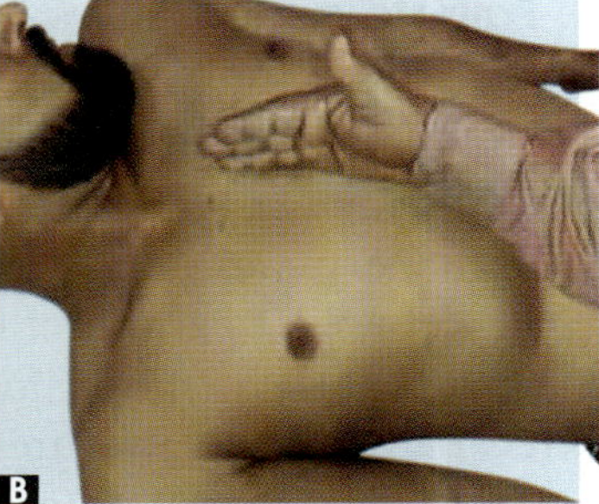

Fig. 3.154: Palpation of left parasternal heave–by heel of palm [A] and ulnar border of hand [B]

PERCUSSION OF THE STERNUM OR BASE OF THE HEART — CASE 75

Q. Three cardinal rules of percussion:

See page 79.

Q. Why percussion is not done routinely in CVS (i.e. cardiac percussion)?

1. Not much informative (has been replaced by chest X-ray and echocardiography).
2. Dislodgement of thrombi may occur in a case of MS, acute myocardial infarction (AMI) or atrial fibrillation. Thus, it may precipitate systemic embolism.
3. The major part of heart is surrounded by resonant lung, which may give rise to ambiguous results.
4. It is a cumbersome method in female patients.

Q. Situations where cardiac percussion is still helpful:

1. Pericardial effusion (cardiac dullness is increased).
2. Emphysema (cardiac dullness is lost).
3. Dextrocardia.

- There is loss of cardiac dullness in left-sided pneumothorax too.

Q. Percussion note over sternum:

It is resonant because aerated lungs are present behind the sternum.

Q. How the sternum is percussed?

Sternum may be directly percussed by percussing finger (like the percussion of clavicle). Here, the sternum itself acts as pleximeter finger. Actually in clinical practice, the method described below is followed for percussion of the sternum.

Q. How to percuss the base of the heart?

1. Ask the patient to sit. Percussion is usually done in the 2nd ICS.
2. First place the pleximeter finger in the *aortic area* parallel to right sternal border.
3. The line of percussion in the aortic area will be perpendicular to right sternal border and go on percussing up to the middle of the sternum (i.e. go from right to left).
4. Now place the pleximeter finger in the *pulmonary area* parallel to left sternal border. The line of percussion in the pulmonary area will be perpendicular to left sternal border and percuss up to the middle of the sternum where you left (i.e. now go from left to right).
5. One may percuss the aortic and pulmonary areas by the above method and may stop the percussion after reaching right and left borders of the sternum, respectively. Then percussion of the sternum may be done directly (alternative method).
6. Listen the percussion note carefully. Thereafter, percussion may be done in the 3rd ICS.

- **The above mentioned method may be used for percussion of base of the heart or percussion of the sternum or 'mediastinal percussion' (Fig. 3.155).**

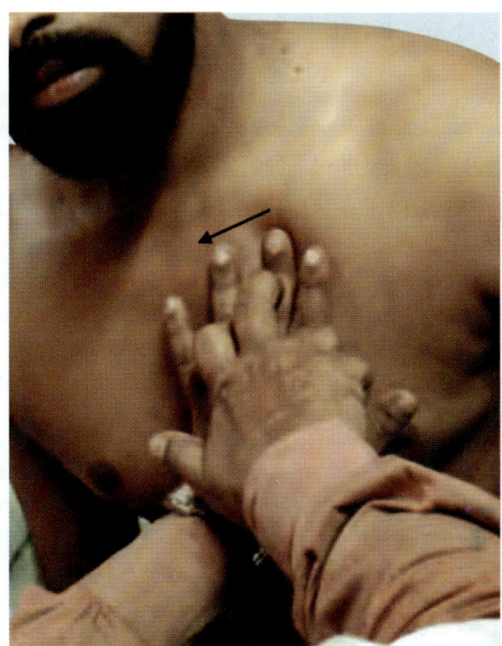

Fig. 3.155: Demostration of **mediastinal percussion**

Q. Dullness over pulmonary area:

1. Aneurysm of the aorta.
2. Any mediastinal mass.
3. Massive pericardial effusion.
4. Pulmonary hypertension.

Q. Dullness over sternum:

Sternum is dull on percussion due to superior and anterior mediastinal mass like:

1. Lymphoma.
2. Bronchogenic carcinoma.
3. Thymoma.
4. Aortic aneurysm.
5. Retrosternal goitre.
6. Teratodermoid.
7. Metastatic carcinoma, and
8. Oesophageal cysts.

Clinical Wisdom

If a dull note is obtained over the sternum, immediately look for any venous prominence in the neck or swelling of the face and arm, i.e. for the signs of 'SVC syndrome'. SVC syndrome is an indirect evidence of the presence of mediastinal mass. Never forget to percuss the sternum in a patient with generalised lymphadenopathy (e.g. mediastinal adenopathy in lymphoma).

Q. How will you percuss the heart?

Cardiac percussion is not routinely practised nowadays for reasons mentioned earlier.

1. At first, find out the upper border of liver dullness along the right MCL.
2. Now to choose your space of percussion for the delineation of right border of heart, select 'one space higher' the upper border of liver dullness. Keeping the pleximeter finger parallel to the arbitrary right border of heart, lightly *percuss from right to left*. Actually, percussion is done in the 3rd and 4th ICS (avoid percussion over ribs). As soon as the dull note is obtained (due to heart), mark it and then join the points. This is the **right border of heart**.
3. Now, localise the apex.
4. For the **left border of heart**, percuss along (or parallel to) the 'left acromio-xiphoid line' (an imaginary line from left-sided tip of the acromion process to the xiphisternum) in the 2nd, 3rd and 4th ICS. Join the points of dullness with the apex.
5. Lastly, percuss the base of the heart to delineate the **upper border** (left 2nd and 3rd ICS). Percussion is done parallel to prasternal line (line in between MCL and lateral sternal line).
6. The **lower border** of heart is not percussed as its dullness is intermingled with hepatic dullness.

- Normally right border remains retrosternal; if the dullness is parasternal, think of pericardial effusion, aneurysm of the ascending aorta (Potain's sign), dextrocardia, mediastinal mass, etc. Left border usually remains along the apex beat; if it is outside the apex beat, think of pericardial effusion. Remember, *normally the left 2nd ICS is resonant and the left 3rd ICS is dull on percussion*; if the 2nd ICS gives dull note, think of pericardial effusion, mediastinal mass, aortic aneurysm, pulmonary hypertension.
- Cardiac dullness is also increased in cardiomegaly due to any cause (left border will be corresponding to apex). In pericardial effusion, left border will be outside the apex.

Clinical Wisdom

In case of loss of either of liver or cardiac dullness, exclude the presence of right- or left-sided pneumothorax respectively; if both the dullness are lost, think of presence of emphysema.

AUSCULTATION OF DIFFERENT AREAS OF HEART: CASE 76

Q. Auscultation of the mitral area (*see* Fig. 1.5):

1. First you have to **localise the apex beat** (i.e. the mitral area) by proper method of palpation (read the section on 'Mitral incompetence'). Mitral area corresponds to cardiac apex which is present in the left 5th ICS, 1/2" inside the left MCL.
2. Now auscultate the mitral area in dorsal decubitus position and then in **left lateral position** (apex comes closure to the chest wall) and at the height of **expiration**. Conventionally, first use the **diaphragm** of stethoscope and **then the bell**.
3. In case of a faint diastolic murmur, you may allow the patient to do mild exercise (if the present condition of the patient permits to do so, i.e. if there is no dyspnoea, CCF, arrhythmia, cyanosis, etc). Allow the patient to sit and touch both feet with both of his hands, and lie down, consecutively for five to six times. The murmur of MS becomes louder and prominent after mild exercise (before doing the exercise, you may take permission of the examiner).
4. In the presence of mitral systolic (pansystolic) murmur, you may auscult the left axilla and inferior angle of left scapula for radiation of MI murmur (always take the permission of the examiner because you are shifting your stethoscope from the mitral area).
5. Comment on murmur, heart sounds (especially on S_1), any split, click, opening snap or pericardial rub.

- If the apex beat could not be localised properly, auscultate the area 'below the left nipple' (in a young adult); usually the nipple lies in the 4th intercostal space.

Q. Auscultation of the aortic area (*see* Fig. 1.14):

1. The right 2nd ICS (close to the sternum) is the aortic area.
2. Allow the patient to **sit and lean forward**. Now auscultate the aortic area at the height of **expiration** (as left-sided events are pronounced in expiration) with the **diaphragm** of stethoscope.

3. If you have to confirm the radiation of murmur to carotids (AS) or towards the neoaortic area (AI), you have to take the permission of the examiner.
4. Comment on murmur, heart sounds (especially on A_2) or any other sounds like split, click, rub, etc.

Q. Auscultation of the pulmonary area (Fig. 3.156):

1. The left 2nd ICS (close to the sternum) is the pulmonary area.
2. Patient will **sit and lean forward** and auscultation is done with the **diaphragm** of stethoscope, at the height of **inspiration** (as right-sided events are pronounced in inspiration).
3. Comment on murmur, heart sounds (especially on P_2) or any split of S_2.

Q. Auscultation of the tricuspid area (Fig. 3.157):

1. The left 4th ICS (close to the sternum) is the tricuspid area.
2. Auscultation is done with the **diaphragm** of stethoscope, at the height of **inspiration** with the patient **lying in supine or right lateral position**. Comment on murmur or heart sounds.

Q. Auscultation of the neoaortic area (aortic II area) (Fig. 3.158):

The left 3rd ICS (close to the sternum) is known as neoaortic area or **Erb's point**. Often the early diastolic mumur of Al is best audible in the neoaortic area. The area should be auscultated in **sitting and leaning forward position** with the **diaphragm** of stethoscope, and at the height of **expiration**. Neoaortic area should be auscultated in every patient as a routine.

Q. Points to note during auscultation of CVS:

1. Heart sounds
2. Murmur.
3. Splitting of heart sounds, ejection click, opening snap, and
4. Others: Pericardial rub, pericardial knock, prosthetic valve sounds, tumour plop, etc.

Q. Sequence of auscultation of heart (*see* **Fig. 1.4**)**:**

Apex → proceed along the left border of sternum, i.e. tricuspid area → pulmonary area → then auscultate aortic area → neoaortic area → auscultate different areas, with dynamic manoeuvres (page 44), if required.

But majority of clinicians prefers to examine or write in the following way: apex → pulmonary area → aortic area → tricuspid area → neoaortic area.

- Lastly, one may auscultate over the carotid arteries (supravalvular AS) and the left axilla (MI).

Q. Basic points to note in a murmur:

Murmurs are abnormal cardiac sounds produced by turbulent blood flow (laminar flow is distorted to turbulent flow) moving through the abnormal valves (MS, MI, etc.), normal valves (pregnancy, severe anaemia), great vessels (any arterial stenosis will produce bruit) or blood passing through an abnormal channel (VSD, ASD, etc.). The points noted in a murmur are:

1. Where best audible or point of maximum intensity (enumerate the area).
2. Timing in cardiac cycle (systole, diastole or continuous).
3. Character (e.g. blowing, harsh, musical, rumbling, honking, squeaking) and pitch.
4. Radiation or direction of selective propagation (radiation indicates the direction of blood flow).
5. Intensity (grading; if thrill is present, it is grade 4 or 4+). Is it associated with thrill?
6. Change with respiration.

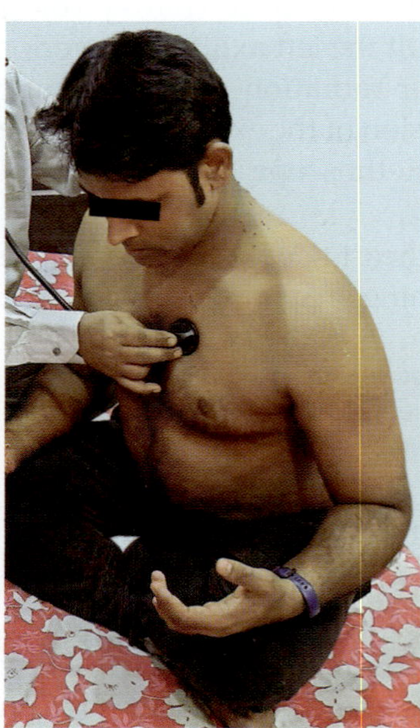

Fig. 3.156: Auscultation of **pulmonary area**

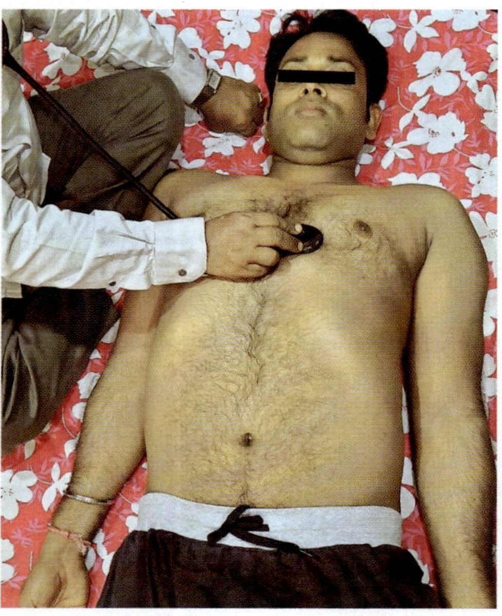

Fig. 3.157: Auscultation of **tricuspid area**

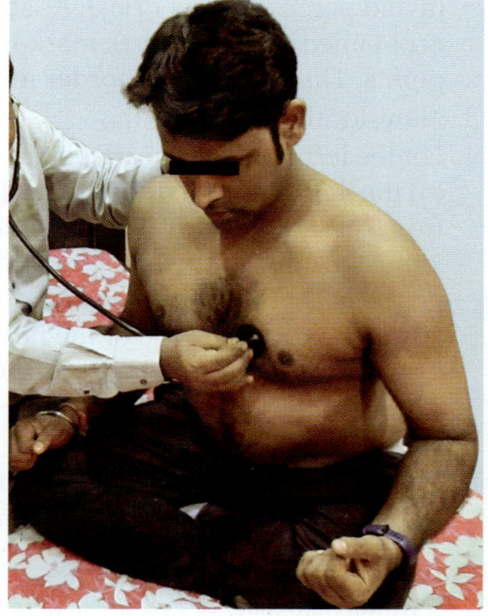

Fig. 3.158: Auscultation of **neoaortic area**

7. Change with posture.
8. Change after exercise.
9. Whether best audible with the diaphragm or the bell of stethoscope.
10. Dynamic auscultation (page 44).

- Always try to describe a murmur with these TEN POINTS.
- 'Pitch' of a murmur is determined by the flow of blood, i.e. low-pitch indicates low-velocity flow and high-pitch indicates high-velocity flow.
- Systole is the interval between S_1 and S_2, while diastole lies in between S_2 and S_1. Systolic murmurs coincide with carotid upstroke and diastolic murmurs precede (or follow) the carotid upstroke.

Clinical Wisdom

As **radiation** of a murmur is along the direction of blood flow, the intensity remains same as in the source. **Conduction** of a murmur travels through a media (i.e. anatomical continuity) like chest wall or bones, and thus its intensity decreases away from the source. It is better to avoid the term conduction of a murmur.

Q. Explanation of effects of respiration or posture on murmur:

Effects of respiration: During inspiration the intrapleural pressure becomes more negative and thus, more blood comes in the right atrium. So, during inspiration there is increase in the stroke output of the right heart and reduction in the stroke output of the left heart. Similarly, stroke output of the left heart increases on expiration. So the murmurs originating from the right side of the heart become louder and prominent on inspiration, and that from the left side of the heart become more intense on expiration.

Effects of posture: In the left lateral position, the apical area (mitral area) comes closer to the chest wall, so does the base of the heart in sitting and leaning forward position. It is why the murmurs in those areas become more intense on adopting the said postures.

Bell or diaphragm of stethoscope: Low-pitched sound, e.g. murmur of MS and TS are best auscultated by the bell of stethoscope. All other murmurs are best heard with the diaphragm of stethoscope.

Clinical Wisdom

Murmurs are produced by different mechanisms like jet impact, microbubbles formation or eddies generated around the jet.

PERICARDIAL RUB — CASE 77

Q. Characteristics:

It is a leathery sound produced by the rubbing of inflamed visceral and parietal pericardium:

1. Superficial, scratchy or leathery, inconstant or evanescent (varies from hour to hour, or day to day), high-pitched, to-and-fro sound (mimics the sound of husking machine); 'close to the ear' quality.
2. Usually best heard on the left side of lower sternum at 4th and 5th ICS (may be heard over the entire precordium): Here lies the bare area of heart, i.e. part of heart not covered by the lung.
3. Intensity of the sound increases when patient sits and leans forward (thus, always auscultate in sitting position of the patient) at the end of expiration.
4. Intensifies by pressing the chest piece (diaphragm) of stethoscope.
5. It may have presystolic, systolic and early diastolic components.
6. **Sound continues even after holding the breath.**
7. May be associated with chest pain.
8. Usually there is no transmission (i.e. localised).
9. At times it is palpable: The 'tactile fremitus' (palpable pericardial rub).

Q. What is your case?

This patient is suffering from acute dry pericarditis and there is presence of pericardial rub (describe the characteristics). *The hallmark of diagnosis of pericarditis is pericardial rub.*

Q. Causes of acute pericarditis:

1. Idiopathic (without any obvious cause).
2. Viral (H/o fever, cough, etc. Commonly Coxsackie B virus infection).
3. Tuberculous (H/o haemoptysis, anorexia, night sweats, etc).
4. Pyogenic (high rise of temperature with toxic features) or amoebic.
5. Acute rheumatic fever (arthritis, pancarditis, subcutaneous nodules).
6. Uraemia (oedema, anaemia, oliguria and usually painless pericarditis).
7. Myxoedema (delayed ankle jerk, hoarseness of voice).
8. Acute myocardial infarction (acute chest pain with collapse) during acute attack, or Dressler's syndrome (after few days to weeks, following an attack of myocardial infarction).
9. Collagen vasular diseases like SLE, systemic sclerosis (skin rash, arthralgia).
10. Neoplastic or post-irradiation (H/o radiation, lymphadenopathy).
11. Post-traumatic, post-surgical pericarditis.
12. Drug-induced (hydralazine, procainamide, INH).

- 1, 2 and 3 are most common causes, especially in India.

Q. Describe the chest pain in pericarditis:

Pain is an important but not invariable symptom in pericarditis. *Pain is absent in* slowly developing tuberculous, hypothyroid, neoplastic, post-irradiation or uraemic pericarditis. There are three types of pain:

1. Pleuritic (steady and constrictive), i.e. due to associated pleurisy and caused by direct extension

of infection and thus, the pain is aggravated by inspiration, coughing, sneezing, jolting, change of posture, etc. The rub is known as 'pleuro-pericardial rub'.
2. Steady constricting retrosternal pain which radiates in either of both arms, shoulders and neck like acute myocardial infarction.
3. Often the pain is present characteristically in the centre of the chest or left precordial, referred to the back, arms and shoulder.

- The pain of pericarditis is due to associated pleurisy or inflammation of the lower 1/3rd of the parietal pericardium (visceral pericardium is pain-insensitive) supplied by phrenic nerve. The pain varies with breathing and posture, and is often relieved by sitting up and leaning forward but increased by lying supine. The pain may last for hours or days, and is not relieved by nitrates.

Q. Investigations you like to perform:

a. Blood: TC, DC, ESR, cholesterol, urea, creatinine, ASO titre, T_4 and TSH, SGOT (AST).
b. Mantoux test: For tuberculous aetiology.
c. ECG: **ST-segment elevation with concavity upwards (saddle-back appearance)**, and flattening or inversion of T-waves.
d. Chest X-ray (in upright posture):
   1. To exclude tuberculosis in the lungs.
   2. To exclude bronchogenic carcinoma or lymphoma (mediastinal widening).
   3. Enlarged cardiac shadow may indicate very early pericardial effusion.
e. Echocardiogram: May be helpful in detecting thickening of pericardium and early effusion.
f. CT and cardiac MRI: Diagnoses thickened (>4 mm) or inflamed pericardium.

- ECG changes of acute myocardial infarction is ST-segment elevation with convexity upwards

Q. D/D of pericardial rub:

1. Systolic murmur.
2. Early diastolic murmur of aortic incompetence.
3. Continuous murmur.
   [(No. 1–3) Consistent in character, audible in all positions, soft/musical/machinery sound, pain is not associated with]
4. Artefact.
5. Hamman's sign.

Q. What is Hamman's sign?

It is a rhythmical, crunching sound heard over the precordium, which is synchronous with the heart beat. This sign is found in pneumomediastinum (or mediastinal emphysema). The sound is best audible in left lateral position. Always search for subcutaneous emphysema meticulously.

Q. Changes appearing if pericardial effusion develops:

A. Symptoms: Patient will complain of heaviness (retrosternal oppression) in the precordium, dyspnoea, palpitations, swelling of feet or whole body, dry cough, etc. Constitutional symptoms like fever, weight loss may persist.

B. Signs:

1. Orthopnoea (sometimes, patient bends forward in sitting position mimicking the position adopted by Mohammedans during prayer).
2. Face: Puffy.
3. Pulse: Tachycardia, low volume, pulsus paradoxus (especially in acutely developing pericardial effusion); other points in pulse are within normal limit.
4. Cyanosis: If present, mainly of *peripheral in type*.
5. Neck veins: Engorged and may be pulsatile; Kussmaul's sign may be present (rare).
6. BP: Systolic BP is low.
7. Oedema: Pitting in nature.
8. Heart:
   a. Bulging of precordium with intercostal fullness.
   b. Apical impulse: Neither visible nor palpable.
   c. Cardiac dullness is increased on percussion. If apex beat is palpable, it will be feeble and will remain within the outer border of cardiac dullness. Percussion note over the sternum and left 2nd ICS is dull. *Tympanicity on Traube's space percussion is retained.*
   d. Heart sounds become faint or muffled. Pericardial friction rub is not always abolished.
9. Lungs: No adventitious sound is heard. Presence of **Ewart's sign** which is,
   a. Dullness on percussion,
   b. Increased vocal resonance, and
   c. Bronchial breath sound (tubular).
   All the features are due to compression collapse of the left lung by massive pericardial effusion and is found at the inferior angle of left scapula (i.e. base of left lung).
10. Alimentary system:
    a. Liver: Enlarged, soft and tender (congestive hepatomegaly).
    b. Ascites: May be present.
11. ECG: Low voltage QRS complexes (vide page 393), electrical alternans (rare).
12. Chest X-ray (PA view): Enlarged cardiac silhouette, globular or 'pear-shaped heart,' oligaemic lung fields and positive Rotch's sign. Echocardiography confirms the diagnosis. CT and cardiac MRI are superior to echocardiography in selective cases.

- Pulsus paradoxus and Kussmaul's sign are hallmarks of **cardiac tamponade** (commonly from tuberculosis, malignancy, post-surgical or traumatic). In cardiac tamponade, there is collection of fluid in the pericardial sac in an amount sufficient to produce serious obstruction to inflow of blood to the ventricles and thus, results in acute heart failure (there is decrease in stroke volume due to impaired cardiac contraction). The amount of fluid may be as small as 250 mL when the fluid collects rapidly or it may be more than 1000 mL in slowly developing effusions. It is a medical emergency and pericardiocentesis is lifesaving.

- Three distinct signs are characteristic of acute cardiac tamponade. They are low arterial BP (i.e. hypotension), distended neck vein, and distant and muffled heart sounds **(Beck's triad)**.
- Haemorrhagic pericardial effusion is common in tuberculosis, trauma, aortic dissection, metastatic carcinoma, use of anticoagulants and rupture of the heart.

Q. Uraemic pericarditis: What to do?

If pericardial rub is heard in a patient of uraemia, immediately send the patient for dialysis.

Q. Treatment of acute pericarditis:

1. Rest in bed.
2. NSAID: Indomethacin (25 mg, thrice daily, orally after meal) or aspirin may be used.
3. Glucocorticoid: Prednisolone 20–80 mg daily in selected cases (immune-mediated or relapsing pericarditis); does not accelerate cure, only gives symptomatic relief. If there is no response to corticosteroid, azathioprine or colchicine may be tried.
4. Treatment of the underlying cause (e.g. antibiotics, antituberculosis drugs).

- The patient is observed frequently for the development of pericardial effusion.

Clinical Wisdom

In a suspected case with pericardial rub, ask the patient to **hold the respiration**. One should do this to differentiate pericardial rub from left-sided pleural rub. *After breath holding, pericardial rub continues but pleural rub stops*. Occasionally during inspiration, pericardial rub intensifies and this component is known as 'pleuro-pericardial rub'.

Pericardial rub usually disappears when pericardial effusion develops.

SHAPE OF THE CHEST — CASE 78

Q. Mention the common chest deformities:

1. Kyphoscoliosis.
2. Barrel-shaped chest.
3. Pigeon chest (pectus carinatum).
4. Funnel chest (pectus excavatum).
5. Alar chest (pterygoid chest).
6. Unilateral or bilateral, depression or fullness of the chest.
7. Deformity associated with ankylosing spondylitis, straight back syndrome, thoracoplasty operation (in this procedure, some ribs are resected on one side of chest to achieve collapse of the lung), severe chest trauma, or absence of part of chest wall (e.g. ribs, pectoralis muscle or clavicle).

- Defects in the chest wall may be described in a better way like:
  - Defects in sternum: Pectus carinatum, pectus excavatum.
  - Defects in spine: Kyphosis, scoliosis, lordosis, straight back syndrome, ankylosing spondylitis.
  - Defects in costal cartilage: Rachitic rosary, scorbutic rosary, costochondritis.

Q. Kyphosis and scoliosis (Fig. 3.159):

A. KYPHOSIS means exaggerated anterior curvature of the spine with an *increased convexity posteriorly* (round back or hunchback—like the shape of the letter 'K'). SCOLIOSIS means *lateral bending* of the vertebral column (like the shape of the letter 'S'). The combination of the two is known as **kyphoscoliosis** (Fig. 3.160).

These are abnormalities of alignment of the dorsal and lumbar spines. In severe kyphoscoliosis, they may lead to asymmetry of the chest wall resulting in restricted expansion of the chest wall, maldistribution of ventilation and blood flow in the lungs. Ultimately type II respiratory failure, pulmonary hypertension, RVF and chronic cor pulmonale develop.

B. Common causes of kyphoscoliosis are:

1. Congenital.
2. Vertebral diseases like ankylosing spondylitis, senile osteoporosis (Dowager's hump or widow's hump), osteoarthritis, rheumatoid arthritis, rickets, etc.
3. Caries spine (Pott's disease): With 'gibbus' (acute angulation in the spine) formation.
4. Neurological causes: Neurofibromatosis, Friedreich's ataxia, syringomyelia, poliomyelitis and cerebral palsy.
5. Occupational (e.g. porters carrying weight on the back), traumatic or postural (tall persons).
6. Miscellaneous: Marfan's syndrome, Turner's syndrome, after thoracoplasty, etc.

- Extensive unilateral fibrosis or collapse of the lung in childhood may give rise to scoliosis.

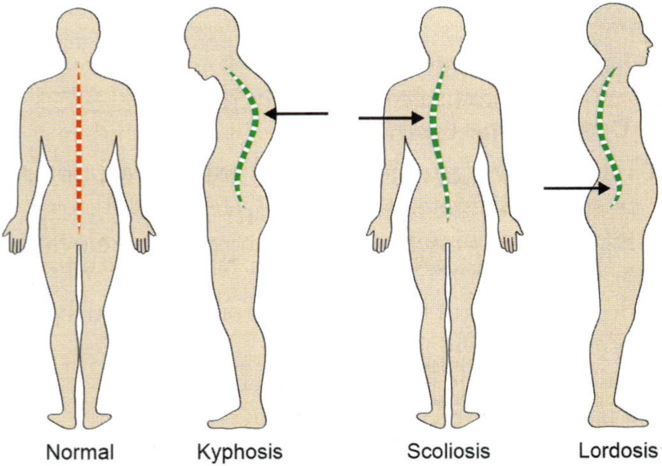

Fig. 3.159: Different **spinal deformities**

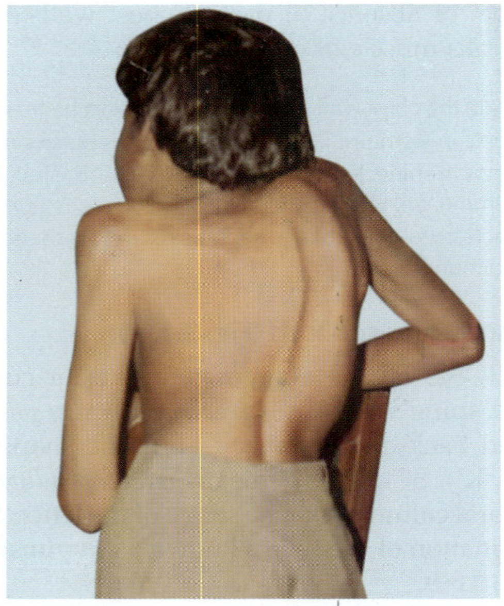

Fig. 3.160: **Kyphoscoliosis** with **winging of the scapula**

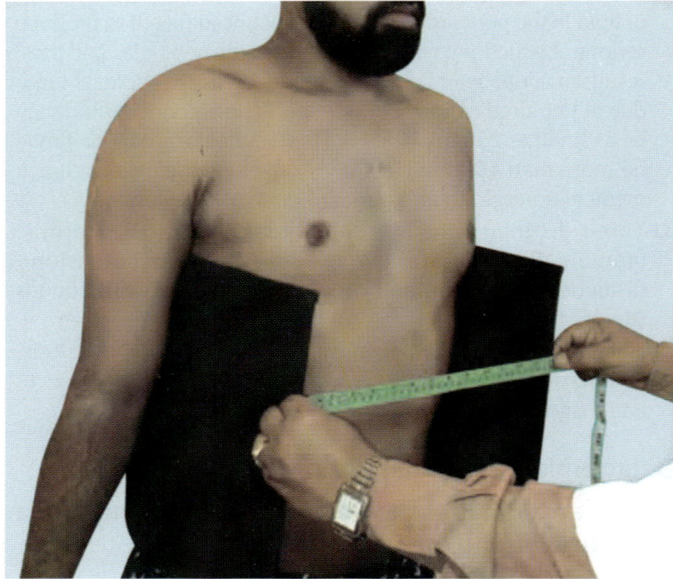

Fig. 3.161A: Measurement of **transverse diameter of chest**

C. The common form of scoliosis with convexity to the right side displaces the apex beat towards the concavity, i.e. to the left side. Trachea may be displaced in simple scoliosis. It should be remembered that the *commonest cause of displacement of the apex beat is deformity of thoracic cage, usually scoliosis.*

D. Method of diagnosis:
   1. Scoliosis: The patient will stand erect with fully exposed chest and the observer looks for scoliosis from his back. It is observed whether the convexity is present in left or right side. Afterwards, it may be corroborated by palpation of the spine.
   2. Kyphosis: The observer inspects the back from the sides in profile, i.e. a tangential view from both sides are necessary. The patient will stand erect with fully exposed chest. In kyphosis, there is an increase in the antero-posterior diameter of the chest.

- [LORDOSIS means *exaggerated inward curvature of lumbar spine* (swayback) or lumbar spine is more convexed anteriorly. Exaggerated lumbar lordosis is commonly seen in advanced pregnancy (hyperlordosis), obesity, secondary to hip joint disorders, muscular dystrophy, in large abdominal tumours or massive ascites].
- In health, there are cervical and lumbar lordosis, and thoracic and sacral kyphosis.

Q. Describe the normal chest:

1. Elliptical in cross section, i.e. transverse: antero-posterior diameter = 7:5 (Figs 3.161A and B).
2. Bilaterally symmetrical and without undue elevation or depression.
3. Both the sides of the chest move simultaneously and symmetrically.
4. Subcostal angle is 90° or less than 90° (males having a narrower angle than females).
5. The intercostal spaces (ICS) are broader anteriorly than posteriorly.

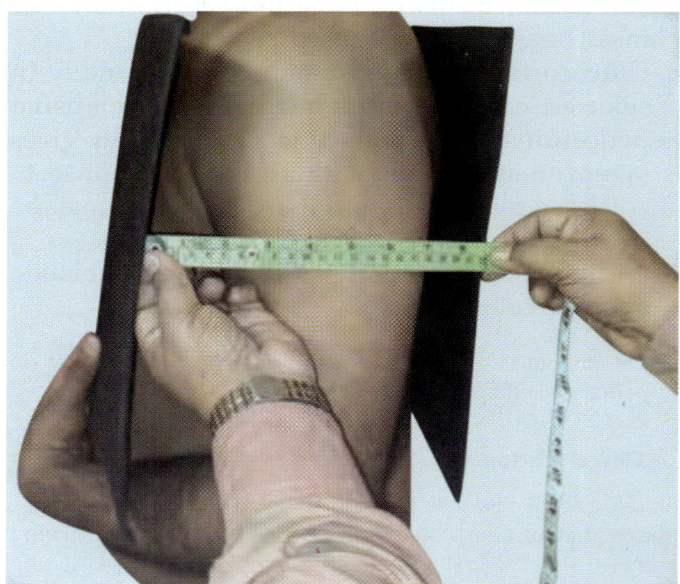

Fig. 3.161B: Measurement of **AP diameter of chest**

Q. Barrel-shaped chest (Fig. 3.162):

1. Antero-posterior diameter of the chest is increased (AP:TR = 1:1) and it is circular in cross section.
2. The whole chest is relatively fixed in full inspiration.
3. Intercostal spaces (ICS) are full, ribs are less obliquely set and wide apart.
4. There may be exaggerated kyphosis of thoracic vertebrae.
5. Fullness of supraclavicular fossae.
6. The chest tends to move upwards in one piece.
7. Wide subcostal angle (>90°).
8. Prominence of sternal angle.
9. Rarely encircling prominent veins are seen in the lower part of the chest.

   Cause: Severe obstructive airway disease or emphysema (i.e. hyperinflated lungs).

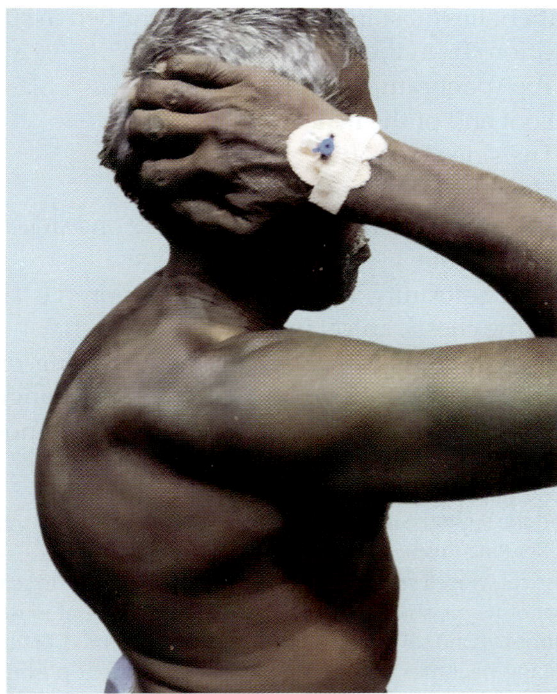

Fig. 3.162: **Barrel-shaped chest** in COPD

Q. Pigeon chest (pectus carinatum) (Fig. 3.163):

1. Triangular chest (in cross section) with forward protrusion of sternum, which resembles a pigeon's breast.
2. Rachitic rosary (beaded appearance of the costochondral junction; best demonstrated in the 4th, 5th and 6th ribs).
3. Harrison's sulcus (linear depression or sulcus present transversely from the sides of the xiphoid process to the midaxillary line as a result of repeated strong contractions of diaphragm).
   Causes:
   a. Childhood bronchial asthma.
   b. Repeated lung infections since childhood.
   c. Rickets (soft pre-pubertal bones).
   d. Idiopathic.

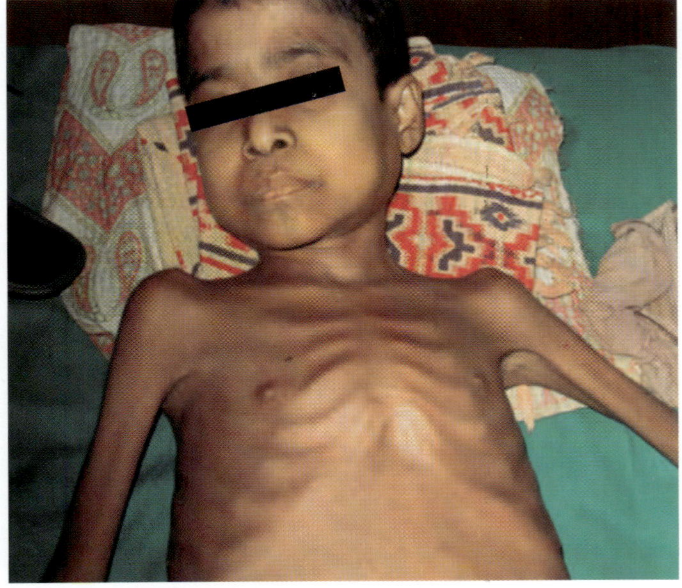

Fig. 3.163: **Pectus carinatum** or **pigeon chest.** Rachitic rosary and Harrison's sulcus are seen in a patient of **rickets**

Q. Funnel chest (pectus excavatum) (Fig. 3.164):

1. Curving backwards (i.e. depression) of the body of the sternum, usually the lower part.
2. Antero-posterior diameter < transverse diameter.
3. Undue prominence of the costochondral junction.
   Causes:
   a. Repeated lung infections since childhood.
   b. In shoe-makers (cobbler's chest).
   c. Congenital.
   d. Marfan's syndrome.

Clinical Wisdom

Pectus excavatum may give rise to displaced apex beat to the left and a 'benign' systolic murmur due to right ventricular outflow tract obstruction; and the cardiac shadow may be enlarged in X-ray chest (PA view) as a result of sternal compression (Pomfret's heart). There may be restrictive type lung function defect, if very severe.

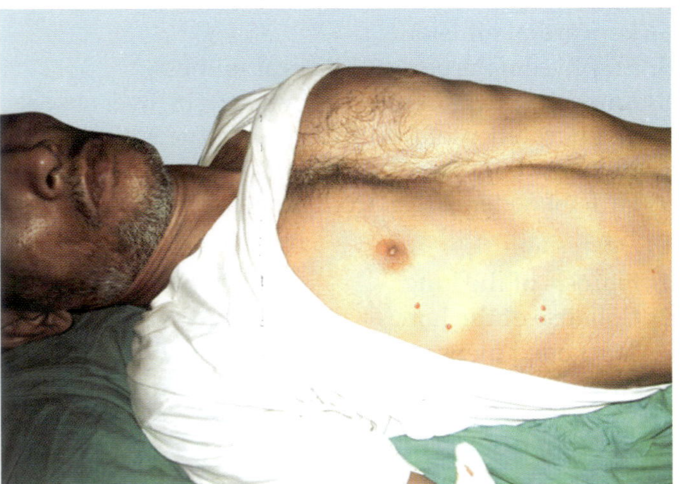

Fig. 3.164: **Pectus excavatum** or **funnel chest**

Q. Alar chest:

1. Drooping of both the shoulders.
2. Winging of both the scapulae (i.e. prominent vertebral borders of scapulae).
3. Chest is narrow and tubular; often loosely termed as 'flat chest'.
   Cause: It is found in tall and thin built normal persons; often known as phthinoid chest.

- Shield-like chest: Broad chest with widely placed nipples, and is found in Turner's syndrome.
- Flail chest: Found in multiple rib fractures where the affected area (fractured portion) moves inwards on inspiration, and outwards on expiration (paradoxical movement of chest).
- Frozen chest: Restricted movement of the chest (e.g. ankylosing spondylitis).
- Hidebound chest: Restriction of chest movement due to tight skin in scleroderma.

Q. Cross-sectional view in different types of chest deformities:

1. Normal: Elliptical.
2. Barrel-shaped chest: Circular
3. Pigeon chest: Triangular.

Q. D/D of rachitic rosary:

Scorbutic rosary (seen in scurvy): The costochondral junctions are prominent, painful and appear sharp as well as angular; due to posterior subluxation or pushing in of the sternum.

Rachitic rosary: The bead-like prominence at costochondral junctions are non-tender, dome-shaped and semicircular. Rosary means 'a chain of roses'.

Q. Fullness or depression of the chest:

A. Fullness:

1. Massive pleural effusion.
2. Empyema thoracis.
3. Pneumothorax.
4. Hydropneumothorax or pyopneumothorax.
5. Bronchogenic carcinoma.
6. Pericardial effusion.
7. Emphysema produces bilateral fullness.
8. Empyema necessitans, aortic aneurysm, liver abscess, or encysted pleural effusion produces 'localised' fullness.
9. Parietal oedema (e.g. from amoebic liver abscess).

B. Depression:

1. Fibrosis of the lung.
2. Collapse of the lung.
3. Thickened pleura or pleural adhesions.
4. After rib resection in thoracotomy, mastectomy.

Q. Straight back syndrome:

The back becomes straight due to loss of normal throacic kyphosis and thus, the antero-posterior diameter of the chest is reduced. The heart may be compressed between the sternum and the spine.

Q. 'Inspection' for shape and movement of the chest:

A. Inspection of the chest is best done in standing or sitting (if standing is not possible) position, in good daylight with proper exposure (by stripping) of front and back of the chest. The breasts should preferably be covered in females. The patient should stand absolutely straight. Sitting means the patient will sit on a stool. The chest is inspected from:
   1. Front.
   2. Back.
   3. The sides in profile.
   4. Looking from above (standing behind the patient), over the shoulders for inspection of the upper part of the chest.

   If standing or sitting is not possible for a severely ill patient, then inspect the chest in lying down position (patient lies 'absolutely straight' in the bed in supine position) from the:
   1. Top (panoramic view).
   2. Foot end of the bed.
   3. The sides in profile.
   4. Head end of the bed.
   5. Back (try to turn the patient to any one side).

B. Points to note:
   1. Any deformity, fullness or depression (i.e. shape of the chest), apical impulse, etc.
   2. Back (winging of the scapulae, drooping of the shoulder, kyphoscoliosis, gibbus, skin changes).
   3. Whether both the sides of the chest are moving simultaneously and symmetrically.

- Read the 'Scheme of examination' of respiratory system under the heading 'Inspection'.
- Classical **winged scapula** is found in paralysis of nerve to serratus anterior (C_{5-7}), sometimes in facio-scapulo-humeral muscular dystrophy, and severe malnutrition **(Figs 3.46 and 3.160)**. The winging becomes more prominent if the patient pushes the outstretched arm against a wall or against examiner's hand **(Fig. 3.165)**. The patient also feels difficulty in raising the arm above the level of the shoulders.
- Kyphosis, intercostal suction and chest deformities (e.g. barrel-shaped chest) are best observed from the sides in profile.

Q. In general survey, how do you examine 'Respiration'?

Respiration should always be described by these 5 points:

A. Rate: Normal respiratory rate in a relaxed adult is 14–18 breaths/min (eupnoea) though a wide variation occurs in health; at birth the rate is about 40/min. The variations are:
   a. Increased rate: Tachypnoea (read the section on 'Bronchial asthma').
   b. Decreased rate: Bradypnoea (read the section on 'Bronchial asthma').

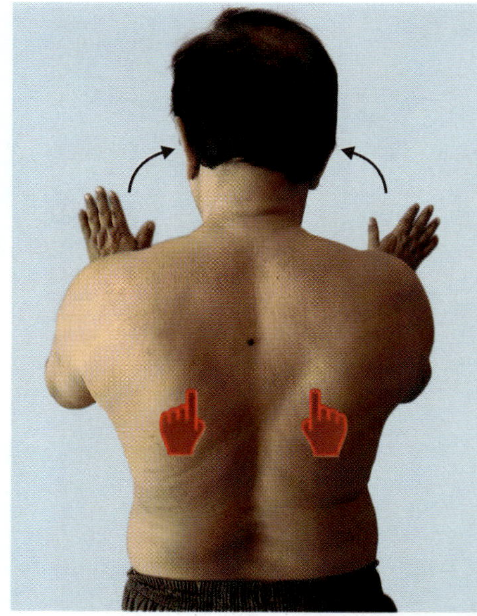

Fig. 3.165: Muscle power testing of **serratus anterior**. Winging of the scapula is unmasked while doing the test

- **Rate of Respiration** is counted surreptitiously (without the knowledge of the patient), by placing the hand in the epigastrium or with the fingers held on the radial pulse to avoid patient's attention to breathing while observing the chest movements (Fig. 3.166). The rate is counted for a full minute.

B. Rhythm: Changes in rhythm are diagnosed by inspecting the rise and fall of anterior chest wall. There may be wide variations in health.
   a. Irregularly irregular or Biot's breathing: The respiration is sometimes slow, sometimes rapid, sometimes superficial, sometimes deep but without any constant relation of succession between the two types, with pauses at irregular intervals. Actually, there are 3–4 respirations without waxing and waning, followed by a pause (similar to atrial fibrillation in pulse). This is most commonly seen in meningitis, especially in children.
   b. Regularly irregular or Cheyne-Stokes respiration (read the section on 'Bronchial asthma').
   c. Miscellaneous: Kussmaul's breathing, stertorous breathing, apneustic breathing, prolonged inspiration or prolonged expiration (obstruction of upper or lower respiratory tract, respectively).

C. Type: Diagnosed by inspecting the movement of the chest wall and abdomen. The variations are:
   a. Thoracic: Adult women, anxiety, peritonitis, huge ascites, hysteria, diaphragmatic palsy.
   b. Abdominal: Adult men, young children, pleurisy, ankylosing spondylitis, intercostal muscle paralysis.
   c. Abdomino-throacic: Young children, sometimes in adult men.
   d. Paradoxical respiration: Diaphragmatic palsy.

- In females, intercostal muscles play more (so, thoracic type) and in males, diaphragm plays more (so, abdominal type) in normal respiration.
- Females with predominantly abdominal type respiration: Any painful condition in chest (e.g. pleurisy, chest trauma), pneumothorax, etc.
- Males with predominantly thoracic type respiration: Any painful condition in abdomen (e.g. acute peritonitis), huge ascites, etc.

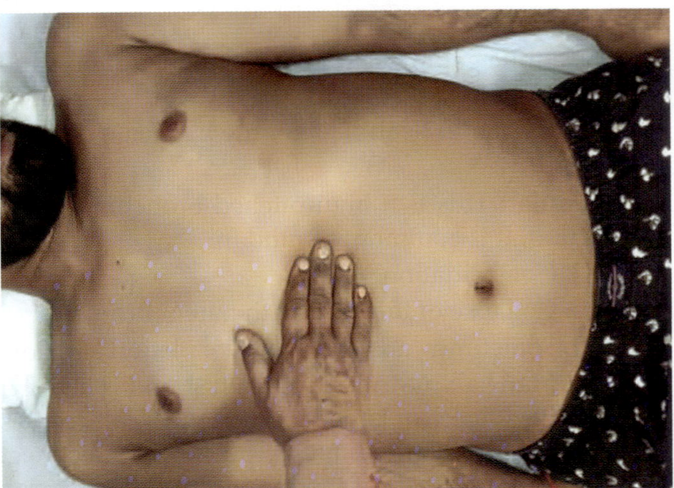

Fig. 3.166: **Respiratory rate** calculation

D. Depth: Inspect the excursion of chest wall. The diagnosis needs clinical experience. The variations are:
   a. Shallow: Narcotic poisoning, panic attacks.
   b. Deep: Hyperpnoea, hyperventilation, e.g. in metabolic acidosis.

E. Breathing pattern: Wheezing or stridor, shallow breathing, air hunger, sighing, gasping, mouth-breathing or purse-lip respiration.

Clinical Wisdom

While examining the 'Respiration', one may comment on movement of accessory muscles of respiration or intercostal suction, if present.

AUSCULTATION OF THE CHEST — CASE 79

Q. What will you do if asked to auscultate the chest?

If anyone is asked to auscultate the chest, he/she has to auscultate for both the respiratory system and CVS.

During auscultation of left side of the chest, one has to be careful for both the systems and during auscultation of right side of the chest, only respiratory system will serve the purpose. Auscultate over front (inflaclavicular area to lower costal margin), sides (axillary and infra-axillary areas) and back (supra-, inter- and infrascapular areas) avoiding auscultation over bones (clavicle, sternum and scapula). Always compare with the other side.

If a particular area of the chest (suppose, the area below the right nipple) is asked to be auscultated, one must take the permission of the examiner for auscultation over the identical site on left side of the chest for observations regarding vocal resonance (always say vocal resonance as normal, increased or decreased after comparing with the other side).

A. **For respiratory system**, the description will be in the order of:
   1. Breath sounds (page 420).
   2. Vocal resonance (page 88), and
   3. Adventitious (or added) sounds (pages 95–96, 421).

B. **For CVS**, the description goes like this:
   1. Heart sounds: S_1, S_2, any S_3 or S_4 (quality, intensity, splitting, etc.) (pages 12–13, 33–34, 44).
   2. Murmurs (pages 412–413).
   3. Pericardial rub, ejection click, opening snap, pericardial knock, etc. (pages 14, 30, 333, 413).

- In the respiratory system, auscultation over trachea is not at all necessary.

Q. During auscultation of the chest, direction given to the patient:

As a clinician, stand on the right side of the patient. Place the stethoscope firmly over the chest, preferably on a sitting patient. Before auscultation, the patient is asked to:

a. Turn the face to the left side (so that the patient cannot breathe on the clinician's face).
b. Breathe through open mouth (to prevent noise from partially closed nose).
c. Breathe regularly and deeply, but without any noise.

- Demonstrate the open mouth respiration to the patient for easy understanding.

Q. How to classify the breath sounds (Fig. 3.167)?

Breath sounds: These are the sounds produced by the passage of air through the tracheo-bronchial tree up to the alveoli. Gas turbulence in the major airways is responsible for inspiratory sound and elastic recoil of the lung for expiratory sound. The intensity of the sound depends on acoustic density of conducting medium. The breath sounds are divided into three types (mainly two types: vesicular and bronchial):

A. Vesicular breath sound

1. Definition: It is the sound produced by the passage of air, in and out of the aleveoli (vesicles) during inspiration and expiration.
2. Characteristics:
   i. 'Rustling' (sound like dry leaves blown by the wind) in character.
   ii. Intensity of inspiration is more than that of expiration.
   iii. Duration of inspiration is greater than that of expiration (I:E = 3:1).
   iv. No gap in between inspiration and expiration.

- As the normal lung tissue selectively filters out some higher frequencies, the breath sound becomes quieter, and results in **vesicular breath sound (the normal breath sound over the chest in health)**.
- The normal ratio of inspiratory to expiratory phase (I : E) is 1:2 to 1:3.

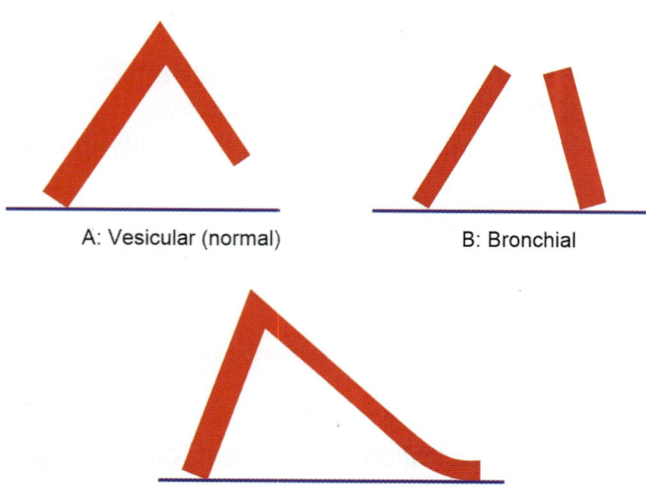

Fig. 3.167: Diagrammatic representation of **breath sounds**

3. Classical sites (in health): Inframammary, infra-axillary and infrascapular regions.
4. Common variations:
   a. Diminished vesicular: Thick chest wall, obesity, thickened pleura, pleural effusion, pneumothorax, hydropneumothorax, empyema thoracis, fibrosis of the lung, emphysema, etc.
   b. Vesicular breath sound with prolonged expiration: Bronchial asthma, chronic bronchitis and emphysema. In this type of respiration, the duration of inspiration and expiration becomes more or less equal.
   c. Harsh vesicular:
      i. Intensities of inspiration and expiration are increased.
      ii. Usually pathological.
      iii. Found in compensatory emphysema, or forced breathing.
   d. Cogwheel or jerky: Patients who are hysterical, very nervous or crying during auscultation.
   e. Absent breath sound: Pneumothorax, massive pleural effusion, hydropneumothorax, collapse with obstructed bronchus, grossly thickened pleura, pneumonectomy, etc.

- Bilateral reduction in intensity of breath sound (i.e. diminished air entry) is found in emphysema.

B. Bronchial breath sound

1. Definition: It is the sound produced by the passage of air through the tracheo-bronchial tree. Bronchial breath sound is audible in situations where sound generated in central airways (i.e. trachea) is transmitted more or less unchanged through the lung substances having undermentioned pathology (e.g. consolidation) with a patent bronchus.
2. Characteristics:
   i. 'Blowing', 'hollow' or 'aspirate' in character.
   ii. Intensity of expiration is more than that of inspiration.
   iii. Duration of expiration is usually equal to inspiration (I:E =1:1).
   iv. Definite gap present in between inspiration and expiration.
3. Classical site (in health): Over the trachea.
4. Types:
   a. Tubular: This is a high-pitched bronchial breath sound. It is commonly found in:
      i. Consolidation.
      ii. Collapse of the lung with patent bronchus.
      iii. Sometimes, above the level of pleural effusion.
      iv. Many a time, tubular breath sound is heard if the trachea or large bronchus physically comes near the stethoscope by push-pull effect (e.g. apical fibrosis of the lung from tuberculosis): Loosely termed as 'pulled trachea syndrome'.

b. Cavernous: It is a low-pitched bronchial breath sound classically heard over a superficial, big, empty cavity connected with a patent bronchus e.g. tuberculous cavity, lung abscess.

c. Amphoric: It is a low-pitched bronchial breath sound with tones and overtones, or with a metallic tone. The sound mimics the whistling sound produced by blowing air across the mouth of a small glass bottle. This is classically seen in:

i. Bronchopleural fistula (open pneumothorax), and

ii. Occasionally in a big cavity connected with a small bronchus.

- **Conditions associated with bronchial breath sound will produce quantitative increase in vocal resonance, i.e. bronchophony and whispering pectoriloquy.**
- In obstructed main bronchus, bronchial breath sound may not be heard over consolidation or collapse.

C. ***Bronchovesicular breath sound*** (obsolete though few old school clinicians still prefer it).

1. Definition: This is a mixture of two breath sounds where the expiration is mainly of bronchial and inspiration is predominantly of vesicular in character, and there is no gap in between inspiration and expiration.
2. Classical sites (in health):
   a. Right infraclavicular area (here, trachea is in direct contact with the lung whereas in the left infraclavicular area, the aorta, oesophagus and internal carotid artery seperate the trachea from the lung).
   b. Interscapular area at the back (root of the lung).
3. Clinical associations:
   a. Consolidation in the stage of resolution.
   b. Partial collapse of the lung.
   c. Cavity in the lung.

Q. Caution adopted during auscultation of respiratory system:

1. *Always try to auscultate with the diaphragm of stethoscope* to avoid time consumption and practical difficulty; as most of the normal lung sounds are low-pitched, the bell is preferred over the diaphragm by some clinicians.
2. Ask the patient to cough:
   a. To clear the throat (if throat sounds appear).
   b. To note the changes in crepitations (often helps in differentiation with pleural rub).
   c. For auscultating post-tussive crepitations (especially in tuberculous cavity).
3. Press the diaphragm of stethoscope in patients with pleural rub to note the local tenderness and enhancement of the intensity of pleural rub.

Q. What is Valsalva manoeuvre?

This is an attempted **forced expiration** in closed glottis when the mouth is shut and the nose is held closed. This manoeuvre increases the intrathoracic pressure and thus obstructs the venous return in the right atrium. Classical example is the straining exerted during defecation or blowing conch shell.

Clinical applications:

1. To make the abdominal or thoracic wall veins prominent (also to see venous flow) with the help of Valsalva manoeuvre while the patient sits in his bed.
2. During the Valsalva manoeuvre: Tachycardia, overshoot of BP and bradycardia occur sequentially in health, which can be appreciated clinically. This phenomenon is found to be absent in CCF, ASD and autonomic neuropathy.
3. Murmur of mitral valve prolapse syndrome (MVPS) and HOCM increases during Valsalva manoeuvre.
4. As a vagotonic procedure to abolish supraventricular ectopic beats.
5. To terminate bouts of hiccough as a simple househould remedy.
6. Analysis of eustachian tube dysfunction.
7. This manoeuvre makes uterine prolapse, inguinal hernia and varicocele more apparent clinically.

- Antonio Maria Valsalva (1666–1723) was an anatomist and surgeon from Italy.

Q. What is Muller's manoeuvre?

It is just the opposite of the Valsalva manoeurve (i.e. reversed Valsalva). This manoeuvre is an attempted **forced inspiration** in closed glottis when the mouth is shut and the nose is held closed. This manoeuvre decreases the intrathoracic pressure. Classical example is a drowning man.

It helps to evaluate the level and degree of upper airway narrowing in obstructive sleep apnoea.

PLEURAL RUB — CASE 80

Q. Characteristics of pleural rub (adventitious sound):

It is a leathery or creaking sound produced by the rubbing of inflamed and roughened, visceral and parietal pleura due to acute dry fibrinous pleurisy; normally both pleural surfaces glide silently over one another. It is the third adventitious sound in respiratory system after rhonchi and crepitations. The pleural rub is:

1. Superficial (the sound seems to be very close to the ear), scratchy or grating in quality.
2. Biphasic (heard during inspiration and expiration both).
3. Better heard on pressing the chest piece of stethoscope over the chest wall.
4. Localised: Generally heard over the antero-inferior part of lateral chest wall or in the lower part of back

of chest as the movement of visceral over the parietal pleura is maximum in these regions.

5. Neither there is any alteration after coughing nor any variation with change of posture.
6. Patient may complain of pain in the chest and local tenderness may be elicited.
7. Disappears when breath is held.
8. At times it is palpable: The 'friction fremitus'.

- The sound is just like rubbing hairs or bending a stiff leather.

Q. Differential diagnosis of pleural rub:

A. It should be **differentiated from coarse crepitations** (which is also biphasic) by the following points. Crepitations are:
   i. Not intensified on pressing the stethoscope.
   ii. Modified or diminished after coughing.
   iii. May be auscultated over a widespread area, and
   iv. Discontinuous; not superficial, not associated with pain or tenderness.

B. Pericardial rub (pericardial rub continues after holding the breath).

C. Hepatic or splenic rub: Often very difficult to differentiate, and is audible over enlarged liver and enlarged spleen respectively. Hepatic and splenic rub are inaudible if the patient holds his breath.

- Occasionally, after pressing the stethoscope in an uneven chest (with prominent ribs), pleural rub-like sound is produced due to friction of moist, sweaty chest wall with the diaphragm of stethoscope. Put the chest piece in a new place near the previous one after wiping off the sweat.
- In a hairy chest wall, avoid friction of hair by moistening the chest wall with sprinkled water and henceforth apply the chest piece firmly over the chest. Be careful about the *false added sounds* evoked by auscultation over hairy skin, shivering of a cold patient or sounds produced by rubbing of clothes against the tube of shethoscope.

Q. What is your diagnosis?

Acute dry pleurisy.

Q. Causes of acute dry pleurisy:

1. Pulmonary tuberculosis
2. Pneumonic consolidation.
3. Bronchogenic carcinoma.
4. Pulmonary infarction.
5. Bornholm disease (epidemic pleurodynia).
6. Amoebic liver abscess.
7. Collagen vascular diseases.
8. Subdiaphragmatic abscess.
9. Bronchiectasis.
10. Injury to the chest wall.
11. Pleural metastases.
12. Mesothelioma of pleura (rare).

- 1, 2, 3 and 4 are most common and important causes.

Q. Classical chest pain of acute dry pleurisy (pleuritic pain):

1. Sharp, stabbing, cutting or tearing localised pain.
2. It increases on coughing, sneezing, deep inspiration, pressure from outside, jolting or bending.
3. Localised pain (usually non-radiating).
4. The pain is usually non-exertional but may increase after exercise (due to tachypnoea).
5. When the diaphragmatic pleura is involved, the pain may be referred to the tip of shoulder (as central part of the diaphragm is supplied by phrenic nerve, C_{3-5}) or to the epigastrium (as domes of the diaphragm are supplied by lower intercostal nerves).
6. The pain is diminished by holding the chest or holding the respiration (i.e. by taking shallow respiration).
7. Associated with pleural rub.

- Pleuritic chest pain is often associated with pyrexia and dry cough. See also page 67.

Clinical Wisdom

Lung parenchyma is pain-insensitive and as such if the pleura is not involved, it does not give rise to any pain. Parietal pleura is pain-sensitive (supplied by intercostal and phrenic nerve), while visceral pleura is pain-insensitive (supplied by autonomic nervous system).

Q. Decubitus in different diseases of pleura:

A. Pneumothorax: Patient prefers to lie on the affected side. It allows maximum expansion of the normal lung.

B. Pleural effusion: Patient prefers to lie on the side of effusion as it allows maximum expansion of the unaffected lung. Pleural fluid may compress the mediastinum and produce discomfort, if the patient lies on the normal side.

C. Acute dry pleurisy:
   1. Majority of patients lie on the affected side (if there is absence of overlying sensitive skin). In this way they splint their chest wall with the surface of the bed.
   2. Few patients lie on the opposite side because the overlying skin is very sensitive and the patient cannot keep contact with the bed.

Q. Describe different types of 'decubitus' in clinical medicine:

Decubitus means posture or attitude of the patient in bed assumed by him/her in most of the time of day and night. The different **variations** are:

1. Of choice: The patient is comfortable in any position in bed (also known as 'dorsal decubitus' or 'supine' position). Remember, a normal person is comfortable in any position in bed.
2. Propped-up: Propped-up position with a back-rest is found in patients suffering from dyspnoea.

The back-rest can be adjusted according to the requirement of the patient, e.g.

- Mild dyspnoea: Adopts 45°
- Moderate dyspnoea: Adopts 60°
- Severe dyspnoea or orthopnoea: Adopts 90° (i.e. patient sits in bed).

Dyspnoea is basically due to respiratory and cardiovascular ailments (cardio-respiratory embarrassment). Gastrointestinal cause like massive ascites, and neurological causes like diaphragmatic palsy, respiratory muscles palsy, myasthenia gravis may also produce dyspnoea. *Propped-up decubitus relieves dyspnoea because,*

a. The excursion of diaphragm occurs better in erect posture.
b. Erect posture diminishes the venous return and thus dyspnoea of cardiac origin becomes less.
c. While in recumbency, the increase in intrathoracic blood volume elevates pulmonary venous and capillary pressure which ultimately increase the pulmonary closing volume and diminishes vital capacity. This is corrected on assuming erect posture.

3. Stooping forward position (Mohammedan's prayer position) on a cardiac table: Seen in severe dyspnoea of pericardial effusion, acute severe asthma, cardiac asthma and COPD. It is also observed in acute pericarditis or acute pancreatitis patients to get relief of pain in this way. Patients with acute pancreatitis is partly relieved by lying down with knees drawn towards the chest.
4. Squatting: Fallot's tetralogy is the commonest cyanotic congenital heart disease where squatting is observed. As soon as the patient becomes dyspnoeic, he adopts squatting posture to relieve from dyspnoea. Squatting increases the peripheral resistance (i.e. pressure in aorta increases) and thus reduces the right-to-left shunting through VSD.
5. Trepopnoea: See page 93.
6. Platypnoea: See page 93.
7. Lateral decubitus: See the question above (decubitus adopted in diseases of pleura); patient of liver abscess prefers to lie on the left side.
8. Listless attitude or where the patient lies still in bed: This attitude is usually seen in peritonitis (abdominal wall movement causes intense pain), anginal pain, coma and hysteria.
9. Curled-up: Observed in renal colic and biliary colic; restless or tossing: In colics, AMI.
10. Head end down (usually adjusted by placing bricks or wooden blocks in the foot end of bed): Adopted in the treatment of bulbar palsy, after lumbar puncture, after spinal anaesthesia, balanced traction in orthopedics, in treatment of sinus bradycardia developed from AMI, hypotension, deep venous thrombosis in legs, and in postural drainage of bronchiectasis and lung abscess (lower lobes).
11. Decubitus of herniplegia: The affected arm remains flexed, adducted and semipronated, and the affected lower limb adopts extended, adducted and plantiflexed attitude. As a whole, the affected side shows less movement while the patient is in bed.
12. Opisthotonus, pleurothotonus and emprosthotonus: Respectively, they are bending of the body like an arc in backward direction (hyperextension), laterally to one side, and forward direction (hyperflexion). These bending postures are seen in tetanus and strychnine poisoning.
13. Dorsal decubitus position with a pillow placed below the legs (pedal oedema, cellulitis of foot) or below the popliteal fossa (acute inflammation of knee joint, e.g. in rheumatic and rheumatoid arthritis, haemophilia).
14. Decerebrate posture: Extended elbows and wrists, with arms pronated; there is tonic extension and plantiflexion of the lower extremity, associated with head retraction and jaw clenching. The lesion lies at upper brainstem level (i.e. midbrain or upper pons), disconnecting cerebral hemispheres from brainstem.
15. Decorticate posture: Flexed elbows and wrists, with arms supinated; lower extremities show tonic extension. It is seen in bilateral hemispherical lesion above midbrain.
16. Supine (dorsal decubitus) position with flexion of knees (e.g. peritonitis) or flexion of thighs (e.g. psoas abscess/haematoma, appendicitis/diverticulilis).
17. Neck extended with head buried in pillow: Meningitis.
18. Prone position: Colics, moderate-to-severe respiratory distress in ARDS, to get some comfort in ankylosing spondylitis and abdominal aortic aneurysm (eroding vertebra and producing back pain).
19. Knee-elbow position: Pain of chronic pancreatitis is reduced on assuming this posture.

Q. Medical (non-surgical) causes of pain abdomen:

1. Basal pneumonia (diaphragmatic pleurisy).
2. Acute myocardial infarction (inferior wall infarction commonly).
3. Diabetic ketoacidosis (may be due to acute gastric dilatation and/or pancreatitis).
4. Henoch-Schönlein purpura (vasculitis).
5. Adrenal crisis.
6. Sickle cell anaemia (vaso-occlusive crisis).
7. Acute intermittent porphyria (autonomic neuropathy).
8. Intercostal herpes zoster (pre-herpetic eruption produces radicular pain) (Fig. 3.168).
9. Caries spine or cord compression (radicular pain); collapse of the vertebra (referred pain).
10. Polyarteritis nodosa (vasculitis).
11. Allergic pain, or hereditary angio-oedema (C_1 esterase inhibitor deficiency).

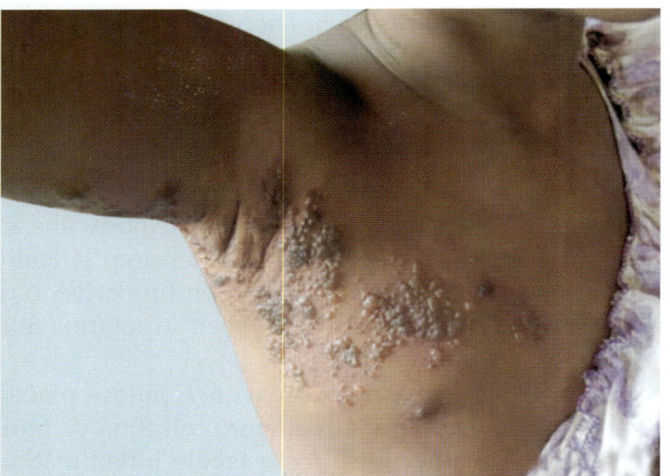

Fig. 3.168: Herpes zoster infection (Shingles) involving the thoracic dermatomes (due to reactivation of latent varicella zoster virus from the dorsal root ganglion of sensory nerves)

12. Hyperlipidaemia (familial).
13. Hypercalcaemia.
14. Abdominal angina (due to chronic mesenteric ischaemia).
15. Chronic lead poisoning (colic).
16. Familial Mediterranean fever.
17. Localised tetanus of anterior abdominal wall muscle.
18. Functional gastrointestinal disorders.
19. Tabetic crisis (probably due to autonomic neuropathy; not seen nowadays).

- Peptic ulcer, acute pyelonephritis and acute pancreatitis may also be considered.
- **Endocrine causes of pain abdomen** are: (i) Diabetic ketoacidosis, (ii) Adrenal crisis, (iii) Hyperparathyroidism, and (iv) Cushing's syndrome.

Q. Pain abdomen associated with shock:

1. Acute pancreatitis.
2. Peptic ulcer complicated by bleeding or perforation.
3. Acute myocardial infarction (inferior wall infarction).
4. Diabetic ketoacidosis.
5. Acute mesenteric ischaemia.
6. Dissection of abdominal aorta.
7. Rupture of amoebic liver abscess.
8. Adrenal crisis.
9. Acute intermittent porphyria.
10. Strangulation of hernia.
11. Ruptured ectopic pregnancy.
12. Septic abortion.

Q. Absent pleural rub after few days—reasoning behind:

Either the patient is cured, or developed pleural effusion.

Q. Management of pleural rub:

1. Rest in bed.
2. Relief of chest pain by:
   a. Hot fomentation.
   b. Splinting of the chest wall with leukoplast.
   c. Analgesics (NSAIDs).
   d. Sedatives.
3. Treatment of the underlying aetiology.

Q. Identification points:

1. Sometimes, pleural rub may be confused with pericardial rub (in left-sided pleurisy). Pleural rub stops after holding the breath but pericardial rub continues.
2. It should be differentiated from coarse crepitations by the points discussed above.

Clinical Wisdom

To diagnose pleural rub, remember these 3 points:

1. Hold the breath (pleural rub disappears while pericardial rub continues).
2. Ask the patient to cough (D/D with crepitations; pleural rub does not alter with cough).
3. Press the chest piece of stethoscope (pleural rub intensifies or patient may complain of pain).

EXAMINATION OF THE TONGUE — CASE 81

Q. Examination of the tongue in clinical practice?

A. Ask the patient to 'show the tongue' by protruding it outside the oral cavity:

The patient is unable to protrude the tongue in case of short frenum (known as 'tongue-tie' or ankyloglossia), malignancy of the tongue and also in bilateral paralysis of the tongue (XIIth nerve palsy). Sluggish and slow protrusion are seen in mental retardation.

B. Movement of the tongue:

1. **'Trombone tongue':** Rapid forward and backward movement of the tongue is characteristic of general paralysis of insane (GPI or neurosyphilis); may be seen in Parkinson's disease.
2. Ask the patient to protrude the tongue: The patient protrudes it momentarily and takes it back within the oral cavity instantaneously (lizard tongue): Seen in rheumatic chorea (Jack-in-the-box tongue).
3. 'Chewing tongue': Seen in athetosis, as if the patient is chewing something.
4. Irregular and continual rotatory movements of the tongue may be seen in extrapyramidal syndromes (dyskinesia) induced by drugs like phenothiazines, metoclopramide, levodopa.
5. Rolling movements of tongue are found in cretins, mongols, and as part of tics.
6. Ask the patient to protrude the tongue out of the oral cavity and look for fine **tremor**: Characteristically found in anxiety neurosis, thyrotoxicosis, chronic alcoholism, etc.
7. Ask the patient to keep the tongue relaxed in the floor of the mouth and look for **fasciculation;** it is seen in MND, bulbar palsy or LMN palsy of XIIth cranial nerve (Fig. 3.169A).

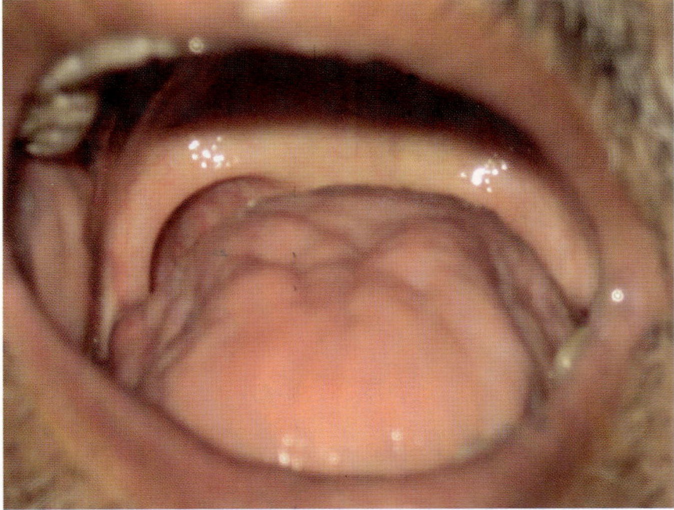

Fig. 3.169A: Flaccid and wasted **tongue with fasciculation** in bulbar palsy from chronic motor neurone disease

8. Observe for lingual myoclonus (with palatal myoclonus), forced deviation of tongue (as part of focal seizure), and tics and habit spasm.

C. Size of the tongue:

Normally tongue should fit comfortably in mouth.

1. Large tongue or **macroglossia** (with impression of teeth in sides) is seen in:
   i. Acromegaly.
   ii. Myxoedema.
   iii. Cretinism.
   iv. Down syndrome (Fig. 3.169B).
   v. Primary amyloidosis (Fig. 2.27).
   vi. Mucopolysaccharidosis, e.g. Hurler syndrome.
   vii. Haemangioma or lymphangioma of tongue.
   viii. von Gierke's disease (glycogen storage disease).
   ix. Angioneurotic oedema.
   x. Pseudomacroglossia: Enlarged tonsils, low palate.
2. Small tongue or **microglossia** is seen in:
   i. Cerebral diplegia.
   ii. Motor neurone disease (MND).
   iii. Bulbar and pseudobulbar palsy.
   iv. Wasting of the tongue.

- **Acute swelling of the tongue** is found in bite, infection, angioneurotic oedema, haemophilia, pemphigus.

D. Colour and morphological changes:

1. Dry tongue: Dehydration, mouth breathing, xerostomia, after administration of atropine.
2. Moist tongue: Sialorrhoea in post-encephalitic parkinsonism, heavy metal poisoning.
3. Pale tongue: Anaemia (severe).
4. Blue tongue (*see* Figs 3.5 and 3.6): Central cyanosis, meth- or sulphaemoglobinaemia (mainly the sides of the tongue), intake of blue coloured food material.
5. Yellow tongue: Jaundice (the undersurface), intake of yellow coloured sweets.
6. Bluish-red tongue: Polycythemia.
7. **Magenta-coloured tongue** (a bit pinkish) (*see* Fig. 3.51): Riboflavin deficiency.
8. Black tongue (Fig. 3.170A): After ingestion of bismuth, liquorice, charcoal; Addison's disease, malabsorpton, Peutz-Jeghers syndrome.
9. Blotting paper like pallor (with black pigmentation in the margin): Seen in hookworm infestation.
10. White or greyish coating or 'furred' tongue: Smoking, chronic debility, acute tonsillitis, sore throat, etc. 'Fur' is common in heavy smokers.
11. **Bald tongue:** There is total loss or atrophy of papillae, and is classically seen in pellagra, pernicious anaemia (Hunter's glossitis), iron deficiency anaemia (Fig. 3.170B), tropical sprue and syphilis.
12. **'Raw-beefy tongue':** Red, swollen and painful tongue. It is found in pellagra and vitamin B_{12} deficiency (Fig. 3.170C).
13. **'Angry-looking' tongue:** Central coating with red tip and margins (enteric fever).

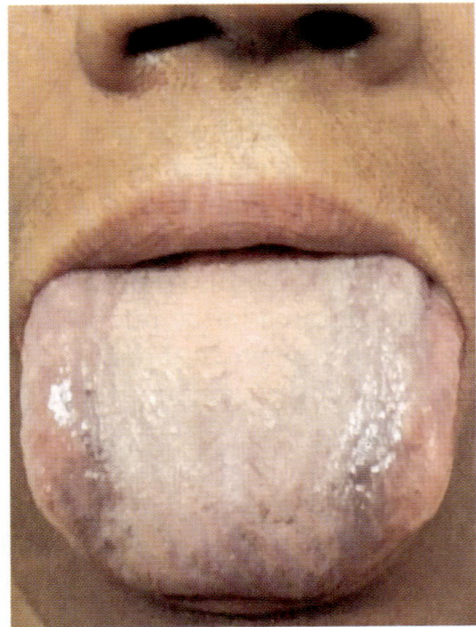

Fig. 3.169B: **Macroglossia** in Down syndrome

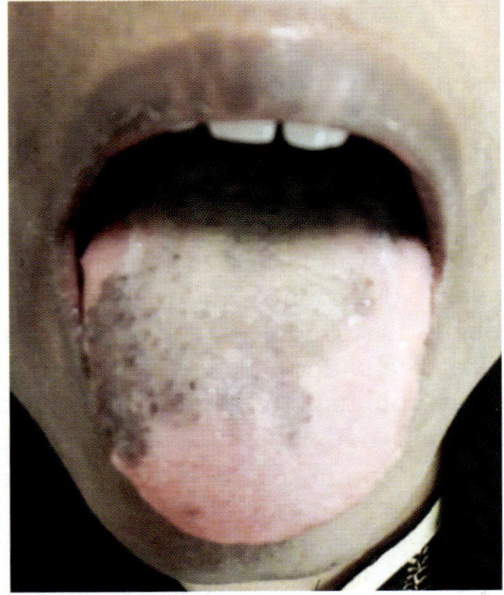

Fig. 3.170A: **Black tongue** in Addison's disease

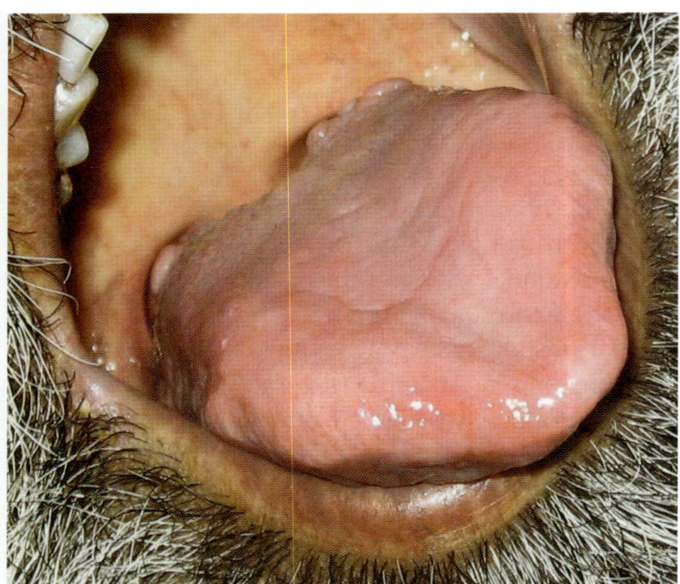

Fig. 3.170B: **Bald tongue** in iron deficiency anaemia (also called atrophic glossitis)

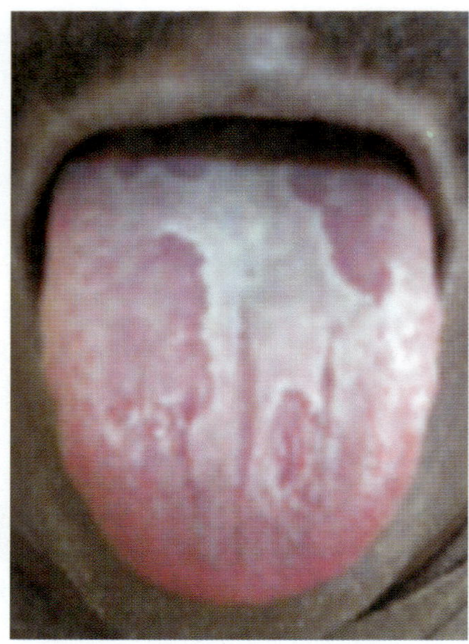

Fig. 3.171A: Denuded 'migratory' red patches in **geographic tongue**. It has no clinical significance

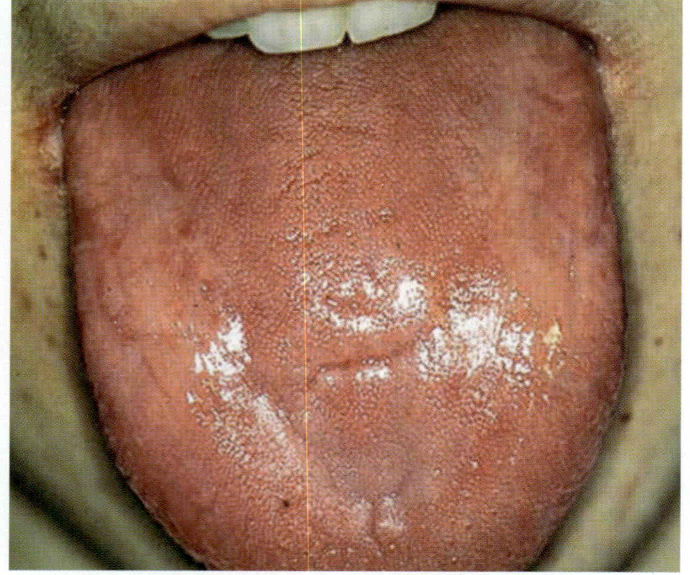

Fig. 3.170C: **Raw-beefy tongue** in pernicious anaemia

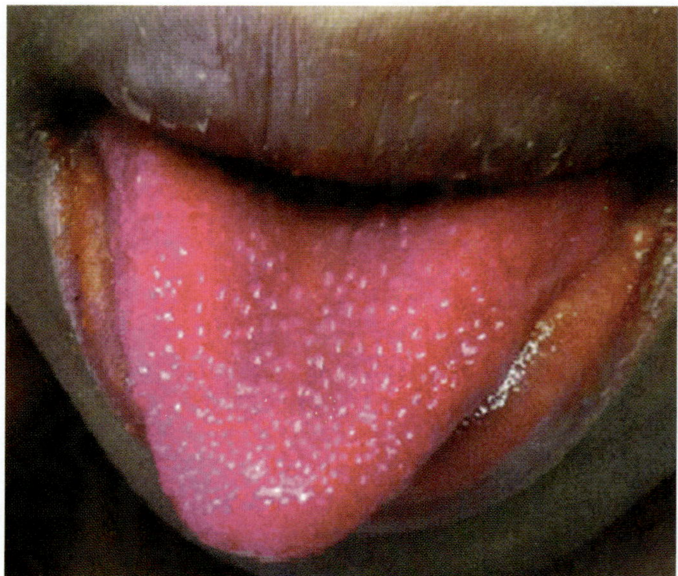

Fig. 3.171B: **Strawberry tongue** in Kawasaki disease

14. 'Black hairy' tongue (patchy blackening): Produced due to failure of keratin layer of the filiform papillae to desquamate normally. It is found in staining by tobacco, food, chromogenic organism, fungal infection, after use of penicillins and tetracyclines, or since birth.
15. 'Geographic' tongue (Fig. 3.171A): Denuded red patches 'wandering' or migrating (look like boundaries of a country map) across the surface of the tongue due to rapid loss and regrowth of filiform papillae. The pattern changes within few days. It is an asymptomatic inflammatory condition and though looks odd, it has no clinical significance.
16. Strawberry tongue: Hypertrophy of fungiform papillae with changes in filiform papillae, and are seen in scarlet fever, Kawasaki disease (Fig. 3.171B) and toxic shock syndrome. The tongue looks red with papillae standing out as white dots.

    Raspberry tongue is common in early stage of scarlet fever.
17. 'Scrotal tongue': Deep horizontal fissures in the tongue where debris may collect; usually inherited and is of no clinical significance. Fissured tongue is common in Down syndrome.
18. Median rhomboid glossitis (Fig. 3.171C) A lozenge-shaped denuded area in the middle of the tongue posteriorly. It is a congenital abnormality and should be differentiated from carcinoma of the tongue as it feels nodular.
19. White patches on the tongue: Due to thrush (Fig. 3.171D) (i.e. moniliasis due to immunosuppressive therapy, diabetes and AIDS; can be scraped), or other fungal infection, leukoplakia (premalignant; cannot be scraped), hairy leukoplakia (e.g. AIDS) and chronic superficial glossitis, etc.

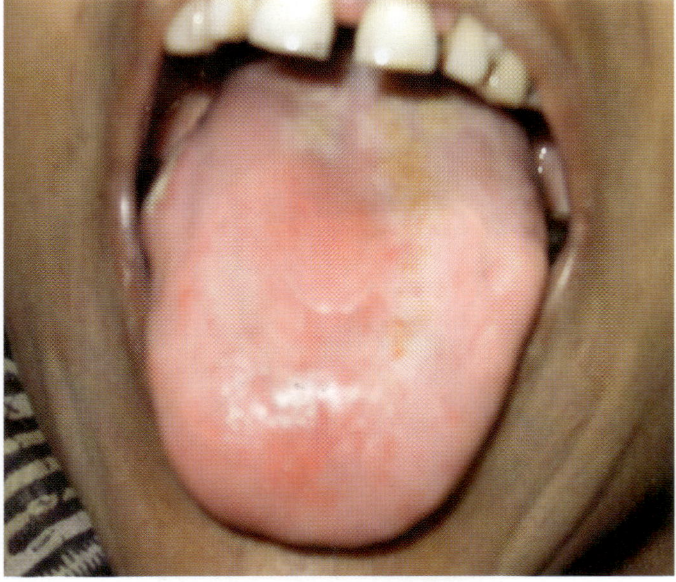

Fig. 3.171C: Median **rhomboid glossitis**

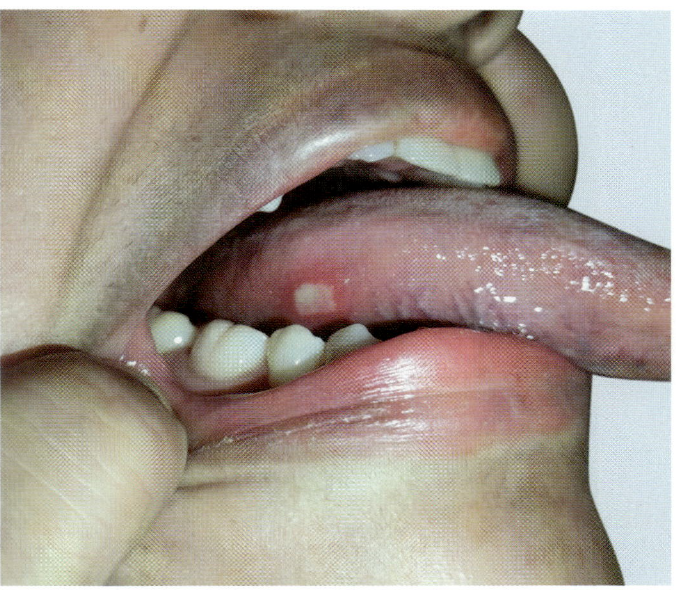

Fig. 3.172A: Shallow, painful **aphthous ulcer in tongue** with a white centre and inflammatory halo

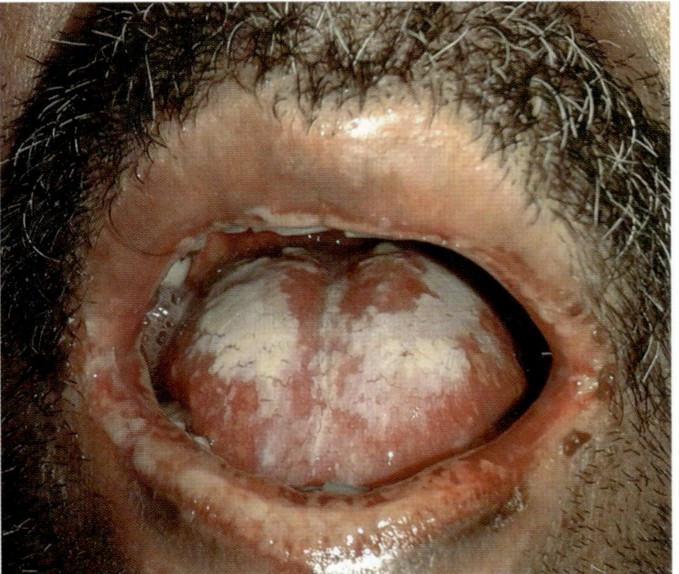

Fig. 3.171D: White patches in tongue due to candidosis (thrush)

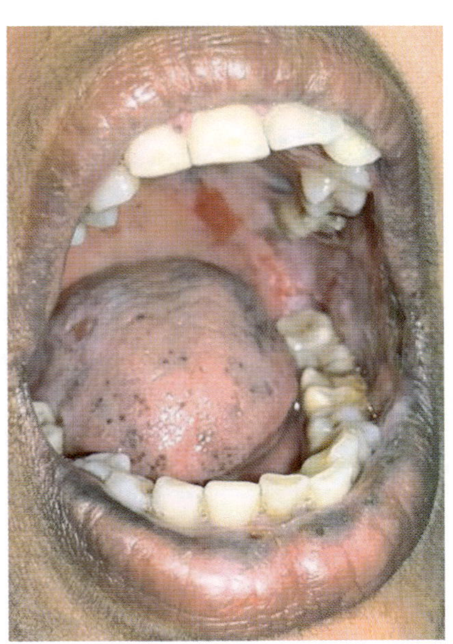

Fig. 3.172B: Methotrexate-induced **ulcers in tongue** and buccal mucosa

20. Ulcers in the tongue: Aphthous ulcer (single or multiple painful ulcers) (Fig. 3.172A), frenal ulcer (in frenum), tuberculous ulcer (in dorsum), malignant ulcer (anywhere in the tongue), snail-track ulcer (in dorsum) in secondary syphilis, ulcers due to lichen planus, ulcers at the margins (by ill-fitted dentures) or ulcers from Behcet's disease (mimicking aphthous ulcer) are not uncommon. Syphilitic and lichen planus ulcers are painless, while others are painful. Recurrent ulcers are common in Behcet's disease, lichen planus, SLE, pempigus, aphthous ulcer and neutropenia. Drugs may also be responsible for an ulcer in mouth (e.g. methotrexate) (Fig. 3.172B).
21. Bite mark in the tongue: Accidental bite during eating or after convulsions.
22. **Spastic tongue** with pointed tip (without any fasciculation): In pseudobulbar palsy.
23. **Flaccid tongue** with rounded tip and the tongue sits on the floor of the mouth like a mushroom (i.e. grossly wasted), often with fasciculation: In bulbar palsy.
24. Growth in the tongue (with halitosis): In squamous cell carcinoma of the tongue.
25. Mushroom-like tongue: Sore tongue with white slough, seen in corrosive poisoning.
26. Horny tongue (crocodile tongue): Tongue with cornification of the mucosa.
27. Dry, red tongue with atrophy of the papillae and fissures: Seen in Sjögren's syndrome (Fig. 3.172C).
28. Hairy leucoplakia: Painless white corrugated lesion on sides are due to Epstein-Barr virus infection, especially in AIDS (Fig. 3.172D).

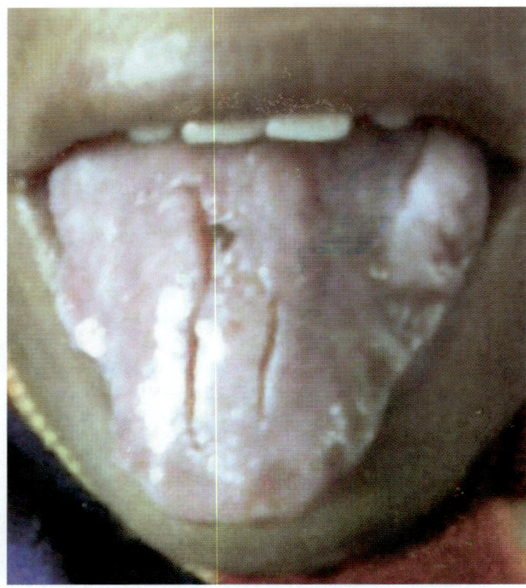

Fig. 3.172C: **Tongue** in **Sjögren's syndrome**

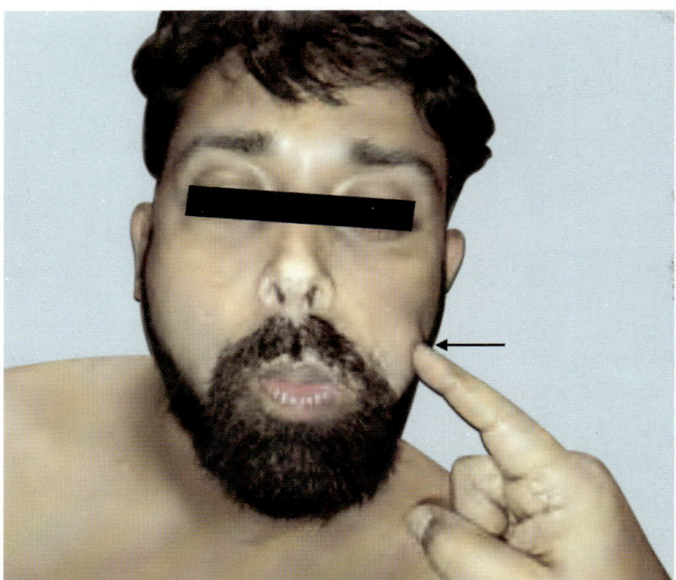

Fig. 3.173: Demonstration of power testing of **tongue muscles**

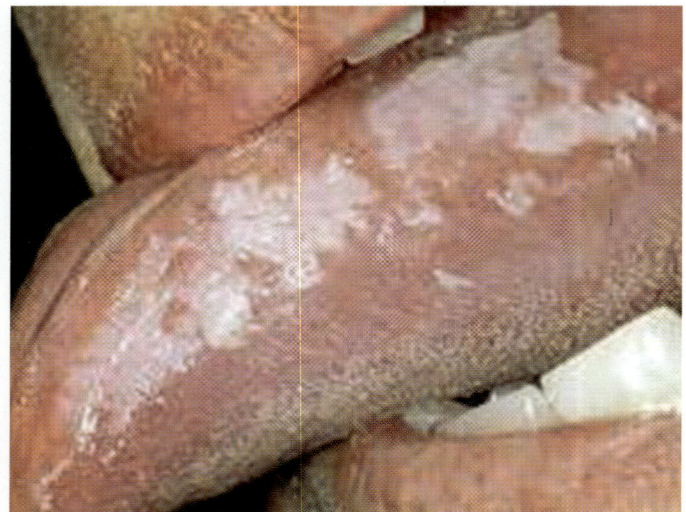

Fig. 3.172D: **Hairy leucoplakia**—white patches on the side of the **tongue** due to HIV infection

E. Deviation of the tongue: Ask the patient to protrude his tongue,

1. In UMN lesion of XIIth cranial nerve: Deviated to the opposite side.
2. In LMN lesion of XIIth cranial nerve: Deviated to the same side.

F. Power of the tongue: Ask the patient to move the tongue inside the oral cavity at random and to press the cheeks with the tongue when resistance is applied in the cheeks from outside (Fig. 3.173).

G. Taste sensation: Taste sensation of anterior 2/3rd of the tongue is carried by the facial nerve and that of posterior 1/3rd is carried by the glossopharyngeal nerve. Sugar or saccharin, common salt, vinegar and quinine are used to test the primary taste sensations like sweet, salt, sour and bitter, respectively. Sensations perceived by the tongue are sweet at the tip, sour at the margins, bitter at the back and salt by any part of the tongue. The fifth sub-modality of taste sensation is umami (savori taste in meat, soy sauce, etc.), tested by glutamate or amino acids. Loss of taste sensation is *ageusia* (as reduction of taste sensation is *hypogeusia*) and may result from lesions in any part of the peripheral and central pathways of taste fibres.

Directly ask the patient for recent loss of taste or any abnormal taste sensation. Explain the test procedure to the patient. Now to test the taste sensation, ask the patient to close his eyes, hold the tongue with a swab and wipe off saliva, and then put the substance on the anterior 2/3rd of the protruded tongue on each side in turn. Ask him to identify the substance. Each time mouth is washed and a new substance is applied. Bitter sensation is tested last.

Test for taste sensation of posterior 1/3rd of the tongue is difficult and thus done by using a galvanic current of 2–4 mA, which produces a metallic taste when touched in the tongue.

Clinical Wisdom

Disorders of taste sensation are due to lesion in VIIth and IXth cranial nerves, inability to appreciate flavors (diseases of nasal mucosa), and aura phase of epilepsy.

Q. What are the causes of halitosis, sialorrhoea and xerostomia?

1. **Halitosis** (malodorous breath): Common causes are bad oral hygiene, smoking, decomposed food debris collected in between teeth, stomatitis, gingivitis, caries tooth, sinusitis, atrophic rhinitis, any tumour of nasal passage, carcinoma of the tongue, bronchiectasis, lung abscess (often foetid), diabetic ketoacidosis (sweetish smell of acetone), hepatic (like dead mouse) and renal failure (fishy ammoniacal), gastro-colic fistula and intestinal obstruction (with foul smelling belching).

2. **Sialorrhoea** or ptyalism (hypersalivation) occurs during pregnancy, carcinoma of the tongue or mouth, stomatitis, caries tooth, Wilson's disease (drooling), acid or alkali poisoning, post-encephalitic parkinsonism, bulbar palsy, schizophrenia, hydrophobia; in arsenic, mercury or lead poisoning.
3. **Xerostomia** (dry mouth) is common in fear, anxiety, dehydration, high fever, mouth breathing during sleep, drug-induced (diuretics, anticholinergics, antidepressants), Sjögren's syndrome, as a complication of polyuria, irradiation for head and neck carcinoma, and psychogenic. Decrease in production of saliva (xerostomia) may be complicated by caries tooth, halitosis and candidosis of the oral cavity.
4. **Aphthous ulcers** (aphthae or canker sores) are small, non-contagious, painful sores inside mouth as a result of stress, acidic food (e.g. citrous food), minor injury to inside mouth, SLE, Behcet's disease, coeliac disease, IBD (e.g. ulcerative colitis) and AIDS.
5. **Pigmented lesions within the oral cavity** are seen in Addison's disease, Peutz-Jeghers syndrome, haemochromatosis, melanoma and chronic lead poisoning (with blue line or Burtonian line in the gum) (Fig. 3.174).

Clinical Wisdom

Tongue may be regarded as mirror of dysfunction of all the systems; previously tongue was known as the mirror of GI tract only.

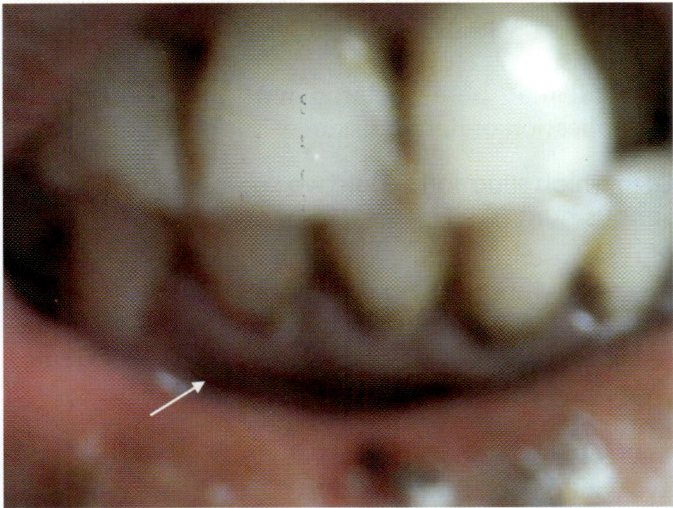

Fig. 3.174: Blue line in the gum in chronic lead poisoning

VISIBLE PERISTALSIS — CASE 82

Q. Significance:

Usually no peristaltic wave is seen in the abdomen in health. Visible peristalsis signifies mechanical obstruction of intestine (pathological). As a normal finding, it is occasionally seen in children with thin abdominal wall or in adults where the abdominal musculature has been thinned out by repeated pregnancy, long-continued ascites or in elderly patients with lax abdominal wall (physiological).

Q. Localisation of obstruction:

Obstruction is generally seen in one of these three places like stomach, small gut or large gut, and the site of obstruction is determined by analysing the peristaltic waves.

a. *Stomach:* Visible peristalsis is seen due to obstruction at pylorus [Children—congenital hypertrophic pyloric stenosis (CHPS), adult—pyloric stenosis from chronic duodenal ulcer, old age—pyloric growth may produce gastric outlet obstruction] and the wave moves in the upper abdomen from left to right hypochondrium, occasionally through the umbilical region. These waves are golf-ball like and generally not more than 2–3 waves are seen at a time.
b. *Small gut* (Fig. 3.175)*:* The peristaltic waves are seen as 'ladder pattern' (zigzag fashion) in the periumbilical region and there may be 10–12 waves formation per minute.
c. *Large gut:* If the obstruction is located in transverse colon, the waves are seen moving from right to left hypochondrium (opposite to pyloric obstruction). These are larger in size, i.e. cricket-ball like. The waves are seen in the right or left flank in case of obstruction of ascending or descending colon, respectively.

Q. How to evoke peristalsis at the bedside in a suspected case?

In a suspected case of intestinal obstruction, peristalsis can be induced by:

1. Flicking, stroking or gentle massage of the anterior abdominal wall, or
2. Drinking a large amount of water (1–2 glasses), or
3. Pouring few drops of ether or alcohol over the abdomen.

Regarding inspection of waves, a 'tangential view' is always better for slow waves. A light across the

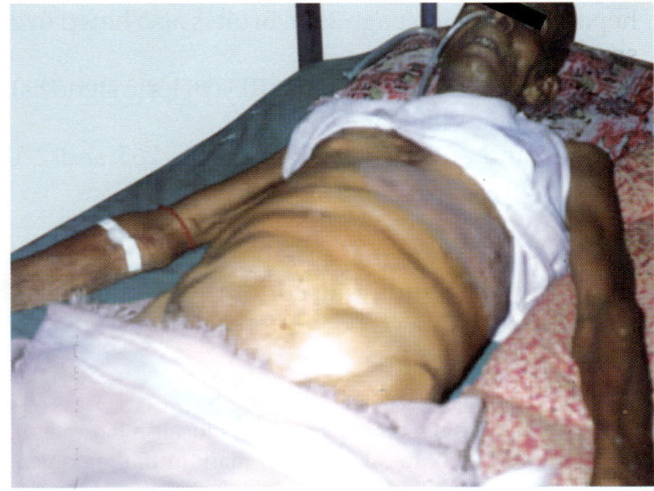

Fig. 3.175: Ladder-pattern **visible peristalsis** in acute small intestinal obstruction

patient's abdomen may detect peristaltic movements by alterations in the pattern of shadows cast over the abdomen. Small intestinal peristalsis may be occasionally seen normally through divarication of recti or in incisional hernia through abdominal scar.

Q. Common causes of gut obstruction:

a. Stomach: Pyloric stenosis, carcinoma of the stomach.
b. Small gut: Adhesions and external hernias.
c. Large gut: Colonic carcinoma, sigmoid diverticulitis and volvulus.

Q. Common causes of gut obstruction in India:

Think of round worm infestation in children and intestinal tuberculosis in any age group.

Q. Clinical confirmation, if peristalsis is seen in upper abdomen:

Give the patient a quick shake and carefully listen for succussion splash (e.g. pyloric stenosis).

Q. Confirmation of diagnosis of intestinal obstruction:

After careful history taking and meticulous clinical examination (by symptoms and signs like pain abdomen, vomiting, abdominal fullness, constipation or obstipation, and complicated by dehydration and electrolyte imbalance), the physician should do a straight **X-ray of the abdomen in erect posture**, where observation of multiple fluid levels will confirm the diagnosis (normally there may be fluid levels in: i) stomach, ii) lower duodenal flexure, and at iii) ileocaecal junction). *More than three fluid levels clinch the diagnosis of intestinal obstruction.*

Q. Importance of auscultation over abdomen:

1. Peristalsis: Normal sound (vide page 106); increased in intestinal obstruction, absent in paralytic ileus.
2. ***Bruit:*** Especially in renal artery stenosis (best heard just above the umbilicus, about 2 cm on either side of midline) (*see* **Fig. 1.55**), coarctation of aorta and aortoarteritis of abdominal aorta (systolic bruit); hepatic bruit (vide page 265). Bruit is also heard over small aortic aneurysm.
3. Succussion splash: Vide page 105 (pyloric stenosis).
4. Venous hum: Vide page 430.
5. Hepatic and splenic rub: Vide pages 265 and 270, respectively.
6. Ausculto-percussion: Vide page 105.
7. Uterine souffle (pregnancy).
8. Foetal heart sounds (auscultate with the bell of stethoscope).

Clinical Wisdom

In a patient with visible peristalsis, always localise the 'site of obstruction' and look for: 1) Incision mark in the abdomen (adhesion from past abdominal operation), 2) Succussion splash, and 3) Borborygmi (intestinal obstruction).

PROMINENT VEINS WITH VENOUS HUM — CASE 83

Q. What is venous hum?

It is synonymous with bruit heard in arteries. One may call it venous murmur. It is produced as a result of enormous blood flow through the veins.

Q. Common sites for venous hum:

Commonly heard as a continuous humming sound over prominent veins (i.e. collaterals) seen in the epigastrium or dilated veins seen around the umbilicus in cirrhosis of liver (pathological) (*see* **Fig. 1.41**). Sometimes, it is heard above either clavicle (in neck) in a child or during pregnancy (physiological). The cervical venous hum (Devil's murmur or Pontain's murmur) in adults (pathological) is often audible in hyperkinetic circulatory states, e.g. severe anaemia, thyrotoxicosis, etc.

Q. Jugular venous hum or cervical venous hum:

It is commonly seen in children. The hum is best audible at the medial part of supraclavicular fossa, just lateral to sternomastoid, with the head turned to opposite direction. *It is physiological in a child* and more common in right side.

Q. Characteristics of venous hum:

1. Soft and low-pitched.
2. Often continuous with early diastolic accentuation.
3. Best heard in sitting or erect position with the bell of stethoscope, which may disappear on lying down.
4. Best audible in inspiration.
5. Disappears on pressing the bell of stethoscope (so, **place the bell lightly** over a prominent vein), and after Valsalva manoeuvre. It is accentuated by exercise.
6. Thrill may be associated with and detected by application of light pressure.

Q. In which situation should we search for abdominal venous hum (*see* Fig. 1.41)?

In the presence of dilated abdominal veins, we search for venous hum. The combination of dilated abdominal wall veins (caput medusae) and a loud venous hum, due to large amount of flowing blood, heard over dilated paraumbilical veins is called Cruveilhier-Baumgarten syndrome. This syndrome may originate due to congenital patency of umbilical vein but more usually to a well-compensated cirrhosis.

Q. Direction of blood flow in these prominent abdominal veins (see question above):

Blood flow is always away from the umbilicus as it is dealing with a case of 'portal hypertension'.

Q. D/D of venous hum:

a. In the epigastrium: Hepatic bruit (over liver) or continuous murmur (e.g. coarctation of aorta).
b. In the upper chest or supraclavicular area (left side): Patent ductus arteriosus.

Q. How these abdominal wall veins are formed in portal hypertension?

Dilated and tortuous veins suggest venous obstruction. These are formed due to blood passing through a large umbilical or paraumbilical vein in the falciform ligament **from the** left branch of portal vein **to the** superior epigastric, internal mammary or inferior epigastric veins present in the abdominal wall (i.e. opening of anastomotic channels between portal and systemic veins).

Q. How these abdominal wall veins are formed in IVC obstruction?

These are dilated anastomotic channels formed between the superficial epigastric and circumflex iliac vein **below**, and the lateral thoracic veins **above**, carrying blood from long saphenous vein to axillary vein. This is why the direction of blood flow is from below upwards.

Q. Conditions associated with dilated chest wall veins:

1. SVC obstruction (commonest).
2. Severe congestive cardiac failure.
3. IVC obstruction (not uncommon).
4. Localised venous prominence: underlying pleural malignancy or empyema thoracis.
5. Extreme cachexia (due to loss of subcutaneous fat) and sometimes in lean and thin persons.
6. Thrombophlebitis of anterior thoracic vein (Mondor's disease): Rare.

Q. How to know the presence of dilated and tortuous abdominal/chest wall veins (Fig. 3.176)?

1. The patient is asked to **sit** with legs hanging from the bed (never examine in lying down position).
2. Now the patient is asked to **cough** or to perform the **Valsalva manoeuvre**. Cough makes the veins prominent transiently while the Valsalva retains the prominence of veins so long the manoeuvre is continued.
3. Proper light is necessary (patient facing the window) for demonstration.

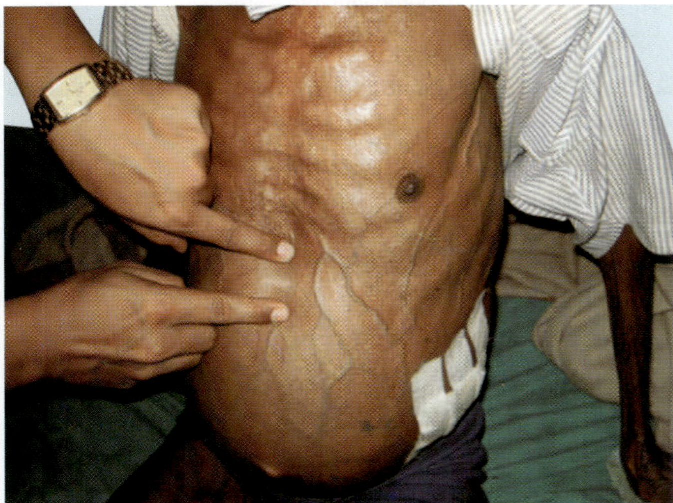

Fig. 3.176: Detection of direction of venous blood flow—a sitting patient with legs hanging from bed, and by selecting a tributory-free vein while the patient is performing **Valsalva manoeuvre** to make the veins more prominent

Q. Detection of direction of venous blood flow (Harveys' sign) (Fig. 3.176):

Method:

1. Make the veins prominent by adopting the above mentioned method. A straight, tributory-free, long segment of vein (preferably one inch or more) is selected for examination.
2. Stand on the right side of the patient and place the index finger of both hands side by side over the vein; the left above the right one. Now start milking the vein by movement of two index fingers in opposite direction.
3. The two ends of the bloodless vein is blocked with the pressure given by two index fingers. The left index finger is now removed and the rapidity of venous filling from above is noted. The same procedure is repeated after removal of the right index finger and the rapidity of venous filling from below is observed. The rapidity of venous filling indicates the direction of blood flow.

Q. Venous flow in different conditions (Fig. 3.177):

a. **Normally:** Away from the umbilicus (but one cannot see any venous prominence in health).
b. **Portal hypertension:** Away from the umbilicus (both above and below the umbilicus).
c. **IVC obstruction:** As a whole, the flow is from below upwards, i.e.
   i. Above the umbilicus: Upwards and away from the umbilicus.
   ii. Below the umbilicus: Towards the umbilicus.
d. **SVC obstruction:** From above downwards as a whole.

- [in **extrahepatic portal vein obstruction or EHO**, flow of blood is towards the umbilicus (rarely seen)].

Q. Diagnosis of these pathological conditions at bedside (Table 3.10):

The classical direction of venous flow helps in the diagnosis and the added features are:

1. Portal hypertension: Pedal oedema follows **ascites; splenomegaly; prominent veins** are mainly present in the epigastrium and umbilical area (*see* Fig. 1.39).
2. IVC obstruction: Ascites with bipedal oedema (with oedema of buttocks and groin) may be present **but ascites follows oedema**. Prominent veins are seen over the abdomen, flanks and back; absence of splenomegaly (*see* Fig. 2.3).
3. SVC obstruction: Tortuous and prominent veins are present in the chest, upper arm with **facial**

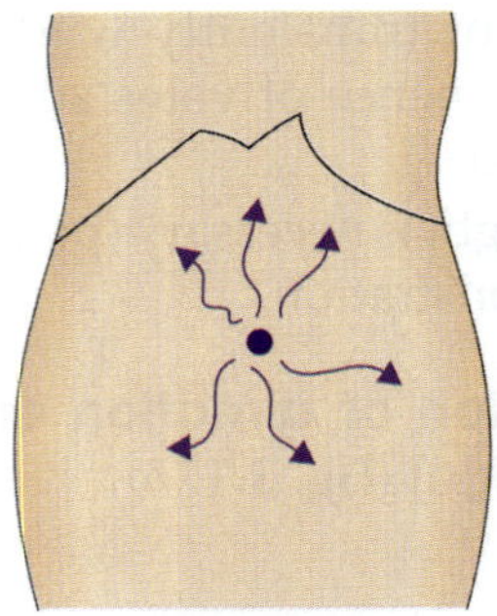
Normal
Direction of flow is away from the umbilicus (no venous prominence is seen in health)

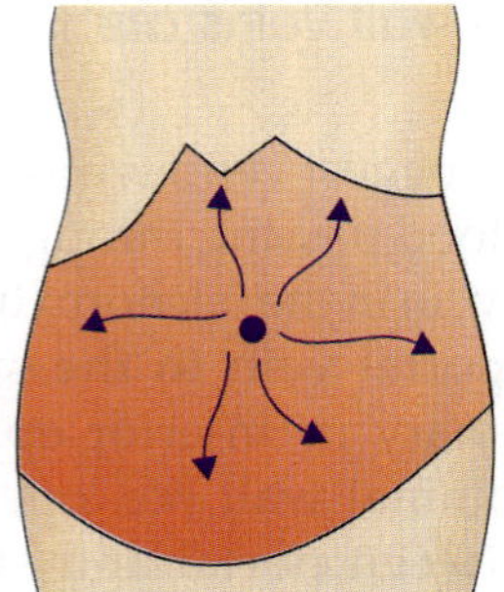
Portal hypertension
Direction of flow is always away from the umbilicus (both above and below the umbilicus)

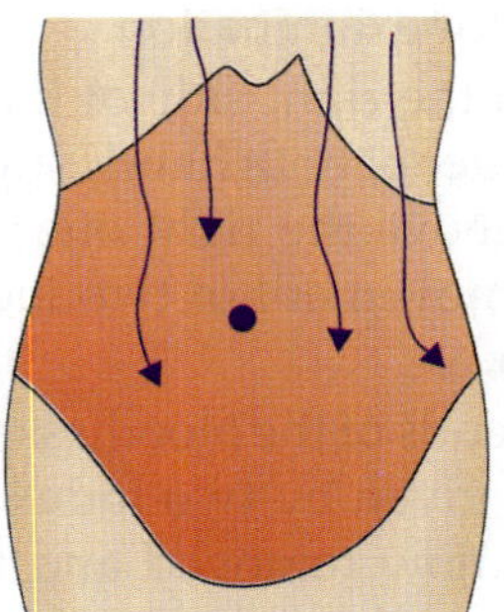
SVC obstruction
Direction of flow is from 'above downwards' whether it is above or below the umbilicus (mainly the chest wall veins are seen)

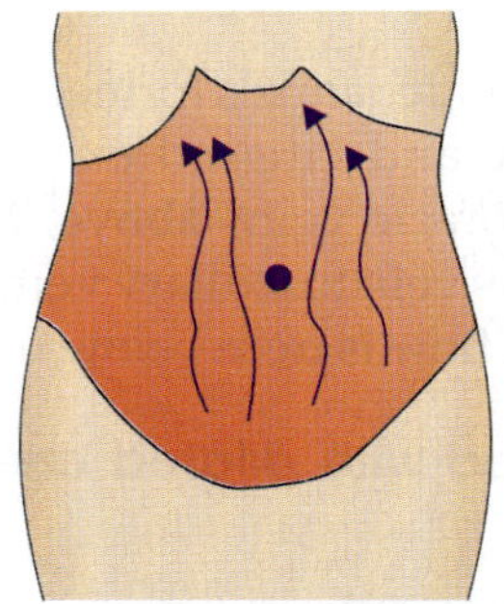
IVC obstruction
Direction of flow is from 'below upwards' whether it is above or below the umbilicus

Fig. 3.177: Abdominal wall veins

Table 3.10: Differentiation between portal hypertension and IVC obstruction

Features	*Portal hypertension*	*IVC obstruction*
1. H/o haematemesis or melaena	May be present	Absent
2. Sites of venous prominence	Epigastrium and periumbilical	Abdomen, flanks, back, lower limbs
3. Direction of flow of blood	Away from the umbilicus	From below upwards
4. Ascites	Precedes oedema; ascites is commonly seen	Follows oedema; ascites is uncommon
5. Splenomegaly	Commonly present	Usually absent
6. Venous hum	May be present	Absent
7. Aetiology	Commonly cirrhosis of liver	Commonly abdominal or pelvic tumour, hypercoagulable states

puffiness, chemosis of conjunctiva, and **engorged and non-pulsatile neck veins**; often the patient is in respiratory distress (*see* **Fig. 2.2**).

Q. 'Visible vein' versus 'engorged vein':

Sometimes, veins are visible normally in thin built persons (often in fair-skinned individuals) and is usually present at the skin level, i.e. flushed with the skin (not of clinical significance). But the engorged vein is a bit raised from the skin surface, which may be confirmed by tangenital application of light. Palpate the vein lightly by index finger and draw your inference. Visibility of a vein does not mean that it is pathological engorgement though tortuosity indicates its pathological nature undeniably.

Q. Thrombophlebitis versus phlebothrombosis versus varicose veins:

Thrombophlebitis: Superficial vein thrombosis is thrombophlebitis and is characterised by:

1. The involved vein is palpable as a tender cord with induration, redness and increased local temperature (**Fig. 3.178**).
2. The linear appearance is characteristic.
3. It commonly results from IV cannulation for IV infusion or blood transfusion.

Phlebothrombosis (*see* **Fig. 1.35**)***:*** It is the deep vein thrombosis (DVT) and is characterised by:

1. Pain or tight feeling of calf muscle with swelling, redness and non-pitting oedema of ankle or leg.
2. Common sites of DVT are calf muscle veins, popliteal, femoral and iliac veins.

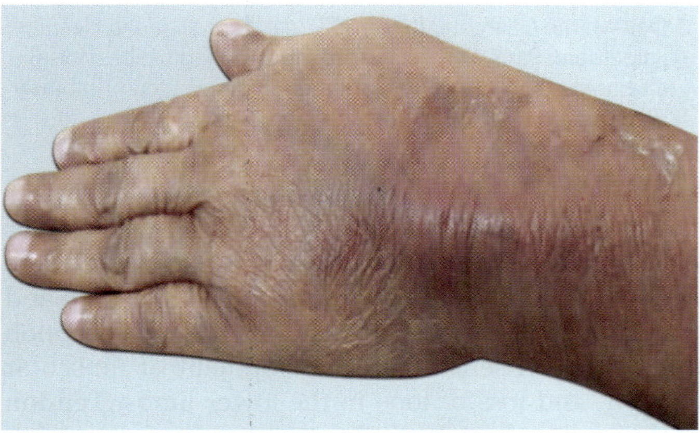

Fig. 3.178: **Thrombophlebitis** after IV fluid therapy

3. Moses' sign (tenderness in calf muscles) and Homan's sign (calf pain on dorsiflexion of foot) are positive. The local part feels warm.
4. Procoagulant states (e.g. antithrombin III ↓), prolonged immobility or long air travel are provocating factor.
5. *It is a medical emergency* and needs urgent treatment to prevent pulmonary thromboembolism (Fig. 3.179).

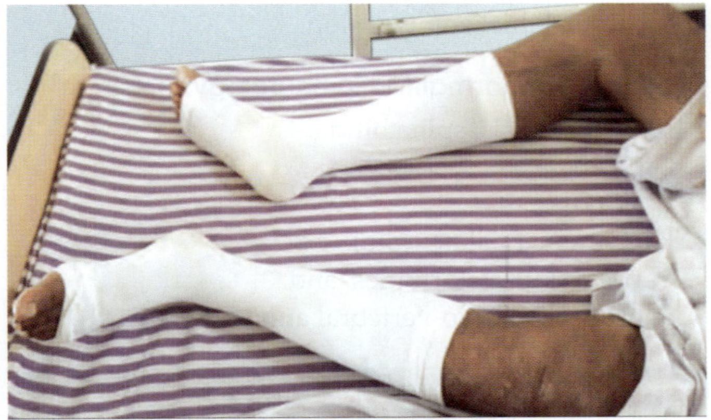

Fig. 3.179: Deep vein thrombosis **(DVT) prophylaxis**

Varicose veins (Fig. 3.180A and B): Characterised by:

1. Large, dilated and tortuous veins appearing in legs in persons habituated with prolonged standing (e.g. traffic police, security guards).

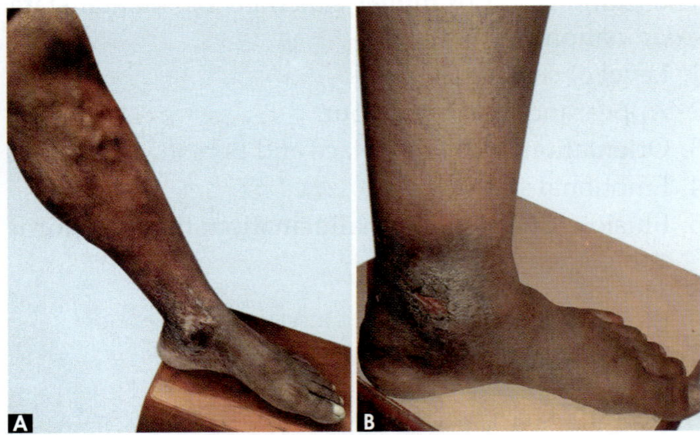

Fig. 3.180: **Varicose veins** (A) and **varicose ulcer** (B) are seen over lower extremity

2. Varicose veins are often complicated by cramping pain in legs, *varicose ulcer (over medial malleolus)*, thrombophlebitis and oedema.

Clinical Wisdom

For obvious reason, it is preferable to choose a vein below the umbilicus for demonstration of venous flow in abdominal wall veins. Engorged and tortuous veins always indicate some underlying pathology.

PES CAVUS — CASE 84

Q. Definition:

This is a fixed deformity of foot where both feet are more or less symmetrically 'high-arched' i.e. there is gross exacerbation of the medial longitudinal arch of the feet. It may result from weakness of intrinsic muscles (lumbricals and interossei) of the foot which in turn may be due to poliomyelitis, spina bifida, etc. Pes cavus may be associated with clawing of the toes (Fig. 3.181). It is just opposite to pes planus (flat foot) defronity (Fig. 3.182).

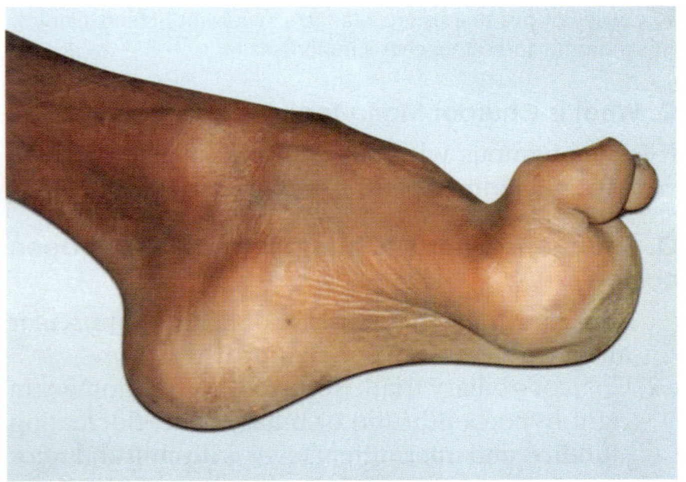

Fig. 3.181: **Pes cavus** (claw foot). The foot is high-arched; callosity has developed in the sole

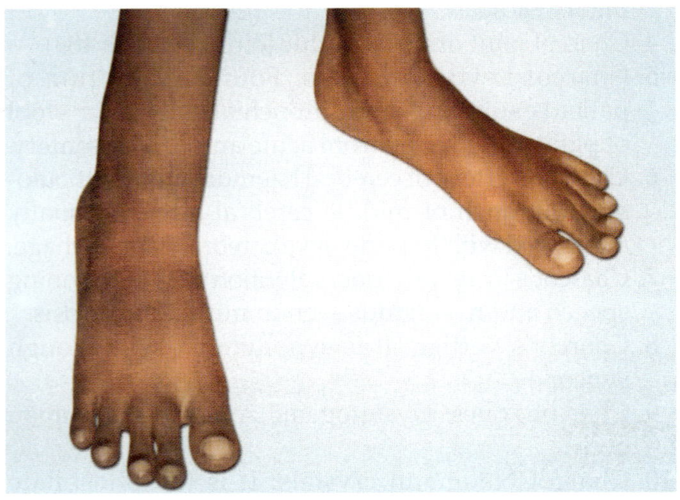

Fig. 3.182: **Flat foot deformity** (pes planus) in Marfan's syndrome

Q. Method of demonstration at the bedside:

It is done by any one of the undermentioned procedures:

1. Ask the patient to stand on the floor and observe that only toes, webs and heel touch the floor surface.
2. Take a foot-print on a white paper after painting the foot by lac-dye or any colouring agent.
3. After immersing the feet in water (wet test), ask the patient to walk barefooted and watch the footprints on the floor.

Q. Diseases associated with pes cavus (claw foot or cocking of toes):

Claw feet results from wasting of small muscles of feet due to any cause. The causes are:

1. Friedreich's ataxia (with hammer toes).
2. Peroneal muscular atrophy.
3. Syringomyelia.
4. Poliomyelitis (old).
5. Spina bifida.
6. Cerebral palsy.
7. Familial neuropathies, e.g. Refsum's disease.
8. Congenital.

- Causes of **pes planus** are Marfan's syndrome, Ehlers-Danlos syndrome and osteogenesis imperfecta.

Q. What is Charcot-Marie-Tooth disease?

It is synonymous with peroneal muscular atrophy (a variety of hereditary sensori-motor neuropathy).

Q. Situations where "Charcot's" name has been coined?

1. Charcot-Marie-Tooth disease or peroneal muscular atrophy (hereditary polyneuropathy).
2. Charcot's biliary triad: Recurrent pain abdomen (in right hypochondrium) or biliary colic, fluctuating jaundice, and intermittent fever with chill and rigor (due to acute cholangitis) in patients suffering from stone in CBD.
3. Charcot's intermittent hepatic fever due to cholangitis, principally in the affection of intrahepatic biliary radicles.
4. Charcot joint or neuropathic joint (*see* page 484).
5. Charcot-Leyden crystals: Found in sputum of patients suffering from bronchial asthma or stool of patients suffering from acute amoebic dysentery.
6. Charcot's artery of cerebral haemorrhage (lenticulo-striate branch of middle cerebral artery): Usually associated with hypertensive cerebral haemorrhage.
7. Charcot's (cerebral) triad: Intention tremor, scanning speech and nystagmus seen in multiple sclerosis.
8. Charcot's vertigo: It is synonymous with 'cough syncope'.
9. Charcot zones: Hysterogenic zones in the human body.
10. Charcot-Neumann crystals: It is the phosphate crystals present in semen.

- Jean-Martin Charcot (1825–1893) was a physician in Hospital Salpetriere, Paris, France. He described hysteria, tabes dorsalis and ankle clonus for the first time. Sigmund Freud, Babinski and Tourette were his students.

Q. What is Friedreich's ataxia?

It is an autosomal recessive form of spinocerebellar degeneration. The patient usually presents between the ages of 5 and 15 years, with clumsiness in walking and trunk ataxia. Gradually there is loss of proprioception and vibration sense with development of muscular atrophy, and loss of tone in the lower limbs. **Tendon reflexes are lost but plantar response remains extensor.** The degenerative process ascends upwards, and affects speech (dysarthria) and movements of the eyes (nystagmus). Optic atrophy (30%) may be seen. Kyphoscoliosis, high arched palate and pes cavus may be evident. It may be associated with diabetes mellitus and cardiomyopathy. The patient is wheelchair bound by the age of 20. Diagnosis is made by positive family history and clinical findings.

Q. Diagnosis of spina bifida occulta:

Over the lower back, there may be:

1. Tuft of hair (Satyre's tail).
2. Dimpling of the skin.
3. Dilated vessels or naevus.
4. Fibrofatty tumour, or
5. Cicatricial thickening of skin.

Q. Skeletal abnormalities in neurology:

1. Kyphoscoliosis, spina bifida.
2. Gibbus.
3. Pes cavus.
4. High arched palate (rare).
5. Various skull deformities, and
6. Short neck (cranio-vertebral anomaly).

TESTS OF HIGHER FUNCTIONS — CASE 85

Q. How to test the patients for assessment of 'Higher functions' (Fig. 3.183)?

The examination of higher functions or 'mental state examination' are:

1. Level of consciousness.
2. Appearance and behaviour.
3. Orientation with time, place and person.
4. Emotional state.
5. Illusion, delusion and hallucination; thought (form and content).
6. Memory.
7. Intelligence.
8. Speech and language with handedness.

A synopsis of each function is described below:

a. Appearance and behaviour: Look for alertness, attitude and conduct. Observe the condition of hair, dress and cleanliness. Poor self-care, e.g. lack of shaving, bad body odour or dirty dresses are seen in severe depression, schizophrenia or dementia. Assess how the patient behaves with the interviewer.

b. Orientation with time, place and person Ask the patient about the time, day and month of the year (i.e. time), where he is present now, either at hospital or home (i.e. place), and what is his name, address and occupation (i.e. person).

c. Emotional state: Try to assess the mood of the patient, i.e. normal (calm and composed), depressed ('really fed up', despairing and hopeless), or manic state (euphoric, cheerful and silly). Look for objective assessment (e.g. anxious, angry or hostile) by observing the patient weeping, laughing or showing irritability. For example, precipitant cry or laughter, i.e. emotional incontinence is common in pseudobulbar palsy, while lack of inhibition is seen in frontal lobe lesion.

d. Thought: Attention should be given to patient's thought process (form and content). Elevated mood with all kinds of grandiose ideas (i.e. unrealistic sense of superiority) are common in GPI (neurosyphilis), and sudden onset of fear or depression prior to an epileptic attack are common of temporal lobe origin.

e. Illusion: False beliefs, which is corrected after proper explanation, e.g. mirage in the desert.

   Delusion: False beliefs, which can never be corrected in spite of evidences to the contrary, e.g. a rope is misinterpreted as a snake in spite of proper explanation.

   Hallucination: False perception of special sensation (e.g. visual, auditory, gustatory or olfactory) in the absence of any sensory stimulus, e.g. humming in the ears in the absence of any disease or focus of origin.

- **Other tests are described below and next section** (Case 86). Other higher function disorders are apraxia and agnosia (vide section of 'Cerebellar disorder').

Q. Different types of memory:

1. Short-term memory, immediate recall or rote memory.
2. Recent memory, and
3. Past memory, long-term or remote memory.

Q. What are the different components of memory?

Memory is the ability to register and retain new information, and may be arbitrarily divided into 4 parts:

1. Registration (defect found in manic states, senile dementia).
2. Retention (defect found in frontal lobe lesion, GPI).
3. Recall (defect found in epilepsy, Korsakoff's psychosis, post-traumatic states), and
4. Reproduction (defect found in CVA).

Q. How to test the memory function at the bedside?

Clinically 3 forms of memory are tested at the bedside:

a. ***Short-term memory:*** Memory which lasts upto 30 seconds and is tested by:
   i. Whether the patient can repeat 'seven digits forwards' or 'five digits backwards' (digit span test).
   ii. Ask the patient to spell 'India' backwards (a good test for 'working memory').
   iii. Give him a telephone number and ask the number after 30 seconds or so.

b. ***Recent memory:*** It is the memory of events occurred within minutes, weeks, months and is an index of the severity of organic brain disease, which is usually tested by:
   i. Ask the morning news what he has read in the newspaper or seen in television.
   ii. Give him the names of three different objects and ask it after 3–5 minutes.
   iii. Ask him about the name of the visitors who met him last evening.

c. ***Past memory:*** This part of memory (events occurred years back) is relatively resistant to the effects of neurological insults. It is examined by:

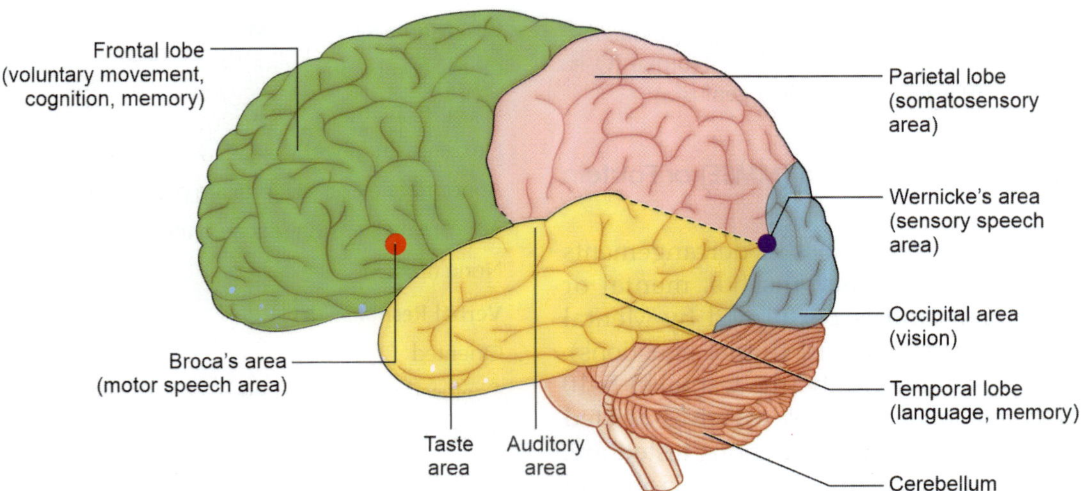

Fig. 3.183: Cerebral hemispheres (functional areas of cerebrum)

i. Ask the patient some important events in life, e.g. date of birth, date of marriage, etc.
ii. Ask him the date of 'Independence day of India'.
iii. Ask him the name of the first Prime Minister of India.

- In Wernicke-Korsakoff syndrome, the recent memory is lost with intact past memory, whereas the past memory is affected in dementia (e.g. in the late stage of Alzheimer's disease).
- Immediate recall or short-term memory is called as 'working memory' by some neurologists.

Q. Causes of emotional lability or 'emotional incontinence':

1. Cerebral atherosclerosis.
2. Multi-infarct dementia.
3. Pseudobulbar palsy.
4. Disseminated sclerosis.

Q. Tests of 'intelligence':

Intelligence is a total assessment of judgement, reasoning, arithmatic ability, etc. and is tested by:

i. Calculation: Serial 7-subtraction test (i.e. 100, 93, 86, 79, 72....), i.e. the arithmatic ability.
ii. Judgement: Ask the patient what will you do if you see a house set on fire, or a stamped and addressed envelope lying on the road in front of your house?
iii. Insight: Observe his awareness about the illness for which he has been admitted.
iv. Reasoning: Can he tell the difference between 'poverty and dishonesty', 'child and dwarf'?
v. Abstract thinking: Ask him the meaning of proverbs like 'all that glitters is not gold'.
vi. Attention: It is tested by tapping the finger with repetition of a particular number, told by examiner.
vii. Concentration: Ask the patient to count backwards from 20 to 1.

- Intelligence quotient (IQ) = $\frac{\text{Mental age}}{\text{Chronological age}} \times 100$
- Mental retardation (assessed by IQ): Mild (50–70), moderate (35–49), severe (20–34), and profound (<20). Normal IQ is 90–109, whereas ≥140 is regarded as 'near genius'.

Q. Mini-mental State Examination (MMSE) or Folstein test:

This is a 'simple bedside test' to assess derrangements in the **cognitive (higher) functions** (i.e. mental or intellectual functions), and is performed by Mental Status Questionnaire (MSQ; by 10 simple questions). The results are scored numerically (the test takes 5–10 minutes and is scored out of 30; scores <21 are associated with cognitive impairment). The functions tested are: 1. Orientation, 2. Registration, 3. Attention and calculation, 4. Recall, and 5. Language.

Q. How do you classify the level of consciousness clinically?

Disorder of arousal can be categorised by the following way:

a. **Conscious:** Relates to the person who is alert, attentive and co-operative. Actually, it is a state of awareness of one's self and environment.
b. **Confused:** It denotes incapacity of the patient to think with customary speed and clarity (i.e. disorientation). The patient is conscious but often talks irrelevantly.
c. **Drowsy:** The patient is sleepy but can be aroused easily by external stimulus.
d. **Stupor:** The patient who appears to be asleep, can be aroused only by painful stimulus (pinching or supraorbital pressure).
e. **Semicoma:** When the patient responds only to internal stimulus (e.g. the patient may shake his body with fullness of urinary bladder) but not to external painful stimulus.
f. **Coma:** No response by internal or external stimuli, and the patient is deeply unconscious.

- **Alert** means normal state of arousal. The degree of coma or the level of consciousness (e.g. in head injury) is assessed nowadays (as the terminology like drowsy, stuporose, semicoma are ill-defined) by **Glasgow Coma Scale (GCS)** but GCS can never be a substitute for thorough neurological examination. Circle the best scores from eye opening, motor response and verbal response, and compute the total **(Table 3.11)**.

Q. What is dementia?

It means loss of reasoning or more particularly, a deterioration of all intellectual and cognitive functions,

Table 3.11: Glasgow Coma Scale (clinical grading of coma)

Assessment area	Score
Eye Opening (E)	
Spontaneous	4
To speech	3
To pain	2
None	1
Best Motor Response (M)	
Obeys commands	6
Localises pain	5
Flexion withdrawal	4
Abnormal flexion (decorticate posture)	3
Abnormal extension (decerebrate posture)	2
None (flaccid)	1
Verbal Response (V)	
Oriented	5
Confused and disoriented	4
Inappropriate words	3
Incomprehensible sounds	2
No response	1

Clinical Wisdom

Coma scores = E + M + V: Fully conscious = 15 (maximum score), and deeply comatose = 3 (minimum score); scores >11 having 5–10% likehood of death, while scoring 3 or 4 have 85% chance of dying. Ocular movements and pupillary reflexes are not part of assessment. GCS is helpful for nurses and paramedical staffs too.

- Read 'brain death' from standard textbook of medicine.

without clouding of consciousness or disturbance of perception, and is due to chronic progressive degenerative disease of brain. In **dementia**, the patient is awake and alert but not aware.

- **Organic brain syndrome (OBS)** is an abnormal mental state with diffuse impairment of brain along with alteration in orientation, judgement, memory and affect. Two most important types of OBS are delirium (acute) and dementia (chronic), that is to say, disorder of cogntition can be acute (i.e. delirium) and chronic (i.e. dementia).

Delirium is an acute confusional state with excitement and hyperactivity due to acute or subacute brain failure, where impairment of attention is accompanied by abnormality of perception and mood; there is increased motor activity, tremulousness and hallucination (±).

Q. 'Released reflexes' in dementia:

In infancy, developmental assessment is very often done by the presence (so called, 'primitive reflexes') or absence of these reflexes. In late infancy, these reflexes disappear as cortical control develops. In few pathological conditions in adults, these reflexes are released from the control of higher centres and thus, may be elicited. The examples are:

(i) Dementia, (ii) Organic confusional states, and (iii) Sometimes in contralateral frontal lobe lesion. The reflexes are:

1. **Grasp reflex:** Stroke the palmar surface of the patient's hand on its 'radial' aspect (region between the thumb and the index finger) by a distally moving stimulus. The patient immediately grasps the object and is unable to relax his grasp voluntarily. It is classically seen in contralateral frontal lobe lesion.
2. Forced groping reflex: Sometimes, if the palmar surface ('radial' aspect) of patient's hand is lightly touched (patient's eyes are closed), the fingers close upon the object, and the hand and arm move towards the stimulus.
3. **Avoiding reflex:** It is the tendency of the patient's hand to move away from palmar stroking when an object is touched on the 'ulnar' side of the hand. It is commonly seen in contralateral parietal lobe disease.
4. **Palmo-mental reflex:** Scratch the thenar eminence with a pin, key or finger, and there will be puckering of the chin due to contraction of the ipsilateral mentalis muscle. It may suggest contralateral frontal lobe lesion, pyramidal lesion or diffuse cerebral disease (may be seen normally in some elderly individuals). This reflex usually have no localising value.
5. Sucking reflex: The contact of an object with the lips or corner of the mouth evokes the movements of the lips, tongue and jaw concerned in sucking.
6. Rooting reflex: The lips follow the stimulating object when it is touched on the lips.
7. Snout reflex: A gentle tap of the examiner's knuckle against the centre of patient's closed upper lips will produce pouting of the lips due to reflex puckering of orbicularis oris.
8. **Glabellar tap reflex (Myerson's sign)** (*see* **Fig. 1.54B**)**:** Normally after repeated tapping of the glabella by standing behind the patient, there are only three or four blinks before the response is inhibited. But in parkinsonism and senile dementia, the response goes uninhibited, i.e. a blink follows after each tap.

Q. Common causes of loss of memory (dementia):

1. Transient: Following concussion, epilepsy.
2. Cerebral atherosclerosis (multi-infarct dementia).
3. Alzheimer's disease, Pick's disease.
4. Tumour affecting frontal lobe or corpus callosum.
5. Alcoholism.
6. Chronic subdural haematoma.
7. Pellagra, vitamin B_{12} deficiency.
8. Hypothyroidism.
9. Wilson's disease.
10. Wernicke-Korsakoff syndrome.
11. 'Normal pressure' hydrocephalus.
12. Huntington's disease.
13. AIDS.
14. Renal failure, hepatic failure.
15. Parkinson's disease.
16. Dialysis dementia.

- Dementia is of two types: Primary (No. 3) and secondary (others except No. 3).

SPEECH DISORDERS — CASE 86

Q. What is speech?

It is the symbolic expression of thought process in spoken words or written words.

Q. Types of speech disorders:

1. Aphasia or dysphasia (defect in higher centre with difficulty in language function)—Dysphasia is 'partial' speech defect while aphasia is 'complete' speech defect.
2. Dysarthria (defect in articulation, commonly due to neuromuscular or muscular disorders resulting in impaired coordination of facio-lingual muscles)—Slurring, mumbling, etc.

3. Dysphonia (disorder of phonation due to abnormality in the vocal cord)—e.g. hoarseness, aphonia.

- **Mutism** means inability to speak while **aphonia** is inability to produce sounds.

Q. Prerequisites before testing speech:

1. Level of consciousness.
2. Handedness (right or left).
3. Mother language.
4. Intelligence level (education, etc).
5. Deaf or not, and
6. Vision.

- So, speech disturbance may be due to: 1. Deafness, 2. Dementia/ depression (severe), 3. Dysphasia (motor or sensory), 4. Dysarthria, 5. Dysphonia.

Q. Where the 'speech area' (i.e. dominant hemisphere) lies in the brain?

In the right-handed person, it is present in the left hemisphere (95%). In a left-handed person, it is present in the left hemisphere in 60% cases. In ambidextrous persons too, the left hemisphere is the dominant one. Dominant hemisphere also controls language and mathematical functions. The speech areas are distributed as follows:

a. Motor or Broca's area (area 44 and 45) is situated in the posterior part of inferior frontal lobe (spoken word) and in the posterior part of middle frontal lobe (written word). Broca's area (after Pierre Paul Broca) controls the fluency and expression of speech.
b. Sensory or Wernicke's area (area 22) is situated in the posterior end of superior temporal lobe and adjoining parietal region. It controls the comprehension of spoken and written words, i.e. decoding of sounds into language formation.

- Shaking hands with the patient will determine the handedness. Also ask him/her directly, whether he/ she is right or left-handed.

Q. Types of dysphasia or aphasia:

1. Expressive aphasia or nonfluent aphasia:

i. Motor or Broca's aphasia: Commonest variety. The patient is unable to speak although there is no paralysis of tongue or lips.

ii. Agraphia: Inability to write although there is no paralysis of hand muscles.

2. Sensory, receptive, Wernicke's aphasia or fluent aphasia:

i. Word deafness: Though the patient can hear the sound, he is unable to analyse its meaning.

ii. Word blindness: The patient can see that something is written but he cannot recognise the words. His mother language appears as a foreign language to him.

3. Global aphasia: This is the combination of 1 and 2, i.e. there is defective comprehension as well as production of speech.

Q. Speech evaluation at the bedside:

Look for:

1. Spontaneous speech, i.e. listen the articulation, content, comprehension and fluency.
2. Ask for naming simple objects like pen, coin, book, etc. (i.e. naming ability).
3. Ask the patient to repeat words or phrases (i.e. repetition).
4. Instruct the patient to read aloud and to write a simple sentence.

Q. Enumerate a 'word' with polysyllabic utterance:

'PATAKA' (polysyllabic consonents with vowel):
Pa—labial,
Ta—lingual,
Ka—guttural (of the throat).

Q. How to examine an aphasic patient?

1. Ask the patient his name. If he keeps mum, then it is the task of the physician to determine the variety of aphasia: expressive or receptive type.
2. Now, write 'show me your tongue' on a white paper and show the paper to the patient. If he protrudes his tongue, then it is a case of expressive aphasia (comprehension is perfect and word blindness is not present) and if he does not protrude the tongue, probably you are dealing with a case of sensory aphasia or global aphasia. This test may be done by showing the examiner's protruding tongue to the aphasic patient.

Q. What is the commonest cause of aphasia?

Ischaemic cerebrovascular disease (CVA) is the commonest cause of aphasia. Cerebral haemorrhage causes aphasia less often than thrombosis because haemorrhage occurs deep in the white matter of the hemisphere, more often than in the cortex or subcortical regions. The patient with motor aphasia is often hemiplegic (right-sided hemiplegia with speech area in the left, as most of the persons are right-handed).

Intracranial tumour is the commonest cause of aphasia during the first half of adult life.

Q. What is nominal aphasia?

The patient fails to name the common objects like pen, pencil, coin, etc. (produced in front of him) though he can tell the use of it. If he is told the actual name of the object, he immediately accepts it gladly.

Site of lesion: In between the angular gyrus and the posterior part of superior temporal gyrus.

Q. What are the different dysarthrias?

The normal requisites for production of syllables are:

- Articulation: Labial, lingual and palatal muscles.
- Phonation: Larynx.
- Resonance: Nasopharynx.
- Along with normal respiration.

The different types of dysarthria are:

1. Spastic (UMN) dysarthria: Difficulty in uttering the words but the words pronounced will be distinct. There is difficulty in pronouncing 'b', 'p' or 't'. It is commonly seen in pseudobulbar palsy.
2. Flaccid (LMN) dysarthria: There is much difficulty in uttering the words and the uttered words will be slurred and indistinct. Often there is added nasal intonation ('egg' is pronounced as 'eng'). This type is commonly seen is bulbar palsy, alcoholism, etc.
3. Scanning or staccato speech (or ataxic speech): Read the section on 'cerebellar disorder'.
4. Slow, monotonous speech without any fluctuation (i.e. lacking accents): Seen in parkinsonism.
5. Lalling speech (voice): Commonly seen in children, cretinism, Down syndrome and mental retardation (i.e. baby speech).
6. Stammering speech: Usually congenital (developmental) in nature, when the patient stammers.
7. Fatiguing speech: Myasthenia gravis.

- For speech testing, ask the patient to pronounce 'British Constitution' or 'West Register Street'.
- In a patient of hemiplegia, dysphasia is due to involvement of dominant hemisphere, and dysarthria is usually due to UMN type of affection of VIIth and/or XIIth cranial nerves.
- Ill-fitted dentures are very common cause of dysarthria.
- VIIth nerve palsy = labial dysarthria, XIIth nerve palsy = lingual dysarthria.

Q. What is dysphonia?

Dysphonia is commonly due to laryngitis, tumour of the vocal cord or bilateral adductor paralysis (the voice becomes hoarse). In this disorder of vocalisation, the fault lies in the vocal cord.

Q. How to diagnose hysterical aphonia?

The hysteric aphonic patient (commonly a female) whispers but cannot talk aloud. Ask the patient to cough or give a painful stimulus. These two menoeuvres will definitely produce a sound.

- Echolalia—repetition of examiner's word, palilalia—repetition of terminal words of own speech, jargon aphasia—using meaningless neologisms (non-existant new words) making no sense at all, phonation—production of vocal sounds without formation of words, paraphasia—rearrangement or substitution in the component of speech, e.g. dat for hat, agraphia—inability to write, alexia—inability to read, and perseveration—repeated use of particular words or phrases.
- Flaccid dysarthria, scanning and monotonous speech may be given in the examination.

TREMOR — CASE 87

Q. What is tremor?

These are involuntary, repetitive, oscillatory movements of a part of the body around a fixed point due to alternate contraction and relaxation of groups of muscles with their antagonists.

Q. How do you classify tremor clinically?

a. According to relationship with posture:
   1. Static tremor,
   2. Essential, postural or action tremor,
   3. Intention tremor, and
   4. Flapping tremor.

b. According to amplitude:
   1. Fine, and
   2. Coarse tremor.

Q. How will you examine a patient for tremor?

At first, look for the presence of any **static tremor** (tremor at rest or during relaxation). This is classically seen in parkinsonism. In the hand, it is described as 'pill-rolling' or 'cigarette making' tremor. This very obvious tremor is characterised by:

1. At the onset, wrist and elbows are semiflexed, fingers flexed at MCP joints and extended at interphalangeal joints with abduction of the thumb. The oscillations of the fingers and thumb in two planes produce the 'pill-rolling' effect (flexion-extension at wrist and fingers, pronation-supination in forearm along with abduction-adduction of thumb and complex combinations).
2. It is a static tremor and does not increase at the goal point of action.
3. Coarse in nature (4–6/second).
4. More prominent in hands and can be controlled temporarily by willed movements.
5. Worse during anxiety or emotion, and is supposed to decrease on activity. It disappears during sleep.
6. If may involve the head, jaw, tongue, legs and even the trunk.

- Other features of parkinsonism like hypokinesia, rigidity, flexed posture and festinant gait will be present. There may by 'drum-beating' or 'bread-cutting' tremor present in parkinsonism.

Now, look for the presence of any **postural** or **action tremor**. The patient is asked to outstretch his hands with separated fingers (a paper or thin piece of cardboard may be placed over the outstretched fingers) for the appearance of tremor, if present. This type of tremor is seen in anxiety, thyrotoxicosis, chronic alcoholism, by application of drugs (salbutamol, sympathomimetics, tricyclic antidepressants) or in familial tremor. It is characterised by:

1. Fine in nature (7–10/second).

2. Disappears at rest, and appears in precise and accurate movements
3. May also be seen in tongue, lips and head.

❍ Familial tremor is often relieved by intake of alcohol. Task-specific tremor is a type of action tremor which occurs while performing a specific skilled task, like 'writing tremor'.

Next the patient is examined for the presence of any **intention tremor.** This is classically seen in cerebellar disease, and rarely in severe parkinsonism. It is characterised by:

1. Coarse in nature (4–6/second).
2. Tremor appears at the goal point of an action (i.e. absent at rest and at the beginning of any movement). The patient is asked to hold a glass of water which is kept on the table or to do the 'finger nose test'. The movement becomes clumsy before he reaches the target.
3. Sometimes, there is tremor seen in head (titubation).

❍ Other signs of cerebellar disease like hypotonia, nystagmus, 'past pointing', etc. will be present.

Lastly, examine the patient for the presence of any **flapping tremor** (asterixis or bat's-wing tremor). This is elicited by three different manoeuvres (it is a coarse tremor at 4–6/second):

1. By asking the patient to outstretch his arms with the hands extended at wrists and MCP joints, and to keep the limbs in this position for 20 seconds, when jerky forward movements of hand occurs every 2–3 seconds **(Fig. 3.184)**, or
2. By keeping the upper limb in bed with forearm fixed, the wrist is passively extended by holding the fingers. After few seconds, the pressure is released and the patient is instructed to keep the hand in the extended position (*classical method*) **(Fig. 3.185)**. The response is described as follows.

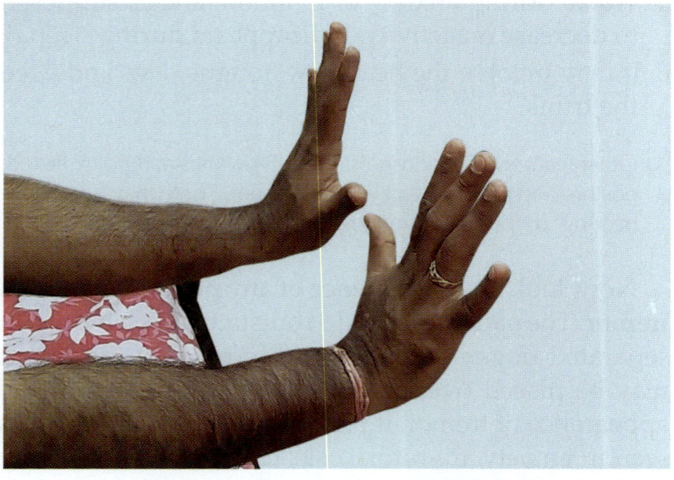

Fig. 3.184: Demonstration of **flapping tremor**

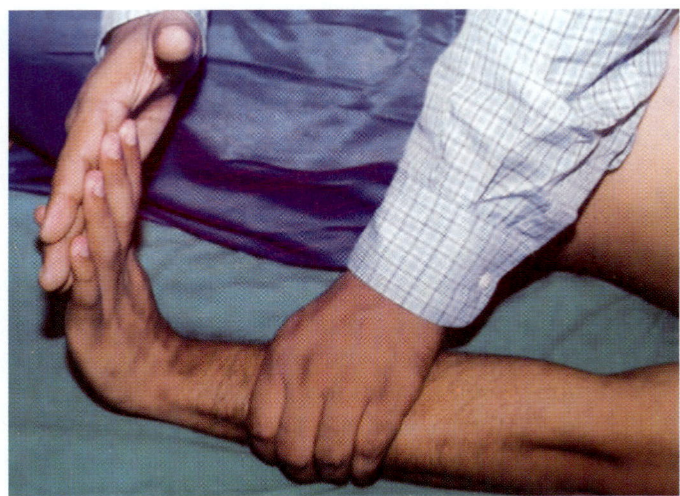

Fig. 3.185: Eliciting **flapping tremor** (classical method)

3. Ask the patient to squeeze the physician's extended fingers: Flapping tremor is said to be present as indicated by repeated intensification and relaxation of the intensity of the squeeze ("milkmaid's grip").
   Response: There is rapid flexion-extension movements at the MCP joints which are often accompanied by lateral movements of the digits and the hand ultimately falls (looks like 'good-bye'). This type of tremor is due to impaired inflow of joint and other afferent information to the brainstem reticular formation which results in lapses in sustained posture, i.e. there is development of neuromuscular incoordination between flexor and extensor muscles. Flapping tremor is a type of negative myoclonus and is classically seen in:
   i. Hepatic pre-coma ('liver flap')–Commonest.
   ii. Renal failure.
   iii. Respiratory failure (carbon dioxide narcosis).
   iv. Severe cardiac failure.
   v. Hypnotic poisoning, and
   vi. Toxic encephalopathies

❍ Flapping tremor is absent in hepatic coma. Patient's understanding is required to demonstrate it.

Q. What are the other sites (other than hands) you will exemine next?

1. **The tongue:** The patient is asked to protrude the tongue out of the oral cavity for at least 1/2 minute (fasciculation in the tongue is seen when the tongue is relaxed in the floor of the mouth, and not protruded).
2. Head (and neck): Titubation.
3. Jaw, lips, trunk or lower limbs.

❍ **One must examine tremor both in hands and tongue.**

Q. Common causes of tremor:

A. Fine (7–10/second):

1. Anxiety, nervousness, fear, fatigue.
2. Senile tremor.
3. Thyrotoxicosis.
4. Chronic alcoholism.
5. Drugs like salbutamol or terbutaline.
6. Familial (benign essential tremor).
7. General paralysis of insane (GPI).

B. Coarse (4–6/second):

1. Static tremor of parkinsonism.
2. Intention tremor of cerebellar disease or multiple sclerosis.
3. Flapping tremor of hepatic failure.
4. Uraemia.
5. Sometimes, senile tremor.
6. Wilson's disease.
7. Rubral tremor.

Q. Types of tremor:

1. Static.
2. Action.
3. Intention
4. Flapping.
5. Senile.
6. Physiological (anxiety).
7. Familial.
8. Hysterical.

- **Hysterical tremor** (variable and does not fit with other types): Occurs at rest, very fast and violent involving a limb or whole body, and while distracted by the examiner, it disappears.
- **Rubral tremor:** A coarse tremor arising out of lesions of the red nucleus (e.g. multiple sclerosis, cerebral infarction) which occurs at rest, posture and action.

Q. Commonest cause of tremor in clinical practice:

Physiological tremor due to anxiety, fear or nervousness.

Q. Identification points (facies) for aetiological diagnosis of tremor:

See the face of the patient and observe for:

1. Exophthalmos: Thyrotoxicosis.
2. Flushed face with parotid swelling: Chronic alcoholism.
3. Masked facies: Parkinsonism.
4. Anxious face: Anxiety neurosis.
5. Very old person: Senile tremor or parkinsonism.
6. K-F ring with jaundice: Wilson's disease (asterixis).
7. Alae nasi moving (i.e. the patient is breathless): Drug-induced (sulbutamol).

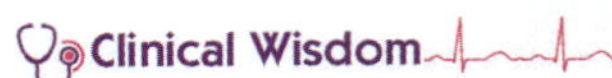

If you are asked to show tremor, start with demonstration for the method of postural or action tremor, i.e. the patient is asked to outstretch his hands.

PTOSIS — CASE 88

Q. Definition:

Drooping of one or both upper eyelids. 'Ptosis' is derived from the Greek word meaning 'to fall'.

Q. What are the types of ptosis?

a. Congenital or acquired.
b. Unilateral or bilateral.
c. Complete or partial.
d. True or pseudo.

- Recently, ptosis is divided into 5 types: blepharoptosis (eye surgery, old trauma), mechanical (oedema of upper eyelid), aponeurotic (cataract surgery), myogenic (myasthenia gravis, myopathies), and neurogenic (IIIrd cranial nerve palsy or Horner's syndrome).

Q. How to recognise partial ptosis?

By the narrowing of the palpebral fissure, when the clinician stands in front of the patient and the patient looks forward.

Q. Common causes of ptosis:

1. Oculomotor nerve paralysis (usually complete, may be partial), e.g. diabetes, multiple sclerosis.
2. Horner's syndrome (always partial or pseudoptosis).

- No. 1 and 2 are principal causes of ptosis.

3. Myasthenia gravis (worsens as day progresses).
4. Myotonia dystrophica; ocular or oculo-pharyngeal myopathy.
5. Congenital (the upper eyelid is smooth and devoid of any cutaneous folds, and with compensatory head posture, i.e. head tilts slightly backwards).
6. Snake bite (Elapidae group).
7. Botulism.
8. Periodic paralysis.
9. Tabes dorsalis (partial): Not seen nowadays.
10. Hysterical.
11. Oedema or tumour of upper eyelid, enucleation of eyeball.
12. Temporal arteritis.
13. Trauma, intraocular surgery, long-term use of contact lens or Wernicke's encephalopathy.

- Congenital ptosis may be unilateral or bilateral. Acquired ptosis is usually **unilateral** in IIIrd nerve palsy, Horner's syndrome, senility, traumatic and hysterical conversion reaction. It is **bilateral** in tabes dorsalis, myopathy or disorders of myoneural junction.
- Unilateral ptosis is a recognised finding in cluster headache, syringobulbia and cavernous sinus thrombosis.
- 'Narrow palpebral fissure' results from ptosis and pseudoptosis, enophthalmos and blepharospasm.

Q. What is the opposite phenomenon of ptosis?

Retraction of the upper eyelid, i.e. spasm of the Muller's muscle in thyrotoxicosis due to sympathetic overactivity.

Q. Nerve supply of the upper eyelid:

There are two muscles in the upper eyelid like,

1. Levator palpebrae superioris (LPS): Supplied by IIIrd cranial nerve.
2. Muller's (tarsal) muscle: Supplied by sympathetic trunk.

Clinical Wisdom

Muller's muscle arises from the undersurface of LPS muscle. The LPS, its aponeurosis and the Muller's muscle are responsible for upper eyelid resting position and elevation. 'Complete' ptosis—the ptotic eyelid covers the pupil completely, and 'partial' ptosis—upper eyelid droops but does not cover the pupil completely. Remember, normally the upper eyelid covers upper 1/3rd of cornea.

Q. Test the power of LPS musole or upper eyelid, or test for ptosis:

a. First step: Stand in front of the patient face to face, and ask him to look upwards or elevate the upper eyelid voluntarily.
b. Second step: Now push down the frontal belly of occipitofrontalis muscle of forehead by your left hand (it is done to eliminate its elevating action on the upper eyelid). Again ask the patient to look upwards.
c. Third step: If the patient can elevate the upper eyelid, now you may apply little resistance by your right index finger over the upper eyelid and ask the patient to look upwards again (obviously with eliminating the action of forehead muscle). Compare with the other side.

- If the patient cannot elevate the upper eyelid voluntarily, it is useless to do the next steps.

Q. What is pseudoptosis?

In a patient of Horner's syndrome, (i.e. damage to the cervical sympathetic fibres) though there is 'partial' drooping of the upper eyelid, the ptosis is often corrected on looking upwards voluntarily (due to intact IIIrd nerve) and thus, it is known as pseudoptosis (i.e. false ptosis).

Q. Features of IIIrd cranial nerve palsy (Fig. 3.186):

1. Usually, it is unilateral 'complete ptosis' (as there is complete ptosis in one eye, patients do not complain of diplopia; patients are not able to open the affected eye voluntarily).
2. Lateral or divergent squint (due to unopposed action of lateral rectus). The patient is unable to move the eye upwards, downwards and medially.
3. Fixed (loss of light and accommodation reflex) and dilated pupil.

- Diplopia is complained by the patient as soon as the affected upper eyelid is elevated by fingers.

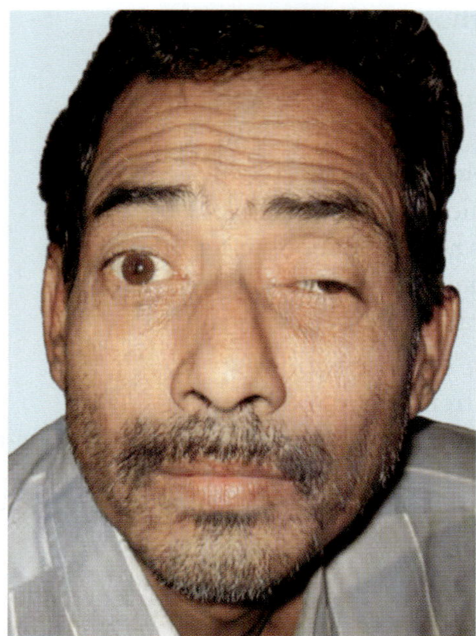

Fig. 3.186: Left-sided partial ptosis with lateral squint due to **IIIrd cranial nerve palsy (recovering)**; increased **wrinkling of forehead** is noted to overcome the drooping of upper eyelid

Q. Components of Horner's syndrome (Fig. 3.187A):

Horner's syndrome results from damage to the cervical sympathetic fibres (Table 3.12). Usually it is unilateral:

1. Pseudoptosis (diagnosed by narrowing of palpebral fissure; it is partial ptosis and is due to paralysis of Muller's muscle).
2. Miosis (constriction of the pupil, as cervical sympathetic supplies the dilator pupillae): The pupil shows reaction to light.
3. Anhidrosis (involves ipsilateral half of the face and neck, front and back of upper chest, arm).

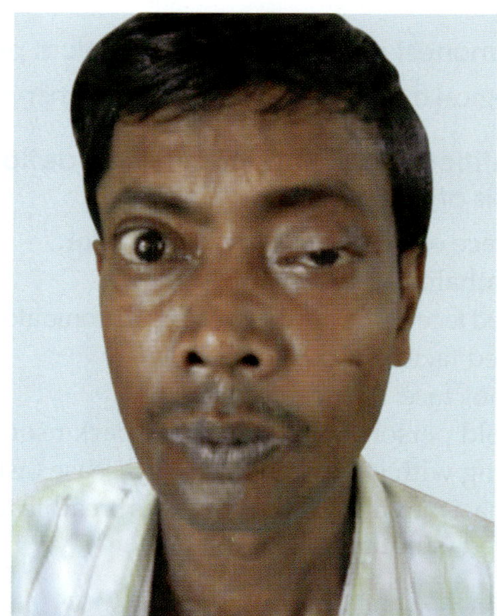

Fig. 3.187A: Recently developed left-sided **partial ptosis** (without squint) due to cervical sympathetic palsy **(Horner's syndrome)** in bronchogenic carcinoma in a chronic smoker. Miosis was evident

Table 3.12: Differentiation between IIIrd nerve palsy and Horner's syndrome-induced ptosis

IIIrd nerve palsy	Horner's syndrome
1. Usually complete ptosis	1. Partial ptosis
2. Dilated pupil	2. Constricted pupil
3. Squint	3. No squint
4. Extraocular muscle palsy present	4. Extaocular muscles—normal

4. Enophthalmos (sympathetic supply maintains the tone of the eyeball): Shrunken eye.
5. Loss of ciliospinal reflex (in health, when the skin of the sides of neck is pinched or scratched, there is reflex dilatation of pupil and this reflex is abolished in Horner's syndrome).

- There is bloodshot conjunctiva due to loss of vasoconstrictor activity in Horner's syndrome.
- Johann F. Horner (1831–1886) was Professor of Ophthalmology, Zurich, Switzerland.

Q. Bedside diagnosis of congenital ptosis (Fig. 3.187B):

1. Isolated partial ptosis (may be bilateral).
2. Ptosis since childhood.
3. No deviation of eyeball (i.e. no squint).
4. Heterochromia of iris may be present.

Q. Trace the pathway of ocular sympathetic fibres:

1st order of neurones of sympathetic fibres descend from hypothalamus → brainstem → intermediolateral horn of spinal cord at C_8, T_1 level → 2nd order of neurones start and go up to superior sympathetic ganglion → 3rd order of neurones from there carried around carotid artery → ophthalmic division of Vth nerve → nasociliary nerve → long ciliary nerve → oculopupillary fibres → supply dilator pupillae and Muller's muscle of upper eyelid.

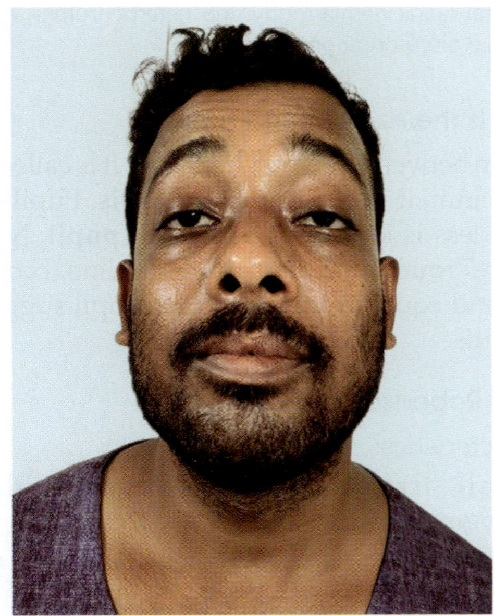

Fig. 3.187B: Congenital ptosis; slight backwards head tilt with wrinkling of forehead is evident

Q. Can you test the Muller's muscle?

No. It is an involuntary muscle.

Q. Ptosis and pupil:

1. Ptosis and dilated pupil: IIIrd nerve palsy.
2. Ptosis with constricted pupil: Horner's syndrome.
3. Ptosis with normal-sized pupil: Myasthenia gravis, myotonia dystrophica, botulism (in majority), snake bite, and rarely in infarction or ischaemia of IIIrd nerve (e.g. vasculitis, migraine or diabetes).

Q. What is 'Tabetic facies'?

This is the classical facies of tabes dorsalis and is characterised by (very rare):

1. Bilateral partial ptosis (as a result of paralysis of Muller's muscle),
2. Presence of compensatory wrinkling in the forehead (to overcome the partial ptosis),
3. Elevated eyebrows, and
4. Associated Argyll Robertson pupill.

- Increased furrowing in the forehead may be seen in any long-standing ptosis.

Q. Speciality of ptosis in myasthenia gravis (Fig. 3.188):

Ptosis may be unilateral or commonly bilateral, and appears towards the end of the day after repeated use of the upper eyelid (fluctuating ptosis with diurnal variation). Ptosis is corrected dramatically by the IV injection of 2 mg of edrophonium chloride (Tensilon test) as edrophonium is a rapidly acting acetylcholinesterase inhibitor. There is **no alteration in the pupillary reflex or size of the pupil.** Sustained upward gaze for 2 minutes leads to increase ptosis.

Q. Bedside tests for myasthenia gravis:

1. Maintain sustained upward gaze of eyes (ceiling test): Observe the appearance of ptosis.

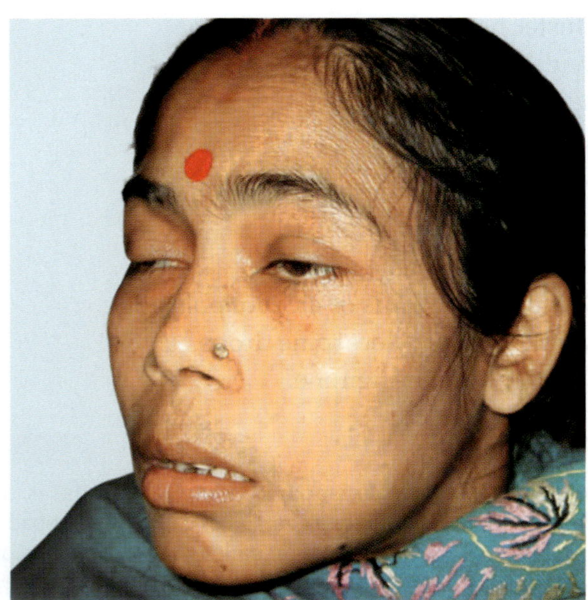

Fig. 3.188: Bilateral partial ptosis (right > left) in **myasthenia gravis**

2. Counting sign: Ask the patient to count up to 20 in one breath. The patient starts counting normally but the voice becomes slurred and unintelligible after counting few numbers due to development of muscle fatigue.
3. Ask the patient to close the eyes tightly and to do it repeatedly: Eye closure becomes weaker after repetition and white sclera is exposed (Peek sign).

- Myasthenia means fatigable weakness which is worse on exercise, itself a neuromuscular junction disorder.

Q. Dilatation (mydriasis) of pupil:

Constrictors of the pupil are supplied by parasympathetics (via oculomotor nerve), while the dilator fibres are controlled by sympathetic nervous system. Changes in the size of the pupil do not affect vision.

A. Unilateral

1. 3rd nerve palsy.
2. Adie's pupil or myotonic pupil.
3. Optic atrophy.
4. Acute congestive glaucoma.
5. Head injury.
6. Tentorial herniation (same side).

B. Bilateral

1. Childhood, anxiety, fear.
2. Application of mydriatic (atropine).
3. Dhatura poisoning.
4. Deep coma.
5. Severe raised intracranial tension.
6. Cerebral anoxia, brainstem death.

Q. Constriction (miosis) of pupil:

A. Unilateral

1. Horner's syndrome.
2. Iridocyclitis.
3. Cluster headache.
4. Ocular trauma.
5. Aphakia (i.e. no lens).

B. Bilateral

1. Old age (senile miosis), bright sunlight.
2. Argyll Robertson pupil, iritis.
3. Pontine haemorrhage.
4. Organophosphorus or alcohol poisoning.
5. Application of pilocarpine drops.
6. Overdose of neostigmine.

Clinical Wisdom

Commonest cause of **anisocoria** (unequal pupils) is the application of mydriatic to one eye. Other causes are idiopathic or physiological (12% population), unilateral IIIrd nerve lesion, unilateral lesion in the sympathetic trunk, blindness in one eye (larger pupil in blind eye), encephalitis, iritis, severe head injury, Holmes-Adie pupil, etc.

- Points 3, 4, 5 of (B) in constriction of pupil, morphine/opioids/ barbiturate overdose, heat stroke may produce **pin-point pupil**.
- **Irregular pupils** are due to iridocyclitis, coloboma, neurosyphilis and following eye operation. Sometimes, it is seen in normal healthy subjects.

Q. How to differentiate between patients with pin-point pupil [points 3 and 4 of (B) of question above]:

a. Pontine haemorrhage: There is coma, hyperpyrexia and long tract signs (i.e. signs of pyramidal tract lesion).
b. Organophosphorus poisoning: It is diagnosed by history of consumption of poison, absense of long tract signs and signs of respiratory depression. The patient may be unconscious but there is absense of pyrexia.

Q. Causes of Horner's syndrome (according to site of lesion):

The site of lesion may be in:

1. Cerebral hemisphere: Massive infarction of one hemisphere.
2. Brainstem: Lateral medullary syndrome (vascular), multiple sclerosis (demyelinating), pontine glioma (SOL), syringobulbia, encephalitis.
3. Spinal cord (lower cervical): Syringomyelia (bilateral Horner's syndrome), glioma, ependymoma.
4. Spinal cord (T_1 root lesions): Cervical rib, trauma, Klumpke's paralysis, aortic aneurysm.
5. Cervical sympathetic chain: Pancoast's tumour **(Fig. 3.187A)**, enlarged cervical lymph nodes, mediastinal mass, thoracic surgery, trauma.
6. Carotid artery: Thrombosis, spasm in migraine (temporary or intermittent Horner's syndrome).
7. Others: Congenital, idiopathic.

- Congenital Horner's syndrome may be associated with ipsilateral facial hemiatrophy and heterochromia of iris (i.e. grey-blue discolouration of iris).

Q. What is the size of normal pupil?

It varies in between 3–5 mm. If <3 mm, it is called **miosis** and if >5 mm, it is known as **mydriasis**. Pupillary size 1 mm or less is known as **pin-point pupil**. Normally pupils are 'round and regular' in outline, centered in the iris, and equal in size. Irregular pupil suggests old iridocyclitis.

Q. Argyll Robertson pupil:

A. Characteristics:

a. Small, irregular and unequal pupil; often depigmented.
b. Usually bilateral involvement but more marked on one side.
c. Accommodation reflex present but light reflex lost.
d. Dilates slowly to mydriatics.

B. Site of lesion: Peri-aqueductal grey matter (pretectal region of mesencephalon). Probably there is damage of both colliculo-nuclear and sympathetic fibres.

C. Clinical associations:
   1. Neurosyphilis (classically seen).
   2. Diabetes mellitus.
   3. Wernicke's encephalopathy.
   4. Multiple sclerosis.
   5. Brainstem encephalitis.
   6. Amyloidosis.
   7. Pinealomas.
   8. Sarcoidosis.

Q. What is 'reversed' Argyll Robertson pupil?

The pupil reacts to light but not to accommodation reflex. This rare phenomenon may be seen in post-encephalitic parkinsonism and diphtheria.

Q. Myotonic or Adie's pupil (Holmes-Adie pupil):

It is characterised by delayed or absent pupillary reaction to light or to accommodation, but once constricted the pupil dilates very very slowly. It is a unilateral defect and the affected pupil is larger. The lesion is due to malfunction of ciliary ganglion.

- **'Hippus'** is rhythmic constriction and dilatation of pupil, either spontaneously or in response to light. It is not of much clinical importance.

Q. Marcus Gunn pupil:

While doing light reflex, when the source of light is moved from normal eye to affected eye, after a short time the affected pupil will dilate paradoxically. It indicates an optic nerve lesion (afferent lesion) and often known as relative 'afferent pupillary defect'. Marcus Gunn was a scottish ophthalmologist.

Q. Describe the pathway of light reflex:

Light falls on retina—optic nerve—optic chiasma—optic tract—superior colliculi at midbrain (pretectal area)—2nd order of neurone starts from here and goes to the Edinger-Westphal (EW) nucleus bilaterally—preganglionic fibres go to the ciliary ganglion through the oculomotor nerve and its branch to the inferior oblique muscle—postganglionic fibres from ciliary ganglion supply the sphincter pupillae and ciliaris muscle through short ciliary nerve.

Q. Describe the pathway of accommodation reflex:

Light falls on retina—optic nerve—optic chiasma—optic tract—lateral geniculate body—optic radiation—calcarine cortex of the occipital lobe (visual cortex)—frontal eyefield area or 'area 8' through superior longitudinal association tract—from here cortico-mesencephalic fibres descend to the oculomotor nuclei at midbrain as follows:

1. Nucleus for medial rectus: Produces medial convergence of eyeball.
2. EW nucleus: Produces miosis.
3. Nucleus of Perlia: Contraction of ciliaris muscle and thus, anterior convexity of lens increases.

- From oculomotor (EW) nucleus, the pathway for accommodation reflex is the same as light reflex.

Q. How to test for light reflex (Fig. 3.189A)?

When light falls on one eye, there is constriction of both the pupils. The pupillary reaction on the stimulated side is called 'direct' light reflex, and the pupillary constriction of the opposite eye is known as 'consensual' light reflex. The method of examination goes like below:

1. Pencil torch is used with good power of illumination.
2. The patient is asked to look straight forward at a distant object and the *light is thrown suddenly in one eye from sides* (to avoid the accommodation reflex). The pupil constricts briskly over about half a second.
3. For **direct** light reflex, opposite eye should be closed by the hollow of the other palm. Direct light reflex should be tested preferably in a dark room.
4. For **consensual** light reflex, one hand of the patient is placed over the nose (like a curtain) to prevent the spillage of light to the other eye. Both the eyes are kept open. When light falls on one eye, observe the pupillary constriction of the other eye (i.e. consensual light reflex).
5. The afferent pathway—optic nerve, efferent pathway—oculomotor nerve, centre—ciliary ganglion, response—constriction of both the pupils.

- For both direct and consensual light reflexes, each eye is tested separately.
- **Light reflex is interpreted as brisk/sluggish/absent.**

Q. Mechanism of consensual light reflex:

As the fibres leaving one optic tract enter both the EW nucleus, there is genesis of consensual light reflex.

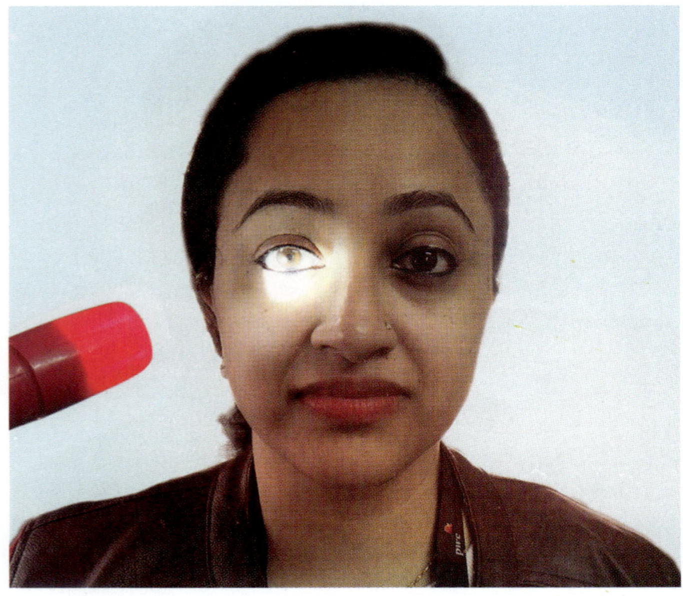

Fig. 3.189A: Testing of **light reflex**

Q. How to test for accommodation reflex or convergence reflex (Fig. 3.189B)?

The patient is first allowed to look at a distant object and then to ask him to look at examiner's finger quickly which is placed near his nose (e.g. at 15 cm from the eyes). The responses are:

1. Miosis (bilateral).
2. Medial convergence of the eyeball (bilateral).
3. Increased anterior convexity of lens (not clinically evident).
4. Enophthalmos (not clinically evident).

- Afferent pathway—optic nerve, efferent pathway—oculomotor nerve, centre—oculomotor nuclei at midbrain.

Q. How will you test the integrity of intraocular muscles (i.e. sphincter and dilator pupillae)?

By light (direct and consensual) and accommodation reflex.

Q. Identification points:

1. In the presence of ptosis, **miosis indicates Horner's syndrome and mydriasis indicates oculomotor palsy**. Ptosis due to Horner's syndrome is partial, and most of the cases it is unilateral.
2. Lateral squint with complete ptosis indicates oculomotor palsy.
3. Wrinkling of the forehead points towards long-standing ptosis.
4. Abnormal fatigability of muscles after repeated use indicates myasthenia gravis (in a case of ptosis).
5. Facies characterised by ptosis, 'hatchet face' with 'swan neck', frontal baldness, cataract with atrophy of temporalis and sternomastoid muscles indicate myotonia dystrophica.

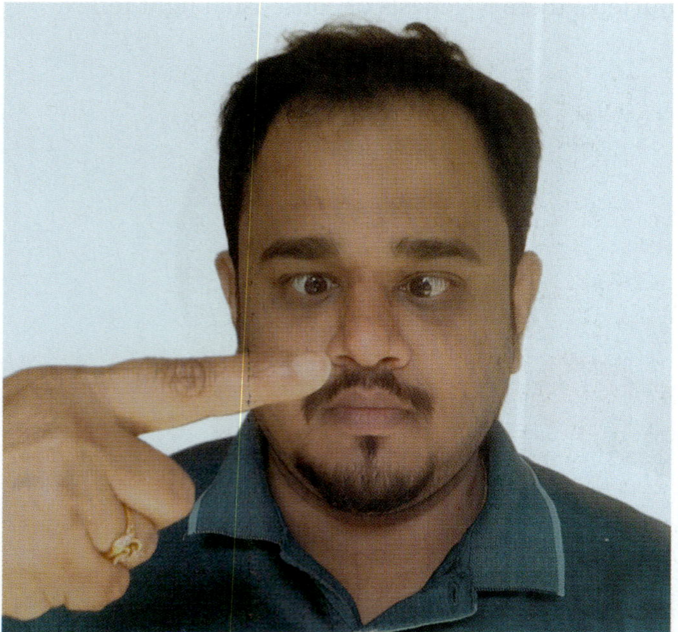

Fig. 3.189B: Testing of **accommodation reflex**

SQUINT — CASE 89

Q. What is squint?

In squint, abnormality of ocular movement is such that the visual axes do not meet at the point of fixation or it is a failure of the normal coordination of the ocular axes. 'Manifest squint' is noticeable when both the eyes are kept open while 'latent squint' is detected only by covering one eye.

Q. Types of squint:

Squint or strabismus is of two types:

1. Concomitant (non-paralytic): There is no paralysis of extraocular muscles.
2. Paralytic: Due to weakness of one or more of the extraocular muscles.
   i. Divergent squint: Due to paralysis of MR (medial rectus).
   ii. Convergent squint: Due to paralysis of LR (lateral rectus).

- Upward or downward paralytic squint is rare.

Q. Nerve supply of extraocular (extrinsic) muscles:

Muscles directly associated with the eye include extraocular and intraocular muscles.

A. There are six **extraocular muscles** that move the eyeball, e.g.:
   a. Lateral rectus (LR): VIth cranial nerve (abducens).
   b. Superior oblique (SO): IVth cranial nerve (trochlear).
   c. Other four muscles (MR, IO, SR, IR): IIIrd cranial nerve (oculomotor).

- IO: Inferior oblique, SR: Superior rectus, and IR: Inferior rectus.
- These muscles move the eyeball upwards (SR, IO), downwards (IR, SO), medially (MR) and laterally (LR).

B. **Intraocular (intrinsic) muscles:** (i) Sphincter pupillae and ciliaris: Supplied by IIIrd cranial nerve, (ii) Dilator pupillae: Supplied by sympathetic trunk.

Clinical Wisdom

Orbicularis oculi (closes the eye) and LPS (elevates the upper eyelid) have no relation with eyeball movement.

Q. Testing of IIIrd, IVth and VIth cranial nerves:

It is customary to test these three nerves at a time under the following headings:

I. Upper eyelid:
   a. Ptosis, and
   b. Lid retraction (due to sympathetic overactivity).

II. Position of the eyeball at rest:
   a. Squint,
   b. Exophthalmos,
   c. Enophthalmos,

d. Hypertelorism (may be associated with intracranial congenital abnormalities), and
e. Conjugate deviation.

III. Movement of the eyeball:
   a. Voluntary, and
   b. Involuntary: Nystagmus.

IV. Pupil:
   a. Size,
   b. Shape, and
   c. Reaction
      i. Light reflex,
      ii. Consensual light reflex,
      iii. Accommodation reflex.

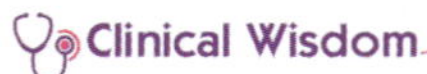

Clinical Wisdom

To summarize, test for: 1. LPS muscle and ptosis (eyelids), 2. Movement of each extraocular muscle (eyeballs), 3. Pupil with reflexes, and 4. Nystagmus.

- Lid retraction, enophthalmos, hypertelorism have no relation with IIIrd, IVth or VIth nerve palsy.
- One should search for arcus senilis (may have atheromatous cerebral vessels) and K-F ring (neurologic form of Wilson's disease) while examining the cornea and iris.
- **Retraction of upper eyelid** (thyrotoxicosis, Claude Bernard syndrome, big eye globe, scar of upper eyelid, short tendon of LPS) and **retraction of lower eyelid** (ectropion, proptosis, early stage of Bell's palsy, ocular myopathy) should be carefully looked for.

Q. Rings around cornea:

1. Arcus senilis (Fig. 3.8): Arcus is present in periphery of cornea and is white or greyish in colour; it usually starts in the lower pole of cornea and gradually affects the upper pole. It represents deposition of phospholipid and cholesterol in corneal tissue, and is generally present above the age of 50 years (no significance in elderly people). Arcus senilis is not unduly associated with atherosclerosis, hypertension, myocardial infarction, diabetes mellitus or stroke; it does not affect vission. If arcus is present <50 years, there is a possibility of underlying hyperlipidaemia **(arcus juvenilis)**.

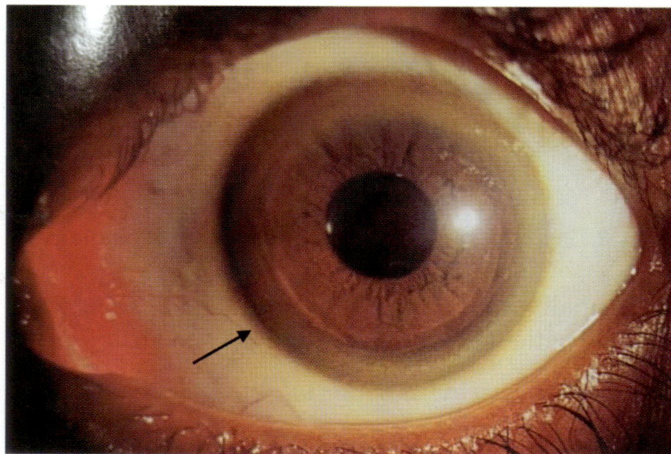

Fig. 3.189C: K-F ring seen in **Wilson's disease**

2. Kayser-Fleischer (K-F) ring (Fig. 3.189C): It is formed by the deposition of golden-brown pigment of copper in the Descemet's membrane of cornea in Wilson's disease (hepatolenticular degeneration). The ring is broader superiorly and inferiorly than it is laterally and medially. The vision is not hampered by its presence. Though the ring may be seen in naked-eye examination, slit-lamp examination by an ophthalmologist is usually necessary for its confirmation. Prolonged cholestasis may give rise to 'K-F like' ring around cornea.
3. Band keratopathy: Corneal calcification, which occurs at the lateral and medial margins of cornea in long-standing hypercalcaemia, e.g. in hyperparathyroidism, may be confused with K-F ring.

Q. How to test for voluntary movements of the eyeball?

It is important to remember that the recti are elevators and depressors alone when the eye is in abduction, and obliques act similarly (elevation and depression) when the eye is in adduction. Obliques do the opposite function (i.e. inferior oblique elevates the eyeball).

Stand in front of the patient and ask him, not to move his head. He is then instructed to follow your finger which is kept at a distance of 50 cm, and placed

Table 3.13: Testing for voluntary movements of eyeball

Position of examiner's finger	Muscles working
1. Above his head in the midline	1. SR and IO (both eyes)
2. Below his head (finger kept at the level of chest) in the midline	2. IR and SO (both eyes)
3. Laterally to the left	3. LR (left eye) and MR (right eye)
4. Laterally to the right	4. MR (left eye) and LR (right eye)
5. Above his head but placed laterally	5. SR (same eye) and IO (opposite eye)
6. Below his head but placed laterally	6. IR (same eye) and SO (opposite eye)
7. Straight ahead	7. All extraocular muscles

- No. 5 and 6 are done on both the sides for each eye. It is better to test individual muscle of each eye by an 'H'-pattern of ocular motility assessment (Table 3.13 and Fig. 3.190).

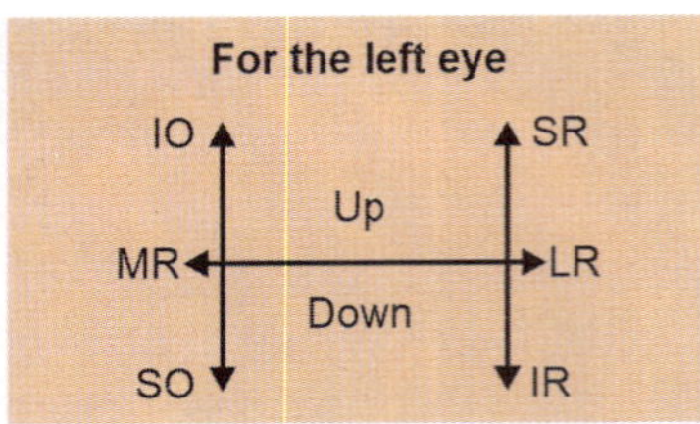

Fig. 3.190: Testing for **voluntary movements of single eye**

sequentially from position 1–7 described in **Table 3.13**. Ask the patient to report for double vision (diplopia).

Function of each extraocular muscle:

- LR–Abduction
- MR–Adduction
- SR–Elevator in abduction
- IR–Depressor in abduction
- SO–Depressor in adduction
- IO–Elevator in adduction

Clinical Wisdom

In the presence of IIIrd nerve palsy, IVth nerve cannot be tested properly as SO muscle cannot adduct due to MR palsy. Try to see the intorsion or internal rotation of the eyeball in that situation as a function of SO muscle in an attempted downward movement of eye.

Q. Different voluntary movements of the eyeball:

The three components of voluntary movements are:

1. Pursuit (following movements): The movements of the eyeball described above, i.e. slow and smooth eye movements following a target.
2. Saccadic (searching movements or sudden, jerky eye movements directed to a target): These are rapid, programmed, conjugate fixation movements. Ask the patient to focus his eyes rapidly to the ceiling fan, then to the window and next to the switch-board and so on.
3. Reflex ocular movements: To see whether both the eyes are moving simultaneously or not, on examiner's command, i.e. the conjugate deviation (i.e. oculocephalic and oculovestibular movement).

- LMN lesion of IIIrd, IVth or VIth cranial nerve (i.e. nucleus or nerve lesion) produces paralysis of individual or group of eye muscles. UMN lesion leads to paralysis of conjugate gaze (gaze palsy or supranuclear ophthalmoplegia) rather than individual muscle paralysis.

Q. Gaze palsies—common aetiology:

A. Vertical gaze palsy:
   a. Downward: Progressive supranuclear palsy.
   b. Upward: Perinaud's syndrome.

B. Horizontal gaze palsy: Cerebrovascular accidents with pontine lesion.

Q. Why there is no diplopia in non-paralytic squint?

In case of paralytic squint, the image on the paralysed side does not fall on the macula and thus diplopia or double vision occurs; whereas in non-paralytic squint, the image formed by the defective eye is either rejected or suppressed by the occipital cortex and thus, there is no diplopia. Diplopia is maximum if the eye is moved in the direction of weak muscle **(Table 3.14)**.

- There are two images in diplopia—true and false. The true image remains closure to the eye (clear image) and the false image is projected outside the true image (blurred image). diplopia is maximum (i.e. seperation of images) in the direction of the action of paralysed muscle. Diplopia may be horizontal, vertical or oblique.
- Remember, 'uniocular diplopia' (diplopia with one eye closed) is a rare phenomenon and mostly occurs due to eye disorders like incipient stage of cataract, subluxation of lens, peripheral iridectomy, astigmatism, keratoconus or hysteria.

Q. Causes of IIIrd, IVth and VIth cranial nerve palsy:

A. ***Isolated oculomotor (IIIrd cranial nerve) palsy:***

   1. Posterior communicating artery aneurysm.
   2. Tuberculous meningitis.
   3. Diabetes mellitus.
   4. Traumatic.
   5. Ophthalmoplegic migraine.
   6. Neoplastic diseases (e.g. pituitary SOL).
   7. Multiple sclerosis.
   8. Vascular disease (e.g. vasculitis).
   9. Wernicke's encephalopathy.
   10. Myasthenia gravis (i.e. autoimmune).
   11. Meningioma at wing of sphenoid.
   12. Congenital.
   13. Postoperative.
   14. Upper brainstem stroke.
   15. Cavernous sinus thrombosis.

B. ***Isolated trochlear (IVth cranial nerve) palsy:***
   Isolated lesion is rare, e.g. in trauma (head injury),

Table 3.14: Clinical differentiation between two types of squint

Features	Paralytic	Non-paralytic
1. Onset	Acquired at any age	Present since childhood
2. Movements	Restricted	Good in all directions
3. Diplopia	Present	Absent
4. Vision	Normal in both eyes	Deviating eye has defective vision

- **Diplopia** or double vision (i.e. binocular diplopia—diplopia occurs when both eyes are open) results from loss of parallel visual axes, and is commonly due to IIIrd, IVth, VIth nerve palsy, myasthenia gravis and myopathies (e.g. thyrotoxicosis).

diabetes mellitus, meningitis, etc. It is almost always involved with IIIrd or VIth nerve paralysis in multiple sclerosis, Wernicke's encephalopathy.

C. *Isolated abducens (VIth cranial nerve) palsy:*

1. Increased intracranial tension (it is a 'false localising sign'; VIth nerve is commonly affected due to its long intracranial course) (**Fig. 3.191**).
2. Diabetes mellitus.
3. Traumatic.
4. Brain tumour (SOL), nasopharyngeal carcinoma, acoustic neuroma.
5. Basal meningitis or encephalitis.
6. Gradenigo's syndrome (unilateral headache, otitis media, VIth nerve palsy with mastoid infection).
7. Lesion in cavernous sinus (aneurysm, meningioma).
8. Multiple sclerosis.

- **Combined IIIrd, IVth and VIth nerve palsies** are common in upper brainstem stroke, cavernous sinus thrombosis, superior orbital fissure syndrome (i.e. Tolosa-Hunt syndrome), multiple sclerosis and diabetes mellitus.
- Symptoms of **extraocular muscle paralysis** are diplopia, squint and vertigo.

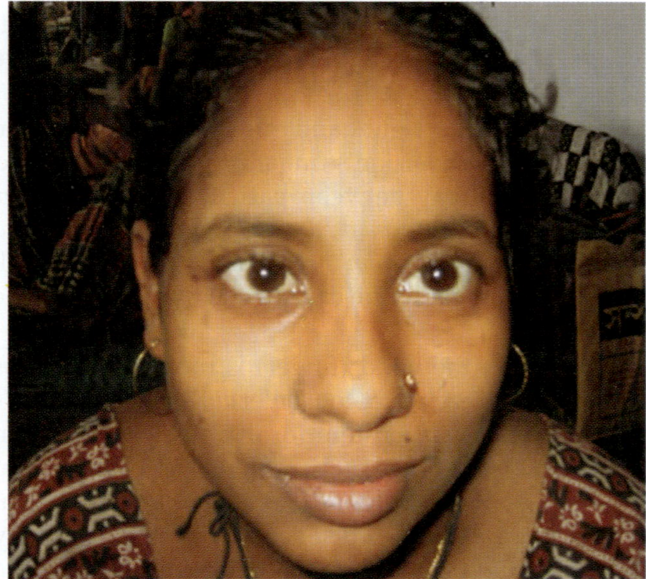

Fig. 3.191: **Squint** developed as a result of bilateral **VIth nerve palsy**. Here, it is a **false localizing sign** due to raised intracranial tension (from meningitis)

Q. Causes of 'multiple' cranial nerve palsy:

1. Basal meningitis (tuberculous, pyogenic or carcinomatous).
2. Malignancy: ICSOL (glioma) or secondary metastases to brain.
3. Diabetes mellitus.
4. Vasculitis.
5. Tuberculoma affecting brainstem.
6. Sarcoidosis.
7. Paget's disease.
8. Myasthenia gravis.
9. Polyneuritis cranialis (e.g. Lyme disease, leprosy).
10. Herpes zoster.
11. Variant of GB syndrome.

- **Plus** cavernous sinus thrombosis and superior orbital fissure syndrome.

Q. Symptoms due to isolated IVth nerve palsy:

In superior oblique palsy, the patient has impaired downward movement of eyeball, i.e. he feels difficulty in going downstrairs or reading newspapers. The patient overcomes this difficulty by tilting his head (head tilt) slightly to opposite direction.

Q. Features due to isolated VIth nerve palsy:

There are absence of abduction of eye, convergent squint due to unopposed action of MR, and diplopia on looking to the side of paralysis (i.e. on lateral gaze).

Q. What is ophthalmoplegia?

Ophthalmoplegia is the paralysis or weakness of one or more eye muscles.

1. Internal ophthalmoplegia: Occurs as a result of paralysis of sphincter pupillae and ciliaris muscle due to IIIrd nerve palsy. The pupil will be dilated and fixed, i.e. there will be absence of direct and consensual light reflex as well as accommodation reflex.
2. External ophthalmoplegia: Occurs due to IIIrd, IVth or VIth nerve palsy (e.g. cavernous sinus thrombosis or metastases at orbital apex); and extraocular muscle paralysis due to myasthenia gravis, ocular myopathy and exophthalmos.

   Combination of No. 1 and 2 is total ophthalmoplegia.
3. Internuclear ophthalmoplegia (INO): Lesion in the medial longitudinal fasciculus (MLF), interrupting connections between nucleus of LR of the same side and nucleus of MR of the opposite side, anywhere in between the midbrain and the pons will produce difficulty in adduction in one eye and nystagmus in the abducting eye, and the side of lesion is on the side of impaired adduction. It is commonly due to multiple sclerosis.

- Temporary ophthalmoplegia may be due to migraine, myasthenia gravis and temporal arteritis.
- **Ophthalmoplegia with sparing of pupil** is seen in diabetes, myopathy and myasthenia gravis.
- **Painful ophthalmoplegia:** Tolosa-Hunt syndrome, cavernous sinus thrombosis, orbital cellulitis and pituitary apoplexy.

Q. Points to note during optic nerve (IInd cranial nerve) examination:

1. Acuity of vision (measures efficacy of the central or macular vision).
2. Field of vision (assess the function of central and peripheral retina).

3. Colour vision (assess the function of retinal cones, macular field and optic nerve), and
4. Fundoscopy (to examine optic nerve head and fundus).

- According to some clinicians, 'pupillary reflexes' are within optic nerve examination.

Q. Neuroanatomy of optic nerve:

Optic nerve is a purely sensory nerve.

Retina → optic nerve → optic chiasma (here, nasal fibres from each retina, representing the temporal field, decussate. Temporal fibres from each retina remain on the same side) → optic tract → lateral geniculate body (some preganglionic fibres project to superior colliculi at midbrain) → optic radiation projects through posterior limb of the internal capsule → to calcarine cortex of the occipital lobe. Fibres carrying the upper and lower visual fields pass respectively through the white matter of temporal and parietal lobe; the right half of the visual field is represented in the left calcarine cortex and *vice versa* for the left half of the visual field. Macular vision is represented in the occipital poles.

Q. How to test for visual acuity or acuity of vision?

It is a test of IInd cranial nerve and it denotes the macular function. The clinical method goes like:

1. First examine the eye for any local pathology, i.e. corneal opacity, etc.
2. One eye is tested at a time (other eye is closed by the hollow of the palm).
3. Ask the patient to count the beams in the ceiling or blades in the fan (distant object testing).
4. Now ask for finger counting (near object testing).
5. If finger counting is not possible, put a lighted torch in the eye and examine for PL/PR (perception of light/projection of rays). Perception of light is absent in total blindness.

- Ideally, distant vision is tested by SNELLEN'S TEST TYPE CHART and near vision by JAEGER'S CHART. The patient should wear the spectacles (if any) during the bedside test.
- Normal visual acuity by Snellen's chart is 6/6; visual acuity of <1/60 is measured by finger counting, PL, PR, or movement of hands. In clinical practice, **loss of visual acuity** is commonly due to cataract, refractive error, corneal and vitreous opacities, or diseases of optic nerve or visual pathways.

Q. How to test for field of vision?

'Field of vision' is the field within which all objects are visible when the vision is fixed to a particular object present in that field. This is tested by **'confrontation perimetry'** (Fig. 3.192).

1. First test the acuity of vision.
2. Sit opposite the patient (face to face) at the same level; distance between the patient and the examiner will be one meter. The examiner should have a normal visual field.
3. If the left eye is to be tested, ask the patient to cover his right eye with the hollow of his right palm; ask him to look straight at your right eye and not to take his own eye off yours (the patient should not move his head). Cover your left eye with the hollow of your left palm and look steadily at the patient's left eye (in this way of testing, slight movement of patient's eye can be easily detected).
4. Now place your right hand out to its full extent (the test object is physician's finger or ideally a large red hat-pin) midway between patient's face and your own. It is better to *move the finger during testing and the finger is brought from the periphery to the centre*. Ask the patient whether he can see the movement of the finger.
5. In this way, the hand (finger) is moved in various directions: i.e. each of the four outer quadrants of patient's visual field—superotemporal (2 o'clock position of hand), superonasal (10 o'clock), inferotemporal (4 o'clock), and inferonasal (8 o'clock) for testing of the left eye. Bring the test object from the periphery into the field of vision (i.e. centrally) *in a curved fashion*. Use your own field of vision for the purpose of comparison. Lastly, test the field of the right eye of the patient.

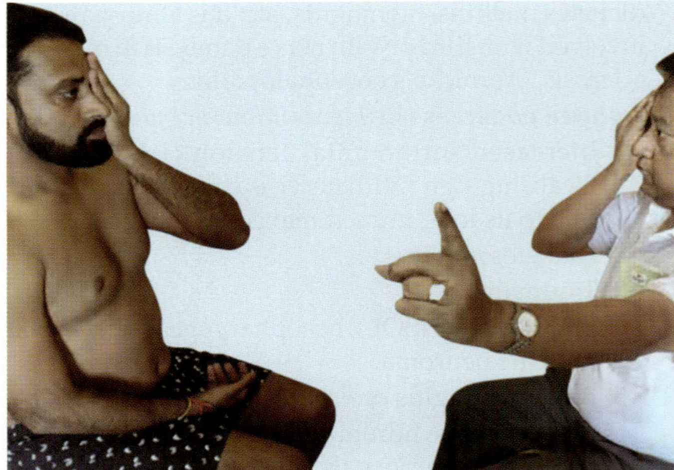

Fig. 3.192: **Confrontation test** (visual field examination) of right eye

- In a non-cooperative patient, a shiny object is moved from the periphery to the centre and ascertain whether the patient is able to see it, or move your hand quickly towards patient's face and observe the reflex blinking of both eyes (menace reflex), as confrontation method is not possible here (this method can also be applied in a patient who is unable to sit in the bed). Ideally, the field of vision is mapped by using a BJERRUM'S SCREEN PERIMETER (perimetry). One may detect the **blind spot** or physiological scotoma (corresponds to absence of photoreceptors where the optic nerve leaves the eye) by confrontation method. Preferably remove both the examiner's and patient's spectacles (if any) while testing the field by confrontation method.

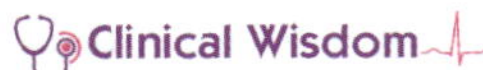

Clinical Wisdom

'Tubular or tunnel vision' (concentric narrowing of the field of vision) is characteristic of terminal glaucoma, advanced retinitis pigmentosa, papilloedema, quinine amblyopia and hysteria.

'Cortical blindness' is a feature of vasospasm of posterior cerebral artery, anoxic encephalopathy, hypertensive encephalopathy, subarachnoid haemorrhage and migraine.

Q. How to test for colour vision?

The **primary colours** are red, green and blue. Roughly, it can be assessed by asking the patient the colour of his shirt or pant, room-wall, ceiling fan, bed-cover, etc. The patient with defective colour vision can not identify the colours correctly.

Ideally it should be assessed by ISHIHARA'S CHART (pseudo-isochromatic plates consisting of multicoloured dots). The commonest defect in colour vision is red-green anomaly (X-linked recessive). Acquired defect may be seen after use of ethambutol or chloroquine. Total colour blindness is rare.

Q. Causes of papilloedema, optic atrophy and optic neuritis:

A. Papilioedema (oedema or swelling of the papilla, i.e. the optic disc) (Fig. 3.193A):

1. Increased intracranial tension (CVA, SOL, cerebral oedema, meningitis, hydrocephalus).
2. Malignant hypertension.
3. Circulatory block (in CSF).
4. Benign intracranial hypertension (steroid withdrawal, hypervitaminosis A).
5. Cavernous sinus thrombosis (Fig. 3.146A).
6. Superior vena caval syndrome.
7. Systemic disorders (vasculitis, chronic hypercapnia, COPD, hyperviscosity syndrome).
8. Miscellaneous: Guillain-Barré syndrome, severe anaemia, central retinal vein occlusion, disc infiltration (leukaemia, sarcoidosis).

- Papilloedema is usually **bilateral**. **Unilateral** papilloedema is seen in central retinal vein occlusion, Foster-Kennedy syndrome, lymphomatous/leukaemic deposits in one eye, and early stage of bilateral papilloedema.

B. Optic neuritis:

1. Multiple sclerosis, Devic's disease (optic neuritis with demyelination of the spinal cord).
2. Vitamin B_1 or B_{12} deficiency.
3. Meningitis, encephalitis, tuberculosis, HIV, syphilis.
4. Toxins: Tobacco, lead, alcohol (ethyl or methyl), and drugs: INH, ethambutol, quinine.
5. Diabetes mellitus, vasculitis, collagen vascular diseases.

- Optic neuritis is of two types: Papillitis (inflammation of optic nerve head) and retrobulbar neuritis (inflammation of retrobulbar portion of optic nerve).

C. Optic atrophy (Fig. 3.193B):

1. Multiple sclerosis (Devic's disease).
2. Toxins—Tobacco, methyl alcohol, ethambutol, chloroquine, etc.
3. Syphilitic optic neuritis.
4. Glaucoma.
5. Anterior ischaemic optic neuritis.
6. Head injury.
7. Retinitis pigmentosa, chorioretinitis.
8. Leber's optic atrophy (familial).
9. Friedreich's ataxia.

Optic atrophy is of two types. **Primary optic atrophy** is secondary to optic neuritis, and **secondary optic atrophy** develops from papilloedema/papillitis. A third variety of optic atrophy is 'consecutive' optic atrophy (a controversial term) resulting from primary retinal diseases (e.g. retinitis pigmentosa, glaucoma, chorioretinitis and central retinal artery occlusion).

- On **fundoscopy**—optic disc (colour, shape, blood vessels, physiological cup, margin), retinal blood vessels, macula and periphery of retina are seen. The visible part of retina is know as 'fundus'. Fundoscopy should be routinely done irrespective of patient's complaints.

Clinical Wisdom

Enquire **visual disturbances** like diplopia, blurred vision (e.g. macular degeneration in the elderly), haloes (coloured lights seen around a bright light, e.g. in corneal oedema), oscillopsia (e.g. objects appear to oscillate and is common in nystagmus affecting primary gaze), flashes and floaters (i.e. the patient complains of something floating within the eye in vitreous degeneration), or loss of vision.

Loss of vision may be sudden (temporary or permanent) or gradual. Temporary visual loss (sudden) is due to migraine, amaurosis fugax and multiple sclerosis. Sudden permanent visual loss is due to retinal artery/retinal vein occlusion, ischaemic optic neuropathy (from giant cell arteritis and traumatic optic neuropathy). Gradual visual loss is commonly caused by cataract, age-related macular degeneration, pituitary tumour or meningioma compressing the optic nerve or chiasma.

Q. Fundoscopy in different pathological conditions:

i. Papilloedema (Fig. 3.193A): The disc is pink (hyperaemic), blurring of disc margin (nasal margin first), cessation of normal venous pulsation, obliteration of physiological cup, disc engorgement with dilated vessels, and small haemorrhages surrounding the disc.

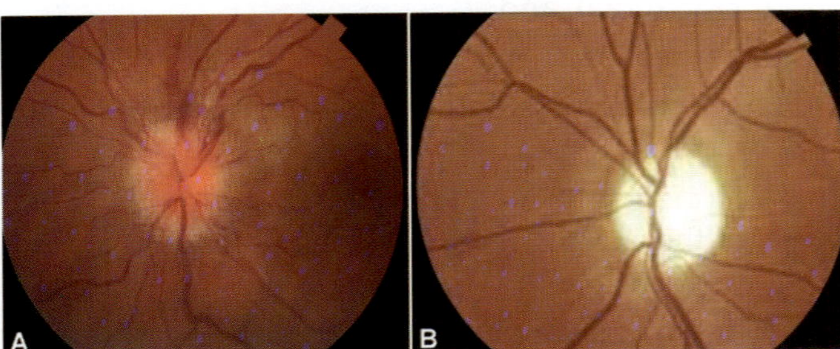

Fig. 3.193: (A) Ophthalmoscopy–**papilloedema**; (B) Ophthalmoscopy—**optic atrophy**

ii. Optic atrophy (Fig. 3.193B): The disc looks pale white (due to loss of nerve fibres); the margin is sharp in primary atrophy while it is blurred in secondary atrophy. The arteries are attenuated in primary variety (Kestenbaum's sign). No change in retina in primary variety but few exudates and haemorrhages may be seen in retina in secondary variety.

iii. Retrobulbar neuritis: Though the patient is blind, the disc is absolutely normal (i.e. the patient cannot see anything and the doctor cannot see any pathology).

Q. Precautions adopted in testing olfactory nerve:

Ideal test objects (non-irritating substances) are—oil of peppermint, oil of cloves, tincture of asafoetida or oil of lemon. But in the examination, the students should test it by common bedside familiar substances like soap, tooth paste, fruit, coffee beans, lemon peel, scent, etc. Irritating substances like ammonia stimulates trigeminal nerve too, and are better to be avoided. The precautions adopted are:

1. Exclude local changes first (i.e. nasal catarrh, patency of the nostrils, polyp, deviated nasal septum).
2. Examine each nostril separately after occluding other nostril by digital pressure.
3. Avoid irritating substances like ammonia (they stimulate the trigeminal nerve and may interfere with interpretation of smell sensation).
4. Eyes remain closed during testing. Ask the patient to identify the substance with two sniffs.
5. The test is usually carried out with two or more substances familiar to the patient.

- *Anosmia* (absense of sense of smell) is usually due to lesion in the olfactory bulb; *parosmia* or perverted smell (pleasant odour seems offensive) results from hysteria; *olfactory hallucination* (usually of unpleasant nature) is found in temporal lobe epilepsy. *Cacosmia* (foul smell) is found in atrophic rhinitis, and *hyperosmia* (increased acuity of smell) in migraine. Commonest cause of bilateral anosmia is coryza. Other causes of anosmia are sinusitis, local injury of cribriform plate, basal meningitis, subarachnoid haemorrhage, zinc deficiency and ageing.
- **Neuroanatomy:** The olfactory and optic nerves are actually made up of central nervous tissue rather than peripheral nerves. The olfactory nerve carries the sense of smell. The axons of the bipolar sensory cells in the olfactory epithelium passes through cribriform plate → to reach the second order of neurones in olfactory bulb → the olfactory bulb neurones project to the olfactory centres (uncus and parahippocampal gyrus).

Q. Identification points (squint):

1. First determine the type, i.e. paralytic or non-paralytic squint by testing the voluntary movement of the eyeball (test all extraocular muscles).
2. Ask for diplopia and the duration of squint.
3. See the pupil. If there is dilatation of pupil (and ptosis) in the paralysed eye, the squint is due to oculomotor palsy (divergent squint due to unopposed action of lateral rectus).
4. If the patient complains of diplopia (obviously paralytic squint), usually the outer image is a false one (and indistinct too) and it disappears on covering the affected eye.

NYSTAGMUS — CASE 90

Q. What is nystagmus?

These are rhythmic, involuntary and jerky movements (oscillations) of the eyeball when they are fixed on an object. Nystagmus signifies the disturbance in ocular posture and informally called 'dancing eyes'.

Q. How to test for nystagmus?

1. Examine the patient under good illumination. At first, test the power of extraocular muscles to eliminate their weakness or paralysis (in that situation, nystagmoid movements will appear).
2. Now ask the patient to look forward. Observe for pendular nystagmus.
3. Ask the patient to fix his head or fix the patient's head by one of your hand.
4. Now the patient is asked to fix his vision towards your index finger (held at about 60 cm distance) which is kept at least for 5 seconds, laterally to the right side and then to the left side in turn (your finger must be placed within the binocular vision of the patient; do not go for extreme abduction to avoid nystagmoid movement). It is the examination of nystagmus in the horizontal plane.
5. Next place your finger above and below his head to examine nystagmus in the vertical plane.
6. Observe nystagmus in both eyes.

Q. How will you describe the nystagmus (if present)?

Nystagmus is usually described under these 6 points:

1. **Pendular** (equal horizontal movement on each side like the swing of a pendulum of wall-clock) or **jerky** (amplitude is more in any one side, i.e. it has a fast and a slow component).
2. **Direction** of the nystagmus: The direction of the faster component of the oscillations is the 'direction' of the nystagmus.
3. **Plane in which nystagmus is being tested** (i.e. direction of gaze which evoke nystagmus):
   i. Horizontal, and
   ii. Vertical.
4. **Plane in which oscillatory movements of nystagmus is occurring**:
   i. Horizontal (side to side, to- and- fro movement of the eyeball in the horizontal plane).
   ii. Vertical (up and down movement of the eyeball in the vertical plane), and
   iii. Rotatory (oscillatory movement of the eyeball is circular in character).

5. **Amplitude:**
   i. Fine (<1 mm),
   ii. Medium (1–3 mm), and
   iii. Coarse (>3 mm).
6. **Grading or degree** (discussed below).

Q. Causes of pendular nystagmus:

Pendular nystagmus is almost always binocular and horizontal, and sometimes associated with head-nodding. The to-and-fro oscillations are equal in speed and amplitude in both directions. **Pendular nystagmus appears when the patient looks forward.** The common causes (due to low vision) are:

i. Miner's nystagmus (who works in dim light of coal-mines for long duration).
ii. Errors of refraction: The ocular fixation is defective.
iii. Amblyopia (if present in early life, impairs fixation of vision), e.g. high infantile myopia.
iv. Familial nystagmus, albinism, retinitis pigmentosa.

Q. Causes of jerky nystagmus:

The eyes drift in one direction and then quickly move in the other. **Jerky nystagmus is always found on fixation of the gaze laterally.**

i. Cerebellar nystagmus: Direction (fast phase) of the nystagmus is *towards the side* of lesion.
ii. Labyrinthine nystagmus: Direction (fast phase) of the nystagmus is *towards the opposite side* of lesion.
iii. Brainstem lesion: Very often 'rotatory', e.g. in brainstem glioma, multiple sclerosis, etc.
iv. Upper spinal cord lesion: Vertical nystagmus, e.g. Arnold-Chiari malformation.
v. Toxic nystagmus: Induced by drugs like benzodiazepines, phenytoin, phenothiazines, barbiturates and sometimes in alcoholics.

- **Vertical nystagmus:** *Downbeat* (i.e. fast phase downwards and slow phase upwards) in cranio-vertebral junction abnormality, e.g. Arnold-Chiari malformation, and *upbeat* nystagmus (i.e. fast phase upwards and slow phase downwards) in lesion of cerebellar vermis.

Q. What is positional nystagmus (Dix-Hallpike's test)?

Method: The patient is asked to sit upright, close to the edge of examination table. Now turn his head 45° to one side. Next the patient is laid back rapidly with his head extended 30° over the end of the table (eyes should be kept open). Intense vertigo with nystagmus appears (affected side down) in vestibular dysfunction. It is the rough assessment of the vestibular function of VIIIth cranial nerve. After a short interval, the test is repeated with the head extended and rotated to the other side. Positional nystagmus is also seen in posterior fossa tumour.

Q. What is optokinetic nystagmus?

This is commonly seen when an individual looks out of the window of a moving train. There is a slow and a fast phase in it. It is a physiological nystagmus and its absence indicates parietal lobe lesion.

Q. What is see-saw nystagmus?

In this condition, one eye raises up and turns in, while the other eye falls and turns out. It is common in parasellar tumour.

Q. What are nystagmoid movements?

These are rhythmic movements of the eyeball when the eyeball is extended laterally beyond the limit of binocular vision. **Brief duration** and **irregularity** of these movements distinguish them from the true nystagmus. There are usually 4 or less oscillations in the nystagmoid movement. Often this movement is monocular.

Q. What is the grading or degree of nystagmus?

For example:
Grade 1: Nystagmus with fast component to left, when the patient looks towards the left.
Grade 2: Nystagmus with fast component to left, when the patient looks straight ahead.
Grade 3: Nystagmus with fast component to left, when the patient looks towards the right.

Q. What do you mean by 'nystagmus to the left'?

It does not refer to the direction of gaze in which nystagmus occurs but it indicates the direction of fast component to the left (i.e. 'direction' of the nystagmus).

- Nystagmus is routinely tested during examination of the IIIrd, IVth and VIth cranial nerves. Always fix the head of the patient. Test for nystagmus in different planes.

Q. Few other abnormal involuntary movements (non-nystagmus oscillations) of eyes:

1. Oculogyric crisis—Involuntary upward conjugate deviation of eyeballs, which can be transient or persisting for hours. It is commonly due to parkinsonism or drug-induced extrapyramidal syndrome (EPS).
2. Skew deviation of eye—One eye is down and medial while the other eye goes up and lateral; seen in acute cerebellar lesion.
3. Ocular bobbing—Periodic brisk downward movement of both eyes, and is a feature of pontine lesion. *Ocular dipping* is brisk upward and slow downward movement of both eyes.
4. Opsoclonus—Coarse, irregular, disorganised, chaotic, dancing and non-rhythmic oscillations of eyeball occurring in both vertical and horizontal plane, and persisting for a long period. It is often found in cerebellar lesion, encephalitis or brainstem damage.
5. Ocular flutter—Pendular horizontal oscillations on fixing gaze on an object; a feature of cerebellar lesion.

Q. Tests of VIIIth cranial nerve:

The VIIIth cranial nerve has a vestibular and cochlear component. The former is concerned with equilibrium and balance, and the latter with hearing. In VIIIth nerve lesion, the patient usually complains of dizziness or vertigo, tinnitus (ringing in the ears) or deafness.

A. *Cochlear functions* (function of hearing): First examine the external acoustic canal using a torch and auroscope (look for wax, tympanic membrane). Hearing should be tested in each ear in turn.

a. Whisper test: First, test for the whispering distance. In health, a person is able to hear the whisper from a distance of approximately 60 cm (approximate intensity 15 dB); it is better to stand behind the patient. First whisper from a distance of 60 cm and gradually move closure (15 cm), or test either by the ticking sound of a wrist-watch (watch test) or by rubbing fingers in the ear; the other ear should be occluded by finger pressure on the tragus. The distance is compared on both sides.

b. If the patient does not understand whispered words, speak loudly from a distance of 15 cm, and gradually come closer to the patient by telling a combination of number and letters. Normal conversational voice should be heard from 15 cm. Both the tests are crude tests.

c. Rinne's test and Weber's test: Read from 'Bedside Clinics in Medicine, Part II'.

B. *Vestibular functions:* Function of equilibrium:

a. Observe for jerky nystagmus: fast phase is away from the side of lesion.

b. Positional nystagmus (*see* above for Dix-Hallpike's test).

c. Caloric test: Read from any standard ENT text-book.

- **Deafness** is of two types:
  - I. Conductive deafness: As a result of impacted wax, damage to tympanic membrane, otosclerosis, CSOM, etc. (i.e. diseases of the external auditory meatus, middle ear and eustachian tube).
  - II. Sensorineural deafness: Due to damage of cochlear nerve and organ of Corti, presbycusis (i.e. hearing loss by natural ageing), Ménière's disease, acoustic neuroma, drugs like aminoglycosides, fracture of petrous part of temporal bone, pontine lesion, etc.
- **Vertigo** is of two types:
  - I. Central: Brainstem ischaemia or infarction, multiple sclerosis, cerebellitis, acoustic neuroma, aura of epilepsy, migraine.
  - II. Peripheral: Ménière's disease, acute labyrinthitis, vestibular neuronitis, benign positional vertigo, post-traumatic vertigo, drugs (anticonvulsants, streptomycin), psychogenic (no nystagmus and may be associated with agoraphobia).
- **Tinnitus** may be due to Ménière's disease, labyrinthitis, acoustic neuroma or aspirin-induced.

Clinical Wisdom

The hearing sensitivity can only be acurately assessed by non-invasive and painless audiometry.

BELL'S PALSY — CASE 91

Q. What is your diagnosis?

This is a case of left-sided LMN type of facial palsy, probably Bell's palsy.

- Sir Charles Bell (1774–1842) was a Scottish surgeon at Middlesex Hospital, London, UK; Professor of Surgery, Edinburgh afterwards.

Q. Why do you say 'probably' ?

I say 'probably' because I am not allowed to know the history (exposure to cold, etc.) and the initial symptoms (pain behind the left ear).

- Facial paralysis may be supranuclear (UMN type), and nuclear/infranuclear (LMN type).

Q. Why do you say so?

Because the **left side of face** on **inspection** shows:

1. Smoothening of furrows in the forehead.
2. Wide palpebral fissure [due to loss of tone of the lower eyelid and unopposed action of the levator palpebrae superioris (LPS)]: Lagophthalmos or unequal palpebral fissure in comparison to other side.
3. Asymmetry of blinking.
4. Abnormality in volitional or reflex movement like smiling or crying.
5. Watering from the eye or epiphora (due to loss of capillary action as the punctum is no more in contact with conjunctiva).
6. **Bell's phenomenon** (Fig. 3.194) (the eyeball rolls upwards and inwards during attempted forced

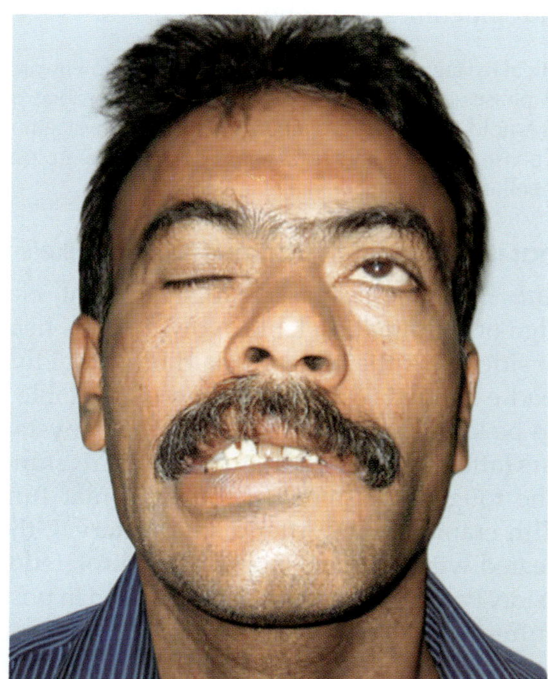

Fig. 3.194: Left-sided **Bell's palsy**. Deviation of face to the right side occurs on showing the teeth as well as **Bell's phenomenon** is noted on forced closure of eyes

eye closure. It is a normal as well as protective phenomenon, and is preserved in LMN type palsy only).

7. Loss of nasolabial fold or flattening of the fold.
8. Angle of the mouth is drawn to right side when the patient is asked to show his upper teeth (a very important bedside test).
9. Drooping of the angle of the mouth (left side).
10. Flapping in and out of the cheek on left side during respiration due to the paralysis of buccinator.
11. Saliva dribbles (drooling of saliva) from the left angle of the mouth with difficulty in spitting.
12. Inability to blow or whistle properly (air escapes from the left side of the mouth).

- An important complaint by the patient is collection of food materials in the affected vestibule during eating. The patient may also complain of numbness and stiffness of the cheek on the affected side though the sensory functions of face remain absolutely intact.
- The patient may complain of slurred speech for obvious reasons (i.e. weakness of facial muscles).
- Bell's palsy is the sudden onset of unilateral LMN type VIIth cranial nerve palsy.

Clinical Wisdom

Bell's palsy does not lead to ptosis.

Q. Test the individual muscle of face (Fig. 3.195):

Test the muscles on both sides of face and observe the weakness on left side (in this index patient).

1. Ask the patient to wrinkle his forehead by raising eyebrows (either the patient will do it on your command or keeping the head fixed, ask him to look at your index finger which is placed above his head): Frontal belly of occipitofrontalis (muscle for surprize) (Fig. 3.195A).
2. Ask the patient to frown: Corrugator superciliaris (small muscles at the medial end of eyebrows).
3. Ask him to close both eyes 'forcibly' and you try to open the eyelids by your fingers (both eyes must

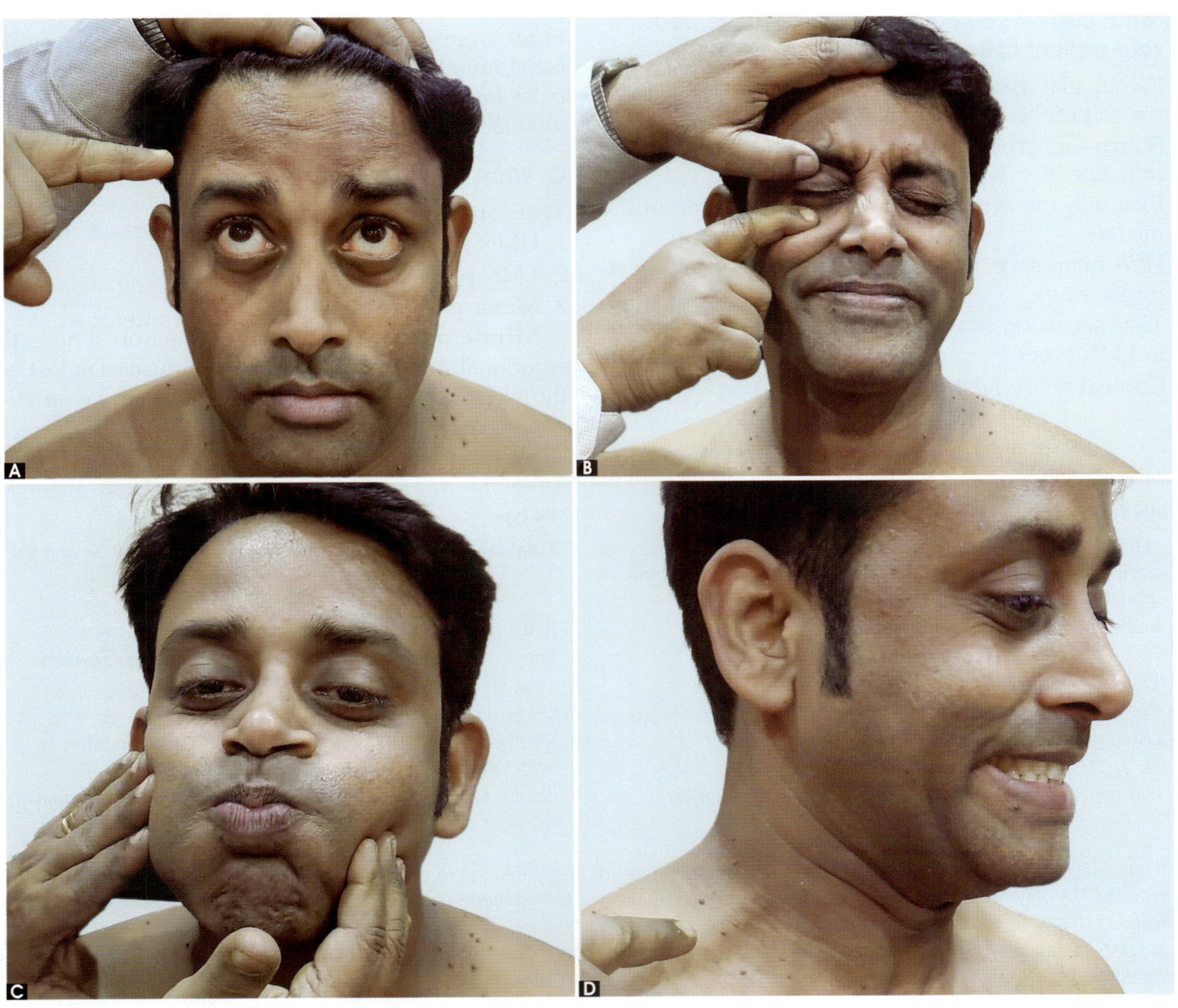

Fig. 3.195: Facial muscles testing: A. Frontal belly of occipitofrontalis; B. Orbicularis oculi; C. Buccinator; D. Platysma

be examined for comparison): Orbicularis oculi (Fig. 3.195B).
4. Ask him to show his upper teeth, or smile: Levator anguli oris, zygomatic major and minor, depressor anguli oris, buccinator and risorius (Fig. 3.194).
5. Ask him to blow or whistle, or inflate the mouth with air: Orbicularis oris and buccinator.
6. Ask him to puff cheeks out: Buccinator (in paralysis, air escapes from the affected side) (Fig. 3.195C).
7. Ask the patient to purse his lips shut: Only orbicularis oris.
8. Ask the patient to retract and depress the angle of the mouth with clenching of teeth (or ask the patient to try to touch the chin to the sternum against resistance): Folds of platysma (muscle for grinning) may be seen in the neck (Fig. 3.195D).

- There may be apparent deviation of the tongue to the healthy side on protrusion.
- The muscle mentalis (muscle for doubt) helps the lips to pout.
- No. 1, 2 and 3 are ideal tests for **'upper face'** and No. 4 for **'lower face'**.

Q. What else do you want to examine at the bedside in your patient of Bell's palsy?

1. Parotid gland enlargement (parotid tumour may give rise to LMN type facial palsy).
2. Search for herpes zoster at external auditory meatus or palate (Ref: Ramsay Hunt syndrome).
3. Examine the tympanic membrane (exclude otitis media).
4. Hyperacusis, i.e. increased sensitivity to sound (test for hearing).
5. Taste sensation of anterior 2/3rd of the tongue (lost in LMN type).
6. Corneal reflex: Lost in LMN type.
7. Plantar response (mentioned in Table 3.15).
8. Evidence of cerebellar signs: If present on the side of facial palsy, the lesion is probably present at the cerebello-pontine angle (e.g. acoustic neuroma). In **cerebello-pontine angle tumour**, features of involvement of ophthalmic division of Vth (loss of corneal reflex), VIIth and VIIIth cranial nerves lesion as well as ipsilateral cerebellar signs along with pyramidal signs are elicited.
9. Examination of VIIIth cranial nerve (affected in acoustic neuroma).

Q. Examination within the oral cavity in Bell's palsy:

1. Food materials present within the vestibule of mouth on the affected side, and
2. Loss of taste sensation (if nerve to chorda tympani is affected).

Q. Why the upper face escapes in UMN palsy?

The upper part of VIIth nerve nucleus (so the upper facial muscles or upper face) is innervated by corticobulbar fibres from both cerebral hemispheres whereas the lower part of VIIth nerve nucleus (so the lower face) receives fibres from opposite hemisphere only. As the upper facial muscles have dual supply, they escape in UMN palsy but LMN is the final common pathway and thus, total face is affected in LMN palsy.

Q. What is mimic facial palsy?

There are three types of facial palsy:
1. UMN palsy.
2. LMN palsy, and
3. Mimic palsy

Mimic palsy is a rare phenomenon where the emotional movement of the facial muscles is lost but the voluntary movements are preserved, i.e. *in other*

Table 3.15: Differentiation between UMN and LMN type of VIIth nerve palsy

UMN type	LMN type
1. **'Upper face' escapes** (or forehead spared): (frontal belly of occipitofrontalis, corrugator superciliaris and upper part of orbicularis oculi escape paralysis)	1. **Total face (i.e. upper plus lower face) is involved** on one side
2. **Bell's phenomenon: Never occurs**	2. **Bell's phenomenon: Present**
3. Facial muscles are not atrophied	3. There may be fasciculation or muscle atrophy on affected side
4. Taste sensation is preserved	4. Taste sensation may be lost
5. Corneal reflex: Preserved	5. Corneal reflex: Lost
6. Usually associated with same-sided hemiplegia	6. May be an isolated phenomenon (Bell's palsy) and if associated with hemiplegia, it is always crossed
7. Plantar response on the paralysed side of face: Extensor	7. Plantar response on the paralysed side of face: Flexor (may be extensor on the opposite side)

- 'Upper face' i.e. forehead wrinkling, frowning, and eye closure and blinking are unaffected in UMN palsy. UMN palsy of face is seen in CVA patients along with same-sided hemiplegia. In drowsy CVA patients, supraorbital pressure evokes grimace of face which helps in diagnosis of UMN facial palsy.
- In **UMN facial palsy:** Causes weakness of the lower part of face on the opposite side. In **LMN facial palsy:** Causes unilateral complete weakness of face which is same-sided.
- 'Upper face' and 'lower face' are divided by an arbitrary horizontal line passing through outer and inner angles of both the eyes.

words, facial palsy or asymmetry is visible only on emotional movements, e.g. in laughing or weeping. This is seen in frontal lobe lesion because the UMN fibres concerned with emotion have a different course and is separate from the pyramidal tract.

As LMN is the final common pathway, LMN facial palsy affects the voluntary, emotional as well as associated movements.

In UMN facial palsy (obviously with hemiplegia), the paralysed angle of the mouth will be retracted during laughing (emotional movement) and during forcible closure of the eyes (associated movement).

Summary:

a. UMN facial palsy: No mimic palsy (i.e. emotional movements are preserved).
b. Frontal lobe lesion: Contralateral mimic palsy (commonly seen in multiple sclerosis).
c. LMN facial palsy (e.g. Bell's palsy): All movements lost.

- So, **UMN palsy** includes the classic UMN type paralysis and rare mimic palsy, **LMN palsy** includes both nuclear and infranuclear lesion.

Q. Neuroanatomy and course of facial nerve:

The VIIth cranial nerve nucleus is situated in the lowermost part of the pons, lateral to the VIth nerve nucleus. After originating from the nucleus, the VIIth nerve fibres hook round the VIth cranial nerve nucleus and come out of the substance of pons at the cerebello-pontine angle. The facial nerve now courses at the base of the brain with VIIIth cranial nerve and nervus intermedius (also known as intermediate nerve of Wrisberg, which contains the taste fibres and courses along with the facial nerve in the opposite direction up to the geniculate ganglion). The facial nerve, along with VIIIth cranial nerve, then enters the petrous part of temporal bone through internal acoustic meatus; from here VIIth nerve follows a separate course.

The facial nerve now enters another bony canal, called 'facial canal', at the bend of which there is a ganglion known as geniculate ganglion, from which nervus intermedius starts. Here facial nerve gives greater superficial petrosal nerve, which innervates the lacrimal gland. The nerve then courses vertically downwards, and gives 'nerve to stapedius' muscle and only 6 mm above the stylomastoid foramen, it gives chorda tympani branch (it carries taste fibres from anterior 2/3rd of the tongue). The facial nerve then emerges out through stylomastoid foramen and enters deep into the parotid gland to be divided into two divisions, the upper one temporofacial (temporal, zygomatic and upper buccal), and the lower one cervicofacial (lower buccal, mandibular and cervical) branches to supply the individual muscle of the face, scalp and platysma.

Q. Different symptoms of facial nerve paralysis:

1. Facial asymmetry and deviation of face.
2. Defective eye closure (lagophthalmos).
3. Epiphora (watering from the eye).
4. Drooling of saliva.
5. Difficulty in spitting.
6. Difficulty in speeeh (dysarthria).
7. Collection of food in the affected vestibule.
8. Loss of taste sensation.

Q. Bedside tests of VIIth nerve:

1. Motor part (follow the question, 'Test the individual muscle of face').
2. Sensory part (test the taste sensation of anterior 2/3rd of the tongue).
3. Reflexes (corneal reflex, glabellar tap, palmo-mental reflex).

Q. Causes of VIIth nerve palsy (LMN type)—mostly 'unilateral':

a. At pons: Vascular, neoplasm, demyelination, abscess, brainstem encephalitis, syringobulbia.
b. At cerebello-pontine angle: Meningioma, acoustic neuroma.
c. At facial canal: Spread of infection from middle ear (CSOM), Ramsay Hunt syndrome (affection of geniculate ganglion by herpes zoster), fracture of base of the skull.
d. At or above stytomastoid foramen: Bell's palsy.
e. At periphery: Parotid tumor, trauma to parotid gland, sarcoidosis, leukaemic or lymphomatous deposits to parotid gland, leprosy, GB syndrome.

Q. Causes of 'bilateral' facial palsy of LMN type (facial diplegia):

1. Acute infective polyneuritis (GB syndrome).
2. Leprosy (Fig. 3.107).
3. Sarcoidosis (Heerfordt syndrome).
4. Forceps delivery (trauma).
5. Leukaemia (ALL) or lymphoma.
6. Bilateral Bell's palsy (rare).
7. Bilateral otitis media or mastoiditis.
8. Diphtheria.
9. Lyme disease.
10. Seroconversion phase of HIV infection.
11. Pontine glioma.
12. Skull base trauma.

Clinical Wisdom

Myasthenia and myopathy produce facial weakness; there is no involvement of facial nerve.

- Melkersson syndrome: Triad of facial palsy (recurrent), recurrent facial oedema (e.g. lips) and fissured tongue.

Q. D/D of alteration of facial contour:

1. Hemiatrophy (e.g. linear scleroderma).
2. Hemihypertrophy (Fig. 3.196).
3. Residual Bell's palsy.
4. Lipodystrophy.
5. Unilateral facial oedema (postural).
6. Paget's disease, fibrous dysplasia.
7. Absence of condyle of mandible (congenital).
8. Massive swelling of parotid glands.
9. Acromegaly.
10. Micrognathia.

Q. How do you diagnose bilateral UMN type of facial palsy?

In bilateral UMN type of lesion, the total face is paralysed (upper 1/2 of face does not escape). **Bilateral UMN type of lesion is diagnosed by** (differentiate from bilateral LMN type facial palsy):

1. Mask like facies.
2. Brisk jaw jerk.
3. Presence of glabellar reflex.
4. Bell's phenomenon—usually absent.
5. Intact emotional fibres, and
6. Associated bilateral long tract signs.

- **Bilateral UMN type facial palsy** is seen in diffuse cerebral atherosclerosis, pseudobulbar palsy (e.g. MND) and double hemiplegia. Loss of spontaneous facial movements are not uncommon in parkinsonism.
- Isolated **unilateral UMN facial palsy** is rare but may be seen in CVA and multiple sclerosis.

Q. Definition of Bell's palsy:

It is an 'acute', idiopathic, unilateral (commonly) LMN type of facial nerve involvement due to non-suppurative inflammation (viral, e.g. often herpes simplex) of the nerve within the facial canal, at or above the stylomastoid foramen.

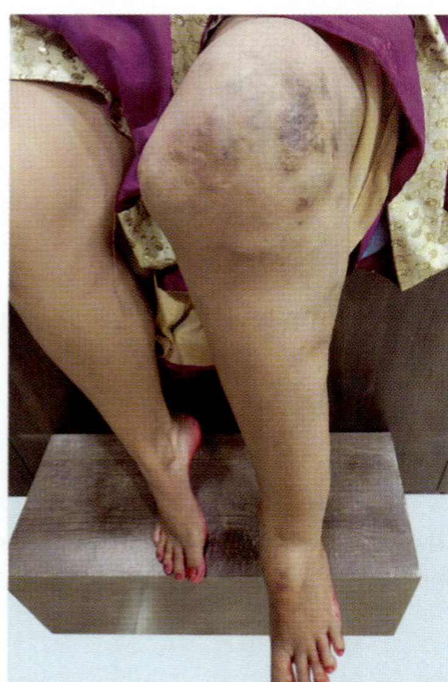

Fig. 3.196: **Hemihypertrophy** seen in different congenital syndromes (e.g. Klippel-Trenaunay syndrome)

Inflammation or oedema strangulates the nerve at the stylomastoid foramen and precipitates the paralysis. Exposure to cold or chill predisposes to Bell's palsy (there may be positive H/o travelling by bus or train, sitting by the side of an open window) with H/o pain behind the ear at the onset.

Bell's palsy affects all ages and both sexes. There is sudden unilateral facial weakness, which may be associated with loss of taste sensation and hyperacusis. There is no objective sensory loss in face. *It is primarily diagnosed on clinical grounds.*

Bell's palsy varies from simple conduction block to severe axonal degeneration of facial nerve.

Q. How do you assess the progressing lesion in Bell's palsy?

1. The inflammation may involve the nerve to chorda tympani: There is loss of taste sensation (hypogeusia) in the anterior 2/3rd of the tongue (chorda tympani arises from the facial nerve about 6 mm above the stylomastoid foramen).
2. Nerve to stapedius may be involved: The patient will complain of hyperacusis due to paralysis of stapedius muscle (sound on the paralysed side seems unusually loud).

- These two features indicate a bad prognosis in Bell's palsy.
- In facial nerve lesion distal to stylomastoid foramen, taste sensation and lacrimation remain intact.

Q. Syndromes in nuclear type of facial palsy:

Millard-Gubler syndrome: Paralysis of VIth cranial nerve (LMN type) ± VIIth cranial nerve palsy (LMN type) with contralateral hemiplegia (crossed hemiplegia).

Foville's syndrome: Ipsilateral paralysis of conjugate gaze ± VIIth cranial nerve palsy (LMN type) with contralateral hemiplegia (crossed hemiplegia).

Q. Clinical features in lesion at the geniculate ganglion:

It is known as **Ramsay Hunt syndrome** which is the affection of geniculate ganglion by herpes zoster (*Shingles*) (Fig. 3.168) infection. The clinical features are:

1. Fever with chill and bodyache.
2. LMN type of ipsilateral facial palsy (identical to Bell's palsy).
3. Loss of taste sensation in the anterior 2/3rd of the tongue (on affected side).
4. Hyperacusis (on affected side).
5. Herpetic rashes on tympanic membrane, external auditory canal, pinna (producing severe earache), and occasionally over pharynx, soft palate and tongue.

Q. How do you elicit corneal reflex (Fig. 3.197)?

Method: The patient is asked to see into the distance or at the ceiling. The cornea at its conjunctival margin is touched lightly with a damp (wet) cotton wool which is twisted into a fine hair. If the reflex is present, there is

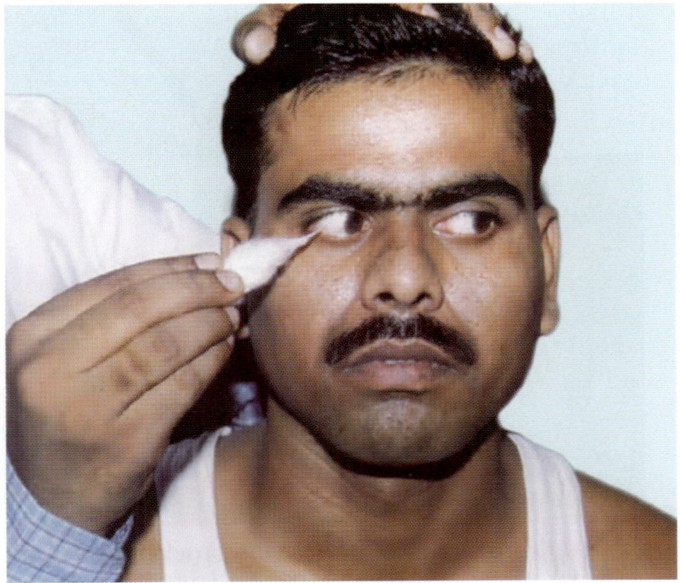

Fig. 3.197: Demonstrating **corneal/conjunctival reflex**

simultaneous prompt closure of both the eyes. Each eye should be tested one by one. The cornea is stimulated from the side to avoid 'menace reflex' (reflex closure of the eyes, if an object is brought to the patient directly from the front).

Afferent path: Vth cranial nerve (ophthalmic division).

Efferent path: VIIth carnial nerve.

Centre: Pons

Response: Closure of both the eyes.

- Never touch the central part of cornea because corneal ulceration may develop in the presence of corneal anaesthesia. In the absence of cotton, blowing a puff of air into each cornea will serve the purpose. This reflex is also known as **conjunctival reflex**. Loss of corneal reflex is an early sign of sensory involvement of trigeminal nerve in cerebello-pontine angle tumour and herpes zoster ophthalmicus (Fig. 3.198).

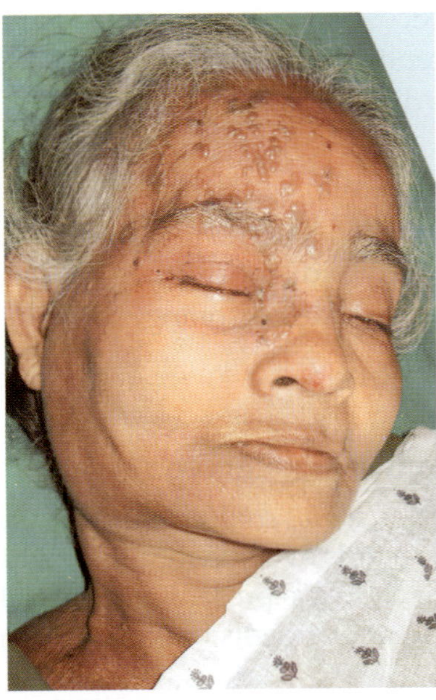

Fig. 3.198: **Herpes zoster ophthalmicus** of right side. There is risk of corneal scarring and secondary panophthalmitis

- While eliciting the corneal reflex, prompt closure of ipsilateral eye (eye being examined) is known as direct corneal reflex whereas closure of contralateral eye is known as consensual corneal reflex.

Q. Investigations your like to perform:

The clinical picture of Bell's palsy is unique by its own. But one may perform:

1. Appropriate diagnostic tests to rule out alternate diagnosis (e.g. CT scan of brain to rule out UMN facial palsy, i.e. CVA).
2. EMG study for prognostication.

Q. Management of Bell's palsy:

1. **Prednisolone:** A course beginning with 60–80 mg daily, orally during the first 5 days and then tapered over the next 5 days may be of some help; ideally started within 72 hours.
2. Aspirin or any other **NSAID** may be given for relief of pain and inflammation.
3. Eye padding is done during sleep and local antibiotic drop is instilled in the eye, if signs of congestion is seen (to prevent exposure keratitis).
4. Proper mouth wash and rinsing of mouth are advised after each meal.
5. Gentle massage over the paralysed muscles is advised.
6. Splint is used to prevent drooping of the lower part of face (by leukoplast).
7. Facial exercise is advised (massage, in front of a mirror) or **consult physiotherapist.**
8. Galvanic current stimulation of the paralysed muscles may be of some help.
9. If not improved at all within 6 weeks, surgical decompression may be done at the stylomastoid foramen (majority of clinicians say that the indications for operation are still not clear). Suturing upper and lower eyelid (tarsorrhaphy) may be done if eye closure is not at all possible.
10. Parenteral vitamin B_1, B_6 and B_{12} may be given; oral or parenteral methylcobalamin may be of some help.
11. Recently, acyclovir (400 mg five times a day for 10 days) or valacyclovir (1000 mg daily for 5–7 days) is tried, although the evidence for giving antivirals is poor (i.e. may not alter recovery).
12. Cosmetic surgical procedures in residual palsy.

- Bell's palsy usually recover (70–80%) spontaneously within 2–12 weeks; <10% may have residual weakness.

Q. Causes of 'facial pain':

1. Trigeminal neuralgia.
2. Postherpetic neuralgia.
3. Costen's syndrome (TM joint osteoarthritis).
4. Clusture headache.
5. Tolosa-Hunt syndrome.

6. Carotidynia.
7. Temporal arteritis.
8. Dental abscess.
9. Impacted wisdom teeth.
10. Acute maxillary sinusitis.

Q. Features of incomplete recovery from VIIth nerve palsy:

1. Residual paralysis on the affected side of face.
2. Hemifacial spasm (irregular, painless clonic unilateral spasm of facial muscles).
3. Crocodile tears or Bogorad's syndrome (unilateral lacrimation during chewing foods): Rare.
4. Unwanted facial movements (e.g. closure of eyes with movement of mouth).

Q. Complications of Bell's Palsy:

1. Exposure keratitis or conjunctivitis.
2. Hemifacial spasm (long-standing palsy).
3. Crocodile tears (aberrant recovery).
4. Facial contracture.
5. Jaw winking (movement of angle of mouth with eye closure).
6. Social embarrassment.

Q. Bad prognostic factors:

1. Complete palsy at the beginning.
2. Delayed recovery.
3. Associated co-morbidities, e.g. hypertension or diabetes.
4. Hyperacusis, or loss of taste sensation.
5. Severe axonal degeneration on electrophysiological study (i.e. EMG) after 10 days.

Q. Identification points:

Observe the face for a) asymmetry, b) symmetry of blinking and eye closure, and c) spontaneous movements. Lastly, ask the patient to show his upper teeth when the angle of the mouth is drawn to the healthy side (Fig. 3.194). Try to test the taste sensation, if possible.

- Read the examination of taste sensation from the chapter on 'Examination of the tongue'.
- Recurrent facial palsy may be a feature of multiple sclerosis, diabetes mellitus and Melkersson syndrome.

Clinical Wisdom

Facial nerve supplies all muscles of the face and scalp, except levator palpebrae superioris.

CHOREA — CASE 92

Q. What is chorea?

These are brief, rapid, jerky, explosive, non-repetitive, quasi-purposive (subjectively purposeful but objectively

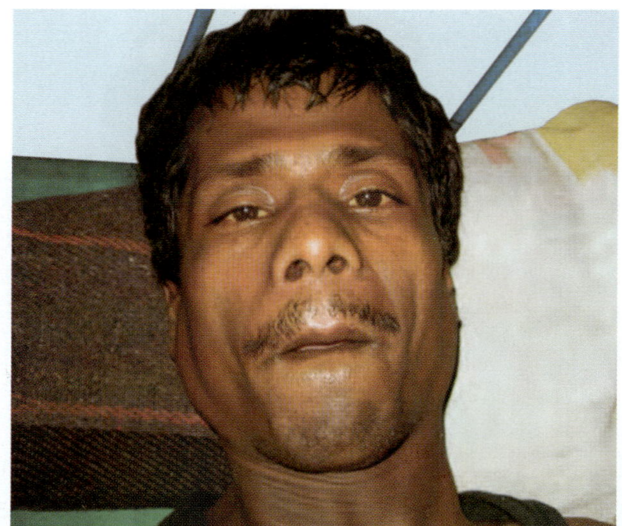

Fig. 3.199: A patient of **chorea** at the onset of choreiform movement

purposeless), unsustained involuntary movements chiefly involving the face, tongue and limbs (Fig. 3.199). The movements are totally irregular in time, rhythm, character and place of occurrence. Chorea literally means 'a dance'.

Q. Types of chorea:

1. Sydenham's chorea or Saint Vitus' dance (rheumatic).
2. Huntington's disease (autosomal dominant disorder of early middle life with dementia).
3. Chorea gravidarum (during pregnancy).
4. Senile chorea (follow vascular lesion in old age; mainly affects oral-buccal-lingual muscles).
5. Chorea mollis (with hemiplegia).

Other aetiology:

6. Drugs: OC pills, L-dopa, phenytoin, phenothiazines.
7. Systemic lupus erythematosus (SLE) and anti-phospholipid syndrome.
8. Polycythemia vera.
9. Thyrotoxicosis.
10. Post-encephalitic.
11. Wilson's disease.
12. Alcohol.
13. Hypernatraemia.
14. Lacunar infarction.
15. Hypoparathyroidism.
16. Carbon monoxide poisoning.
17. Kernicterus.
18. HIV-related.

Q. How to demonstrate chorea?

The diagnosis is made on clinical grounds. Ask the patient to raise up the hands over his shoulders and to maintain the posture. If chorea is present, patient will start rapid as well as jerky movements of the upper limbs.

- Very often emotion, agitation or excitement (e.g. a sudden slap over patient's face) increases chorea; it disappears during sleep.

Q. Six cardinal features in chorea:

1. **Hypotonia** (though an extrapyramidal disorder): Assessed by decreased resistance to passive movement. It is the only extrapyramidal lesion with hypotonia.
2. Patient will tend to pronate the outstretched hands (and sway outward) while extending the arms above the head The **'pronator sign'**.
3. Ask the patient to grasp or squeeze the examiner's hand or finger tightly. There is waxing and waning of the grip: This is known as **"milkmaid's grip"** or **'milking sign'**, and is due to irregular repetitive contraction of fingers.
4. The patient is asked to stretch out the hand and spread the fingers: Elbow is hyperextended, forearm is hyperpronated, wrist joint is flexed, metacarpophalangeal joints are extended with separation of the fingers **(dinner-fork deformity)**. This is a manifestation of hypotonia. This will be more obvious, if the patient is asked to raise up the hands above his head. This is also known as **'spooning sign'**.
5. Knee jerk: Pendular (due to hypotonia) and often the jerk is called **'hung-up reflex'** (when choreiform movements are superimposed on a tendon reflex).
6. Ask the patient to protrude the tongue: The patient protrudes it momentarily and takes it back within the oral cavity instantaneously **(lizard tongue)**. The tongue, when projected, looks like a 'bag of worms' (wormian tongue) due to continuous movements. Typical grimacing of face with protrusion of tongue often clinches the diagnosis.

- Clinical triad of chorea are: hypotonia, choreiform movement and mental instability.

Q. What is athetosis and tics?

Athetosis **(Table 3.16)**: These are slow, sinuous, purposeless, writhing involuntary movements usually involving the distal part of a limb (athetosis means 'instability of posture'). The movements are best seen in fingers, hands, toes, feet and tongue (snake charmer's movement). Athetosis is a slower form of chorea.

Tics: Simple, normal movements which are repeated unnecessarily (seemingly purposive) to become a social embarrassment. These are stereotyped movements like head-nodding, shrugging shoulders, eye blinking or grimacing of face. Tics may be seen in anxiety states. They can be briefly suppressed by the patient.

Aetiology of athetosis are:

1. Post-hemiplegic (infantile).
2. Wilson's disease (bilateral athetosis).
3. Kernicterus.
4. Overdose of L-dopa, phenothiazines.
5. Birth injury (perinatal anoxia).
6. Encephalitis.
7. Cerebral palsy.
8. Degenerative brain disease.

Q. What is 'pure chorea'?

Chorea is a delayed manifestation of rheumatic fever (Jones major criteria) and other manifestations may not be present when chorea appears. Arthritis always subsides before the appearance of chorea. Sydenham's chorea appears after a long latent period (up to several months) from the antecedent streptococcal infection. When no previous rheumatic manifestations are observed, the cases are known as 'pure chorea'.

- **Hemichorea:** Choreiform movements restricted to one half of the body and is seen after stroke, vascular malformations and cerebral neoplasms (contralateral lesion). Usually chorea is bilateral.

Q. Drugs used in the treatment of chorea:

1. Phenobarbitone.
2. Clonazepam.
3. Chlorpromazine.
4. Haloperidol.
5. Sodium valproate.
6. Tetrabenazine.
7. Risperidone.
8. Quetiapine.

Q. What are the differential diagnosis of chorea?

1. Athetosis.
2. Dyskinesia (mainly affects the pharyngeal, perioral and neck muscles, and produces axial tortional movements. This movement disorder is mainly drug-

Table 3.16: Differentiation between chorea and athetosis

Features	Chorea	Athetosis
1. Lesion	1. Caudate nucleus	1. Putamen
2. Tone	2. Hypotonia	2. Hypertonia (rigidity)
3. Basic pattern	3. Rapid, continually interrupted and never proceeding to completion	3. Slow movements, extension and pronation plus flexion and supination of the arm*
4. Effect of excitement	4. Often increased	4. No effect
5. Parts involved	5. Both distal and proximal part	5. Usually distal > proximal
6. Tongue	6. Lizard tongue	6. Chewing tongue
7. Deep reflexes	7. Pendular or hung-up reflex	7. Normal

*With alternating flexion an extension of fingers, often clenching the thumb in the grip.

induced, e.g. by metoclopramide, phenothiazines, levodopa, etc).

3. Tics.
4. Hemiballismus (violent ballistic and flinging movement of one side of body with maximum amplitude at the shoulder and hip, sparing the face and trunk. Usually a self-limited condition where the lesion is in subthalamic nucleus of Luys).
5. Myoclonus (sudden, rapid, brief electric shock-like, irregular, jerky involuntary movements of a limb due to contraction of a single muscle or a group of muscles): It may originate from lesion in cortex, subcortex or spinal cord. The common causes are encephalitis, advanced renal or hepatic failure.

Q. What are the other involuntary movements you know?

Other than: 1. Chorea, 2. Athetosis, and 3. Tics (habit spasm), they are:

4. Myoclonus.
5. Convulsions.
6. Tremor.
7. Dyskinesia.
8. Dystonia (abnormally maintained posture).
9. Hemiballismus.
10. Spasmodic torticollis (see below).
11. Myokymia (called 'false or benign fasciculation').
12. Asterixis.
13. Tetany (see the section on 'Fasciculation'), and
14. Muscle cramp or writer's cramp.

- Fasciculation, titubation and opisthotonus are involuntary movements too. Tremor is a very common involuntary movement in clinical practice. Few clinicians do not agree that convulsions and muscle cramp are involuntary movements. **Myokymia** (continuous rippling movements) is not uncommon, e.g. twitching of muscles around eye in day to day practice.
- **Akathisia** is motor restlessness with inability to sit still. There is always an intense urge to move. It is commonly seen in parkinsonism, chorea, thyrotoxicosis or phenothiazine therapy.
- **Restless leg syndrome** or burning feet syndrome (Ekbom syndrome): Intense desire to move the legs due to unpleasant sensation there, especially when the patient attempts to sleep or sits quiet. This is seen in chronic renal failure, peripheral neuropathy (diabetes, alcoholism), pregnancy and iron deficiency anaemia
- **Torticollis** (a form of dystonia) is characterised by abducted and rotated posture of neck.
- **Muscle cramp** (painful shortening of muscles, e.g. in calf muscles) is due to idiopathic (mostly at night), pregnancy, unaccustomed exertion, severe dehydration with dyselectrolytaemia (e.g. hypokalaemia), uraemia, writer's cramp, McArdle's disease and drug-induced (e.g. diuretics).

Q. Chores without hypotonia:

Probably, it is a patient of chorea associated with athetosis (choreoathetosis), e.g. Wilson's disease.

Q. Identification points:

1. Classical movements are already described. When choreiform movements are superimposed on voluntary movements, there may be a 'grotesque' (strange or ugly) look of the posture.
2. Observe the face and movements of the tongue. At rest, the patient is 'unable to sit still'.
3. Inability to perform a voluntary movement in the absence of paralysis.
4. Bizarre gait.
5. Demonstrate six cardinal features (*see* above).

Clinical Wisdom

In a case of chorea, always examine the heart for any valvular lesion; search for exophthalmos, butterfly rash in face, K-F ring in cornea or polycythemia.

FASCICULATION — CASE 93

Q. What is fasciculation?

These are fine, rapid, irregular and inconstant visible twitching movements (or ripples) of large group of muscle fibres or the whole motor unit. **It indicates LMN lesion**.

It is easily seen or felt by the patient, or palpated by the clinician.

Q. What is fibrillation?

These are contractions of a single muscle fibre. It is a state of hyperirritability (denervation hypersensitivity) of single muscle fibre and usually can not be detected in naked eye. It can be diagnosed by electromyography (EMG) and signifies complete denervation of individual muscle fibre.

Q. Methods of bedside demonstration of fasciculation:

1. They may be seen as ripples underneath the skin overlying muscles at rest, or sometimes 'spontaneously' produce clinically visible contractions.
2. If fasciculation is not spontaneous, they may be evoked by mechanical stimulation. Sharply tap (by the conical end of a hammer) over the degenerating muscle (never on fully degenerated muscle) for demonstration of fasciculation. Usually the bigger muscles like biceps, triceps, deltoid, calf muscles are chosen (this procedure is controversial because fasciculation should be spontaneous).
3. Fasciculation of the tongue: Keep the tongue relaxed in the floor of the mouth (never protrude the tongue) for demonstration of fasciculation (Fig. 3.169A).

Q. Significance of fasciculation:

1. It signifies chronic degeneration of anterior horn cells or their homologue cranial nerve nuclei. It is always seen in a muscle which has undergone wasting (i.e. clinically significant). In the absence of

wasting, fasciculation has no significance (benign fasciculation). So **fasciculation is seen in muscles undergoing active degeneration, not totally degenerated yet (wasting but not wasted)**.

2. If fasciculation disappears from a muscle (which showed fasciculation), it signifies that the muscle is totally degenerated, i.e. the anterior horn cells are completely destroyed (prognostically worse).
3. The muscular contraction of this special type of involuntary movement (fasciculation) is of fine amplitude and thereby, it is not able to move the adjoining joint.

- Fasciculation is due to spontaneous firing of surviving axons to innervate the denervated muscle fibres.

Q. Can you see fibrillation in naked eye ?

As previously discussed, it is diagnosed by EMG but sometimes it is clinically evident in tongue (in LMN type of XII th nerve palsy) as tongue has no submucous coat.

Q. Common causes of fasciculation:

1. Chronic motor neurone disease (MND).
2. Cervical spondylosis.
3. Syringomyelia or syringobulbia.
4. Hyperthyroidism.
5. Recovery from facial palsy (Bell's palsy).
6. Intramedullary tumour.
7. Peripheral neuropathy.
8. Acute or recovery phase of poliomyelitis.
9. Hypoxia, hypercapnoea, hypoglycaemia.
10. Organophosphorus poisoning.

- MND (amyotrophic lateral sclerosis) is the commonest cause of fasciculation. Fasciculation may be evoked by voluntary muscular contraction, cooling the muscle by ethyl chloride spray or hyperventilation.
- Benign fasciculation (normal individual), electrolyte imbalance (↓Ca^{++}, ↓Mg^{++}, ↓K^{+}), and No. 9 and No. 10 are non-neurological causes.

Q. What is benign fasciculation?

When fasciculation is present in the absence of muscular wasting, weakness or any abnormality of reflexes, it is known as 'benign fasciculation'. It is commonly seen in anxiety, after exhaustive physical activity and fatigue states. It is often evident in thenar eminences, thighs, around the shoulder joint or orbicularis oculi (myokymia) muscles.

Q. How do you classify chronic motor neurone disease (MND)?

This is a devastating progressive disease of unknown origin which leads to degeneration of anterior horn cells of the spinal cord, motor nuclei of cranial nerves, and the corticospinal and corticobulbar pathways. The disease is characterised by insidious onset with a steadily progressive course, in a middle aged or elderly person. The classification of MND goes like:

a. Progressive muscular atrophy (pure LMN type): Weakness, wasting and fasciculation.
b. Amyotrophic lateral sclerosis (predominant UMN type in lower limbs, and combined LMN plus UMN type in upper limbs): Commonest (see below).
c. Primary lateral sclerosis (pure UMN type): Progressive quadriparesis (rare).
d. Progressive bulbar palsy (medullary lesion; LMN type).
e. Pseudobulbar palsy (cortical or subcortical lesion; UMN type).
f. Mixed type of No. d and e.

- **MND may be given as a long case.**

Q. Describe the 'motor functions' in amyotrophic lateral sclerosis (MND):

A. Nutrition of muscles:
   1. **Wasting of the small muscles of hands (skeleton hand)**, prominence of long flexor and extensor tendons of hands; sometimes, there is presence of claw hand. Knuckles are prominent and interosseous spaces are depressed (Fig. 3.84).
   2. At first there is wasting of the small muscles of hands which is followed by involvement of forearm muscles. Lastly, there is wasting of deltoid, supraspinatus, etc.
   3. There is not much wasting of lower limbs.

B. Tone of muscles:
   Upper limb: Tone is usually decreased (hypotonia).
   Lower limb: Increased (clasp-knife spasticity).

C. Power of muscles: Power is decreased more in upper limb than in lower limb because of the combined UMN and LMN involvement. Small muscles of the hands are weak.

D. Coordination of movements: Normal in both limbs (severe wasting may hamper coordination).

E. Involuntary movements: **Fasciculation is seen predominantly in the upper limbs.** Presence of fasciculation helps in the clinical diagnosis of MND. Never forget to see the tongue for fasciculation.

- There is early weakness of respiratory muscle. Usually there is no bed sore formation due to preserved sensory function.
- Rationality of nomenclature in MND: LMN involvement—muscle atrophy (i.e. amyotrophy), UMN involvement—loss of fibres of lateral column (fibrillary gliosis, i.e. lateral sclerosis).
- The patient presents with cramps, fasciculation, weakness and atrophy of the small muscles of hands and feet in an asymmetric fashion. The course of the disease is through spastic quadriparesis or paraparesis with wasting.

Q. Reflexes and gait in MND:

A. Superficial reflex:
   i. Abdominal reflexes are lost. It is seen that abdominal reflex may not be lost for a considerable

period in MND though there is bilateral UMN lesion.

ii. Cremasteric reflex: Lost

iii. Plantar response: Bilaterally extensor.

B. Deep reflexes:

i. Upper limb: Jerks are brisk in the presence of wasting (clinically very characteristic of amyotrophic lateral sclerosis).

ii. Lower limb: Jerks are brisk, clonus (ankle and pateller) may be seen.

C. Visceral reflexes: Normal.

D. Gait: Spastic gait.

Clinical Wisdom

Small muscles of hands, forearm, deltoid, tongue, facial muscles are involved early. *Higher functions, external ocular muscles, autonomic, cerebellar, extrapyramidal, sensory and sphincteric functions are normal in MND*. So, the disease presents with spasticity, brisk jerks, Babinski's sign in the **lower limb**, and fasciculation, weakness, wasting in the **upper limb**. Electromyography (EMG) is diagnostic (shows chronic partial denervation with fasciculation and fibrillation); nerve conduction velocity (NCV) is usually normal. Male > female; progressive and fatal course within 3–5 years. Riluzole (100 mg/day) may slow progression.

Q. UMN Palsy in lower limb and LMN palsy in upper limb:

1. Amyotrophic lateral sclerosis (MND).
2. Cervical spondylosis.
3. Syringomyelia.
4. Friedreich's ataxia.
5. Cervical extramedullary compression.
6. Patchy arachnoiditis.

Q. What is tetany?

Tetany is increased neuromuscular irritability due to low ionic calcium in blood. Normal serum calcium level is 9–11 mg/dL and the ionic fraction is 4.5–5.6 mg/dL.

Serum calcium <8.5 mg/dL is hypocalcaemia while >11 mg/dL is regarded as hypercalcaemia.

Q. Classical physical signs in tetany:

The increased neuromuscular irritability is tested at the bedside by:

1. **Trousseau's sign:** When the pressure is raised above the systolic BP for 3 minutes, typical 'carpal spasm' appears. There is flexion of MCP joints with extension of interphalangeal joints and the flexed thumb takes its position in between the index and the middle fingers (opposition of thumb). This is known as "main d'accoucheur" or obstetrician's hand (Fig. 3.200). 'Pedal spasm' is less frequently demonstrated. Latent tetany is best recognised by eliciting this sign.
2. **Chvostek's sign:** Tapping the facial nerve (by finger or hammer) in front of the ear will produce twitching of facial muscles.

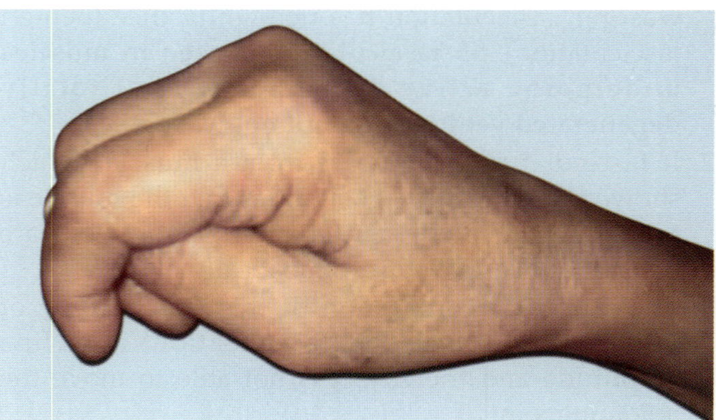

Fig. 3.200: "Main d'accoucheur" or **carpal spasm in tetany**

3. **Erb's sign:** Muscular contractions can be produced by application of subthreshold electrical stimulation (0.5–2.0 milli-amps).
4. **Peroneal sign:** Tapping the peroneal nerve at the neck of fibula will produce plantiflexion and adduction of the foot with extension of knee (pedal spasm).
5. [ECG: Prolonged Q-T interval.]

Clinical Wisdom

Symptoms of tetany are:

1. Irritability.
2. Muscle cramps (carpopedal spasm).
3. Peripheral (hand and feet) and circumoral paraesthesia.
4. Triad of symptoms are common in children, i.e. carpopedal spasm, laryngysmus stridulus (stridor, respiratory distress, cyanosis), and convulsions.
5. Dysphagia, dyspnoea, dysuria, abdominal colic, etc.

Q. Common causes of hypocalcaemia:

1. Malabsorption syndrome (e.g. coeliac disease).
2. Chronic renal failure (CRF).
3. Acute pancreatitis.
4. Hypoparathyroidism or pseudohypoparathyroidism.
5. Rickets and osteomalacia.
6. Hypoalbuminaemia.
7. Alkalosis due to hyperventilation (often hysterical) or persistent vomiting (pyloric stenosis).
8. Citrated blood in massive transfusion.
9. Drugs: Calcitonin, bisphosphonates.

- Low total calcium is not associated with tetany if ionised fraction is normal. Low ionised calcium is associated with tetany irrespective of total calcium level. Transient hypocalcaemia (burn, sepsis) does not develop into tetany.
- Tetany is common in the presence of alkalosis (hyperventilation, persistent vomiting, primary hyperaldosteronism, excess antacid therapy) and hypocalcaemia (mentioned above). Tetany is rare in chronic renal failure because of the presence of metabolic acidosis.
- Causes of **hypercalcaemia** are: Primary hyperparathyroidism, malignant tumours (with bone metastasis), prolonged immobilisation, multiple myelona, ingestion of excess vitamin A or D, milk-alkali syndrome (Burnett syndrome), Paget's disease, thiazide diuretic, Addison's disease, sarcoidosis.

Q. Causes of lock jaw or trismus:

Trismus develops due to sustained involuntary spasm of masseter and temporalis (masticatory muscles) resulting in inability to open the mouth and mastication, and is found in:

1. **Tetanus** (spatula test is positive; trismus is by far the most important early symptom).
2. Impacted wisdom tooth.
3. Peritonsillar abscess (quinsy), dental abscess, Ludwig's angina.
4. Acute follicular tonsillitis.
5. Temporo-mandibular (TM) joint osteoarthritis (Costen's syndrome) or rheumatoid arthritis.
6. Sometimes in drug-induced dyskinesia (metoclopramide, phenothiazines).
7. Sometimes in tetany, strychnine poisoning, cyanide toxicity.
8. Parotitis, mumps.
9. Hydrophiidae group of snake bite.
10. Rabies.
11. Anaesthesia-induced malignant hyperthermia.
12. Hysterical.

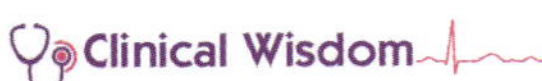

Painful trismus—2, 3, 4 and 8; painless trismus—tetanus and others.

- **Spatula test:** In health, touching the posterior pharyngeal wall by spatula produces reflex opening of mouth. In tetanus, paradoxically mouth closes in such a way that the spatula can not be taken out easily. Thus, spatula test is positive in tetanus and negative in others.
- In scleroderma and submucosal fibrosis of oral cavity, the patient may find difficulty in opening the mouth; but this is not true trismus. Patients cannot close the mouth in subluxation of TM joint.
- **'Facies' in tetanus** (Fig. 3.201)**:** Characteristic risus sardonicus (grimace mimicking 'smile of Satan') due to sustained contraction of facial muscles, and blepharospasm.

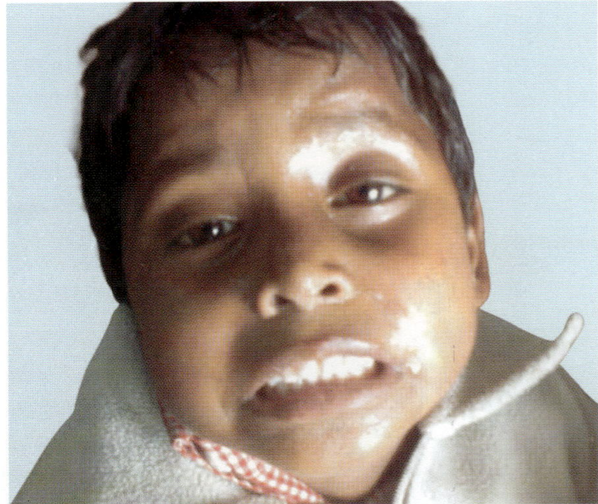

Fig. 3.201: **Tetanus** with a fixed sardonic smile (**risus sardonicus** or 'smile of Satan')—the smile does not reach the eyes

MYOTONIA — CASE 94

Q. What is myotonia?

In certain muscle disease like dystrophia myotonica (an autosomal dominant disorder), the relaxation of the muscle is impaired following a strong contraction (*myotonia*). This continued, involuntary muscular contraction after cessation of voluntary effort (or stimulus), i.e. failure of muscle relaxation, is known as myotonia. Myotonias are also classified as 'channelopathies' as there is defective skeletal muscles cell chloride ion membrane conductance (i.e. defect in muscle membrane ion channel).

Q. Types of dystrophies of the muscle:

There are two types mainly:

1. Muscular dystrophy (Duchenne type, etc.) or myopathy (vide page 468), and
2. Myotonic dystrophy (or dystrophia myotonica).

- The two most common myotonias are myotonic dystrophy and myotonia congenita.

Q. How do you diagnose myotonia at the bedside?

The phenomenon (described below) is most evident when the muscles are cold. Myotonic muscle shows sustained contraction on direct percussion (Fig. 3.202). The different bedside methods are:

1. *Shake hand with the patient* and then let it go suddenly: The patient's grasp is maintained for a moment, then released slowly and gradually, i.e. there is poor hand grip relaxation.
2. Percuss the thenar eminence by a hammer (Fig. 3.202): It shows a peculiar movement of the thumb (opponens movement) and a dimple of contraction appears on thenar eminence which fill up very slowly ('percussion myotonia'); this can also be tested over the wrist extensors.
3. Percuss over the tongue: A dimple of contraction appears which relaxes very slowly.

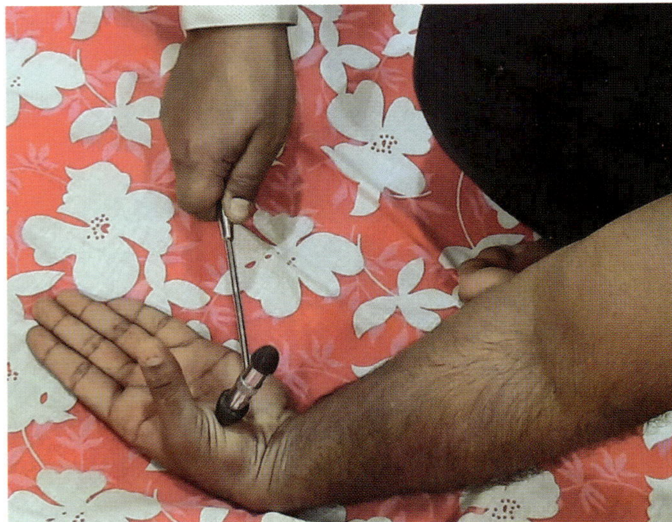

Fig. 3.202: Demonstration of **myotonia**

4. Ask the patient to close the eyes forcibly and then to open the eyes: The patient cannot open the eyes promptly or opens it very slowly after closure.
5. Ask the patient to smile and then to stop it suddenly: Smile remains fixed in face for a longer duration.

Q. Clinical features of myotonic dystrophy:

Males are affected more than females, and usually becomes evident between 20–50 years. The patient complains of progressive muscle wasting and weakness.

1. Myotonia.
2. Ptosis (partial) with smooth forehead (apathetic monk face).
3. Proximal muscle wasting with distal limb muscles weakness.
4. Long, lean and triangular facial structure (typical 'hatchet faced' and 'swan neck' appearances are due to atrophy of temporalis/masseter/facial muscles, and sternomastoid muscle at neck, respectively) **(Fig. 3.203)**; a weak and expressionless face.
5. Cataracts.
6. Frontal baldness.
7. Mental retardation (mild).
8. Testicular atrophy.
9. Alopecia.
10. Dysarthria due to weak palatal, pharyngeal and tongue muscles.
11. Others: Gynaecomastia, cardiac conduction defects, cardiomyopathy, arrhythmias, mitral valve prolapse, glucose intolerance, insulin resistance, decreased oesophageal and colonic motility, small pituitary fossa, low serum IgG, poor tolerance to general anaesthetics.

- **Diagnosis is essentially clinical.** Serum CK level may be normal or mildly elevated, EMG is diagnostic and shows evidence of myotonia (waxing and waning of potentials to produce a characteristic sound on loud speaker, known as *dive-bomber-effect)*, while muscle biopsy shows type I fibres with increased number of nuclei, ring fibres and sarcolemmal masses.

Q. Drugs used in the treatment of myotonia:

1. Phenytoin.
2. Mexiletine.
3. Quinine and
4. Procainamide.

Q. How to test the temporalis muscle?

First inspect the suprazygomatic region for the muscle bulk of **temporalis**. In weakness of temporalis, the temporal fossa above the zygoma will be hollow. Now ask the patient to clench his teeth **(Fig. 3.204)**. Inspect (above the zygoma) and palpate the temporalis muscle on both sides. Paralysed muscles will be less prominent and active muscle will stand out.

Masseter, another muscle supplied by the Vth cranial nerve, is tested in the same way. Paralysis of masseter results in flattening of the angle of the jaw. Again ask the patient to clench his teeth. Look for the prominence of masseter and palpate it, which stands out as corrugated hard mass at the angle of the jaw. Masseter, and temporalis to a lesser extent elevate the jaw (jaw closure).

- The other muscles supplied by the Vth cranial nerve are lateral and medial pterygoids. Individually, lateral or medial **pterygoids** help in jaw opening and its side to side movement **(Fig. 3.205)**. When both the pterygoids act, they help in jaw opening and its protrusion. They are tested by asking the patient to depress the jaw and to move it from side to side; then to do the test against resistance offered by you by placing your hand under the chin and sides of the chin from time to time. In unilateral pterygoid palsy, on attempted jaw opening, the

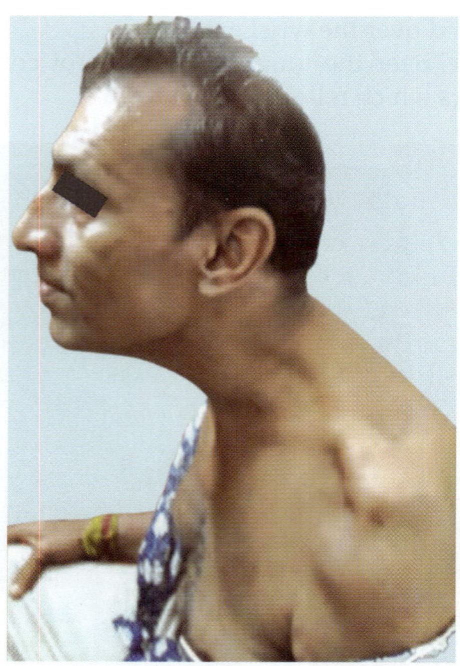

Fig. 3.203: Swan neck appearance in **myotonia dystrophica**

Fig. 3.204: Power testing of **muscles of mastication**

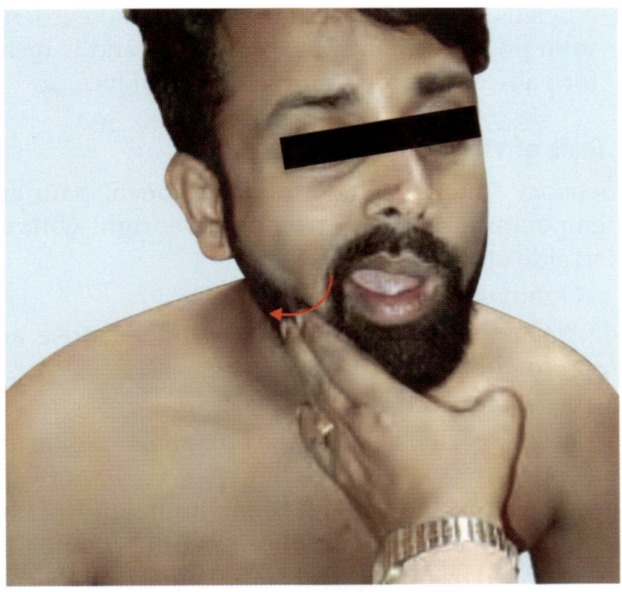

Fig. 3.205: Muscle power testing of **pterygoid**

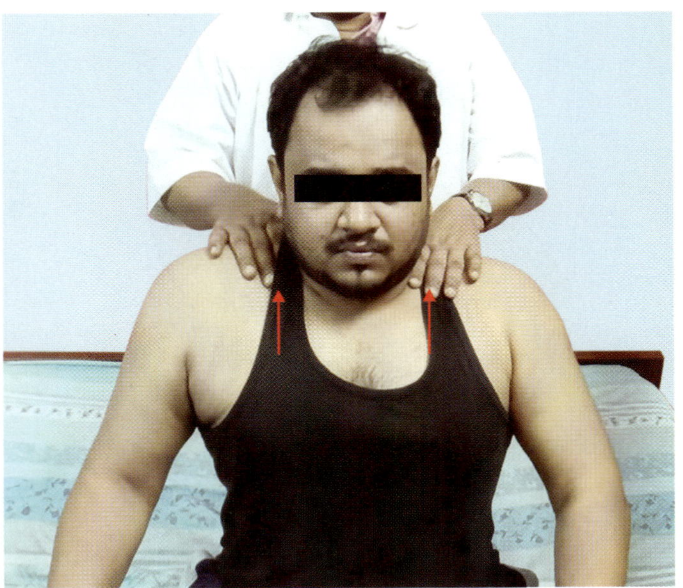

Fig. 3.207: Muscle power testing of **trapezius**

jaw will deviate (appraised by noting the relation between upper and lower incisor teeth) towards the paralysed side being pushed by the healthy pterygoids (as geniglossus muscle in tongue).

- Jaw opening is done by pterygoids, mylohyoid and anterior belly ot digastric muscle.

Q. How do you test the sternomastoids?

1. Individual sternomastoid (Fig. 3.206A): To test the right sternomastoid, ask the patient to turn the chin to left side against resistance by placing your hand on left side of patient's face; the sternomastoid present on the right side becomes prominent on chin movement, if healthy. Compare the test with the other side.
2. Both sternomastoids (Fig. 3.206B): Ask the patient to press the chin downwards against the examiner's resistance. Both stenomastoids will become prominent which can be corroborated both by inspection and palpation of the muscles in neck.

- *In bilateral sternomastoid weakness, head will drop backwards.* Two muscles which are supplied by the XIth cranial nerve are trapezius and sternomastoid. Test the **trapezius** by asking the patient to shrug his shoulders, against your resistance (first demonstrate the 'shrugging' to the patient and then press both shoulders downwards simultaneously from BEHIND) (Fig. 3.207).
- Accessory nerve (XIth cranial nerve) has two parts: Cranial (arising from the caudal part of nucleus ambiguus) and spinal (arising from upper five cervical segments). Cranial part, with vagus nerve, supplies pharyngeal and laryngeal muscles, while spinal part supplies sternomastoid and trapezius muscle. While **examining accessory nerve**, first observe for wasting and fasciculation of sternomastoid and trapezius, and then examine for drooping of the shoulder (trapezius) and turning head to right and left (sternomastoid). Lastly, palpate them to assess their bulk, and test their powers (described above).

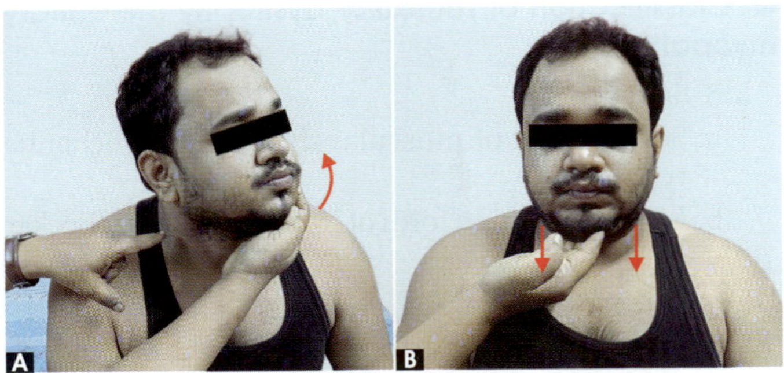

Fig. 3.206: Muscle power testing of **sternomastoids**—unilateral (A) and bilateral (B)

Q. Weakness of neck muscles (so called, 'broken neck' sign) are seen in:

Dropped head syndrome results from weakness of extensors of neck.

1. Snake bite (Elapidae group).
2. Organophosphorus poisoning.
3. Motor neurone disease ('head drop').
4. GB syndrome.
5. Myaesthenia gravis and myopathies.

Q. Neuroanatomy of the trigeminal nerve:

It is the largest cranial nerve. Sensation of face is provided through three branches of trigeminal nerves (Fig. 3.208), e.g.

i. Ophthalmic branch (V_1): Supplies conjunctiva, cornea, mesial part of the skin of the nose as far as the tip, upper eyelids, forehead and scalp as far as the vertex.
ii. Maxillary nerve (V_2): Supplies lower eyelids, upper cheek, temple, sides of nose, upper lip, roof of pharynx, gum/teeth/palate of upper jaw.
iii. Mandibular division (V_3): Supplies the ear, lower part of face (except the angle of mandible supplied by C_2 segment), lower lip, lower teeth and the epithelium of anterior 2/3rd of the tongue.

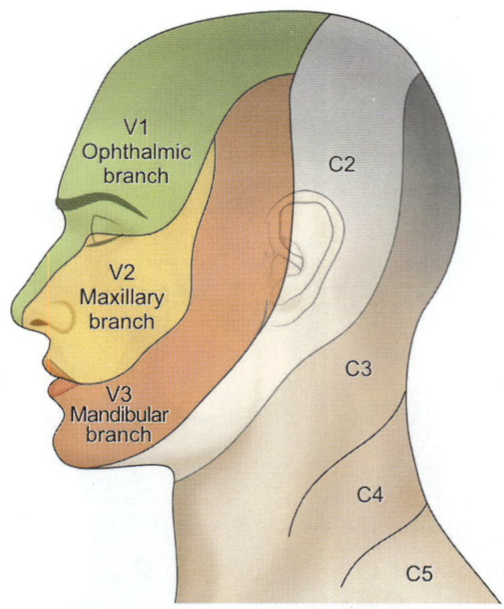

Fig. 3.208: Sensory distribution of **trigeminal nerve**

The motor branch supplies the **'muscles of mastication'**, i.e. masseter, temporalis, lateral and medial pterygoids (Fig. 3.209). It also supplies anterior belly of digastric, mylohyoid, tensor tympani and tensor veli palatini (not examined clinically).

The nuclei of trigeminal nerve are arranged like:

i. Principal nucleus (motor and sensory) at pons: The motor branch conveys through V_3 to innervate muscles of mastication; sensory nucleus is meant for touch, joint-position sense).
ii. Mesencephalic nucleus: Carries unconscious proprioceptive information from palate, temporomandibular joint and muscles of mastication, e.g. governs how much pressure is required to break a chicken bone during mastication.
iii. Nucleus of spinal tract of trigeminal nerve extends from pons to C_2 level of spinal cord, and is meant for pain and temperature sensation of face.

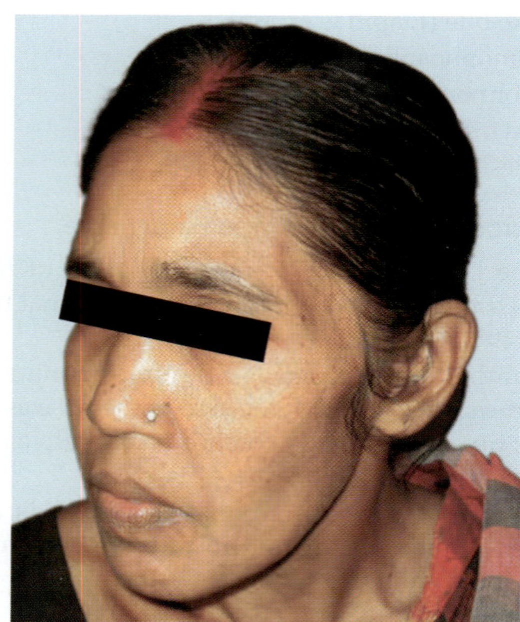

Fig. 3.209: Motor component of **Vth cranial nerve paralysis** resulting in wasting of muscles of mastication, e.g. temporalis (suprazygomatic portion) and masseter (infrazygomatic portion)

Q. Tests of Vth cranial nerve:

1. Sensory functions: Test for light touch, pain and temperature sensation (compare the right with the left side of face).
   a. Ophthalmic division:
      i. On the both sides of root of the nose and forehead.
      ii. Test for corneal reflex.
   b. Maxillary division: On the both malar region and upper lip.
   c. Mandibular division: On the both sides of chin (always avoid the angle of mandible which is supplied by C_2 segment of the spinal cord by great auricular nerve).
2. Motor functions: Test the power of temporalis, masseter and pterygoids (i.e. muscles of mastication).
3. Reflex: Demonstrate the jaw jerk.

Q. Clinical pearls in trigeminal nerve:

1. Bruxism: Involuntary and forceful teeth grinding during sleep.
2. Trismus: Sustained involuntary spasm of masseter and temporalis, commonly seen in tetanus.
3. Jaw tremor: In parkinsonism.
4. Complex partial seizure: Chewing and masticatory movement of lower jaw.
5. Jaw claudication: Giant cell arteritis.
6. Jaw fatigability: Myasthania gravis.
7. Pain in lower jaw: From ischaemic heart disease (IHD).

MYOPATHY — CASE 95

Q. What is muscular dystrophy or myopathy?

These are genetically determined abnormality characterised by progressive degeneration of group of muscles without involvement of the nervous system (generally, myopathy describes diseases of voluntary muscles).

Q. Classification of muscular dystrophy (hereditary myopathy):

I. X-linked:
   a. Severe form of muscular dystrophy (Duchenne type).
   b. Milder or benign form of X-linked disease (Becker type).
II. Autosomal recessive:
   a. Limb-girdle type (usually scapulo-humeral, rarely pelvi-femoral).
   b. Congenital variety.

III. Autosomal dominant:
   a. Facio-scapulo-humeral (Landouzy-Dejerine type).
   b. Distal myopathy (Gower type).
   c. Ocular or oculo-pharyngeal.
   d. Myotonic dystrophy.

Q. Why do you say Duchenne type of myopathy (DMD)?

1. Male patient (due to X-linked inheritance, females carry the disease and males are the victims): Starts in infancy and childhood (3–5 years) with H/o frequent fall and delayed motor activity (e.g. walking), rare after puberty.
2. Positive family history (as it is X-linked disease, oblique transmission is present and maternal uncle, uncle or nephew are affected): If you are allowed to take the history.
3. Insidious onset with gradually progressive course.
4. Mental retardation, cardiomyopathy or kyphoscoliosis (may be present).
5. Positive Gowers' sign (*see* below).
6. Difficulty in climbing upstairs and getting up from sitting position (due to involvement of pelvi-femoral muscles, i.e. **proximal muscles**); pelvic muscles involvement > shoulder muscles.
7. **Pseudohypertrophy** in few muscles and atrophy in others.
8. **Sensory system, bladder function, reflexes (superficial and deep): All are normal.** There is no fasciculation (to differentiate it from MND).
9. Waddling gait.

- Deep reflexes are normal till the late stage.
- At 8–10 years, walking requires use of braces; by the age of 12 years, the patient is wheel chair-bound. Few patients survice upto 20 years.

Q. Classification of muscle diseases:

A. Acquired:

1. Inflammatory myopathies: Polymyositis, dermatomyositis, inclusion body myositis.
2. Endocrine and toxic myopathies: Cushing's syndrome, thyroid disease (both hyper- and hypothyroid), hypokalaemia, hypocalcaemia, alcohol abuse, steroids/fibrates.
3. Myasthenic: Myasthenia gravis, Lambert-Eaton myasthenic-myopathic syndrome.

B. Genetic:

1. Dystrophic: See the classification of muscular dystrophy (*see* above).
2. Myotonic: Myotonic dystrophy, myotonia congenita.
3. Channelopathies: Hypokalaemic/hyperkalaemic/normokalaemic periodic paralysis.
4. Metabolic myopathies: Myophosphorylase deficiency (McArdle's disease), mitochondrial diseases, malignant hyperpyrexia.

Clinical Wisdom

Disorders of neuromuscular transmission are myasthenia gravis, Lambert-Eaton syndrome, botulism, periodic paralysis (↓K^+, ↑K^+), Elapidae snake bite, stiffman syndrome and drugs (e.g. organophosphorus insecticides).

Q. What are the X-linked disordes?

1. Haemophilia (*see* **Fig. 1.62**).
2. G_6PD deficiency.
3. Christmas disease.
4. Duchenne muscular dystrophy.
5. Ocular albinism.
6. Colour blindness.
7. Hunter's syndrome.
8. Hypophosphataemic rickets.
9. Nephrogenic diabetes insipidus.
10. Lesch-Nyhan syndrome.

- **Y-linked single gene disorder** is manifested by 'hairy ears' in male. Other Y-linked disorders are XY female with the Y chromosome lacking the SRY (sex-region determining Y factor) gene or XY male having the SRY gene.
- X-linked disorders affect males while females are the carrier. Rarely a female can suffer from haemophilia (when the mother is carrier and the father suffers from haemophilia /or the patient suffers from Turner's syndrome [45, XO]/or by Lyon hypothesis, where there is inactivation of one X-chromosome).

Q. Pseudohypertrophy versus true hypertrophy:

'Hypertrophy' means increase in size, bulk and volume of the muscle.

A. Pseudohypertrophy:

These are the large muscles as a result of deposition of fibrofatty tissue. The muscles look bulkier than normal muscles and they are doughy in feel (elastic feel is lost). When asked to contract, they are not hard and globular. The muscles are strikingly weak in spite of their large size. They are hypotonic and the deep reflexes may be dull (reflexes involving the muscles). Muscles affected by pseudohypertrophy in DMD are:

1. Calf muscles (**Fig. 3.210**), 2. Glutei, 3. Quadriceps, 4. Deltoid, and 5. Infraspinatus.

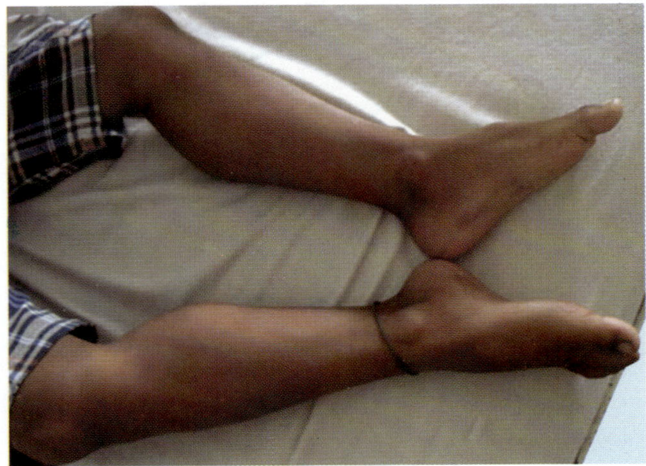

Fig. 3.210: Calf muscles pseudohypertrophy in Duchenne muscular dystrophy

Atrophy is also observed in DMD, and is classically seen in 1. Pectoralis major (parchment paper-like), 2. Latissimus dorsi, and 3. Biceps.

B. True hypertrophy:

Large muscles, elastic in feel; when asked to contract, they are hard and globular. These muscles are stronger then normal-sized muscles.

Clinical Wisdom

In DMD, usully there is symmetrical involvement of muscles. Ultimately all the muscles in the body become atrophied. Facial muscles and small muscles of the hands are usually spared in DMD.

Q. Causes of true hypertrophy of muscles:

1. Manual labourers.
2. Athletes.
3. Myotonia.
4. Sometimes, in cysticercosis (in muscle).
5. Acromegaly.
6. Benign hypertrophy of limb muscles.
7. Haemangioma or arteriovenous malformations in muscle.

- **Pseudohypertrophy** of muscles is seen in DMD, hypothyroidism (percussion myoedema is characteristic), glycogen storage disease and rarely in trichinosis.

Q. What is Gowers' rising test (Figs 3.211A and B)?

When the patient is asked to stand from lying down position, he adopts a curious manner of rising. He first rolls over his body and then take support successively on the ground, feet, legs, knees and waist, and finally stands up. It seems that the patient is 'climbing up the legs' and is known as Gowers' rising test or Gower's sign. This sign is not specific for DMD, as it may be found in any condition where the pelvic girdle muscles are weakened

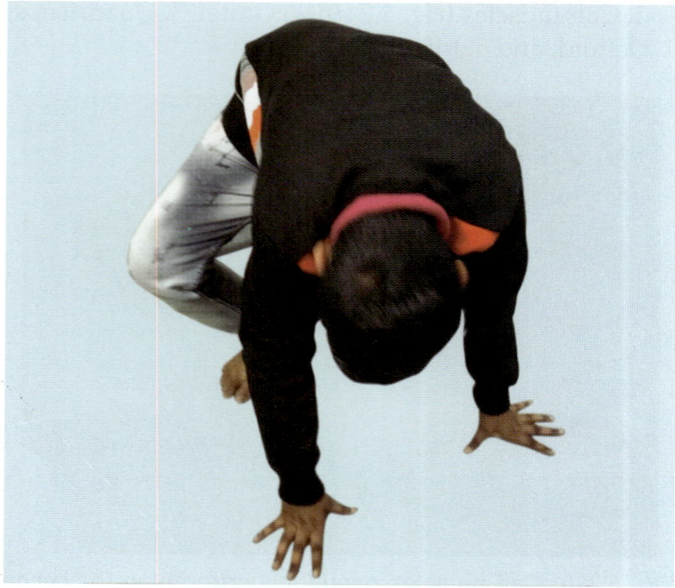

Fig. 3.211A: **Gowers' sign** in Duchenne type of myopathy

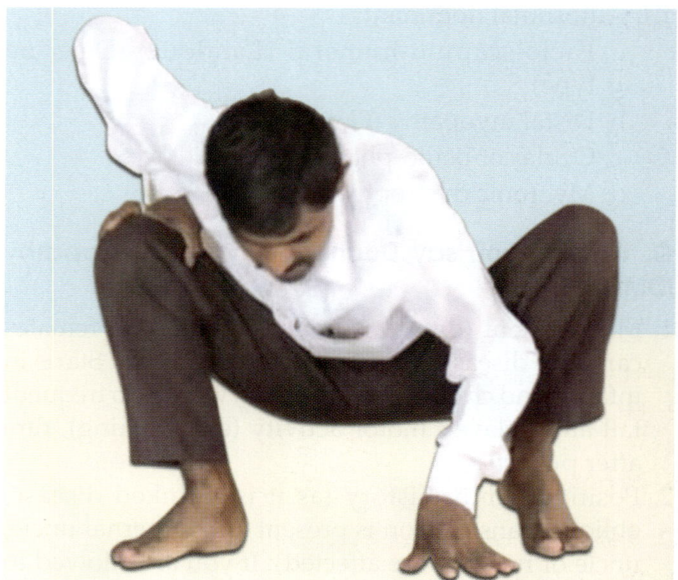

Fig. 3.211B: **Gowers' sign** in muscular dystrophy (Becker type)

and thus, it may be observed in polymyositis, spinal muscular atrophy and other myopathies (e.g. endocrine myopathy).

- Sir William R Gowers (1845–1915) was a British clinical neurologist, born to a bootmaker in London.

Q. What is waddling gait?

It is like the 'gait of a duck'. The body is first tilted backwards, with an increase of lumbar lordosis. The feet are placed wide apart and the body sways from side to side as soon as the patient starts stepping. The hip tilts down when the leg is being lifted. The heel and toes are brought down simultaneously. *It is due to weakness of the proximal pelvic muscles* and is specially seen in myopathy. Causes of waddling gait are:

1. Duchenne muscular dystrophy.
2. Pregnancy (advanced).
3. Congenital dislocation of hip (bilateral).
4. Often in huge ascites or morbid obesity.
5. Osteomalacia.
6. Hip dysplasia or bilateral Perthes' disease.

Q. Causes of proximal muscle weakness:

1. Muscular dystrophy.
2. Polymyositis and dermatomyositis.
3. Diabetic amyotrophy.
4. GB syndrome.
5. Neuralgic amyotrophy.
6. Radicular lesion, e.g. cervical spondylosis.
7. Sometimes in fulminant myasthenia gravis.
8. Thyrotoxic myopathy or Cushing's syndrome.
9. Metabolic myopathy, e.g. hypokalaemia.
10. Drug-induced: Corticosteroid, statins.
11. Malignancy.
12. Osteomalacia.
13. Porphyric and HIV neuropathy.

Q. Causes of distal muscle weakness:

1. Wasting of the small muscles of hands (*see* page 342).
2. Polyneuropathy (familial or acquired).
3. Distal myopathy of Gowers.
4. Sometimes in myotonic dystrophy.
5. Charcot-Marie-Tooth disease.
6. Inclusion body myositis.
7. Welander's distal myopathy.

Q. Causes of recurrent muscle weakness:

1. Myasthenia gravis.
2. Hypokalaemic periodic paralysis.
3. Hyperkalaemic periodic paralysis.
4. Normokalaemic periodic paralysis.

Q. Aetiology of painful muscles:

1. Post-exercise.
2. Polymyalgia rheumatica.
3. Poly- or dermatomyositis.
4. Fibromyalgia.
5. Myositis (infection).
6. Post-convulsions.
7. Hypovitaminosis D.
8. Drugs (statins, penicillamine).

Q. Causes of wasting of muscles:

1. LMN lesion due to any cause.
2. UMN lesion: There is disuse atrophy only.
3. Muscular dystrophy.
4. Disseminated malignancy.
5. Diabetes mellitus.
6. Thyrotoxicosis.
7. Malnutrition.
8. Disseminated tuberculosis.
9. AIDS (slim disease).
10. Anorexia nervosa.

- Causes of unilateral wasting of leg—old poliomyelitis, diabetic amyotrophy, disuse due to severe arthritis, prolapsed intervertebral disc, cerebral palsy.

Q. Power testing of different muscles involved in DMD:

1. Calf muscles (gastrocnemius and soleus) (Fig. 3.212): Patient lies supine with legs extended. Ask the patient to plantiflex the foot against resistance (keep the ankle fixed by holding it firmly).
2. Quadriceps (Fig. 3.213): Patient lies supine; first bend the knee and then ask the patient to straighten the leg when resistance is applied over the shin.
3. Glutei: For test of gluteus maximus, ask the patient to lie supine; raise the patient's foot off the bed and ask him to push it down against your resistance; knee must be kept extended.
   Other method: Patient lies prone and raises the thigh against resistance (Fig. 3.214). Gluteus maximus helps in hip extension while gluteus medius and minimus help in hip abduction (Fig. 3.215).

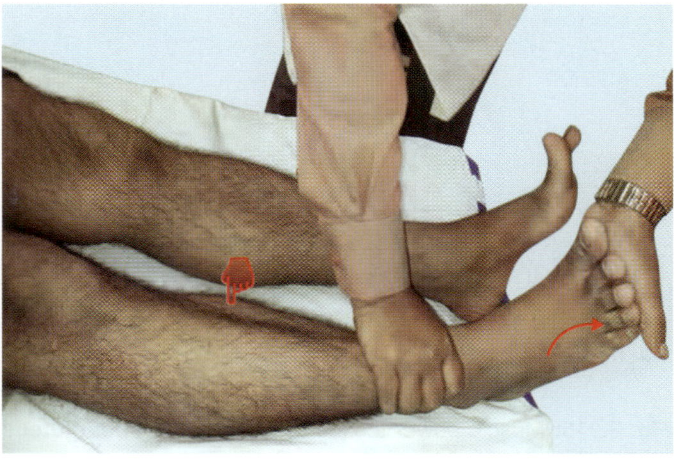

Fig. 3.212: Muscle power testing of **calf muscles** (gastrocnemius and soleus) against resistance

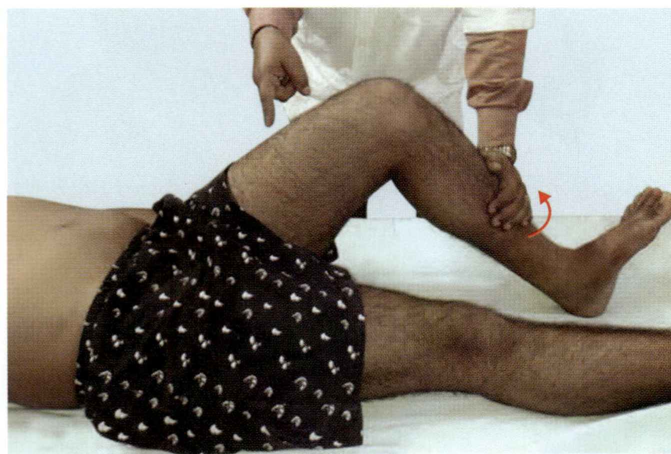

Fig. 3.213: Muscle power testing of **quadriceps femoris** against resistance

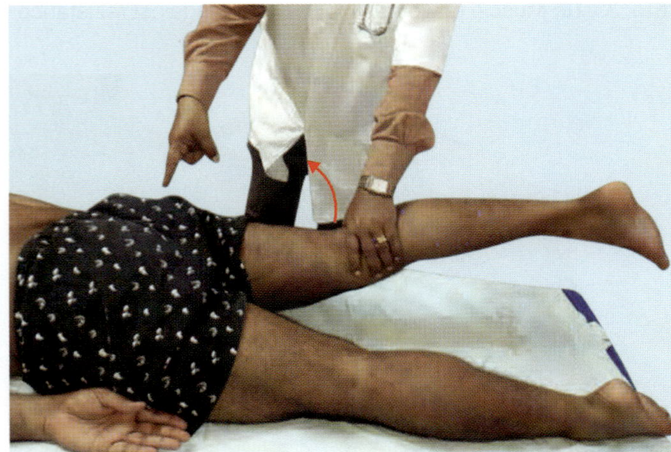

Fig. 3.214: Muscle power testing of **gluteus maximus** muscle against resistance

4. Deltoid: First abduct the patient's arm to 15° and tell him to keep his arm in that position. Now ask him to abduct his arm up to 90° against your resistance (Fig. 3.216) [supraspinatus abducts the first 15° (Fig. 3.217)].

- From 90° to rest, shoulder abduction is done by trapezius and serratus anterior.

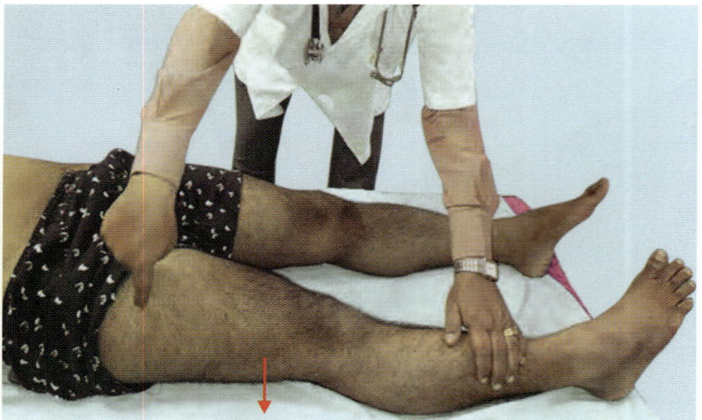

Fig. 3.215: Muscle power testing of **gluteus medius, gluteus minimus and tensor fascia lata** against resistance

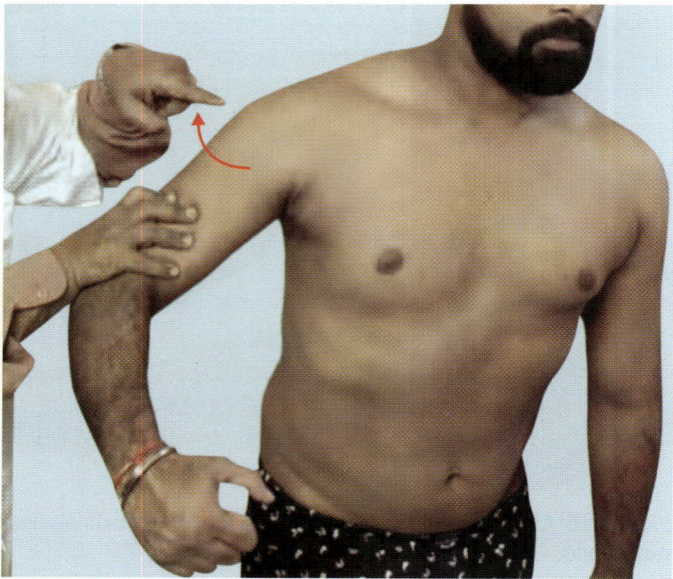

Fig. 3.216: Muscle power testing of **deltoid** against resistance

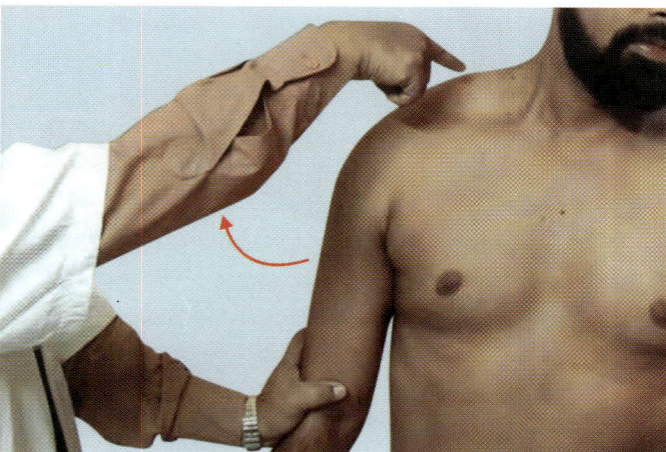

Fig. 3.217: Muscle power testing of **supraspinatus** against resistance

5. Infraspinatus: The examiner stands behind the patient. The patient is asked to tuck his elbow into his side with the forearm placed at right angle. He is now asked to rotate the limb outwards against your resistance (elbow will be placed against the side throughout the test) (Fig. 3.218).

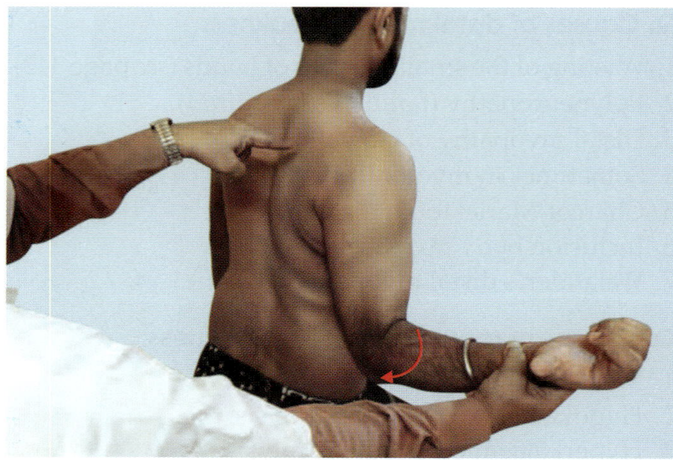

Fig. 3.218: Muscle power testing of **infraspinatus** against resistance

6. Latissimus dorsi: Palpate the posterior axillary folds from behind when the patient coughs. Compare the contraction on both sides; or ask the patient to clasp his hands behind his back and you offer resistance to the downward and backward movement (stand behind the patient) (Fig. 3.219).
7. Pectoralis major: Standing in front of the patient, ask him to clap his hands together and you attempt to keep them apart. The contraction of pectoralis can be seen (Fig. 3.220).

Clinical Wisdom

Hamstrings muscles: The patient lies supine with knee flexed at 90°. Ask the patient to pull the heel towards buttock while you resist it by holding the leg at ankle. The test can also be done in prone position of the patient (figure in Case 96). Other muscles testing:

- Biceps (Fig. 3.221): The patient flexes the elbow with forearm at supinated position. Hold the wrist, stabilise the elbow, and resist flexion. Observe the biceps is contracting.
- Brachioradialis (Fig. 3.222): The patient flexes the elbow with forearm at mid-prone position. Hold the wrist, stabilise

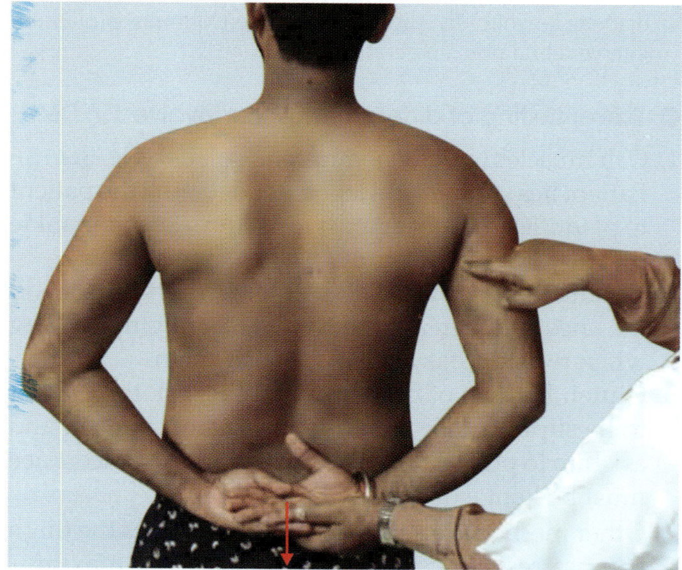

Fig. 3.219: Muscle power testing of **latissimus dorsi** against resistance

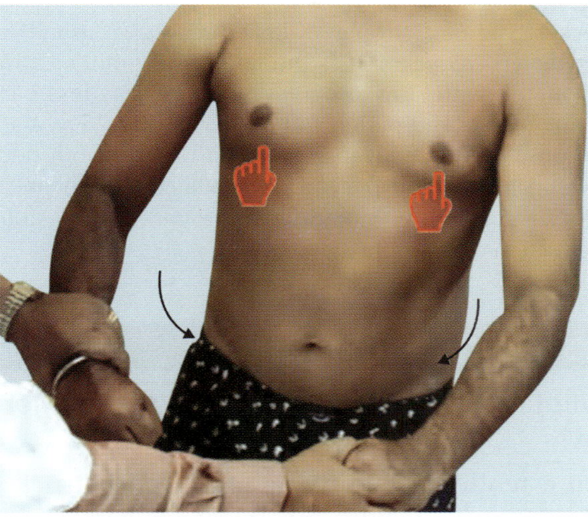

Fig. 3.220: Muscle power testing of **pectoralis major** against resistance

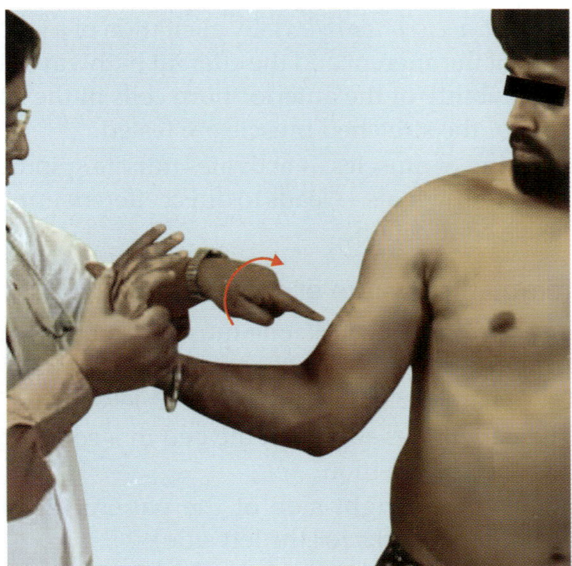

Fig. 3.221: Muscle power testing of **biceps** against resistance

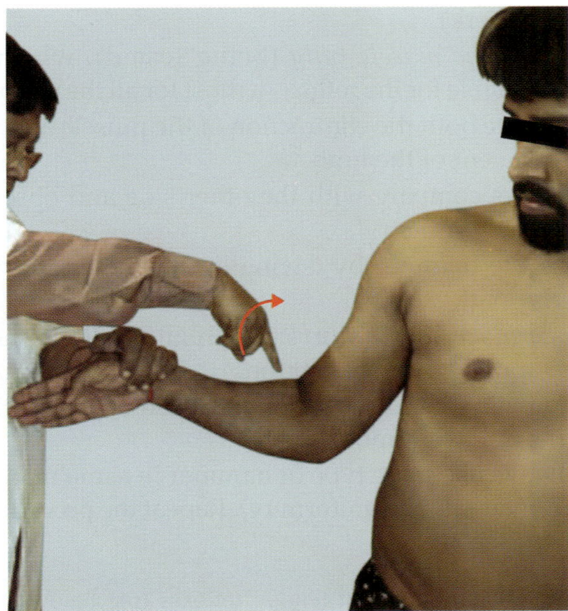

Fig. 3.222: Muscle power testing of **brachioradialis** against resistance

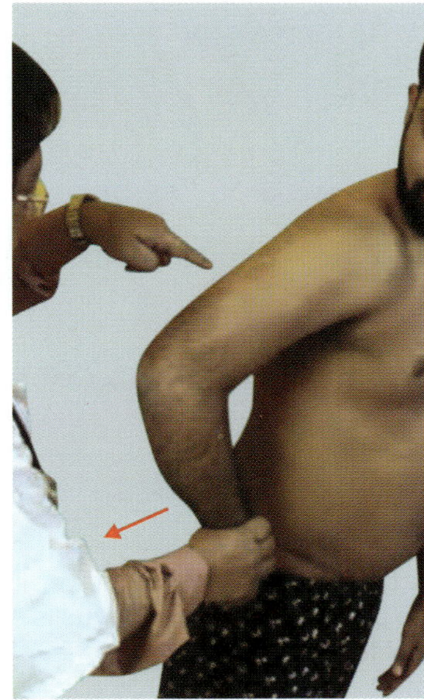

Fig. 3.223: Muscle power testing of **triceps** against resistance

at elbow, and resist flexion. Observe the muscle belly of brachioradialis at upper forearm.

- Triceps (Fig. 3.223): Ask the patient to hold the arm out with the elbow semi-extended. Now, hold at the wrist, stabilise at elbow and resist the extension of forearm. Now palpate the contracted triceps muscle at the back of arm.

- **While testing the 'power' of muscles:** Before testing, always try to demonstrate the movement to the patient rather than explaining it verbally. Always remember that the patient does not know anatomy. Now:
  i. Expose the muscle fully.
  ii. Ask the patient to contract the muscle against your resistance.
  iii. See the muscles contracting
  iv. Feel the strength of contraction, and
  v. Compare with your own strength or what you judge to be normal.
- There are two methods of testing muscle power:
  i. **Isometric testing:** The patient is asked to contract the muscle powerfully and to maintain the contracted position while the examiner tries to keep it in original position. In isometric testing, there is no shortening of muscle.
  ii. **Isotonic testing:** The patient is asked to contract the muscle and the examiner opposes the movement at the initial part of contraction.

Isometric method is more sensitive and detects minor degree of weakness though *isotonic testing is commonly practised* method in neurology.

Q. D/D you will consider in this case:

1. Different causes of proximal muscle weakness.
2. Peripheral neuropathy: Sensory changes, distal involvement, loss of deep reflexes.
3. Motor neurone disease: Adults with asymmetrical wasting and fasciculation.
4. Post-poliomyelitis (Fig. 3.224): Jerks lost with asymmetrical atrophy (characteristics of poliomyelitis: post-febrile, asymmetrical, non-progressive, without any sensory loss and with LMN signs).

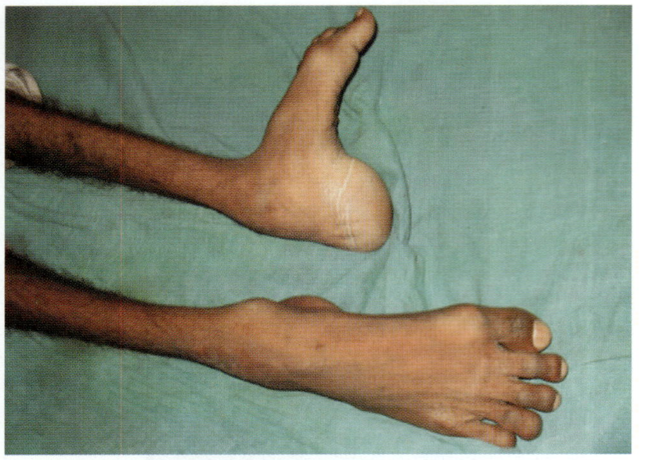

Fig. 3.224: LMN type paralysis of both lower limbs (producing paraplegia) due to **poliomyelitis**; **pes cavus** is due to atrophy of intrinsic muscles of feet

Q. How do you like to investigate myopathy?

1. Enzyme study: Serum aldolase and creatine kinase (CK) are raised. Normal value of aldolase is 1.5–8.1 units/litre and CK is 55–170 units/litre. Enzymes are often increased by 100–200 times than normal.
2. Electromyography (EMG) shows myopathic pattern.
3. Muscle biopsy: 'Confirms' the diagnosis of myopathy (select a symptomatic muscle for biopsy). It shows islands of muscular degeneration as well as regeneration in the ocean of fibrofatty tissue, without any cellular infiltration. There is diminished dystrophin (a protein present on inner surface of sarcolemma, essential for cell membrane stability) level in muscle tissue, determined by immunochemical staining.
4. CSF study and nerve conduction velocity (NCV) are normal.
5. ECG changes: Tachycardia, tall R waves in right precordial leads, deep Q waves in left precordial leads, bundle branch block due to cardiac involvement (cardiomyopathy).
6. Molecular genetic testing.

Q. Do you know its management?

No specific management of muscular dystrophy is available. Few neurologists advocate prednisolone (0.75 mg/kg) for up to 3 years of age for slow progression of the disease. Active exercise, passive physiotherapy, orthopedic measures are often helpful. Usually death occurs in second decade of life due to pneumonia, respiratory failure, cardiomyopathy or cardiac failure.

Q. Identification points:

1. Male child.
2. Waddling gait and positive Gowers' sign (ask the patient for demonstration).
3. Pseudohypertrophy (principally the calf muscles) plus atrophy of muscles.
4. Proximal muscles weakness (ask the patient to get up from sitting position).

- **Becker type** of dystrophy (X-linked recessive) usually starts between 5–25 years. It is the late onset, 'milder form' of myopathy with slow progression as well as less cardiac involvement. The patients are chair-bound 25 years after the onset and may even survive up to 5th or 6th decade. Investigations and management are similar to Duchenne type.
- DMD is caused by mutation of the gene responsible for production of the protein dystrophin.

JERKS AND CLONUS — CASE 96

Q. What is jerk, deep reflex, stretch reflex or tendon reflex?

When a tendon is lightly stretched and struck by a single sharp blow with a soft rubber hammer, there is brief contraction of that muscle, which is known as deep tendon reflex (DTR). The tendon reflex is a '*monosynaptic' stretch reflex* (note: superficial reflexes are *polysynaptic nociceptive reflex*). By elicitation of a jerk, the integrity of the afferent and the efferent pathways along with excitability of the anterior horn cells in the spinal segment of the stretched muscle are tested.

Stretching of muscles → activates muscle spindles → sends afferent signals → leads to direct efferent impulses → muscle contraction.

Q. Prerequisites before elicitation of a jerk:

Before elicitation of a jerk, one must be cautious about following:

1. Use a hammer with firm and flexible shaft.
2. The patient lies supine in the bed in a comfortable and relaxed position.
3. Stand on the right side of the patient (even for elicitation of jerks for the left side).
4. *Explain the procedure to the patient.* Reassure that it will not hurt him.
5. *Tap the tendon, not the muscle belly* (especially in triceps jerk).
6. *Expose the muscle fully* (being tested), which is responsible for the reflex—a must for all the reflexes.
7. Observe both the contraction of the muscle and the movement of the limb.
8. Always compare with the other side and observe for the 'symmetry'.
9. Use the hammer by 'swinging movement' of the wrist joint.
10. *Sudden, single and sharp blow* with sufficient threshold are applied over the tendon.
11. Genitalia should be properly covered while eliciting jerks of lower limbs.
12. Always use same type of hammer in same manner (i.e. maintain the uniformity). Repeat the procedure, if necessary).

- While eliciting different tendon reflexes (*see* below), the position of the limb is maintained in such a way that the tendon to be tapped is slightly stretched.

Q. Jerks commonly examined in clinical neurology with localising value:

Root values and peripheral nerves concerned in different jerks are given below:

1. Ankle jerk ($S_{1,2}$): Medial popliteal nerve.
2. Knee jerk ($L_{2,3,4}$): Femoral nerve.
3. Biceps jerk ($C_{5,6}$): Musculocutaneous nerve.
4. Triceps jerk ($C_{6,7}$): Radial nerve.
5. Supinator jerk ($C_{5,6}$): Radial nerve.
6. Jaw jerk: Trigeminal nerve.

Q. Ankle jerk:

1. Conventional method **(Fig. 3.225)**: The patient lies supine. The thigh is abducted and externally rotated with partial flexion of the knee (for the lower limb to be examined). Now dorsiflex the foot (and slightly evert the foot too) with the left hand and apply a sharp tap on tendo-Achilles. A quick contraction of calf muscles with plantiflexion of foot occur.
2. Special method **(Fig. 3.226)**: The patient takes kneel-down position on a chair with both feet hanging out of the chair. Sharp tap is applied over tendo-Achilles

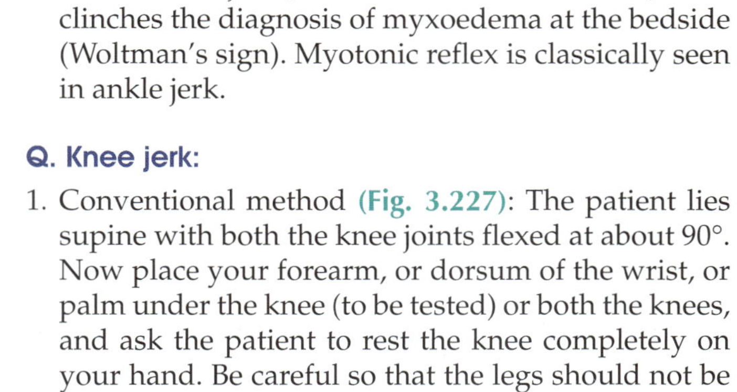

on both sides in turn (do not passively dorsiflex the foot). Calf muscles contract and plantiflexion of foot results. It is done specially on myxoedema patients to observe the delayed relaxation time (myotonic reflex). Careful observation of delayed relaxation time in ankle jerk (due to ↓ muscle metabolism) often clinches the diagnosis of myxoedema at the bedside (Woltman's sign). Myotonic reflex is classically seen in ankle jerk.

Q. Knee jerk:

1. Conventional method **(Fig. 3.227)**: The patient lies supine with both the knee joints flexed at about 90°. Now place your forearm, or dorsum of the wrist, or palm under the knee (to be tested) or both the knees, and ask the patient to rest the knee completely on your hand. Be careful so that the legs should not be in contact with each other in bed. Feel the quadriceps tendon and apply a sharp tap there. The quadriceps muscle contracts with extension of the knee.

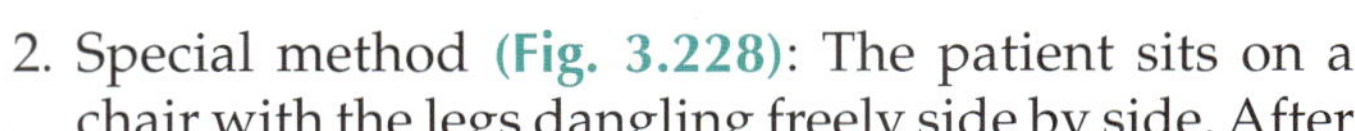

2. Special method **(Fig. 3.228)**: The patient sits on a chair with the legs dangling freely side by side. After

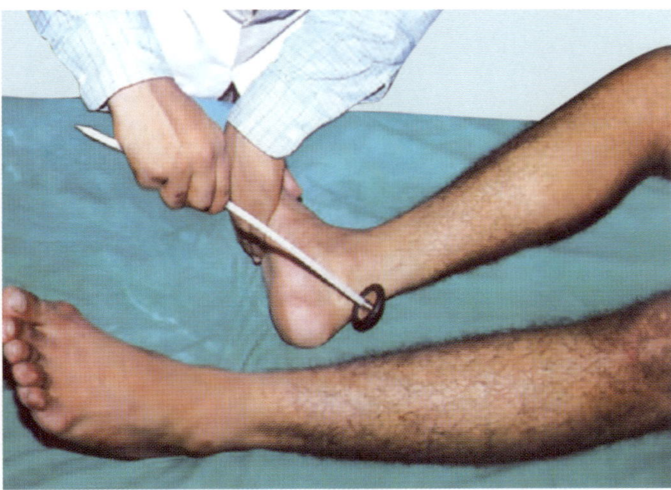

Fig. 3.225: Eliciting **ankle jerk**

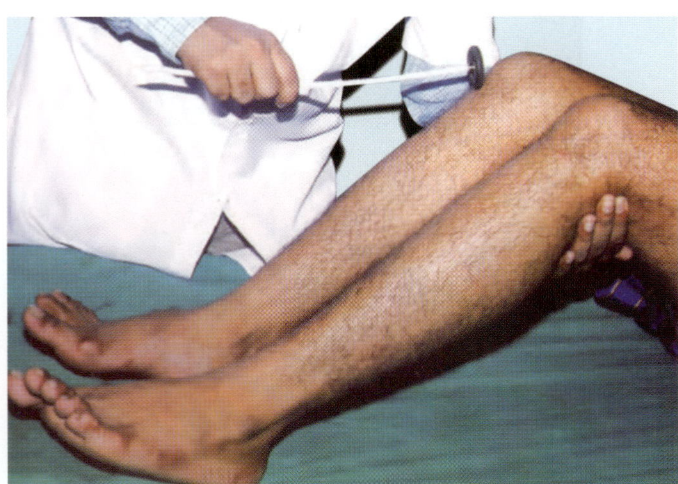

Fig. 3.227: Eliciting **knee jerk**

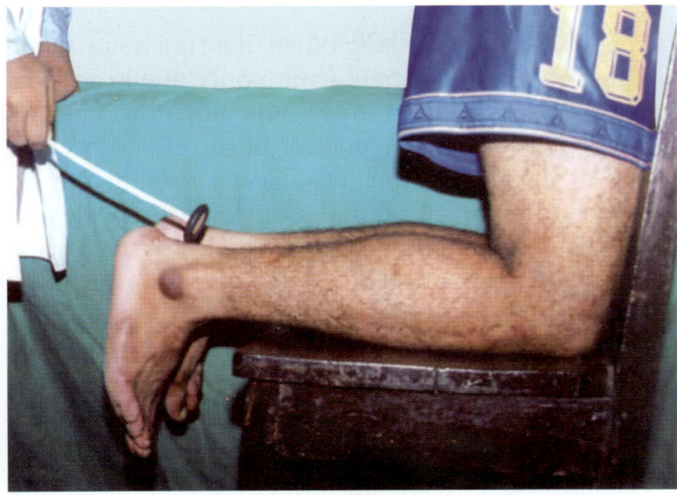

Fig. 3.226: Eliciting **ankle jerk by special method** (on kneeling patient)

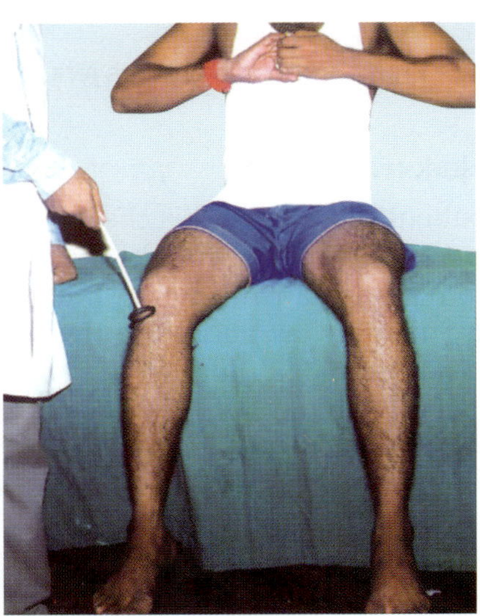

Fig. 3.228: Eliciting **knee jerk by special method** with **'re-inforcement'**

tapping the patellar tendon, look for the pendulous movement of the legs. This is classically seen in cerebellar lesion and sometimes in chorea (indicates hypotonia). Hung-up reflex (the knee may be held in extension for few seconds before relaxing) may be seen by this special method (read the section on 'Cerebellar disorder' for interpretation of pendular knee jerk).

Clinical Wisdom

The 'patella' hammer derives its name from knee jerk (because the patellar tendon is tapped) as it was the first tendon reflex which was regularly practised for neurological examination.

Q. Biceps jerk (Fig. 3.229):

The elbow remains semiflexed at right angle with a semipronated position of the forearm. The limb may rest on patient's abdomen or upon your left hand. Place your left thumb or index finger (*transmitter for blow* from hammer) on the biceps tendon in the antecubital fossa and tap suddenly over your finger. The biceps muscle contracts with flexion of the elbow.

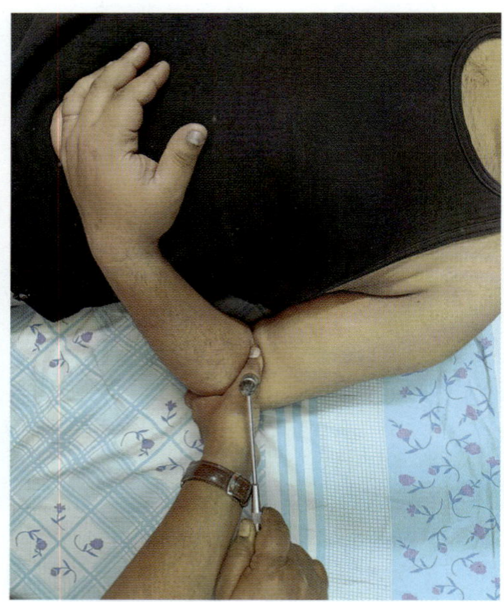

Fig. 3.229: Testing **biceps jerk**

Q. Tricpes jerk (Fig. 3.230):

Place the patient's hand over his chest with the elbow flexed. Support the patient's hand at the wrist by your left hand so that the patient's upper limb does not fall on the bed. Suddenly tap above the olecranon process (strike the triceps tendon, not the belly of the muscle; tap 2" above the elbow) and observe the contraction of triceps with slight extension of the elbow. Muscle contraction after direct hammering is not a stretch reflex.

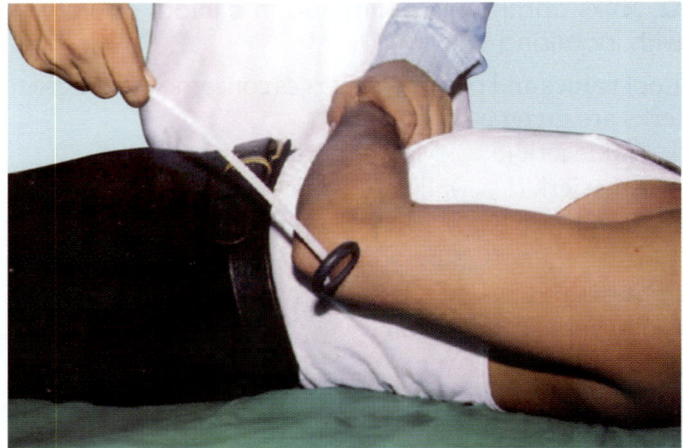

Fig. 3.230: Testing **triceps jerk**

Q. Supinator jerk (Fig. 3.231):

Forearm is semipronated and the elbow is flexed. Hold the patient's hand at wrist (or keep it across the chest or in the patient's lap) and a sharp tap is applied on the styloid process which results in contraction of brachioradialis, supination of the forearm, and flexion of the elbow with minimal flexion of the fingers. As this muscle was previously called supinator longus, the reflex is known as supinator jerk (also referred as radial jerk).

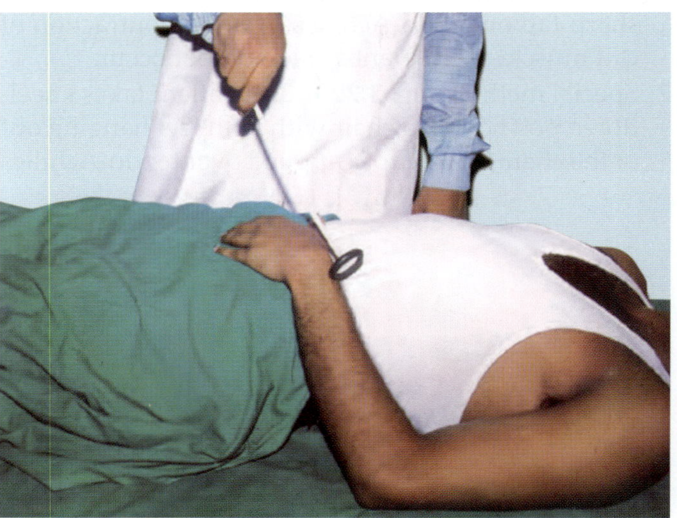

Fig. 3.231: Testing **supinator jerk**

Inversion of supinator jerk: When there is a lesion in the spinal cord at $C_{5,6}$ segment (commonly due to cervical spondylosis resuting in myeloradiculopathy), there is hyperexcitability of the anterior horn cells below this level. So, *during elicitation of supinator jerk*, there is no contraction of brachioradialis but only brisk flexion of the fingers (as $C_{7,8}$ take upperhand) occur; this is inversion of supinator jerk.

Similarly, ***in inversion of biceps jerk*** (lesion at $C_{5,6}$ segment), there is no contraction of biceps *during elicitation of biceps jerk* but one can see the contraction of triceps (as $C_{6,7}$ take upperhand). Inversion of a jerk localises the level of lesion in the spinal cord. Usually, inversion of supinator and biceps jerks are seen in a single patient (i.e. with lesion at $C_{5,6}$ segment), and is most commonly found in cervical spondylosis.

Q. Jaw jerk (Fig. 3.232):

Prerequisites:

1. Preferably the patient should be seated with mouth partially open.
2. Tongue remains inside the mouth.
3. Left thumb or forefinger is placed over the middle of the patient's chin.
4. Strike the hammer lightly on the thumb or forefinger in a downward direction.

The normal response is slight and consists of sudden closure of the mouth due to contractions of masseter and temporalis. *This reflex is just present, or absent in health.* The jaw **jerk is increased in** bilateral UMN (bipyramidal) lesions above the Vth cranial nerve nucleus, e.g. pseudobulbar palsy or multiple sclerosis. Both the afferent and the efferent fibres pass through the trigeminal nerve, and the centre for this reflex lies in the pons. Interpretation regarding mere presence or briskness is often very difficult.

Q. What is finger-flexion jerk (Fig. 3.233)?

Its presence indicates hyperreflexia, and exaggeration or asymmetry suggests UMN lesion on the abnormal side.

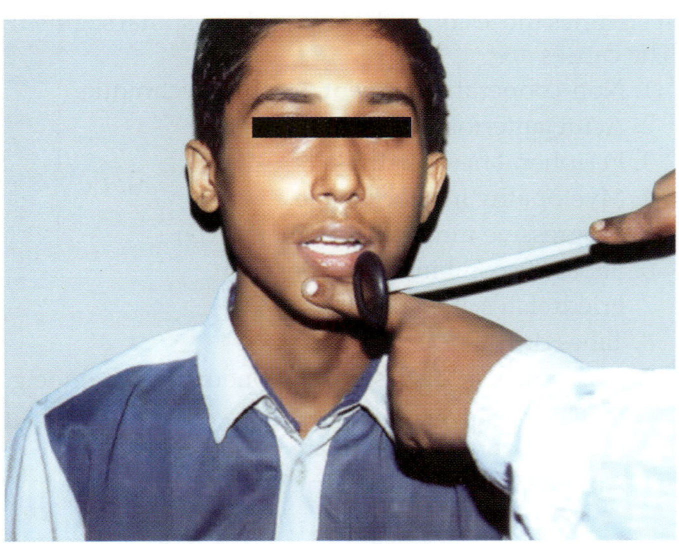

Fig. 2.232: Testing **jaw jerk**

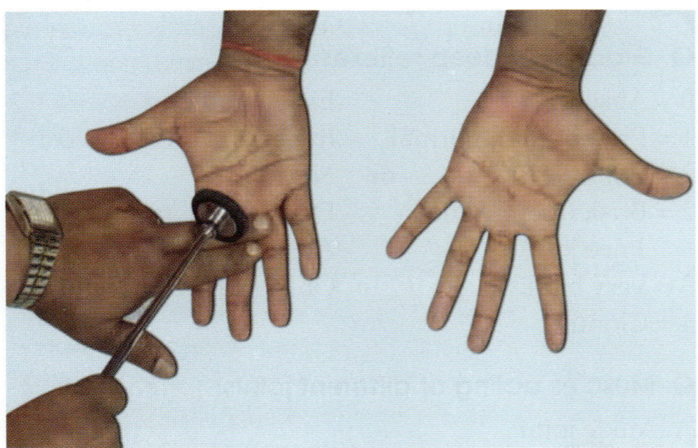

Fig. 2.233: Eliciting **finger-flexion jerk**

The tips of your middle and index fingers are placed across the palmar surfaces of the proximal phalanges of the patient's relaxed fingers. A sudden tap by a hammer on your fingers produces flexion of patient's fingers, but a very brisk contraction indicates hyperreflexia. The root value of this reflex is $C_{7,8}$ and T_1, and the peripheral nerves involved are median and ulnar nerve.

Q. Hoffmann's sign (reflex) (Fig. 3.234):

Flex the DIP joint of patient's middle finger with your index finger and thumb, and now flick it down suddenly. The response is brisk flexion and adduction of the thumb as well as flexion of the tip of other fingers. It is also a manifestation of hyperreflexia. This reflex may not be present in all patients with pyramidal tract lesion and moreover, it may be present in a nervous individual without any organic lesion. If the reflex is seen on one side (unilateral) only, it may have some value as a sign of pyramidal tract lesion. The root value of the reflex is C_8, T_1.

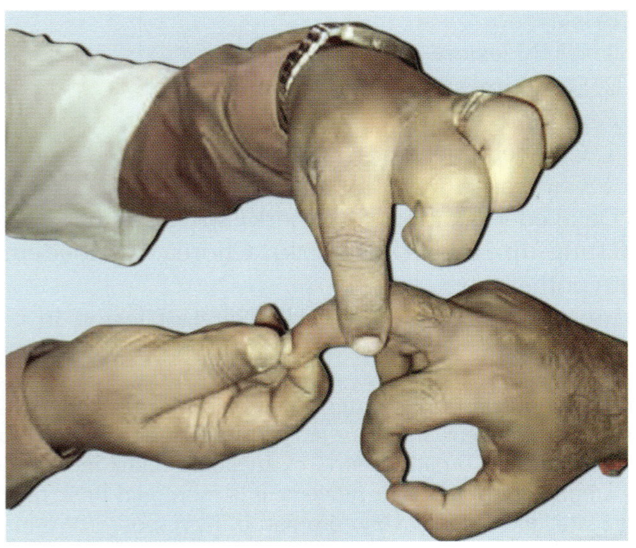

Fig. 2.234: Eliciting **Hoffmann's sign** (reflex)

Q. Wartenberg's sign (Fig. 3.235):

Interlock the flexed fingers of the patient with your flexed fingers and try to pull apart. In health, the thumb remains abducted and extended but in pyramidal tract lesion, the thumb flexes and adducts.

Q. Interpretation of tendon reflexes:

A. Present: In health.

B. Lost or diminished:

   1. LMN lesion (poliomyelitis, syringomyelia, peripheral neuropathy, tabes dorsalis, peroneal muscular atrophy).
   2. UMN lesion in shock stage.

- Isolated loss of a reflex usually suggests radiculopathy. Symmetrical loss of reflex may be found in peripheral neuropathy. Reflexes may be absent if the patient is 'unable to relax'.

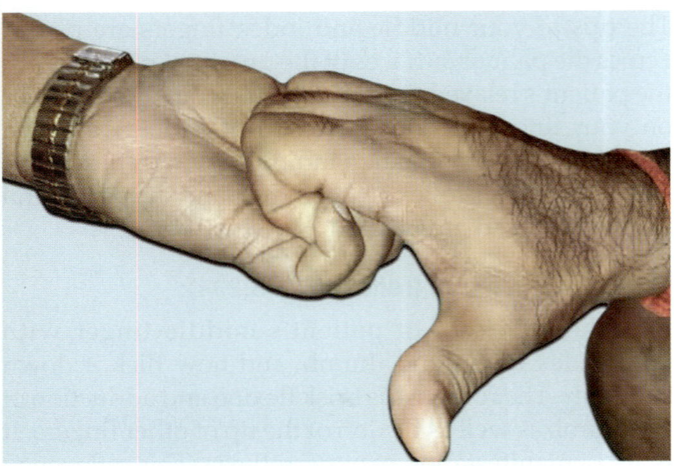

Fig. 2.235: Eliciting **Wartenberg's sign**

C. Exaggerated:
 1. Anxiety neurosis, nervousness, hysteria.
 2. Thyrotoxicosis.
 3. Tetany.
 4. Tetanus.

D. Brisk:
 1. UMN lesion.
 2. Sometimes in hypoglycaemic coma.

E. Pendular:
 1. Cerebellar lesion.
 2. Chorea.

F. Delayed relaxation (ankle jerk): Myxoedema.

G. Hung-up reflex (knee jerk): Chorea, myxoedema, hypothermia.

H. Inversion of supinator jerk: Level of lesion in $C_{5,6}$ spinal segments.

- **Hyperreflexia** means exaggerated or brisk response. For a beginner student, it is very difficult to differentiate between the two. In a broader sense, exaggerated reflex means the 'amplitude' of the limb movement is more and brisk reflex means, the reflex is very 'prompt' in its response. We may conclude that hyperreflexia is only of pathological significance when it is asymmetrical (comparing with the other side) or if associated with other signs of UMN lesion (spasticity, Babinski's sign, etc.)
- **A reflex seems lost or diminished in defect of technique, relaxation, or observation.**
- Sometimes, lesion in the spinal cord may give rise to 'crossed reflex induction', e.g. while eliciting a knee jerk on right side, it may produce a reflex response on the left knee jerk.

Q. What is Jendrassik's manoeuvre?

It is also known as 'reinforcement'. When the deep reflexes or jerks are not elicited by routine manoeuvre, reinforcement is applied for augmentation of response. It is done by distraction of patient's attention. Ask the patient:

1. To make a fist with the contralateral hand, or
2. To interlock the fingers of two hands together and then pull them as hard as possible (Fig. 3.228), or
3. To clench the teeth, or
4. To push the knees hard together.

It is very important to remember that this phenomenon lasts for less than a second. So the patient is asked to do the manoeuvre almost synchronously with the tapping of the tendon (the procedure must be demonstrated to the patient before tapping the tendon). Reinforcement (to make some strong voluntary muscular effort) acts by:

a. Increasing the excitability of the anterior horn cells, and
b. Increasing the recruitment of gamma-fibres, i.e. increasing the sensitivity of the muscle spindle primary sensory endings to stretch (*increased gamma fusimotor drive*).

- **Always perform the Jendrassik's manoeuvre before declaring a tendon reflex 'absent'.**
- For upper limb reflexes: 1, 3, 4, for lower limb reflexes: 2, 3.

Q. Causes of delayed relaxation of ankle jerk:

1. Myxoedema (the contraction phase is delayed too)—Commonest cause, 2. Gross pedal oedema, 3. Hypothermia, 4. Obesity, 5. Parkinsonism, 6. Anorexia nervosa, 7. Advanced age.

Q. Causes of loss of knee jerk:

It signifies the lesion at the level of $L_{2,3,4}$ spinal segment. The causes are:

1. Non-cooperative patient or faulty technique.
2. Acute anterior poliomyelitis.
3. Peripheral neuropathy.
4. Myelopathy in shock stage.
5. Progressive musclar atrophy (MND).
6. Subacute combined degeneration.
7. Friedreich's ataxia.
8. Tabes dorsalis.
9. Sometimes in diseases of myoneural junction (e.g. myasthenic crisis).
10. Muscular dystrophy in late stages.
11. Ankylosis of the knee joint.

- In case of loss of deep reflex restricted to one limb only, one should not forget acute anterior poliomyelitis, entrapment neuropathy, leprosy and diabetic mononeuropathy.

Q. Grading of deep reflexes:

0 = Absent		Exaggerated or hyperactive +++
1 = Present (as a normal ankle jerk)	**or**	Normal ++
2 = Brisk (as a normal knee jerk)		Diminished +
		Absent–
3 = Very brisk		Only with reinforcement ±
4 = Clonus		

Q. Muscles acting of different joints:

A. Ankle joint:
 a. Dorsiflexion: Tibialis anterior (Fig. 3.236).

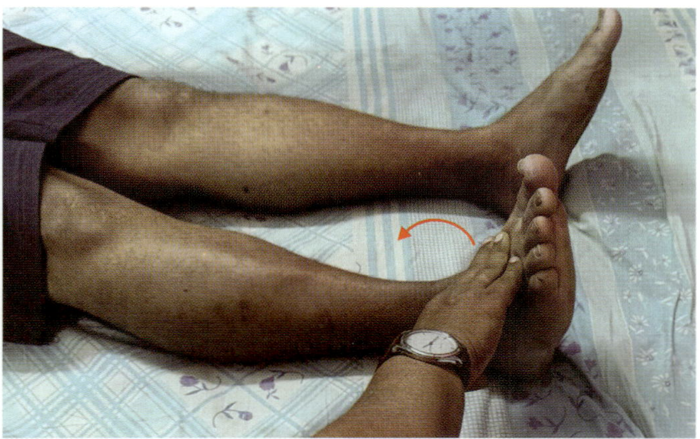

Fig. 3.236: Muscle power testing of **tibialis anterior** against resistance

b. Plantiflexion: Gastrocnemius and soleus (calf muscles) (Fig. 3.212).
c. Inversion: Tibialis anterior and tibialis posterior (Figs 3.236 and 3.237).
d. Eversion: Peroneus muscles.

B. Knee joint:
a. Extension: Quadriceps femoris (i.e. three vasti muscles like vastus lateralis, vastus medialis and vastus intermedius + rectus femoris) (Fig. 3.213).
b. Flexion: Hamstring muscles (biceps femoris, semimembranosus and semitendinosus) (Fig. 3.238).

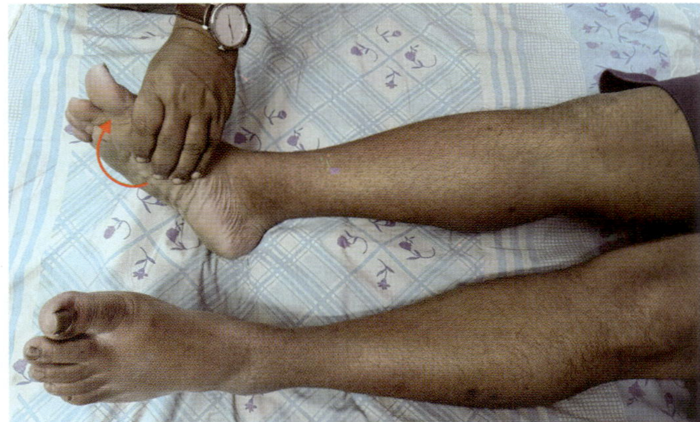

Fig. 3.237: Muscle power testing of **tibialis posterior** against resistance

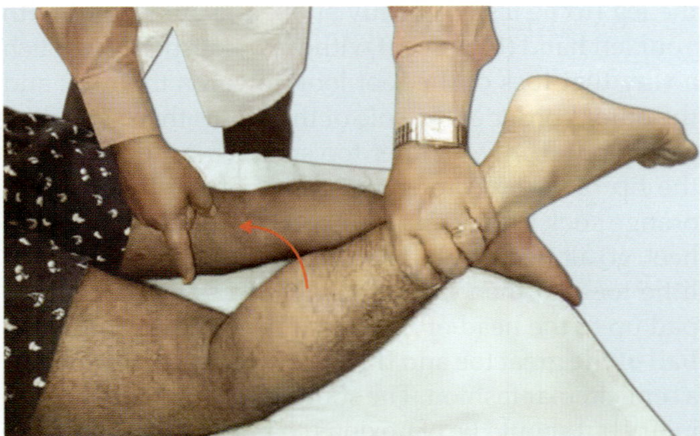

Fig. 3.238: Muscle power testing of **hamstring muscles** against resistance

C. Hip joint:
a. Extension: Gluteus maximus mainly (Fig. 3.214).
b. Flexion: Iliopsoas (Fig. 3.239).
c. Adduction: Adductor muscles (adductor longus, brevis and magnus).
d. Abduction: Gluteus medius and minimus, tensor fascia lata (Fig. 3.215).

D. Elbow: Flexion (biceps brachii), extension (triceps brachii); **wrist** (flexor and extensor muscles); **hand** grip (long flexors).

E. Small muscles of hand and foot (finer movements).

Q. Muscles acting on neck, shoulder and trunk:

A. Neck:

a. Extension: Trapezius and paravertebral muscles.
b. Flexion: Sternocleidomastoid, scalene, longus colli, longus capitis, rectus capitis, platysma.

B. Shoulder:

a. Extension: Latissimus dorsi, teres major and minor, posterior deltoid.
b. Flexion: Pectoralis major, anterior deltoid, coraco-brachialis, biceps brachii (weakly assist).
c. Abduction: supraspinatus, deltoid (middle fibres), trapezius, serratus anterior.
d. Adduction: Pectoralis major, latissimus dorsi, teres major, triceps brachii (long head).

C. Trunk (vide page 136):

Stabilizing the body in everyday tasks, protection of viscera, assist essential body activities (e.g. breathing), rotation of body and helping elevation of head in supine position.

The abdominal part of anterior trunk muscles are rectus abdominis, external and internal oblique, transversus abdominis, pyramidalis.

Q. What is clonus?

It is the rhythmical, involuntary contraction of a muscle or group of muscle in response to sudden, passive and sustained stretching. Clonus is always associated with brisk tendon reflex, spasticity and Babinski's sign. It is

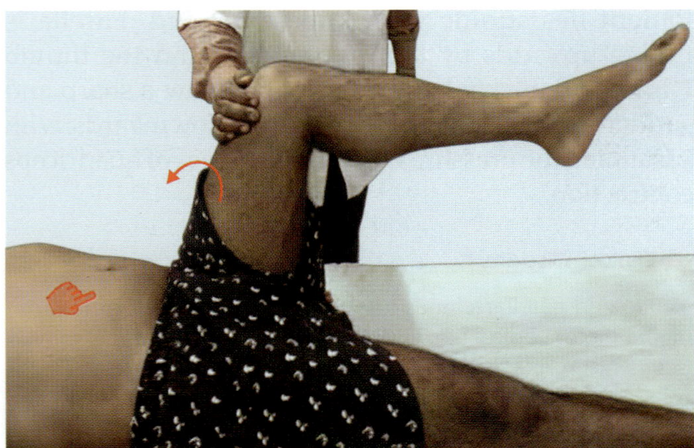

Fig. 2.239: Muscle power testing of **Iliopsoas muscle** against resistance

a very reliable sign of pyramidal tract lesion. There are two types of clonus:

1. Sustained clonus (true clonus).
2. Unsustained clonus (pseudoclonus).

Q. Sites for clonus in clinical neurology:

1. Ankle clonus.
2. Patellar clonus (or knee clonus).
   (No. 1–2): Routinely practised in clinical neurology.
3. Jaw clonus (elicit the jaw jerk to see a series of closure and opening of the mouth).
4. Wrist clonus (elicited by sudden passive hyper-extension of the wrist with maintaining the stretch on long flexors of the palm, which will evoke clonic movement of palm at wrist).

Q. Ankle clonus (Fig. 3.240):

Patient lies supine. Support the **flexed knee** (both knee and ankle resting in 90° flexion) with your left palm by placing it in popliteal fossa in such a way that heel rests gently on the bed. Now suddenly dorsiflex the foot by grasping the forepart of it with your right hand. A series of contraction and relaxation of calf muscles are seen if a steady pressure is maintained on the foot by the right hand.

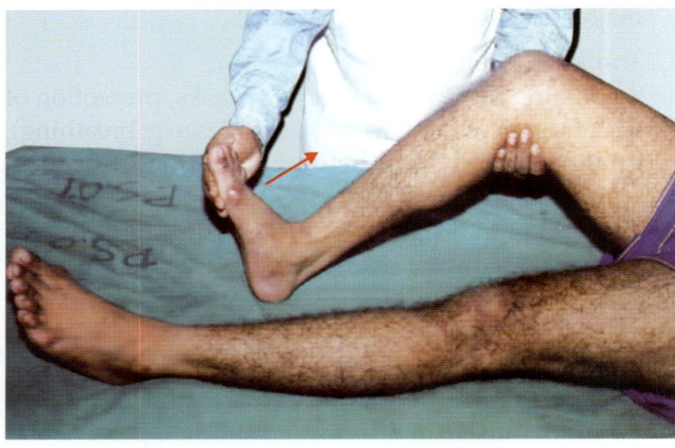

Fig. 3.240: Eliciting **ankle clonus**

Q. Patellar clonus (Fig. 3.241):

Patient lies supine with **knee extended**. Patella is pulled upwards by the index finger and the thumb with a fold of skin behind the palm. Now a sharp and sudden displacement of the patella downwards with sustaining the pressure will produce series of quadriceps contraction.

Clinical Wisdom

Ankle and patellar clonus are produced as a result of loss of upper motor control (i.e. UMN lesion) over $S_{1,2}$ and $L_{2,3,4}$ spinal segments, respectively.

Q. Pseudoclonus:

1. The clonus is not sustained inspite of a steady pressure.

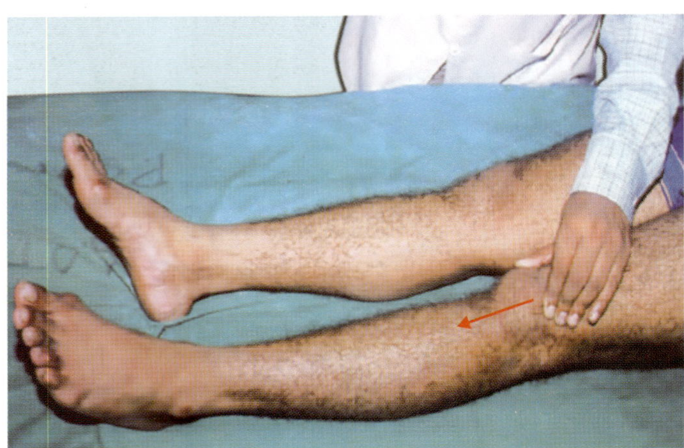

Fig. 3.241: Eliciting **patellar clonus**

2. Irregular in rate (usually less than 6 at a time) and rhythm.
3. It is commonly seen in anxiety, tense persons, often in hysteria and thyrotoxicosis.
4. Plantar response is always flexor.

- Many a time, the boundary between true and pseudoclonus is not very clear.

Clinical Wisdom

It you are in doubt whether the clonus is true or pseudo, immediately do the following:

1. Plantar response will be extensor in true clonus and flexor in pseudoclonus.
2. Examine the pulse for any abnormality (high volume in thyrotoxicosis, tachycardia in anxiety) and look for fine tremor (anxiety, thyrotoxicosis)—if present, indicates pseudoclonus.

- **Never forget to examine a patient for clonus if there is presence of brisk tendon reflex.**

PLANTAR RESPONSE (REFLEX) CASE 97

Q. Method of elicitation (Fig. 3.242):

One should learn how to elicit this superficial reflex properly. At first, educate the patient about the procedure. The patient lies supine with extended legs and relaxation of the muscles of the lower limbs. Hold the leg (to be tested) firmly above the ankle joint with your left hand (to prevent withdrawal response) in such a way that toes of the foot look towards the roof; and the outer border of the sole of the foot is then scratched gently but firmly (neither too speedy nor too slow) by the tip of a key (preferable), stick of the hammer, an orange stick (ideal) or a blunt needle. Starting from the heel, go along the lateral border of the sole towards the little toe and then turn medially across the metatarsal pad up to the head of 2nd metatarsus **(never touch the ball of the great toe and the flexor creases of the toes)** in a semicircular fashion. The stimulus should not produce injury but should be of noxious character (a combination of pressure, pain and touch) since this is a 'nociceptive reflex'. A strong stimuli is needed in the presence of thick

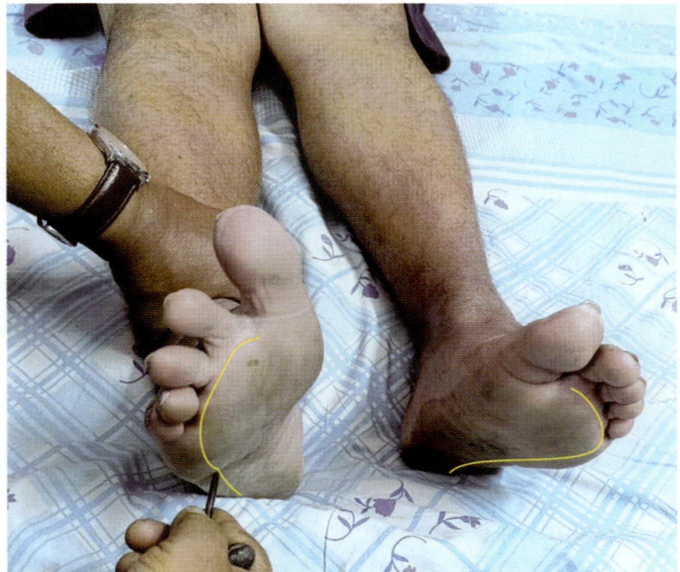

Fig. 3.242: Elicitation of **plantar response**

sole of the patient. Stop stimulating the sole as soon as you get the first movement of the great toe. One may do the test once or twice, and not for multiple times. Now do the test on the other side. Plantar response is a spinal reflex arc modified by the pyramidal tract.

It is the most important and most frequently misinterpreted reflex in the body.

Q. What is the 'normal' plentar response?

The normal response of this age-old sign in neurology is 'flexor' in type and is manifested by:

1. Flexion of all the five toes.
2. Dorsiflexion and inversion of the foot (with a stronger stimulus).
3. Contraction of adductors of the thigh, sartorius and tensor fascia lata (minimal response).

- While eliciting plantar response in a normal healthy person: Slight stimulus—No. 3 occurs, slightly stronger stimulus—No. 1 and 2 occur, even on still stronger stimulus—withdrawal of the limb occurs.

Q. Precautions taken before eliciting plantar response:

1. Assess the thickness of the sole (by touching it): Thick sole may be responsible for 'no response'.
2. Look for any deformity of great toe: Move the great toe, and confirm that it is moving freely and is not rigid (e.g. hallux rigidus, rheumatoid arthritis).
3. Knee must be extended.
4. Sole should be made warm (e.g. by rubbing with your palm, especially in winter season).
5. Leg should lie straight (do not allow rotation of thigh) and heels should rest on the bed.
6. One may assess the power of extensor hallucis longus before doing the test (Fig. 3.19) (optional).
7. Ask the patient whether sensation in sole is intact or not (may confirm by touching the sole with your palm).

Q. What is the root value of this reflex?

It is the sacral spinal nerve S_1.

Q. Why the lateral aspect of the sole is stimulated?

1. Probably the receptors for extensor plantar response are present there in abundance and thus, even in minimal UMN lesion, extensor plantar response is obtained by stimulating the lateral aspect of the sole.
2. If the medial aspect of the sole is stimulated, it may elicit flexion (even in the presence of UMN lesion) of all the toes as part of the grasp reflex, itself a different phenomenon.

Q. What are the different plantar responses?

Usually there are 5 types of responses:

1. Flexor.
2. Extensor (up-going toe).
3. Equivocal.
4. No response.
5. Withdrawal response.

Q. Briefly describe the different responses:

A. **Flexor:** Normal response; already described.

B. **Extensor** (extensor plantar response is also known as "Babinski's sign"). The responses are:
   1. Dorsiflexion (extension) of the great toe (movement occurs at the metatarsophalangeal joint) which usually precedes all other movements mentioned below.
   2. Fanning (spreading out) and extension of outer four toes.
   3. Dorsiflexion of the ankle, and flexion of the knee and the hip.
   4. Contraction of tensor fascia lata.

In 1896, Babinski first described this sign. Josef Jules Francois Felix Babinski (1857–1932) was a French physician cum neurologist. This sign is regarded as THE SIGN in clinical neurology.

C. **Equivocal**, i.e. incomplete response or variable response. When the full components of the extensor response is not manifested, e.g. (i) only fanning of outer four toes is seen without any movement of the great toe, or (ii) the hemiplegic side does not show any response and the healthy side shows flexor response (sometimes seen in early cases of CVA), or (iii) asymmetry of 'flexor' response on both sides. *Remember, today's equivocal response may be tomorrow's extensor response.*

D. **No response** (mute or zero response): After striking the sole of the foot, there is no movement of any of the toes.

E. **Withdrawal response:** Often withdrawal response is seen in anxious individuals or in normal persons with hyperaesthetic/sensitive sole. It is seen that the initial normal flexor response is quickly followed by mass extension of toes with withdrawal of the entire leg.

- The afferent nerve of this reflex (plantar response) is tibial nerve; the efferent nerve is tibial nerve for flexor response and peroneal nerve for extensor response.
- Babinski's sign is the most senstive, delicate and reliable sign of corticospinal tract lesion.
- In hemiplegia or paraplegia (i.e. UMN lesion), the plantar response remains extensor lifelong.
- 'Crossed' extensor response: On unilateral stimulation of the sole in a case of bilateral cerebral or spinal cord lesion, bilateral extensor response can be evoked (e.g. in severe spastic paraplegia).

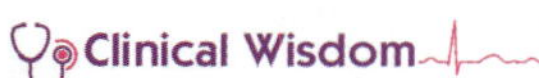

Clinical Wisdom

An extensor plantar response should be reproducible.

Q. Significance of presence of Babinski's sign:

It signifies pyramidal tract lesion with or without anatomical discontinuity. The causes are:

1. **Pyramidal tract lesion** (i.e. UMN lesion above the S_1 level of the spinal cord).
2. Children below 1 year of age (due to lack of myelination of pyramidal tract).
3. Deep coma due to any cause.
4. Deep sleep.
5. Deep anaesthesia, neuroleptics or narcotic overdose; hypnosis; drugs (e.g. barbiturates).
6. Metabolic encephalopathy.
7. Often in hypoglycaemia (even in the absence of coma).
8. Immediately after the attack of generalised convulsions or epilepsy (post-ictal phase).
9. Electroconvulsive therapy.
10. Physical exhaustion (e.g. marathon runner).
11. Apnoea phase of Cheyene-Stokes respiration.

Clinical Wisdom

Except 1, all are the causes of lesion in pyramidal tract without anatomical discontinuity, and thereby produce transient plantar extensor response. No. 8, 9 and 10 are due to exhaustion of corticospinal tract.

Q. 'Reinforcement test' of plantar response, if any:

1. Rotating the patient's head to opposite side.
2. Knee must be extended during the test.
3. Apply warmth to the cold skin of the sole.

Q. 'No response' or loss of plantar response reasons behind:

1. Faulty technique.
2. Thick sole.
3. Coldness of the feet.
4. Stage of 'neural shock'.
5. Peripheral neuropathy.
6. Myelopathy involving S_1 segment.
7. Paralysis of dorsiflexors of the foot.
8. Hallux valgus or hallux rigidus.

Q. What are the 'plantar equivalence'?

In case of widespread and severe UMN lesion, the reflexogenic receptor zone over the lower limb may be greatly widened and an 'extensor' plantar response may be evoked by different techniques. This is the basis of multiple signs or plantar equivalance. They are:

1. **Oppenheim's sign** (Fig. 3.243)**:** Heavy pressure is applied by the thumb and index finger from above downwards to anterior surface of tibia (to its medial side). The extensor response usually occurs towards the end of the stimulation.
2. **Gordon's reflex:** Squeezing or applying deep pressure to calf muscles produce extensor plantar response.
3. **Schaeffer's sign:** Extensor plantar response is evoked after applying deep pressure to tendo-Achilles.
4. **Chaddock's sign:** Extensor response is seen after striking the skin around the lateral malleolus in a circular fashion
5. **Bing sign:** Pricking the dorsum of foot or the great toe by a pin produces extensor response.
6. **Moniz sign:** Extensor response is seen after forceful passive plantar flexion of ankle.
7. **Gonda sign:** Extensor resopnse is elicited after forceful stretching or snapping of distal phalanx of either of the 2nd or 4th toe.
8. **Brissaud's reflex:** It is the contraction of tensor fascia lata as a part of extensor response (palpate the upper and lateral part of thigh for appreciation). *This is helpful in patients with amputated or absent great toe, or complete paralysis of extensors of toes.*

- 1, 2, 3 and 4 are commonly practised 'alternative methods' to elicit plantar response.
- **These reflexes are useful** in non-cooperative patients or when the soles are extremely sensitive or the soles are wounded/ injured.

Q. What is Rossolimo's sign?

Method: Either tap the ball of the foot (by percussing the plantar surface of the ball of the great toe with a hammer) or flick the distal phalanges of the toes into

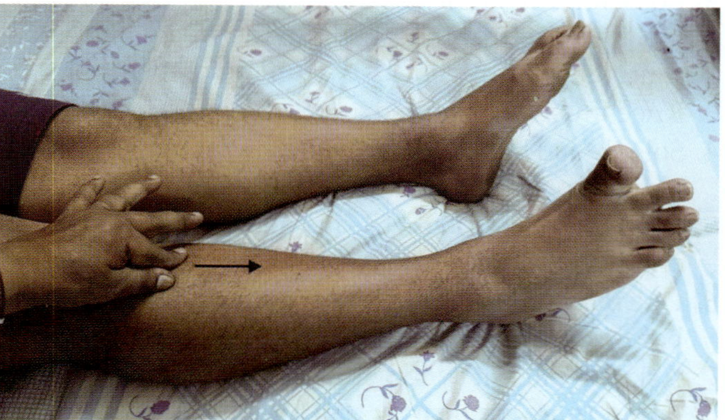

Fig. 3.243: Elicitation of **Oppenheim's sign**

extension, and then allow them to fall back into their normal position.

Response: Pyramidal tract lesion, manifested by plantiflexion of all the five toes (only sign with UMN lesion, manifested by plantiflexion of great toe). It is the homologue of Hoffmann's sign of upper limb.

Q. Plantar response is extensor with loss of ankle jerk:

In UMN lesion, plantar response is extensor and ankle jerk is brisk. But this may not happen in:

1. Subacute combined degeneration (SCD) of the spinal cord.
2. Taboparesis (GPI plus tabes dorsalis).
3. Friedreich's ataxia.
4. Cauda-cona lesion (cauda equina lesion with lesion in conus medullaris).
5. Combined cervical and lumbar spondylosis.
6. Rarely in the stage of spinal shock.

Q. Plantar response is flexor with brisk ankle jerk:

1. Sometimes in anxiety and thyrotoxicosis (exaggerated deep reflex).
2. Hepatic pre-coma.

Q. Why the ball of the great toe is not touched while eliciting plantar response?

During the elicitation of plantar response, one should stop scratching the sole at the head of 2nd metatarsus. If the ball of the great toe is scratched, there may be dorsiflexion of the great toe (by direct stimultion) in the absence of any UMN lesion. It is why the root value of the plantar resonse is only the 1st sacral segment (S_1) of the spinal cord.

Clinical Wisdom

The first movement of the great toe is important. Extension of great toe after a brief initial flexion is not extensor response. Remember, there is nothing called negative or positive Babinski's sign.

Pseudo-Babinski's sign may be seen in plantar hyperaesthesia, chorea or dystonic posture of great toe.

TROPHIC CHANGES (NEUROGENIC) CASE 98

Q. What are the trophic changes?

1. Trophic changes in the skin and appendages (i.e. hairs and nails).
2. Trophic ulcers, and
3. Charcot joint (neuropathic joint).

Q. Changes in the skin and appendages:

1. Dry, rough and cold skin.
2. Pigmentation.
3. Local cyanosis or local oedema.
4. Hypohydrosis (lack of sweating).
5. Hypotrichosis (fall of hairs).
6. Brittle nails.

Q. Sites examined for trophic changes:

Denudation of skin with ulcer **(bed sore)** (Fig. 3.244) formation over the bony prominences is seen:

1. On the lateral malleolus.
2. Back of the heel of foot.
3. Shoulder girdles.
4. Over the sacrum (classical bed sore).

- Bed sore or pressure sore may form in a patient with prolonged recumbency (with or without urinary or fecal incontinence), especially without change of posture.

Q. What is trophic ulcer or perforating ulcer?

The perforating ulcers are usually present **over the heel** or **ball of the great toe** (Fig. 3.245). During walking, heel is touched first in the ground and thus, it is a common site for pressure sore formation. The patients with foot drop touches the ground with the ball of the toes (leprosy, diabetes mellitus) and thus, trophic ulcer forms there. In syringomyelia and tabes dorsalis, the ulcer is usually situated in the heel (as no foot drop is there). Trophic ulcer is usually painless.

- 'Tropical ulcer' (totally different from trophic ulcer) is a chronic form of callous ulcer with its edge raised and undermined. It often refuses to heal.

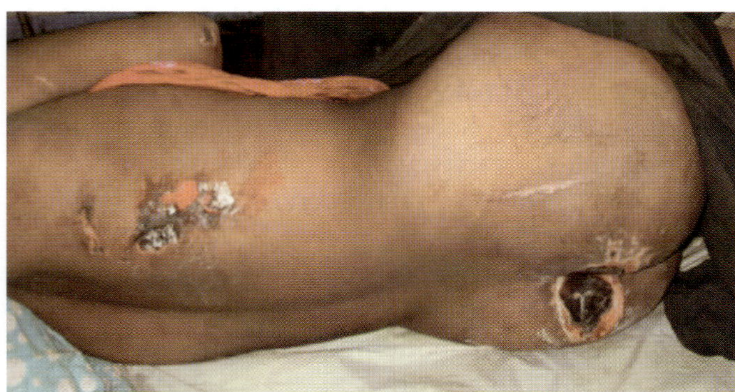

Fig. 3.244: **Bed sores** (trophic changes) with exposed deeper tissues are seen over buttock and inferior angle of right scapula in a paraplegic patient

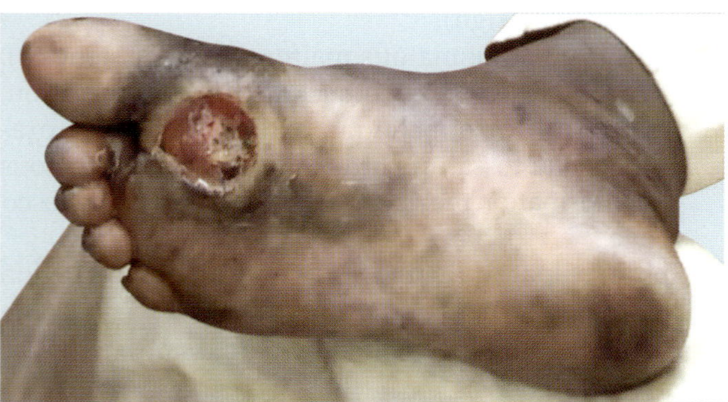

Fig. 3.245: **Perforating ulcer** over ball of the great toe in a case of peripheral neuropathy with foot drop

Q. Common causes for trophic ulcer in feet:

Same as the causes of Charcot joint or neuropathic joint (*see* Case 99).

- Peripheral nerve injury (in legs) and spina bifida may give rise to trophic ulcer in feet.

Q. Aetiopathogenesis of trophic changes:

1. Loss of muscular action upon the circulation.
2. Vasomotor paralysis due to destruction of the vasoconstrictor (sympathetic) fibres, and
3. Partly due to disuse.

- **Search for trophic changes in hemiplegia, paraplegia and peripheral neuropathy patients.**
- **Autonomic nervous system (ANS)** may be involved in hypothalamic disorders, diabetes mellitus or spinal lesions. The points noted during examination of ANS are: Sleep disorder (insomnia or somnolence, sleep apnoea), temperature regulation, genital dysfunction (impotence or amenorrhoea), sweating (diminished or excessive), postural or orthostatic hypotension (syncope or fainting), trophic changes (e.g. ulcer), Horner's syndrome, bladder and bowel dysfunction (urinary incontinence or urgency, diarrhoea or constipation), pupillary areflexia.

Q. Points to note in examination of cranium and spine in neurology:

A. **Cranium** (inspection, palpation, percussion and auscultation):
   1. Microcephaly (cerebral palsy), macrocephaly (hydrocephalus, Paget's disease) or turricephaly (tower-like peaked appearance due to synostosis of sutures), dolichocephaly (long antero-posterior diameter), brachycephaly (short antero-posterior diameter) or oxycephaly (cone-shaped and pointed head).
   2. Haematoma, elevation, fracture or depression, scar mark, secondaries in skull, mass in multiple myeloma, scalp tenderness, tender temporal artery (i.e. giant cell arteritis).
   3. Fontanelle (tense fontanelle is seen in hydrocephalus and raised intracranial tension).
   4. Sutures (springing of the sutures is seen in hydrocephalus).
   5. Cracked-pot sound in hydrocephalus, on percussion (Macewen sign).
   6. Bruit (in angiomatous malformation or stenosis): Carotid artery bruit in neck at carotid bifurcation, vertebral or subclavian artery bruit at supra-clavicular fossa, and bruit in cerebral arteriovenous malformation may be heard over cranium or closed eye.

B. **Spine** (palpate the spine from cervical to sacral region for any tenderness or deformity):
   1. Any tenderness (elicited by percussion).
   2. Kyphoscoliosis.
   3. Gibbus (e.g. caries spine, metastasis, trauma) (*see* Fig. 1.22).
   4. Spina bifida occulta [by inspecting the tuft of hair (Satyre's tail), dimpling of skin, fibrofatty tumour or dilated vessels over the sacrum].
   5. Short neck (cranio-vertebral anomaly) and low hairline.
   6. Bruit heard over spine in vertebral angiomatous malformations.
   7. Examine the movement of spine by asking the patient to bend forward, backward and sideways.

Clinical Wisdom

One must examine the spine in all neurological cases, especially in paraplegia.

CHARCOT JOINT — CASE 99

Q. What is Charcot joint (Fig. 3.246A and B)?

This is a chronic, progressive degenerative arthropathy (also known as **neuropathic joint**) resulting from disturbance in the sensory innervation of the involved joint. The characteristics are:

1. Huge swelling of knee, hip, ankle or shoulder joint **(most common site is knee joint)**.
2. Painless (most characteristic).
3. Disorganised, deformed and destroyed joint.
4. Increased mobility (rarely, genu recurvatum may be produced) of the joint and thus, easy dislocation is possible: Unstable or subluxation of the joint.
5. Loose bodies may be palpated in the joint cavity and crepitus may be felt with new bone formation (osteophytes).

Q. What are the common causes of neuropathic joint?

Neuropathic joint commonly develops from:

1. Leprosy (commonly affects the upper extremity).
2. Diabetes mellitus (tarsal and metatarsal joints mostly affected).
3. Syringomyelia (shoulder, elbow and wrist joints mostly involved).
4. Tabes dorsalis (knee, hip and ankle joints commonly affected).
5. Hereditary sensory neuropathy or after repeated intra-articular injection of steroid (rare).

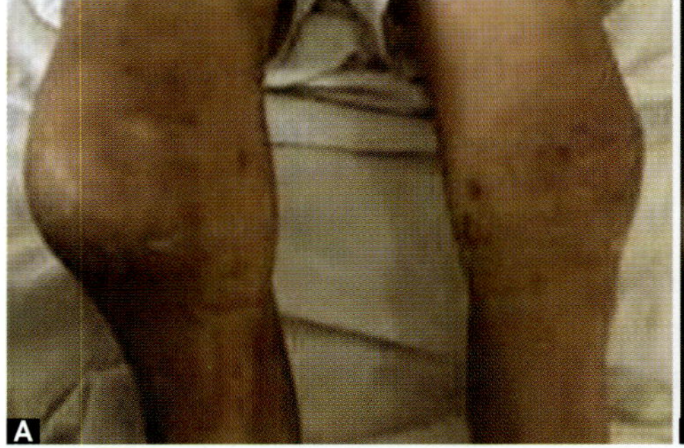

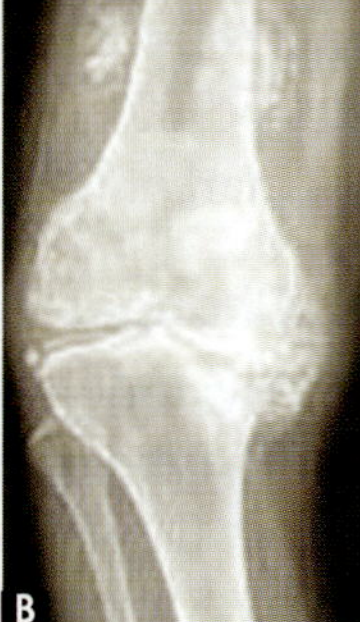

Fig. 3.246: (A) Painless and swollen knee (Charcot joint) in diabetes mellitus; (B) X-ray of same destroyed joint

Q. Most important neurological sign tested in a patient of Charcot joint:

Posterior column sensations, i.e. joint, position, muscle, vibration and pressure senses are lost here. Charcot joint is the complication of chronic loss of proprioception.

Q. Pathophysiology of development of Charcot joint:

There are two theories:

1. Loss of proprioception → leads to recurrent trauma → damage goes unnoticed by the neuropathic patient → ultimately leads to progressive destruction, degeneration and disorganisation of the joint.
2. Hyperaemia results from neurally mediated vascular reflex → leads to increased osteoclastic bone resorption.

Q. Basic principles of testing sensory functions:

Sensory evaluation is the most unreliable part of neurological examination as it is subjective (i.e. examiner has to rely on patient's reports) and is difficult to quantify. Basic principles of testing are:

1. Explain the patient clearly what is going to be tested; patient's cooperation and alertness are essential. Try to gain confidence by proper understanding.
2. Anatomical knowledge of sensory system (e.g. dermatomes) is essential for proper interpretation.
3. *First test with eyes open and then with eyes closed.*
4. Always compare the sensory function with the opposite side for symmetry.
5. First apply the sensory stimulus to the area of altered sensation and delineate its borders by testing from abnormal to normal area. Ask the patient to say 'yes', if he feels anything.
6. Test from less sensitive to more sensitive area.
7. A hairy area may be shaved before testing.
8. Test the spinal segments or **dermatomes** sequentially (e.g. in the lower limb, first examine the L_1 segment and then proceed downwards for L_{2-5} segments and again upwards for S_{1-4} segments present in different places in the said limb) (Fig. 3.247).

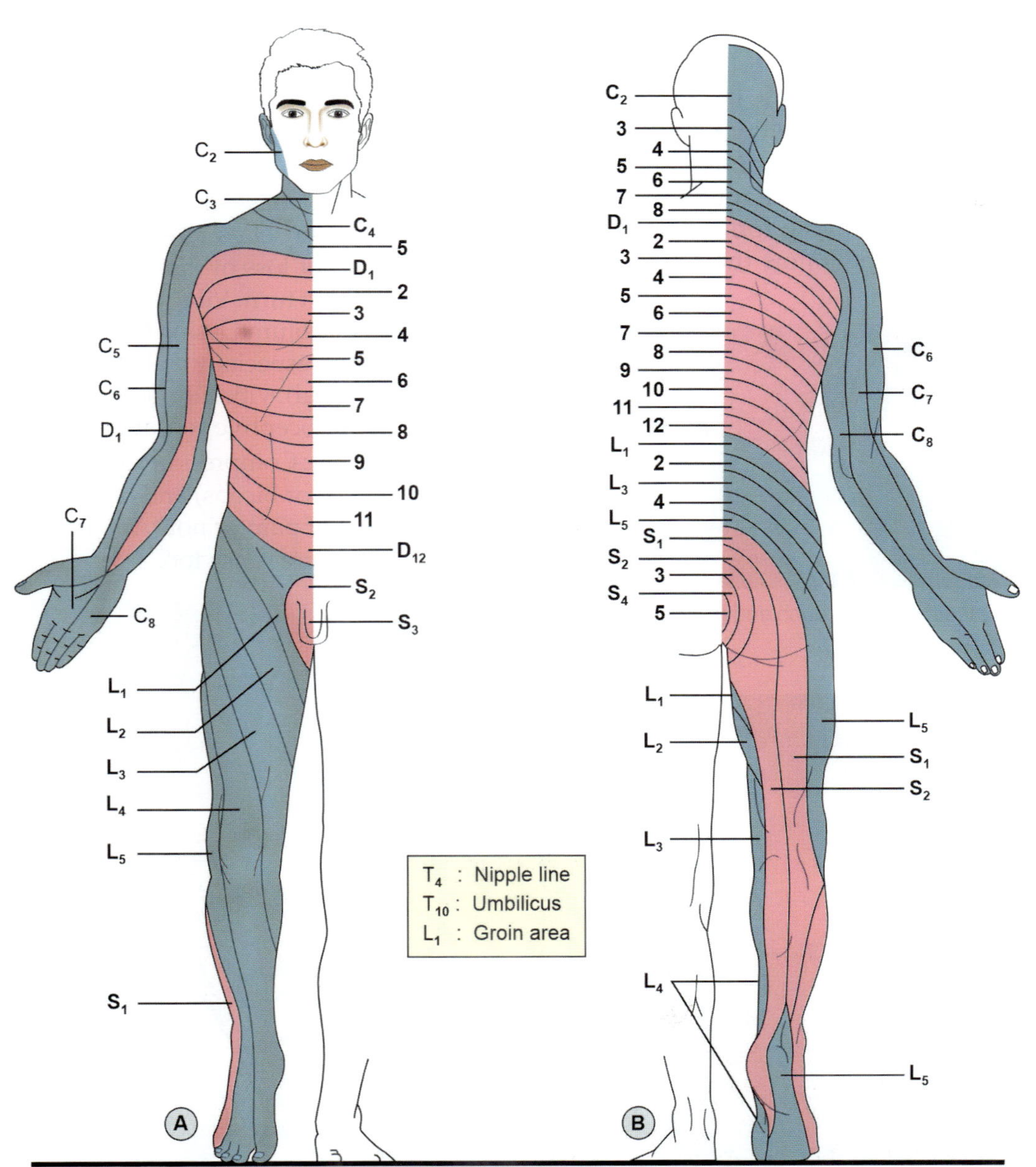

Fig. 3.247: **Dermatomes** of body: (A) Front view; (B) Back view

- Cervical (C_1) has no cutaneous supply, which only supplies meninges.

Superficial or exteroceptive sensations (spinothalamic tract functions) tested are:

a. Touch (Fig. 3.248A): *Fine touch* is tested with a small piece of cotton wool which is twisted into fine hair while *crude touch* may be tested by the wider side of a cotton wool or the tip of index finger. Fine touch sensation may be evaluated over toes, metatarsal heads, heels, and dorsum of feet with a 10-g monofilament (Semmes-Weinstein monofilament, used as a semi-quantitative test of sensory loss), especially in a patient of diabetes. Compare either side for symmetry.

b. Pain (Fig. 3.248B): Usually tested by a pin (avoid heavy pressure; use both ends of the pin separately, i.e. the patient should say sharp for the sharp end and blunt for the head end of the pin); select the presternal area for baseline sharpness before testing a limb; ask whether the quality of sensation becomes sharper or painful (hyperaesthesia), or feels blunter (hypoaesthesia).

c. Temperature (Fig. 3.249): Actually it is tested by two test tubes containing cold (5°–10°C) and hot (40°–45°C) water touched on face, forearms, hands, trunk and legs in a random sequence; a rough assessment is done by the metal of tuning fork or stethoscope (cold), or by rubbing the palms (hot) as a clinical bedside routine. A normal person can appreciate even a difference of 1°C.

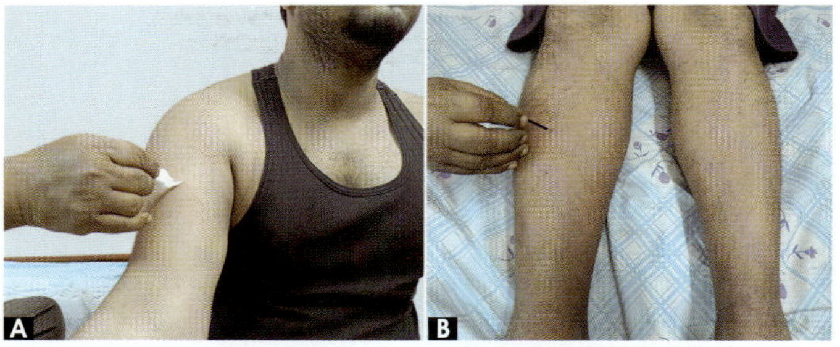

Fig. 3.248: Sensory testing for (A) touch and (B) pain sensation

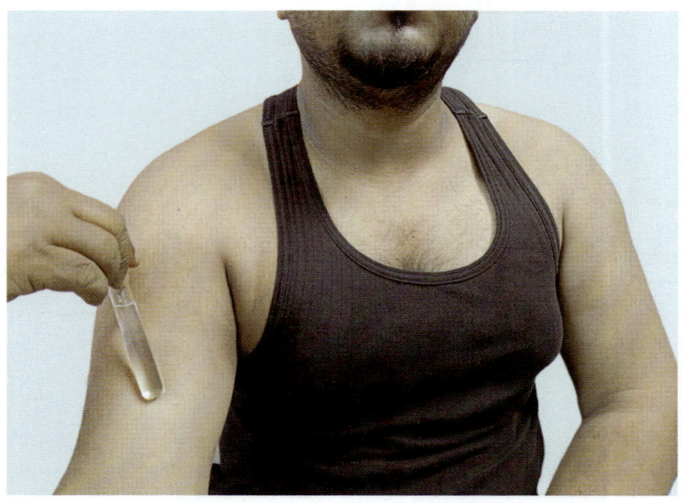

Fig. 3.249: Sensory testing for **temperature sensation**

- Deep pain sensation is tested by squeezing the calf muscles, tendo-Achilles or testes.

Q. How to test for deep and cortical sensations?

Deep or proprioceptive sensations (posterior column functions) tested are:

A. Vibration sense (Fig. 3.250): It is the test of repeated touch sensation in quick succession. First keep the vibrating tuning fork (128 cycles/sec) over the sternum so that the patient can identify the sense of vibration or buzzing (not the touch sensation). On a particular site, vibration sense should be perceived minimally for 10 seconds. Instruct the patient to close his eyes. For the *lower limb*, hold the vibrating fork sequentially over the great toe, dorsum of foot, medial malleolus, tibial shaft (shin) and tuberosity, and anterior superior iliac spine. In the *upper limb*, the fork is kept sequentially over DIP and PIP joints of forefinger, dorsum of hand, wrist joint, olecranon process and over the shoulder tip. In the *trunk*, it is tested by placing the fork over ribs, sternum, clavicles and vertebral spines. Always compare with the other side. From time to time, judge the patient by stopping vibrating fork with your hands. The rule goes like this—if the distal vibration sensation persists, it is useless to examine the proximal parts but in case of loss of distal sensation, always move proximally in turn. Vibration sense is commonly lost in posterior column lesion (tabes dorsalis), peripheral neuropathy (especially diabetes mellitus) and old age (physiological). Vibration sense is lost earlier than the other proprioceptive sensations.

B. Muscle sense: Compress or squeeze big muscle bellies (calf, triceps or biceps) and note whether the patient complains of pain or not (Abadie's sign). This is the test of pressure sense too.

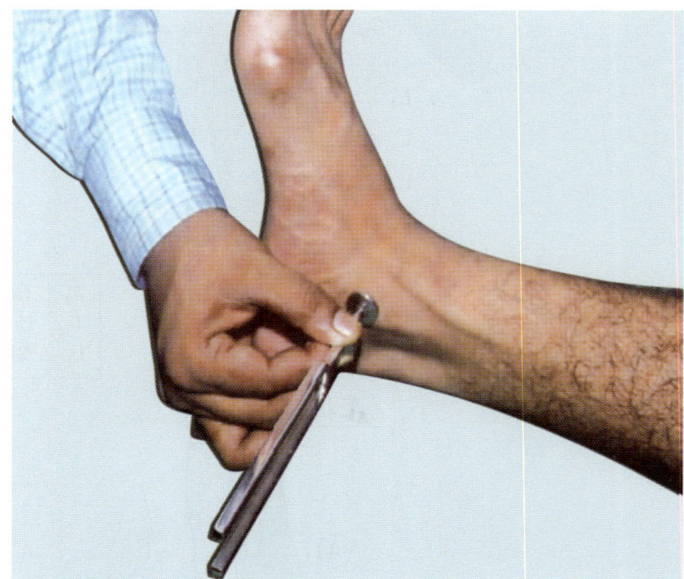

Fig. 3.250: Testing **vibration sensation** at the ankle

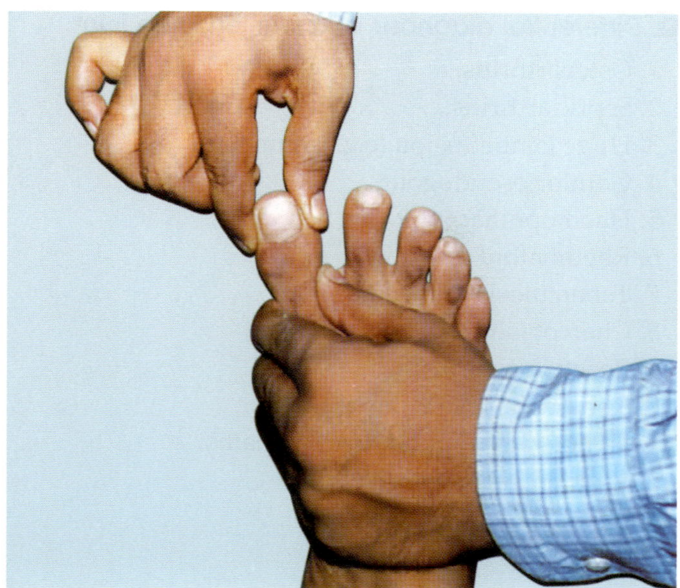

Fig. 3.251: Testing **joint-position sense**

C. Joint and position sense (Fig. 3.251): First, explain the patient about the test with movements of joints ('it is up' or 'it is down'). Now, ask the patient to close the eyes. For examination of the lower limb, grasp the proximal phalanx of great toe by your left hand, and hold the *medial and lateral borders of the distal phalanx* with the thumb and index finger of your right hand so that pressure above and below does not reveal the direction of movement. Move the distal phalanx up and down at random (15°–30°) and ask the patient whether any movement is perceived by him or not (joint sense), and to identify the direction of movement (position sense). In health, movements of <10° can be perceived at all normal joints. In the upper limb, this test can be done in the index finger. Perform the test on the other limb too. If there is impaired joint sense in small joints, test the big joints in turn. Caution should be taken during the test so that your fingers should not rub against the patient's other toes. *At least four wrong answers* should be received before declaring the joint sensation impaired or lost. Position sense can also be tested by instructing the patient to keep one limb in a particular position and then ask him to keep the opposite limb in the similar position.

Cortical sensations (parietal lobe functions) tested are:

A. One point (tactile) localisation (Fig. 3.248A and B): Ask the patient to localise accurately parts of his body when touched by a cotton wool or pin (eyes remain closed).

B. Two point discrimination: It is tested by the use of blunt compass, two-point discriminator or divider (eyes remain closed). In health, a minimum distance of 2–3 mm on the lips, 3–5 mm on the finger tips, 2–3 cm on the dorsum of hands, or 3–4 cm on the dorsum of the foot can be recognised as two different stimuli. Explain the test to the patient and try to measure the minimum distance at which two separate points can be identified.

C. Stereognosis: Small objects of various size, e.g. coins, match box, pencil, key (i.e. familiar objects) are placed in the patient's palm and asked to identify while the eyes remain closed. Recognition of size, shape, weight and form of a common object, and identification of it by touch and manipulation is known as *stereognosis*. Patient's failure is known as astereognosis. Impaired or lost stereognosis is a feature of parietal lobe lesion.

D. Graphaesthesia: Draw letter, number, diagram or circle with a blunt object, or with your index finger over the patient's back, thigh or forearm (eyes remain closed). A normal person can easily identify the letter or number written on the skin surface (graphaesthesia). This is lost in affection of parietal lobe.

E. Sensory extinction (sensory inattention, sensory neglect, perceptual rivalry): Homologous points on two sides of the body are pricked with a pin separately (eyes remain closed). If the patient can identify the pin prick in both the situations, the previous points are now pricked 'simultaneously'. In unilateral parietal lobe lesion, the sensation on the opposite side is not perceived by the patient.

- Cortical sensations are carried to contralateral parietal lobe through peripheral nerves via posterior column. If peripheral nerves or primary sensations are at jeopardy, it is useless to test cortical sensations.
- See page 164 for different sensations carried through spinothalamic tract and posterior column.

Q. What are the patterns of different sensory disturbances?

Sensory modalities should be tested in search of a pattern consistent with spinal cord, spinal root or peripheral nerve abnormalities.

1. Peripheral neuropathy: Symmetrical 'glove and stocking' paraesthesia or anaesthesia (i.e. graded sensory loss), affecting the distal parts more; involves all modalities of sensations.
2. Nerve root lesion: Pain is often felt more than the loss of touch sensation; dermatomal pattern of sensory loss in the distribution of nerve roots.
3. Complete section of the spinal cord: Loss of all modalities of sensations below the level (i.e. with a definite sensory level); a narrow zone of hyperaesthesia on the top of anaesthetic zone. 'Sacral sparing' may be present in few cases of high cord compression.
4. Hemisection of the spinal cord (Brown-Sequard syndrome) Vide page 149.
5. Cauda-cona (cauda equina plus conus medullaris) lesion: 'Perianal anaesthesia', i.e. all modalities of sensations are lost involving lower sacral segments. In cauda equina lesion, there is asymmetric sensory loss in lower limbs.
6. Anterior spinal artery syndrome, e.g. in anterior spinal artery thrombosis there is loss of pain, crude

touch and temperature on both the sides below a level, with preservation of proprioception; there is flaccid and areflexic paraplegia. Remember, spinal cord is supplied by one anterior spinal artery and two posterior spinal arteries.

7. Posterior spinal artery syndrome: It is just the opposite of the anterior spinal artery syndrome. There is loss of joint, position and vibration sense below a particular level with preservation of touch, pain and temperature; there is absence of motor deficit. It is commonly seen in tabes dorsalis.
8. Central cord lesion, e.g. in syringomyelia (syrinx is a fluid-filled cavity within the spinal cord), there is affection of spinothalamic tract due to involvement of fibres crossing the cord from both sides in the anterior commissure though it spares the posterior column. Thus, touch sensation persists but pain and temperature sensations are lost (dissociated anaesthesia). The sensory loss is in shawl-like distribution ('sleeve jacket' anaesthesia).
9. Mid-brainstem lesion: Ipsilateral sensory loss in face with contralateral sensory loss on the body (i.e. crossed sensory loss). There is loss of touch, pain and temperature sensations as a result of affection of trigeminal tract or nucleus, and lateral spinothalamic tract.
10. Thalamic lesion: Contralateral loss of all modalities of sensations (position sense is affected more) on one side of face and body. There may be history of spontaneous, disabling type of pain i.e. hyperpathia (thalamic pain).
11. Parietal lobe syndrome: Loss of tactile localisation and tactile discrimination, presence of astereognosis, graphaesthesia and sensory inattention (i.e. loss of cortical sensations).

- **Dissociated sensory loss** (a sign of spinothalamic tract involvement with sparing of posterior column), i.e. loss of pain and temperature with preservation of touch (fine) sensation is found in:
  1. Anterior spinal artery thrombosis.
  2. Syringomyelia, haematomyelia, hydromyelia, intramedullary tumour.
  3. Posterior inferior cerebellar artery syndrome (or lateral medullary syndrome).
  4. Brown-Sequard syndrome (hemisection of spinal cord).
  5. Leprosy neuropathy (small fibre neuropathy).

Q. What other signs will you search in a patient with Charcot joint?

Always search for trophic ulcers in the heel or ball of the great toe in a patient with Charcot joint.

Q. Radiological features of Charcot joint (Fig. 3.246B):

1. Osteopenia (bone density is less).
2. Sharp cortical margin.
3. Severe disruption and disorganisation of the joint.
4. Inappropriate new bone formation; loose bodies.

Q. Differential diagnosis of a swollen knee joint:

1. Osteoarthritis.
2. Septic arthritis.
3. Huge joint effusion (e.g. traumatic).
4. Gout or pseudogout.
5. Haemophiliac joint.
6. Rheumatoid arthritis.
7. Tuberculosis of the knee joint.
8. Charcot joint.
9. Reactive arthritis.
10. Rheumatic fever.
11. Seronegative spondyloarthropathy.
12. Psoriatic arthritis.

- Except 8, all are painful joints.

Q. Management of Charcot joint:

Treatment is usually conservative.

1. Treatment of the underlying disorder.
2. Stabilisation (or immobilisation) of the joint is done by braces and splints.
3. In case of diabetes mellitus, prevent weight bearing in the foot for 2 months to prevent severe disease (trophic ulcer, etc.); proper shoe-wear.
4. Lastly, fusion of a very unstable joint may be done. Palmidronate or calcitonin supplements may be of some help.

Clinical Wisdom

In a suspected patient of Charcot joint:
1. Test the joint for pain sensation (by moving the joint).
2. Test for posterior column sensations.
3. Always search for trophic ulcers in foot.

ABNORMAL GAIT — CASE 100

Q. What is gait?

It is the posture of the patient during walking (decubitus means posture of the patient in bed).

Q. Precautions taken before examination of gait:

The pattern of gait very often gives *a clue to neurological disorder*. Normal body posture and locomotion require integration of motor and sensory system, extrapyramidal system, visual information, intact labyrinthine function and proprioception—the last one is the most important. One should ascertain the following facts before the examination of gait:

1. Examine the stance. Is the patient able to walk? Any deviation? Any tendency to fall?
2. Exclude the disease of joints and bone, or surgical causes producing disorders in gait (say, osteoarthritis of the hip).
3. Legs should be adequately exposed (i.e. at least upto the knee). Feet should be bare.

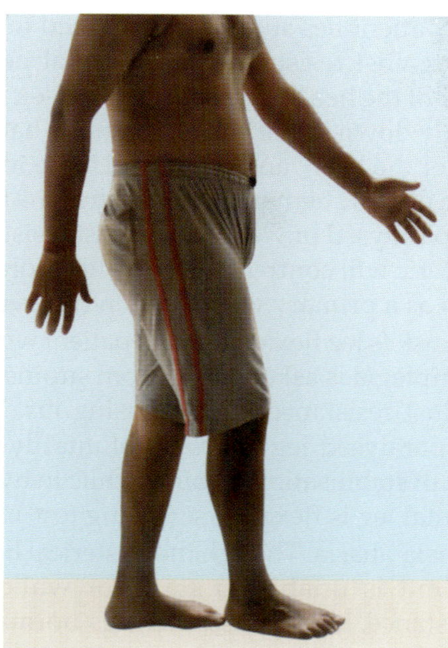

Fig. 3.252: Demonstration of **tandem gait** (heel to toe walking)

4. The patient is asked to walk freely in the room, and then along a straight line (crack or glass placed in floor-mosaic); and then to turn and walk back in the original position.
5. Look for ease of turning, stopping, and movement of arms and legs.
6. The patient may be asked to walk on toes or on heels. 'Tandem gait' (heel to toe gait, i.e. heel of one foot is touched by toes of other foot) should always be examined. Tandem literally means 'one behind another' (Fig. 3.252).
7. Ability of jumping and hopping may be observed.
8. Assure the patient of his safety by your close presence.

- During walking look meticulously for posture (e.g. stooped), arm swinging, associated involuntary movements, pain complained, fall towards one side, turning around, symmetry of steps and width of the base.

Q. What is stance?

It is known as 'attitude of the patient on standing'. The bipedal stance is examined by asking the patient to stand erect with feet close to each other. First examine with eyes open, then with eyes closed. Observe for any unsteadiness, swaying, deviation or tendency to fall. Often the patient is asked to stand on one foot at a time, then to stand on toes, and then on heels. The patient may be pulled abruptly backwards from the shoulders while noting his balance (i.e. postural reflex). Stance in different disease are:

1. Hemiplegic stance: The patient stands with extended and adducted lower limb with plantiflexed foot on the affected side, keeping the body weight on the healthy side. The affected upper limb is typically flexed, adducted and semipronated, and there is flexion of the wrist, MCP and IP joints with slight adduction of the thumb.
2. Wide base stance: The patient stands with legs and feet placed wide apart to keep balance of the body weight, and is classically seen in alcoholics, sensory ataxia, myopathy and peripheral neuropathy.
3. Stance with unilateral cerebellar disease: The affected-sided shoulder is held at a lower level and the body weight is thrown on the healthy side. 'Head tilt' is observed towards the affected side.
4. Stance in parkinsonism: The patient stands in a general attitude of flexion (typical 'stoop'). The head is slightly flexed on the trunk and there is general flexion of the spine. All the limbs are held in flexion in all the joints and the hands may exhibit static tremor.
5. Lordotic stance: In proximal pelvic muscles weakness (e.g. myopathy), the patient can stand erect with an exaggerated lumbar lordosis. In weakness of erector spinae muscles (e.g. spinal muscular atrophy), the patient also stands with a lordotic stance.
6. Hysterical stance: The patient starts swaying which starts in hips instead of ankles but never falls on the ground. The effects are same whether the eyes are open or remain closed (false-positive Romberg's sign).

Q. Different types of gait:

1. Hemiplegic or spastic gait: This is seen in hemiplegic patients (UMN lesion) after recovery. The patient walks on a narrow base, the hemiplegic limb is held stiffly, and does not flex at the knee and hip. While the patient drags his affected foot, the foot is raised from the ground by tilting the pelvis and the leg is swung forward forming a semicircle or an arc—known as 'circumduction' of the leg. The outer side of the sole of the shoe is worn (as there is plantiflexion on the affected side). The affected arm is carried in a flexed, adducted and internally rotated position and does not swing naturally. The hemiplegic gait is essentially a spastic gait.
2. Scissors or spastic paraplegic gait: The patient stands with crossed legs (often with a stick in one hand). Each leg is advanced slowly and stiffly with restricted motion at the knee and hip. He steps one limb in front of the other in a semicircular fashion ('scissoring' of gait), mimicking to walk on toes. It is found in patients with spastic paraplegia and cerebral diplegia; in bilateral pyramidal tract lesion, there is adductor spasm of thigh, resulting the legs crossing each other.
3. Stamping gait: This is the gait of posterior column lesion or sensory ataxia, and is classically seen in tabes dorsalis. The patient stands on a broad base with careful watch on the ground. He raises his foot suddenly to abnormally high level (as he does not know where the foot is), jerks them forward and bring them on the ground with a stamp (the heel touches the ground first and one may find a trophic ulcer in the heel) due to lack of proprioceptive

sensation. These patients are severely ataxic with eyes closed (ataxia is more at night). Romberg's sign is present in patients with stamping gait.

4. High-stepping gait or equine gait: This type of gait is found in patients with foot drop and is commonly seen in peripheral neuropathy, acute anterior poliomyelitis or common peroneal nerve palsy. This is just like the gait of sensory ataxia where the patient elevates his legs to a high level and bring them on the ground with a slapping noise. As there is foot drop, toes touch the ground first (trophic ulcer is found over the ball of the great toe) though a high-stepping attitude is adopted by the patient in order to avoid injury to the toes.
5. Festinant gait: It is the gait of parkinsonism (read the section on 'Parkinsonism'). It is worthwhile to remember that a patient of parkinsonism may run better than walk or walk backward better than forward.
6. Waddling gait: The walking becomes a 'waddle', i.e. the pelvis being poorly supported by each leg. It is seen is proximal pelvic muscle weakness. Read the section on 'Myopathy'.
7. Reeling, staggering, drunken or ataxic gait: This is seen in cerebellar ataxia and alcoholic intoxication. The patient walks on a broad base, the unsteady feet are planted widely apart and placed irregularly. The patient sways from side to side. The steps are uncertain, some are shorter and some are longer than intended, and the patient tends to fall or deviate to the side of cerebellar lesion. The ataxia is equally severe whether the eyes are open or closed. Tandem walking is virtually impossible. Read the section on 'Cerebellar disorder'.
8. Prosthetic gait: This is the gait with an artificial limb.
9. Limping gait: This type of gait is adopted due to joint diseases (e.g. tuberculosis of the hip), talipes equinovarus or any painful condition in the lower extremities (even in Achilles tendonitis or heel pain).
10. Hysterical or functional gait: The patient often walks with bent knees or trunk. This is a bizarre gait with combination of all the varieties (hemiplegic, paraplegic, ataxic, etc.) and does not resemble any known pattern of organic disease. The patient drags the affected leg with an exggerated delay, while the typical circumduction is absent; but walks normally in the absence of an observer. He/she never falls during walking. Hysterical hemiplegia patient should be examined for (to differentiate from organic hemiplegia):
    a. The patient lies supine and is asked to raise one leg against resistance. In a normal person, the back of the heel of the contralateral leg is pressed firmly down in the bed (examiner's hand placed under the heel), and the same is true in a patient with organic hemiplegia when he/she tries to lift the paralysed or weak leg against resistance. The hysteric will contract the good leg more strongly than as a primary willed action **(Hoover's sign)**.
    b. Babinski's leg flexion test: If a patient with organic hemiplegia is asked to sit (from supine position) against resistance without using his/her arms, the paralysed leg flexes involuntarily owing to lack of stabilisation of joints while in hysteria the normal leg is flexed first ('rising test').
    c. Astasia-abasia: Though the hysterical hemiplegic patient is unable to stand or walk without assistance, he/she uses his legs normally while in bed.
11. Others:
    a. 'Marche a petit pas' (after the Russian ballet master): In bilateral corticospinal lesions (diffuse cerebrovascular disease) short, stamping steps occur with bilateral spasticity and extensor plantar response. The rapid steps resemble a ballet dancer on her points. It is found in bilateral frontal lobe disease, pseudobulbar palsy, Alzheimer's disease and normal pressure hydrocephalus.
    b. Jaunting gait is seen in chorea. Patient's knee may give way momentarily resulting in a fall.
    c. Arthritis and muscular pain make walking stiff and slow (antalgic gaint). Gait of ankylosing spondylitis mimics parkinsonism (with a bit stooping forward).

- There is another Hoover's sign in internal medicine where the patients with advanced COPD show paradoxical inward movement of rib cage with each inspiration.

Clinical Wisdom

Broad-base gait: Cerebellar ataxia, posterior column lesion (i.e. sensory ataxia) and waddling gait.
Narrow-base gait: Hemiplegia, spastic paraparesis, parkinsonism.

Q. Different varieties of gait:

1. Neurogenic–1, 2, 3, 4, 5 and 7
2. Myogenic–6
3. Prosthetic–8
4. Arthrogenic–9
5. Psychogenic–10

"Success is not final, failure is not fatal: it is the courage to continue that counts"
—**Sir Winston Churchill (1874–1965)**, *British Statesman*

Appendix

THE EXAMINATION HALL (IMPORTANT TIPS)

1. Be smart, gentle, polite and courteous in your gesture. Do not rush, be patient. Remember, a lot of physical and mental stress is responsible for underperformance.
2. You should look confident and professional in attitude. Show confidence in your body language and behaviour. Never show overconfidence but have faith on yourself.
3. Be precise. Listen the question carefully and then answer 'to the point'. Speak out clearly, slowly and concisely in a confident voice. Be optimistic and free from any tension.
4. Do not hesitate to revise the diagnosis. Do not try to be clever but be careful. While you are in the viva table or case presentation, converse in a moderate speed, in a loud and clear voice with good fluency.
5. Be methodical. Remember, mostly the errors are made by making cursory and incomplete physical examination than due to lack of knowledge and skill.
6. While examining a patient, you should have a fine and gentle touch with an eagle's eye. Show respect to your patients as well as examiners (try to wish at the beginning and also at the end).
7. Nothing succeeds like thorough preparation though you may not know everything—so prepare yourself for the 'unexpected'. Do not panic and leave the anxiety out of the door.
8. Neither argue with your examiner nor interrupt him/her. Do not be biased. Do not agree to anything you are not sure of. Always try to be alert and focused (key of success).
9. Try to answer in order, i.e. from more common to less common causes, and avoid rare ones. Perform systematically in your (case) presentation.
10. Remember, the difference between success and failure is marginal.

INSTRUMENTS TO CARRY FOR MEDICINE PRACTICAL EXAMINATION (CHECK-LIST)

1. Stethoscope (preferably double-tube).
2. Sphygmomanometer (mercury or aneroid type)—It is better to have your own instrument.
3. Hammer (preferably round head with flexible shaft).
4. Pencil torch (with fully charged batteries).
5. Pins (for testing of pain sensation and blanching reaction in spider naevi).
6. Cotton (for testing of corneal reflex and touch sensation).
7. Measuring tape (for measurement of expansion of chest, abdomen in ascites, neck in thyroid enlargement, height, head circumference in hydrocephalus and assessment of nutrition).
8. Tuning fork (128 or 256 cycles/second for vibration sense, and 256 or 512 cycles/second for cochlear function).
9. Skin pencil and rulers/scales (e.g. two small 15-cm rulers for measurement of JVP).
10. Divider or compass (for two point discrimination)—Optional.
11. Tongue depressor.
12. Clinical thermometer.
13. Two one-rupee coin (for coin percussion in the chest and test for stereognosis).
14. Glass slides (for examination of capillary pulsation, spider naevi and haemorrhagic spots).
15. Wrist watch (not digital and with a 'second hand')—A must.
16. Cotton wrapped in a broom-stick or throat swab stick (for gag reflex).
17. Test tubes (two) for hot and cold sensation (optional), goniometer (optional).
18. Four small glass containers for taste sensation (containing solutions of sugar, common salt, vinegar and quinine), soap/clove/coffee or camphor balls for smell sensation, ribbons (red, green and blue-coloured) for colour vision, gloves (e.g. to palpate an ulcer or per rectal examination)—Optional.

19. Cardboard or clipboard (for history writing), two pieces of cardboard for AP and TR diameter of chest.
20. Ophthalmoscope, log book, thesis/dissertation (for postgraduate students).
21. Admit card (hall ticket/call letter), apron (with clearly visible nameplate, roll number or ID card), pen, pencil, sharpener, eraser, a blunt-ended key (for eliciting plantar response), face mask and small hand sanitizer bottle. **Positive attitude** and **self-confidence** are your shield in examination hall.
22. **Try to follow**—Wear formal clothes with polished shoes, clean and neat apron with a clean shave (if you are a boy) and hair tied up in a ponytail (if you are a girl).

Clinical Wisdom

Do not hesitate to ask for a back-rest (for neck vein examination), gauze pieces (for examination of tongue or penis), or weighing machine. Switch off your mobile phone or all electronic gadgets while in the examination hall.

THE HISTORY SHEET (IN LONG CASE)

1. Prefix the patient's name by Sri/Mr/Mrs/Miss.
2. Write sequentially upto differential diagnosis. Relevant investigations are optional.
3. 'All the systems' should be written. Usually the time alloted in a 'long case' is 45 minutes.
4. Be alert of these four things: the allotted case may be unpredictable, the patient may be non-cooperative, the limited time periods for long and short case examination, and the liking/disliking of the examiners. In the history and clinical examination, stress the important points (e.g. by underlining them).
5. Blood pressure should always be measured because it is part and parcel of general survey (mandatory—supine, optional—standing position, i.e. to diagnose 'postural drop').
6. Do not write the facts which you have not enquired or examined but remember if any test/fact is not written, it is granted that it is not done.
7. A beautiful handwriting influences the examiner. Spelling mistakes create a bad impression.
8. Try to avoid abbreviations; remember, MS means mitral stenosis as well as multiple sclerosis.
9. If anaemia, cyanosis or jaundice is present, mention the degree or type whichever is applicable. If any system has no abnormality, it is better to write 'within normal limit' or 'no abnormality detected' against the subheadings of the respective system. In case of build or nutrition, the term 'average' is preferred to 'normal'. If the facies is inconclusive, write 'nothing suggestive'.
10. Write the summary meticulously. Many examiners give stress on summary. A good summary will speak for yourself.

THE 'MODEL' DISTRIBUTION OF MARKS IN GENERAL MEDICINE (MBBS)

The basic format is described below. This may vary from university to university:

General medicine: Full marks 300.

1. Theory: Paper I + II = 60 + 60 (total 120).
2. Internal assessment: 60 (theory 30+ practical/oral 30).
3. Oral (including instruments, X-ray, CT scan, ECG, emergency medicine, charts, flying oral): Usually 4 oral tables, carrying 5 marks in each: Total 20.
4. Clinical/practical (bedside): total 100 (one long case 60 + one short case 30 + two spot cases 10).

- Marks distributed in long case (60) as follows: History taking 15+ demonstration of signs 30+ discussion 15.

Clinical Wisdom

Criteria to pass in the examination:
- Aggregate 50%, i.e. 150 marks
- Theory and oral (including internal assessment) 50%, i.e. 100 marks
- Practical (bedside clinics) 50%, i.e. 50 marks

- One should get 50% in internal assessment to pass in the examination. Each theory paper usually contains 2 long questions (one deals with basic and allied, and other, with clinical problem), short questions and short notes. In many universities, MCQs have been added.
- Theory paper
  Paper I: Cardiology, gastrointestinal and hepatobiliary system, genitourinary, deficiency disorder, tropical diseases, rheumatology, genetics and immunology.
  Paper II: Respiratory system, endocrinology, haematology, neurology, infectious diseases including HIV, psychiatry, dermatology including STD.
- Acute cases like acute severe asthma, LVF are usually not given in the examination.

Long case (45 minutes) comprises of history writing + demonstration of signs + relevant discussion.

Short case (15 minutes) means general survey and examination of one particular system (nothing to be written).

Spot cases (1–3 minutes each) means spotting the diagnosis (with examiner observing) and mentioning the justification.

Clinical Wisdom

Check the website of National Medical Commission (NMC) and local University regularly.

ADDENDUM

OSCE (Objective Structured Clinical Examination)—to judge 'clinical skills' by giving a clinical senario, which is a common practice in MD, DNB and MRCP examination. UGs (MBBS group) should start the rehearsal with their teachers (yet to be started).

In **DNB** examination there are OSCE (25 stations), *viva voce* (4 stations: on drugs, ECG, ABG, EEG, X-ray, PFT, capnography, instruments, emergency, therapeutics, recent advances, research methodology), ward round cases (4 real case scenarios) and clinical cases (2). In **MD** examination, semilong cases are given.

NExT (National Exit Test) will start soon and has two parts: NExT 1 and 2. NExT 1 is the online theory examination (with 540 MCQs) which will give entry to internship and to get a PG seat; the theory examination will be governed by Central Board of NMC (National Medical Commission). NExT 2 is purely a practical/clinical/*viva voce* examination controlled by respective Health University, which will give the license to practice Medicine with an MBBS certificate. OSCE is included in NExT 2. The subjects to be dealt with in NExT examination are Medicine, Surgery, Gynae and Obstetrics, Pediatrics, Orthopedics, Eye and ENT (total 7).

Artificial Intelligence (AI) looks to be the future of the world. It is the human intelligence processes by machines, especially computer system. AI seems to be very promising in healthcare system. Try to build-up some idea about it.

Route of success: Try to practice mock examination in front of your teacher/mentor or even a friend. Be systematic, plan ahead, set realistic goals and keep motivating yourself.

THE PATH OF SUCCESS

1. For true success ask yourself these four questions: Why? Why not? Why not me? Why not now?—James Allen (a British philosophical writer who was famous for his inspirational books and poetry).
2. Strategic planning, creative visualisation and willpower to succeed in the face of all odds; sufficient preparations with hardcore sincerity. Stick to the time limit.
3. Ability to build-up good relationship between the patient and the examinee, and the examiner and the examinee.
4. Ability to express, and to have confidence as well as common sense, and
5. Good luck.

THE REFERENCES/SUGGESTED READING

1. Hutchison's Clinical Methods.
2. Macleod's Clinical Examination.
3. Harrison's Principles of Internal Medicine.
4. Davidson's Principles and Practice of Medicine.
5. Kumar and Clark's Clinical Medicine.
6. Talley and O'Connor's Clinical Examination.
7. Bates' Guide to Physical Examination and History Taking.
8. Sapira's Art and Science of Bedside Diagnosis.
9. Chamberlain's Symptoms and Signs in Clinical Medicine: An Introduction to Medical Diagnosis.
10. Charles Seward's Bedside Diagnosis.
11. Ferri's Clinical Advisor.
12. Oxford Handbook on Clinical Medicine by JJ Murray Longmore.
13. Pappworth MH's A Primer of Medicine.
14. DeGowin and DeGowin's Bedside Diagnostic Examination.
15. Cecil Textbook of Medicine.
16. Bedside Cardiology by Jules Constant.
17. Bickerstaff's Neurological Examination in Clinical Practice.
18. Neurological Differential Diagnosis by John Patten.
19. Adams and Victor's Principles of Neurology.
20. The Washington Manual of Medical Therapeutics.
21. Sherlock's Diseases of the Liver and Biliary System.
22. Crofton and Douglas: Respiratory Disease.
23. Oxford Textbook on Medicine.
24. Colour Atlas of Dermatology by LK Bhutani.
25. CURRENT Medical Diagnosis and Treatment (CMDT).
26. Color Atlas and Text of Clinical Medicine by Charles Forbes and William Jackson.
27. Medicine update [published every year by Association of Physicians of India (API)].
28. Progress in Medicine [published every year by Association of Physicians of India (API)].
29. API Textbook of Medicine.

Index

Craniotabes 386

G

H

T

U

V

W

X

Y

Z